Evidence-based Cardiology

Second edition

Volume III

Provided as a service to medical education by

Evidence-based Cardiology

Second edition

Volume III

Edited by

Salim Yusuf
Heart and Stroke Foundation of Ontario Research Chair,
Senior Scientist of the Canadian Institute of Health Research
Director of Cardiology and Professor of Medicine, McMaster
University, Hamilton Health Sciences, Hamilton, Canada

John A Cairns
Dean, Faculty of Medicine, University of British Columbia,
Vancouver, Canada

A John Camm
Professor of Clinical Cardiology and Chief, Department of
Cardiological Sciences, St George's Hospital Medical
School, London, UK

Ernest L Fallen
Professor Emeritus, McMaster University, Faculty of Health
Sciences, Hamilton, Canada

Bernard J Gersh
Consultant in Cardiovascular Diseases and Internal Medicine,
Mayo Clinic; Professor of Medicine, Mayo Medical School,
Rochester, Minnesota, USA

BMJ Books is an imprint of the BMJ Publishing Group
Chapter 27 (Rihal) All figures are © Mayo Foundation

Second edition first published in 2003
First edition published in 1998
Second impression 1999
by BMJ Books, BMA House, Tavistock Square,
London WC1H 9JR

www.bmjbooks.com

British Library Cataloguing in Publication Data
A catalogue record for this book is available from the British Library

ISBN 0 7279 1714 5

Typeset by Newgen Imaging Systems (P) Ltd.
Printed and bound by MPG Books, Bodmin, Cornwall

Contents

Contributors

Walter Ageno
Department of Medicine
University of Insubria
Varese, Italy

Craig S Anderson
Clinical Trials Research Unit
University of Auckland
Auckland, New Zealand

Jeffrey L Anderson
Department of Medicine
University of Utah
Cardiology Division, LDH Hospital
Salt Lake City, USA

Bert Andersson
Department of Cardiology
Sahlgrenska University Hospital
Göteborg, Sweden

David G Benditt
Professor of Medicine
Co-Director Cardiac Arrhythmia Center
University of Minnesota Medical School
Minneapolis, Minnesota, USA

CR Benedict
Professor of Medicine
Department of Internal Medicine
Division of Cardiology
The University of Texas Medical School
Houston, Texas, USA

Jeffery A Breall
University of Indiana
Indianapolis, USA

Blasé A Carabello
Department of Medicine
Medical University of South Carolina
Charleston, USA

John F Carlquist
LDS Hospital
Division of Cardiology and University of Utah
Department of Medicine
Salt Lake City
Utah, USA

Jack M Colman
Associated Professor Toronto Congenital Cardiac Center for Adults
University Health Network and Mount Sinai Hospital
University of Toronto
Toronto, Canada

Patrick J Commerford
Helen and Morris Mauerberger
Professor of Cardiology
Department of Medicine
University of Cape Town
and
Cardiac Clinic
Groote Schuur Hospital
Cape Town, South Africa

Heidi M Connolly
Consultant, Cardiovascular Diseases and Internal Medicine
Associate Professor of Medicine
Mayo Medical School
Mayo Clinic
Rochester, USA

Stuart J Connolly
Division of Cardiology and Population Health Research Institute
McMaster University
Hamilton, Canada

Deborah Cook
Professor, Department of Medicine
McMaster University
Hamilton, Canada

Harry JGM Crijns
Academische Ziekenhuis Groningen,
Groningen, the Netherlands

Eugene Crystal
Division of Cardiology and Population Health Research Institute
McMaster University
Hamilton, Canada

Daniel J Diver
Cardiac Catheterization Laboratory
Georgetown University Medical Center,
Washington, USA

Paul Dorian
St Michael's Hospital
University of Toronto
Toronto, Canada

David T Durack
Becton Dickinson Microbiological Systems
Sparks, USA

Andrew J Einstein
Department of Medicine
University of Medicine and Dentistry of New Jersey
Robert Wood Johnson Medical School
New Brunswick, USA

Perry M Elliot
St George's Hospital Medical School
London, UK

Cengiz Ermis
Fellow in Clinical Cardiac Electrophysiology
Cardiac Arrhythmia Center
University of Minnesota Medical School
Minneapolis, Minnesota, USA

John K French
Cardiology Department
Green Lane Hospital
Auckland, New Zealand

Jeffrey S Ginsberg
Department of Medicine
McMaster University
Hamilton, Canada

Neil R Grubb
Department of Cardiology
Royal Infirmary of Edinburgh
Edinburgh, UK

Jack Hirsh
Department of Medicine
Hamilton Health Sciences, Research Center
McMaster University
Hamilton, Canada

Desmond G Julian
Department of Cardiology
University of Newcastle-upon-Tyne
Newcastle-upon-Tyne, UK

Clive Kearon
Department of Medicine
McMaster University
Hamilton, Canada

Sanjaya Khanal
Cardiac Catheterization Laboratory
Henry Ford Heart and Vascular Institute
Detroit, USA

Peter Kowey
Professor of Medicine
Jefferson Medical College
Philadelphia
and
Chief of Electrophysiology
Mainline Arrhythmia
Philadelphia, USA

Roberto Latini
Department of Cardiovascular Research
Mario Negri Institute
Milano, Italy

Keith G Lurie
Professor of Medicine Co-Director
Cardiac Arrhythmia Center
University of Minnesota Medical School
Minneapolis, Minnesota, USA

Benedito Carlos Maciel
Associate Professor of Medicine
Cardiology Division
Internal Medicine Department
Medical School of Ribeirão Preto
University of São Paulo
Brazil

Aldo P Maggioni
ANMCO Research Centre
Florence, Italy

José A Marin-Neto
Full Professor and Head
Cardiology Division
Internal Medicine Department
Medical School of Ribeirão Preto,
University of São Paulo
Brazil

Bongani M Mayosi
Cardiac Clinic
University of Cape Town
Cape Town, South Africa

RS McKelvie
Division of Cardiology and Population Health
Research Institute
McMaster University
Hamilton, Canada

William J McKenna
St George's Hospital Medical School
London, UK

Barry McKeown
Advanced Trainee in Cardiology
The Heart Research Institute of Western Australia
Sir Charles Gairdner Hospital
Perth, Western Australia

Lionel H Opie
Heart and Research Unit and Hypertension Clinic
Department of Medicine
Medical School
Observatory
Cape Town, South Africa

Jan Östergren
Department of Medicine,
Karolinska Hospital
Stockholm, Sweden

Paul J Pearson
Michigan Heart and Vascular Institute
Minnesota, USA

Barbara A Pisani
Loyola University Medical Center
Maywood, USA

Dominic Raco
Division of Cardiology
McMaster University
Hamilton, Canada

Shahbudin H Rahimtoola
University of Southern California
and Keck School of Medicine at USC
Los Angeles, California, USA

Charanjit S Rihal
Division of Cardiovascular Diseases and
Internal Medicine
Mayo Clinic
Rochester, USA

Scott Sakaguchi
Associate Professor of Medicine
Cardiac Arrhythmia Center
University of Minnesota Medical School
Minneapolis, Minnesota, USA

Sanjeev Saksena
Director, Cardiovascular Institute, AHS (East)
Clinical Professor of Medicine
RWJ Medical School
New Brunswick, USA

Irina Savelieva
St George's Hospital Medical School
Department of Cardiology
Cranmer Terrace, Tooting
London, UK

Hartzell V Schaff
Division of Thoracic and Cardiovascular Surgery
Mayo Clinic and Mayo Foundation
Rochester, Minnesota, USA

Nicola E Schiebel
Department of Emergency Medicine
Mayo Clinic and Mayo Foundation
Rochester, USA

Marcus Vinícius Simões
Associate Professor of Medicine
Cardiology Division
Internal Medicine Department
Medical School of Ribeirão Preto
University of São Paulo
Brazil

Maarten M Simoons
Thoraxcenter
Erasmus University
Rotterdam, the Netherlands

Samuel C Siu
Toronto Congenital Cardiac Center for Adults
University Health Network and Mount Sinai Hospital
Toronto, Canada

Peter Sleight
University Department of Cardiovascular Medicine
John Radcliffe Hospital
Oxford, UK

Karl Swedberg
Department of Medicine
Sahlgrenska University Hospital/Östra
University of Göteborg
Göteberg, Sweden

Jesper Swedenborg
Department of Surgery
Division of Vascular Surgery
Karolinska Hospital
Stockholm, Sweden

Rajesh Thaman
St George's Hospital Medical School
London, UK

Pierre Theroux
Department of Medicine
Montreal Heart Institute
Montreal, Canada

Peter L Thompson
Clinical Professor of Medicine and Public Health
University of Western Australia
and
Cardiologist, Sir Charles Gairdner Hospital
Perth, Western Australia

William D Toff
Division of Cardiology
University of Leicester
Leicester, UK

Gianni Tognoni
Department of Cardiovascular Research
Mario Negri Institute
Milano, Italy

Michael L Towns
Becton Dickinson Microbiology Systems
Sparks, USA

Zoltan G Turi
MCP Hahnemann University Medical School
Philadelphia, USA

Alexander GG Turpie
Department of Medicine
McMaster University
Hamilton, Canada

Isabelle C Van Gelder
Thorax Center
Department of Cardiology
University Hospital
Groningen, the Netherlands

James L Velianou
Division of Cardiology
McMaster University
Hamilton, Canada

James A Volmink
Global Health Council
Washington, USA

W Douglas Weaver
Division of Cardiovascular Medicine
Heart and Vascular Institute
Detroit, USA

Harvey D White
Cardiology Department
Green Lane Hospital
Auckland, New Zealand

Roger D White
Department of Anesthesiology
Mayo Clinic
Rochester, USA

Ronald R van der Wieken
Ouze Lieve Vrouwe Gasthuss
Amsterdam, the Netherlands

James S Zebrack
Cardiology Division
Salt Lake Regional Hospital
Salt Lake City, USA

Preface to the Second edition

"Where is the knowledge in all that information?
Where is the wisdom in all that knowledge?"

W H Auden

The recent proliferation of carefully controlled large scale clinical trials, their meta-analyses and selective observational studies has contributed to the remarkable strides made in the management of cardiovascular disease. One of the prophesies stated in the first edition of this textbook has come to pass – namely, that management guided by external evidence is an evolving process as newer and more effective treatment modalities come to light. While successful as a critical approach for managing patients, evidence-based medicine is nevertheless a work in progress which, if allowed to rest on its laurels, will "by nature be threatened with impending obsolescence". In addition to keeping abreast of new information, there is a need to integrate and distill the information into coherent recommendations. Authors were therefore instructed to provide their recommendations including those based on qualitative judgments. The recognition of new developments in a rapidly changing dynamic field combined with the overwhelmingly positive worldwide response to the first edition have prompted the publication of this second edition.

This edition is again dedicated to providing a comprehensive compendium of best evidence for the diagnosis and management of a wide variety of cardiovascular disorders. To avoid critical information gaps as meaningful new data emerge, the text contains several new features. Because our concepts of what constitutes evidence-based medicine is subject to change we have included a completely revised introductory chapter. Appended to the printed text is a CD Rom that permits ready access to new information and periodic updates by way of a dedicated and active website. In addition, there will be available a compact hand-held (PDA) version of the text. There are new chapters on clinical trials and meta-analysis; fetal origins of cardiovascular disease; genetics; diet and cardiovascular disease; obesity; and cardiopulmonary resuscitation. Several chapters have been completely rewritten and most have undergone substantial revision. Finally, the layout of the text has been reformatted for better handling, portability, readability and affordability.

In preparing this edition the editors and contributors have subscribed to the principle that the best external evidence found in these pages are not to be considered as hierarchical choices but rather should be used judiciously with other forms of evidence be they pathophysiologic, observational or experiential. No effort has been spared in the preparation of this edition and to this end invaluable assistance has been accorded us by Judy Lindeman at McMaster University and Mary Banks and Christina Karaviotis at BMJ Books.

Salim Yusuf
John A Cairns
A John Camm
Ernest L Fallen
Bernard J Gersh

Preface to the First edition

"... if a man declares to you that he has found facts that he has observed and confirmed with his own experience, be cautious in accepting what he says. Rather, investigate and weigh this opinion or hypothesis according to requirements of pure logic, without paying attention to this contention that he affirms empirically."

MOSES MAIMONIDES. *ca.* 1195

Thus did the great physician Maimonides make a plea for an evidence-based approach to medicine by admonishing his followers to seek common ground between objectivism and empiricism. If Maimonides had lived in the year 1785, he would likely have read William Withering's *An Account of the Foxglove*, a compendium of Withering's personal observations on the clinical effect of the digitalis leaf. At first blush, Maimonides would cry foul at such flagrant empiricism, demanding to know the whole of the inception cohort. It turns out that Withering, instead of selecting specific cases which would have "... spoken strong in favour of the medicine, and perhaps been flattering to my own reputation" went on to say in his Preface "I have therefore mentioned every case in which I have prescribed the foxglove, proper or improper, successful or otherwise ..." thus heralding a genuine, albeit retrospective, cohort study. It took 212 years before Withering was ultimately vindicated by the results of the first large scale randomized placebo controlled trial of digoxin (*N Engl J Med* 1997; **336**: 526). Sixty-eight hundred patients with congestive heart failure, in sinus rhythm, were randomized to receive digoxin (avg dose 0·25 mg/day) or placebo in addition to ACE inhibitors and diuretics. Over a three-year period there was no statistical difference in overall mortality but digoxin proved to be effective in reducing hospitalizations due to worsening heart failure.

The advent of large scale prospective randomized clinical trials has strengthened the external evidence upon which management decisions can be made with some confidence. We have come to rely on so-called external best evidence as critical guideposts for establishing minimal criteria for treatment of many cardiovascular disorders. In the process, some myths based on putative mechanisms have been dispelled while insights into the efficacy of new treatments have been more rapidly facilitated. On the other hand there is a danger of righteous complacency which, if unchecked, could lead to a slavish dependency on statistical bottom lines and, ultimately, to "cook book" medicine. It is the intent of this textbook to present a proper balance between "objectivism and empiricism". In this regard, the very first chapter begins by defining the practice of evidence-based cardiology as "... integrating individual clinical expertise with the best available external clinical evidence from systematic research".

The textbook has four principal components. An introductory general section addresses important topics in clinical epidemiology, as applied both to the bedside and to a population. This section includes: critical appraisal of data; clinical trials methodology;

quality of life measurements; health economics; and methods of decision analysis, all in the context of current clinical practice. Next follows a section on preventive strategies based on evidence that should enable the practicing physician to advise, with confidence, on risk factor modification and quality of life issues for selected patients. There follows a section on a broad range of specific cardiovascular disorders that highlight management issues based on current best evidence. Finally, the section on clinical applications is an attempt to put a clinical face on evidence derived from population statistics through the use of "live" clinical cases. Here, an attempt is made judiciously to couple external evidence with clinical expertise and a sound knowledge of cardiovascular pathophysiology. There is understandably a wide range of the kinds of evidence available to support different practices and treatments. The editors have chosen not to constrain the authors into rigid and uniform formats for each chapter. While several of the chapters have the level of evidence/recommendations graded, or key messages highlighted, a uniform format would not have been appropriate for every chapter.

This textbook is designed for a wide audience. Since cardiovascular disease comprises more than fifty percent of adult medicine, there is something here for everyone in clinical practice and at all levels of medical undergraduate and postgraduate training. Its emphasis on practical applications of research methodology and critical appraisal of data covering a cross-section of clinical topics should invite interest among those engaged in population studies, biostatistics, clinical epidemiology and health economics as well as those involved in healthcare decision analysis, quality assurance committees and stakeholders responsible for healthcare planning.

Because this textbook relies so heavily on current best evidence, it is by nature threatened with impending obsolescence. To ensure that this does not happen, the editors, in concert with the publisher, have agreed to issue up-dates periodically in the form of special supplements or updated editions, so that the text can be continually revised in accordance with emerging relevant data. In this context, it is well to bear in mind that good science always proceeds hesitantly through a series of tenuous conclusions. And so any recommendation made on the basis of available best evidence is subject to revision as we probe deeper into the mysterious nature of disease processes. One may ask of the large scale clinical trial "Why did it require more than 10,000 patients to show incontrovertible evidence that the experimental drug is effective?" Aye, there is the scientific question!

The editors wish to acknowledge the herculean efforts of Catherine Wright and Karin Dearness who kept everyone on track and offer a special appreciation to Mary Banks for her editorial expertise, patience and support.

Salim Yusuf
John A Cairns
A John Camm
Ernest L Fallen
Bernard J Gersh

Glossary

Abbreviations commonly used in this book

ABI	ankle brachial pressure index
ACC	American College of Cardiology
ACE	angiotensin-converting enzyme
AED	automated external defibrillator
AF	atrial fibrillation
AHA	American Heart Association
AMI	acute myocardial infarction
APSAC	anisoylated plasminogen streptokinase activator complex
APTT	activated partial thromboplastin time
ARR	associated risk reduction
AS	aortic stenosis
ASD	atrial septal defect
ASMR	age standardized mortality rate
BBB	bundle branch block
BMI	body mass index
CABG	coronary artery bypass grafting
CAD	coronary artery disease
CBVD	cerebrovascular disease
CCB	calcium-channel blockers
CCU	coronary care unit
CEE	conjugated equine estrogen
CHD	coronary heart disease
CHF	congestive heart failure
CI	confidence interval
CK-MB	creatinine kinase MB isoenzyme
CPP	coronary perfusion pressure
CPR	cardiopulmonary resuscitation
CT	computerized tomography
CYA	cyclophosphamide
DA	dopamine
DALY	disability adjusted life years
DHP	dihydropyridines
DM	diabetes mellitus
DVT	deep vein thrombosis
ECG	electrocardiogram
EEG	electroencephalogram
EGF	epidermal growth factor
EMF	endomyocardial fibrosis
EOA	effective orifice area
EPS	electrophysiologic studies
FGF	fibroblast growth factor
FS	fractional shortening
GPI	glycoprotein inhibitor
HCM	hypertrophic cardiomyopathy
HDL	high density lipoprotein (HDL_2)
HMG-CoA	3-hydroxy-3-methylglutaryl-coenzyme A
HOCM	hypertrophic obstructive cardiomyopathy
HRT	hormone replacement therapy
IC	intracoronary
ICD	implantable cardioverter defibrillator
ICH	intracerebral hemorrhage
IDC	idiopathic dilated cardiomyopathy
IDL	intermediate density lipoprotein
IE	infective endocarditis
IFN-γ	interferon gamma
IGF	insulin-like growth factor
IGT	impaired glucose tolerance
IL	interleukin
IM	intramuscular
INR	international normalization ratio
IQR	interquartile range
IV	intravenous
LAE	left atrial enlargement
LBBB	left bundle branch block
LDL	low density lipoprotein
LDL-C	low density lipoprotein cholesterol
LMWH	low molecular weight heparin
Lp(a)	lipoprotein
LQTS	long QT syndrome
LV	left ventricular
LVE	left ventricular enlargement
LVEF	left ventricular ejection fraction
LVH	left ventricular hypertrophy
MCP	monocyte chemoattractant protein
MHC	major histocompatibility complex
MHS	Milan Hypertensive Strain
MI	myocardial infarction
MPA	medroxyprogesterone acetate
MRI	magnetic resonance imaging
MUFA	monounsaturated fatty acid
NA	not available
NHLBI	National Heart Lung Blood Institute
NINDS	National Institute of Neurologic Disease and Stroke
NNT	number needed to treat
NSAIDs	non-steroidal anti-inflammatory drugs
NSTEMI	non-ST-segment elevation myocardial infarction
NYHA	New York Heart Association
OR	odds ratio
P	probability
PAI	plasminogen activator inhibitor
PCI	percutaneous coronary intervention
PCR	polymerase chain reaction
PDGF	platelet derived growth factor
PE	pulmonary embolism
PET	positron emission tomography
PPCM	peripartum cardiomyopathy
PSVT	paroxysmal supraventricular tachycardia
PTA	percutaneous transluminal angioplasty
PTCA	percutaneous transluminal coronary angioplasty

PUFA	polyunsaturated fatty acid		TEE	transesophageal echocardiography
PVC	premature ventricular complex		t-FA	*trans* fatty acid
RCT	randomized controlled trial		TGF	transforming growth factor
RFLP	restriction fragment length polymorphisms		TIA	transient ischemic attack
ROSC	return of spontaneous circulation		TIMI	Thrombolysis in Myocardial Infarction
RRR	relative risk reduction		TMP	TIMI myocardial perfusion
rtPA	recombinant tissue plasminogen activator		TNF	tumor necrosis factor
RV	right ventricular		TNK	tenecteplase
RVEF	right ventricular ejection fraction		tPA	tissue plasminogen activator
RVF	right ventricular enlargement		TTE	transthoracic echocardiography
RVH	right ventricular hypertrophy		UK	urokinase
SAECG	signal-averaged ECG		*v*	versus
SC	subcutaneous		VF	ventricular fibrillation
SK	streptokinase		VPD	ventricular premature depolarization
SMC	smooth muscle cells		VSD	ventricular septal defect
SFA	saturated fatty acid		VT	ventricular tachycardia
SFA	superficial femoral artery		VTE	venous thromboembolism
STEMI	ST-segment elevation myocardial infarction		VUI	venous ultrasound imaging
TEA	thromboendarterectomy			

Grading of recommendations and levels of evidence used in *Evidence-based Cardiology*

GRADE A

Level 1a   Evidence from large randomized clinical trials (RCTs) or systematic reviews (including meta-analyses) of multiple randomized trials which collectively has at least as much data as one single well-defined trial.

Level 1b   Evidence from at least one "All or None" high quality cohort study; in which ALL patients died/failed with conventional therapy and some survived/succeeded with the new therapy (for example, chemotherapy for tuberculosis, meningitis, or defibrillation for ventricular fibrillation); or in which many died/failed with conventional therapy and NONE died/failed with the new therapy (for example, penicillin for pneumococcal infections).

Level 1c   Evidence from at least one moderate-sized RCT or a meta-analysis of small trials which collectively only has a moderate number of patients.

Level 1d   Evidence from at least one RCT.

GRADE B

Level 2   Evidence from at least one high quality study of non-randomized cohorts who did and did not receive the new therapy.

Level 3   Evidence from at least one high quality case–control study.

Level 4   Evidence from at least one high quality case series.

GRADE C

Level 5   Opinions from experts without reference or access to any of the foregoing (for example, argument from physiology, bench research or first principles).

A comprehensive approach would incorporate many different types of evidence (for example, RCTs, non-RCTs, epidemiologic studies, and experimental data), and examine the architecture of the information for consistency, coherence and clarity. Occasionally the evidence does not completely fit into neat compartments. For example, there may not be an RCT that demonstrates a reduction in mortality in individuals with stable angina with the use of β blockers, but there is overwhelming evidence that mortality is reduced following MI. In such cases, some may recommend use of β blockers in angina patients with the expectation that some extrapolation from post-MI trials is warranted. This could be expressed as Grade A/C. In other instances (for example, smoking cessation or a pacemaker for complete heart block), the non-randomized data are so overwhelmingly clear and biologically plausible that it would be reasonable to consider these interventions as Grade A.

Recommendation grades appear either within the text, for example, **Grade A** and **Grade A1a** or within a table in the chapter.

The grading system clearly is only applicable to preventive or therapeutic interventions. It is not applicable to many other types of data such as descriptive, genetic or pathophysiologic.

Part IIIa

Specific cardiovascular disorders: Stable coronary artery disease

Bernard J Gersh and John A Cairns, Editors

Grading of recommendations and levels of evidence used in *Evidence-based Cardiology*

GRADE A

Level 1a   Evidence from large randomized clinical trials (RCTs) or systematic reviews (including meta-analyses) of multiple randomized trials which collectively has at least as much data as one single well-defined trial.

Level 1b   Evidence from at least one "All or None" high quality cohort study; in which ALL patients died/failed with conventional therapy and some survived/succeeded with the new therapy (for example, chemotherapy for tuberculosis, meningitis, or defibrillation for ventricular fibrillation); or in which many died/failed with conventional therapy and NONE died/failed with the new therapy (for example, penicillin for pneumococcal infections).

Level 1c   Evidence from at least one moderate-sized RCT or a meta-analysis of small trials which collectively only has a moderate number of patients.

Level 1d   Evidence from at least one RCT.

GRADE B

Level 2   Evidence from at least one high quality study of non-randomized cohorts who did and did not receive the new therapy.

Level 3   Evidence from at least one high quality case–control study.

Level 4   Evidence from at least one high quality case series.

GRADE C

Level 5   Opinions from experts without reference or access to any of the foregoing (for example, argument from physiology, bench research or first principles).

A comprehensive approach would incorporate many different types of evidence (for example, RCTs, non-RCTs, epidemiologic studies, and experimental data), and examine the architecture of the information for consistency, coherence and clarity. Occasionally the evidence does not completely fit into neat compartments. For example, there may not be an RCT that demonstrates a reduction in mortality in individuals with stable angina with the use of β blockers, but there is overwhelming evidence that mortality is reduced following MI. In such cases, some may recommend use of β blockers in angina patients with the expectation that some extrapolation from post-MI trials is warranted. This could be expressed as Grade A/C. In other instances (for example, smoking cessation or a pacemaker for complete heart block), the non-randomized data are so overwhelmingly clear and biologically plausible that it would be reasonable to consider these interventions as Grade A.

Recommendation grades appear either within the text, for example, **Grade A** and **Grade A1a** or within a table in the chapter.

The grading system clearly is only applicable to preventive or therapeutic interventions. It is not applicable to many other types of data such as descriptive, genetic or pathophysiologic.

26 Anti-ischemic drugs

Lionel H Opie

A major problem ... is the lack of sufficient data comparing antianginal and placebo treatment.[1]

The major anti-ischemic drugs are, in historical order of appearance, the nitrates, the β adrenergic blockers, the calcium-channel antagonists, the metabolic modifiers, and the potassium-channel openers. In addition, there is increasing evidence that the angiotensin converting enzyme (ACE) inhibitors and the statin lipid lowering drugs have indirect anti-ischemic properties. Preservation of endothelial function may also be an indirect anti-ischemic procedure. The antiplatelet agents, including aspirin, clopidogrel, and the GPIIb/IIIb receptor blockers, as well as the antithrombotics and thrombolytics, will not be considered here but in the following section of Part III on acute ischemic syndromes. Special attention will be paid to the potential effect of the standard anti-ischemic drugs not just in giving symptomatic relief of angina, but, in keeping with the aim of this book, on hard outcome end points such as re-infarction and mortality.

What is ischemia?

Ischemia of the myocardium is probably the most important cause of cardiovascular and total mortality and morbidity in Western societies. Although there are many definitions, in the end they come down to an inadequate blood supply to the myocardium.[2] The Greek *ischo* means "to hold back" and *haima* means "blood". The word "ischemia" was, it seems, first used by Rudolf Virchow in 1858, to describe a situation in which limitation of blood flow resulted from an increased resistance to blood flow. The "modern" concept of supply-demand imbalance as a cause of ischemia dates back to observations made nearly two hundred years ago on the exercising limb[3]:

> If we call into vigorous action a limb around which we ... applied a ligature, we find then that the member can only support its action for a very short time; for now its supply of energy and its expenditure do not balance each other.

Myocardial ischemia therefore exists when the reduction of coronary flow is so severe that the supply of oxygen is inadequate for the demands of the tissue, which is the generally accepted situation in acute effort angina. Ischemia is often distinguished from infarction, the latter reflecting prolonged irreversible ischemia with myocardial cell death. Therefore the ischemia is also the underlying situation in unstable angina and the very early phase of the clinical syndrome of acute myocardial infarction (AMI), when reperfusion can still reverse the ischemic myocardial damage. Myocardial ischemia is also thought to contribute, together with the underlying anatomical substrate, to the potentially lethal ventricular arrhythmias found in patients with ischemic heart disease.

Myocardial ischemia may also occur chronically, as proposed for hibernation. In the latter case, the proposal is that the myocardium has undergone a chronic adaption to ischemia by downregulation of contraction. The simplified concept is "little blood, little work".[4]

Therefore, there is a wide spectrum of conditions in which myocardial ischemia is clinically relevant (Table 26.1) and for which anti-ischemic drugs can be used. As will be argued, the hard evidence for their long-term benefit is, in general, strikingly absent.

Safety and efficacy

General aspects

Safety and efficacy are ultimately linked: the more pronounced the beneficial effects of a therapeutic regimen, the greater the degree of side effects that may be tolerated. A drug that significantly prolongs life, such as alteplase or streptokinase in AMI, is recommended for use despite an increased incidence of hemorrhagic stroke, because the balance of mortality plus stroke favors the use of the drug. There exists a hierarchy for the significance of end points, the most important primary end point being prolongation of life, with a secondary end point being an improved quality of life, either by reduction of morbidity or by relief of symptoms such as anginal pain. Tertiary end points are those that neither improve the quantity nor the quality of life, but which are expected to prevent disease by reducing risk factors, examples being the treatment of mild asymptomatic arterial hypertension.

Evidence for the first of these end points is, in general, scant in relation to the anti-ischemic drugs. Information gathered in one situation is not necessarily directly relevant to another. Thus, for example, the benefits of β blockade in post-MI prevention[5] do not necessarily show that these

Table 26.1   The clinical spectrum of acute ischemia and the various drugs used

Clinical syndrome	Pathophysiology	Drug therapy	Outcome in RCTs
Effort angina	Imbalance of oxygen supply–demand, transient	Nitrates, β blockers, calcium antagonists, metabolic modifiers, K-channel openers	None for nitrates or metabolic modifiers, limited for β blockers and calcium antagonists, positive for K-opener
Unstable angina, acute NSTE coronary syndrome	As above, prolonged	As above, antithrombins, antiplatelet agents	None for anti-ischemic drugs
Threatened MI	As above prior to start of cell necrosis	β blockade	Possible benefit for β blockade, harm for nifedipine
Ischemic arrhythmias	Ischemia-induced rise in cyclic AMP and cell calcium; increased I_f in Purkinje fibers; lipid changes	β blockade	Indirect evidence strongly favors β blockade, but no RCTs have been directed towards ischemic arrhythmias

Abbreviations: I_f, "funny current"; MI, myocardial infarction; NSTE, non-ST elevation; RCTs, randomized controlled trials

drugs also prolong life in stable effort angina. The present author agrees with Hjemdahl et al[1] that the pathophysiologic situation in patients with symptomatic angina is often very different from that in the post-MI setting. In MI, there is a zone of dead tissue, and depending on its size there will be reactive remodeling in the rest of the ventricle, introducing a different pathophysiologic situation and predisposing to left ventricular (LV) failure. Also, the presence of viable and non-viable myocardium creates electrical inhomogeneity that predisposes to re-entry with risks of lethal ventricular arrhythmias. Furthermore, the possibility of the coexistence of stunning, hibernation, and preconditioning, collectively called *the new ischemic syndromes*, all predispose to a highly complex and multifarious spectrum that constitutes ischemic LV dysfunction.[6] Although some of these abnormalities may be found in chronic stable angina because there may be coexisting previous MI, nonetheless the predominant and basic pathology is in the one case transient myocardial ischemia causing effort angina, and in the other case dead tissue with reactive ventricular remodeling. Of note, a sizable portion of patients in studies on chronic stable angina – up to one third – have had previous infarcts.[1] Post-MI angina therefore merits specific consideration, but again outcome studies are missing.

How is safety assessed? The hierarchy of evidence

Safety is not well defined but could be regarded as the absence of significant adverse effects when the drug is used

with due regard for its known contraindications.[7] Safety implies the added assurance that there are no hidden dangers in the legitimate use of the drug. Evidence for safety, like evidence for efficacy, can come from a variety of sources. There is a hierarchy of evidence regarding safety, starting from anecdotal case reports as the least reliable, followed by case series, case–control studies, cohort studies, going through to more coherent information with emphasis on large controlled randomized trials (RCTs) and carefully conducted meta-analyses of these trials. These lead to acceptance of the overall evidence as favoring a position where the benefit and the safety of a drug group is well established (which is the most reliable evidence).[7] For example, in the case of calcium antagonists, most of the earlier evidence on adverse effects comes from case–control or cohort studies or small RCTs. Such data are subject to serious intrinsic problems of the methodology, which can generate hypotheses without providing proof or otherwise. On the other hand, in the case of β blockers, there is concordant evidence for benefit in the data on post-MI patients from many large trials,[5] and a very large observational study on over 200 000 patients.[8]

Are there safety concerns regarding calcium antagonists and β blockers?

A number of safety concerns have been raised in relation to calcium antagonists, and to some extent also to β blockers. Many of these are based on case–control or cohort studies, which are not a reliable source of information.[7,9] There are major contradictions between the various studies. The question of cancer and gastrointestinal hemorrhage as possible side effects is reviewed by the WHO-ISH committee, and by Opie *et al*[7] without a causative association being found.[10] In the case of cancer, one small cohort study is outweighed by two bigger negative studies.[11,12] In the case of hemorrhage, the evidence is incomplete and not supported by prospective studies. In general, it is the short-acting calcium antagonists,[13] and in particular short-acting nifedipine, that have been associated with adverse effects.[7,14]

There is long-standing good evidence that short-acting instant release (IR) nifedipine in capsule form can increase mortality in acute ischemic syndromes[7,15,16] so that it is contraindicated in unstable angina or early phase MI unless accompanied by β blockade. It follows that:

- the mechanism of the adverse effects of IR nifedipine is very probably by reflex adrenergic activation;
- even in stable effort angina, neither short-acting nifedipine nor any other short-acting dihydropyridine should be used in the absence of an accompanying β blocker.

Indirect data from a meta-analysis of effort angina[17] could also suggest that any short-acting dihydropyridine should be avoided in effort angina. Experience in unstable angina would, however, suggest that combination with β blockade would be safe. **Grade B**

Safety concerns have also been raised in relation to β blockers. Case–control studies suggest an increased incidence of sudden cardiac arrest or death in hypertensive patients treated by β blockade.[18,19] In a prospective observational study on 12 550 hypertensive patients over 6 years,[20] those taking calcium antagonists or ACE inhibitors were at no increased risk of diabetes versus hypertensive patients not receiving therapy, whereas with β blockers there was a 28% increase (RR 1·28, 95% CI 1·04–1·57). Although the potential weakness of observational studies must again be emphasized, other short-term studies have shown that β blockade added to thiazide therapy for hypertension has a hyperglycemic effect.[21]

Safety *v* safe use

Whenever a serious side effect of any given drug becomes known, and acted on, then that safety issue should be obviated so that the drug becomes safer. For example, β blockers are no longer given to patients with pre-existing excess bradycardia, sick sinus syndrome, or asthma. In that sense, the increased mortality long known in relation to the use of IR nifedipine in acute ischemic syndromes is a safety issue that should already have been overcome by the appropriate warnings.

RCTs

Calcium antagonists and β blockers in effort angina

Regarding trials with outcome end points, the major studies are two relatively small RCTs comparing calcium antagonists with β blockers in effort angina, neither trial having a placebo arm. In the APSIS[22] study, slow release verapamil was compared with metoprolol, the main prognostic end points being a combination of morbidity and mortality (total and cardiovascular), and non-fatal cardiovascular complications including MI, revascularization, stroke, and peripheral vascular events, as well as treatment failure. These end points did not differ significantly between the treatments, nor were side effects or quality of life indices different between the two drugs. Because of the very low death rate, which was about 2% per year of follow up, it is impossible to exclude that either drug might be better than the other, or that one or the other drugs might be better or worse than placebo (not tested). Studies to settle the mortality issue are unlikely to be undertaken, so we must evaluate the combined end points actually tested. On present evidence there are not enough data to conclude that either the calcium antagonists or the β blockers differ one from the other, or from placebo.

TIBET[23] compared slow release nifedipine (twice daily formulation) with atenolol. As there were three treatment arms including the combination of these drugs, and only 682 patients in total to start with, there were only 450 patient-years in each group. Outcome was assessed by a combination of end points considered either "hard" (cardiac mortality, MI, or unstable angina) or "soft" (revascularization or treatment failure). Thus the major conclusion of this study is that it is underpowered for hard end points and even for combined hard and soft end points. The firm conclusion is the poor tolerance of nifedipine tablets.

The more recent Stanford meta-analysis[24] added 59 short-term studies in which cardiac death or MI were reported during the use of β blockers or calcium antagonists for effort angina, giving 116 extra events, still with no differences between the outcomes and an odds ratio very close to unity.

In addition there are two placebo-controlled trials, ASIST and PREVENT. The ASIST[25] study is the only one in mild effort angina or silent ischemia that compares a β blocker, atenolol, with placebo. Patients with moderate to severe angina were excluded. Over 1 year, atenolol gave better event-free survival, using a mixed bag of end points, including death, resuscitation, non-fatal MI, hospitalization for unstable angina, aggravation of angina, and revascularization. There were only a few serious events and the most evident difference was that there was less aggravation of angina with atenolol (9 of 152 *v* 26 of 154 with placebo, *P*=0·003). This trial, therefore, tells us that atenolol is antianginal, which is not surprising. PREVENT makes roughly a similar message for the long-acting dihydropyridine (DHP), amlodipine, which reduced unstable angina and revascularizations when added to existing treatment, which often included a β blocker.[26]

The combined message emerging from APSIS, TIBET, ASIST, and PREVENT is this: the real problem is that the incidence of hard end points, such as mortality, infarction, or unstable angina, is so low in chronic stable effort angina that vast trials would be needed to show beyond doubt that calcium antagonists or β blockers do more than relieve symptoms. For example, it can be estimated that a study of 600 total deaths in effort angina, even with a risk reduction of one quarter, would need about 30 000 patients in a long-term trial (60 000 if the end point is cardiac mortality) to show any differences between calcium antagonists and β blockers. Trials of this size are, in the view of the present author, unlikely ever to be undertaken. Rather, it makes much more sense to select high-risk patients (see section on nicorandil) with clusters of risk factors, such as age, male gender, hypertension, smoking, and hypercholesterolemia. Alternatively, trials carefully designed to establish whether or not two treatments have an equivalent effect may be considered because fewer numbers are required than in megatrials.[27] From the point of view of evidence-based medicine, and except for nicorandil the data currently available are insufficient.

Therefore the author has argued that the choice of drug between β blocker and calcium-channel blocker should be geared to the needs and the pathophysiology of the individual patient.[28] For example in a middle-aged man athletically active and anxious to avoid impotence, a calcium-channel blocker would be first choice. **Grade B** In a person with a compromised myocardium or with a previous MI, a β blocker appropriately titrated would be first choice. **Grade A** In someone at high risk of MI, antihypertensive therapy started with a β blocker is somewhat safer than starting with a calcium-channel blocker, while, if the major aim is prevention of stroke and hence intellectual integrity, a calcium-channel blocker may be preferable (Figure 26.1).[29]

Combination therapy: calcium antagonist added to β blocker in higher risk effort angina

ACTION is a large trial testing the outcome efficacy of long-acting nifedipine (GITS, gastro-intestinal tract system) in higher risk patients with chronic effort angina.[30] It is powered both for efficacy (death, AMI, heart failure, stroke) and for safety (death, AMI, stroke). Of the 7720 entrants, 78% were already taking β blockade. Therefore this trial is chiefly going to tell us about changes in hard end points when nifedipine GITS is added to a β blocker. Extrapolating from what little is already known from unstable angina, but with only 48 hour re-infarction as the outcome, the combination of nifedipine with a β blocker is likely to improve

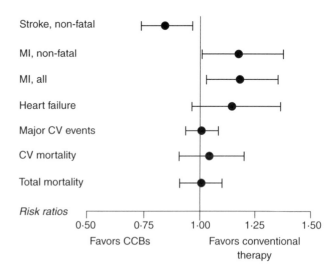

Figure 26.1 Outcomes in a meta-analysis of hypertension trials, comparing calcium-channel blocker (CCB)-based therapy *v* therapy conventional therapy (starting with either diuretic or β blocker). Note decrease ($P = 0 \cdot 013$) in non-fatal stroke, the increase in non-fatal myocardial infarction (MI) ($P = 0 \cdot 036$), and unchanged cardiovascular (CV) and total mortality. Figure corrected from error in original publication of Opie and Schall.[29]

outcome. The trail will terminate in late 2003. There may be enough of a difference in the subgroup of those not receiving a β blocker to help judge on the efficacy of long acting nifedipine alone.

Nitrates in effort angina

There are no such trials reported and none is being planned. Nitrates therefore remain strictly in the realm of agents that provide symptomatic relief, without evidence for outcome benefit. **Grade C** Theoretically, the reflex tachycardia that they invoke might adversely affect the long-term outcome in ischemic states. Equally theoretically, their capacity to act as nitric oxide donors might protect the vascular endothelium and provide protective preconditioning.[31]

Unstable angina as an example of prolonged ischemia

This condition has two major components: acute myocardial ischemia and a disturbance of the thrombotic mechanism. Antianginal drugs therefore constitute only part of the therapy. In contrast to the good data on the benefit of heparin and aspirin, and now on clopidogrel, there is again no good evidence for the benefit of nitrates in unstable angina. Compared with intravenous diltiazem, intravenous nitroglycerin was less effective on short-term end points such as refractory angina and MI.[32] Furthermore, there was still a benefit in favor of diltiazem-treated patients at 1 year of follow up.[33] Regarding long-term outcome with nitrates in unstable angina, there has been only one trial, which compared transdermal nitroglycerin with placebo therapy over 4 months, each arm receiving in addition conventional medical treatment. Outcome events such as death, MI or refractory angina were similar in the nitrate and placebo arms.[34]

There is a difference in the safety profile of the dihydropyridines (DHPs) and the non-DHPs (such as verapamil and diltiazem). Of the DHPs, only IR nifedipine has been well tested, with an adverse outcome in two trials. In the HINT study,[27] IR nifedipine was inferior to placebo with MI within 48 hours as an end point (OR 2·0, 95% CI 1·1–3·6) so that the trial was stopped,[35] while in the other study[36] there was an increase in early mortality. The heart rate-increasing effect of IR nifedipine[36] was probably the result of adrenergic activation because a benefit for the addition of IR nifedipine to prior β blockade was shown in both these trials and also by Gerstenblith *et al.*[37] By contrast, the non-DHP diltiazem was successfully used in comparison with a nitrate, both agents being given intravenously with a relative risk of 0·49 in favor of diltiazem for short-term events, chiefly recurrent pain.[32] Diltiazem decreased the heart rate whereas the nitrate increased it. Although there has been no similar trial with verapamil, several smaller trials suggest efficacy.[38–40] While it is possible that long-acting DHPs such as amlodipine that do not increase the heart rate might be safe in unstable angina, no such trials are likely to be done. The conclusion from the safety point of view is that the non-DHP diltiazem is best tested without the trial being large enough to yield outcome data, that verapamil may be similar in its effects though even less well tested, and that the DHPs as a group are relatively contraindicated in the absence of β blockade, with short-acting nifedipine (and nicardipine) totally contraindicated.

In the case of β blockade, there are no good studies in unstable angina, the only one available showing an insignificant trend to short-term benefit as measured by the decrease in recurrent ischemia or MI within 48 hours.[35] Neither of two older studies had hard end points.[41,42]

Prinzmetal's variant angina

This type of angina at rest is caused by coronary spasm and is specifically relieved by calcium antagonists. There are no outcome studies with hard end points, perhaps because the condition is potentially fatal and therefore placebo-controlled trials would be impossible. Some of the studies with remission of attacks as end point are reviewed by Opie and Maseri.[43] **Grade B** Short-acting agents are standard. Of these, nifedipine should not be used unless the diagnosis is firm and it is sure that the patient does not have unstable angina or threatened MI.

Threatened infarction

In this situation where ischemia is threatening to develop into infarction, IR nifedipine had adverse short-term (2 week) effects in a relatively small randomized trial, in which mortality was increased from 0 of 82 placebo patients to 7 of 89 nifedipine patients ($P = 0·018$).[15] By contrast, in another relatively small trial with propranolol started intravenously within 4 hours of the onset of symptoms of AMI and then continued orally, there were fewer completed infarcts as shown by a limitation of blood enzyme rise,[42] and the incidence of ventricular fibrillation was less.[44] **Grade B** When given in a pilot study to patients with clinically threatened MI, atenolol reduced eventual infarction but, as the authors point out, the small numbers mean that the statistics are far from robust.[45] These small trials do not provide definitive information but are in agreement with the general concept that adrenergic activation is harmful in threatened infarction[42] so that β blockade is the preferred mode of therapy. This recommendation is, however, not based on good trial data.

Postinfarct effort angina

Two large RCTs suggest that long-term post-AMI therapy by instant release capsular nifedipine in standard doses is not beneficial or possibly harmful.[16,46] **Grade A** The presumed mechanism is reflex sympathetic stimulation. Angina was not a specific end point. Even though evidence from cohort studies is contradictory,[47,48] this agent is far from ideal for post-MI patients with angina.

Only one of the post-MI trials with calcium antagonists specifically reported on the incidence of angina pectoris in a subgroup of the postinfarct DAVIT II study,[49] in which verapamil 360 mg/day was started 7–15 days following infarct and continued for up to 18 months. Verapamil was significantly antianginal.[50] Regarding the outcome of the DAVIT II study as a whole, in the verapamil group there was a reduction (RR 0·80, 95% CI 0·64–0·99) in the combined end point predetermined as death and/or re-infarction. Although total mortality did not fall, the RR was also 0·80 (95% CI 0·61–1·05), and the lack of significance could possibly be ascribed to the relatively small numbers involved. Regarding heart failure, analysis of predetermined subgroups, undertaken before the code was broken, showed that in patients without prior heart failure during their stay in the coronary care unit, there was a mortality reduction ($P = 0·024$). There was no effect of verapamil, either beneficial or harmful, in those with prior (not concurrent) heart failure. However, subgroup analysis even with predetermined end points is open to criticism. **Grade B**

Regarding diltiazem, the MDPIT post-MI study, in which diltiazem was given as 240 mg/day for a mean of 25 months, did not report on effort angina.[51] An earlier study in which diltiazem was given for 14 days after non-Q wave infarction found no difference in the incidence of chest pain "recognized as angina pectoris".[52] Outcome evidence that this drug increases cardiac events (cardiac deaths and/or non-fatal infarction) in post-MI patients with congestive heart failure cannot be disputed.[51] **Grade A**

Regarding β blockers, there is impressive evidence that these drugs prolong life in post-MI patients.[5] Furthermore, in a very large observational study on over 200 000 post-MI patients, mortality was reduced by about 40% in all subgroups of those receiving β blockers, including those with prior revascularization.[8] **Grade A** Therefore, although there appear to be no formal trials on antianginal properties in post-MI patients, the large number of post-MI trials and the many patients studied, mean that these drugs have more overall compelling evidence in their favor in the postinfarct situation than does verapamil and much more compelling evidence than for the DHP calcium antagonists. First principles suggest it is likely that they are exerting their benefit at least in part by an anti-ischemic effect, although benefits on remodeling and postinfarct heart failure are a reasonable alternative.[53,54]

Ischemic arrhythmias

The Cape Town hypothesis is that β blockers have a ventricular antiarrhythmic effect in AMI by limiting metabolic changes, such as increased levels of cyclic AMP in the ischemic tissue.[55] Nonetheless, other modes of action are possible, for example by inhibition of the current I_f that initiates pacemaker activity in injured Purkinje cells. A meta-analysis has shown that β blockade is effective when given as prophylactic antiarrhythmic therapy in the context of AMI, and that it reduces mortality with an odds ratio of 0·81 in 55 trials.[56] Further evidence for outcome benefit for β blockers, as in postinfarct patients, comes from the Cardiac Arrhythmia Suppression Trial (CAST) in which prior β blockade therapy was associated with a one third reduction in arrhythmic death or cardiac arrest.[54] By contrast, calcium antagonists had a slightly increased relative risk, albeit not of statistical significance. Yet these findings do not prove that the β blockers were acting as anti-ischemic agents, and only provide indirect evidence that β blockers are safe when deliberately chosen as anti-ischemic drugs in other clinical situations.

Calcium antagonists in stable angina after angioplasty

There still is no convincing evidence that pharmacologic therapy by any of the anti-ischemic drugs alters the incidence of restenosis. There is some evidence from a meta-analysis that calcium antagonists as a group may help to prevent restenosis,[57] which should mean lessened effort angina – a possibility that was not reported. In one specific study over 6 months, twice daily verapamil reduced restenosis following percutaneous transluminal coronary angioplasty (PTCA), but only in patients with stable angina.[58] **Grade B** β blockers appear to be untested in this situation.

Congestive heart failure and effort angina

There are no studies with this combination as a predetermined end point. In view of the consistent benefit that accrues to patients with heart failure, already receiving a diuretic and an ACE inhibitor when a β blocker is carefully phased in, such added therapy can be expected to improve angina. However, direct evidence is missing. **Grade C**

ACE inhibitors as potential anti-ischemic drugs

There are at least four potentially anti-ischemic mechanisms whereby ACE inhibitors may operate. First, angiotensin II is known to facilitate sympathetic adrenergic transmission, also in humans.[59] Second, ACE inhibitors, by formation of bradykinin, indirectly promote the formation of nitric oxide, which in turn inhibits myocardial oxygen consumption.[60] Third, ACE inhibitors are potentially antihypertensive and thereby reduce the afterload. Fourth, in 15 hypertensive patients of whom 11 had effort angina, ACE inhibitors improved coronary flow reserve after long-term therapy.[61] The mechanism may be by reversal of endothelial dysfunction. Not surprisingly, these agents have a documented antianginal effect in hypertensive patients with angina[62,63] without, however, any outcome data. In patients with low ejection fractions, below 35%, chronic therapy by enalapril in the Studies of Left Ventricular Dysfunction (SOLVD) trials led to less hospital admissions for unstable angina, and therefore might well have reduced stable effort angina, but the data are not clear on this point.[64] In the SAVE study there was an unexpected reduction in recurrent MI in the group given captopril.[65]

The hypothesis that ACE inhibitors can protect against manifestations of ischemic heart disease in those at high risk was tested in HOPE,[66] in which one of the predetermined secondary or other outcomes was reduction of revascularization (RR 0·85, 95% CI 0·77–0·94) and of worsening angina (RR 0·89, 95% CI 0·82–0·96). However, what is controversial is the mechanism: is it just blood pressure reduction,[67] or an additional explanation specific to ACE inhibition such as an increased formation of bradykinin? Objective anti-ischemic effects can be found in hypertensive but not normotensive people.[68] **Grade A** In "standard" angina of effort, without hypertension or heart failure, ACE inhibitors have an inconstant effect, as reviewed elsewhere.[69] Logically, the expected benefit would be more in patients with more severe ischemia and a greater activation of the adrenergic and renin–angiotensin systems.[70]

Metabolic modifiers

Trimetazidine and ranolazine are antianginals that act metabolically, probably through multiple mechanisms including partial fatty acid oxidation. While there is no doubt about their antianginal efficacy, supported by the recent oral presentation of data on 800 patients in the case of ranolazine, there are no outcome trials.

Nicorandil

This antianginal drug acts through several mechanisms including nitric oxide formation and potassium channel opening, the latter leading to preconditioning and to an antiadrenergic effect during experimental ischemia.[71] In a large prospective trial on higher risk patients with stable effort angina,[72] the primary composite end point was achieved, namely a reduction of coronary heart disease death, nonfatal MI, or unplanned hospitalization for cardiac chest pain. The secondary end point, coronary heart disease death or non-fatal MI, showed a strong trend to reduction without significance being reached. This trial is remarkable because it shows that a trial testing hard end point reduction in effort angina can be undertaken. Nicorandil is thus, in the view of the present author, the only antianginal that has strong evidence-based data in its favor. It is licensed in the UK, Japan, and several other countries, but not in the USA. **Grade A**

Statins as potential anti-ischemic drugs

Statins have made a considerable difference to the mortality of patients with ischemic heart disease in several studies. In the West of Scotland Coronary Prevention Study (WESCOPS), pravastatin was able to reduce hard end points in middle-aged hypercholesterolemic men without prior MI. In this group, the occurrence of angina pectoris was highly correlated ($P < 0.0001$) with the primary end point, which was definite coronary heart disease death or non-fatal MI.[73] Therefore, in hypercholesterolemic males with angina, statins are able to reduce hard end points. That they have a direct anti-ischemic effect is shown by reduction of ST segment deviations on 48 hour Holter traces in patients with stable angina pectoris, documented coronary artery disease and pre-existing antianginal therapy, the latter not being

specified.[74] **Grade A** Statin therapy can improve endothelial function, measured in the brachial artery, within 3 days in high-risk patients (elderly patients).[75] Formal prospective proof that cholesterol lowering by a statin has clinical antianginal efficacy is provided by the MIRACL study (Myocardial Ischemia Reduction with Aggressive Cholesterol Lowering) in which a high daily dose of atorvastatin (80 mg/day) reduced symptomatic ischemia and hospitalization in patients within 16 weeks of an acute coronary syndrome.[76]

Diuretics as potential anti-ischemic drugs

Short-term diuretic therapy has an antianginal effect, possibly by reduction of the left ventricular preload.[77] No outcome data are available. Some case–control studies on hypertensive patients have suggested increased mortality on diuretics when given in high doses and without potassium supplementation.[18,19]

Conclusions

There are few if any satisfactory outcome studies available with the conventional antianginal drugs in effort angina. There are no trials at all on nitrates, and only rather small trials comparing β blockers and calcium antagonists. Some indirect evidence suggests that the ACE inhibitors may have antianginal properties. Statins are indirectly antianginal. Adequately powered outcome trials in patients with cardiac death and non-fatal MI as end points in effort angina would require mega-trials in view of the low incidence of these events. It would be more practicable to select high-risk categories or to aim trials at showing drug equivalence. Thus in higher risk patients with effort angina, the relative new antianginal nicorandil gave a positive outcome with a reduction in the primary end point of coronary heart disease death, non-fatal MI and hospitalization, or unplanned cardiac chest pain. In unstable angina, where ischemia is prolonged, there are no good trials showing that nitrates, β blockers or calcium antagonists – all commonly used drugs – have outcome benefit. Although β blockers have good evidence favoring their use as prophylactic antiarrhythmic drugs in AMI, with a reduction in mortality shown by meta-analysis, it is not certain that they are acting as anti-ischemic drugs in this situation.

> ### Key points
> - Standard anti-ischemic drugs (nitrates, β blockers, calcium antagonists) relieve anginal pain but their effect on outcome in effort angina is not known. Two relatively small trials and a meta-analysis suggest equivalence between calcium antagonists and β blockers. It is desirable but

unlikely that mega-trials will be conducted to settle this issue.

- Nicorandil is a relatively new anti-anginal with hard outcome data in its favor when tested in higher risk patients with effort angina.
- Likewise in unstable angina, outcome data for the anti-ischemic agents are lacking.
- An exception is short-acting nifedipine, which in two trials in acute ischemic syndromes has increased mortality, probably by reflex adrenergic activation.
- The closer the patient is to AMI, the stronger are the data for the safety of β blockers.
- In the postinfarct phase the data for safety and efficacy of β blockers are especially strong. The only calcium antagonist with good evidence for safety is verapamil, but without mortality benefit in the relatively small trials conducted.
- In acute ischemic ventricular arrhythmias, there is indirect evidence for the prophylactic effect of β blockers on mortality, even though there is no formal trial.
- Indirect evidence suggests that angiotensin converting enzyme inhibitors have some anti-ischemic properties without clear evidence for antianginal efficacy except in hypertensive patients. A large prospective study shows that ramipril protects from worsening angina in high-risk patients.
- In one trial, early use of high-dose statin following an acute coronary syndrome reduced symptomatic ischemia within 16 weeks.

References

1. Hjemdahl P, Eriksson SV, Held C, Rehnqvist N. Prognosis of patients with stable angina pectoris on antianginal drug therapy. *Am J Cardiol* 1996;**77**:6D–15D.

2. Hearse DJ. Myocardial ischaemia: can we agree on a definition for the 21st century? *Cardiovasc Res* 1994;**28**:1737–44.

3. Burns A. Observations on some of the most frequent and important diseases of the heart; on aneurysm of the thoracic aorta; on preternatural pulsation in the epigastric region; and on the unusual origin and distribution of some of the large arteries of the human body. Edinburgh: Bryce, 1809.

4. Rahimtoola SH. The hibernating myocardium. *Am Heart J* 1989;**117**:211–21.

5. Yusuf S, Peto R, Lewis J, Collins R, Sleight P. Beta blockade during and after myocardial infarction: an overview of the randomized trials. *Prog Dis Cardiovasc Dis* 1985;**27**:335–71.

6. Opie LH. The multifarious spectrum of ischemic left ventricular dysfunction: relevance of new ischemic syndromes. *J Mol Cell Cardiol* 1996;28:2403–14.

7. Opie LH, Yusuf S, Kübler W. Current status of safety and efficacy of calcium-channel blockers in cardiovascular diseases. A critical analysis based on 100 studies. *Prog Cardiovasc Dis* 2000;**43**:171–96.

8. Gottlieb SS, McCarter MJ, Vogel RA. Effect of beta-blockade on mortality among high-risk and low-risk patients after myocardial infarction. *N Engl J Med* 1998;**339**:489–97.

9. Yusuf S, Garg R, Zucker D. Analyses by the intention-to-treat principle in randomized trials and databases. *PACE* 1991;**14**:2078–82.

10. WHO-ISH Committee. Ad Hoc Subcommittee of the Liaison Committee of the World Health Organisation and the International Society of Hypertension. Effects of calcium antagonists on the risks of coronary heart disease, cancer and bleeding. *J Hypertens* 1997;**15**:105–15.

11. Jick H, Jick S, Derby LE, Vasilakis C, Myers M. Calcium-channel blockers and risk of cancer. *Lancet* 1997;**349**:525–8.

12. Olsen JH, Sorensen HT, Friis S, McLaughlin JK, Steffensen FH. Cancer risk in users of calcium-channel blockers. *Hypertension* 1997;**29**:1091–4.

13. Alderman MH, Cohen H, Roque R, Medhaven S. Effect of long-acting and short-acting calcium antagonists on cardiovascular outcomes in hypertensive patients. *Lancet* 1997;**349**: 594–8.

14. Pahor M, Guralnik JM, Corti M, Foley DJ, Carbonin P, Havlik RJ. Long term survival and use of antihypertensive medications in older persons. *J Am Geriat Soc* 1995;**43**:1191–7.

15. Muller J, Morrison J, Stone P *et al.* Nifedipine therapy for patients with threatened and acute myocardial infarction: a randomized, double-blind, placebo-controlled comparison. *Circulation* 1984;**69**:740–7.

16. SPRINT II Study. Goldbourt U, Behar S, Reicher-Reiss H *et al.* Early administration of nifedipine in suspected acute myocardial infarction. The Secondary Prevention Reinfarction Israel Nifedipine Trial 2 Study. *Arch Intern Med* 1993;**153**: 345–53.

17. Glasser SP, Clark PI, Lipicky RJ, Hubbard JM, Yusuf S. Exposing patients with chronic, stable, exertional angina to placebo periods in drug trials. *JAMA* 1991;**265**:1550–4.

18. Hoes AW, Grobbee DE, Lubsen J, Man in 't Veld AJ, van der Does E, Hofman A. Diuretics, β-blockers, and the risk for sudden cardiac death in hypertensive patients. *Ann Intern Med* 1995;**123**:481–7.

19. Siscovick DS, Raghunathun TE, Psaty BM. Diuretic therapy for hypertension and the risk of primary cardiac arrest. *N Engl J Med* 1994;**330**:1852–7.

20. Gress TW, Nieto J, Shahar E, Wofford MR, Brancati FL. For the Atherosclerosis Risk in Communities Study. Hypertension and antihypertensives therapy as risk factors for type 2 diabetes mellitus. *N Engl J Med* 2000;**342**:905–12.

21. Swislocki ALM, Hoffman BB, Reaven GM. Insulin resistance, glucose intolerance and hyperinsulinemia in patients with hypertension. *Am J Hypertens* 1989;**2**:419–23.

22. Rehnqvist N, Jjemdahl P, Billing E, Bjokander I, Eriksson SV. Effects of metoprolol vs verapamil in patients with stable angina pectoris. The Angina Prognosis Study in Stockholm (APSIS). *Eur Heart J* 1996;**17**:76–81.

23. Dargie HJ, Ford I, Fox KM. On behalf of the TIBET Study Group. Total Ischaemic Burden European Trial (TIBET) Effects of ischaemia and treatment with atenolol, nifedipine SR and their combination on outcome in patients with chronic stable angina. *Eur Heart J* 1996;**17**:104–12.

24. Heidenreich PA, McDonald KM, Hastie T *et al.* Meta-analysis of trials comparing β-blockers, calcium antagonists, and nitrates for stable angina. *JAMA* 1999;**281**:1927–36.

25. Pepine C, Cohn PF, Prakash C *et al.* Effects of treatment on outcome in mildly symptomatic patients with ischemia during

daily life. The Atenolol Silent Ischemia Study (ASIST). *Circulation* 1994;**90**:762–8.

26. Pitt B, Byington R, Furberg C *et al.* Effect of amlodipine on the progression of atherosclerosis and the occurrence of clinical events. *Circulation* 2000;**102**:1503–10.

27. Hampton JR. Alternatives to mega-trials in cardiovascular disease. *Cardiovasc Drugs Ther* 1996;**10**:759–65.

28. Opie LH. First line drugs in chronic stable effort angina – the case for newer, longer-acting calcium-channel blocking agents. *J Am Coll Cardiol* 2000;**36**:1967–71.

29. Opie LH, Schall R. Evidence-based evaluation of calcium-channel blockers (CCBs) for hypertension. Equality of mortality and cardiovascular risk relative to conventional therapy. *J Am Coll Cardiol* 2002;**39**:315–22 (correction in press).

30. Lubsen J, Poole-Wilson PA, Pocock SJ *et al.* Design and current status of ACTION: a coronary disease trial investigating outcome with nifedipine GITS. *Eur Heart J* 1998;**19**:1202.

31. Bolli R. Cardioprotective function of inducible nitric oxide synthase and role of nitric oxide in myocardial ischemia and preconditioning: an overview of a decade of research. *J Mol Cell Cardiol* 2001;**33**:1897–918.

32. Göbel EJ, Hautvast RW, van Gilst WH *et al.* Randomised, double-blind trial of intravenous diltiazem versus glyceryl trinitrate for unstable angina pectoris. *Lancet* 1995;**346**:1653–7.

33. Göbel EJ, van Gilst WH, de Kam PJ, ter Napel MGJ, Molhoek GP, Lie KI. Long-term follow-up after early intervention with intravenous diltiazem or intravenous nitroglycerin for unstable angina pectoris. *Eur Heart J* 1998;**19**:1208–13.

34. Ardissino D, Merlini PA, Savonitto S, Demicheli G, Zanini P. Effect of transdermal nitroglycerin on N-acetylcysteine, or both, in the long-term treatment of unstable angina pectoris. *J Am Coll Cardiol* 1997;**29**:941–7.

35. HINT Study. Early treatment of unstable angina in the coronary care unit, a randomised, double-blind placebo controlled comparison of recurrent ischemia in patients treated with nifedipine or metoprolol or both. The Netherlands Inter-university Nifedipine Trial. *Br Heart J* 1986;**56**:400–13.

36. Muller J, Turi Z, Pearl D *et al.* Nifedipine and conventional therapy for unstable angina pectoris: a randomized, double-blind comparison. *Circulation* 1984;**69**:728–33.

37. Gerstenblith G, Ouyang P, Achuff SC, Bulkley BH, Becker LC. Nifedipine in unstable angina. A double-blind, randomized trial. *N Engl J Med* 1982;**306**:885–9.

38. Mauritson DR, Johnson SM, Winniford MD, Cary JR, Willerson JT. Verapamil for unstable angina at rest: a short-term randomized, double-blind study. *Am Heart J* 1983;**106**:652–8.

39. Mauri F, Marfici A, Briaghi M, Cerri P, de Biase AM. Effectiveness of calcium antagonist drugs in patients with unstable angina and proven coronary artery disease. *Eur Heart J* 1988;**9**:158–63.

40. Capucci A, Bassein L, Bracchetti D, Carini G, Maresta A. Propranolol v. verapamil in the treatment of unstable angina. A double-blind cross-over study. *Eur Heart J* 1983;**4**:148–54.

41. Fischl SJ, Herman MV, Gorlin R. The intermediate coronary syndrome. Clinical, angiographic and therapeutic aspects. *N Engl J Med* 1973;**288**:1193–8.

42. Norris RM, Sammel NL, Clarke ED, Smith WM. Protective effect of propranolol in threatened myocardial infarction. *Lancet* 1978;**2**:907–9.

43. Opie LH, Maseri A. Vasospastic angina. In: Krebs R, ed. *Treatment of cardiovascular disease by Adalat (nifedipine).* Stuttgart: Schattauer, 1986.

44. Norris RM, Brown MA, Clarke ED, Barnaby PF, Geary GG. Prevention of ventricular fibrillation during acute myocardial infarction by intravenous propranolol. *Lancet* 1984:883–6.

45. Yusuf S, Sleight P, Rossi R *et al.* Reduction in infarct size, arrhythmias and chest pain by early intravenous beta blockade in suspected acute myocardial infarction. *Circulation* 1983;**67**(Suppl. I):I-32–I-41.

46. SPRINT Study. Secondary Prevention reinfarction Israeli Nifedipine Trial. A randomized intervention trail of nifedipine in patients with acute myocardial infarction. *Eur Heart J* 1988;**9**:354–64.

47. Braun S, Boyko V, Behar S *et al.* Calcium antagonists and mortality in patients with coronary artery disease: a cohort study of 11 575 patients. *J Am Coll Cardiol* 1996;**28**:7–11.

48. Koenig W, Lowel H, Lewis M, Hormann A. Long-term survival after myocardial infarction: relationship with thrombolysis and discharge medication. Results of the Augsburg myocardial infarction follow-up study. *Eur Heart J* 1996;**17**: 1199–206.

49. Jespersen CM, Hansen JF, Mortensen LS. Danish Study Group on Verapamil in Myocardial Infarction. The prognostic significance of post-infarction angina pectoris and the effect of verapamil on the incidence of angina pectoris and prognosis. Results of the Survival and Ventricular Enlargement trial. *Eur Heart J* 1994;**15**:270–6.

50. DAVIT Study. Danish Study Group of Verapamil in Myocardial Infarction. Verapamil in acute myocardial infarction. *Eur Heart J* 1984;**5**:516–28.

51. MDPIT Study. The Multicenter Diltiazem Postinfarction Trial Research Group. The effect of diltiazem on mortality and reinfarction after myocardial infarction. *N Engl J Med* 1988;**319**: 385–92.

52. Gibson RS, Boden WE, Theroux P, Strauss HD, Pratt CM. Diltiazem and reinfarction in patients with non-Q-wave myocardial infarction. *N Engl J Med* 1986;**315**:423–9.

53. Lichstein E, Hager D, Gregory JJ, Fleiss JL, Rolnitzky L, Bigger JT. Relation between beta-adrenergic blocker use, various correlates of left ventricular function and the chance of developing congestive heart failure. *J Am Coll Cardiol* 1990;**16**: 1327–32.

54. Kennedy HL, Brooks MM, Barker AH, Bergstrand R, Huther ML. β-blocker therapy in the cardiac arrhythmia suppression trial. *Am J Cardiol* 1994;**74**:674–80.

55. Lubbe WH, Podzuweit T, Opie LH. Potential arrhythmogenic role of cyclic adenosine monophosphate (AMP) and cytosolic calcium overload: implications for prophylactic effects of beta-blockers in myocardial infarction and proarrhythmic effects of phospodiesterase inhibitors. *J Am Coll Cardiol* 1992;**19**:1622–33.

56. Teo KK, Yusuf S, Furberg CD. Effects of prophylactic antiarrhythmic drug therapy in acute myocardial infarction. *JAMA* 1993;**270**:1589–95.

57. Hillegass WB, Ohman M, Leimberger JD, Califf RM. A meta-analysis of randomized trials of calcium antagonists to reduce restenosis after coronary angioplasty. *Am J Cardiol* 1994;**73**: 835–9.

58. Hoberg E, Kubler W. Prevention of restenosis after PTCA: role of calcium antagonists. *J Cardiovasc Pharm* 1991;**18** (Suppl. 6):S15.

59.Lyons D, Webster J, Benjamin N. Angiotensin II. Adrenergic sympathetic constriction action in humans. *Circulation* 1995; **91**:1457–60.

60.Zhang X, Xie Y-W, Nasjletti A, Xu X, Wolin MS, Hintze TH. ACE inhibitors promote nitric oxide accumulation to modulate myocardial oxygen consumption. *Circulation* 1997;**95**: 176–82.

61.Motz W, Strauer BE. Improvement of coronary flow reserve after long-term therapy with enalapril. *Hypertension* 1996; **27**:1031–8.

62.Akhras F, Jackson G. The role of captopril as single therapy in hypertension and angina pectoris. *Int J Cardiol* 1991;**33**: 259–66.

63.Stumpe KO, Overlack A. On behalf of the Perindopril Therapeutic Safety Study Groups (PLUTS). A new trial of the efficacy, tolerability and safety of angiotensin-converting enzyme inhibition in mild systemic hypertension with concomitant diseases and therapies. *Am J Cardiol* 1993;**71**:32E–37E.

64.Yusuf S, Pepine CJ, Garces C, Pouleur H, Salem D. Effect of enalapril on myocardial infarction and unstable angina in patients with low ejection fractions. *Lancet* 1992;**340**: 1173–8.

65.Pfeffer MA, Braunwald E, Moye LA, Basta L, Brown EJ, Cuddy TE. Effect of captopril on mortality and morbidity in patients with left ventricular dysfunction after myocardial infarction. Results of the Survival and Ventricular Enlargement Trial. *N Engl J Med* 1992;**327**:669–77.

66.HOPE Investigators. Yusuf S, Sleight P *et al.* Effects of an angiotensin-converting enzyme inhibitor, ramipril, on cardiovascular events in high-risk patients. *N Engl J Med* 2000; **342**:145–53.

67.Staessen JA, Wang J-G, Thijs L. Cardiovascular protection and blood pressure reduction: a meta-analysis. *Lancet* 2001;**358**: 1305–15.

68.Prasad A, Mincemoyer R, Quyyumi AA. Anti-ischemic effects of angiotensin-converting enzyme inhibition in hypertension. *J Am Coll Cardiol* 2001;**38**:1116–22.

69.Opie LH. *Angiotensin converting enzyme inhibitors: scientific basis for clinical use, 3rd ed.* New York: Author's Publishing House, 1999.

70.Remme WJ, Kruyssen DA, Look MP, Bootsma M, de Leeuw PW. Systemic and cardiac neuroendocrine activation and severity of myocardial ischemia in humans. *J Am Coll Cardiol* 1994;**23**:82–91.

71.Miura T, Kawamura S, Tatsuno H *et al.* Ischemic preconditioning attenuates cardiac sympathetic nerve injury via ATP-sensitive potassium channels during myocardial ischemia. *Circulation* 2001;**104**:1053–8.

72.IONA Study Group. Effect of nicorandil on coronary events in patients with stable angina: the Impact Of Nicorandil in Angina (IONA) randomised trial. *Lancet* 2002;**3509**:1262–9.

73.WESCOPS Study. The West of Scotland Coronary Prevention Study Group. Baseline risk factors and their association with outcome in the West of Scotland Coronary Prevention Study. *Am J Cardiol* 1997;**79**:756–62.

74.van Boven AJ, Jukema W, Zwinderman AH, Crijns HJ, Lie KI, Bruschke AV. Reduction of transient myocardial ischemia with pravastatin in addition to the conventional treatment in patients with angina pectoris. *Circulation* 1996;**94**: 1503–5.

75.Tsunekawa T, Hayashi T, Kano H *et al.* Cerivastatin a hydroxy-methylgutaryl coenzyme A reductase inhibitor, improves endothelial function in elderly diabetic patients within 3 days. *Circulation* 2001;**104**:376–9.

76.Schwartz GG, Olsson AG, Ezekowitz MD *et al.* Effects of atorvastatin on early recurrent ischemic events in acute coronary syndromes. the MIRACL study: a randomized controlled trial. *JAMA* 2001;**285**:1711–18.

77.Parker JD, Parker AB, Farrell B, Parker JO. Effects of diuretic therapy on the development of tolerance to nitroglycerin and exercise capacity in patients with chronic stable angina. *Circulation* 1996;**93**:691–6.

27 Impact of revascularization procedures in chronic coronary artery disease on clinical outcomes: a critical review of the evidence

Charanjit S Rihal, Dominic Raco, Bernard J Gersh, Salim Yusuf

Coronary artery disease (CAD) is the leading cause of death worldwide and a major determinant of morbidity, use of healthcare resources, and lost productivity from illness. Since the original descriptions of surgical[1] and percutaneous[2] revascularization, the number of revascularization procedures has increased yearly (Figure 27.1). By 1998, 1 202 000 cardiac catheterizations, 926 000 percutaneous transluminal coronary angioplasty (PTCA) procedures, and 553 000 coronary artery bypass graft (CABG) operations were being performed annually in the USA alone.[3] An equivalent number are likely being performed in the rest of the world. Because the immediate risks of invasive procedures must be balanced against future potential benefits, it is important to critically evaluate the evidence supporting the use of these procedures, and to define the types of patients most likely to benefit and those unlikely to have any substantial benefit.

Considered empirically, there are three broad potential reasons to recommend myocardial revascularization:

- to alleviate symptoms caused by myocardial ischemia;
- to improve the likelihood of long-term survival; and
- to reduce the risk of future non-fatal cardiac events such as myocardial infarction, serious arrhythmias, or congestive heart failure.

Within these categories, the potential and magnitude of benefit must be balanced against the intrinsic risk of invasive procedures. These considerations require thorough knowledge of both the technical aspects and the pertinent evidence, in particular relative efficacies with respect to outcomes of interest, estimation of individual risk-to-benefit ratios, and an understanding of the limitations and potential harm of each procedure. This chapter reviews the evidence comparing CABG surgery, PTCA, stents, and medical therapy for chronic CAD with respect to both fatal and non-fatal clinical outcomes. By building a conceptual framework, this chapter attempts to place the evidence from more recent trials of percutaneous revascularization into the context of previous trial data that compared CABG with medical therapy. Limitations of the available data and application to clinical practice are also discussed.

CABG surgery versus medical therapy

The first generation of randomized clinical trials of chronic CAD tested CABG surgery against medical therapy. Three moderate sized, prospective randomized studies conducted two decades ago provide the bulk of the data: the European Coronary Surgery Study (ECSS), the Veterans Administration (VA) Coronary Artery Bypass Surgery Cooperative Study Group, and the Coronary Artery Surgery Study (CASS).[4–6] These trials and numerous retrospective studies from associated registries demonstrated that the benefits of CABG were proportional to the long-term risk among patients who

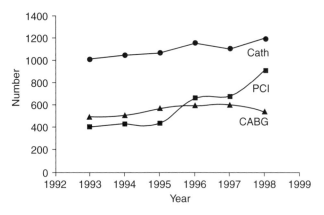

Figure 27.1 Annual growth in number of invasive cardiac procedures performed in the USA 1993–1998. Data are from the annual National Hospital Discharge Surveys 1993–1998. National Center for Health Statistics, Hyattsville, Maryland (www.cdc.gov/nchs). Values represent total number of discharges, not patients, with the indicated procedure listed as the primary procedure. Because federal, military, and Veterans Affairs hospitals are not included, the numbers may be underestimated. CABG, coronary artery bypass graft surgery (ICD-9 Code 36.1); Cath, catheterization; PCI, percutaneous coronary intervention.

received medical therapy.[5–7] Although both the VA study and CASS failed to demonstrate a difference in overall mortality between the medical and surgical groups that was statistically significant, subgroups in which CABG appeared to be superior to medical therapy were identified early. These subgroups included patients with left main CAD,[8,9] so-called left main equivalent disease,[10] and three vessel disease with left ventricular dysfunction.[11] Because each trial was relatively small (350–400 patients per treatment arm), only the ECSS trial demonstrated a decrease in mortality overall that was statistically significant.[4,9]

The three major trials (CASS, VA, and ECSS) plus four smaller trials (50 patients per treatment arm), in which patients were followed for 10 years, have been subjected to meta-analysis.[7] In all, 2649 patients randomly allocated to CABG or medical therapy were included. Original clinical and angiographic data were collected and analyzed according to uniform definitions. Enrolled patients had stable angina pectoris, whereas those with medically refractory or unstable angina generally were not included. The baseline angiographic and clinical characteristics are listed in Table 27.1. Of note, the majority had three vessel (50·6%) or left main CAD (6·6%), most of the patients were between 40 and 60 years old, almost all were male, and only 20% had an ejection fraction less than 50%. About half of the patients were taking β adrenergic blockers, but only 3·2% were receiving antiplatelet drugs at enrollment.

Mortality

Cumulative mortality after initial medical therapy or initial CABG over 12 years of follow up is shown in Figure 27.2. Because of the perioperative mortality associated with CABG, 1 year mortality was not different between the groups and a net benefit in favor of CABG was not observed for 2 to 3 years (Figure 27.2). The advantage in favor of an initial strategy of CABG substantially widened at 5 to 7 years, before narrowing again by 10 to 12 years. At 5, 7, and 10 years, 10·2%, 15·8%, and 26·4% of patients, respectively, assigned to CABG had died, compared with 15·8%, 21·7%, and 30·5% of their medically assigned counterparts. Risk reductions were significant at all three time points (relative risk [RR], 0·61, 0·68, 0·83), even though 40% of patients initially assigned to medical treatment had delayed CABG surgery by 10 years. Because such crossovers tend to occur in the highest risk medical patients (left main coronary artery or three vessel disease, unstable angina), these trials may underestimate the real benefits of CABG surgery compared with medical therapy alone, and this underestimation would be greatest among high-risk subsets. This tendency for the relative – but not the absolute – benefit to converge is likely due to high rates of crossover to surgery among the highest risk medical patients, the development of graft atherosclerosis, and progression of underlying native vessel disease.

Table 27.1 Clinical and angiographic characteristics of patients enrolled in randomized trials of CABG versus medical therapy

Characteristic[a]	% of patients
Age distribution (years)	
≤40	8·5
41–50	38·2
51–60	46·0
>60	7·3
Ejection fraction (n = 2474)	
<40	7·2
40–49	12·5
50–59	28·0
≥60	52·3
Male	96·8
Severity of angina	
none	11·2
class I or II	53·8
class III or IV	35·0
History	
myocardial infarction	59·6
hypertension	26·0
heart failure	4·0
diabetes mellitus	9·6
smoking (n = 1949)	83·5
current smokers (n = 2298)	45·5
ST-segment depression > 1 mm	
resting (n = 2423)	9·9
exercise (n = 1985)	70·5
Drugs at baseline	
β blockers (n = 2308)	47·4
antiplatelet agents (n = 1195)	3·2
digitalis (n = 2319)	12·9
diuretics (n = 1940)	12·6
Number of vessels diseased	
left main coronary artery	6·6
one vessel[b]	10·2
two vessels[b]	32·4
three vessels[b]	50·6
Location of disease	
proximal left anterior descending	59·4
left anterior descending diagonal	60·4
circumflex	73·8
right coronary	81·6

Abbreviation: CABG, coronary artery bypass graft
[a] Data on some characteristics are not available for all patients.
[b] Without left main artery. (From Yusuf *et al*[7] by permission of *The Lancet* Ltd.)

Significant heterogeneity of treatment effect was observed between various angiographic and clinical subgroups (Table 27.2). In general, the survival advantage of CABG over medical therapy was proportional to the

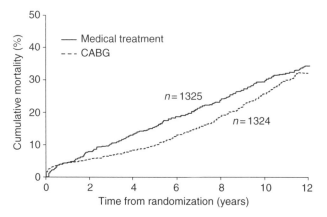

Figure 27.2 Overall survival after random allocation to medical treatment or coronary artery bypass graft (CABG). (From Yusuf *et al*[7] by permission of *The Lancet* Ltd.)

number of diseased coronary arteries (three vessel RR, 0·58; $P < 0·001$, or left main RR, 0·32; $P = 0·004$), particularly if the left anterior descending artery was involved (RR, 0·58). Although the relative benefits were similar regardless of left ventricular function (RR, 0·61 if normal and 0·59 if abnormal), the *absolute* benefit was greater among patients with an abnormal ejection fraction, because the risk of death was twice as high in this group (5 year medical mortality rate of 25·2% with an ejection fraction <50% *v* 13·3% if it was >50%). Similarly, absolute (and to some extent relative) mortality benefits were greater among patients with evidence of myocardial ischemia (abnormal exercise test results or severe angina).

To put the relative and absolute benefits of CABG further into the perspective of baseline risk, a score stratified by clinical and angiographic markers was developed. This indicated that patients at high risk (5 year medical mortality, 23%) experienced a clinically and statistically highly significant

Table 27.2 Outcomes of various subgroups in medical therapy versus CABG trials at 5 years

Subgroup	Overall number		Medical therapy mortality rate (%)	Odds ratio (95% CI)	P for CABG v medical treatment	P for interaction
	Deaths	Patients				
Vessel disease						
one vessel	21	271	9·9	0·54 (0·22–1·33)	0·180	0·19
two vessels	92	859	11·7	0·84 (0·54–1·32)	0·450	
three vessels	189	1341	17·6	0·58 (0·42–0·80)	<0·001	
left main artery	39	150	36·5	0·32 (0·15–0·70)	0·004	
No LAD disease						
one or two vessels	50	606	8·3	1·05 (0·58–1·90)	0·880	0·06
three vessels	46	410	14·5	0·47 (0·25–0·89)	0·020	
left main artery	16	51	45·8	0·27 (0·08–0·90)	0·030	
overall	112	1067	12·3	0·66 (0·44–1·00)	0·050	
LAD disease present						
one or two vessels	63	524	14·6	0·58 (0·34–1·01)	0·050	0·44
three vessels	143	929	19·1	0·61 (0·42–0·88)	0·009	
left main artery	22	96	32·7	0·30 (0·11–0·84)	0·020	
overall	228	1549	18·3	0·58 (0·43–0·77)	0·001	
LV function						
normal	228	2095	13·3	0·61 (0·46–0·81)	<0·001	0·90
abnormal	115	549	25·2	0·59 (0·39–0·91)	0·020	
Exercise test status						
missing	102	664	17·4	0·69 (0·45–1·07)	0·100	0·37
normal	60	585	11·6	0·78 (0·45–1·35)	0·380	
abnormal	183	1400	16·8	0·52 (0·37–0·72)	<0·001	
Severity of angina						
class 0, I, II	178	1716	12·5	0·63 (0·46–0·87)	0·005	0·69
class III, IV	167	924	22·4	0·57 (0·40–0·81)	0·001	

Abbreviations: CABG, coronary artery bypass graft; CI, confidence interval; LAD, left anterior descending; LV, left ventricle. (From Yusuf *et al*[7] by permission of *The Lancet* Ltd.)

improvement in survival (RR, 0·50; $P = 0.001$). Those at moderate risk (5 year medical mortality, 11·5%) also benefitted (RR, 0·63; $P = 0.05$), but the absolute benefits were smaller. No evidence of a survival benefit was observed among those at low risk (5 year medical mortality, 5·5%; RR, 1·18; $P = 0.70$).

Myocardial infarction and other non-fatal end points

Registry studies have suggested a favorable effect on late myocardial infarction only among the highest risk subsets, such as patients with three vessel disease and severe angina pectoris.[12] In the meta-analysis, no overall effect of CABG on subsequent infarction could be demonstrated, primarily because of an excess of infarction in the perioperative period (10·3% incidence of death or myocardial infarction at 30 days) among those assigned to surgery.[7] Although the risk of subsequent myocardial infarction was lower during extended follow up, this was not statistically significant (24·4% incidence of death or myocardial infarction at 5 years for the CABG group v 30·7% for the medical group).[7] Most trials did not prospectively collect data on rehospitalization for unstable angina, stroke, quality of life, or cost.

Recent trials

Few randomized data from the modern era compare CABG surgery with medical therapy. The Asymptomatic Cardiac Ischemia Pilot (ACIP) prospectively assigned 558 patients with asymptomatic ischemia to one of two medication strategies or to routine revascularization with CABG or PTCA.[13,14] Despite the relatively small sample size, mortality (1·1% v 6·6% and 4·4% for the two medical groups, $P < 0.02$), and death or myocardial infarction (4·7% revascularization v 12·1% and 8·8%, $P < 0.04$) was significantly lower after 2 years of follow up among the patients assigned to routine revascularization.[15] Rates of non-protocol revascularization procedures and hospital admission were also lower among the routine revascularization group (29% of medically assigned patients "crossed over" to invasive procedures).

The Medicine, Angioplasty, or Surgery Study (MASS) prospectively enrolled 214 patients with proximal left anterior descending artery stenoses to CABG surgery with an internal thoracic arterial conduit ($n = 70$), to PTCA ($n = 72$), or to medical therapy alone ($n = 72$). Rates of death (one in each group) or non-fatal myocardial infarction (one CABG, two PTCA) were very low over a mean 3 year follow up. After 3 years, 98% of patients assigned to CABG and 82% assigned to PTCA were free of angina, compared with only 32% of those in the medical group; however, 21 patients (29%) in the PTCA group required repeat procedures. No patient in any treatment group had severe angina (class III or IV).

Because previous trials have systematically tended to exclude elderly patients, precise estimates of relative risks and benefits are not available and must be extrapolated from other data. A recently published Swiss study focused on elderly patients. Patients older than 75 years (mean age, 80 years; 44% women) who had chronic, severe angina pectoris were randomly assigned to either an invasive approach or continued medical therapy.[16] Of 155 patients assigned to the invasive approach, 80 received PTCA, 33 CABG surgery, and 34 continued medical treatment. A third of the medical group required non-protocol revascularization for symptom control. By 6 months, angina severity and quality of life measures had improved in both groups but to a significantly greater extent in the invasive group. In the invasive group, 16·3% of patients had either died or had a non-fatal infarction, compared with 15·5% in the medical group. A greater proportion of the medical group (49% v 9·8%) required hospital admission during the ensuing 6 months. Although this was a relatively small trial, the findings affirmed the role of revascularization in improving symptoms and quality of life among elderly patients, the most important goal of treatment in this group.

Although the findings described above were derived from relatively small trials, they suggest that among patients with evidence of myocardial ischemia, modern revascularization techniques may be more effective than previously thought. These data point to a need for larger, more definitive randomized trials that test current revascularization techniques against modern medical therapy so that reliable estimates of effect of size on clinical outcomes with narrower confidence intervals can be made.

Conclusions

The available data suggest that a strategy of early CABG surgery improves long-term survival in a broad spectrum of patients at moderate to high risk with medical therapy. Relative reductions in mortality risk of about 40% over 5 years can be expected in comparison with the alternative of medical therapy. Absolute benefits are proportional to the risk expected with medical therapy. Clinical and angiographic markers of risk, including severity of CAD, left ventricular dysfunction, and myocardial ischemia, can identify patients in various risk strata. The benefits of CABG are greatest among those who are at highest risk with medical therapy (5 year mortality greater than 20%).

Limitations of first generation randomized clinical trials

During the last two decades, advances have occurred in both surgical and medical treatments that potentially could alter the results if trials were repeated today. These advances include the use of left internal thoracic artery conduits that have long-term patency rates markedly superior to venous bypass grafts, and aggressive lipid lowering and chronic antiplatelet therapies.[17,18] The CABG surgery versus medical therapy trials were confined to patients 65 years or younger, but more than 50% of CABG procedures are now performed on patients 65 years or older.[3] Similarly, only CASS enrolled women, whereas women now commonly undergo CABG surgery. The use of internal thoracic conduits was limited to only 14% of the patients in CASS, and this conduit was not used in the other trials. Lipid lowering agents were not widely used, HMG-CoA reductase inhibitors were not available, and aspirin was not widely used in either the medical or surgical groups. High-risk patients, such as those with severe angina and left main coronary artery stenosis, were underrepresented in these trials. These considerations and the results of the small recent trials suggest that the benefits of CABG surgery on clinical outcomes are likely to be larger than in the old randomized trials, especially among subsets of high risk patients.

PTCA versus medical therapy

PTCA was first introduced in the late 1970s as a treatment for single vessel CAD,[2] and it has become one of the most commonly performed major procedures. Most PTCA procedures are still performed for single vessel disease,[19,20] but its role in multivessel disease is expanding, and rates of procedural success and complications[19,20] have been described in large observational databases. Six prospective trials have enrolled patients to strategies of initial medical therapy versus balloon angioplasty.[21–26]

The first of such trials, A Comparison of Angioplasty With Medical Therapy in the Treatment of Single-Vessel Coronary Artery Disease (ACME), was published in 1992,[21] 13 years after the first report of PTCA.[2] In this trial, 212 patients with

stable, single vessel CAD and exercise induced myocardial ischemia were randomly assigned to PTCA or medical therapy. The proportion of patients free of angina at 6 months was greater in the PTCA arm (64% *v* 46%, *P*< 0·01), and the number of monthly anginal episodes was fewer among those with angina despite a low (by current standards) technical success rate of only 80% with PTCA. These patients required fewer medications and had better improvement in treadmill exercise duration (increase, 2·1 *v* 0·5 minutes; *P*< 0·0001) and psychologic wellbeing scores. However, these symptomatic improvements came at a considerable price, which included two emergency CABG operations and five myocardial infarctions. An accompanying trial from the ACME group enrolled 328 patients with double vessel disease and was reported in 1997. In this trial, functional improvement occurred in both the medical and angioplasty treated groups, and without statistically significant differences between the groups.[25]

The largest prospective trial of PTCA versus medical therapy was the multicenter Randomized Intervention Treatment of Angina (RITA) 2 trial.[23] Most of the patients had mild symptoms (80% Canadian Cardiovascular Society class 0 to II), 60% had single vessel CAD, and 33% had two vessel disease; only 6% had marked left ventricular dysfunction. The primary end point of death or myocardial infarction occurred in 6·3% of the PTCA group and 3·3% of the medical therapy group (absolute difference, 3·0%, 95% CI 0·4–5·7; *P*= 0·02). The combined rates of death, myocardial infarction, and non-protocol revascularization were about 25% in both groups by 3 years of follow up, and were primarily due to repeat procedures in the PTCA group and progression of symptoms in the medical group (Figure 27.3). Angina pectoris and treadmill exercise time improved significantly in both groups. Patients with grade 2 or worse angina appeared to benefit more from PTCA; they had a lower incidence of angina and longer treadmill

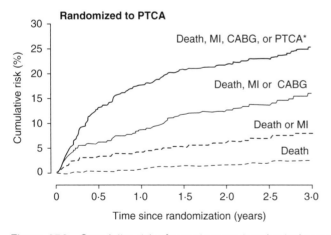
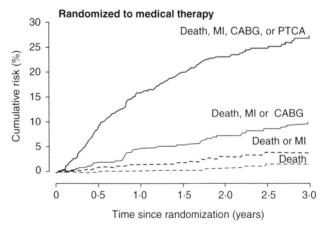

Figure 27.3 Cumulative risk of percutaneous transluminal coronary angioplasty (PTCA) and coronary artery bypass graft (CABG) for myocardial infarction (MI), or death. *denotes PTCA in addition to randomized PTCA. (From RITA-2 Trial participants[23] by permission of *The Lancet* Ltd.)

exercise times than that of the medical therapy group. Patients with mild symptoms at enrollment had no measurable improvement from PTCA. Quality of life measures were assessed at 6 months and at 1 and 3 years with the SF-36 instrument.[1] Both groups experienced improvement, with PTCA producing greater improvement in physical functioning, vitality, and general health at 3 months and 1 year; 33% of the PTCA group and 22% of the medical therapy group rated their health much improved ($P = 0.008$). These improvements were related to breathlessness, angina, and treadmill exercise time. By 3 years, no intergroup differences were observed, which may be explained partly by the 27% crossover to PTCA among the medical therapy group.[27]

The Atorvastatin Versus Revascularization Treatment (AVERT) trial[26] randomly assigned 341 patients with low risk CAD (99% of patients had stable Canadian Cardiovascular Society class 0 to II angina) to percutaneous revascularization plus usual medical care, or to medical care including aggressive therapy with atorvastatin. Over a mean follow up of 18 months, the PTCA group experienced more cardiac events (cardiac death or arrest, revascularization, stroke, or worsening angina) overall than the atorvastatin group (21% *v* 13% for PTCA and atorvastatin groups, respectively, $P = 0.048$). However, a greater proportion of the PTCA group had improvement in anginal symptoms (54% *v* 41%, $P = 0.009$).

The findings of the individual trials are reinforced by a systematic review of PTCA versus medical treatment for stable CAD.[28] The review included data from six randomized clinical trials that enrolled 953 patients given balloon angioplasty and 951 given medication. Treatment with PTCA resulted in significant improvement in angina (RR, 0.70, 95% CI 0.50–0.98); however, patients who had PTCA required CABG more frequently (RR, 1.59, 95% CI 1.09–2.32). No differences in death (RR, 1.32, 95% CI 0.65–2.70) or myocardial infarction (RR, 1.42, 95% CI 0.90–2.25) were observed (Figure 27.4). Because a substantial proportion of patients enrolled in medical arms required PTCA for symptom control, the overall odds of non-protocol PTCA did not differ despite the occurrence of restenosis after initial PTCA (RR, 1.29, 95% CI 0.72–3.36).

Conclusions: PTCA versus medical therapy

On the basis of the results of the above trials, it is evident that among patients with low risk symptomatic CAD (Canadian Cardiovascular Society class II or greater and average mortality of <1% per year), PTCA can improve symptoms and measures of quality of life compared with medication alone. No apparent reduction can be expected in overall mortality, need for subsequent PTCA, myocardial infarction, or CABG (which may be higher than with medical therapy). These data suggest that PTCA is indicated if the desired level of anginal relief and physical activity

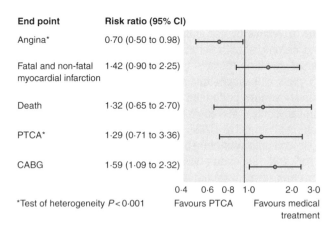

End point	Risk ratio (95% CI)
Angina*	0.70 (0.50 to 0.98)
Fatal and non-fatal myocardial infarction	1.42 (0.90 to 2.25)
Death	1.32 (0.65 to 2.70)
PTCA*	1.29 (0.71 to 3.36)
CABG	1.59 (1.09 to 2.32)

0.4 0.6 0.8 1.0   2.0 3.0
*Test of heterogeneity $P < 0.001$ Favours PTCA   Favours medical treatment

Figure 27.4 Pooled risk ratios for various end points from six randomized controlled trials comparing percutaneous transluminal coronary angioplasty (PTCA) with medical treatment in patients with non-acute coronary heart disease. CABG, coronary artery bypass grafting; $n = 953$ for PTCA and 951 for medical treatment. (From Bucher *et al*[28] by permission of BMJ Publishing Group.)

cannot be achieved with medical therapy. Aggressive lipid lowering therapy is indicated for all patients with stable CAD. With the excess risk of cardiac events seen in several trials, PTCA purely for the treatment of an anatomical coronary artery stenosis or for ischemia without symptoms cannot be recommended. Similarly, PTCA for prevention of myocardial infarction is not indicated.

Theoretic considerations for comparison of CABG, PTCA, and medical therapy

Although PTCA was conceived originally as an alternative to CABG, rates of both PTCA and CABG have increased consistently and in parallel.[3] This and the fact that most PTCA procedures have been performed for single vessel disease suggest that PTCA has been used primarily as an alternative to medical therapy rather than to CABG. More recently, with increased experience and technical advances, the pattern of use of PTCA has increasingly included subsets of patients previously referred for CABG. Several prospective randomized clinical trials have compared multivessel PTCA, CABG, and stents. Before the results of these trials are reviewed (which compare two active invasive therapies without medical or placebo controls), several methodologic issues need to be considered.

Moderate- to high-risk patients

As mentioned above, several outcomes can be assessed in comparing PTCA with CABG: mortality, non-fatal events (such as non-fatal myocardial infarction), symptoms, cost, and surrogate laboratory end points (such as left ventricular function). Because neither PTCA nor CABG has been shown to decrease the incidence of non-fatal myocardial infarction compared with medical therapy, this end point is unlikely to be sensitive to a possible differential effect of the two procedures. Indeed, considering non-fatal infarction in a composite end point may dilute event rates sufficiently to preclude detection (by lowering statistical power). Similarly, inclusion of low-risk subgroups in which CABG has *not* been shown to improve survival compared with medical therapy, such as single vessel disease, would decrease the ability to demonstrate mortality differences. An exception would occur if PTCA were significantly worse than medical therapy or substantially superior to CABG (both of which can be considered unlikely).

It has been demonstrated that CABG is associated with a 30–50% mortality risk reduction in moderate- and high-risk subgroups at 5 years compared with medical therapy. The detection of a difference in relative risk difference of half this magnitude (15–25%) between CABG and PTCA would be clinically relevant. If such a comparison indicated superiority of PTCA over CABG, it could reasonably be concluded that PTCA was superior to both medical therapy (indirect extrapolation) and CABG (direct inference). However, if a 20% difference in the relative risk of mortality in favor of CABG existed, surgical revascularization generally would be preferred over PTCA for such patients if the goal were improvement in prognosis. If the available data from such a comparison were large, the confidence interval of any observed difference would be narrow enough (for example, 20% ± 10%) to suggest that PTCA was superior to medical therapy to a clinically worthwhile extent, an indirect extrapolation that would be necessary in the absence of a medical control arm.

If no difference were observed between CABG and PTCA, it could be concluded that PTCA is equivalent to CABG only if trials were large enough to reliably detect or exclude relative differences in mortality of about 20% (with narrow confidence intervals) and included a large number of patients for whom CABG has been shown to improve prognosis. Because approximately 600 deaths would be needed in the "control" group to exclude a relative risk difference of 20% with 90% power, trials with about 8000 moderate- to high-risk patients would be needed. If a 30% risk difference were considered the smallest clinically important difference, then trials of about 4000 patients would be required. Moreover, in such a comparison, if the confidence limits of any difference included the possibility that PTCA was worse than CABG by 50% (relative risk), it could not be inferred that PTCA had any favorable effect on survival compared with medical therapy.

Low-risk patients

Among low-risk patients (annual mortality <2%), it may be moot to assess mortality differences between PTCA and CABG, because CABG has not been shown to decrease mortality. Conducting a trial to detect clinically important differences in such patients would be extremely difficult because of the large number of patients that would be required. For example, if a control group annual mortality rate of 1% is assumed, 8000 patients would need to be followed for 5 years to detect reliably a 30% risk reduction (or 16 000 patients to detect a 20% risk reduction). In such low-risk patients, any absolute benefit is likely to be too small to justify the costs and risks associated with revascularization. A large difference (for example, a 50% risk reduction that could be demonstrated with about 4000 randomized patients) would be extremely unlikely.

Therefore, among low-risk patients, the most relevant comparison is between PTCA and medical therapy. Such trials are unlikely to demonstrate a difference in mortality between PTCA and medical therapy (unless PTCA were harmful), and symptom improvement is the most relevant outcome of interest. Effects on a combined clinical variable could be compared, potentially including other non-fatal events such as myocardial infarction, severe angina, cost, and need for further revascularization procedures. Non-fatal events in a composite end point would need to be chosen carefully. As mentioned above, neither CABG nor PTCA has been shown to decrease the risk of subsequent non-fatal myocardial infarction, and inclusion of such an end point would dilute relative differences and decrease the likelihood of detecting differences. Both PTCA and CABG are effective in relieving angina and myocardial ischemia, and a relevant composite end point could include death plus severe angina. Such trials are feasible and could provide clinically relevant answers. It must be borne in mind that invasive procedures may increase rates of myocardial infarction, because of periprocedural risks, while decreasing subsequent angina pectoris.

Conclusions

These considerations indicate that to reliably compare the relative effect of PTCA versus CABG and to avoid missing clinically important differences, the following conditions need to be met:

- inclusion of subgroups in which surgery has been shown to be superior to medical therapy;
- inclusion of a sufficient number of patients (that is, adequate statistical power);
- follow up of at least 4–5 years to accrue a sufficient number of end points and to obtain data well beyond the early period when periprocedural events predominate; and
- a high rate of compliance to the original treatment allocation.

If a substantial proportion of patients crossover (30–40% by 5 years), the ability to detect differences in survival decreases markedly.

Trials of PTCA versus CABG

Technologic advances in the last 5–7 years have increasingly allowed wider application of PTCA, and a number of prospective, randomized trials have directly compared PTCA with CABG. A systematic review of eight of these trials[29] has been published.

Single vessel disease

In patients with single vessel CAD, medical therapy generally is indicated first, but revascularization may be indicated for symptom relief. Both PTCA and CABG offer a high rate of procedural success in such patients. Three randomized trials have provided data comparing PTCA and CABG for single vessel disease. The largest of these was the British RITA trial, which included 456 patients with single vessel disease.[30,31] After a median 6·5 years of follow up, no significant difference in death plus myocardial infarction was found (16·7% CABG v 19·3% PTCA, P = 0·56) among patients with single vessel disease. Patients randomly assigned to PTCA required a significantly greater number of repeat interventional procedures (38% v 12%, P = 0·01).

The results of MASS, the only three-way randomization among PTCA, CABG, and medical therapy to date, have been reviewed above. A second, single-center Swiss study was published in 1994.[32] In this trial, 134 patients with isolated proximal left anterior descending coronary artery stenosis were randomly assigned to angioplasty or CABG with a left internal thoracic artery conduit. Over 2·5 years of follow up, only one cardiac death occurred in the CABG group and none in the PTCA group, confirming the generally low-risk status of these patients. No significant difference was found in cardiac death or myocardial infarction (4·5% CABG v 11·7% PTCA, P = 0·21), and the only significant difference between the two groups was a higher rate of repeat revascularization in the PTCA group (34%) because of restenosis. Relief of angina was achieved in a high proportion of each group (more than 95% of patients were in Canadian Cardiovascular Society class I at 1 year), and no difference in the duration of the exercise test was found.

The meta-analysis of Pocock *et al*[29] included 732 patients with single vessel disease. Results of an updated meta-analysis, including the RITA long-term follow up data, are presented in Table 27.3. No significant differences were found in overall mortality. Rates of death or myocardial infarction favored CABG but did not reach statistical significance. Rates of additional revascularization procedures were significantly higher after PTCA.

In summary, the data available suggest that both PTCA and CABG are effective in providing symptom relief for patients with severe single vessel CAD. Rates of myocardial infarction may be higher after PTCA, likely because of periprocedural events; however, because no such difference was found for multivessel disease (see below), caution is needed to avoid overinterpretation of these data. Patients undergoing PTCA unequivocally have a greater likelihood of repeat procedures because of restenosis. If this is acceptable to patients and their physicians, then PTCA offers a simpler and less invasive method of revascularization. Of note, the meta-analysis of CABG versus medical therapy trials suggested a mortality benefit for CABG in one or two vessel disease with involvement of the proximal left anterior descending coronary artery (odds ratio, 0·58, 95% CI 0·34–1·01).[7] These patients have a large area of myocardium at jeopardy and are at higher risk for death than those with other forms of single vessel disease and may represent a group that merits special consideration. For single vessel disease, the current conclusions and recommendations are based on a relatively small number of patients and events (n = 731, with 44 deaths), and the possibility that potentially important differences between therapies were missed cannot be excluded.

Multivessel disease

For multivessel disease, CABG has remained the mainstay of therapy, especially for moderate- and high-risk patients such as those with severe two or three vessel disease with concomitant left ventricular dysfunction. The group of patients with multivessel disease is a heterogeneous group, with marked heterogeneity in the location and extent of anatomical stenosis, clinical symptoms, ventricular function, and coexistent disease. Thus, characteristics of patients enrolled need to be evaluated carefully when comparing trial results.

Nine prospective randomized clinical trials have compared PTCA (that is, balloon angioplasty) with CABG surgery in the treatment of multivessel disease.[24,30,32–38] These trials have enrolled 5200 patients and, although they vary in design, methods, and stage of follow up, they are broadly comparable and it is instructive to consider them together. The main characteristics of these trials are compared in Tables 27.3 and 27.4. All trials shared important features: treatment allocation to PTCA or CABG was randomly assigned, a high degree of compliance with the assigned therapy was achieved (more than 95%), and follow up data describing vital status, incidence of myocardial infarction, and prevalence of angina pectoris (or measures of myocardial ischemia) were collected. No trial individually was powered to detect or to exclude differences in mortality, and various composite clinical end points were used. Length of follow up varied, and in some instances, additional follow up is planned.

The largest of the PTCA versus CABG trials, the Bypass Angioplasty Revascularization Investigation (BARI), was published in 1996.[39] Designed as an "equivalence" trial,

Table 27.3 Main characteristics of nine prospective randomized trials of PTCA versus CABG

	BARI[37]	CABRI[35]	EAST[33]	ERACI[36]	GABI[34]	MASS[24]	RITA[30]	Swiss[32]	Toulouse[38]
Location	North America, multicenter	Europe, multicenter	Emory University (Atlanta, GA), single-center	Argentina, single-center	Germany, multicenter	Brazil, single-center	Britain, multicenter	Switzerland, single-center	France, single-center
Patients screened (n)	25 200	?	5118	1409	8981	?	17 237	?	?
Randomized (%)	1829 (7·3)	1054	392 (7·7)	127 (9·0)	359 (4·0)	214	1011 (4·8)	142	152
Equivalent revascularization required	No	No	No	No	Yes	Yes	Yes	Yes	Yes
Follow up Planned duration (years)	10	5–10	3	3	1	3·5	5	2·5	3
Completed	No	No	Yes	Yes	Yes	Yes	No	Yes	Yes
Primary end point	Mortality, MI	Mortality, non-fatal MI, angina, functional capacity	Combined death, MI, and large thallium defect	Combined death, MI, and angina	Freedom from angina at 1 year (>CCS 2)	Combined cardiac death, MI, refractory angina	Combined death and MI	Death, MI, repeat revascularization	?

Abbreviations: CABG, coronary artery bypass graft; CCS, Canadian Cardiovascular Society; MI, myocardial infarction; PTCA, percutaneous transluminal coronary angioplasty (Adapted from Raco D, Rihal CS, Yusuf S. Randomized trials of percutaneous transluminal coronary angioplasty: comparison of medical and surgical therapy. In: Grech ED, Ramsdale DR, eds. *Practical interventional cardiology.* St. Louis: Mosby, 1997. By permission of Martin Dunitz)

Table 27.4 Patient profiles in nine randomized trials of PTCA versus CABG

	BARI[37]	CABRI[35]	EAST[33]	ERACI[36]	GABI[34]	MASS[24]	RITA[30]	Swiss[32]	Toulouse[38]
Number of stenotic vessels (%)									
one	0	0	0	0	0	100	45	100	–
two	56	58	60	55	81	–	43	–	49
three	43	40	40	45	19	–	12	–	14
Mean ejection fraction (%)	58	63	61	61	?	75	?	?	?
Average age (years)	61	61	62	57	59	56	57	56	?
CCS class 3 or 4 angina (%)	?	65	80	?	65	?	60	89	?
Mammary artery used (% of CABG procedures)	82	?	90	77	37	100	74	100	?
Male:female	74:26	63:37	74:26	54:46	80:20	58:42	81:19	80:20	?
Previous MI (%)	?	41	41	32	47	?	43	0	?

Abbreviations: CABG, coronary artery bypass graft; CCS, Canadian Cardiovascular Society; MI, myocardial infarction
(Adapted from Raco D, Rihal CS, Yusuf S. Randomized trials of percutaneous transluminal coronary angioplasty: comparison of medical and surgical therapy. In: Grech ED, Ramsdale DR, eds. *Practical interventional cardiology*. St. Louis: Mosby, 1997. By permission of Martin Dunitz)

sample size calculations were predicated on an estimated cumulative 5 year mortality of about 5%, with the goal that the upper 95% confidence limit for any observed difference would not exceed 2·5%.[37] Approximately 30% of screened angiograms of patients with multivessel disease were considered eligible and 1829 patients were enrolled. About 40% of these patients had three vessel disease, and 22% had an ejection fraction less than 50%. Assignment to PTCA or CABG was randomly allocated, and follow up was continued for 5 years before the first results were presented. Five year mortality among patients assigned to CABG was 10·7%, and 13·7% among those assigned to PTCA (absolute difference 3·0%, 95% CI $-0·2-6·0$; $P = 0·19$). The study was interpreted as negative because the 22% relative risk reduction in favor of CABG did not reach statistical significance, but the study had less than 40% power to detect the observed difference. Extension of follow up to 7 years demonstrated a mortality advantage to CABG that was nominally significant (15·6% v 19·1% for PTCA, $P = 0·043$).[40] The entire difference appears to be confined to the subgroup of 353 (19% of total enrollees) patients with diabetes mellitus (7 year mortality 23·6% CABG v 44·3% PTCA, $P = 0·0011$). No difference in survival was noted among the remaining 1476 (81%) patients (7 year mortality, 13·6% CABG v 13·2% PTCA, $P = 0·72$). Implications of the findings in the diabetic subgroup are discussed in more detail below; however, considerable caution should be applied to interpretation of these findings unless they are confirmed by other randomized clinical trials.

A systematic review of eight of these trials has been published;[29] however, BARI was published after the initial meta-analysis. Results of updated systematic reviews of all-cause mortality (death or myocardial infarction) and non-protocol revascularization after the initial randomly assigned treatment are presented in Table 27.3. Inclusion of late follow up data, particularly from BARI, yielded a nominally significant difference in total mortality in favor of CABG (11·1% PTCA v 9·5% CABG; odds ratio 1·20, 95% CI 1·00–1·45; $P = 0·05$). The combined end point of death or myocardial infarction, however, did not differ (17·2% PTCA, 16·8% CABG; odds ratio 1·04, 95% CI 0·89–1·20). Rates of repeat procedures were much higher after PTCA (52% v 11%; odds ratio 9·15, 95% CI 7·9–10·6).

Substudies have demonstrated that PTCA and CABG produce similar benefits on quality of life measures and return to employment, and are roughly equivalent in cost over 3–5 years of follow up.[41–44] CABG is associated with more complete revascularization, but differences in degree of revascularization of major lesions are less pronounced.[43]

Conclusions: PTCA (balloon angioplasty) versus CABG

In summary, 5200 patients with multivessel CAD have been enrolled in nine trials of PTCA versus CABG. When long-term follow up data are considered, cumulative mortality rates are lower with CABG than with PTCA, and fewer patients require repeat procedures. However, the initial morbidity is less with PTCA, rates of myocardial infarction are similar, and overall anginal relief is nearly equivalent by 3 years. Restenosis continues to be a major limitation of PTCA. These data suggest that for patients at high risk for death, CABG is preferred. For other patients, PTCA is a reasonable alternative if a higher rate of repeat procedures is acceptable.

Can it be concluded, then, that PTCA and CABG are roughly equivalent modes of revascularization for multivessel disease among angiographically eligible patients, except for the unsolved problem of restenosis? To answer this question, it is necessary to consider the marked heterogeneity of what is termed "multivessel disease". Although discrete lesions of the right coronary and circumflex arteries in a patient who has a normal left ventricle or diffuse three vessel disease in a patient with an ejection fraction of 30% can rightly be classified under the term "multivessel disease", the prognoses, risks, and potential benefits of revascularization vary considerably.

In the recent PTCA versus CABG trials, enrolled patients were relatively low risk: fewer than 20% had left ventricular dysfunction and almost 70% had one or two vessel disease. In the meta-analysis of Pocock *et al*,[29] for example, the observed first year mortality of 2·6% and 1·1% per year thereafter confirms the relatively low-risk status of these patients. (However, no medical control arms were present.) Patients enrolled in BARI had higher observed mortality rates and more closely approximated moderate-risk patients, in part because of the higher proportion of patients with diabetes mellitus. Even in BARI, however, nearly 60% of patients had two vessel coronary artery disease. In contrast, patients enrolled in the earlier CABG versus medical therapy trials had a 20% prevalence of left ventricular dysfunction and 60% had three vessel or left main CAD.[7] Thus, the current PTCA versus CABG trials include a high proportion of patients in whom CABG has *not* been shown to be superior to medical therapy. Moreover, the total enrollment of 5200 patients falls short of the roughly 8000 needed to demonstrate clinically important differences in mortality of 20–30% among low- and moderate-risk patients. It is reasonable to surmise that, if CABG were superior to PTCA in moderate- and high-risk patients, the current PTCA versus CABG trials would have low power to reliably detect significant differences, and that such a difference cannot be ruled out. Large mortality differences on the order of 40–50%, however, are unlikely, given the current data. Also, these trials were performed before the wide use of intracoronary stents, and whether stents may change the observed outcomes is discussed below.

Relative effect of PTCA and CABG in patients with diabetes

BARI findings

On 21 September 1995, the National Heart, Lung, and Blood Institute took the unusual measure of issuing a Clinical Alert to physicians in the United States about the observed superiority of CABG over PTCA among the 353 treated diabetic patients enrolled in the BARI randomized trial.[45] After 5 years of follow up, the cumulative mortality after CABG was 19%

among patients with diabetes compared with 35% for those treated with PTCA ($P < 0·0024$). The findings, however, were unexpected. At the initiation of the trial, patients were categorized into four subgroups for purposes of analysis: by anginal status, left ventricular function, extent of ischemia, and angiographic risk. Patients with diabetes were not among the original four pre-assigned subgroups, but within 1 year after the trial began, the Data and Safety Monitoring Board requested that these patients be monitored separately.[46] The magnitude of the difference favoring CABG met the pre-specified significance criteria ($P < 0·005$) for subgroup analyses and led to the Clinical Alert.

The recently published 7 year outcome data have extended these observations.[40] Among the patients with diabetes in the BARI randomized trial, estimated 7 year survival was 76·4% after CABG and 55·7% after PTCA ($P = 0·0011$). The difference in outcome was confined to diabetic patients who received at least one internal mammary arterial graft (7 year survival 83·2%, $n = 140$), whereas diabetic patients who received only saphenous vein grafts had a 7 year survival (54·5%, $n = 33$), similar to those who had PTCA (55·5%, $n = 170$).[40] Long-term follow up from the much smaller Emory Angioplasty versus Surgery Trial (EAST) that included 59 patients with diabetes was consistent with these results, although it did not attain statistical significance (8 year survival, 75·5% after CABG and 60·1% after PTCA; $P = 0·23$).[47] Of course, the key question is whether the BARI outcomes among diabetic patients were real or only a play of chance. Several lines of evidence suggest it is real, and they have been reviewed in detail.[46]

In a combined analysis from the BARI trial and registry of 641 diabetic patients and 2962 non-diabetic patients, 5 year death (20% *v* 8%) and Q wave myocardial infarction (8% *v* 4%) rates were significantly higher among those with diabetes.[48] Multivariate analysis identified insulin treated diabetes, heart or renal failure, black race, and older age as most strongly associated with high overall mortality.[49] The only significant interaction term was between treatment and insulin treated diabetes ($P = 0·042$).[49] Overall, CABG did not have a protective effect against the incidence of Q wave myocardial infarction; however, CABG greatly decreased the risk of death among diabetic patients when infarction occurred (RR 0·09, 95% CI 0·03–0·29; $P < 0·001$). This effect may account for up to 50% of the overall reduction in mortality after CABG observed in the diabetic subgroup of BARI.

An independent, angiographic case–control study has suggested a significantly higher propensity for the development of new coronary vascular lesions among patients with diabetes, both when previously instrumented (16·9% *v* 12·7% of non-diabetic arteries) and *de novo* (13·2% *v* 7·3%).[50] Unpublished 5 year angiographic follow up data from BARI 1 (Frye RL, read at the American College of Cardiology 50th Annual Scientific Sessions, Orlando, Florida, 20 March 2001) have suggested similar findings. These data suggest that

CABG, particularly with internal mammary artery conduits, confers a protective shield against the complications of progression of the underlying vascular disease in patients with diabetes. Whether intensive medical therapy for diabetes can influence progression of macrovascular complications in this group is not known.

The results of the BARI subgroup have not been reproduced in other large trials, and observational data sets and caution must be exercised in the interpretation of the BARI diabetic data.[51–55] Retrospective analysis of small subgroups may overestimate or even misdirect the treatment effect. A Duke University study of 3230 patients (24% with diabetes), selected for similarity to BARI enrollees, found that diabetes was a marker of a worse prognosis after both CABG and PTCA, but with no clear superiority of one procedure over the other.[52]

The largest database study of patients with diabetes undergoing revascularization is from Emory University, where 2639 such patients with multivessel coronary artery disease who underwent PTCA or CABG between 1981 and 1994 were examined. CABG was superior only among the 889 patients treated with insulin, but confidence intervals were wide (hazard ratio for mortality after PTCA 1·35, 95% CI 1·01–1·79 compared with CABG). This finding is consistent with the BARI trial, in which CABG superiority was more pronounced among patients with diabetes who were taking insulin.[54] In the BARI observational registry, which accompanied the randomized trial, a clear difference in outcomes after CABG or PTCA was not observed.[53] Five year mortality among diabetic patients after PTCA ($n=182$) was 14·4% and 14·9% after CABG ($n=117$; RR 1·10, $P=0·86$).[54] Significant differences in adverse socioeconomic and angiographic characteristics (such as number of significant lesions and presence of diffuse disease) between patients treated with PTCA or CABG were present. Generally, patients who had PTCA had fewer adverse risk factors than those assigned to CABG. After adjustment for these differences, the hazard ratio for mortality after PTCA rose to 1·41 but did not attain significance (95% CI 0·60–3·29).

Conclusions: revascularization in patients with diabetes

In both trials and observational data sets, diabetes mellitus is clearly a marker for high risk and, in comparison with non-diabetic patients, the prognosis is worse after either PTCA or CABG. In the largest randomized trial of PTCA versus CABG, patients with diabetes who received internal mammary artery grafts had better outcomes than those treated with PTCA. However, large non-randomized registry data suggest equivalent outcomes after either procedure as long as the sicker patients are triaged to surgery. One conclusion that may resolve the apparent dilemma is that selected patients with diabetes, such as those with favorable

angiographic characteristics, may do as well with PTCA and CABG, whereas those with more diffuse or advanced coronary artery disease do better with CABG as initial therapy. Because 5200 patients have been enrolled in trials of PTCA versus CABG surgery, collaborative meta-analysis based on individual patient data may allow more definitive characterization of outcomes after revascularization among diabetic patients. It remains to be determined whether the use of stents, particularly in combination with parenteral antiplatelet drugs and aggressive metabolic management, will change these conclusions.

Although no prospective randomized trial of myocardial revascularization in patients with diabetes exists, the BARI 2 trial will test the hypothesis that revascularization for diabetic patients early in the stages of CAD may significantly decrease 5 year mortality. This study will incorporate strict metabolic and risk factor control and test both insulin-providing and insulin-sensitizing agents.

Effect of stents on outcome after revascularization

Since first approved by the US Food and Drug Administration in 1993, coronary stents have been adopted rapidly and widely as the main method of percutaneous revascularization, although the pace of adoption has outstripped the pace of the accompanying clinical investigation and regulatory approval.[56,57] Likely, more than 1 000 000 patients now receive intracoronary stents in the USA annually, with an equivalent number in the rest of the world, primarily Europe.

The first indication for stents was for the treatment of severe coronary artery dissection with acute or threatened vessel closure. The National Heart, Lung and Blood Institute 1985–86 PTCA registry documented the risks of balloon angioplasty before the development of stents. Abrupt vessel closure occurred in 6·8% of all procedures, with 32% of these patients requiring emergency CABG and 42% having a myocardial infarction; the case fatality rate was 5%.[58] A prospective multicenter registry of 518 patients with acute or threatened vessel closure after PTCA treated with stents was reported in 1993.[59] Successful stent deployment occurred in 95·4% of cases. The rates of inhospital emergency CABG and myocardial infarction among these patients with severe coronary artery dissections were 4·3% and 5·5%, respectively, markedly lower than the historical control rates mentioned above. Although not randomized, this study and others[60] established the role of stents in the treatment of arterial dissections after PTCA.

Numerous prospective, randomized trials published over the past 10 years have compared elective stenting to balloon angioplasty under various circumstances. These studies have enrolled patients with various lesion types, including elective procedures for single discrete lesions in vessels of 3·0 mm or larger,[61–71] restenosis lesions after previous balloon angioplasty,[72] lesions of saphenous vein grafts,[73] small caliber vessels,[74–77] and chronic total occlusions.[78–84] The effect of stents versus balloon angioplasty on the clinical outcomes of death, death or myocardial infarction, and repeat procedures, and the angiographic outcome of restenosis are shown in Table 27·5. In total, almost 7000 patients have been randomly allocated in published trials of stent versus balloon angioplasty, including 4694 who had systematic angiographic follow up. As shown in Table 27·5, overall mortality was low (1·5% v 1·9% for stent versus balloon angioplasty patients, respectively; odds ratio 0·83, 95% CI 0·57–1·21), as were death or myocardial infarction rates (6·1% v 6·5%; odds ratio 0·93, 95% CI 0·77–1·14). The impact of stenting on clinical end points was related to the need for repeat revascularization (14·7% after stenting v 23·9% after balloon angioplasty; 9·2% absolute risk reduction; odds ratio 0·53, 95% CI 0·46–0·60). A significant decrease in the incidence of angiographic restenosis was

found (27·5% v 42·2%; odds ratio 0·50, 95% CI 0·44–0·57) among patients who had systematic follow up angiography (26·6% stent v 41·6% PTCA; odds ratio 0·48, 95% CI 0·42–0·56).

As with any rapidly evolving therapy, advances have occurred in techniques of stenting – for example, high pressure inflations[85] and improved antiplatelet therapy with oral[86,87] and parenteral antiplatelet[69] agents – that have allowed wider application.

A novel approach to the further optimization of results – the use of local drug delivery to inhibit the restenotic process after intracoronary stenting – is being evaluated in multiple trials. The first published trial tested a metal stent coated with the macrolide antibiotic sirolimus, an immunosuppressive agent that is a potent inhibitor of lymphocyte and smooth muscle cell proliferation.[88] In animal studies, sirolimus has been shown to be a potent inhibitor of restenosis.[89] The trial enrolled 238 patients with standard clinical indications for stenting and randomly assigned them to receive stents

Table 27.5 Summary of meta-analyses of revascularization for chronic coronary artery disease

PTCA[a] v CABG

Variable	PTCA (%)	CABG (%)	Trials (n)	Patients (n)	OR (95% CI)
Single vessel disease					
All cause mortality	5·6	6·4	3	732	0·86 (0·47–1·59)
Death or MI	15·0	11·7	3	732	1·33 (0·87–2·05)
Repeat revascularization	33·8	8·1	3	732	4·73 (3·32–6·77)
Overall					
All cause mortality	16·2	14·6	9	5200	1·14 (0·98–1·34)
Death or MI	17·2	16·8	9	5200	1·04 (0·89–1·20)
Repeat revascularization	52·6	13·1	9	5200	8·24 (7·14–9·52)

Stents v PTCA

Variable	Stents (%)	PTCA (%)	Trials (n)	Patients (n)	OR (95% CI)
Mortality	1·5	1·9	21	6929	0·83 (0·57–1·21)
Death or MI	6·1	6·5	21	6929	0·93 (0·77–1·13)
Repeat revascularization	14·7	23·9	21	6929	0·53 (0·44–0·57)
Angiographic restenosis > 50%	27·5	42·2	20	4694	0·50 (0·77–1·33)

Stents v CABG

Variable	Stents (%)	CABG (%)	Trials (n)	Patients (n)	OR (95% CI)
Mortality	5·5	5·6	5	3218	0·98 (0·72–1·34)
Death or MI	7·9	8·9	4	2764	0·87 (0·67–1·14)
Repeat revascularization	19·0	4·5	5	3218	5·00 (3·83–6·51)

Abbreviations: CABG, coronary artery bypass graft; CI, confidence interval; MI, myocardial infarction; OR, odds ratio; PTCA, percutaneous transluminal coronary angioplasty

[a] Meta-analyses were performed using RevMan 5·0 software (Cochrane Collaboration). To accrue the largest number of events possible, data used represent the longest term follow up available for each trial included, whether published or presented orally; 1 was added to all zero cells. Data are presented in summary form only. Details of each meta-analysis are beyond the scope of the current review.

coated with a sirolimus-polymer matrix or uncoated stents. Results were assessed by routine angiography at 6 months. None of the patients who received a sirolimus-coated stent had restenosis, as defined by at least 50% stenosis within the stent, compared with 26·6% of those who had a bare metal stent ($P < 0.001$). After 1 year of clinical follow up, there were no episodes of stent thrombosis, and 5·8% of the sirolimus group experienced an adverse cardiac event (death, MI, CABG, or revascularization of the original target vessel) compared with 28·8% of control stent group ($P < 0.001$). Although the decrease in restenosis rate and the corresponding reduction in need for further procedures are striking, the trial was only a relatively small single study with follow up limited to 1 year. Whether potent intra-arterial immunosuppression will have unanticipated long-term problems related to impaired arterial healing is unknown.

Several prospective randomized trials have compared multivessel stenting with multivessel CABG, although follow up periods remain short. The Arterial Revascularization Therapy Study (ARTS)[90] enrolled 1205 patients with multi-vessel disease (average, 2·7 treated lesions) to either stenting or CABG. At 12 months of follow up, 2·5% of the 600 stent patients and 2·8% of the 605 CABG patients had died. Kaplan–Meier estimated rates of the irreversible end points of death, stroke, or myocardial infarction at 1 year were 9·5% for the stent group and 11·2% for the CABG group (RR 0·92, 95% CI 0·62–1·35; $P = 0.65$). Stent patients required more follow up procedures than those assigned to CABG, with cumulative event rates at 1 year of 26·2% for the stent group and 12·2% for the CABG group (absolute difference, 14%). Within the stent group, the incremental 16·7% event rate at 1 year attributable to repeat revascularization was about half of the corresponding 33·7% 1 year repeat revascularization rate after balloon angioplasty in a meta-analysis of the balloon versus CABG trials,[29] and was consistent with the findings of the stent versus balloon trials described above. For comparison, 1 year rates of repeat revascularization after CABG have remained constant: 3·3% in the meta-analysis and 3·5% in ARTS.

Data from four other trials of stents versus CABG have been published or presented, including Stents or Surgery (Sigwart U, read at the American College of Cardiology 50th Annual Scientific Sessions, Orlando, Florida, 20 March 2001), a multicenter European study of nearly 1000 patients; Argentine Randomized Trial of PTCA Versus Coronary Artery Bypass Surgery in Multivessel Disease (ERACI) II,[91] a multi-center Argentinian study of 450 patients; and Stenting versus Internal Mammary Artery (SIMA),[92] a Swiss–Italian study of 123 patients. Findings are summarized in the accompanying meta-analyses in Table 27.3 and are consistent with those of ARTS. Data from Angina With Extremely Serious Operative Mortality Evaluation (AWESOME),[93] a prospective random-ized clinical trial conducted at 16 Veterans Affairs Medical Centers that assigned 454 patients with refractory angina and

markers of high risk to either percutaneous coronary inter-vention or CABG, are included because a high proportion of the patients in the percutaneous coronary intervention group received stents. Together, these randomized clinical trials have enrolled 3218 patients. No significant differences in mortality (5·45% after percutaneous coronary intervention v 5·61% after CABG; odds ratio 0·98, 95% CI 0·98–1·34), or death or myocardial infarction (7·9% after percutaneous coro-nary intervention v 8·9% after CABG; odds ratio 0·87, 95% CI 0·67–1·14) were found. The need for repeat proce-dures remains higher after stenting (19% v 4·5% after CABG; odds ratio 5·54, 95% CI 3·83–6·51), although lower than the rates reported earlier after multivessel balloon angioplasty.

Longer follow up and accrual of events is necessary before final conclusions can be drawn. Similarly, the num-ber of patients with diabetes enrolled was small and no specific conclusions can be drawn yet.

Miscellaneous interventional device trials

Numerous devices have been developed to allow or facili-tate percutaneous revascularization. After balloon angio-plasty, the directional atherectomy catheter was the first such device, gaining FDA approval in 1990. This device allows cutting and removal of coronary plaque in a con-trolled ("directional") manner. The hypothesis was that plaque removal would cause less trauma to the artery, incite a less vigorous neointimal response, and, ultimately, signifi-cantly decrease rates of restenosis and repeat procedures. Although marginal benefits regarding angiographic restenosis were observed in some trials (CAVEAT, BOAT),[94,95] this was not so in others (CCAT).[96] Worrisome increases in rates of myocardial infarction, death, and other major complications were noted in several trials (BOAT, CAVEAT, CAVEAT-II).[97,98] The rapid ease of use and rapid adoption of intracoronary stents have made directional atherectomy a so-called niche device, used only for particular anatomic circumstances.

Rotational atherectomy is another procedure that can be used for performing lesion debulking. It is performed with a high-speed rotating, diamond-tipped abrasive burr. The device allows recanalization of heavily calcified lesions or fibrotic lesions as well as debulking. No tissue is removed, and the device pulverises atherosclerotic plaque into tiny particles that pass through the microcirculation and are removed by the reticuloendothelial system. The device is associated with a rel-atively high incidence of poor flow after use and non-Q wave myocardial infarction and has had no particular benefit on restenosis (ERBAC).[99–101] Currently it is used primarily to facil-itate stent deployment when this would otherwise be impossi-ble because of severe calcification or fibrosis of the target lesion.

Intracoronary brachytherapy, or the local delivery of radi-ation to inhibit the restenotic process, was approved for the treatment of in-stent restenosis, a vexing problem that is difficult to treat initially and has high recurrence rates. Two competing systems, one capable of delivering beta radiation, and the other, gamma radiation, have been widely used. These devices have been demonstrated to significantly lower the rates of subsequent recurrent restenosis (14·6% v 60·8% in pooled data from three studies totalling 442 patients) and adverse cardiac events (24·5% v 70% P<0·001).[102–6] A triple-blind design with dummy radiation sources was used in some studies.[104] A delayed risk of stent thrombosis, particularly when a new stent was placed at the time of the procedure, was observed in follow up (6·2% of brachytherapy patients with a new stent v 0·7% of control patients with a new stent).[102] Avoidance of placement of new stents and continuation of dual antiplatelet therapy with aspirin and clopidogrel for 6–12 months has largely obviated this problem. If local drug-elution essentially eliminates or greatly reduces the incidence of in-stent restenosis, utilization of coronary brachytherapy is expected to decrease.

Database studies

Prospective randomized trials provide the highest level of evidence for clinical decision making; nonetheless,

information from trials frequently must be supplemented and enhanced by observational studies. Long-term survival for 9263 patients with angiographically documented CAD has been reported recently from Duke University Medical Center.[107,108] Although treatment assignment was non-random, the 97% complete follow up of this consecutive series has provided insight into the outcomes after various treatments (2449 patients, medical only; 2924, PTCA; and 3890, CABG), with concurrent controls. Nine risk strata based on the number and extent of diseased coronary arteries were identified (left main CAD and stenoses less than 75% were excluded). Long-term survival comparisons between treatments were assessed with Cox proportional hazards models and Kaplan–Meier survival analysis. CABG was significantly associated with improved long-term outcomes in comparison with medical therapy for patients in moderate-and high-risk strata (for three vessel disease [n = 2771]: odds ratio, 0·44, 95% CI 0·42–0·80) (Figure 27.5). PTCA, however, was superior to medical therapy only among low-risk strata.[108] In comparison with PTCA, CABG was associated with improved outcomes among high-risk strata, namely, all patients with three vessel disease and two vessel disease with

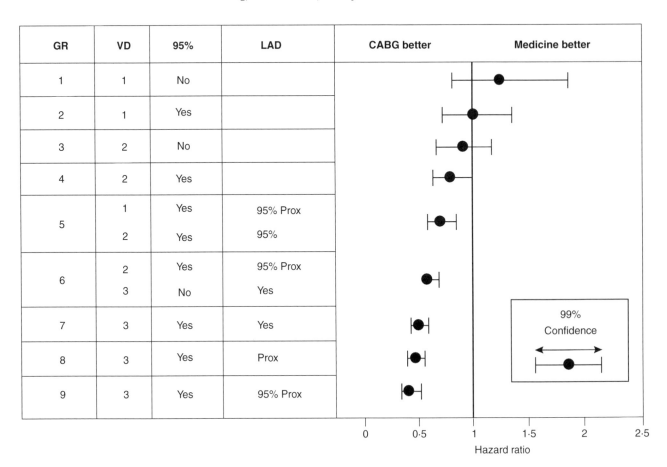

Figure 27.5 Adjusted hazard ratios comparing coronary artery bypass graft (CABG) and medicine for the nine coronary anatomy groups. GR, group; LAD, left anterior descending coronary artery; Prox, proximal; VD, number of diseased vessels; 95%, ≥95% coronary artery stenosis. (From Jones *et al*[108] by permission of Mosby-Year Book, Inc.)

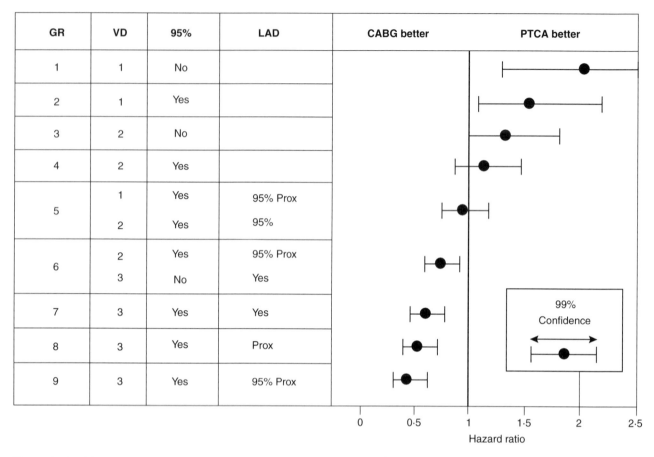

Figure 27.6 Adjusted hazard ratios comparing coronary artery bypass graft (CABG) and percutaneous transluminal coronary angioplasty (PTCA) for the nine coronary anatomy groups. GR, group; LAD, left anterior descending coronary artery; Prox, proximal; VD, number of diseased vessels; 95%, ≥95% coronary artery stenosis. (From Jones *et al*[108] by permission of Mosby-Year Book, Inc.)

95% involvement of the proximal left anterior descending coronary artery. Conversely, adjusted hazard ratios demonstrated superiority of PTCA over CABG among low-risk patients (Figure 27.6) and a trend toward superiority among moderate-risk patients.

These prospective observational data are broadly consistent with the previously presented framework placing PTCA versus CABG trials in the context of CABG versus medical therapy trials. Although a definitive benefit of CABG over medical therapy for one and two vessel disease could not be demonstrated in the randomized trials (with the possible exception of proximal left anterior descending CAD), non-significant trends favoring CABG were found. The relatively low number of observed events (113 deaths over 5 years) in these trials may have precluded detection of even a large benefit (type II error). The Duke observational data extended the randomized trials and, by virtue of the much larger number of events (related to the larger number of patients and longer duration of follow up), allow further characterization of possible treatment differences. As with any non-randomized study, important limitations related to intrinsic biases in patient

selection remain, and definitive conclusions require performance of larger randomized trials. For example, determination of time zero is a problem and deaths occurring while awaiting revascularization were assigned to medical therapy, which would tend to inflate event rates among medical patients.

Limitations of current data

In an evolving field, all trials designed to address specific clinical questions at a specific time should be interpreted in the context of relevant changes in the procedures and complementary treatments. This is especially notable for the CABG versus medical therapy trials performed 20 to 25 years ago. The wide application of antiplatelet, antihyperlipidemic, and ACE inhibitor therapy in current practice may substantially mitigate the published results. Temporal changes in angioplasty and surgical techniques are continuing and, in some cases, accelerating. The development of new interventional devices designed to deal with procedural complications, specific high-risk lesions, or previously unapproachable lesions has broadened the feasibility of percutaneous procedures. Coronary stents have decreased the incidence of both emergency and late CABG and lower restenosis. New adjunctive medical therapies such as platelet IIb/IIIa receptor antagonists reduce the risk of non-fatal myocardial infarction and emergency CABG with interventional procedures. CABG, too, has undergone considerable technologic advances. Internal thoracic arterial conduits with excellent long-term patency are now widely used. Improved myocardial preservation techniques, adjunctive medical therapies, and less invasive surgical approaches have been developed.

Specific methodologic concerns also exist about the available data. All the trials discussed above compared two active treatments and were not placebo controlled, decreasing the chances of detecting differences among arms. Invasive or surgical trials are logistically very complex, tend to be small compared with drug therapy trials, and are inherently open label. The possibility of missing potentially important differences, even when one exists, is always higher for small trials. Although systematic reviews, preferably based on individual patient data, can provide some redress, larger definitive trials (along with meta-analysis of their results) are preferable. In trials of invasive treatments, crossover to the other therapy occurs with increasing frequency during the course of follow up, necessitating consideration of therapeutic strategies rather than specific treatments. As with many large surgical trials, applicability of results to medical centers with lower volume and different levels of experience remains unproven.[109–111]

The greatest limitation of the currently available data is the low statistical power to detect potential differences in clinical outcomes, in particular the PTCA trials, whereas PTCA rates have grown dramatically. This situation could be rectified partly by long-term follow up of the trials that have been completed, accompanied by a collaborative meta-analysis based on individual patient data. Even if this were done, however, the lack of large trials incorporating all three major approaches to patients with coronary artery disease – medical, interventional, and surgical – would limit comprehensive comparisons to observational databases.[107]

Summary: overview of the evidence for myocardial revascularization in patients with chronic stable angina

CABG surgery versus medical therapy

- Among patients with medically refractory angina pectoris, CABG is indicated for symptom improvement. **Grade A1a**
- Among patients with medically stable angina pectoris, CABG is indicated for left main coronary artery or three

vessel disease, regardless of left ventricular function, for prolongation of life. **Grade A1a**
- CABG may be indicated for prolongation of life if the proximal left anterior descending coronary artery is involved, regardless of the number of diseased vessels. **Grade A1c**

Percutaneous coronary intervention versus medical therapy

- Among patients with medically refractory angina pectoris, PTCA is indicated for symptom improvement. **Grade A**
- In the absence of symptoms or myocardial ischemia, PTCA is not indicated merely for the presence of an anatomical stenosis. **Grade A**
- Stents are indicated for the treatment of arterial dissections with abrupt or threatened vessel closure after balloon angioplasty. **Grade B**
- Electively placed stents are superior to balloon angioplasty for reducing the need for repeat procedures and, likely, the risks of periprocedural myocardial infarction and emergency CABG surgery. **Grade A1a**

Percutaneous coronary intervention versus CABG

- For single vessel disease, both PTCA and CABG provide excellent symptom relief, but repeat revascularization procedures are required more frequently after PTCA. **Grade A**
- For multivessel disease, the higher the baseline risk of the patient, the more CABG is to be preferred. **Grade A1c** This includes both diabetic and non-diabetic patients with three vessel or diffuse disease or with left ventricular dysfunction. The following caveats should be considered:
  - Large differences in mortality (40–50%) between PTCA and CABG are unlikely, but smaller differences in mortality (on the order of 20–30%) cannot be excluded given the available data.
  - CABG is associated with more complete revascularization and superior early relief of angina, but these differences are lessened after 3–5 years.
  - No significant differences in rates of myocardial infarction have been demonstrated.
  - Repeat revascularization procedures are required significantly more often after PTCA, an effect partly mitigated by the use of stents.
  - The cost, quality of life, and return to work are initially more favorable with PTCA than CABG, but these variables roughly equalize over 3–5 years.

References

1. Favaloro RG. Saphenous vein autograft replacement of severe segmental coronary artery occlusion: operative technique. *Ann Thorac Surg* 1968;**5**:334–9.
2. Gruntzig AR, Senning A, Siegenthaler WE. Nonoperative dilatation of coronary-artery stenosis: percutaneous transluminal coronary angioplasty. *N Engl J Med* 1979;**301**:61–8.
3. Hall MJ, Popovic JR. *1998 Summary: National Hospital Discharge Survey. Advance data from Vital and Health Statistics; no. 316.* Hyattsville, Maryland: National Center for Health Statistics, 2000.
4. European Coronary Surgery Study Group. Long-term results of prospective randomised study of coronary artery bypass surgery in stable angina pectoris. *Lancet* 1982;**2**:1173–80.
5. The VA Coronary Artery Bypass Surgery Cooperative Study Group. Eighteen-year follow-up in the Veterans Affairs Cooperative Study of Coronary Artery Bypass Surgery for stable angina. *Circulation* 1992;**86**:121–30.
6. Alderman EL, Bourassa MG, Cohen LS *et al.* Ten-year follow-up of survival and myocardial infarction in the randomized Coronary Artery Surgery Study. *Circulation* 1990;**82**: 1629–46.
7. Yusuf S, Zucker D, Peduzzi P *et al.* Effect of coronary artery bypass graft surgery on survival: overview of 10-year results from randomised trials by the Coronary Artery Bypass Graft Surgery Trialists Collaboration. *Lancet* 1994;**344**:563–70.
8. Caracciolo EA, Davis KB, Sopko G *et al.* Comparison of surgical and medical group survival in patients with left main coronary artery disease. Long-term CASS experience. *Circulation* 1995;**91**:2325–34.
9. European Coronary Surgery Study Group. Prospective randomised study of coronary artery bypass surgery in stable angina pectoris. Second interim report by the European Coronary Surgery Study Group. *Lancet* 1980;**2**:491–5.
10. Caracciolo EA, Davis KB, Sopko G *et al.* Comparison of surgical and medical group survival in patients with left main equivalent coronary artery disease. Long-term CASS experience. *Circulation* 1995;**91**:2335–44.
11. Passamani E, Davis KB, Gillespie MJ, Killip T. A randomized trial of coronary artery bypass surgery. Survival of patients with a low ejection fraction. *N Engl J Med* 1985;**312**: 1665–71.
12. Myers WO, Schaff HV, Fisher LD *et al.* Time to first new myocardial infarction in patients with severe angina and three-vessel disease comparing medical and early surgical therapy: a CASS registry study of survival. *J Thorac Cardiovasc Surg* 1988;**95**:382–9.
13. Chaitman BR, Stone PH, Knatterud GL *et al.* Asymptomatic Cardiac Ischemia Pilot (ACIP) study: impact of anti-ischemia therapy on 12-week rest electrocardiogram and exercise test outcomes. The ACIP Investigators. *J Am Coll Cardiol* 1995;**26**:585–93.
14. Rogers WJ, Bourassa MG, Andrews TC, *et al.* Asymptomatic Cardiac Ischemia Pilot (ACIP) study: outcome at 1 year for patients with asymptomatic cardiac ischemia randomized to medical therapy or revascularization. The ACIP Investigators. *J Am Coll Cardiol* 1995;**26**:594–605.
15. Davies RF, Goldberg AD, Forman S *et al.* Asymptomatic Cardiac Ischemia Pilot (ACIP) study 2-year follow-up: outcomes of patients randomized to initial strategies of medical therapy versus revascularization. *Circulation* 1997;**95**: 2037–43.
16. The TIME Investigators. Trial of Invasive versus Medical Therapy in Elderly Patients with Chronic Symptomatic Coronary-Artery Disease (TIME): a randomised trial. *Lancet* 2001;**358**:951–7.
17. The Scandinavian Simvastatin Survival Study. Randomised trial of cholesterol lowering in 4444 patients with coronary heart disease: the Scandinavian Simvastatin Survival Study (4S). *Lancet* 1994;**344**:1383–9.
18. West of Scotland Coronary Prevention Study. Identification of high-risk groups and comparison with other cardiovascular intervention trials. *Lancet* 1996;**348**:1339–42.
19. Detre K, Holubkov R, Kelsey S *et al.* One-year follow-up results of the 1985–1986 National Heart, Lung, and Blood Institute's Percutaneous Transluminal Coronary Angioplasty Registry. *Circulation* 1989;**80**:421–8.
20. Detre K, Holubkov R, Kelsey S *et al.* Percutaneous transluminal coronary angioplasty in 1985–1986 and 1977–1981. The National Heart, Lung, and Blood Institute Registry. *N Engl J Med* 1988;**318**:265–70.
21. Parisi AF, Folland ED, Hartigan P. A comparison of angioplasty with medical therapy in the treatment of single-vessel coronary artery disease. Veterans Affairs ACME Investigators. *N Engl J Med* 1992;**326**:10–16.
22. Sievers B, Hamm CW, Herzner A, Kuck KH. Medical therapy versus PTCA: a prospective, randomized trial in patients with asymptomatic coronary single vessel disease (abstract). *Circulation* 1993;**88**(Suppl. 1):I-297.
23. RITA-2 trial participants. Coronary angioplasty versus medical therapy for angina: the second Randomised Intervention Treatment of Angina (RITA-2) trial. *Lancet* 1997;**350**:461–8.
24. Hueb WA, Bellotti G, de Oliveira SA *et al.* The Medicine, Angioplasty or Surgery Study (MASS): a prospective, randomized trial of medical therapy, balloon angioplasty or bypass surgery for single proximal left anterior descending artery stenoses. *J Am Coll Cardiol* 1995;**26**:1600–5.
25. Folland ED, Hartigan PM, Parisi AF. Percutaneous transluminal coronary angioplasty versus medical therapy for stable angina pectoris: outcomes for patients with double-vessel versus single-vessel coronary artery disease in a Veterans Affairs cooperative randomized trial. Veterans Affairs ACME Investigators. *J Am Coll Cardiol* 1997;**29**:1505–11.
26. Pitt B, Waters D, Brown WV *et al.* Aggressive lipid-lowering therapy compared with angioplasty in stable coronary artery disease. Atorvastatin versus Revascularization Treatment Investigators. *N Engl J Med* 1999;**341**:70–6.
27. Pocock SJ, Henderson RA, Clayton T, Lyman GH, Chamberlain DA. Quality of life after coronary angioplasty or continued medical treatment for angina: three-year follow-up in the RITA-2 trial. Randomized Intervention Treatment of Angina. *J Am Coll Cardiol* 2000;**35**:907–14.
28. Bucher HC, Hengstler P, Schindler C, Guyatt GH. Percutaneous transluminal coronary angioplasty versus medical treatment for non-acute coronary heart disease: meta-analysis of randomised controlled trials. *BMJ* 2000;**321**:73–7.
29. Pocock SJ, Henderson RA, Rickards AF *et al.* Meta-analysis of randomised trials comparing coronary angioplasty with bypass surgery. *Lancet* 1995;**346**:1184–9.

30. Coronary angioplasty versus coronary artery bypass surgery: The Randomized Intervention Treatment of Angina (RITA) trial. *Lancet* 1993;**341**:573–80.

31. Henderson RA, Pocock SJ, Sharp SJ *et al.* Long-term results of RITA-1 trial: clinical and cost comparisons of coronary angioplasty and coronary-artery bypass grafting. Randomised Intervention Treatment of Angina. *Lancet* 1998; **352**:1419–25.

32. Goy JJ, Eeckhout E, Burnand B *et al.* Coronary angioplasty versus left internal mammary artery grafting for isolated proximal left anterior descending artery stenosis. *Lancet* 1994; **343**:1449–53.

33. King SB III, Lembo NJ, Weintraub WS *et al.* A randomized trial comparing coronary angioplasty with coronary bypass surgery. Emory Angioplasty versus Surgery Trial (EAST). *N Engl J Med* 1994;**331**:1044–50.

34. Hamm CW, Reimers J, Ischinger T, Rupprecht HJ, Berger J, Bleifeld W. A randomized study of coronary angioplasty compared with bypass surgery in patients with symptomatic multivessel coronary disease. German Angioplasty Bypass Surgery Investigation (GABI). *N Engl J Med* 1994;**331**:1037–43.

35. CABRI Trial Participants. First-year results of CABRI (Coronary Angioplasty versus Bypass Revascularisation Investigation). *Lancet* 1995;**346**:1179–84.

36. Rodriguez A, Boullon F, Perez-Baliño N, Paviotti C, Liprandi MI, Palacios IF. Argentine Randomized Trial of Percutaneous Transluminal Coronary Angioplasty versus Coronary Artery Bypass Surgery in Multivessel Disease (ERACI): in-hospital results and 1-year follow-up. ERACI Group. *J Am Coll Cardiol* 1993;**22**:1060–7.

37. Williams DO, Baim DS, Bates E *et al.* Coronary anatomic and procedural characteristics of patients randomized to coronary angioplasty in the Bypass Angioplasty Revascularization Investigation (BARI). *Am J Cardiol* 1995;**75**:27C–33C.

38. Puel J, Karouny E, Marco F *et al.* Angioplasty versus surgery in multivessel disease: immediate results and in-hospital outcome in a randomized prospective study (abstract). *Circulation* 1992;**86**(Suppl. 1):I-372.

39. The Bypass Angioplasty Revascularization Investigation (BARI) Investigators. Comparison of coronary bypass surgery with angioplasty in patients with multivessel disease. *N Engl J Med* 1996;**335**:217–25.

40. The BARI Investigators. Seven-year outcome in the Bypass Angioplasty Revascularization Investigation (BARI) by treatment and diabetic status. *J Am Coll Cardiol* 2000;**35**: 1122–9.

41. Pocock SJ, Henderson RA, Seed P, Treasure T, Hampton JR. Quality of life, employment status, and anginal symptoms after coronary angioplasty or bypass surgery. 3-year follow-up in the Randomized Intervention Treatment of Angina (RITA) Trial. *Circulation* 1996;**94**:135–42.

42. Zhao XQ, Brown BG, Stewart DK *et al.* Effectiveness of revascularization in the Emory Angioplasty versus Surgery Trial. A randomized comparison of coronary angioplasty with bypass surgery. *Circulation* 1996;**93**:1954–62.

43. Weintraub WS, Mauldin PD, Becker E, Kosinski AS, King SB III. A comparison of the costs of and quality of life after coronary angioplasty or coronary surgery for multivessel coronary artery disease. Results from the Emory Angioplasty versus Surgery Trial (EAST). *Circulation* 1995;**92**:2831–40.

44. Rodriguez A, Ahualli P, Pérez Baliño N *et al.* Argentine Randomized Trial of Percutaneous Transluminal Coronary Angioplasty Versus Coronary Artery Bypass Surgery in Multivessel Disease (ERACI): late cost and three years follow up results (abstract). *J Am Coll Cardiol* 1994;**23**:469A.

45. Ferguson JJ. NHLI BARI clinical alert on diabetics treated with angioplasty. *Circulation* 1995;**92**:3371.

46. Kelsey SF. Patients with diabetes did better with coronary bypass graft surgery than with percutaneous transluminal coronary angioplasty: was this BARI finding real? *Am Heart J* 1999;**138**:S387–93.

47. King SB III, Kosinski AS, Guyton RA, Lembo NJ, Weintraub WS. Eight-year mortality in the Emory Angioplasty versus Surgery Trial (EAST). *J Am Coll Cardiol* 2000;**35**:1116–21.

48. Detre KM, Lombardero MS, Brooks MM *et al.* The effect of previous coronary-artery bypass surgery on the prognosis of patients with diabetes who have acute myocardial infarction. Bypass Angioplasty Revascularization Investigators. *N Engl J Med* 2000;**342**:989–97.

49. Brooks MM, Jones RH, Bach RG *et al.* Predictors of mortality and mortality from cardiac causes in the Bypass Angioplasty Revascularization Investigation (BARI) randomized trial and registry. For the BARI Investigators. *Circulation* 2000;**101**: 2682–9.

50. Rozenman Y, Sapoznikov D, Mosseri M *et al.* Long-term angiographic follow-up of coronary balloon angioplasty in patients with diabetes mellitus: a clue to the explanation of the results of the BARI study. Balloon Angioplasty Revascularization Investigation. *J Am Coll Cardiol* 1997;**30**:1420–5.

51. Kurbaan AS, Bowker TJ, Ilsley CD, Sigwart U, Rickards AF. Difference in the mortality of the CABRI diabetic and nondiabetic populations and its relation to coronary artery disease and the revascularization mode. *Am J Cardiol* 2001; **87**:947–50.

52. Barsness GW, Peterson ED, Ohman EM *et al.* Relationship between diabetes mellitus and long-term survival after coronary bypass and angioplasty. *Circulation* 1997;**96**:2551–6.

53. The BARI Investigators. Influence of diabetes on 5-year mortality and morbidity in a randomized trial comparing CABG and PTCA in patients with multivessel disease: the Bypass Angioplasty Revascularization Investigation (BARI). *Circulation* 1997;**96**:1761–9.

54. Detre KM, Guo P, Holubkov R *et al.* Coronary revascularization in diabetic patients: a comparison of the randomized and observational components of the Bypass Angioplasty Revascularization Investigation (BARI). *Circulation* 1999;**99**: 633–40.

55. Weintraub WS, Stein B, Kosinski A *et al.* Outcome of coronary bypass surgery versus coronary angioplasty in diabetic patients with multivessel coronary artery disease. *J Am Coll Cardiol* 1998;**31**:10–19.

56. Pepine CJ, Holmes DR Jr. Coronary artery stents. American College of Cardiology. *J Am Coll Cardiol* 1996;**28**:782–94.

57. Topol EJ. Coronary-artery stents – gauging, gorging, and gouging. *N Engl J Med* 1998;**339**:1702–4.

58. Detre KM, Holmes DR Jr, Holubkov R *et al.* Incidence and consequences of periprocedural occlusion. The 1985–1986 National Heart, Lung, and Blood Institute Percutaneous Transluminal Coronary Angioplasty Registry. *Circulation* 1990;**82**:739–50.

59. George BS, Voorhees WD III, Roubin GS *et al.* Multicenter investigation of coronary stenting to treat acute or threatened closure after percutaneous transluminal coronary angioplasty: clinical and angiographic outcomes. *J Am Coll Cardiol* 1993; **22**:135–43.

60. Herrmann HC, Buchbinder M, Clemen MW *et al.* Emergent use of balloon-expandable coronary artery stenting for failed percutaneous transluminal coronary angioplasty. *Circulation* 1992;**86**:812–19.

61. Versaci F, Gaspardone A, Tomai F, Crea F, Chiariello L, Gioffre PA. A comparison of coronary-artery stenting with angioplasty for isolated stenosis of the proximal left anterior descending coronary artery. *N Engl J Med* 1997;**336**:817–22.

62. Serruys PW, de Jaegere P, Kiemeneij F *et al.* A comparison of balloon-expandable-stent implantation with balloon angioplasty in patients with coronary artery disease. Benestent Study Group. *N Engl J Med* 1994;**331**:489–95.

63. Fischman DL, Leon MB, Baim DS *et al.* A randomized comparison of coronary-stent placement and balloon angioplasty in the treatment of coronary artery disease. Stent Restenosis Study Investigators. *N Engl J Med* 1994;**331**:496–501.

64. George CJ, Baim DS, Brinker JA *et al.* One-year follow-up of the Stent Restenosis (STRESS I) Study. *Am J Cardiol* 1998; **81**:860–5.

65. Kiemeneij F, Serruys PW, Macaya C *et al.* Continued benefit of coronary stenting versus balloon angioplasty: five-year clinical follow-up of Benestent-I trial. *J Am Coll Cardiol* 2001; **37**:1598–603.

66. Serruys PW, van Hout B, Bonnier H *et al.* Randomised comparison of implantation of heparin-coated stents with balloon angioplasty in selected patients with coronary artery disease (Benestent II). *Lancet* 1998;**352**:673–81.

67. Betriu A, Masotti M, Serra A *et al.* Randomized comparison of coronary stent implantation and balloon angioplasty in the treatment of de novo coronary artery lesions (START): a four-year follow-up. *J Am Coll Cardiol* 1999;**34**:1498–506.

68. Lincoff AM, Califf RM, Moliterno DJ *et al.* Complementary clinical benefits of coronary-artery stenting and blockade of platelet glycoprotein IIb/IIIa receptors. Evaluation of Platelet IIb/IIIa Inhibition in Stenting Investigators. *N Engl J Med* 1999;**341**:319–27.

69. The EPISTENT Investigators. Randomised placebo-controlled and balloon-angioplasty-controlled trial to assess safety of coronary stenting with use of platelet glycoprotein-IIb/IIIa blockade. Evaluation of Platelet IIb/IIIa Inhibitor for Stenting. *Lancet* 1998;**352**:87–92.

70. Eeckhout E, Stauffer JC, Vogt P, Debbas N, Kappenberger L, Goy JJ. Comparison of elective Wiktor stent placement with conventional balloon angioplasty for new-onset lesions of the right coronary artery. *Am Heart J* 1996;**132**:263–8.

71. Witkowski A, Ruzyllo W, Gil R *et al.* A randomized comparison of elective high-pressure stenting with balloon angioplasty: six-month angiographic and two-year clinical follow-up. On behalf of AS (Angioplasty or Stent) trial investigators. *Am Heart J* 2000;**140**:264–71.

72. Erbel R, Haude M, Hopp HW *et al.* Coronary-artery stenting compared with balloon angioplasty for restenosis after initial balloon angioplasty. Restenosis Stent Study Group. *N Engl J Med* 1998;**339**:1672–8.

73. Savage MP, Douglas JS Jr, Fischman DL *et al.* Stent placement compared with balloon angioplasty for obstructed coronary bypass grafts. Saphenous Vein De Novo Trial Investigators. *N Engl J Med* 1997;**337**:740–7.

74. Park SW, Lee CW, Hong MK *et al.* Randomized comparison of coronary stenting with optimal balloon angioplasty for treatment of lesions in small coronary arteries. *Eur Heart J* 2000; **21**:1785–9.

75. Kastrati A, Schomig A, Dirschinger J *et al.* A randomized trial comparing stenting with balloon angioplasty in small vessels in patients with symptomatic coronary artery disease. ISAR-SMART Study Investigators. Intracoronary Stenting or Angioplasty for Restenosis Reduction in Small Arteries. *Circulation* 2000;**102**:2593–8.

76. Koning R, Eltchaninoff H, Commeau P *et al.* Stent placement compared with balloon angioplasty for small coronary arteries: in-hospital and 6-month clinical and angiographic results. *Circulation* 2001;**104**:1604–8.

77. Doucet S, Schalij MJ, Vrolix MC *et al.* Stent placement to prevent restenosis after angioplasty in small coronary arteries. *Circulation* 2001;**104**:2029–33.

78. Sirnes PA, Golf S, Myreng Y *et al.* Stenting in Chronic Coronary Occlusion (SICCO): a randomized, controlled trial of adding stent implantation after successful angioplasty. *J Am Coll Cardiol* 1996;**28**:1444–51.

79. Rubartelli P, Niccoli L, Verna E *et al.* Stent implantation versus balloon angioplasty in chronic coronary occlusions: results from the GISSOC trial. Gruppo Italiano di Studio sullo Stent nelle Occlusioni Coronariche. *J Am Coll Cardiol* 1998;**32**:90–6.

80. Buller CE, Dzavik V, Carere RG *et al.* Primary stenting versus balloon angioplasty in occluded coronary arteries: the Total Occlusion Study of Canada (TOSCA). *Circulation* 1999;**100**: 236–42.

81. Hancock J, Thomas MR, Holmberg S, Wainwright RJ, Jewitt DE. Randomised trial of elective stenting after successful percutaneous transluminal coronary angioplasty of occluded coronary arteries. *Heart* 1998;**79**:18–23.

82. Sievert H, Rohde S, Utech A *et al.* Stent or angioplasty after recanalization of chronic coronary occlusions? (The SARECCO Trial.) *Am J Cardiol* 1999;**84**:386–90.

83. Hoher M, Wohrle J, Grebe OC *et al.* A randomized trial of elective stenting after balloon recanalization of chronic total occlusions. *J Am Coll Cardiol* 1999;**34**:722–9.

84. Lotan C, Rozenman Y, Hendler A *et al.* Stents in total occlusion for restenosis prevention. The multicenter randomized STOP study. The Israeli Working Group for Interventional Cardiology. *Eur Heart J* 2000;**21**:1960–6.

85. Colombo A, Hall P, Nakamura S *et al.* Intracoronary stenting without anticoagulation accomplished with intravascular ultrasound guidance. *Circulation* 1995;**91**:1676–88.

86. Schomig A, Neumann FJ, Kastrati A *et al.* A randomized comparison of antiplatelet and anticoagulant therapy after the placement of coronary-artery stents. *N Engl J Med* 1996;**334**: 1084–9.

87. Leon MB, Baim DS, Popma JJ *et al.* A clinical trial comparing three antithrombotic-drug regimens after coronary-artery stenting. Stent Anticoagulation Restenosis Study Investigators. *N Engl J Med* 1998;**339**:1665–71.

88. Morice MC, Serruys PW, Sousa JE *et al.* A randomized comparison of a sirolimus-eluting stent with a standard stent for coronary revascularization. *N Engl J Med* 2002; **346**:1773–80.

89. Gallo R, Padurean A, Jayaraman T *et al.* Inhibition of intimal thickening after balloon angioplasty in porcine coronary arteries by targeting regulators of the cell cycle. *Circulation* 1999;**99**: 2164–70.

90. Serruys PW, Unger F, Sousa JE *et al.* Comparison of coronary-artery bypass surgery and stenting for the treatment of multivessel disease. *N Engl J Med* 2001;**344**:1117–24.

91. Rodriguez A, Bernardi V, Navia J *et al.* Argentine Randomized Study: Coronary Angioplasty with Stenting Versus Coronary Bypass Surgery in Patients with Multiple-Vessel Disease (ERACI II): 30-day and one-year follow-up results. ERACI II Investigators. *J Am Coll Cardiol* 2001;**37**:51–8.

92. Goy JJ, Kaufmann U, Goy-Eggenberger D *et al.* A prospective randomized trial comparing stenting to internal mammary artery grafting for proximal, isolated de novo left anterior coronary artery stenosis: the SIMA trial. Stenting vs Internal Mammary Artery. *Mayo Clin Proc* 2000;**75**:1116–23.

93. Morrison DA, Sethi G, Sacks J *et al.* Percutaneous coronary intervention versus coronary artery bypass graft surgery for patients with medically refractory myocardial ischemia and risk factors for adverse outcomes with bypass: a multicenter, randomized trial. Investigators of the Department of Veterans Affairs Cooperative Study 385, the Angina With Extremely Serious Operative Mortality Evaluation (AWESOME). *J Am Coll Cardiol* 2001;**38**:143–9.

94. Topol EJ, Leya F, Pinkerton CA *et al.* A comparison of directional atherectomy with coronary angioplasty in patients with coronary artery disease. The CAVEAT Study Group. *N Engl J Med* 1993;**329**:221–7.

95. Baim DS, Cutlip DE, Sharma SK *et al.* Final results of the Balloon vs Optimal Atherectomy Trial (BOAT). *Circulation* 1998; **97**:322–31.

96. Adelman AG, Cohen EA, Kimball BP *et al.* A comparison of directional atherectomy with balloon angioplasty for lesions of the left anterior descending coronary artery. *N Engl J Med* 1993;**329**:228–33.

97. Elliott JM, Berdan LG, Holmes DR *et al.* One-year follow-up in the Coronary Angioplasty Versus Excisional Atherectomy Trial (CAVEAT I). *Circulation* 1995;**91**:2158–66.

98. Holmes DR Jr, Topol EJ, Califf RM *et al.* A multicenter, randomized trial of coronary angioplasty versus directional atherectomy for patients with saphenous vein bypass graft lesions. CAVEAT-II Investigators. *Circulation* 1995;**91**:1966–74.

99. Reifart N, Vandormael M, Krajcar M *et al.* Randomized comparison of angioplasty of complex coronary lesions at a single center. Excimer Laser, Rotational Atherectomy, and Balloon Angioplasty Comparison (ERBAC) Study. *Circulation* 1997;**96**: 91–8.

100. Reisman M, Harms V, Whitlow P, Feldman T, Fortuna R, Buchbinder M. Comparison of early and recent results with rotational atherectomy. *J Am Coll Cardiol* 1997; **29**:353–7.

101. MacIsaac AI, Bass TA, Buchbinder M *et al.* High speed rotational atherectomy: outcome in calcified and noncalcified coronary artery lesions. *J Am Coll Cardiol* 1995;**26**:731–6.

102. Sapirstein W, Zuckerman B, Dillard J. FDA approval of coronary-artery brachytherapy. *N Engl J Med* 2001;**344**:297–9.

103. Waksman R, White RL, Chan RC *et al.* Intracoronary gamma-radiation therapy after angioplasty inhibits recurrence in patients with in-stent restenosis. *Circulation* 2000;**101**: 2165–71.

104. Leon MB, Teirstein PS, Moses JW *et al.* Localized intracoronary gamma-radiation therapy to inhibit the recurrence of restenosis after stenting. *N Engl J Med* 2001;**344**:250–6.

105. Verin V, Popowski Y, de Bruyne B *et al.* Endoluminal beta-radiation therapy for the prevention of coronary restenosis after balloon angioplasty. The Dose-Finding Study Group. *N Engl J Med* 2001;**344**:243–9.

106. Teirstein PS, Massullo V, Jani S *et al.* Three-year clinical and angiographic follow-up after intracoronary radiation: results of a randomized clinical trial. *Circulation* 2000;**101**:360–5.

107. Mark DB, Nelson CL, Califf RM *et al.* Continuing evolution of therapy for coronary artery disease: initial results from the era of coronary angioplasty. *Circulation* 1994;**89**:2015–25.

108. Jones RH, Kesler K, Phillips HR III *et al.* Long-term survival benefits of coronary artery bypass grafting and percutaneous transluminal angioplasty in patients with coronary artery disease. *J Thorac Cardiovasc Surg* 1996;**111**:1013–25.

109. Ellis SG, Omoigui N, Bittl JA *et al.* Analysis and comparison of operator-specific outcomes in interventional cardiology. From a multicenter database of 4,860 quality-controlled procedures. *Circulation* 1996;**93**:431–9.

110. Ellis SG, Weintraub W, Holmes D, Shaw R, Block PC, King SB III. Relation of operator volume and experience to procedural outcome of percutaneous coronary revascularization at hospitals with high interventional volumes. *Circulation* 1997;**95**: 2479–84.

111. Jollis JG, Peterson ED, Nelson CL *et al.* Relationship between physician and hospital coronary angioplasty volume and outcome in elderly patients. *Circulation* 1997;**95**: 2485–91.

28 Adjunctive medical therapy in percutaneous coronary intervention

James L Velianou, Ronald R van der Wieken, Maarten M Simoons

Introduction

The introduction of percutaneous transluminal coronary angioplasty (PTCA) has proven to be a major step forward in the treatment of coronary heart disease. Unfortunately, the gain has not come without a price: frequent and serious complications can occur, acute as well as chronic. In 1977, when Gruentzig introduced PTCA, it was clear that the technique required pharmacologic support. Since then, the development of adjunctive therapy has come a long way. Great progress has been made, but some major problems still wait to be resolved.

The goal of this chapter is to provide the reader with a general overview of adjunctive therapy directed primarily against acute complications, and the pathophysiologic principles involved in percutaneous coronary interventions (PCI).

Key points

Acute complications of PCI
- Intimal dissection with or without thrombus
- Plaque rupture with thrombus
- Spasm
- Perforation
- Distal embolization

Acute complications

The complications in the key points box can each lead to abrupt vessel closure. This occurs in 6·8–8·3% of PTCA procedures and is responsible for a sizeable mortality (up to 1·7%), acute myocardial infarction (1·3–8·6%), emergency bypass surgery (1·3–3·6%), and emergency re-PTCA (4·5%).[1–5] Abrupt vessel closure usually happens in the catheterization laboratory, with the great majority taking place within 6 hours post-PTCA. If it is not possible to open the vessel rapidly, major problems can be expected: persisting anginal pain and myocardial infarction, hemodynamic instability and arrhythmias. Rather unexpectedly, these difficulties can also arise with the abrupt re-closure after opening a chronically occluded vessel. The incidence of abrupt vessel closure is more frequent in unstable coronary syndromes and in angiographically complicated lesions.

Intimal dissection is caused by intravascular maneuvering of guidewires, balloons or other devices. It occurs in a wide variety, from minor and acceptable to major and occlusive. It is usually but not always accompanied by thrombus formation. At present, the only feasible therapy for a significant dissection is mechanical. The most widely used therapy used to be prolonged balloon inflation at the site of the dissection, preferably with a perfusion catheter, but this has to a large extent been replaced by the application of stents.[6,7]

Plaque rupture results from pressure applied to an atherosclerotic lesion. The fibrous cap of the plaque ruptures, uncovering highly thrombogenic plaque contents, in many ways resembling the events in the acute coronary syndromes. This probably happens in a large number of angioplastic maneuvers, often without deleterious consequences. It is only harmful if excessive flow limitation and thrombus formation takes place, leading to coronary occlusion or near occlusion. Antiplatelet strategies usually prevent thrombus formation to a large extent. However, it may still occur and treatment often proves to be difficult. Though often used, thrombolysis in the form of intracoronary urokinase,[8] streptokinase or intravenous or intracoronary rTPA has not been proven to be effective in a randomized fashion. Furthermore, it may complicate an ensuing emergency bypass operation. It is likely that abciximab can be helpful in these often-awkward situations and it is indeed frequently used for this indication, but its beneficial effect has not yet been demonstrated in a randomized trial.[9]

Spasm can be caused by the mere touch of the intracoronary guidewire. Isolated spasm, without dissection or plaque rupture, can rarely lead to abrupt vessel closure. More often, spasm is associated with dissection and/or plaque rupture. Antispasmodic therapy usually consists of intracoronary nitroglycerin.[10,11] In refractory cases a calcium antagonist can be given.[12,13]

Chronic sequelae

Restenosis is an indirect sequela of angioplastic trauma to the endovascular structures. Six months after successful conventional angioplasty, it is angiographically present in approximately 40% of cases. Causal factors of chronic restenosis are shown in the key points box.

Key points

Events leading to chronic restenosis
● Elastic recoil
● Formation of mural thrombus
● Intimal proliferation and synthesis of intracellular matrix
● Pathological arterial remodeling

Many drugs have been named as potentially valuable in the prevention of chronic restenosis. A host of trials have been conducted but only a few have reported a positive outcome. It was shown in a double-blind, placebo-controlled, randomized trial that probucol, an antioxidant, was effective in reducing the restenosis rate.[14] One month before PTCA, 317 patients were randomly assigned to receive one of four treatments: placebo, probucol (500 mg bid), multivitamins (30 000 IU of betacarotene, 500 mg of vitamin C, and 700 IU of vitamin E, bid), or both probucol and multivitamins (bid). Patients were treated for 4 weeks before and 6 months after angioplasty. Follow up angiography 6 months after PTCA showed restenosis in 20·7% in the probucol group, 28·9% in the combined treatment group, 40·3% in the multivitamin group, and 38·9% in the placebo group. The difference between the probucol and non-probucol groups is statistically highly significant ($P = 0.003$). More recently, a double-blind, placebo-controlled, randomized trial of folate treatment revealed a reduction in restenosis. A total of 205 patients were randomized after successful PCI to folate treatment (folic acid 1 mg, vitamin B_{12} 400 micrograms and pyridoxine 10 mg) or placebo for a total of 6 months. Follow up angiography was carried out at 6 months (or earlier if clinically indicated). The rate of restenosis was significantly reduced in the folate group (19·6% v 37·6%, $P = 0.01$), as was the need for revascularization (10·8% v 22·3%, $P = 0.047$).[15] These results need confirmation in other trials before probucol or folate treatment can be advocated as an indispensable adjunct to PTCA.

Pharmacologic suppression of restenosis is, however, still under intense research. Trials are presently being conducted with new pharmacologic agents, systemically or locally delivered. Promising new strategies include drug-eluting stents. Stents alone have been successful, at least in large vessels.[16,17] Effects in smaller coronary arteries are awaited, but seem to be less promising. Stenting prevents recoil and pathological remodeling to a large extent, but leaves formation of mural thrombus and intimal proliferation unhampered. Stenting is therefore at best a partial remedy to the problem of chronic restenosis, reducing the incidence of restenosis but not abolishing it. However, drug-eluting stents may provide the ability to localize therapy without systemic effects. Rapamycin, an anti-rejection drug, has shown the most promise to date. The recent RAVEL study, a double-blind, placebo-controlled, randomized trial of rapamycin drug-eluting stent versus bare stents revealed a significant decrease in both restenosis (0% v 26·6%,

$P < 0.001$) and major adverse events (5·8% v 28·8%, $P < 0.001$) at 6 months. A total of 238 patients were randomized of which 88·7% underwent 6 month angiograms.[18] However promising these agents appear, more studies are required to fully evaluate the efficacy, safety and cost effectiveness of drug-eluting stents.

Thrombus, platelets, and thrombin

Thrombus formation

This plays a leading role in abrupt vessel closure and may be of importance in chronic restenosis. The composition of arterial thrombi ("white thrombi"), with their predominance of platelets, shows that thrombocytes are central in angioplasty-related thrombus formation and acute vessel occlusion. A second agent of great importance is thrombin.

Platelets, physiology, and pathophysiology

The properties of platelets relevant to the formation of thrombus are shown in the key points box and are discussed in some detail below. Platelets are produced by the megakaryocyte. Through processes yet unexplained, this cell fragments into many platelets, which are disk-shaped cells with a diameter of 2–3 μm derived from the cytoplasm of the megakaryocyte without a nucleus. They do contain platelet-specific granules and a dense tubular system as well as a skeleton consisting of actin. The surface has a host of receptors for a wide variety of agents all playing a role in the very complex processes of adhesion, aggregation, and release of granules.

Normally, platelets are in contact solely with the other blood components and the endothelial lining of the blood vessels. Any other contact is inducive to platelet adhesion, with the potential to escalate to aggregation. As long as the endothelial lining of the blood vessels is intact, platelets are not activated. This does not mean that they are inert. Platelets produce substances responsible for the maintenance of the integrity of the vessel walls.

Platelets are normally heterogeneous, both physically and functionally. Younger platelets seem to be larger and more responsive to thrombin than older ones.[19] The lifespan of the platelet is 7–10 days. They are not distributed evenly throughout the lumen; the arterial flow pattern is such that platelets tend to concentrate near the wall, while red blood cells are present predominantly in the central part of the vessel.

Key points

Platelet properties relevant to thrombus formation
● Adhesion
● Aggregation
● Synthesis and release of prostaglandins, thromboxane, and intracellular granules

Adhesion

Platelets contacting surfaces other than erythrocytes, leukocytes or intact endothelium can adhere to them. They adhere to subendothelial structures, macrophages, activated leukocytes, and endothelial cells activated by inflammatory cytokines, and through the expression of membrane integrins, a subset of the glycoprotein receptors situated on the platelet membrane. The main endothelial adhesive protein is the von Willebrand factor, but many others can play a role. Adhesion denotes the deposition of thrombocytes on a surface perceived as foreign, involving a monolayer of platelets and, at least theoretically, having the effect of providing a more natural environment for the other blood corpuscles. Often, however, aggregation ensues.

The most frequently encountered foreign structure is subendothelial tissue that is exposed when endothelium is damaged, for example, during angioplasty. The level of platelet adherence is dependent on the nature of the foreign structure; deeper seated structures are a stronger stimulus than those just under the endothelial lining,[20] and on the presence of the von Willebrand factor. The von Willebrand factor can bind to certain types of collagen and form complexes that bind to the platelet membrane glycoprotein GP IIb and thus cause adhesion.[21] Adhesion involves one single layer of thrombocytes only.

On adhesion, contact with subendothelial collagen can initiate the following physiologic events:

- intracellular platelet granules are released into the extracellular space;
- P-selectin, a platelet membrane glycoprotein, expresses itself on the platelet surface, mediating adhesion to white blood corpuscles;
- activation of the intraplatelet eicosanoid pathway, starting with the emanation of arachidonic acid;
- a profound change in the shape of the platelets, from a smooth disc to a spiculated structure.

These reactions together constitute the activation of the platelets which leads to platelet aggregation, a process that accelerates itself considerably in a short passage of time.

Aggregation

More extensive vessel damage induces platelets to aggregate. Activation and ensuing aggregation can be caused by many factors including adenosine diphosphate (ADP) and serotonin, which are produced (among many others) by the release of platelet granules, thromboxane A_2 (TXA_2), which is generated in the interior of the platelet as an end product of the eicosanoid pathway, and platelet activating factor, which is produced by injured endothelial cells. Adrenaline, noradrenaline, and thrombin (most powerful) also activate platelets, and vice versa; platelet activation catalyzes the conversion of prothrombin to thrombin, thereby accelerating the process of activation and aggregation. Fibrillar collagen, which is exposed when the vessel is damaged, not only promotes adhesion, but also induces aggregation.

After the specific agents have made contact with the platelet membrane, the platelet changes in shape from disc to spiculated sphere. This change in shape is regulated by a skeleton of actin situated interior to the plasmalemma. The filopodial projections that constitute the spiculae probably facilitate contact between GP IIb/IIIa, the receptor on the platelet surface which is the final common pathway responsible for aggregation, and crucial proteins: fibrinogen and von Willebrand factor. In the next stage the GP IIb/IIIa receptor changes in conformation, allowing fibrinogen and von Willebrand factor to bind simultaneously to the GP IIb/IIIa receptors on the surface of two platelets, thus creating a link between them. This usually irreversible linkage is called aggregation. A plug of linked platelets constitutes a thrombus and may obstruct a vessel lumen.

Synthesis and release of prostacyclin, thromboxanes, and intracellular granules

The eicosanoid pathway exists in endothelial cells as well as in the interior of the platelet. Arachidonic acid is converted by cyclo-oxygenase to endoperoxides that form prostacyclin in the endothelial cells but generate TXA_2 in the platelet. TXA_2 enhances aggregation, and is a vasoconstrictor; prostacyclin, on the other hand, has strong vasodilatory and antiaggregant properties. Platelets contain at least three different types of intracellular storage granules. These granules contain a host of substances that can be liberated from the activated platelets by an exocytotic mechanism.[22] The various materials are able to potentiate platelet aggregation and blood coagulation and increase vascular permeability.

Thrombin

Thrombin is the second major player in the pathogenesis of acute coronary thrombosis. It is at the center of reactions essential to thrombus formation. It can activate platelets strongly and independently.[23] Thrombin can cause the release of the von Willebrand factor from endothelium, and facilitates the activation of factor V and VIII and the transition of fibrinogen to fibrin. It promotes the formation of a fibrin mesh around thrombi. Thrombin is abundantly generated during angioplasty.[24]

Antiaggregatory strategies

Four major classes of antiaggregatory agents can be discerned:

- cyclo-oxygenase inhibitors, for example, aspirin;
- thienopyridines, for example, ticlopidine, clopidogrel;

- glycoprotein IIb/IIIa inhibitors, for example, abciximab (Reopro), eptifibatide (Integrilin) and tirofiban (Aggrastat);
- thrombin inhibitors, for example, heparin, LMWH and hirudin.

Aspirin

Platelet aggregability can be inhibited to some extent by aspirin. In thrombocytes, aspirin irreversibly inhibits cyclooxygenase and thereby the generation of TXA_2 which is an aggregation promotor. Aspirin thus inhibits platelet aggregation and thrombus formation. However the production of antiaggregatory prostacyclin is also reduced in the endothelium. Possibly this unfavorable side effect becomes more pronounced with higher doses of aspirin, rendering the lower doses relatively more effective.[25] Aspirin leaves other platelet activation pathways untouched. It is therefore a relatively weak antiaggregatory agent.

Aspirin has been used as premedication to angioplasty since its debut in 1977 and is a universally used adjunctive,[26] but with few prospective trials ever having proven the efficacy. In one trial, a daily dose of 990 mg aspirin combined with dipyridamole (225 mg daily) showed no effect on restenosis compared to placebo, but periprocedural infarctions were significantly less in the treatment group.[27] Among the 376 randomized patients, there were periprocedural Q wave infarctions in 6·9% in the placebo group and 1·6% in the active drug group, the difference reaching statistical significance ($P = 0·0113$). A retrospective angiographic study also showed a clear periprocedural advantage of aspirin and dipyridamole.[28] After doubts had been raised concerning the contribution of dipyridamole to the antithrombotic action of aspirin,[29] this drug disappeared from the adjunctive armamentarium.

The optimal daily dosage of aspirin with a reliable effect in angioplasty is not known. In the USA, 325 mg is usual, while in Europe 100 mg or 80 mg is accepted. The higher dosages (over 100 mg) are associated with more, predominantly gastrointestinal, side effects but not convincingly with greater efficacy. Aspirin is rapidly absorbed from the stomach and upper small intestine. Following ingestion, peak plasma levels are reached 20 minutes after ingestion.[30] Clinically relevant inhibition of platelet aggregation requires 80–90% blockade of TXA_2 synthesis.[31] With daily oral dosages of 80 mg it takes 48 hours to develop this effect on TXA_2 production and aggregation.[32] In higher dosages effective inhibition is reached earlier. It is therefore advisable to start oral aspirin at a low dose at least 48 hours before the angioplasty. Often time is lacking to prepare the patient along these lines. If an immediate procedure has to be performed and the patient is not on aspirin, chewing of enteric coated aspirin results in a sufficient antiplatelet effect after 30 min.[33] Intravenous injection of 250 or 500 mg aspirin results in an even more immediate platelet inhibition, however this is not readily available in many countries.[34]

Ticlopidine and clopidogrel

Ticlopidine is metabolized to an as yet unknown substance, which inhibits ADP-induced platelet aggregation but has no effect on TXA_2-induced aggregation. It leads to a remarkable prolonging of the bleeding time. An effect on platelet aggregation is demonstrable only after 3–5 days of medication.

Ticlopidine has proven its usefullness in conjunction with aspirin in the prevention of acute and subacute stent thrombosis. This complication occurs after insertion of an intracoronary stent in 2–8% of cases, usually between days 2 and 14 with a peak between days 5 and 7 after stent placement. Very extensive regimens, consisting of vitamin K antagonists, dipyridamole, and dextran as well as aspirin and heparin, did not positively influence this complication and led to unacceptable bleeding complications.[16] However, the combination of aspirin and ticlopidine achieved a significant decrease of stent thrombosis as well as bleeding complications.[35] Simultaneously, significant improvement of stent delivery technique such as high pressure implantation also affected results. Until recently, the standard of practice was to administer ticlopidine daily, beginning 7 days before scheduled stent placement. If a stent is inserted as a bailout procedure or because of a suboptimal result, it is customary to start the drug immediately after the procedure. It is continued for 30 days in a regimen of 250 mg bid. The main untoward but reversible effect is bone marrow depression, especially of the neutrophil granulocytes, occurring in less than 2% of patients.[36] In less than 1%, thrombocytopenia is encountered. Two weeks after starting ticlopidine, a white blood cell and thrombocyte count should be performed.

However, clopidogrel is now utilized for most patients treated by PCI in North America and Europe. While in many respects similar to ticlopidine (though it differs in its chemical structure and shares no common metabolites), it displays a lesser tendency to bone marrow depression and other adverse side effects, prompting its use in lieu of ticlopidine.[37] Multiple studies of clopidogrel versus ticlopidine have been carried out.[38–47] Initially, evidence for clopidogrel use in PCI came from non-randomized, single center registries.[38–44] These centers initially had altered their practices from ticlopidine to clopidogrel due to the belief that the benefits of the two drugs would be similar, but the side effects of ticlopidine were significantly worse. Moderate-sized randomized trials were subsequently carried out comparing ticlopidine (plus aspirin) and clopidogrel (plus aspirin) in PCI. These included the Clopidogrel Aspirin Stent International Cooperative Study (CLASSICS), the Ticlid Or Plavix Post-Stent (TOPPS) trial and another by Muller *et al.*[45–47] CLASSICS was the largest study and the only one that was double-blinded. None of these individual studies revealed any significant differences in terms of 30 day major adverse cardiac events. A meta-analysis of these registries and trials reveals that clopidogrel is associated with a lower adverse cardiac event rate (2·1% v 4·0%, OR 0·51; P = 0·001) and mortality (0·48% v 1·09%, OR 0·44; P = 0·001) at 30 days.[48] Overall, given the totality of evidence, clopidogrel appears as effective if not more effective at reducing adverse events in standard PCI.

Patients with unstable angina or non-ST elevation myocardial infarction undergoing PCI are a known higher-risk subset with regard to adverse cardiac events. Pretreatment with 300 mg and continued treatment after one month with 75 mg per day of clopidogrel (in addition to aspirin) prior to PCI in the CURE-PCI study decreased adverse cardiac events at both 30 days (adjusted relative risk 0·65, P = 0·01) and long-term follow up at 12 months (adjusted relative risk 0·72, P = 0·03).[49]

IIb/IIIa receptor blockers

Although there are many ways to activate the platelet, all converge into the same final common pathway, the IIb/IIIa receptor. Blockade of this receptor impedes aggregation to a very large extent, if not completely, with all modes of platelet activation using the final common pathway.

Presently, IIb/IIIa blockers are known in four forms:

- a chimeric monoclonal antibody (derived from murine antibodies), abciximab, which is commercially available;
- naturally occurring snake venom polypeptides. These non-enzymatic peptides have a low potency and short half life, diminishing their therapeutic value;[50]
- synthetic peptides, for example, integrilin and tirofiban;
- non-peptide IIb/IIIa inhibitors, which have not been efficacious until now.

Relevant large scale clinical investigations have been conducted with abciximab, integrilin, and tirofiban.

Abciximab was tested in the CAPTURE, EPILOG, EPIC and EPISTENT trials. All were prospective, multicenter, randomized, double-blind, placebo-controlled, Phase III studies, with over 8500 patients. Table 28.1 shows the main results of these studies.

EPIC studied 2099 patients at increased risk for ischemic complications during or after PTCA[51]: unstable angina and/or recent non-Q wave infarction, acute Q wave infarction within 12 hours of symptom onset, and clinical and angiographic characteristics predictive of increased risk of ischemic complications according to AHA Medical/Scientific Statement Guidelines.[52] Patients were randomized to one of the following regimens:

- placebo bolus + infusion;
- abciximab bolus 0·25 mg/kg IV + 12 hour infusion of placebo;
- abciximab bolus 0·25 mg/kg IV + 12 hour infusion of abciximab 10 migrograms/min.

Treatment started at least 10 min before PTCA, all patients received 325 mg aspirin orally and 10 000–12 000 IU heparin intravenously. Abciximab dosages were devised to reach a receptor blockade of at least 80%. Patients were followed for 30 days, 6 months and 3 years post-procedure. The 30 day composite end point, as in the other two studies, comprised death from any cause, acute infarction or the need for urgent coronary intervention and was statistically significantly reduced by 34·8% in the group treated with bolus and infusion of abciximab as compared to placebo bolus and infusion (P = 0·008). Thirty days emergency repeat PTCA was necessary in 6% of the placebo group and in 1% of the bolus plus infusion group (P = 0·002). At 6 months and after 3 years, the 30 day benefits were sustained.

Thrombocytopenia (<100 000/ml) was seen more often in the bolus plus infusion than in the placebo group (respectively 5·2% and 3·4%; P = 0·01). Of the patients who received abciximab, 6·5% developed human antichimeric antibody, mostly in low titers; none showed allergic reactions. Major hemorrhagic complications immediately after angioplasty, predominantly involving the access site, were higher in the abciximab treated patients. Hemorrhage was especially prominent in patients with a body weight under 75 kg receiving abciximab bolus plus infusion, suggesting that the fixed dose heparin was to blame.

This concept was tested in EPILOG.[53] A total of 2792 patients undergoing elective angioplasty were allocated among three regimens. In the EPIC trial an abciximab regimen was used almost similar to the bolus plus infusion in two of the three groups: one with standard dose heparin (100 IU/kg with a maximum of 10 000 IU) and one with low dose heparin (70 IU/kg, with a maximum of 7000 IU). A third cohort received placebo with standard dose heparin. In all groups additional heparin was administered to keep ACT above 300 seconds.

It was demonstrated that the efficacy of abciximab was preserved under the low dose regimen of heparin. It was also shown that the rate of major bleeding could be reduced to acceptable values: 2·0% in the low dose heparin group versus 3·1% and 3·5% in the heparin-only and the standard heparin with abciximab groups respectively (P = NS). Minor bleeding was 3·7% in the heparin-only group, 4·0% in the low dose heparin with abciximab and 7·4% in the standard heparin and abciximab group (P = 0·01). In this study, too, the benefit of abciximab was preserved after 6 months: primary end points after 30 days were reached in 11·7% in the heparin-only group, 5·2% in the standard dose heparin with abciximab group, and 5·4% in the low dose heparin with abciximab group (P < 0·0001).

In the CAPTURE trial, 1265 patients with refractory unstable angina were randomized to abciximab (bolus and infusion 18 hours preceding angioplasty) or placebo. Abciximab was given as a bolus and an infusion during 18–24 hours preceding the PTCA procedure. This infusion was stopped 1 hour after PTCA. Heparin was administered prior to randomization, until at least 1 hour after PTCA and

Table 28.1   Main results of CAPTURE, EPILOG, EPIC and EPISTENT trials

	CAPTURE (Refractory angina)			EPIC (High-risk PTCA)					EPILOG (Elective PTCA)					EPISTENT (PCI with STENT)				
	Placebo	Abciximab	P value	Placebo	Bolus	P value	Bolus + infusion	P value	Placebo	Abciximab+ low heparin	P value	Abciximab+ normal heparin	P value	Stent + placebo	Stent + abciximab	P value	PTCA + abciximab	P value
	$n = 635$	$n = 635$		$n = 696$	$n = 695$		$n = 708$		$n = 939$	$n = 918$		$n = 935$		$n = 809$	$n = 794$		$n = 796$	
30 day MAE	15·9%	11·3%	0·012	12·8%	11·5%	ns	8·3%	0·008	11·7%	5·4%	<0·001	5·2%	<0·001	10·8%	5·3%	<0·001	6·8%	ns
Mortality	1·3%	1·0%	ns	1·7%	1·3%	ns	1·7%	ns	0·8%	0·3%	ns	0·4%	ns	0·6%	0·3%	ns	0·8%	ns
Myocardial infarction	8·2%	4·1%	0·002	8·6%	6·2%	ns	5·2%	0·01	8·7%	3·7%	<0·001	3·8%	<0·001	4·5%	9·6%	<0·05	5·3%	<0·05
Emergency revascularization	10·9%	7·8%	0·054	7·8%	6·4%		4·0%	0·003	5·2%	2·3%	0·001	1·6%	<0·001	2·2%	1·5%	ns	1·45%	ns
Major bleeding	1·9%	3·8%	0·043	6·6%	11·1%	0·003	14·0%	<0·001	3·1%	2·0%	ns	3·5%	ns					
6 month MAE	30·8%	31·0%	ns	35·1%	32·6%	ns	27·0%	0·001	25·8%	22·8%	ns	22·3%	0·004					
3 year MAE	–			47·2%	41·1%	0·009												

Abbreviations: CAPTURE, C7E3 Anti Platelet Therapy in Unstable Refractory Angina; EPIC, Evaluation of C7E3 to Prevent Ischemic Complications; EPILOG, Evaluation in PTCA to Improve Long-term Outcome with abciximab GP IIb/IIIa blockade; EPISTENT, Evaluation of Platelet IIb/IIIa Inhibitor for Stenting; MAE, major adverse events, comprising death, myocardial infarction, urgent revascularization of any sort, in percentages

adjusted to keep APTT between 2·0 and 2·5 times normal or an ACT of 300 s.[54]

It should be noted that EPILOG and CAPTURE were terminated early, interim analyses demonstrating a significant reduction in end points in the abciximab treated groups.

The relative reduction of primary end points was of the same magnitude as in EPIC. The difference in primary end points between CAPTURE (placebo v active drug: 15·9% v 11·3%; P= 0·012) and EPIC (12·8% v 8·3%; P= 0·008) can be explained by inclusion of more severely unstable patients in CAPTURE ("refractory" v "high risk"). The significance of the difference in regimens – abciximab being administered before and during angioplasty in CAPTURE, and during and after in EPIC – is not clear.

Stent use was low in these early studies. However, practice patterns changed with increased stent use and less PTCA alone or "plain old balloon angioplasty" (POBA). The Evaluation of Platelets IIb/IIIa Inhibitor for Stenting (EPISTENT) was initiated to evaluate the use of abciximab in PCI with stent implantation.[55] A total of 2399 patients were randomized to one of three treatment arms; stent plus abciximab, PTCA plus abciximab or stent plus placebo. Patients were otherwise treated with standard medications including aspirin, ticlopidine, and heparin. The primary end point was a composite of death, myocardial infarction and the need for urgent target revascularization in the first 30 days. Patients randomized to the stent/abciximab therapy had a lower event rate compared to stent/placebo (5·3% v 10·8%, P< 0·001, hazard ratio 0·48) and PTCA/abciximab (5·3% v 6·9%, P= 0·007, hazard ratio 0·63). Major bleeding complications were not significantly different, but this study was not powered to detect this. The benefits of abciximab appear to be maintained over time.[56] Debate over the implications of the results continues to occur. Many of the events prevented were troponin and CK rises which may or may not be an accurate surrogate of mortality. As with any therapeutic intervention, higher-risk patients probably benefit most from abciximab. In the case of PCI, diabetic patients appear to benefit both in the short-term and longer follow up. However, evidence from EPISTENT is a substudy analysis with different baseline characteristics. Other non-randomized studies have confirmed the 30 day but not the long-term results.[57]

Eptifibatide was tested in the IMPACT II study,[58] which involved 4010 patients undergoing angioplasty or atherectomy. The incidence of major ischemic complications or emergency revascularization at 24 hours was lower in two groups treated with integrilin (135 micrograms/kg bolus plus 0·5 micrograms/ kg/min or 0·75 micrograms/kg/min, both for 20–24 hours) than in the placebo treated patients, but this was not statistically significant after 30 days (11·4% v 9·2% v 9·9% respectively for placebo, low-dose, and high-dose eptifibatide; P= 0·063 placebo v low-dose eptifibatide). There was no difference in the occurrence of major bleeding. The IMPACT II study displayed statistically

non-significant results. However, it was felt that platelet inhibition was not optimal. The Enhanced Suppression of the Platelet IIb/IIIa Receptor with Integrilin Therapy (ESPRIT) trial compared eptifibatide to placebo in stable patients undergoing PCI with stent.[59] Patients in this study were deemed appropriate not to necessarily need GP IIb/IIIa inhibitor, therefore considered lower risk than patients in the abciximab trials. Furthermore, patients were excluded if they were pretreated with clopidogrel greater than 24 hours. The ESPRIT study utilized a significantly higher dose of eptifibatide (2 boluses 180 micrograms/kg 10 min apart plus 2·0 micrograms/kg/min for 18–24 hours). The primary end point was the composite of death, myocardial infarction, urgent target vessel revascularization and bailout glycoprotein IIb/IIIa inhibitor use at 48 hours. ESPRIT was terminated early due to efficacy. The primary end point was reduced in the eptifibatide group (6·6% v 10·5%, P= 0·0015). There appeared to be continued benefit out to 6 months.[60] However, many of the events in the ESPRIT trial were arguably of borderline significance such as enzymatic rise and bailout use of glycoprotein IIb/IIIa inhibitor.

Tirofiban was tested in the RESTORE (Randomized Efficacy of Tirofiban for Outcomes and Restenosis) study in 2139 patients with unstable angina or acute myocardial infarction, undergoing PTCA or atherectomy. Tirofiban (bolus of 10 micrograms/kg + 0·15 micrograms/kg/min for 36 hours) was compared with placebo, both groups receiving aspirin and heparin. At 30 days, the incidence of a composite end point of death, acute infarction, urgent or emergent PTCA or CABG was 10·5% in the placebo group and 8·0% in the tirofiban group (P= 0·052). Here also, the incidence of major bleeding did not differ significantly.[61] The RESTORE study did not conclusively prove that tirofiban provided protection from adverse events peri-PCI. However, since there were differences between the small-molecule inhibitors (eptifibatide and tirofiban) and monoclonal antibodies (abciximab) in both structure and cost, a direct comparison was carried out. The TARGET (do Tirofiban And ReoPro Give similar Efficacy Trial) was designed as a non-inferiority trial of tirofiban and abciximab. This was a double-blind, double-dummy randomized trial of 4809 patients undergoing PCI with stent. Primary end point was a composite of death, non-fatal myocardial infarction, and urgent target vessel revascularization at 30 days. A significantly higher number of patients treated with tirofiban reached the primary end point (7·6% v 6·0%, P= 0·038). Importantly, pretreatment with clopidogrel was associated with fewer adverse events in both treatment arms.[62]

Comparison of abciximab, eptifibatide, and tirofiban shows that abciximab is probably the most effective in reducing ischemic complications. This can be possibly explained by the tightness of the abciximab-IIb/IIIa binding, while eptifibatide and tirofiban are loosely bound. Also, actual dosages of the small molecule GP IIb/IIIa inhibitors may be inadequate. Furthermore, it is probable that only abciximab also binds to the vitronectin receptor (which shares an epitope with IIb/IIIa), extending its blocking capacities. Unfortunately, a direct comparison of abciximab and eptifibatide is not currently available.

Antithrombins

The most widely used thrombin antagonist is heparin. In its unfractionated form, it has been used in PTCA since its introduction. Its effect on peri-procedural complications has never been demonstrated unequivocally.

Heparin is not a simple substance but consists of a combination of agents that all bind to antithrombin III (ATIII). Its molecular weight is 15 000. Through a reversible binding with ATIII, a naturally occurring inhibitor of activated blood coagulation factors,[63,64] heparin converts ATIII from a slow inhibitor to a rapid inhibitor of factors XIIa, XIa, IXa, Xa, and thrombin. Thrombin is more sensitive to the effects of heparin than is Xa and in keeping with this, unfractionated heparin exerts its action mainly through inhibition of thrombin-induced activation of factors V and VIII.[65] For thrombin inhibition it is necessary that both thrombin and ATIII bind to heparin. This requires a minimum chain length of 18 monosaccharides.

Heparin also comes in fractionated forms. These low molecular weight heparins (LMWH) have a molecular weight of 4000–5000 and a chain length >18 monosaccharides. These LMWH, when compared to the heavier components of unfractionated heparin, are more prone to bind to ATIII. They cannot bind to thrombin but they retain anti-Xa activity. The heavier components, on the other hand, are probably responsible for heparin-associated thrombocytopenia and possibly for some platelet activation. LMWH can be administered subcutaneously once daily.

In accordance with the better binding to ATIII, LMWH are more effective than unfractionated heparin in the prevention of deep venous thrombosis.[66] Hopes for a better safety profile did not materialize: in a meta-analysis of 62 studies with a total of over 20 000 patients, it was shown that LMWH are associated with a higher bleeding risk than heparin.[67]

In the treatment of unstable angina, LMWH were proven valuable in various trials as compared to unfractionated heparin, without excessive bleeding.[68–70] LMWH inhibits *in vitro* smooth muscle cell migration and proliferation without affecting endothelial cell growth.[71] However, *in vivo*, one LMWH, enoxaparin, did not show any effect on the incidence of restenosis nor did another,[72] reviparin, compared to unfractionated heparin in patients undergoing PTCA.[73] Reviparin was not associated with a decrease in the incidence of bleeding complications nor did it show any advantage in the occurrence of acute complications during and after PTCA. Further studies have been carried out by the National Investigators Collaborating on Enoxaparin

(NICE) utilizing enoxaparin with (NICE-4) and without (NICE-1) abciximab. These were registries, but the results appear promising. Presently, there are no compelling evidence-based arguments to replace unfractionated heparin with LMWH as an adjunctive to PTCA.

Heparin is a relatively weak antiplatelet agent, in part because it does not inhibit the other platelet activators that operate independently from thrombin. Also, it tends to bind to the platelet surface, thus increasing platelet activity.[74,75] Furthermore, thrombin is incorporated into a developing thrombus and binds to fibrin. This fibrin bound thrombin can generate activated factors V and VIII, producing additional thrombin and promoting thrombus growth.

The heparin-ATIII complex is a potent inhibitor of free thrombin but only weakly inhibits fibrin bound thrombin. Heparin therefore can only inhibit but not completely prevent the growth of thrombi.[76,77] Moreover, heparin can only exert its influence in the presence of adequate levels of antithrombin III.

Direct thrombin inhibitors have been developed to circumvent the need for antithrombin III. Hirudin is a natural antithrombin, produced by the salivary glands of the European leech. A recombinant form is equipotential. Both inhibit all known functions of thrombin,[50] at least theoretically overcoming many of the disadvantages of heparin. However, in contrast to heparin, thrombin generation is left intact. In the HELVETICA (Hirudin in a European Trial versus Heparin in the Prevention of Restenosis after PTCA) trial hirudin was compared with heparin in patients with unstable angina undergoing PTCA.[78] This study in 1141 patients was designed to evaluate the effect of hirudin on chronic restenosis. In the occurrence of early cardiac events, a clear advantage could be attributed to hirudin: after 96 hours a combination of death, myocardial infarction, bypass surgery and second angioplasty occurred in 11% of the group treated with heparin, 7·9% in the intravenous hirudin group and 5·6% in the intravenous and subcutaneous hirudin group ($P = 0·023$). There was a particular benefit in patients in Braunwald class III angina;[79] in patients who had angina at rest during the 48 hours before randomization, the event rate was 21·6% in the heparin group as compared with 5·3% in the patients receiving intravenous hirudin and 12·3% among the patients receiving intravenous and subcutaneous hirudin ($P = 0·006$). After 7 months, however, there was no difference in major end points between the three cohorts, nor was there any difference in the angiographic degree of restenosis. Bleeding complications did not differ significantly. It was argued that the hirudin dosage was sufficient to limit acute thrombin mediated platelet aggregation and thus could affect acute complications, but insufficient to produce an adequate level of anticoagulation to influence restenosis.

In the GUSTO IIb study, in acute myocardial infarction, immediate angioplasty was performed in a subgroup. Patients were randomized to heparin and hirudin and to immediate angioplasty and thrombolysis. No beneficial effect of hirudin over heparin was found.[80]

Hirulog is a synthetic peptide designed on the structure of hirudin. Its effectiveness in angioplasty was studied in a prospective double-blind randomized trial of 4098 patients with unstable angina who were treated with either heparin or bivalirudin (hirulog).[81] No difference was demonstrated in short- and long-term complications. Bivalirudin was associated with a lower incidence of major hemorrhage.

At present, neither a direct thrombin inhibitor nor LMWH can be advocated to take the place of heparin in PTCA.

Recommendations

Preventive

Aspirin is indispensable as an adjunct to PTCA. It is safe, cheap, and effective as well as easy to administer. It should be given in a single daily dose of at least 80 or 100 mg for at least 3 days before PTCA. It should be continued afterwards indefinitely. **Grade A1a**

If a stent is inserted, ticlopidine (250 mg bid) or clopidogrel (75 mg od) preferably starting 7 days before and continuing at least 2–4 weeks after the procedure should be added to the regimen. **Grade A1a**

Heparin is the thrombin inhibitor of choice in all PTCA procedures; dosage is a bolus of 70–100 IU/kg bodyweight or 5000 IU IV at the start of the procedure, with repeated bolus injections during procedure to maintain therapeutic APTT (around 70 sec) or ACT (above 200 sec). It is still not clear as to the ideal ACT, but clear heparin required for PCI. Other anticoagulants such as LMWH or direct thrombin inhibitors can also be utilized during PCI, but there is still no significant evidence they are more efficacious than standard heparin. **Grade A1a**

In high-risk procedures, as in unstable angina or angiographically complicated lesions (type B2, C), abciximab should be considered, before PCI, followed by a 12 hour infusion. Heparin should be rigorously weight adjusted. Abciximab, eptifibatide or tirofiban can be considered for lower risk PCI, but overall absolute benefit may not be significant. **Grade A1a**

Therapeutic

Spasm can be countered with nitroglycerin or nifedipine. **Grade B2**

Acute or threatened closure due to dissection/thrombus can be treated with thrombolytics or glycoprotein IIb/IIIa inhibitors, but there is weak evidence that this is useful. **Grade B2**

References

1. Myler RK, Shaw RE, Stertzer SH *et al.* Lesion morphology and coronary angioplasty: current experience and analysis. *J Am Coll Cardiol* 1992;**9**:1641–52.

2. Detre KM, Holmes DR, Holubkov R *et al.* Incidences and consequences of periprocedural occlusion: the 1985–1986 National Heart, Lung, and Blood Institute Percutaneous Transluminal Coronary Angioplasty Registry. *Circulation* 1990;**82**:739–50.

3. De Feyter PJ, van den Brand M, Laarman GJ *et al.* Acute coronary artery occlusion during and after percutaneous transluminal coronary angioplasty: frequency, prediction, clinical course, management and follow up. *Circulation* 1991;**83**:927–36.

4. Lincoff AM, Popma JJ, Ellis SG *et al.* Abrupt vessel closure complicating coronary angioplasty: clinical angiographic, and therapeutic profile. *J Am Coll Cardiol* 1992;**19**:926–35.

5. Ellis SG, Roubin GS, King SB III *et al.* Angiographic and clinical predictors of acute closure after native vessel coronary angioplasty. *Circulation* 1988;**77**:372–9.

6. Roubin GS, Cannon AD, Agrawol SK *et al.* Intracoronary stenting for acute and threatened closure complicating PTCA. *Circulation* 1992;**85**:916–21.

7. Scott NA, Weintraub WS, Carlin SF *et al.* Recent changes in the management and outcome of acute closure after PTCA. *J Am Coll Cardiol* 1993;**71**:1159–63.

8. Schachinger V, Kasper W, Zeiker AM. Adjunctive intracoronary urokinase therapy during PTCA. *J Am Coll Cardiol* 1996;**77**:1174–8.

9. Velianou JL, Strauss BH, Kreatsoulas C, Pericak D, Natarajan MK. Evaluation of the role of abciximab (Reopro) as a rescue agent during percutaneous coronary interventions: in-hospital and six-month outcomes. *Cathet Cardiovasc Intervent* 2000;**51**:138–44.

10. Margolis JR, Chen C. Coronary artery spasm complicating percutaneous transluminal angioplasty: role of intracoronary nitroglycerin. *Z Kardiol* 1989;**78**(Suppl. 2):41–7.

11. Fischell TA, Derby G, Tse TM, Stadius ML. Coronary artery vasoconstriction routinely occurs after PTCA: a quantitative arteriographic analysis. *Circulation* 1988;**78**:323–4.

12. McIvor ME, Undemir C, Lawson J, Reddinger J. Clinical effects and utility of intracoronary diltiazem. *Cathet Cardiovasc Diagn* 1995;**35**:287–91.

13. Pomerantz RM, Kuntz RE, Diver DJ, Safian RD, Baim DS. Intracoronary verapamil for the treatment of distal microvascular coronary artery spasm following PTCA. *Cathet Cardiovasc Diagn* 1991;**24**:283–5.

14. Tardif JC, Cote G, Lesperance J *et al.* Probucol and multivitamins in the prevention of restenosis after coronary angioplasty. *N Engl J Med* 1997;**337**:418–19.

15. Schnyder G, Roffi M, Pin R *et al.* Decreased rate of coronary restenosis after lowering of plasma homocysteine levels. *N Engl J Med* 2001;**345**:1593–600.

16. Serruys PW, de Jaegere P, Kiemeney F *et al.* A comparison of balloon-expandable stent implantation with balloon angioplasty in patients with coronary artery disease (Benestent I). *N Engl J Med* 1994;**331**:489–95.

17. Fischman DL, Leon MB, Baim DS *et al.* A randomized comparison of coronary stent placement and balloon angioplasty in the treatment of coronary artery disease (STRESS). *N Engl J Med* 1994;**331**:496–501.

18. Morice M-C, Serruys PW, Sousa JE *et al.* A randomized comparison of sirolimus-eluting stent with a standard stent for coronary revascularization. *N Engl J Med* 2002;**346**:1773–80.

19. Peng JP, Friese P, Heilmann E, George JN, Burstein SA, Dale GL. Aged platelets have an impaired response to thrombin. *Blood* 1994;**83**:161–6.

20. Kehrel B. Platelet-collagen interactions. *Semin Thromb Hemost* 1995;**21**:123–9.

21. Stel HV, Sakariassen KS, de Groot PG *et al.* Von Willebrand factor in the vessel wall mediates platelet adherence. *Blood* 1985;**65**:85–90.

22. Heptinstall S, Hanley SP. Blood platelets and vessel walls. In: Walter Bowie EJ, Sharp AA, eds. *Hemostasis and thrombosis.* London: Butterworths, 1985.

23. Coughlin SR, Vu TK, Hung DT, Wheaton VI. Characterization of a functional thrombin receptor: issues and opportunities. *J Clin Invest* 1992;**89**:351–5.

24. Marmur JD, Merlini PA, Sharma SK *et al.* Thrombin generation in human coronary arteries after percutaneous transluminal balloon angioplasty. *J Am Coll Cardiol* 1994;**24**:1484–91.

25. Verheugt FWA, van der Laarse A, Funke Kupper AJ *et al.* Effects of early intervention with low-dose aspirin (100 mg) on infarct-size, reinfarction and mortality in anterior wall acute myocardial infarction. *Am J Cardiol* 1990;**66**:267–70.

26. Antiplatelet Trialists' Collaboration. Collaborative overview of randomised trials of antiplatelet therapy. II. Maintenance of vascular graft or arterial patency by antiplatelet therapy. *BMJ* 1994;**308**:159–68.

27. Schwartz L, Bourassa MG, Lesperance J *et al.* Aspirin and dipyridamole in the prevention of restenosis after percutaneous transluminal coronary angioplasty. *N Engl J Med* 1988; **318**:1714–19.

28. Barnathan ES, Sanford Schwartz J, Taylor L *et al.* Aspirin and dipyridamole in the prevention of acute coronary thrombosis complicating coronary angioplasty. *Circulation* 1987;**76**: 125–34.

29. Fitzgerald GA. Dipyridamole. *N Engl J Med* 1987;**316**: 1247–57.

30. Hirsh J, Dalen J, Fuster V, Harker LB, Salzman EW. Aspirin and other platelet-active drugs: the relationship between dose, effectiveness, and side effects. *Chest* 1992;**102**: 327–36.

31. Reilly IAG, Fitzgerald GA. Aspirin in cardiovascular disease. *Drugs* 1988;**35**:154–76.

32. Ridker PM, Hebert PR, Fuster V *et al.* Are both aspirin and heparin justified as adjuncts to thrombolytic therapy for acute myocardial infarction? *Lancet* 1993;**341**:1574–7.

33. Jimenez AH, Stubbs ME, Tofler GH, Winther K, Williams GH, Muller JE. Rapidity and duration of platelet suppression by enteric coated aspirin in healthy young men. *Am J Cardiol* 1992;**69**:258–62.

34. Husted SE, Kristensen SD, Vissinger H, Mann B, Schmidt EB, Nielsen HK. Intravenous acetyl-salicylic acid – dose related effects on platelet function and fibrinolysis in healthy males. *Thromb Haemost* 1992;**68**:226–9.

35. Schomig A, Neumann FJ, Kastrati A *et al.* A randomized comparison of platelet and anticoagulant therapy after the placement of coronary-artery stents. *N Engl J Med* 1996; **334**:1084–9.

36. Bonita R. Epidemiology of stroke. *Lancet* 1992;**339**:342–4.

37. CAPRIE Steering Committee. A randomised, blinded, trial of clopidogrel versus aspirin in patients at risk of ischaemic events (CAPRIE). *Lancet* 1996;**348**:1329–39.

38. Calver AL, Blows LJ, Harmer S *et al.* Clopidogrel for the prevention of major cardiac events after coronary stent implantation: 30-day and 6-month results in patients with smaller stents. *Am Heart J* 2000;**140**:483–91.

39. Mishkel GJ, Aguirre FV, Ligon RW, Rocha-Singh KJ, Lucore CL. Clopidogrel as adjunctive antiplatelet therapy during coronary stenting. *J Am Coll Cardiol* 1999;**34**:1884–90.

40. Allier PL, Aronow HD, Cura FA *et al.* Short-term mortality lower with clopidogrel than ticlopidine following coronary artery stenting. *J Am Coll Cardiol* 2000;**35** (Suppl. 66A):

41. Berger PB, Bell MR, Rihal CS *et al.* Clopidogrel versus ticlopidine after intracoronary stent placement. *J Am Coll Cardiol* 1999;**34**:1891–4.

42. Moussa I, Oetgen M, Roubin G *et al.* Effectiveness of clopidogrel and aspirin versus ticlopidine and aspirin in preventing stent thrombosis after coronary stent implantation. *Circulation* 1999;**99**:2364–6.

43. Dangas G, Mehran R, Abizaid AS *et al.* Combination therapy with aspirin plus clopidogrel versus aspirin plus ticlopidine for prevention of subacute thrombosis after successful native coronary stenting. *Am J Cardiol* 2001;**87**:470–2.

44. Plucinski DA, Scheltema K, Krusmark J, Panchyshyn N. A comparison of clopidogrel to ticlopidine therapy for the prevention of major adverse events at thirty days and six months following coronary stent implantation. *J Am Coll Cardiol* 2000;**35** (Suppl. 67A):

45. Bertrand ME, Rupprecht HJ, Urban P, Gershlick AH. Double-blind study of the safety of clopidogrel with and without a loading dose in combination with aspirin compared with ticlopidine in combination with aspirin after coronary stenting: the Clopidogrel ASpirin Stent International Cooperative Study (CLASSICS). *Circulation* 2000;**102**:624–9.

46. Taniuchi M, Kurz HI, Lasala JM. Randomized comparison of ticlopidine and clopidogrel after intracoronary stent implantation in a broad patient population. *Circulation* 2001;**104**: 539–43.

47. Muller C, Buttner HJ, Petersen J, Roskamm H. A randomized comparison of clopidogrel and aspirin versus ticlopidine and aspirin after the placement of coronary-artery stents. *Circulation* 2000;**101**:590–3.

48. Bhatt DL, Bertrand ME, Berger PB *et al.* Meta-analysis of randomized and registry comparisons of ticlopidine with clopidogrel after stenting. *J Am Coll Cardiol* 2002;**39**:9–14.

49. Mehta SR, Yusuf S, Peters RJ *et al.* Clopidogrel in Unstable angina to prevent Recurrent Events trial (CURE) Investigators. Effects of pretreatment with clopidogrel and aspirin followed by long-term therapy in patients undergoing percutaneous coronary intervention: the PCI-CURE study. *Lancet* 2001; **358**:527–33.

50. Verstraete M, Zoldhelyi P. Novel antithrombotic drugs in development. *Drugs* 1995;**49**:856–84.

51. The EPIC Investigators. Use of a monoclonal antibody directed against the platelet glycoprotein IIb/IIIa receptor in high-risk coronary angioplasty. *N Engl J Med* 1994;**330**: 956–61.

52. AHA Medical/Scientific Statement Guidelines for percutaneous transluminal coronary angioplasty. 1993;**88**: 2987–3007.

53. The EPILOG Investigators. Effect of the platelet glycoprotein IIb/IIIa receptor inhibitor abciximab with lower heparin dosages on ischemic complications of percutaneous coronary revascularization. *N Engl J Med* 1997;**336**: 1689–96.

54. The CAPTURE Investigators. Refractory unstable angina; reduction of events by treatment with abciximab prior to coronary intervention. *Lancet* 1997;**349**:1429–35.

55. Randomised placebo-controlled and balloon-angioplasty-controlled trial to assess safety of coronary stenting with use of platelet glycoprotein-IIb/IIIa blockade. The EPISTENT Investigators. Evaluation of Platelet IIb/IIIa Inhibitor for Stenting. *Lancet* 1998;**352**:87–92.

56. Topol EJ, Mark DB, Lincoff AM *et al.* Outcomes at 1 year and economic implications of platelet glycoprotein IIb/IIIa blockade in patients undergoing coronary stenting: results from a multicenter randomised trial. EPISTENT Investigators. Evaluation of Platelet IIb/IIIa Inhibitor for Stenting. *Lancet* 1999;**354**:2019–24.

57. Velianou JL, Mathew V, Wilson SH, Barsness GW, Grill DE, Holmes DR Jr. Effect of abciximab on late adverse events in patients with diabetes mellitus undergoing stent implantation. *Am J Cardiol* 2000;**86**:1063–8.

58. Tcheng JE, Lincoff AM, Sigmon KN, Califf RM, Topol EJ. Platelet glycoprotein IIbIIIa inhibition with Integrelin during percutaneous coronary intervention: the IMPACT II Trial (Integrilin to Manage Platelet Aggregation to Prevent Coronary Thrombosis II). *Circulation* 1995;**92**(Suppl. 1): 543.

59. The ESPRIT Investigators. Novel dosing regimen of eptifabitide in planned coronary stent implantation (ESPRIT): a randomized, placebo-controlled trial. *Lancet* 2000;**356**: 2037–44.

60. O'Shea JC, Hafley GE, Greenberg S *et al.* Platelet glycoprotein IIb/IIIa integrin blockade with eptifibatide in coronary stent intervention: the ESPRIT trial: a randomized controlled trial. *JAMA* 2001;**285**:2468–73.

61. Effects of platelet glycoprotein IIb/IIIa blockade with tirofiban on adverse cardiac events in patients with unstable angina or acute myocardial infarction undergoing coronary angioplasty. The RESTORE Investigators. Randomized Efficacy Study of Tirofiban for Outcomes and REstenosis. *Circulation* 1997;**96**:1445–53.

62. Topol EJ, Herrmann HC, Powers ER *et al.* TARGET Investigators. Comparison of two platelet glycoprotein IIb/ IIIa inhibitors, tirofiban and abciximab, for the prevention of ischemic events with percutaneous coronary revascularization. *N Engl J Med* 2001;**344**:1888–94.

63. Rosenberg RD, Rosenberg JS. Natural anticoagulant mechanisms. *J Clin Invest* 1984;**74**:1–6.

64. Salzman EW, Rosenberg RD, Smith MH, Lindon JN, Favreau L. Effect of heparin and heparin fractions on platelet aggregation. *J Clin Invest* 1980;**65**:64–73.

65. Ofusu FA, Hirsh J, Esmon CT *et al.* Unfractionated heparin inhibits thrombin-catalysed amplifications of coagulation more efficiently than those catalysed by Xa. *Biochem J* 1989;**257**: 143–50.

66. Kakkar VV, Murray WJG. Efficacy and safety of low molecular weight heparin (CY216) in preventing postoperative venous thrombo-embolism: a cooperative study. *Br J Surg* 1985;**72**: 786–91.

67. Rosendaal FR, Nurmohamed MT, Buller HR, Dekker E, Vandenbroucke JP. Low molecular weight heparins in the prophylaxis of venous thrombosis: a meta-analysis. *Haemost Thromb* 1991;**65**:927.

68. Gurfinkel EP, Manos EJ, Mejail RI *et al.* Low molecular weight heparin versus regular heparin or aspirin in the treatment of unstable angina and silent ischemia. *J Am Coll Cardiol* 1995;**26**:313–18.

69. Klein W, Buchwald A, Hillis SE *et al.* Comparison of low-molecular weight heparin with unfractionated heparin acutely and with placebo for 6 weeks in the management of unstable coronary artery disease (FRIC). *Circulation* 1997; **96**:61–8.

70. FRISC Study Group. Low-molecular weight heparin during instability in coronary artery disease. *Lancet* 1996;**347**:561–8.

71. Roth D, Betz E. Kultivierte Gefasswandzellen des Menschen. *Vasa* 1992;**35**:125–7.

72. Faxon DP, Spiro TE, Minor S *et al.* Low molecular weight heparin in prevention of restenosis after angioplasty. Results of the Enoxaparin Restenosis (ERA) trial. *Circulation* 1994; **90**:908–14.

73. Karsch KR, Preisack MB, Baildon R *et al.* Low molecular weight heparin (Reviparin) in PTCA: results of a randomized, double-blind unfractionated heparin and placebo-controlled, multicenter trial (REDUCE trial). *J Am Coll Cardiol* 1996; **28**:1437–43.

74. Coller BS. Antiplatelet agents in the prevention and therapy of thrombosis. *Annu Rev Med* 1992;**43**:171–80.

75. O'Reilly RA. Anticoagulant antithrombotic and thrombolytic drugs. In: Gilman AG, Goodman LS, Rall TW, Murad F, eds. *The pharmacological basis of therapeutics*, 7th edn. New York: Macmillan, 1985.

76. Hirsh J, Fuster V. Guide to anticoagulant therapy. I. Heparin. *Circulation* 1994;**89**:1449–68.

77. Hull RD, Delamore T, Genton E *et al.* Warfarin sodium versus low dose heparin in the long term treatment of venous thromboembolism. *N Engl J Med* 1979;**301**:855–8.

78. Serruys PW, Herrman JR, Simon R *et al.* for the HELVETICA Investigators. A comparison of hirudin with heparin in the prevention of restenosis after coronary angioplasty. *N Engl J Med* 1995;**333**:757–63.

79. Braunwald E. Unstable angina: a classification. *Circulation* 1989;**80**:410.

80. Angioplasty Substudy Investigators. The global use of strategies to open occluded coronary arteries in acute coronary syndromes (GUSTO IIb). A clinical trial comparing primary coronary angioplasty with tissue plasminogen activator for acute myocardial infarction. *N Engl J Med* 1997;**336**:1621–8.

81. Bittl JA, Strony J, Brinker JA *et al.* Treatment with Bivalirudin (Hirulog) as compared with heparin during coronary angioplasty for unstable or postinfarction angina. *N Engl J Med* 1995;**333**:764–9.

29 Restenosis: etiologies and prevention

Giuseppe Sangiorgi, David R Holmes, Robert S Schwartz

Introduction

Percutaneous coronary interventions have revolutionized the treatment of coronary atherosclerosis, creating an alternative strategy to medical and surgical therapy for myocardial ischemia and acute coronary events. The concept was that atherosclerotic plaque can be fractured, removed or ablated within the vessel by different device technologies. However, it was quickly understood that following the intervention, a healing response, known as restenosis, significantly reduced the long-term success of the procedure.

Restenosis is a substantial medical problem, both because it occurs in 40–50% of patients undergoing coronary revascularization procedures, with increased patient morbidity, but also for the significant burden of medical costs,[1,2] which is estimated to be of nearly $2·0 billion per year.[3] Restenosis may be effectively treated by repeat angioplasty. However, further interventional procedures entail additional cost, and the redilated lesions are more prone to the development of restenosis than native lesions.

Because of this unacceptably high restenosis rate and the huge health cost implications, it is not surprising that in the past ten years or so there have been intense efforts to elucidate the pathophysiologic mechanisms of this process and, most importantly, extensive clinical trials aimed at a wide array of strategies to prevent restenosis. Today, while the cellular mechanisms and interactions involved in the pathobiology of restenosis have been better understood, and powerful effects have been obtained in some animal models with the use of different drugs and devices, the search for successful therapeutic effects continues, because when transferred into clinical practice, restenosis is still a shadow over the broad use of the interventional techniques. The introduction of the drug-eluting stent has recently offered a light at the end of the tunnel. As we stand on the verge of a "cure" for restenosis, it is interesting to ask, "Why has it taken so long?"

Since the late 1970s, enormous efforts and resources have been directed to the problem of restenosis. Our understanding of restenosis evolved slowly, but major components in the evolution of the restenosis process have been identified, and in the early 1990s several pivotal studies distinguished basic restenosis mechanisms such as early recoil, negative remodeling, and proliferative response to injury.[4,5] Other landmark studies established the concept that the extent of luminal "late loss" at follow up is proportional to the amount of "acute gain" achieved during the initial procedure.[6] Although this strategy provided incremental reduction in restenosis under the philosophy of "bigger is better", the scientific community soon realized that restenosis could not be eliminated using only mechanical devices like bare stents. Thus, the fertile soil for the development of drug-eluting stents was created. This also required the development of predictable animal models to allow precise, quantitative documentation of the *in vivo* response to injury.[7] The initial stent coatings, however, were dismal failures.[8] Only recently, biocompatible materials have been developed that maintain adequate patency in the animal model. Another problem was applying coating to stent struts and then sterilizing the combination without altering the properties of the coating or the drug.

With these aspects kept in mind, this chapter will review four aspects of the restenosis problem. First, it will highlight the mechanisms of restenosis, including neointimal hyperplasia, acute recoil, and vascular remodeling. These, in turn, influence the response of the vessel wall to mechanical injury. Second, the issue of mural thrombus in restenosis will be addressed for both stenting and balloon angioplasty, since blood elements and factors produced by circulating cells play a key role in the initiation and propagation of neointima formation. The importance of antithrombotic agents such as GPIIb/IIIa receptor antagonists in reducing morbidity and mortality after percutaneous transluminal angioplasty (PTCA) and their potential in reducing the restenosis process will be reviewed. Third, emerging concepts in gene therapy and moreover in drug-eluting stents and their clinical trials will be reviewed.

The problem of restenosis

Defining restenosis

Restenosis studies have suffered to various degrees from methodological problems. Since native coronary atherosclerotic and restenotic lesions are both identified and treated with the use of angiography, one would hope that a uniform angiographic definition of restenosis exists. Unfortunately, such definitions are currently lacking, representing a major limitation in comparing different studies.

The numerous angiographic definitions used in clinical studies,[9] and more recently, definitions based on absolute changes in minimal lumen diameter at follow up,[10] have led to confusion and hampered investigations in this field[11] (Box 29.1).

Box 29.1   Angiographic definitions of restenosis

- An increase of ≥30% from immediate postangioplasty diameter stenosis to follow up stenosis
- An initial diameter stenosis <50% after angioplasty, increasing to ≥70% at follow up angiography
- An increase in diameter stenosis at follow up angiography to within 10% of the preangioplasty value
- A loss of >50% of the initial diameter stenosis gain achieved by angioplasty, from immediate postangioplasty to follow up angiography
- A postangioplasty diameter stenosis <50% increasing to >50% at follow up angiography
- A decrease in the minimal lumen diameter at the lesion of >0·72 mm from immediate postangioplasty to follow up angiography
- Cumulative distribution of MLD

Using clinical criteria, restenosis may be defined by evidence of recurrent myocardial ischemia after the revascularization procedure discovered during clinical tests by the presence of symptoms (that is, recurrence of angina, need for target vascular revascularization). Difficulties occur with a discordance between angiography and clinical status. A patient with a lesion fitting the angiographic criteria for restenosis but who is asymptomatic and/or has negative tests for ischemia will likely not be recatheterized on the basis of clinical criteria alone.

Moreover, restenosis has been previously characterized as an "all or none" phenomenon and, by subsequent studies, as a continuous variable that takes place to a different extent in all treated lesions.[12] Many studies have been small, and the timing and methods of follow up have been variable,[1,13] introducing the selection biases and misleading interpretations of the data.

It is clear that a more uniform definition, that includes a combination of angiographic and clinical criteria, and studies with more uniform groups of patients, may provide a more accurate picture of the restenosis phenomenon.[14]

Predicting restenosis

While many clinical studies have been performed to identify correlates of restenosis,[1,13,15–19] the ability to predict an excessive healing response after percutaneous interventions has remained particularly difficult.[20]

Three different categories of variables are related to an increased risk of restenosis. These include clinical patient-related factors, anatomic-related factors, and interventional procedure-related factors. Patient-related variables include older age, male gender, diabetes, hypertension, hyperlipidemia, unstable angina prior to angioplasty, vasospastic angina, and continued smoking after angioplasty. Anatomical and procedural factors include ostial lesions, longer lesions, total occlusions, multilesion and multivessel angioplasty procedures, saphenous vein graft location, left anterior descending location, presence of calcium, balloon-to-artery ratio, suboptimal results with significant residual stenosis, and extent of dissection.

However, no variables have yet been found that predict restenosis with absolute certainty. Of all the factors, the most consistent in predicting a better long-term outcome appears to be a large postprocedural lumen diameter.[21] This finding has led to the current aphorism "bigger is better",[6] which has been widely applied as a therapeutic strategy of angioplasty and which may explain the improved long-term outcome observed with coronary stents or directional atherectomy.[22,23]

Other factors that are not yet fully evaluated may also predict restenosis. Angioscopic observations suggest that coronary thrombus is an important determinant of the late outcome.[24] Recent clinical studies using the glycoprotein IIb/IIIa receptor antagonist 7E3 have shown in support of the role of thrombus a significative reduction in the incidence of restenosis.[25] Experimental evidences suggest that oxidative stress may be important in the restenotic process, and the results of the MVP study[26] indicate that probucol is effective in reducing restenosis by means of low density lipoprotein oxidation prevention, decreasing platelet aggregation and modulation of prostaglandin and leukotriene synthesis.[27–29]

Studying restenosis

Traditionally, animal models are the cornerstone to test strategies aimed at developing treatments for pathologic conditions and for understanding pathophysiologic mechanisms that may cause that particular condition. In this respect, restenosis is no exception and several animal models have been developed during the past decade in an attempt to reproduce restenotic lesions and find a therapeutical strategy to reduce neointimal formation. Unfortunately, although several models of restenosis have been evaluated in the past 15 years, there is no perfect animal model for human restenosis. Common models include the rat carotid air desiccation or balloon endothelial denudation model,[30,31] the rabbit femoral or iliac artery balloon injury model with or without cholesterol supplementation,[32] and the porcine carotid and coronary artery model.[33]

The rat model, based on elastic arteries, does not develop severe stenotic neointimal lesions, and is therefore very permissive in terms of efficacy of pharmacological interventions. The cholesterol-fed rabbit model has been criticized for the high level of hyperlipidemia required for the development of lesions. The latter results in a large macrophage foam cell component, resembling fatty streaks rather than human restenotic lesions. Conversely, the histopathologic features of neointima obtained in porcine models closely resemble the human neointima, and the amount of neointimal thickening is proportional to injury severity. This has allowed the creation of an injury–neointima relationship that can be used to evaluate the response to different therapies. However, the repair process in the pig coronary artery injury model using normal coronary arteries is certainly more rapid and may be different from the response to balloon angioplasty that characterizes human coronary atherosclerotic plaques.

The major limitation in the use of animal models of restenosis is that agents effective in reducing neointima in those models are ineffective when transferred into the clinical arena. Many explanations might support those differences. Different animal species, types of artery, degree of arterial injury, volume of neointima, drug dosages and timing regimens, and atherosclerotic substrate might be considered.

To address this concern, we believe that before transferring the results obtained in animal models into clinical trials, standardization of injury type, the method of measurement, and the dose and timing of drug administration among different animal models is necessary.

Other issues in the study of restenosis are the limitations in the design of restenosis clinical trials. Incomplete angiographic follow up leading to the occurrence of selection and withdrawal biases, followed by inadequate power due to small patient sample leading to the potential of β (type II) errors, are the most common problems. Non-uniform definitions of angiographic restenosis and poor correlation between angiographic and clinical outcome are other problems that need to be resolved when comparing different trial results. Future restenosis studies should utilize composite clinical outcomes as primary end points, with multiple, simultaneous treatment approaches and careful choice of the appropriate regimen. These studies should also include an angiographic or IVUS subset to allow assessment of mechanisms of action, and using these data can help limit sample size necessary to detect efficacy at reducing neointima.

Understanding restenosis

To better understand the mechanisms of restenosis, it is useful briefly to review the potential mechanisms by which coronary interventional procedures increase lumen patency. Since the explanation given by Dotter and Judkins,[34] who ascribed the enlargement of vessel lumen by balloon angioplasty to compression of atheromatous plaque against the arterial wall, several morphologic and histologic observations have been made both in human necropsy studies[35–37] and experimental models.[38] Different mechanisms of action have been identified. The original concept of plaque compression is unlikely to occur because the majority of atherosclerotic plaques are composed of dense fibrocollagenous tissue with hard calcium deposits, and thus, are difficult to compress. However, this mechanism can play a major role in the dilation of newly formed atherosclerotic plaque – that is, soft plaques – or recently formed thrombus.

Subsequent data suggest that the major mechanisms of action of coronary angioplasty are breaking, cracking, and splitting of the intimal plaque with partial disruption of the media and stretching of the plaque-free vessel wall.[39–41] In particular, intravascular ultrasound studies have shown that those mechanisms may vary depending on the histologic plaque composition, with more plaque dissection in calcified lesions and more vessel expansion in non-calcified plaques.[42]

Conversely, directional and rotational coronary atherectomy improve lumen caliber by tissue removal, with little disruption and expansion of the vessel wall. Finally, the mechanism of laser angioplasty is related to atherosclerotic tissue photoablation and dissection associated with vessel expansion.

Based on these clinical and experimental observations, the presumed healing and repair processes leading to arterial restenosis may be categorized as follow: (a) exaggerated cell proliferation at the site of injury; (b) incomplete plaque dissection by balloon angioplasty or incomplete tissue removal by directional coronary atherectomy (DCA), rotational atherectomy, and laser angioplasty; (c) thrombus formation and organization at the site of injury; (d) favorable or unfavorable artery wall remodeling.

Pathobiologic events in restenosis: from growth regulatory factors to cell cycle genes

It has been more than a decade since Essed *et al* first documented intimal proliferation after PTCA as a cause of restenosis.[43] During this interval, enormous progress has been made in defining the pathogenetic mechanisms of human restenotic lesions. At the same time, molecular techniques coupled with increasing understanding of the regulatory events at the level of nucleic acids have been applied to investigation of the restenotic process. Today, there is a general consensus that restenosis involves the interactions of cytokines, growth factors, vascular elements, blood cells, and the extent of injury.

Based on the experiences derived from experimental models, cell culture, human pathologic evidence as well as angiographic, angioscopic, and intravascular ultrasound observations, the sequence of events that take place in the artery and that characterize the restenotic process can be divided into three phases (Figures 29.1 and 29.2). **Grade A**

1. A first phase of elastic recoil, usually occurring within 24 hours of the procedure.

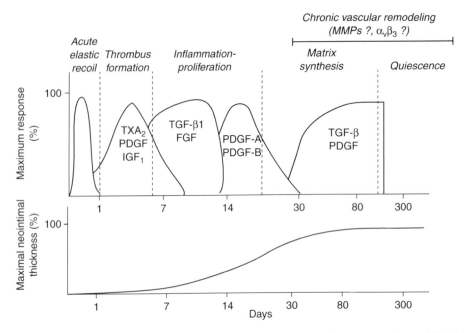

Figure 29.1 Different phases of the restenotic process. The lower panel indicates the increase in neointimal thickening and the upper panel the associated expression of growth factors (for abbreviations see text).

2. A second phase of mural thrombus formation and organization associated with inflammatory infiltrate at the site of vascular injury in the subsequent 2 weeks. In this phase, immediately after stent implantation, activation, adhesion, aggregation, and deposition of platelets and neutrophils occurs. The platelet thrombus formed can even become large enough to occlude the vessel. Within hours the thrombus at the injured site becomes fibrin-rich and also fibrin/red cell thrombus adheres to the platelet mass. From day 3 the thrombus is covered by a layer of endothelial-like cells and intense cellular infiltration begins at the injury site with monocytes (which become macrophages after migration into the mural thrombus) and lymphocytes. In the process these cells progressively migrate deeper into the mural thrombus and vessel wall.

3. A third phase of cell activation, proliferation, and extracellular matrix formation, which usually lasts from 2 to 3 months. In this phase, smooth muscle cells from different vessel wall layers proliferate and migrate and thereafter resorb the residual thrombus until all of it is gone and replaced by neointimal cells. For several weeks proliferative activity can be detected in the endothelial layer, the intimal layer, the medial layer, and in the adventitia. Thereafter a more or less quiescent fourth state will ensue, characterized by further buildup of extracellular matrix.[33,44]

Therefore, several factors may influence the production of excessive neointimal volume, including the amount of

platelet–fibrin thrombus at the injury site, the total number of smooth muscle cells (SMC) within the neointima, and the amount of extracellular matrix elaborated by neointimal cells. Limiting one of those steps, either individually or in combination, might perhaps reduce the neointimal response following mechanical injury (Table 29.1).

Phase I: elastic recoil

The vessel wall itself can participate in acute lumen loss observed in some patients just after coronary interventions by a mechanism termed "recoil". Elastic recoil occurs within minutes to hours following balloon angioplasty and seems to be the consequence of the "spring-like" properties of the non-diseased vascular wall responding to its overstretching.[45–47] Other possible explanations are vasoconstriction due to vessel endothelial disruption[48] or platelet activation and thrombus formation with consequent release of vasoconstrictive substances.[49,50] Whenever the normal wall is significantly stretched, recoil may be the predominant mechanism of restenosis. Different studies, indeed, have shown that this very early vessel wall recoil increases the likelihood of subsequent restenosis with a rate of 73·6% for the lesions that had lumen loss >10% and only 9·8% for lesions that diminished by <10%.[51,52] Early recoil may possibly have a significant importance in restenosis when the vessel has not been severely injured and the lesion consists of SMC. When the vessel wall injury is more severe, thrombus formation with consequent activation of growth factors

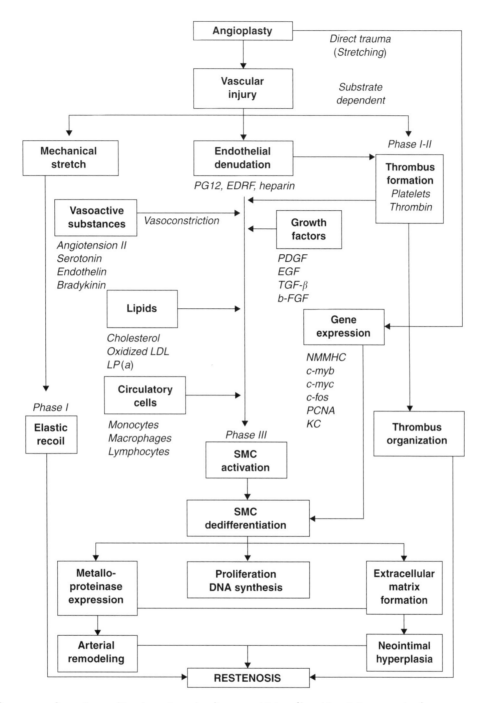

Figure 29.2 Sequence of events resulting in restenosis after vessel injury (for abbreviations see text)

and release of cytokines may be, instead, the predominant mechanism of restenosis.

Prevention of phase I: mechanical v pharmacologic approaches

It is clear that the utilization of methods to minimize the angioplasty injury, reduce the elastic recoil and enlarge the lumen size should result in a lower incidence of restenosis.

Balloon angioplasty allows manipulation of only few parameters that cause injury or recoil. Several studies have evaluated the number of balloon inflations,[53,54] duration of inflation,[53,55–57] inflation pressure,[58–60] and balloon–artery ratio.[54,59,61,62] Although higher inflation pressures and larger balloon size have been related to a small decrease in restenosis rate, they also cause a substantial increase in acute complications such as rate of emergency surgery and myocardial infarction.[59,63]

Table 29.1 Potential therapeutic approaches for the treatment of the different phases of the restenotic process

Response to vessel injury	Potential therapy
Early elastic recoil	Achievement of greater MLD by stents
Thrombus formation	Antithrombotic agents
	Antiplatelet agents
	Rapid re-endothelization
	Molecular therapies
Inflammation	Coated/drug-eluting stents
Neointimal proliferation	
SMC activation	Molecular therapies, coated/ drug-eluting stents
SMC migration	Rapid re-endothelization, MMP inhibitors, coated/drug-eluting stents
SMC proliferation	Antiproliferative agents, brachytherapy, rapid re-endothelization, molecular therapies, coated/drug-eluting stents
ECM formation	Antiproliferative agents, rapid re-endothelization, molecular therapies, coated/drug-eluting stents
Chronic vascular remodeling	Stents

Abbreviations: ECM, extracellular matrix; MLD, minimal lumen diameter; MMP, metalloproteinase; SMC, smooth muscle cells

Coronary stents, by means of their rigid structure, significantly decrease acute recoil. One of the most important advantages of intracoronary stents is that those devices represent the "bigger is better" approach. Stents address restenosis from the direction of greater luminal gain and a decrease in the elastic recoil. By this radial support, the technique results in increased residual lumen and expansion of the artery at the long-term follow up.[6,64] Furthermore, coronary stents limit the exposure of deep vessel wall tissue to blood elements, diminishing the activation of unfavorable rheological factors and allowing a higher anterograde flow through a smooth contoured lumen.

Randomized studies such as the Stent in Restenosis Study (STRESS)[65] and the European Belgian–Netherlands Stent trial (BENESTENT)[22] have both shown a significant decrease in restenosis in the groups with stent placement compared with conventional balloon angioplasty.[22,66] **Grade A** The STRESS investigators reported a 10% decrease in restenosis rate with Palmaz–Schatz stent compared with balloon

angioplasty (32% v 42% respectively), and the BENESTENT trial also demonstrated a 10% decrease in restenosis (22% in the stent group v 32% in the PTCA group), with better event-free survival and fewer revascularization procedures at 8 month follow up. Stenting technique has continued to evolve and other trials have compared conventional balloon angioplasty with contemporary stenting techniques – high pressure deployment,[67] IVUS,[68] reduced anticoagulation,[68] ostial placement,[69] – always demonstrating a reduction of restenosis rate in patients receiving coronary stents.

Grade B The pilot phase of a new study, the BENESTENT-II trial, has shown that the rate of restenosis was impressively reduced to less than 13% when heparin coated stents were placed with high pressure delivery.[70] These results were confirmed by the BENESTENT-II trial,[71] which demonstrated that use of a heparin coated stents plus antiplatelet therapy resulted in better event-free survival at 6 months compared to standard balloon angioplasty. However, with respect to an antiproliferative effect of heparin, data of preclinical studies as well as from the BENESTENT-II trial suggest no reduction of neointimal hyperplasia within the stent in comparison to uncoated stents.[71–74] **Grade A**

Other devices, such as directional atherectomy, rotational atherectomy, and TEC atherectomy, improve lumen patency by tissue removal and are associated with less vessel wall recoil and dissection.[75,76] The CAVEAT-I and the C-CAT trials did not show a significative advantage of atherectomy over conventional balloon angioplasty.[77–79] This was a surprising finding since experimental and clinical studies have shown that a larger final lumen correlates with lower restenosis rates. However, it is important to note that in those trials the final lumen achieved with atherectomy did not differ compared with that obtained by balloon angioplasty. Indeed, a prospective multicenter registry of 199 patients treated by optimal DCA (<15% residual stenosis), the OARS study,[80] demonstrated a 6 month restenosis rate of 28·9% with a target lesion revascularization rate of 17·8% at 1 year follow up. These results have been recently confirmed by the Balloon versus Optimal Atherectomy Trial (BOAT),[81] which randomized 1000 patients with single *de novo*, native vessel lesions to DCA (<20% short-term post-treatment residual stenosis) or PTCA and demonstrated that optimal DCA provided lower angiographic restenosis than conventional PTCA (31·4% v 39·8%, respectively) at 6 month follow up. **Grade B** Other debulking modalities, such as aggressive rotational atherectomy utilized in the STRATAS study, demonstrated a trend toward increasing late loss index, restenosis, and target revascularization.[82]

Phase II: platelet aggregation/thrombus formation and inflammation

As an integral part of the dilation mechanism, coronary angioplasty results in injury to the arterial wall, including endothelial damage with loss of antithrombotic properties (EDRF, PGI2, t-PA), induction of procoagulant factors (thrombin, tissue factor) and inflammatory infiltrate at the site of vascular injury. In addition, rupture of the internal elastic lamina and medial disruption, with exposure of the blood elements to wall constituents like collagen, von Willebrand factor, and extracellular matrix components, stimulates the interaction with platelet surface receptors (primarily glycoprotein Ib and IIb/IIIa integrins), resulting within minutes to hours after the intervention in platelet activation and deep mural thrombus formation[83-86] inaccessible to the action of heparin.[87,88] Experimental and clinical studies have also shown that platelets are activated by contrast medium.[89,90] Activated platelets secrete several substances from their α granules that stimulate vasoconstriction, chemotaxis, and activation of neighboring platelets.[91,92] In addition, platelet aggregation releases or stimulates the production of several factors and cytokines including thrombin, tromboxane A2, serotonin, plasminogen activator inhibitor (PAI-1), platelet derived growth factor (PDGF), transforming growth factor-β (TGF-β), basic fibroblast growth factor (b-FGF), epidermal growth factor (EGF), insulin-like growth factor (IGF-1), interleukin-1, and monocyte chemoattractant protein-1 (MCP-1) (Box 29.2).[93-95] These factors are believed to be responsible for neointimal growth by attracting and stimulating SMC migration and proliferation at the site of injury. (Figure 29.3).[96-99] The severity of the thrombogenic response depends on the degree of vascular injury, the surface area of exposure, the type of substrate exposed in the underlying vessel wall, and the rheological conditions such as shear stress and time of exposure.

Platelet activation leads to the recruitment of glycoprotein IIb/IIIa integrin surface receptors, which mediate platelet aggregation and thrombus formation by binding fibrinogen molecules between adjacent receptors.[93,100,101] Aggregated platelets accelerate the conversion of prothrombin to thrombin, which in turn stimulates further platelet activation.[102] Thrombin is involved in both thrombus formation, upregulation of E-selectin and P-selectin expression on endothelial cells, monocyte and neutrophil migration in the injured wall,[103] and stimulation of endothelin and tissue factor release from endothelial cells with a mitotic effect on SMC.[104] Of interest, there is also evidence that monocyte-macrophage recruitment may contribute to thrombus myofibrotic organization.[105] Genes for the PDGF ligands and receptor components are expressed in normal and injured rat carotid arteries.[106] Basic FGF and FGF receptor Type 1 are both expressed by endothelial cells and SMC after mechanical injury and inhibition of this growth factor reduces neointimal formation.[94,107,108] TGF-β seems to be the principal growth factor involved in the regulation and synthesis of proteoglycans, the major components of the extracellular matrix.[109-111] TGF-β

induces both migration and proliferation of vascular cells and recent evidences suggest that this is an important factor in the vascular remodeling process associated with restenosis.[112,113]

Box 29.2 Extracellular factors involved in restenosis
- Angiotensin-II
- Collagen
- Collagenase
- Colony stimulating factors (CSFs)
- Elastic fibers
- Endothelins (ETs)
- Epidermal growth factor/transforming growth factor α (EGF/TGF-α)
- Fibroblast growth factors, acidic and basic (a-FGF, b-FGF)
- Heparin
- Heparin-binding epidermal growth factor (HB-EGF)
- Insulin-like growth factor 1 (IGF-1)
- Interferon γ (IFN-γ)
- Interleukin-1 (IL-1)
- Low density lipoprotein, oxidized (oxLDL)
- Monocyte-macrophage colony stimulating factor (M-CSF)
- Monocyte chemotactic protein 1 (MCP-1/MCAF-1)
- Nitric oxide/endothelium-derived relaxing factor (NO/EDRF)
- Plasmin
- Plasminogen activator inhibitor (PAI-1)
- Platelet derived growth factor A (endothelium, PDGF-AA)
- Platelet derived growth factor B (smooth muscle cells, PDGF-BB)
- Prostacyclin (PGI$_2$)
- Prostaglandin E
- Proteoglycans
- Thrombin
- Thromboxane A$_2$ (TXA$_2$)
- Tissue plasminogen activator (tPA)
- Transforming growth factor β (TGF-β)
- Tumor necrosis factor α (TNF-α)

Following platelet activation, circulating inflammatory cells adhere to the site of injury and migrate into the thrombus. Neutrophils, lymphocytes, and monocytes have been observed within the mural thrombus 1–5 days following angioplasty in an atherosclerotic rabbit model,[114] and presence of leukocytes and macrophages has been demonstrated by scanning electron microscopy adherent to the luminal surface of stented arteries in different animal models.[115,116] Stent deployment can also cause a foreign body reaction due to deeper arterial injury compared to balloon angioplasty.[117] Karas *et al* found reactive inflammatory infiltrates and multinucleated giant cells surrounding the stent wires at 4 week follow up in a porcine model of coronary injury.[118] Recently, the present authors demonstrated in a large

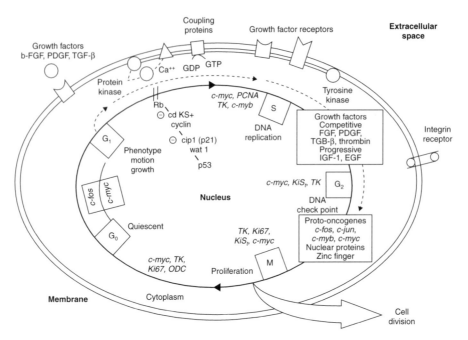

Figure 29.3 Cytoplasmatic and nuclear control points for SMC division and proliferation: CDKS, cyclin-dependent kinases; ODC, ornithine decarboxylase gene; Rb, retinoblastoma protein; TK, tyrosine kinase (for other abbreviations see text)

autopsy series that acute inflammation (mainly composed by neutrophils) linked to the extent and location of vessel injury and that chronic inflammation (lymphocytes and macrophages) was frequently observed around metallic struts at different time points following stent placement in humans.[119] Furthermore, it has been demonstrated that the extent of inflammatory reaction is significantly correlated, both independently and in combination with the degree of arterial injury, with the amount of neointimal formation.[120] The inflammatory response after stent deployment is also related to the material, design, and surface of the stent.[8,121–124]

In summary, the extent of vessel wall injury, amount of thrombus formation, and likelihood of neointimal proliferation are interrelated. Although the relationship of thrombus formation to restenosis remains to be elucidated, evidence suggests that thrombus contributes directly to restenosis by vessel occlusion[125] and indirectly by mediating the release of several factors, which in turn are also involved in the third phase of the restenotic process.[126]

Prevention of phase II: the role of new antithrombotic drugs

Since platelet function and consequent thrombus formation are important in the vascular response to injury, they have been logical targets of several therapeutic strategies. In addition to existing antithrombotic and anticoagulant drugs (that is, heparin and aspirin), antiplatelet therapies to prevent restenosis have been recently boosted by the development

of newer agents that specifically inhibit critical steps in the coagulation cascade and proteins on the surface of platelets. These new drugs include inhibitors of thrombin generators (factor Xa inhibitors),[127,128] thrombin action (direct thrombin inhibitors),[129] or platelet aggregation (Gp IIb/IIIa receptor antagonists).[130]

Although aspirin,[131] dypiridamole,[132] ticlopidine,[133] warfarin,[134–136] thromboxane antagonists,[137–139] and prostacyclin analogs,[140,141] have been shown to be effective in animal models of restenosis, these drugs have failed to show any benefit in clinical practice. **Grade B** However, several factors may confound the interpretation of those studies. For example, differences in the lesion substrate, inappropriate drug doses, or incomplete block of the target, may explain the discrepancy between animal models and human studies. Moreover, while the magnitude of injury and thrombus formation correlate with the degree of neointimal formation in animals, the relationship in humans is by no means established. In addition, specific anticoagulant agents such as heparin,[142–145] low molecular weight heparin,[146,147] hirudin and hirulog,[148–151] did not show any favorable effect either on angiographic or clinical outcome related to restenosis. Recently, dietary fish oils have been demonstrated to inhibit platelet aggregation and thromboxane synthesis.[152] It has also been shown that fish oil intake reduces blood and red cell viscosity and reduces the inflammatory response to injury.[153,154] However, the two largest trials designed to test the hypothesis that restenosis could be reduced by fish oil intake have definitively demonstrated the lack of efficiency of these agents in the clinical arena.[155,156] **Grade A**

Both animal models of restenosis and clinical trials demonstrated a reduction of neointimal proliferation by blocking the platelet Gp IIb/IIIa ($\alpha_{IIb}\beta_3$) or the vitronectin receptors ($\alpha_v\beta_3$).[25,157–160] By using a chimeric 7E3 antibody directed against the platelet membrane IIb/IIIa receptor complex, the EPIC trial demonstrated a reduction in the onset of acute complications and clinical restenosis in high-risk angioplasty.[25] Since this trial was published, other studies have evaluated the effect at 6 month follow up of IIb/IIIa antagonists versus placebo. Unfortunately, IMPACT[161], IMPACT-II[160], RESTORE[162], EPILOG, and CAPTURE trials,[163,164] that studied the efficacy of integrilin, tirofiban, and abciximab, respectively, did not demonstrate a reduction in target vessel revascularization compared to placebo treatment. The EPISTENT trial demonstrated lower need for repeat target vessel revascularization among diabetic patients receiving abciximab compared to placebo,[165,166] as previously noted at 6 months.[167] **Grade A**

Aggarwal *et al* reported results of platelet Gp IIb/IIIa antibody eluting from cellulose polymer coated stents, implanted in iliac arteries of rabbits after balloon injury. There was a significant improvement in patency rates after both 2 hours and 28 days, but no difference in mean neointimal thickness at 28 days.[168] **Grade C** A clinical trial has been planned (UK RESOLVE trial), but thus far clinical results have not been reported. Alt *et al* coated a Palmaz-Schatz stent with a 10 μm layer of biocompatible and biodegradable high molecular weight poly-l-lactic acid and incorporated in this coating recombinant polyethylene glycol (r-PEG)-hirudin and the prostacyclin analog iloprost. Both drugs have antithrombotic and potentially antiproliferative effects. Stents were implanted in the non-overstretch model in sheep and in the overstretch pig model and compared to non-coated controls. At 28 days a greater luminal diameter was seen with a significant reduction of mean restenosis area of 22·9% in the sheep and 24·8% in the pig model, independently of the extent of vascular injury.[169] **Grade C**

Prevention of phase II: the role of anti-inflammatory approaches

The inflammatory reaction in restenosis relates to neointimal formation and arterial remodeling. Therefore, inhibition of the inflammatory response after vascular injury may have some beneficial effects on restenosis.

P-selectin, a protein stored in the α granules of platelets and Weibel–Palades bodies of endothelial cells, and binding to circulating monocytes and leukocytes, plays a crucial role in the early inflammatory response. Manka *et al* reported that apolipoprotein E-deficient mice with targeted disruption of the P-selectin gene exhibited dramatically decreased monocyte infiltration into the arterial wall and significantly decreased neointimal formation in a carotid artery injury

model.[170] Mac-1 (CD11b/CD18, $\alpha_M\beta_2$), a leukocyte integrin, promotes adhesion and transmigration of leukocytes and monocytes at the site of vascular injury. Upregulation of Mac-1 in patients is associated with increased restenosis.[171,172] M1/70, a CD11b blocking Mab, was shown to inhibit neutrophil infiltration and medial SMC proliferation in a balloon denudation model.[173] Administration of recombinant human interleukin-10 (rhuIL-10), an anti-inflammatory cytokine, inhibited monocytes and macrophage infiltration in hypercholesterolemic rabbits, which was associated in turn with dramatic reduction in neointimal hyperplasia.[174] In addition, due to a broad range of anti-inflammatory and immunosuppressive activities, dexamethasone stent coating has been shown to reduce neointima hyperplasia compared to uncoated stents in canine femoral arteries.[175] Tranilast, a novel anti-inflammatory agent, has been shown to interfere with the PDGF-induced proliferation and migration of SMCs. This drug has been evaluated in the largest interventional anti-restenosis trial conducted to date, the Prevention of Restenosis with Tranilast and Its Outcome (PRESTO) trial,[176] which enrolled more than 11 500 patients after successful percutaneous coronary intervention. Unfortunately, this trial provided unequivocal evidence that this compound has no effect on both restenosis and clinical events. **Grade A/C**

Phase III: smooth muscle cell activation and synthesis of extracellular matrix

This final phase of vascular healing is predominantly characterized by neointimal formation due to SMC proliferation and extracellular matrix accumulation produced by the neointimal cells at the injury site.[45,177–180] The healing response is a normal process which is essential in maintaining vascular integrity after an injury to the vessel wall, but varies in the degree to which it occurs. One pathogenetic explanation of restenosis is, indeed, an exaggeration of this healing response.

Phase III could be further divided into three different waves.[44] In the *first wave* (days 1–4 after vessel injury), medial SMC from the site of injury and possibly from adjacent areas are activated and stimulated by the triggering factors mentioned earlier. In addition to mitogenic factors released by endothelial cells, stretching of the arterial wall is a potent stimulus for SMC activation and growth.[181] Once activated, SMC undergo characteristic phenotypic transformation, from a "contractile" to a "synthetic" form,[178] which is responsible for the production of extracellular matrix rich in chondroitin sulfate and dermatan sulfate seen in the first 6 months after injury. The *second wave* (3–14 days after vessel injury) and the *third wave* (14 days to months after vessel injury) are respectively characterized by the migration of SMC through breaks in the internal elastic lamina into the intima, the local thrombus,[182] and

SMC proliferation followed by extracellular matrix formation.[126,183–186] Those events are characterized by complex interactions between growth factors, second messengers, and gene regulatory proteins resulting in phenotypic change from a quiescent state to a proliferative one.[96] The peak of proliferation is observed 4–5 days after balloon injury but the duration of migration is not known, nor is it known whether a phase of cellular replication is required before SMC migration. Few studies have been done to identify the matrix molecules involved in the migration into the intima. Osteopontin is expressed in sites of marked remodeling,[187] and antibodies to osteopontin inhibit SMC migration into the intima after balloon angioplasty.[188] Proteoglycans may also be important for the formation of neointima. CD44, a receptor for hyaluronic acid, seems to play a role in the migration of cells into fibrin or osteopontin.[189,190] SMC migration presumably requires degradation of the basement membrane surrounding the cells. Several metalloproteinases, including tissue type plasminogen activator, plasmin, MMP-2, and MMP-9, may be responsible for this process,[191,192] and the administration of a protease inhibitor reduces SMC migration into the intima.[193] Cell migration is probably initiated by recognition of extracellular matrix proteins by a family of cell surface adhesion receptors known as integrins.[194,195] *In vitro* and *in vivo* studies have demonstrated that the selective blockage of the $\alpha_v\beta_3$ integrin inhibits SMC migration and reduces neointimal formation.[158,196]

Experimental studies have suggested that endothelin-1 (ET-1) and endothelin receptors may also be indirectly implicated in the SMC migration and matrix synthesis.[197–199] Immunohistochemical studies demonstrate a time-dependent increase in endothelin immunoreactivity after balloon angioplasty in the rat model.[200] The administration of endothelin receptor antagonists in different animal models of balloon injury has been shown to be effective in reducing neointimal formation.[197,201,202]

Several *in vitro* studies have suggested that different growth factors, such as PDGF-AA, PDGF-BB, β-FGF, IGF, EGF, FGF, TGF-β, and angiotensin II, may also play a major role in this process.[96,185,203–207] Control of SMC proliferation is regulated by the actions of mitogens (that is, PDGF) and the opposing effect of inhibitors (that is, TGF-β). The growth factors bind to cell surface receptors and initiate a cascade of events which leads to cell migration and division. Components of the cascade include different tyrosine kinases, coupling proteins, and membrane-associated and cytoplasmic protein kinases (see Figure 29.3). On stimulation by growth factors, proto-oncogenes are transiently activated and together with other cell cycle-dependent proteins such as zinc finger proteins, mediate the effects within the nucleus. Several studies have demonstrated that stimulation of SMC *in vitro* is associated with an increase of the proto-oncogenes *c-myc*, *c-myb*, and *c-fos*.[208–210] The ornithine decarboxylase (ODC) gene and the thymidine kinase (TK) messenger RNA are both expressed in stimulating cells and in continuously cycling cells.[210] SMC proliferation may also result from a reduction in an inhibitory factor which normally prevents cell division. Proteins such as p21 are inhibitors of the cyclin-dependent kinases (cdks) which regulate the entry of the cell in the cycle (see Figure 29.3). Stimulation of these proteins, indeed, inhibits SMC proliferation and neointima formation after balloon injury.[211]

As smooth muscle cells decrease their proliferation rate, they begin to synthesize large quantities of proteoglycan matrix. The extracellular matrix production continues for up to 20–25 weeks and over time it is gradually replaced by collagen and elastin, while the SMC turn into quiescent mesenchymal cells. The resulting neointima is composed of a fibrotic extracellular matrix with few cellular constituents. The endothelial cells proliferate and cover the denuded area resulting in a re-endothelization process, and the new endothelium begins to produce large quantities of heparan sulfate and nitric oxide, both of which inhibit SMC proliferation.[86] However, whether SMC proliferation and extracellular matrix production cease after re-endothelization is still unknown at this time.

Prevention of phase III: the past and the future

Multiple experimental and clinical trials[212,213] have been carried out specifically to target what seemed the key in the restenosis process: smooth muscle cell proliferation. To date, with only few exceptions, no pharmacologic or mechanical agent has been conclusively shown to reduce restenosis.

Antiproliferative approaches

The aim of an antiproliferative approach to restenosis is to control and modulate the action of possible mediators of proliferation at any point in the biologic pathway in which they are involved or to enable the cell to respond appropriately to the proliferative stimulus. Two different strategies to inhibit neointima hyperplasia are available:

1. the cytostatic approach, by which regulation and expression of cell cycle modulating proteins at any level along the pathway is performed;
2. the cytotoxic approach, by which proliferating cells are killed and eliminated.

The latter approach has the disadvantage of necrosis induction, associated with inflammation, which may contribute to vessel wall weakening. Hence, the cytostatic approach is conceptually more attractive.

Several antiproliferative agents targeting SMC migration and proliferation have been evaluated, including glucocorticoids, colchicine, somatostatin, hypolipidemic drugs, antineoplastic agents, and angiotensin-converting enzyme (ACE) inhibitors. Both natural and synthetic corticosteroids are potent inhibitors of SMC proliferation, leukocyte migration, and degranulation, PDGF and macrophage derived growth factor release, and matrix production.[214] While experimental and preclinical studies[215–217] have reduced SMC proliferation with the use of local glucocorticoids delivery, three different human trials using oral steroid dosage have failed to shown any reduction in restenosis rate.[131,218,219] **Grade A**

Contradictory results have been obtained as well with antineoplastic agents such as methotrexate, cytarabine, azathioprine, etoposide, vincristine, taxol, and doxorubicin. While some *in vitro* and *in vivo* studies show an attenuation of vascular SMC proliferation,[220,221] other studies show no efficacy in reducing the incidence of restenosis after PTCA.[222–224] Colchicine, which has an antimitotic and anti-inflammatory action in addition to an inhibitory effect on platelet aggregation and release of secretory products, has been shown to reduce restenosis in animals.[225] However, no clinical benefit has been seen with colchicine in two randomized placebo-controlled clinical trials.[226,227] **Grade A** As with other chemotherapeutic agents, the narrow therapeutic index of these drugs may be of concern. However, the recent availability of new local delivery systems (Box 29.3), such as drug eluting stents, has increased interest in the antiproliferative approach and has led to the evaluation of a multitude of compounds with antiproliferative properties. Furthermore, local therapy offers the combined advantages of high local concentrations at the injury site and diminished systemic levels, with decreased risk of adverse effects. The problem of systemic toxicity may be overcome.[228–233]

Box 29.3 Local drug delivery systems
- Double balloon system
- Iontophoretic porous balloon
- Balloon with hydrophilic polyacrylic polymer (hydrogel)
- Channel catheter
- Transport porous catheter
- Dispatch catheter
- Rheolytic system
- Ultrasonic energy and radiofrequency
- Balloon over a stent
- Biodegradable drug eluting polymer stent
- Dacron stent
- Silicone stent
- High molecular weight poly-l-lactic acid stent
- Nitinol stent with polyurethane coating
- Fibrin coated stent
- Stent with cell layer
- Stent with radioactive substance

After verification of an inhibitory effect on neointimal hyperplasia in animal models,[234–236] ACE inhibitors have been extensively studied to assess the clinical effect on restenosis. Unfortunately, two large clinical studies (MERCATOR and MARCATOR), with over 2129 patients enrolled, failed to show any impact on clinical or angiographic restenosis.[237,238] **Grade A** Intensive treatment with cholesterol lowering agents such as the HMG-CoA (3-hydroxy-3methylglutaryl coenzyme A) reductase inhibitors lovastatin, pravastatin, simvastatin, and fluvastatin, reduces intimal hyperplasia in the rat and rabbit models,[224,239,240] probably for serum lipid reduction and decreased platelet aggregation. Despite this promising preliminary data, chronic high-dose lovastatin treatment does not attenuate the incidence of clinical restenosis.[241] Antioxidant agents such as probucol, ascorbic acid and α-tocopherol may be useful in limiting restenosis by reducing platelet aggregation, and modulating prostaglandin and leukotriene synthesis. Both animal[242,243] and clinical[26,244] studies have recently shown a reduction in restenosis with the use of such agents. **Grade B**

Paclitaxel is a cytostatic drug which is extensively used in cancer therapy. It is a micro-tubule stabilizing agent with antiproliferative activity as well as inhibition of migration of smooth muscle cells. *In vitro* studies with cultured human vascular smooth muscle cells (VSMC) and endothelial cells show strong antiproliferative effects on the VSMC.[245] In rabbits an antiproliferative effect was seen at 1 month, which was dose-related. However, in this *in vivo* model more inflammation was seen in the paclitaxel group as well as a poor endothelization.[246] Herdeg *et al* have reported a significant reduction in neointimal stenosis after balloon dilation and subsequent local paclitaxel delivery with a double balloon catheter, compared to balloon dilation alone in rabbit carotid arteries. **Grade C** They observed marked enlargement of vessel size with positive remodeling after paclitaxel treatment (at 7, 28, and 56 days).[247] Phosphorylcholine (PC) coated stent with incorporated angiopeptin has also been tested (Table 29.2). This is a somatostatin analog which is hypothesized to prevent myointimal thickening after vessel injury mainly by inhibiting secretion of growth factors. After balloon injury effective inhibition of intimal hyperplasia has been shown in porcine coronary arteries.[248] In a randomized clinical trial including 553 patients with 742 lesions the incidence of events was significantly reduced in the angiopeptin treatment group, despite no difference in angiographic variables at follow up.[249] **Grade B** De Scheerder *et al* demonstrated the feasibility of loading a polymer coated stent with angiopeptin and significant reduction of neointimal proliferation was found 6 weeks after stenting in porcine coronary arteries.[250] Armstrong *et al* demonstrated in pig coronary arteries using 125-I angiopeptin loaded PC stents that the drug was still detectable in the vessel wall after 28 days.[251] Impressive

Table 29.2 Stent coating and covering categories

Material type	Examples
(In)-organic/ceramic materials	Gold, iridium oxide, silicium carbide, diamond-like carbon, biogold
Synthetic and biologic polymers	PC, PU, PLA, PE, cellulose
Human polymers	Chondroitin sulfate, hyaluronic acid, fibrin, elastin, endothelial cells
Immobilized drugs	Heparin, paclitaxel, abciximab
Eluting, degradable matrices	PLA-hirudin-iloprost, PLA-paclitaxel, PC-angiopeptin, cellulose-abciximab, PU-forskolin, PLA-PC-viral vector, PE-DNA
Covering substances	PTFE, autologous vein

Different materials can be used to cover a stent surface using an array of techniques such as dipping, (plasma) spraying, plating, sputtering, and surface induced mineralization. Some materials have been used as coatings *per se*, while others have been tested as a platform for local drug delivery.
Abbreviations: PC, metacrylyl phosphorylcholine laurylmethacrylate; PE, polyester; PLA, poly-l-lactic acid; PTFE, polytetrafluoroethylene; PU, polyurethane.

results have been demonstrated in the RAVEL trial[252,253] using rapamycin coated stent (Sirolimus). **Grade A** Rapamycin is a potent immunosuppressive agent that inhibits vascular SMC proliferation by blocking cell cycle progression. Significant reduction of arterial proliferative response after systemic administration of rapamycin was already shown in the porcine coronary model by Gallo *et al.*[254] Finally, other drugs, such as tranilast, a novel inflammatory agent, batimastat, a matrix metalloproteinases inhibitor, and nitric oxide-eluting polymer coated stents are currently under investigation and the clinical results are eagerly awaited. In the case of the Batimast-coated stent, preliminary results are negative.

The concept and technique of applying ionizing radiation to the arterial wall (brachytherapy) during percutaneous coronary intervention procedures has emerged and gained considerable momentum,[255–261] including entry in clinical trials.[262,263] Ionizing radiation affects dividing cells by chromosomal damage in the vascular smooth muscle cells, fibroblasts, and, when present, endothelial cells, resulting in the loss of cells' ability to reproduce, with mitotic cell death.[264] Radiation may also reduce neointima proliferation by increasing the rate of apoptosis within the intima.[265] External beam radiotherapy involves the generation of

a beam of radiation from a source external to the patients, for example linear accelerator or ^{60}Co unit. Brachytherapy is a method of delivering radiation to a target organ by placing radioactive sources, for example ^{90}Yt or ^{192}Ir sources, close to or within an organ. This method is well suited (as opposed to external beam radiation) to deliver high doses of radiation to a small defined region. Both γ and β emitters have been utilized in clinical trials of intracoronary radiation therapy.[266–269] However, γ emitters deliver a more uniform dose to the arterial wall than β emitters, but at the cost of increased radiation risk. In addition, radioactive stents, made either by bombardment with subatomic particles, ion implantation of the stents with radioisotopes, or by chemical methods that incorporate the radioactive material into the metallic stents, have been evaluated.[270] Encouraging results from small human clinical studies utilizing both γ and β emitters have set the stage for human clinical trials. The SCRIPPS trial[263] was the first randomized, placebo-controlled clinical trial to evaluate the safety and efficacy of coronary brachytherapy with a γ radiation source (^{192}Ir) in reducing restenosis. At 6 months, the angiographic restenosis rate was 53·6% in the control versus 16·7% in the irradiated group. The clinical benefit was maintained at 2 year follow up with target vessel revascularization of 15·4% as against 44·8% of the placebo group.[271] The GAMMA-1 trial randomized 252 patients with in-stent restenosis to placebo or gamma irradiation. The restenosis rate was 22% in the irradiated arm compared to 51% for the placebo arm.[272]

Several clinical trials (ARREST, Angiorad Radiation for REStenosis trial; ARTISTIC, Angiorad Radiation Therapy for In-Stent Restenosis Intra-Coronary trial; SMART, Smart Artery Radiation Therapy trial; WRIST-SVG, Washington Radiation for In-Stent Restenosis-Saphenous Vein Graft trial) are still ongoing and the results as awaited. BETA CATH, which is the largest multicenter placebo-controlled trial assessing intracoronary β radiation therapy (^{90}Sr/Y source) for restenosis prevention, recently started the enrollment phase. In this trial, clinical end points will be MACE at 8 months, 1 and 2 years follow up. BRIE (Beta Radiation in Europe) is a European trial in 180 patients with encouraging interim results.[270] Finally, European trials on radioactive stents, such as the ^{32}P-Isostent BX^{TM} stent, resulted in an increased restenosis rate (43–50% of the lesions treated) due to neointimal hyperplasia development at the stent edge, the so called "candy wrapper effect".[273]

Growth factor approaches

For the reason that several growth factors have been implicated in the pathogenesis of restenosis, interference with the cellular processes that control cellular migration, replication, and matrix deposition has attracted much interest in the continuous search for pharmacologic agents to reduce the incidence of restenosis.

Angiopeptin, an analog of somatostatin, prevents the mitotic effect of several growth factors, including somatomedin-C, epidermal growth factor, insulin-like growth factor, and PDGF. It inhibits SMC proliferation and reduces neointimal hyperplasia in different experimental models.[274–276] A multicenter trial in which 1246 patients were randomized to receive placebo or three different doses of angiopeptin showed no reduction in clinical events and restenosis rates between the different groups.[277] **Grade A** On the other hand, in a smaller randomized study, angiopeptin treatment reduced restenosis after PTCA (7·5% *v* 37·8% of the placebo group).[278] However, using the same drug regimen, this promising finding was not confirmed by another multicenter European study.[279] Questions remain whether a more prolonged dosing of this agent is needed to affect neointimal growth.

Trapidil is a potent thromboxane-A2 and PDGF antagonist which significantly reduces neointimal formation in animal models of restenosis.[280] The STARC trial randomized 305 patients to receive trapidil versus aspirin and showed a reduction in restenosis rate by 40%, and reduction in clinical symptoms at 6 month follow up in the trapidil treatment group.[281] **Grade B** The efficacy of trapidil in the prevention of restenosis after balloon angioplasty has also been reported in a meta-analysis by Serruys and coauthors.[282] However, results from a randomized trial of trapidil versus aspirin (performed in the stent era) showed no benefit in terms of late restenosis in patients treated systemically with trapidil compared to the aspirin control group.[283]

Molecular approaches

With the growing understanding that the failure of several antiproliferative agents to reduce neointima hyperplasia may be related to the amplification and redundancy present in the membrane and nuclear protein signaling, several attempts have been made to control and transform the gene expression at the molecular level.[284] The mechanisms by which genetic material is transferred into the target tissue include:

1. *in vivo* gene transfer by infusion of naked DNA or antisense oligonucleotides;[285]
2. transport by hybrid liposomes containing viral coat particles;[286]
3. transport by cationic liposomes containing the DNA;[287]
4. via viral vectors using retro- or adenoviruses.[288,289]

Besides the potential safety concern of gene therapy, there are also problems of transfection efficiency and which gene should be delivered. In previous years, in agreement with the restenosis hypothesis, SMC have been the preferential target. In more recent years, however, with the improved knowledge of the pathogenetic mechanisms involved in the restenosis phenomenon, other targets have been selected, including endothelial cells, thrombus formation, growth factors, matrix production, and vascular remodeling.[290–294] In addition, increased extracellular growth inhibitors of SMC proliferation might be another potential approach.[211,295,296] Other future approaches may include enhancement of re-endothelization and repair by cell seeding,[297–300] and photodynamic therapy with light which shows cytotoxic properties on SMC and cell membranes through the production of activated singlet oxygen species.[301–304]

New etiologies in restenosis: the role of chronic vascular remodeling and adventitia

Vascular remodeling, first described in relation to atherosclerosis,[305,306] has assumed great importance as a cause of coronary restenosis in the past few years in non-stented patients.[307] In atherosclerotic vessels a chronic focal enlargement of the artery occurs in response to plaque increase, in order to preserve blood flow.[308–312] Artery size changes also occur following coronary angioplasty[313] and the artery may exhibit three different remodeling responses:

1. compensatory enlargement;[314]
2. absence of compensation;[315] or
3. vascular constriction.[316,317]

Intravascular ultrasound (IVUS) has become an important means to understand the concept of remodeling. IVUS imaging has shown that after PTCA there is an axial plaque redistribution, and that failure to cause dissection is one of the causes of early lumen loss by elastic recoil.[39,42] More recently, serial IVUS studies indicated that the restenotic lesion led to contraction of the artery and late lumen narrowing.[5,318–320] While the mechanisms of chronic remodeling are poorly understood, several explanations have been postulated to explain the late lumen narrowing after PTCA: fibrosis of the vessel wall underlying the lesion, rearrangement of extracellular matrix composition and structure, and response to increased shear stress.[4,321–323] A recent paper suggests that $\alpha_v\beta_3$ may regulate contraction of the vessel wall.[324] The integrins may therefore play a role in active contraction as well as migration of SMC. Animal studies indicate that after PTCA, stretching of the adventitia may result in the proliferation and synthesis of extracellular matrix by myofibroblasts within the adventitia, itself with consequent scar-like contraction and compression of the underlying vascular wall.[325–327] This mechanism, however, does not seem relevant for late lumen narrowing in human coronary arteries subjected to balloon angioplasty.[328]

The potential impact of neointimal hyperplasia and geometric remodeling on restenosis requires further studies. Methods to prevent constrictive remodeling or to promote compensatory enlargement should be investigated. The metallic stent or drugs like cytokalasin B, which seems to function as a biologic stent, may serve this function.[329]

Conclusions: is the end of restenosis possible?

The failure effectively to circumvent the problem of restenosis, after 15 years of research, underscores the complexity of this biological process, which, to date, has not yet been fully understood. The elimination of the intimal healing response to injury is probably not achievable, nor is it desirable, considering that this physiologic response to preserve vascular integrity has been maintained across millions of years in different species. The more we delve into it, the more complex and redundant this process appears.

From the above description of the postulated model of restenosis, although SMC proliferation and neointima formation undoubtedly play a central role in restenosis, it is more likely that multifactorial mechanisms, involving different stimuli, interacting in a synergistic manner, are responsible for the restenosis phenomenon. Given the multimechanistic nature of restenosis, it is too simplistic to expect that a single drug or mechanical device will solve this problem completely. The solution, as the problem, will most likely be multifactorial, possibly involving the use of drug therapy in conjunction with adjunctive second-generation mechanical devices. Of these devices, coronary stents are the most promising, especially for their ability to achieve the best post-treatment luminal size in comparison with other devices.

In the history of medicine, human attempts to interfere with the natural course of a disease by active interventions have often led to undesired consequences. Restenosis is a new disease, one of the many that medicine has encountered trying to solve an old disease. Enormous progress has been made in the past years in understanding the pathogenetic mechanisms of restenosis and in the search for a cure. If the efficacy of drug eluting stents was to be confirmed, this would lead to a repositioning of the indications for percutaneous coronary interventions. Most of the events observed after balloon angioplasty, with or without stent implantation, in recent multicenter trials were linked to the problem of restenosis in the first months of evolution. It may well be that in the future new clinical trials could demonstrate that percutaneous coronary intervention is proven to be superior to surgical revascularization techniques. To some it may seem a nightmare, to us, as interventional cardiologists, and to our patients, it may indeed seem like a dream.

References

1. Califf RM, Fortin DF, Frid DJ *et al.* Restenosis after coronary angioplasty: an overview. *J Am Coll Cardiol* 1991;**17**: 2B–13B.
2. Franklin SM, Faxon DP. Pharmacologic prevention of restenosis after coronary angioplasty: review of the randomized clinical trials. *Coronary Artery Dis* 1993;**4**:232–42.
3. Topol EJ, Ellis SG, Cosgrove DM *et al.* Analysis of coronary angioplasty: practice in the United States with an insurance-claims database. *Circulation* 1993;**87**:1489–97.
4. Glagov S. Intimal hyperplasia, vascular remodeling, and the restenosis problem. *Circulation* 1994;**89**:2888–91.
5. Mintz GS, Popma JJ, Pichard AD *et al.* Arterial remodeling after coronary angioplasty: a serial intravascular ultrasound study. *Circulation* 1996;**94**:35–43.
6. Kuntz RE, Gibson CM, Nobuyoshi M, Baim DS. Generalized model of restenosis after conventional balloon angioplasty, stenting and directional atherectomy. *J Am Coll Cardiol* 1993;**21**:15–25.
7. Schwartz RS, Murpphy JG, Edwards WD *et al.* Restenosis after balloon angioplasty: a practical proliferative model in porcine coronary arteries. *Circulation* 1990;**82**:2190–200.
8. van der Giessen WJ, Lincoff AM, Schwartz RS *et al.* Marked inflammatory sequelae to implantation of biodegradable and nonbiodegradable polymers in porcine coronary arteries. *Circulation* 1996;**94**:1690–7.
9. Holmes DR, Vlietstra RE, Smith HC *et al.* Restenosis after percutaneous transluminal coronary angioplasty (PTCA): a report from the PTCA registry of the National Heart, Lung, and Blood Institute. *Am J Cardiol* 1984;**53**:77C–81C.
10. Serruys PW, Luijten HE, Beat KJ *et al.* Incidence of restenosis after successful coronary angioplasty: a time-related phenomenon. A quantitative angiographic study in 342 consecutive patients at 1,2,3, and 4 months. *Circulation* 1988;**77**:361–71.
11. Serruys PW, Rensing BJ, Hermans WRM, Beatt KJ. Definition of restenosis after percutaneous transluminal coronary angioplasty: a quickly evolving concept. *J Interv Cardiol* 1991; **4**:256–76.
12. Beatt KJ, Luijten HE, de Feyter PJ, van den Brand M, Reiber JH, Serruys PW. Change in diameter of coronary artery segments adjacent to stenosis after percutaneous transluminal coronary angioplasty: failure of percent diameter stenosis measurement to reflect morphologic changes induced by balloon dilation. *J Am Coll Cardiol* 1988;**12**:315–23.
13. Kuntz RE, Keaney KM, Senerchia C, Baim DS. A predictive method for estimating the late angiographic results of coronary intervention despite incomplete ascertainment. *Circulation* 1993;**87**:815–30.
14. Kuntz RE, Baim DS. Defining coronary restenosis: newer clinical and angiographic paradigms. *Circulation* 1993;**88**:1310–23.
15. Renkin J, Melin J, Robert A *et al.* Detection of restenosis after successful coronary angioplasty: improved clinical decision making with use of a logistic model combining procedural and follow-up variables. *J Am Coll Cardiol* 1990;**16**: 1333–40.
16. Weintraub W, Ghazzal Z, Liberman H, Cohen C, Morris D. Long term clinical follow-up in patients with angiographic restudy after successful angioplasty. *Circulation* 1991;**84**: II-364.
17. Weintraub WS, Kosinski AS, Brown CL, King SB. Can restenosis after coronary angioplasty be predicted from clinical variables? *J Am Coll Cardiol* 1993;**21**:6–14.
18. Mick MJ, Piedmonte MR, Arnold AM, Simpfendorfer C. Risk stratification for long-term outcome after elective coronary angioplasty: a multivariate analysis of 5,000 patients. *J Am Coll Cardiol* 1994;**24**:74–84.

19. Melkert R, Violaris AG, Serruys PW. Luminal narrowing after percutaneous transluminal coronary angioplasty: a multivariate analysis of clinical, procedural and lesion related factors, affecting long-term angiographic outcome in the PARK study. *J Invas Cardiol* 1994;**6**:160–71.

20. Peters RJC, Wouter EM, Kok MD *et al.*, for the PICTURE study group. Prediction of restenosis after coronary balloon angioplasty: results of PICTURE (post-intracoronary treatment ultrasound result evaluation), a prospective multicenter intracoronary ultrasound imaging study. *Circulation* 1997;**95**:2254–61.

21. Farb A, Virmani R, Atkinson JB, Anderson PG. Long-term histologic patency after percutaneous transluminal coronary angioplasty is predicted by the creation of a greater lumen area. *J Am Coll Cardiol* 1994;**24**:1229–35.

22. Serruys PW, de Jaegere P, Kiemeneij F *et al.*, for the BENESTENT study group. A comparison of balloon expandable-stent implantation with balloon angioplasty in patients with coronary artery disease. *N Engl J Med* 1994;**331**:489–95.

23. Fischman DL, Leon MB, Baim DS *et al.*, for the Stent Restenosis Study Investigators. A randomized comparison of coronary-stent placement and balloon angioplasty in the treatment of coronary artery disease. *N Engl J Med* 1994;**331**:496–501.

24. Feld S, Ganim M, Carrel ES *et al.* Comparison of angioscopy, intravascular ultrasound imaging and quantitative coronary angiography in predicting clinical outcome after coronary interventions in high risk patients. *J Am Coll Cardiol* 1996;**28**:97–105.

25. Topol EJ, Califf RM, Weisman HF *et al.* Randomised trial of coronary intervention with antibody against platelet IIb/IIIa integrin for reduction of clinical restenosis: results at six months. The EPIC investigators. *Lancet* 1994;**343**:881–6.

26. Tardif JC, Cote G, Lesperance J *et al.* Prevention of restenosis by pre- and post-PTCA probucol therapy: a randomized clinical trial. *Circulation* 1996;**94**(Suppl. I):I-91 (Abstract).

27. Godfried SL, Deckelbaum LI. Natural antioxidants and restenosis after percutaneous transluminal coronary angioplasty. *Am Heart J* 1995;**129**:203–10.

28. Chisolm G. Antioxidants and atherosclerosis: a current assessment. *Clin Cardiol* 1991;**14**:125–30.

29. Schneider J, Berk B, Santoian E *et al.* Oxidative stress is important in restenosis: reduction of neointimal formation by the antioxidant probucol in a swine model of restenosis. *Circulation* 1992;**86**(Suppl. I):I-186.

30. Clowes AV, Karnovsky MJ. Suppression by heparin of smooth muscle cell proliferation in injured arteries. *Nature* 1977;**265**:625–6.

31. Olson LV, Clowes AW, Reidy MA. Inhibition of smooth muscle cell proliferation in injured rat arteries. *J Clin Invest* 1992;**90**:2044–9.

32. Faxon DP, Weber VJ, Haudenschild C, Bottsman SB, McGovern WA, Ryan TJ. Acute effect of transluminal angioplasty in three experimental models of atherosclerosis. *Arteriosclerosis* 1982;**2**:125–33.

33. Schwartz RS, Edwards WD, Huber KC *et al.* Coronary restenosis: prospects for solution and new perspectives from a porcine model. *Mayo Clin Proc* 1993;**68**:54–62.

34. Dotter CT, Judkins MP. Transluminal treatment of atherosclerotic obstruction: desciption of new technique and a preliminary report of its application. *Circulation* 1964;**30**:654–70.

35. Baughman KL, Pasternak RC, Fallon JT, Block PC. Transluminal coronary angioplasty of post mortem human hearts. *Am J Cardiol* 1981;**48**:1044–7.

36. Block PC, Myler RK, Stertzer S, Fallon JT. Morphology after transluminal angioplasty in humans. *N Engl J Med* 1981;**305**:382.

37. Waller BF. Pathology of transluminal balloon angioplasty used in the treatment of heart disease. *Hum Pathol* 1987;**18**:476–84.

38. Sanborn TA, Faxon DP, Haudenschild C, Gottsman SB, Ryan TJ. The mechanism of coronary angioplasty: evidence for formation of aneurysms in experimental atherosclerosis. *Circulation* 1983;**68**:1136–40.

39. Potkin BN, Roberts WC. Effects of coronary angioplasty on atherosclerotic plaque composition and arterial size to outcome. *Am J Cardiol* 1988;**62**:41–50.

40. Kohchi K, Takebayashi S, Block PC *et al.* Arterial changes after percutaneous coronary angioplasty: results at autopsy. *J Am Coll Cardiol* 1987;**10**:592–9.

41. Mizuno K, Kurita A, Imazeki N. Pathologic findings after percutaneous transluminal coronary angioplasty. *Br Heart J* 1984;**52**:588–90.

42. Potkin BN, Keren GN, Mintz GS *et al.* Arterial responses to balloon coronary angioplasty: an intravascular ultrasound study. *J Am Coll Cardiol* 1992;**20**:942–51.

43. Essed CE, van der Brand M, Becker AE. Transluminal coronary angioplasty and early restenosis: fibrocellular occlusion after wall laceration. *Br Heart J* 1983;**49**:393–6.

44. Fuster V, Erling F, Fallon JT, Badimon L, Chesebro JH, Badimon JJ. The three processes leading to post PTCA restenosis: dependence on the lesion substrate. *Thromb Haemostas* 1995;**74**:552–9.

45. Nobuyoshi M, Kimura T, Nosaka H *et al.* Restenosis after successful percutaneous transluminal coronary angioplasty: serial angiographic follow-up of 229 patients. *J Am Coll Cardiol* 1988;**12**:616–23.

46. Sanders M. Angiographic changes thirty minutes following percutaneous transluminal coronary angioplasty: serial angiographic follow-up of 229 patients. *Angiology* 1985;**36**:419–24.

47. Daniel WC, Pirwitz MJ, Willard JE *et al.* Incidence and treatment of elastic recoil occurring in the 15 minutes following successful percutaneous transluminal coronary angioplasty. *Am J Cardiol* 1996;**78**:253–9.

48. Fischell TA, Derby G, Tse TM, Stadius ML. Coronary artery vasoconstriction routinely occurs after percutaneous transluminal angioplasty. *Circulation* 1988;**78**:1323–34.

49. Mabin TA, Holmes DR, Smith HC *et al.* Intracoronary thrombus: role in coronary occlusion complicating percutaneous transluminal coronary angioplasty. *J Am Coll Cardiol* 1985;**5**:198–202.

50. Arora RR, Platko WP, Bhadwar K, Simpfendorfer C. Role of intracoronary thrombus in acute complications during percutaneous transluminal coronary angioplasty. *Cath Cardiovasc Diagn* 1989;**16**:226–9.

51. Rodriguez AE, Santaera O, Larribeau M, Sosa MI, Palacios IF. Early decrease in minimal luminal diameter after successful percutaneous transluminal angioplasty predicts late restenosis. *Am J Cardiol* 1993;**71**:1391–5.

52. Rodriguez AE, Santaera O, Larribeau M *et al.* Coronary stenting decreases restenosis in lesions with early loss in luminal diameter 24 hours after successful PTCA. *Circulation* 1995;**91**:1397–402.

53. Rupprecht HJ, Brennecke R, Bernhard G *et al.* Analysis of risk factors for restenosis after PTCA. *Cath Cardiovasc Diagn* 1990;**19**:151–9.

54. Guiteras V, Bourassa MG, David PR *et al.* Restenosis after percutaneous transluminal coronary angioplasty: the Montreal Heart Institute experience. *Am J Cardiol* 1987;**60**:50B.

55. Staudacher RA, Hess KR, Harris SL, Abu-Khalil J, Heibig J. Percutaneous transluminal coronary angioplasty utilizing prolonged balloon inflations: initial results and six-month follow-up. *Cath Cardiovasc Diagn* 1991;**23**:239–44.

56. Kaltenbach M, Beyer J, Walter S *et al.* Prolonged application of pressure in transluminal coronary angioplasty. *Cath Cardiovasc Diagn* 1984;**10**:213–19.

57. Douglas GS, King SBI, Roubin GS. Influence of methodology of percutaneous transluminal coronary angioplasty on restenosis. *Am J Cardiol* 1987;**60**:29B.

58. Rensing BJ, Hermans WR, Deckers JW, de Feyter PJ, Tijssen JG, Serruys PW. Lumen narrowing after percutaneous transluminal coronary balloon angioplasty follows a near gaussian distribution: a quantitative angiographic study in 1445 successfully dilated lesions. *J Am Coll Cardiol* 1992;**19**:939–45.

59. Meier B, Gruntzig AR, King SBI, Douglas GS, Hollman J, Ischinger T. Higher balloon dilatation pressure in coronary angioplasty. *Am Heart J* 1984;**107**:619–22.

60. Shaw RE, Myler RK, Fishman-Rosen J *et al.* Clinical and morphologic factors in prediction of restenosis after multiple vessel angioplasty. *J Am Coll Cardiol* 1986;**7**:63A.

61. Detre K, Holubkov R, Kelsey S *et al.* Percutaneous transluminal coronary angioplasty in 1985–1986 and 1977–1981; the NHLBI registry. *N Engl J Med* 1988;**318**:265.

62. Mata LA, Bosch X, David PR, Rapold HJ, Corcos T, Bourassa MG. Clinical and angiographic assessment 6 months after double vessel percutaneous coronary angioplasty. *J Am Coll Cardiol* 1985;**6**:1239–44.

63. Roubin GS, Douglas JSJ, King SBI *et al.* Influence of balloon size on initial success, acute complications and restenosis after percutaneous coronary angioplasty: a prospective randomized study. *Circulation* 1988;**78**:557–65.

64. Sangiorgi G, Nunez BD, Keelan E, Berger P, Schwartz RS, Holmes DRJ. Detailed restenosis angiographic analysis after "crackers, stretchers, drillers, shavers and burners". *J Invas Cardiol* 1995;**7**(Suppl. c): (Abstract).

65. Schatz RA, Penn IM, Baim DS *et al.* for the STRESS investigators. Stent Restenosis Study (STRESS): analysis of in-hospital results. *Circulation* 1993;**88**:I-594.

66. Serruys P, Macaya C, de Jaegere P *et al.* Interim analysis of the BENESTENT-trial. *Circulation* 1993;**88**:594.

67. Colombo A, Maiello L, Almagor Y *et al.* Coronary stenting: single institution experience with the initial 100 cases using the Palmaz–Schatz stent. *Cath Cardiovasc Diagn* 1992;**26**:171–6.

68. Colombo A, Hall P, Nakamura S. Intracoronary stenting without anti-coagulation accomplished with intravascular ultrasound guidance. *Circulation* 1995;**91**:1676–88.

69. Versaci F, Gaspardone A, Tomai F, Crea F, Chiariello L, Gioffre PA. A comparison of coronary stenting with angioplasty for isolated stenosis of the proximal left anterior descending coronary artery. *N Engl J Med* 1997;**336**:817–22.

70. Serruys PW, Emanuellsson H, van der Giessen W *et al.* Heparin-coated Palmaz–Schatz stents in human coronary arteries: early outcome of the Benestent-II Pilot Study. *Circulation* 1996;**93**:412–22.

71. Serruys PW, van Hout B, Bonnier H *et al.* Randomised comparison of implantation of heparin-coated stents with balloon angioplasty in selected patients with coronary artery disease (Benestent II). *Lancet* 1998;**352**:673–81.

72. van der Giessen WJ, van Beusekom HMM, Larsson R, Serruys PW. Heparin-coated coronary stents. *Curr Intervent Cardiol Rep* 1999;**1**:234–40.

73. Serruys PW, Kay IP *et al.* Benestent II, a remake of Benestent I? Or a step towards the era of stentoplasty? *Eur Heart J* 1999;**20**:779–81 (Hotline Editorial).

74. Vrolix MC, Legrand VM, Reiber JH *et al.* Heparin-coated Wiktor stents in human coronary arteries (MENTOR trial). *Am J Cardiol* 2000;**86**:385–9.

75. Tanaglia AN, Buller CE, Kisslo KB *et al.* Mechanisms of balloon angioplasty and directional atherectomy as assessed by intracoronary ultrasound. *J Am Coll Cardiol* 1992;**20**:685–91.

76. Kimball BP, Bui S, Cohen EA. Comparison of acute elastic recoil after directional coronary atherectomy vs standard balloon angioplasty. *Am Heart J* 1992;**124**:1459–66.

77. Elliot JM, Berdan LG, Homes DR *et al.* One year follow-up in the coronary angioplasty versus excisional atherectomy trial (CAVEAT I). *Circulation* 1995;**91**:2158–66.

78. Topol EJ, Leya F, Pinkerton CA *et al.* A comparison of patients with coronary artery disease. *N Engl J Med* 1993;**329**:221–7.

79. Adelman AG, Cohen EA, Kimball BP *et al.* A comparison of directional atherectomy with balloon angioplasty in the treatment of coronary artery disease for lesions of the left anterior descending arteries. *N Engl J Med* 1993;**329**:228–33.

80. Simonton CA, Leon MB, Baim DS *et al.* "Optimal" Directional Coronary Atherectomy. Final Results of the Optimal Atherectomy Restenosis Study (OARS). *Circulation* 1998;**97**:332–9.

81. Baim DS, Cutlip DE, Sharma SK *et al.* Final results of the Balloon vs Optimal Atherectomy Trial (BOAT). *Circulation* 1998;**97**:322–31.

82. Whitlow PL, Bass TA, Kipperman RM *et al.* Results of the Study to Determine Rotablator and Transluminal Angioplasty Strategy (STRATAS). *Am J Cardiol* 2001;**87**:699–705.

83. Uchida Y, Hasegawa K, Kawarmura K, Shibuya I. Angioscopic observation of the coronary luminal changes induced by percutaneous transluminal coronary angioplasty. *Am Heart J* 1989;**117**:769–76.

84. Miller DD, Boulet AJ, Tio FO *et al. In vivo* technetium-99 m S12 antibody imaging of platelet al.pha granules in rabbit endothelial neointimal proliferation after angioplasty. *Circulation* 1991;**83**:224–36.

85. den Heijer P, van Dijk RB, Hillege HL, Pentinga ML, Serruys PW, Lie KI. Serial angioscopic and angiographic observations during the first hour after successful coronary angioplasty: a preamble to a multicenter trial addressing angioscopic markers for restenosis. *Am Heart J* 1994;**128**:656–63.

86. Ip JH, Fuster V, Israel D, Badimon L, Badimon J, Chesebro JH. The role of platelets, thrombin and hyperplasia in

restenosis after coronary angioplasty. *J Am Coll Cardiol* 1991;**17**:77B–88B.

87. Weitz JI, Huboda M, Massel D, Maraganore J, Hirsh J. Clot-bound thrombin is protected from inhibition by heparin-antithrombin III but is susceptible to inactivation by antithrombin III-independent inhibitors. *J Clin Invest* 1990;**86**:385–91.

88. Bar-Shavit R, Eldor A, Vlodavsky I. Binding of thrombin to subendothelial extracellular matrix: protection and expression of functional properties. *J Clin Invest* 1989;**84**:1096–104.

89. Chronos NAF, Goodall AH, Wilson DJ, Sigwart U, Buller NP. Profound platelet degranulation is an important side effect of some type of contrast media used in interventional cardiology. *Circulation* 1993;**88**:2035–44.

90. Kolarov P, Tschoepe D, Nieuwenhuis HK, Gries FA, Strauer B, Schultheiss HP. PTCA: periprocedal platelet activation. Part II of the Dusseldorf PTCA Platelet Study (DPPS). *Eur Heart J* 1996;**17**:1216–22.

91. Fukami MH, Salganicoff L. Human platelet storage organelles. *Thromb Haemostas* 1977;**38**:963–70.

92. Holmsen H. Secretable storage pools in platelets. *Annu Rev Med* 1979;**30**:119–34.

93. Le Breton H, Plow EF, Topol EJ. Role of platelets in restenosis after percutaneous coronary revascularization. *J Am Coll Cardiol* 1996;**28**:1643–51.

94. Lindner V, Reidy MA. Expression of basic fibroblast growth factor and its receptor by smooth muscle cells and endothelium in injured rat arteries: an enface study. *Circ Res* 1993;**73**:589–95.

95. Shimokawa H, Ito A, Fukumoto Y *et al.* Chronic treatment with interleukin-1 induces coronary intimal lesions and vasospastic responses in pigs *in vivo. J Clin Invest* 1996;**97**:769–76.

96. Casscells W. Migration of smooth muscle and endothelial cells. Critical events in restenosis. *Circulation* 1992;**86**:723–9.

97. Rekhter MD, O'Brien E, Shah N, Schwartz SM, Simpson JB, Gordon D. The importance of thrombus organization and stellate cell phenotype in collagen I gene expression in human coronary atherosclerosis and restenotic lesions. *Cardiovasc Res* 1996;**32**:496–502.

98. Poole JCF, Cromwell SP, Benditt EP. Behavior of smooth muscle cells and formation of extracellular structures in the reaction of the arterial walls to injury. *Am J Pathol* 1971;**62**:391–413.

99. Jeong MH, Owen WG, Staab ME *et al.* Porcine model of stent thrombosis: platelets are the primary component of acute stent closure. *Cath Cardiovasc Diagn* 1996;**38**:38–43.

100. Plow EF, McEver RP, Coller SW *et al.* Related binding mechanisms for fibrinogen, fibronectin, von Willebrand factor and thrombospondin on thrombin-stimulated human platelets. *Blood* 1985;**66**:724–7.

101. Weiss HG, Hawiger J, Ruggeri ZW, Turitto VT, Thiagarajan P, Hoffmann T. Fibrinogen-independent platelet adhesion and thrombus formation on subendothelium mediated by glycoprotein IIb/IIIa complex at high share rate. *J Clin Invest* 1989;**83**:288–97.

102. Unterberg C, Sandrock D, Nebendhal K, Buchwald AB. Reduced acute thrombus formation results in decreased neointimal proliferation after coronary angioplasty. *J Am Coll Cardiol* 1995;**26**:1747–54.

103. Sugama Y, Malik A. Thrombin receptor 14-aminoacid peptide mediates endothelial hyperadhesivity and neutrophil adhesion by P-selectin-dependent mechanism. *Circ Res* 1992;**71**:1015–19.

104. Shi Y, Hutchinson HG, Hall DG, Zalewsky A. Downregulation of c-myc expression by antisense oligonuleotides inhibits proliferation of human smooth muscle cells. *Circulation* 1993;**88**:1190–95.

105. Moreno P, Falk E, Palacios I, Newell JB, Fuster V, Fallon JT. Macrophage infiltration in acute coronary syndromes: implications for plaque rupture. *Circulation* 1994;**90**:775–8.

106. Majesky MW, Reidy MA, Bowen-Pope DF, Hart CE, Wilcox JN, Schwartz SM. PDGF ligand and receptor genes expression during repair of arterial injury. *J Cell Biol* 1990;**111**:2149–58.

107. Nabel EG, Yang ZY, Plautz G, Forough R, Zhan X *et al.* Recombinant fibroblast growth factor-1 promotes intimal hyperplasia and angiogenesis in arteries *in vivo. Nature* 1993;**362**:844–6.

108. Lindner V, Reidy MA. Proliferation of smooth muscle cells after vascular injury is inhibited by an antibody against basic fibroblast growth factor. *Proc Natl Acad Sci USA* 1991;**88**:3739–43.

109. Chen JK, Hoshi H, McKeehan WL. Transforming growth factor type beta specifically stimulates synthesis of proteoglycan in human adult arterial smooth muscle cells. *Proc Natl Acad Sci USA* 1987;**84**:5287–91.

110. Nikol S, Weir L, Sullivan A, Sharaf B, White CJ *et al.* Persistently increased expression of the transforming growth factor beta 1 gene in human vascular restenosis: analysis of 62 patients with one or more episodes of restenosis. *Cardiovasc Pathol* 1992;**3**:57–62.

111. Nabel EG, Shum L, Pompili VJ *et al.* Direct transfer of transforming growth factor beta 1 into arteries stimulates fibrocellular hyperplasia. *Proc Natl Acad Sci USA* 1993;**90**:10759–763.

112. Shi Y, O'Brien J, Fard A, Zalewski A. Adventitial myofibroblasts contribute to neointimal formation following coronary arterial injury. *Circulation* 1995;**92**:I-34 (Abstract).

113. Shi Y, Pieniek M, Fard A, O'Brien J, Mannion JD, Zalewski A. Adventitial remodeling after coronary arterial injury. *Circulation* 1996;**93**:340–8.

114. Wilensky RL, March KL, Gradus-Pizlo I *et al.* Vascular injury, repair, and restenosis after percutaneous transluminal angioplasty in the atherosclerotic rabbit. *Circulation* 1995;**92**:2995–3005.

115. Rodgers GP, Minor ST, Robinson K *et al.* Adjuvant therapy for intracoronary stents. Investigation in atherosclerotic swine. *Circulation* 1990;**82**:560–9.

116. Whelan DM, van der Giessen WJ, Krabbendam SC *et al.* Biocompatibility of phosporylcholine coated stents in normal porcine coronary arteries. *Heart* 2000;**83**:338–45.

117. Kollum M, Kaiser S, Kinscherf R *et al.* Apoptosis after stent implantation compared with balloon angioplasty in rabbits: role of macrophages. *Arterioscler Thromb Vasc Biol* 1997;**17**:2383–88.

118. Karas SP, Gravanis MB, Santoian EC *et al.* Coronary intimal proliferation after balloon injury and stenting in swine: an animal model of restenosis. *J Am Coll Cardiol* 1992;**20**:467–74.

119. Farb A, Sangiorgi G, Carter AJ *et al.* Pathology of acute and chronic coronary stenting in humans. *Circulation* 1999;**99**:44–52.

120. Kornowski R, Hong MK, Tio FO *et al.* In-stent restenosis: contributions of inflammatory responses and arterial injury to neointimal hyperplasia. *J Am Coll Cardiol* 1998;**31**:224–30.

121. Tanigawa N, Sawada S, Kobajashi M. Reaction of the aortic wall to six metallic stent materials. *Acad Radiol* 1995;**2**:379–84.

122. Rogers C, Edelman E. Endovascular stent design dictates experimental restenosis and thrombosis. *Circulation* 1995;**91**:2995–3001.

123. Edelman E, Seifert P, Groothuis A *et al.* Gold-coated NIR stents in porcine coronary arteries. *Circulation* 2001;**103**:429–34.

124. McKenna CJ, Camrud A, Sangiorgi G *et al.* Fibrin-film stenting in porcine coronary injury model: efficacy and safety compared with uncoated stents. *J Am Coll Cardiol* 1998;**31**:1434–8.

125. Violaris AG, Melkert R, Hermann JPR, Serruys PW. Role of angiographically identifiable thrombus on long-term luminal renarrowing after coronary angioplasty: a quantitative angiographic analysis. *Circulation* 1996;**93**:889–97.

126. Schwartz RS, Holmes DRJ, Topol EJ. The restenosis paradigm revisited: an alternative proposal for cellular mechanisms. *J Am Coll Cardiol* 1992;**20**:1284–93.

127. Yamazaki M. Factor Xa inhibitors. *Drugs Future* 1995;**20**:911–18.

128. Schwartz RS, Holder DJ, Holmes DRJ *et al.* Neointimal thickening after severe coronary artery injury is limited by short-term administration of a factor Xa inhibitor: results in a porcine model. *Circulation* 1996;**94**:2998–3001.

129. Deutsch E, Rao AK, Colman RW. Selective thrombin inhibitors: the next generation of anticoagulants. *J Am Coll Cardiol* 1993;**22**:1089–92.

130. Fitzgerald GA, Meagher EA. Antiplatelets drugs. *Eur J Clin Invest* 1994;**24**:46–9.

131. Hillegas WB, Ohman EM, Califf RM. Restenosis: the clinical issues. In: Topol EJ ed. *Texbook of interventional cardiology*, 2nd edn. Philadelphia, PA: WB Saunders, 1994.

132. Schwartz L, Bourassa MG, Lesperance J *et al.* Aspirin and dipyridamole in the prevention of restenosis after percutaneous transluminal coronary angioplasty. *N Engl J Med* 1988;**318**:1714–19.

133. White C, Knudson M, Schmidt D. Neither ticlopidine nor aspirin-dipyridamole prevents restenosis post PTCA: results from a randomized placebo-controlled multicenter trial. *Circulation* 1987;**76**:IV-213 (Abstract).

134. Thomton MA, Gruentzig AR, Hollman J *et al.* Coumadin and aspirin in prevention of restenosis after transluminal coronary angioplasty: a randomized study. *Circulation* 1984;**69**:721–7.

135. Urban P, Buller N, Kox K, Shapiro L, Bayliss J, Richards A. Lack of effect of warfarin on the restenosis rate or on clinical outcome after balloon coronary angioplasty. *Br Heart J* 1988;**60**:485–8.

136. Bertrandt ME, Allain H, Lablanche JM. Results of a randomized trial of ticlopidine vs placebo for the prevention of acute closure and restenosis after coronary angioplasty: the TACT study. *Circulation* 1990;**82**:190 (Abstract).

137. Serruys PW, Rutsch W, Heyndrickx GR *et al.* Prevention of restenosis after percutaneous transluminal coronary angioplasty with thromboxane A2-receptor blockade. A randomized, double-blind, placebo-controlled trial. Coronary Artery Restenosis Prevention on Repeated Thromboxane-Antagonism Study (CARPORT). *Circulation* 1991;**84**:1568–80.

138. Feldman RL, Bengston JR, Pryor DB, Zimmerman MB, from the GRASP Study Group. Use of a thromboxane A_2 receptor blockers to reduce adverse clinical events after coronary angioplasty. *J Am Coll Cardiol* 1992;**19**:259A.

139. Bove A, Savage M, Deutsch E *et al.* Effects of selective and non-selective thromboxane A2 blockade on restenosis after PTCA: M-Heart II. *J Am Coll Cardiol* 1992;**19**:259A (Abstract).

140. Knudtson ML, Flintoft VF, Roth DL, Hansen JL, Duff HJ. Effect of short-term prostacyclin administration on restenosis after percutaneous transluminal coronary angioplasty. *J Am Coll Cardiol* 1990;**15**:691–7.

141. Raitzner AE, Holman J, Abukhalil J, Demke D. Ciprostene for restenosis revisited: quantitative analysis of angiograms. *J Am Coll Cardiol* 1993;**21**:321A (Abstract).

142. Ellis SG, Roubin GS, Wilentz J, Douglas JSJ, King SB. Effect of 18- to 24-hour heparin administration for prevention of restenosis after uncomplicated coronary angioplasty. *Am Heart J* 1989;**117**:777–82.

143. Ellis S, Roubin G, Wilentz J *et al.* Results of a randomized trial of heparin and aspirin vs. aspirin alone for prevention of acute closure (AC) and restenosis (R) after angioplasty (PTCA). *Circulation* 1987;**76**:213 (Abstract).

144. Dryski M, Mikat E, Bjornsson TD. Inhibition of intimal hyperplasia after arterial injury by heparins and heparinoids. *J Vasc Surg* 1988;**8**:623–33.

145. Lehmann KG, Doria RJ, Feuer JM *et al.* Paradoxical increase in restenosis rate with chronic heparin use, final results of randomized trials. *J Am Coll Cardiol* 1991;**17**:181A (Abstract).

146. Currier JW, Pow TK, Haudenschild CC, Minihan AC, Faxon DP. Low molecular weight heparin (Enoxaparin) reduces restenosis after iliac angioplasty in the hypercholesterolemic rabbit. *J Am Coll Cardiol* 1991;**17**:118B–25B.

147. Faxon D, Spiro T, Minor S *et al.* Low molecular weight heparin in the prevention of restenosis after angioplasty: results of enoxaparin restenosis (ERA) trial. *Circulation* 1994;**90**:908–14.

148. Topol EJ, Bonar R, Jewitt D *et al.* Use of a direct antithrombin, hirulog, in place of heparin during coronary angioplasty. *Circulation* 1993;**87**:1622–9.

149. Serruys PW, Herrman JR, Simon R *et al.* Investigators for the HELVETICA. A comparison of hirudin with heparin in the prevention of restenosis after coronary angioplasty. *N Engl J Med* 1995;**333**:757–63.

150. Heras M, Chesebro JH, Penny WJ, Bailey KR, Badimon L, Fuster V. Effects of thrombin inhibition on the development of acute platelet-thrombus deposition during angioplasty in pigs. Heparin versus recombinant hirudin, a specific thrombin inhibitor. *Circulation* 1989;**79**:657–65.

151. van den Boss AA, Deckers JW, Heyndrickx GR *et al.* Safety and efficacy of recombinant hirudin (CGP 39393) vs heparin in

patients with stable angina undergoing coronary angioplasty. *Circulation* 1993;**88**:2058–66.

152. Thorwest M, Balling E, Kristensen SD *et al.* Dietary fish oil reduces microvascular thrombosis in a porcine experimental model. *Thromb Res* 2000;**99**:203–8.

153. Baumann KH, Hessel F, Larass I *et al.* Dietary omega-3, omega-6, and omega-9 unsaturated fatty acid and growth factor and cytokine gene expression in unstimulated and stimulated monocytes. A randomized volunteer study. *Arterioscler Thromb Vasc Biol* 1999;**19**:59–66.

154. Kuiper KK, Muna ZA, Erga KS, Dyroy E *et al.* Tetra-decylthioacetic acid reduces stenosis development after balloon angioplasty injury of rabbit iliac arteries. *Atherosclerosis* 2001;**158**:269–75.

155. Cairns JA, Gill J, Morton B *et al.*, for the EMPAR collaborators. Fish oils and low- molecular- weight heparin for the reduction of restenosis after percutaneous transluminal coronary angioplasty. The EMPAR study. *Circulation* 1996;**94**:1153–60.

156. Leaf A, Jorgensen MB, Jacobs AK *et al.* Do fish oils prevent restenosis after coronary angioplasty? *Circulation* 1994;**90**:2248–57.

157. Matsuno H, Stassen JM, Vermylen J, Deckmyn H. Inhibition of integrin function by a cyclic RGD-containing peptide prevents neointimal formation. *Circulation* 1994;**90**:2203–6.

158. Choi ET, Engel L, Callow AD, Sun S, Trachtenberg J, Santoro S, Ryan US. Inhibition of neointimal hyperplasia by blocking $\alpha_v\beta_3$ integrin with a small peptide antagonist GpenGRGDSPCA. *J Vasc Surg* 1994;**19**:125–34.

159. The EPIC investigators. Use of monoclonal antibody direct against the platelet glycoprotein IIa/IIIb receptor in high risk coronary angioplasty. *N Engl J Med* 1994;**14**:956–61.

160. Lincoff AM, Tcheng JE, Ellis SG *et al.* IMPACT-II investigators. Randomized trials of platelet glycoprotein IIb/IIIa inhibition with Integrelin for prevention of restenosis following coronary interventions: the IMPACT-II angiographic substudy. *Circulation* 1995;**92**:I-607.

161. Tcheng JE, Harrington RA, Kottke-Marchant K *et al.* Multicenter, randomized, double-blind placebo-controlled trial of the platelet integrin glycoprotein IIb/IIIa inhibition blocker integrelin in elective coronary intervention. *Circulation* 1995;**91**:2151–7.

162. Tcheng JE. Glycoprotein IIb/IIIa receptor inhibitors: putting the EPIC, IMPACT II, RESTORE and EPILOG trials into perspective. *Am J Cardiol* 1996;**78**:35–40.

163. van der Werf F. More evidence for a beneficial effect of platelet glycoprotein IIb/IIIa – blockade during coronary interventions: latest results from the EPILOG and CAPTURE trials. *Eur Heart J* 1996;**17**:325–6 (Editorial).

164. Ferguson J Jr. EPILOG and CAPTURE trials halted because of positive interim results. *Circulation* 1996;**93**:637 (news).

165. Topol EJ, Mark DB, Lincoff AM *et al.* Outcomes at 1 year and economic implications of platelet glycoprotein IIb/IIIa blockade in patients undergoing coronary stenting: results from a multicenter randomized trial. *Lancet* 1999;**354**: 2019–24.

166. Cura FA, Deepak LB, Lincoff AM, Kapadia SR *et al.* Pronounced benefit of coronary stenting and adjunctive platelet glycoprotein IIb/IIIa inhibition in complex atherosclerotic lesions. *Circulation* 2000;**102**:28–34.

167. EPISTENT Investigators. Randomised placebo-controlled and balloon-angioplasty-controlled trial to assess safety of coronary stenting with use of platelet glycoprotein IIb/IIIa blockade: evaluation of Platelet IIb/IIIa Inhibitor for Stenting. *Lancet* 1998;**352**:87–92.

168. Aggarwal RK, Ireland DC, Azrin MA *et al.* Antithrombotic potential of polymer-coated stents eluting platelet glycoprotein IIb/IIIa receptor antibody. *Circulation* 1996;**94**: 3311–17.

169. Alt E, Haehnel I, Beilharz C *et al.* Inhibition of neointima formation after experimental coronary artery stenting: a new biodegradable stent coating releasing hirudin and the prostacyclin analogue Iloprost. *Circulation* 2000;**101**:1453–8.

170. Manka D, Collins RG, Ley K *et al.* Absence of P-selectin but not intercellular adhesion molecule-1, attenuates neointimal growth after arterial injury in apolipoprotein E-deficient mouse. *Circulation* 2001;**103**:1000–5.

171. Inoue T, Sakai Y, Morooka S *et al.* Expression of polymorphonuclear leukocyte adhesion molecules and its clinical significance in patients treated with percutaneous transluminal coronary angioplasty. *J Am Coll Cardiol* 1996;**28**: 1127–33.

172. Mickelson JK, Lakkis NM, Villareal-Levy G *et al.* Leukocyte activation with platelet adhesion after coronary angioplasty: a mechanism for recurrent disease? *J Am Coll Cardiol* 1996;**28**:345–53.

173. Rogers C, Edelman ER, Simon DI. A mAb to the beta2-leukocyte integrin Mac-1 (CD11/CD18) reduces intimal thickening after angioplasty or stent implantation in rabbits. *Proc Natl Acad Sci USA* 1998;**95**:10134–9.

174. Feldman LJ, Aguirre L, Ziol M *et al.* Interleukin-10 inhibits intimal hyperplasia after angioplasty or stent implantation in hypercholesterolemic rabbits. *Circulation* 2000;**101**:908–16.

175. Strecker EP, Gabelmann A, Boos I *et al.* Effect of intimal hyperplasia of dexamethasone released from coated metal stents compared with non-coated stents in canine femoral arteries. *Cardiovasc Intervent Radiol* 1998;**21**:487–96.

176. Holmes DRJ, Fitzgerald P, Goldberg S *et al.* Prevention of Restenosis with Tranilast and its Outcome (PRESTO) protocol: a double-blind, placebo-controlled trial. *Am Heart J* 2000;**139**:23–31.

177. Ueda M, Becker AE, Tsukada T, Numano F, Fujimoto T. Fibrocellular tissue response after percutaneous transluminal coronary angioplasty. An immunocytochemical analysis of the cellular composition. *Circulation* 1991;**83**:1327–32.

178. Nobuyoshi M, Kimura T, Ohishi H *et al.* Morphologic studies: restenosis after percutaneous transluminal coronary angioplasty: pathologic observations in 20 patients. *J Am Coll Cardiol* 1991;**17**:433–9.

179. Garratt KN, Edwards WD, Kaufmann UP, Vlietstra RE, Holmes DR. Differential histopathology of primary atherosclerotic and restenotic lesion in coronary arteries and saphenous vein bypass grafts: analysis of tissue obtained from 73 patients by directional atherectomy. *J Am Coll Cardiol* 1991;**17**: 442–8.

180. van Beusekom H, van der Giessen W, van Suylen R, Bos E, Bosman FT, Serruys PW. Histology after stenting of human saphenous vein bypass grafts: observations from surgically excised grafts 3 to 320 days after stent implantation. *J Am Coll Cardiol* 1993;**21**:45–54.

181.Clowes A, Clowes M, Fingerle J, Reidy M. Kinetics of cellular proliferation after arterial injury V. Role of acute distension in the induction of smooth muscle proliferation. *Lab Invest* 1989;**49**:360–4.

182.Clowes AW, Schwartz SN. Significance of quiescent smooth muscle cell migration in the injured rat carotid artery. *Circ Res* 1985;**56**:139–45.

183.Forrester JS, Fishbein M, Helfant R, Fagin J. A paradigm of restenosis based on cell biology: clues for the development of new preventive therapies. *J Am Coll Cardiol* 1991;**17**:758–69.

184.Clowes AW, Reidy MA, Clowes MM. Kinetics of cellular proliferation after arterial injury. I. Smooth muscle growth in the absence of endothelium. *Lab Invest* 1983;**49**:327–33.

185.Clowes AW, Clowes MM, Fingerle J, Reidy MA. Kinetics of cellular proliferation after arterial injury. V. Role of acute distension in the induction of smooth muscle proliferation. *Lab Invest* 1989;**60**:360–4.

186.Clowes A, Clowes M, Reidy M. Kinetics of cellular proliferation after arterial injury: endothelial and smooth muscle growth in chronically denuded vessels. *Lab Invest* 1986; **54**:295–303.

187.Thayer JM, Giachelli PM, Mirkes PE, Schartz SM. Expression of osteopontin in the head process late in gastrulation in the rat. *J Exp Zool* 1995;**272**:240–4.

188.Liaw L, Lombardi DM, Almeida MM, Schwartz SM. Neutralizing antibodies direct against osteopontin inhibit rat carotid neointimal thickening following endothelial denudation. *Arterioscler Thromb Vasc Biol* 1997;**17**:188–93.

189.Weber GF, Ashkar S, Glimcher MJ, Cantor H. Receptor-ligand interaction between CD44 and osteopontin (Eta-1). *Science* 1996;**271**:509–12.

190.Jain M, He Q, Lee WS *et al.* Role of CD44 in the reaction of vascular smooth muscle cells to arterial wall injury. *J Clin Invest* 1996;**97**:596–603.

191.Bendeck M, Zempo N, Clowes A, Galardy R, Reidy M. Smooth muscle cell migration and matrix metalloproteinase expression after injury in the rat. *Circulation Res* 1994;**75**: 539–45.

192.Schwartz SM. Smooth muscle migration in atherosclerosis and restenosis. *J Clin Invest* 1997;**99**:2814–17.

193.Bendeck MP, Irvin C, Reidy MA. Inhibition of matrix metalloproteinase activity inhibits smooth muscle cell migration but not neointimal thickening after arterial injury. *Circ Res* 1996;**78**:38–43.

194.Ruoslahti E. Integrins. *J Clin Invest* 1991;**87**:1–5.

195.Hynes RO. Integrins: versatility, modulation, and signalling in cell adhesion. *Cell* 1992;**69**:11–25.

196.Samanen J, Ali FE, Romoff T *et al.* Development of a small RGD-peptide fibrinogen receptor antagonist with potent anti-aggregatory activity *in vitro. J Med Chem* 1991;**34**: 3114–125.

197.Douglas S, Ohlstein E. Endothelin-1 promotes neointima formation after balloon angioplasty in the rat. *J Cardiovasc Pharmacol* 1993;**22**(Suppl. 8):S371–3.

198.Helset E, Sildnes T, Seljelid R, Konoski ZS. Endothelin-1 stimulates human monocytes in vitro to release TNFα, IL-1β and IL-6. *Mediat Inflamm* 1993;**2**:417.

199.Scott-Burden T, Resink TJ, Hahn AWA, Vanhoutte PM. Induction of endothelin secretion by angiotensin II: effects on growth and synthetic activity of vascular smooth muscle cells. *J Cardiovasc Pharmacol* 1991;**17**:S96.

200.Wang X, Douglas SA, Louden C, Vickery-Clark LM, Feuerstein GZ, Ohlstein EH. Expression of endothelin-1, endothelin-3, endothelin-converting-enzyme-1, endothelin-A and endothelin-B receptor mRNA following angioplasty-induced neointima formation in the rat. *Circ Res* 1996;**78**: 322–8.

201.Tsjuno M, Hirata Y, Eguchi S, Watanabe T, Chatani F, Marumoi F. Nonselective ETA/ETB receptor antagonist blocks proliferation of rat vascular smooth muscle cells after balloon angioplasty. *Life Sci* 1995;**56**:PL449.

202.Wessale J, Adler A, Novosad E, Burke S, Dayton B, Opgenorth T. Endothelin antagonism reduces neointima formed following balloon injury in rabbit. In: *Fourth International Conference on Endothelin.* London, UK, 1995:153.

203.Ferns GA, Raines EW, Sprugel KH, Motani AS, Reidy MA, Ross R. Inhibition of neointimal smooth muscle accumulation after angioplasty by an antibody to PDGF. *Science* 1991;**253**:1129–32.

204.Clowes AW, Clowes MM, Fingerle J, Reidy MA. Regulation of smooth muscle cell growth in injured artery. *J Cardiovasc Pharmacol* 1989;**14**:S12–15.

205.Nabel EG, Yang Z, Plautz *et al.* rFGF-1 gene expression in porcine arteries induces intimal hyperplasia and angiogenesis *in vivo. Nature* 1993;**362**:844–6.

206.Nabel EG, Liptay S, Yang *et al.* r-PDGF gene expression in porcine arteries induces intimal hyperplasia *in vivo. J Clin Invest* 1993;**91**.

207.Scott-Burden T, Vanhoutte PM. Regulation of smooth muscle cell growth by endothelium-derived growth factors. *Text Heart Inst J* 1993;**21**:91–7.

208.Kindy MS, Sonenshein GE. Regulation of oncogene expression in cultured aortic smooth muscle cells: post-transcriptional control of c-myc m-RNA. *J Biol Chem* 1986;**261**: 12865–8.

209.Simons M, Edelman ER, DeKeyser JL, Langer R, Rosenberg RD. Antisense c-myb oligonucleotides inhibit intimal arterial smooth muscle cell accumulation *in vivo. Nature* 1992; **359**:67–70.

210.Campan M, Desgranges C, Gadeau AP, Millet D, Belloc F. Cell cycle dependent gene expression in quiescent stimulated and asynchronously cycling arterial smooth muscle cells in culture. *J Cell Physiol* 1992;**150**:493.

211.Chang MW, Barr E, Lu MM, Barton K, Leiden JM. Adenovirus-mediated over-expression of the cyclin/cyclin-dependent kinase inhibitor, p21 inhibits vascular smooth muscle cell proliferation and neointima formation in the rat carotid artery model of balloon angioplasty. *J Clin Invest* 1995;**96**:2260–8.

212.Paranandi SN, Topol EJ. Contemporary clinical trials of restenosis. *J Invas Cardiol* 1994;**6**:109–24.

213.Dangas G, Fuster V. Management of restenosis after clinical intervention. *Am Heart J* 1996;**132**:428–36.

214.Berk BC, Gordon JB, Alexander RW. Pharmacologic roles of heparin and glucocorticoids to prevent restenosis after coronary angioplasty. *J Am Coll Cardiol* 1991;**17**:111B–17B.

215.Longenecker JP, Kilty LA, Johnson LK. Glucocorticoid inhibition of vascular smooth muscle cells proliferation: influence of homologous extracellular matrix and serum mitogens. *J Cell Biol* 1984;**98**:534–40.

216. Longeneker JP, Kilty LA, Johnson LK. Glucocorticoid influence on growth of vascular cells in culture. *J Cell Physiol* 1982;**113**:197–202.

217. Stone GW, Rutherford BD, McConahay DR *et al.* A randomized trial of corticosteroids for the prevention of restenosis in 102 patients undergoing repeat coronary angioplasty. *Cath Cardiovasc Diagn* 1989;**18**:227–31.

218. Pepine CJ, Hirshfield JW, MacDonald RG *et al.* A controlled trial of corticosteroids to prevent restenosis after coronary angioplasty. M-HEART Group. *Circulation* 1990;**81**:1753–61.

219. Villa AE, Guzman LA, Chen W, Golomb G, Levy RJ, Topol EJ. Local delivery of dexamethasone for prevention of neointimal proliferation in a rat model of balloon angioplasty. *J Clin Invest* 1994;**93**:1243–9.

220. Voisard R, Dartsch PC, Seitzer U *et al.* The in-vitro effect of antineoplastic agents on proliferative activity and cytoskeletal components of plaque-derived smooth muscle cells from human coronary arteries. *Coronary Artery Dis* 1993;**4**:935–42.

221. Sollott SJ, Cheng L, Pauly RR *et al.* Taxol inhibits neointimal smooth muscle cell accumulation after angioplasty in the rat. *J Clin Invest* 1995;**95**:1869–76.

222. Murphy JG, Schwartz RS, Edwards WD *et al.* Methotrexate and azathioprine fail to inhibit porcine coronary restenosis. *Circulation* 1990;**82**:III-429.

223. Cox DA, Anderson PG, Roubin GS, Chou C-Y, Agrawal SK, Cavender C. Effect of local delivery of heparin and methotrexate on neointimal proliferation in stented porcine coronary arteries. *Coronary Artery Dis* 1992;**3**:237–48.

224. Mullett DW, Topol EJ, Abrams GD, Gallagher KP, Ellis SG. Intramural metrotrexate therapy for the prevention of the neointimal thickening after balloon angioplasty. *J Am Coll Cardiol* 1992;**20**:460–6.

225. Muller D, Ellis S, Topol E. Colchicine and antineoplastic therapy for the prevention of restenosis after percutaneous coronary interventions. *J Am Coll Cardiol* 1991;**17**:126B–31B.

226. O'Keefe J, McCallister B, Bateman T, Kuhnlein D, Ligon R, Hartzler G. Colchicine for the prevention of restenosis after coronary angioplasty. *J Am Coll Cardiol* 1991;**17**:181A (Abstract).

227. Grines CL, Rizik D, Levine A *et al.* Colchicine angioplasty restenosis trial (CART). *Circulation* 1991;**84**:II-365 (Abstract).

228. Wolinsky H, Thung SN. Use of perforated balloon catheter to deliver concentrated heparin into the wall of the normal canine artery. *J Am Coll Cardiol* 1990;**15**:475–81.

229. Santoian EC, Gravanis MB, Schneider JE *et al.* Use of the porous balloon in porcine coronary arteries: rationale for low pressure and volume delivery. *Cath Cardiovasc Diagn* 1993;**31**:240–5.

230. Murphy JG, Schwartz RS, Edwards WD, Camrud AR, Vlietstra RE, Holmes DR Jr. Percutaneous polymeric stents in porcine coronary arteries. Initial experience with polyethylene terephthalate stents. *Circulation* 1992;**86**:1596–604.

231. van der Giessen WJ, Slager CJ, van Beusekom HMM *et al.* Development of a polymer endovascular prosthesis and its implantation in porcine arteries. *J Interv Cardiol* 1992;**5**:175–85.

232. Bier JD, Zalesky P, Li ST *et al.* A new bioabsorbable intravascular stent: *in vitro* assessment of hemodynamic and morphometric characteristics. *J Interv Cardiol* 1992;**5**:187–94.

233. Riessen R, Isner JM. Prospects for site-specific delivery of pharmacologic and molecular therapies. *J Am Coll Cardiol* 1994;**23**:1234–44.

234. Powell JS, Clozel JP, Muller RK *et al.* Inhibitors of angiotensin-converting enzyme prevent myointimal proliferation after vascular injury. *Science* 1989;**245**:186–8.

235. Huber KC, Schwartz RS, Edwards WD, Camrud AR, Bailey K. Effects of angiotensin converting enzyme inhibition on neointimal hyperplasia in a porcine coronary injury model. *Am Heart J* 1993;**125**:695–701.

236. Janiak P, Libert O, Vilaine JP. The role of the renin-angiotensin system in neointima formation after injury in rabbits. *Hypertension* 1994;**24**:671–8.

237. The Multicenter European Research Trial with Cilazapril After Angioplasty to Prevent Transluminal Coronary Obstruction and Restenosis (MERCATOR) Study Group. Does the new angiotensin converting enzyme inhibitor cilazapril prevent restenosis after percutaneous transluminal coronary angioplasty? Results of the MERCATOR Study. *Circulation* 1992;**86**:100–10.

238. Faxon DP, on behalf of the MARCATOR investigators. Angiotensin converting enzyme inhibition and restenosis: the final results of the MARCATOR trial. *Circulation* 1992;**88**:506 (Abstract).

239. Rogler G, Lacknet KJ, Schmitz G. Effects of fluvastatin on growth of porcine and human vascular smooth muscle cells in vitro. *Am J Cardiol* 1995;**76**:114A–6A.

240. Gellman J, Ezekowitz MD, Sarembock IJ *et al.* Effect of lovastatin on intimal hyperplasia after balloon angioplasty: a study in an atherosclerotic hypercholesterolemic rabbit. *J Am Coll Cardiol* 1991;**17**:251–9.

241. Weintraub WS, Boccuzzi SJ, Klein JL *et al.* Lack of effect of lovastatin on restenosis after coronary angioplasty: lovastatin restenosis trial study group. *N Engl J Med* 1994;**331**:1331–7.

242. Lafont AM, Chai Y-C, Cornhill JF, Whitlow PL, Howe PH, Chisolm GM. Effect of alpha-tocopherol on restenosis after angioplasty in a model of experimental atherosclerosis. *J Clin Invest* 1995;**95**:1108–25.

243. Schneider JE, Berk BC, Gravanis MB *et al.* Probucol decreases neointimal formation in a swine model of coronary artery balloon injury. *Circulation* 1993;**88**:628–37.

244. Watanabe K, Sekiya S, Miyagawa M, Hashida K. Preventive effects of probucol on restenosis after percutaneous transluminal coronary angioplasty. *Am Heart J* 1996;**132**:23–9.

245. Haehnel I, Pfeifer U, Resch A *et al.* Differential effect of a local paclitaxel release from a biodegradable stent coating on vascular smooth muscle cells and endothelial cells in a co-culture model (Abstract). *J Am Coll Cardiol* 1999;**33**(Suppl. A):1011–24.

246. Farb A, Heller PF, Shroff S, Cheng L *et al.* Pathological analysis of local drug delivery of paclitaxel via a polymer-coated stent. *Circulation* 2001;**104**:473–9.

247. Herdeg C, Oberhoff M, Baumbach A *et al.* Local paclitaxel delivery for the prevention of restenosis: biological effects and efficacy *in vivo. J Am Coll Cardiol* 2000;**35**:1969–76.

248. Santoian ED, Schneider JE, Gravanis MB *et al.* Angiopeptin inhibits intimal hyperplasia after angioplasty in porcine coronary arteries. *Circulation* 1993;**88**:11–14.

249. Emanuelsson H, Beatt KJ, Bagger JP *et al.* Long-term effects of angiopeptin treatment in coronary angioplasty: Reduction of clincial events but not angiographic restenosis. *Circulation* 1995;**91**:1689–96.

250. De Scheerder I, Wilczek K, van Dorpe J *et al.* Local angiopeptin delivery using coated stents reduces neointimal proliferation in overstretched porcine coronary arteries. *J Invas Cardiol* 1996;**8**:215–22.

251. Armstrong J, Gunn J, Holt CM *et al.* Local angiopeptin delivery from coronary stents in porcine coronary arteries (Abstract). *Eur Heart J* 1999;**20**(Suppl.):366.

252. Morice MC, Serruys PW, Sousa JE *et al.* A randomized comparison of a sirolimus-eluting stent with a standard stent for coronary revascularization. *N Engl J Med.* 2002;**346**:1773–80.

253. Sousa JE, Costa MA, Abizaid A *et al.* Sustained suppression of neointimal proliferation by sirolimus eluting stents: one year angiographic follow-up and intravascular ultrasound follow-up. *Circulation* 2001;**104**:2007–11.

254. Gallo R, Padurean A, Jayaraman T *et al.* Inhibition of intimal thickening after balloon angioplasty in porcine coronary arteries by targeting regulators of the cell cycle. *Circulation* 1999;**99**:2164–70.

255. Schwartz RS, Koval TM, Edwards WD *et al.* Effect of external beam irradiation on neointimal hyperplasia after experimental coronary artery injury. *J Am Coll Cardiol* 1992;**19**:1106–13.

256. Waksman R, Robinson KA, Crocker IR *et al.* Intracoronary low-dose beta-irradiation inhibits neointima formation after coronary artery balloon injury in the swine restenosis model. *Circulation* 1995;**92**:3025–31.

257. Wiedermann JG, Marboe C, Amols H, Schwartz A, Weinberger J. Intracoronary irradiation markedly reduces restenosis after balloon angioplasty in a porcine model. *J Am Coll Cardiol* 1994;**23**:1491–8.

258. Wiedermann JG, Marboe C, Amols H, Schwartz A, Weinberger J. Intracoronary irradiation markedly reduces neointimal proliferation after balloon angioplasty in swine: persistent benefit at 6-month follow-up. *J Am Coll Cardiol* 1995;**25**:1451–6.

259. Waksman R, Robinson KA, Crocker IR, Gravanis MB, Cipolla GD, King SB. Endovascular low-dose irradiation inhibits neointima formation after coronary artery balloon injury in swine. A possible role for radiation therapy in restenosis prevention. *Circulation* 1995;**91**:1533–9.

260. Verin V, Popowski Y, Urban P *et al.* Intra-arterial beta irradiation prevents neointimal hyperplasia in a hypercholesterolemic rabbit restenosis model. *Circulation* 1995;**92**: 2284–90.

261. Liermann D, Boettcher HD, Schopohl B *et al.* Is there a method to prevent intimal hyperplasia after stent implantation in peripheral vessels? *Angiology* 1992;**92**:269–70.

262. Condado JA, Waksman R, Gurdiel O *et al.* Long-term angiographic and clinical outcome after percutaneous transluminal coronary angioplasty and intracoronary radiation in humans. *Circulation* 1997;**96**:727–32.

263. Teirstein PS, Masullo V, Jani S *et al.* Catheter-based radiotherapy to inhibit restenosis after coronary stenting. *N Engl J Med* 1997;**336**:1697–703.

264. Hall EJ, Millers RC, Bvenner DJ. The basic radiobiology of intravascular irradiation. In: Waksman R, ed. *Vascular brachytherapy.* Armonk NY: Futura Publishing Co, Inc, 1999.

265. Sangiorgi G, Kline RW, Bonner JA *et al.* 17 kilovolt beta-radiation induce apoptosis following experimental balloon angioplasty: results in a tissue culture model. In: *Restenosis summit IX*; 1997.

266. Popowski Y, Verin V, Papirov I *et al.* High dose rate brachytherapy for prevention of restenosis after percutaneous transluminal coronary angioplasty: preliminary dosimetric tests of a new source presentation. *Int J Radiat Oncol Biol Phys* 1995;**33**:211–15.

267. Condado JA, Gurdiel O, Espinoza R *et al.* Percutaneous transluminal coronary angioplasty (PTCA) and intracoronary radiation therapy (IRT): a possible new modality for treatment of coronary restenosis. A preliminary report of the first 10 patients treated with intracoronary radiation therapy. *J Am Coll Cardiol* 1995;**38**:228A (Abstract).

268. Liermann D, Bottcher HD, Kollath J *et al.* Prophylactic endovascular radiotherapy to prevent intimal hyperplasia after stent implantation in femoropopliteal arteries. *Cardiovasc Intervent Radiol* 1994;**17**:12–16.

269. Bottcher HD, Schopohl B, Liermann D, Kollath J, Adamietz IA. Endovascular irradiation – a new method to avoid recurrent stenosis after stent implantation in peripheral arteries: technique and preliminary results. *Int J Radiat Oncol Biol Phys* 1994;**29**:183–6.

270. Salame MY, Verheye S, Croker IR *et al.* Intracoronary radiation therapy. *Eur Heart J* 2001;**22**:629–47.

271. Teirstein PS, Massullo V, Jani S *et al.* Two-year follow-up after catheter-based radiotherapy to inhibit coronary restenosis. *Circulation* 1999;**99**:243–7.

272. Leon MB, Tierstein PS, Moses JW. Localized intracoronary gamma-radiation therapy to inhibit the occurrence of restenosis after stenting. *N Engl J Med* 2001;**344**:250–6.

273. Albiero R, Di Mrio C, De Gregorio J. Intravascular ultrasound (IVUS) analysis of beta-particle emitting radioactive stent implantation in human coronary arteries. Preliminary immediate and intermediate-term results of the MILAN study (Abstract). *Circulation* 1998;**98**:I-780.

274. Grant MB, Wargovich TJ, Ellis EA, Caballero S, Mansour M, Pepine CJ. Localization of insulin growth factor I and inhibition of coronary smooth muscle cell growth by somatostatin analogues in human coronary smooth muscle cells: a potential treatment for restenosis? *Circulation* 1994;**89**:1511–17.

275. Lundergan CF, Foegh ML, Ramwell PW. Peptide inhibition of myointimal proliferaion by angiopeptin, a somatostatin analogue. *J Am Coll Cardiol* 1991;**17**:132B–136B.

276. Santoian EC, Schneider JE, Gravanis MB *et al.* Angiopeptin inhibits intimal hyperplasia after angioplasty in porcine coronary arteries. *Circulation* 1993;**88**:11–14.

277. Kent KM, Williams DO, Cassagneau B *et al.* Double blind, controlled trial of the effect of angiopeptin on coronary restenosis following balloon angioplasty. *Circulation* 1993; **88**:506 (Abstract).

278. Eriksen UH, Amtorp, Bagger JP *et al.* Angiopeptin Study Group. Continuous angiopeptin infusion reduces coronary restenosis following coronary angioplasty. *Circulation* 1993;**88**:594 (Abstract).

279. Emanuelsson H, Beatt KJ, Bagger JP *et al.* Long-term effect of angiopeptin treatment in coronary angioplasty: reduction of clinical events but not angiographic restenosis. *Circulation* 1995;**91**:1689–96.

280. Liu MW, Roubin GS, Robinson KA *et al.* Trapidil in preventing restenosis after balloon angioplasty in the atherosclerotic rabbit. *Circulation* 1990;**81**:1089–93.

281. Maresta A, Balducelli M, Cantini L *et al.* Trapidil (triazolopyrimidine), a platelet-derived growth factor antagonist, reduces restenosis after percutaneous transluminal coronary angioplasty: results of the randomized, double-blind STARC study. *Circulation* 1994;**90**:2710–15.

282. Serruys PW, Banz K, Darcis T *et al.* Results of a meta-analysis of trapidil, a PDGF inhibitor. A sufficient reason for a second look at the pharmacologic approach to restenosis. *J Invas Cardiol* 1997;**9**:505–12.

283. Galassi AR, Tamburino C, Nicosia A *et al.* A randomized comparison of trapidil (triazolopyrimidine), a platelet-derived growth factor antagonist, versus aspirin in prevention of angiographic restenosis after coronary artery Palmaz–Schatz stent implantation. *Cath Cardiovasc Interv* 1999;**46**:162–8.

284. Ohno T, Gordon D, San H, Pompili VJ, Imperiale MJ, Nabel GJ, Nabel EG. Gene therapy for vascular smooth muscle cell proliferation after arterial injury. *Science* 1994;**265**:781–4.

285. Chapman G, Lim CS, Gammon RS *et al.* Gene transfer into coronary arteries of intact animals with a percutaneous balloon catheter. *Circ Res* 1992;**71**:27–33.

286. Morishita R, Gibbons GH, Kaneda Y, Ogihara T, Dzau VJ. Novel *in vitro* gene transfer method for study of local modulators in vascular smooth muscle cells. *Hypertension* 1993;**21**:894–9.

287. Mazur W, Ali NM, Geske RS *et al.* Lipofectin-mediated versus adenovirus-mediated gene transfer in vitro and *in vivo*: comparison of canine and porcine models systems. *Coronary Artery Dis* 1994;**5**:779–86.

288. Kahn ML, Lee SW, Dichek D. Optimization of retroviral vector-mediated gene transfer into endothelial cells in vitro. *Circ Res* 1992;**71**:1508–17.

289. French BA, Mazur W, Ali NM *et al.* Percutaneous transluminal *in vivo* gene transfer by recombinant adenovirus in normal porcine coronary arteries, atherosclerotic arteries, and two models of coronary restenosis. *Circulation* 1994;**90**:2402–13.

290. Epstein S, Siegall C, Biro S, Fu Y, Fitzgerald D, Pastan I. Cytotoxic effects of a recombinant chimeric toxin on rapidly proliferating vascular smooth muscle cells. *Circulation* 1991;**84**:778–87.

291. Pickering G, Weir L, Jekanowski J, Isner J. Inhibition of proliferation of human vascular smooth muscle cells using antisense oligonucleotides to PCNA. *J Am Coll Cardiol* 1992;**19**:165A (Abstract).

292. Pickering JC, Bacha P, Weir L, Jekanowski J, Nichols JC, Isner JM. Prevention of smooth muscle cells outgrowth from human atherosclerotic plaque by a recombinant cytotoxin specific for epidermal growth factor receptor. *J Clin Invest* 1993;**91**:724–9.

293. Biro S, Siegall CB, Fu YM, Speir E, Pastan I, Epstein SE. *In vitro* effects of a recombinant toxin targeted to the fibroblast growth factor receptor on rat vascular smooth muscle and endothelial cells. *Circ Res* 1992;**71**:640–5.

294. Casscells W, Lappi DA, Olwin BB *et al.* Elimination of smooth muscle cells in experimental restenosis: targeting of fibroblast growth factor receptors. *Proc Natl Acad Sci USA* 1992;**89**:7159–63.

295. Chang MW, Barr E, Seltzer J *et al.* Cytostatic gene therapy for vascular proliferative disorders with a constitutively active form of the retinoblastoma gene product. *Science* 1995;**267**:518–22.

296. von der Leyen H, Gibbons G, Morishita R *et al.* Gene therapy inhibiting neointimal vascular lesion: *in vivo* transfer of endothelial cell nitric oxide synthase gene. *Proc Natl Acad Sci USA* 1995;**92**:1137–41.

297. Nabel EG, Plautz G, Boyce FM, Stanley JC, Nabel GJ. Recombinant gene expression *in vivo* within endothelial cells on the arterial wall. *Science* 1989;**244**:1342–4.

298. Thompson MM, Budd JS, Eady SL *et al.* Endothelial cell seeding of damaged native vascular surfaces: prostacycline production. *Eur J Vasc Surg* 1992;**6**:487–93.

299. Thompson MM, Budd JS, Eady SL, James RFL, Bell PRF. A method to transluminal seed angioplasty sites with endothelial cells using a double balloon catheter. *Eur J Vasc Surg* 1993;**7**:113–21.

300. Baker JE, Nikolaychick V, Sahota H *et al.* Reconstruction of balloon injured artery with fibrin glue/endothelial cell matrix. *Circulation* 1994;**90**:1–492.

301. Ortu P, LaMuraglia GM, Roberts G, Flotte TJ, Hasan T. Photodynamic therapy of arteries. A novel approach for treatment of experimental intimal hyperplasia. *Circulation* 1992;**85**:1189–96.

302. Eton D, Borhani M, Spero K, Cvaa RA, Grossweiner L, Ahn SS. Photodynamic therapy. Cytotoxicity of aluminium phthalocyanin on intimal hyperplasia: acute and chronic. *J Vasc Surg* 1995;**19**:321–9.

303. Lamuraglia GM, Chandraekar NR, Flotte TJ, Abbott WM, Michaud N, Hasan T. Photodynamic therapy inhibition of experimental intimal hyperplasia: acute and chronic effects. *J Vasc Surg* 1994;**19**:321–9.

304. Tang G, Hyman S, Schneider JH, Giannotta SL. Application of photodynamic therapy to the treatment of atherosclerotic plaques. *Neurosurgery* 1993;**32**:438–43.

305. Mann GV, Spoerry A, Gray M, Jarashow D. Atherosclerosis in the Masai. *Am J Epidemiol* 1972;**95**:26–37.

306. Glagov S, Weisenberg E, Zarins CK, Stankunavicius R, Kolettis GJ. Compensatory enlargement of human atherosclerotic coronary arteries. *N Engl J Med* 1987;**316**:1371–5.

307. Schwartz RS, Topol EJ, Serruys PW, Sangiorgi G, Holmes DR. Artery size, neointima, and remodeling: time for some standards (Editorial). *J Am Coll Cardiol* 1998;**32**:2087–94.

308. Kamiya A, Togawa T. Adaptative regulation of wall shear stress to flow change in the canine carotid artery. *Am J Physiol* 1980;**239**:H14–H21.

309. Zarins CK, Weisenberg E, Kolettis G, Stankunavicius R, Glagov S. Differential enlargement of artery segments in response to enlarging atherosclerosis plaques. *J Vasc Surg* 1988;**7**:386–94.

310. Langille BL, Bendeck MP, Keeley FW. Adaptations of carotid arteries of young and mature rabbits to reduced carotid blood flow. *Am J Physiol* 1989;**256**:H931–H9.

311. Langille BL. Remodeling of developing and mature arteries: endothelium, smooth muscle, and matrix. *J Cardiovasc Pharmacol* 1993;**21**:S11–S17.

312. Clarkson TB, Prichard RS, Morgan TM, Petrick GS, Klein KP. Remodeling of coronary arteries in human and nonhuman primates. *JAMA* 1994;**271**:289–94.

313. Zarins CK, Lu CT, Gewertz BL, Lyon RT, Rush DS, Glagov S. Arterial disruption and remodeling following balloon dilatation. *Surgery* 1982;**92**:1086–95.

314. Kakuta T, Currier JW, Haudenschild CC, Ryan TJ, Faxon DP. Differences in compensatory vessel enlargement, not intimal formation, account for restenosis after angioplasty in the hypercholesterolemic rabbit model. *Circulation* 1994;**89**:2809–15.

315. Kakuta T, Currier JW, Horten K, Faxon DP. Failure of compensatory enlargement, not neointimal formation, accounts for lumen narrowing after angioplasty in the atherosclerotic rabbit. *Circulation* 1993;**88**:I-619 (Abstract).

316. Pasterkamp G, Wensing PJW, Post MJ, Hillen B, Mali WPTM, Borst C. Paradoxical arterial wall shrinkage may contribute to luminal narrowing of human atherosclerotic femoral arteries. *Circulation* 1995;**91**:1444–9.

317. Pasterkamp G, Borst C, Gussenhoven EJ *et al.* Remodeling of *de novo* atherosclerotic lesions in femoral arteries: impact on mechanism of balloon angioplasty. *J Am Coll Cardiol* 1995;**26**:422–8.

318. Kovach JA, Mintz GS, Kent KM *et al.* Serial intravascular ultrasound studies indicate that chronic recoil is an important mechanism of restenosis following transcatheter therapy. *J Am Coll Cardiol* 1993;**21**:484A (Abstract).

319. Mintz GS, Kenneth MK, Pichard AD, Satler LF, Popma JJ, Leon MB. Contribution of inadequate arterial remodeling to the development of focal coronary artery stenoses: an intravascular ultrasound study. *Circulation* 1997;**95**:1791–8.

320. Kimura T, Kaburagi S, Tashima Y, Nobuyoshi M, Mintz GS, Popma J. Geometric remodeling and intimal regrowth as mechanisms of restenosis: observations from serial ultrasound analysis of restenosis (SURE) trial. *Circulation* 1995;**92**:I-76 (Abstract).

321. Libby P, Schwartz D, Brogi E, Tanaka H, Clinton SK. A cascade model for restenosis. A special case of atherosclerosis progression. *Circulation* 1992;**86**(Suppl. III):III-47–III-52.

322. Gibbons GH, Dzau VJ. The emerging concept of vascular remodeling. *N Engl J Med* 1994;**330**:1431–8.

323. Isner JM. Vascular remodeling: honey, I think I shrunk the artery. *Circulation* 1994;**89**:2937–41 (Editorial).

324. Mogford JE, Davies GE, Platts SH, Meininger GA. Vascular smooth muscle alpha(v)beta(3) integrin mediates arteriolar vasodilatation in response to RGD peptides. *Circ Res* 1996;**79**:821–6.

325. Lafont A, Guzman LA, Whitlow PL, Goormastic M, Cornhill JF, Chisolm GM. Restenosis after experimental angioplasty. Intimal, medial, and adventitial changes associated with constrictive remodeling. *Circ Res* 1995;**76**:996–1002.

326. Staab ME, Srivatsa SS, Lerman A *et al.* Arterial remodeling after percutaneous injury is highly dependent on adventitial injury histopathology. *Int J Cardiol* 1997;**58**:31–40.

327. Shi Y, Pieniek M, Fard A, O'Brien J, Mannion JD, Zalewski A. Adventitial remodeling after coronary arterial injury. *Circulation* 1996;**93**:340–8.

328. Sangiorgi G, Taylor AJ, Farb A *et al.* Histopathology of post-percutaneous transluminal coronary angioplasty remodeling in human coronary arteries. *Am Heart J* 1999;**138**:681–7.

329. Kuntz LL, Anderson PG, Schroff RW, Roubin GS. Sustained dilatation and inhibition of restenosis in pig femoral artery injury model. *Circulation* 1994;**90**:I-197 (Abstract).

Part IIIb

Specific cardiovascular disorders: Acute ischemic syndromes and acute myocardial infarction

John A Cairns and Bernard J Gersh, Editors

Grading of recommendations and levels of evidence used in *Evidence-based Cardiology*

GRADE A

Level 1a   Evidence from large randomized clinical trials (RCTs) or systematic reviews (including meta-analyses) of multiple randomized trials which collectively has at least as much data as one single well-defined trial.

Level 1b   Evidence from at least one "All or None" high quality cohort study; in which ALL patients died/failed with conventional therapy and some survived/succeeded with the new therapy (for example, chemotherapy for tuberculosis, meningitis, or defibrillation for ventricular fibrillation); or in which many died/failed with conventional therapy and NONE died/failed with the new therapy (for example, penicillin for pneumococcal infections).

Level 1c   Evidence from at least one moderate-sized RCT or a meta-analysis of small trials which collectively only has a moderate number of patients.

Level 1d   Evidence from at least one RCT.

GRADE B

Level 2   Evidence from at least one high quality study of non-randomized cohorts who did and did not receive the new therapy.

Level 3   Evidence from at least one high quality case–control study.

Level 4   Evidence from at least one high quality case series.

GRADE C

Level 5   Opinions from experts without reference or access to any of the foregoing (for example, argument from physiology, bench research or first principles).

A comprehensive approach would incorporate many different types of evidence (for example, RCTs, non-RCTs, epidemiologic studies, and experimental data), and examine the architecture of the information for consistency, coherence and clarity. Occasionally the evidence does not completely fit into neat compartments. For example, there may not be an RCT that demonstrates a reduction in mortality in individuals with stable angina with the use of β blockers, but there is overwhelming evidence that mortality is reduced following MI. In such cases, some may recommend use of β blockers in angina patients with the expectation that some extrapolation from post-MI trials is warranted. This could be expressed as Grade A/C. In other instances (for example, smoking cessation or a pacemaker for complete heart block), the non-randomized data are so overwhelmingly clear and biologically plausible that it would be reasonable to consider these interventions as Grade A.

Recommendation grades appear either within the text, for example, **Grade A** and **Grade A1a** or within a table in the chapter.

The grading system clearly is only applicable to preventive or therapeutic interventions. It is not applicable to many other types of data such as descriptive, genetic or pathophysiologic.

30 Acute non-ST-segment elevation coronary syndromes: unstable angina and non-ST-segment elevation myocardial infarction

Pierre Theroux, John A Cairns

Introduction and historical perspective

The definition of acute myocardial ischemic syndromes as well as their management has dramatically changed over the past two decades. Not long ago, clinical acute myocardial ischemia was classified as stable angina, Q and non-Q wave myocardial infarction, and unstable angina. The latter encompassed all the highly heterogeneous manifestations of ischemia intermediate between stable angina and myocardial infarction. Fowler proposed the terminology of unstable angina in 1971,[1] following half a century of retrospective observations on the premonitory symptoms of myocardial infarction and of prospective studies of the clinical outcomes. The importance of risk stratification became recognized, at that time focusing on ischemic chest pain patterns and on ST-T abnormalities. A variety of interventions were also attempted to interrupt the disease process and prevent death or myocardial infarction. One of these studies by Wood was prematurely interrupted because of the observation of a greater efficacy of oral anticoagulants versus no anticoagulants observed in a few patients.[2] The term "acute coronary syndromes" was introduced in 1985 by Fuster to highlight the specific pathophysiologic mechanisms that distinguish unstable angina and myocardial infarction from stable coronary artery disease.[3] Pathologic studies by Michael J Davies[4,5] and by Erling Falk[6,7] had then documented the presence of intracoronary thrombus on a ruptured plaque in 95% of patients with unstable angina suffering sudden cardiac death. Thrombi of various ages were described.[6] They could be at multiple sites, typically occurring on lesions of only moderate severity, and were often associated with platelet aggregates in small intramyocardial arteries and microscopic foci of necrosis.[4,5] DeWood documented that an occlusive thrombus was consistently present in angiograms obtained very early after the onset of myocardial infarction.[8] The analyses of angiograms in unstable angina then shifted from descriptions of the severity and extent of atherosclerosis, which could not distinguish unstable angina from stable angina, to morphologic descriptions of the culprit lesion. Complex plaques with fissures and ruptures and partially occlusive thrombi were identified and confirmed by angioscopic studies. The concept of the active vulnerable plaque was established, opening a new era of advances in cell biology and clinical investigation. The science was advanced and oriented by clinical trials that reached a level of unprecedented sophistication, providing the setting for the current evidence-based approach to clinical medicine.

New dimensions and definitions

Unstable angina has achieved the maturity of a syndrome with a well-defined spectrum of clinical manifestations, epidemiology and prognosis, pathophysiology, and options for effective treatment. Delineation of the syndrome has led to unique research opportunities for better understanding of atherosclerosis and mechanisms of plaque activation, and potential patient management. The definition has evolved to become practical by incorporating algorithms for rapid diagnosis, risk stratification, patient orientation, and therapy.

The diagnosis of an acute coronary syndrome implies recognition of a change in the pattern of ischemic chest pain – or equivalent symptoms – to more severe, in the absence of evidence of an extracoronary cause for the increased severity. Thus, the diagnosis of an acute coronary syndrome is first clinical. Current nomenclature has been developed to provide clinicians with a logical framework within which to categorize patients who present with a constellation of clinical symptoms that are compatible with acute myocardial ischemia, and to guide early diagnosis and management. The nomenclature is also helpful for ensuring consistency in clinical trials and in epidemiologic studies. Hence, the acute coronary syndromes are considered to encompass unstable angina, non-ST-segment elevation (non-Q wave) myocardial infarction (NSTEMI), and ST-segment elevation (Q wave) myocardial infarction (STEMI). The designation of possible acute coronary syndrome (ACS) is useful when patients first present, at a point where there is uncertainty about the likelihood of the presence of myocardial ischemia. As ECGs are done and biochemical cardiac markers are assessed over the next few hours, the patient may eventually be characterized as having unstable angina, non-Q wave MI or Q wave MI. Unstable angina has been traditionally classified as new onset angina, increasing angina, rest angina, and recurrent ischemia after myocardial infarction (Table 30.1).[9] Braunwald classified unstable angina by severity of symptoms and clinical circumstances (Table 30.2).[10] Details of timing and duration of pain have been included in these classifications to optimize their specificity. Thus, classification as new onset angina and increasing angina requires a component of severity, and rest pain a component of duration.

The clinical management first requires a search for ST-segment elevation, the presence of which or a new left bundle branch block, mandates consideration for immediate reperfusion therapy.[10] In the absence of ST-segment elevation, the working diagnosis is non-ST-segment elevation acute coronary syndrome.[11] Table 30.1 summarizes the clinical manifestations, Table 30.2 the Braunwald classification, and Figure 30.1 an early and highly practical diagnostic scheme. Most ST-segment elevation will evolve to a Q wave myocardial infarction. Most non-ST-segment elevation ACS will eventually be diagnosed as unstable angina or non-ST-segment elevation MI according to the absence or presence of an elevation of the various markers of cell necrosis. Accordingly, all patients with suspect symptoms should be evaluated clinically and should have a 12-lead ECG as soon as possible – immediately if ischemic pain is present. The availability of troponin T and troponin I has increased the sensitivity of the diagnosis of myocardial infarction and has sharpened the distinction between unstable angina and myocardial infarction.[12] The troponins are highly sensitive and specific markers of cell damage and permit the diagnosis of cell necrosis and myocardial infarction in up to 30% of patients who would otherwise be diagnosed as having unstable angina based on normal CK-MB blood values.[13]

The new insights into disease have modified previous statistics on the incidence and prognosis of unstable angina versus myocardial infarction. Thus myocardial infarction is more frequently diagnosed with the use of the troponins. However, the non-ST-segment elevation MI is often small, does not affect ejection fraction, and is considered and managed more like unstable angina. Epidemiological data may include ST- and non-ST-segment elevation MI in a single category, whereas clinical data reflect on one hand STEMI and, on the other, unstable angina and NSTEMI.

Table 30.1   Clinical presentation of ACS

Rest angina	Angina occurring at rest and prolonged, usually >20 minutes
New onset angina	New onset angina of at least CCS class III severity
Increasing angina	Angina that has become distinctly more frequent, longer in duration, or lower in threshold (that is, increased by greater than or equal to 1 CCS class to at least CCS class III severity)
Early post-MI ischemia	Ischemic chest pain recurrent within 30 days after MI

Source: adapted from Braunwald *et al*[24]

Table 30.2   Braunwald classification of unstable angina

	Clinical circumstances		
Severity	A: Develops in presence of extracardiac condition that intensifies myocardial ischemia (secondary unstable angina)	B: Develops in absence of extracardiac condition (primary unstable angina)	C: Develops within 2 weeks after acute myocardial infarction (postinfarction unstable angina)
New onset of severe angina or accelerated angina: no rest pain	IA	IB	IC
Angina at rest within past month but not within preceding 48 h (angina at rest, subacute)	IIA	IIB	IIC
Angina at rest within 48 h (angina at rest, acute)	IIIA	IIIB	IIIC

Source: reproduced with permission from Braunwald[10]

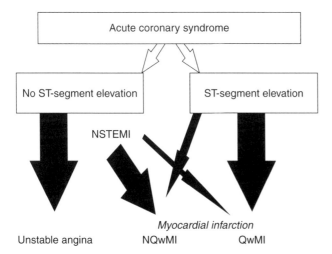

Figure 30.1 Nomenclature of acute coronary syndromes (ACS). The spectrum of clinical conditions that range from unstable angina to non-Q wave AMI and Q wave AMI is referred to as acute coronary syndrome. Patients with ischemic discomfort may present with or without ST-segment elevation on the ECG. Most patients who present with non-ST-segment elevation ACS will eventually be classified as having unstable angina or non-Q wave MI. The distinction between these two diagnoses is ultimately made based on the presence or absence of a cardiac marker detected in the blood. Only a minority of patients with non-ST-elevation MI will develop Q wave MI. Most patients with ST-segment elevation will evolve to develop Q wave MI. Adapted with permission from Antman and Braunwald.[11]

Incidence and prognosis

It is estimated that the number of consultations for chest pain in emergency departments in the USA approximates 5 500 000 yearly.[14] In the 1990s, hospital discharges for unstable angina exceeded 700 000 annually, about equal to those for MI, one third of which were of the non-Q wave type.[15,16] In 1996, a total of nearly 1 500 000 patients were hospitalized for unstable angina or NSTEMI, exceeding the number of hospitalizations for STEMI.

There is evidence that the incidence of acute coronary syndromes defined as unstable angina and non-ST-segment elevation has been increasing, whereas that of ST-segment elevation MI has been decreasing. Epidemiologic data using the WHO MONICA criteria for the diagnosis of Q wave myocardial infarction from Halifax county (Canada),[17] Turku (Finland), Oxfordshire (England),[18] Denmark,[19] the Netherlands,[20] France, and northern Italy showed that the mortality rates from Q wave MI have decreased by more than 30% between 1975 and 1995, two thirds of the decline being attributable to reduced incidence and one third to decreased hospital mortality. These decreases were observed in women as well as men.

On the other hand, the number of patients hospitalized for a non-ST-segment ACS exceeds that of ST-segment elevation MI and statistics suggest that the magnitude of the excess is increasing. In the ENACT registry of 3092 patients from 29 European countries performed in the mid-1990s, the admission diagnosis was unstable angina/NSTEMI in 46%, myocardial infarction in 39%, and a suspected ACS in 14% (ratio 1·2:1) and is similar across Europe.[21] The Global Registry of Acute Coronary Events (GRACE) extended the data collection to 10 693 patients recruited between 1999 and 2001 from North and South America, Australia, New Zealand, and Europe. Two thirds of admitted patients had unstable angina/non-ST-segment elevation ACS, and one third STEMI.[22]

A large epidemiologic study of 5 832 residents from metropolitan Worcester, Massachusetts has shown that the incidence of Q wave MI progressively decreased between 1975/78 (incidence rate = 171/100 000 population) and 1997 (101/100 000 population).[23] By contrast, the incidence of non-Q wave MI has progressively increased during the same period (62/100 000 population in 1975/78 and 131/100 000 population in 1997). While the hospital mortality of Q wave MI has progressively declined from 24% in 1975/78 to 14% in 1997, that of non-Q MI has remained constant at 12%. These trends persisted after adjusting for potentially confounding prognostic factors. Therefore, despite impressive declines in the incidence of Q wave MI and the inhospital and long-term mortality, the incidence of non-Q wave MI has been increasing with unchanged mortality rates compared to about 22 years ago.

The shifts in the clinical manifestations of acute coronary syndromes correspond to changes in patterns of practice and referral in accordance with the emphasis on primary and secondary prevention and earlier intervention. Public education programs may also favor early diagnosis, referral, and treatment. Figure 30.2 describes the distribution of admission diagnoses in the Coronary Care Unit of the Montreal Heart Institute, a referral center, over the past decade. There is a major shift in the distribution of admissions from STEMI to non-ST-segment elevation ACS, as well as an increase in the total number of admissions.

Natural history

Patients admitted for an ACS experience 10 times more events in the short term than patients with stable angina and several-fold more than individuals with high cholesterol values and no known coronary disease. The natural history of unstable angina/NSTEMI is determined by the severity and extent of coronary artery disease, the presence of comorbid conditions, age, and the ischemic pain pattern which may range from the simple onset of new angina, to profound and prolonged episodes of angina at rest,

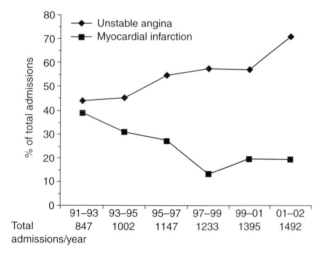

Total admissions/year: 91–93 847, 93–95 1002, 95–97 1147, 97–99 1233, 99–01 1395, 01–02 1492

Figure 30.2 This figure describes the distribution of admission diagnosis in the Coronary Care Unit of the Montreal Heart Institute, a referral center, over the past decade. The total number of patients admitted through the past decade has nearly doubled. A major shift has occurred, however, in the distribution of ST-segment elevation versus non-ST-segment elevation ACS. Patients with a non-ST-segment elevation ACS now represent more than two thirds of patients admitted in the CCU, while the incidence of ST-segment elevation MI has decreased from 40% to 20% of admissions. This phenomenon is observed in most hospitals in industrialized countries.

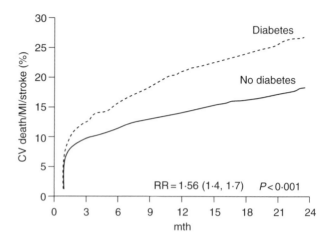

Figure 30.3 Kaplan-Meier event curves for diabetic and non-diabetic patients for total cardiovascular death, MI, stroke, and new onset of congestive heart failure for a 24 month follow up period after an episode of non-ST-segment elevation ACS. Data from the OASIS Registry study reproduced with permission from Malmberg *et al.*[25]

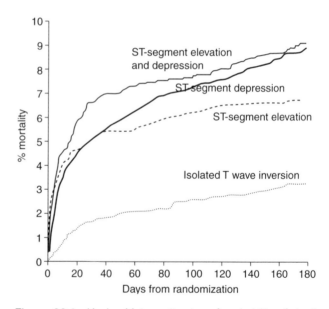

Figure 30.4 Kaplan-Meier estimates of probability of death at 6 months by ECG changes at admission. The event rate was highest inhospital in patients with ST-segment elevation MI. However, by 6 months, mortality in patients with ST depression exceeded that of patients with ST elevation. Data from the GUSTO-II study, reproduced with permission from Savonitto *et al.*[26]

accompanied by LV dysfunction and resistance to medical therapy.[24] The risk of the disease is highest in the first few days, decreases over the following weeks and months, and eventually becomes similar to the prognosis of patients with stable angina. The long-term prognosis is influenced by the severity of the underlying disease. In the OASIS registry, the incidence of events was 10% at one month and increased steadily in the following 2 years to reach more than 20% after 24 months (Figure 30.3), higher in diabetic patients and in patients with previously known coronary artery disease.[25] In the GUSTO-II study, the inhospital mortality rate was highest, as expected, in patients with STEMI; however, increasing mortality during follow up in patients with ST-segment depression eventually exceeded that of patients with ST elevation after 6 months, reaching 8·7% as against 6·8% (Figure 30.4).[26] The empirical concept that NSTEMI represents an unresolved acute coronary syndrome at risk of being completed by a recurrent MI may therefore be partially true in many patients, and is likely explained by an underlying disease process that remains active. This is supported by data showing that markers of inflammation and of activation of coagulation may remain elevated months past the acute phase of an episode of acute coronary syndrome.[27,28] It is difficult to evaluate the effect of advances in treatment on the natural history of unstable angina/NSTEMI, since the

diagnostic criteria have evolved concurrently. Recent randomized trials have shown an impressive decrease in MI and death. Prior to the routine prescription of bed rest, nitrates and β blockers for unstable angina, the rate of MI after one month was in the range of 40% and of death, 25%.[29] By the 1970s these rates had fallen to about 10%

and 2%. In 1979–80, a study of all patients hospitalized with unstable angina in Hamilton, Canada over a period of one year noted inhospital and 1 year mortalities of 1·5% and 9·2% respectively.[30] By the time of the re-evaluation of heparin in the late 1980s, study inclusion criteria had shifted toward patients at somewhat higher risk, and some trials included patients with NSTEMI. In these trials, the rates of the composite outcome of death or non-fatal myocardial infarction by 5 days were about 10%.[31,32] These rates fell to the range of 4% with the addition of heparin to aspirin, and fell further with enoxaparin and the glycoprotein IIb/IIIa antagonists. The event rates at 30 days in recent trials with new antithrombotic therapies and an invasive management strategy are shown in Figure 30.5.[33–44]

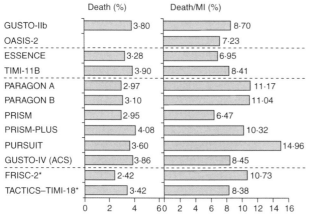

*Invasive management trials, 6 month follow up

Figure 30.5 Rates of death and of death or myocardial infarction in contemporary trials that evaluated new antithrombotic drugs and routine invasive treatment strategy in patients with non-ST-segment ACS. Data are the average of events in the intervention and control groups. The interventions resulted in a reduction in rates of death ranging from −5% to 36% and in rates of death or myocardial infarction ranging from −8% to 27%.[33–44]

Risk stratification

A gradient in risk exists in ACS from relatively benign to severe; accordingly, patient management should be guided by clinical risk stratification. The high-risk features for death and ischemic events present at admission, or developing rapidly, have been identified in many registries and clinical trials. Registry studies look at a broad spectrum of patients with acute chest pain, while clinical trials enroll more selected populations predefined by entry criteria in a specific study. Recent registries have focused mainly on regional differences in application of drug therapy and interventional procedures,[21,22,25] whereas trials have evaluated specific predictors, biased by entry criteria of the trials. Nevertheless, important common determinants of risk have been identified by the two approaches. These include older age, presence of ST-segment shifts, elevation of the cardiac markers, and recurrent ischemia (Table 30.3). Ejection fraction is not available in the majority of patients but is known to be a potent predictor of prognosis in all manifestations of coronary artery disease. Cardiac risk factors are in general poor predictors of acute risk in patients with an ACS but are useful for the evaluation of the likelihood of coronary artery disease and its prognosis.[45] The rate of the progression of the severity of chest pain is clinically recognized as suggesting a more rapidly evolving coronary stenosis. There is a gradient in risk from new onset, to crescendo, to prolonged rest angina.[9] Women and the elderly are more likely to have atypical presentations. The prognosis for patients who have atypical symptoms at the time of their infarction can be worse than that of patients with more typical symptoms.[46] Women enrolled in clinical trials are in general older than men and have more risk factors such as diabetes and hypertension. The proportion of women with ST-segment elevation is less than in men but their prognosis is then worse. Women who present with a non-ST-segment elevation acute syndrome less often have an elevation of the cardiac markers and have a better prognosis. The odds for infarction and death in the GUSTO-IIb study in women compared to men was 0·65 (95% CI 0·49–0·87; $P = 0.003$),[47] and in the non-invasive strategy arm of the FRISC-II study 0·64 (95% CI 0·43–0·97; $P = 0.03$).[48] Coronary angiography in general revealed less severe coronary artery disease for women than for men.[48] Diabetes is present in 20–25% of patients

Table 30.3 Determinants of prognosis

Determinants of short-term prognosis

Confirming the diagnosis of ACS	Clinical pattern of pain
	ST-T ischemic changes
	Troponin T or I elevation
	Hemodynamic or electrical instability
Other major determinants	Older age
	Left ventricular dysfunction
	Recent myocardial infarction
	Recurrent ischemia
	Diabetes
	Previous myocardial infarction
	Previous CABG
	Previous aspirin use
	Depression

Determinants of long-term prognosis

	Left ventricular dysfunction
	Diabetes
	Extensive coronary artery disease
	Strongly positive provocative testing
	Elevated CRP levels
	Depression

enrolled in trials in ACS. Diabetes carries a major negative impact on morbidity and mortality in the setting of ACS and after percutaneous interventions and coronary artery bypass grafting. In the OASIS registry, diabetes was an important and independent predictor of 2 year mortality (RR 1·57; 95% CI 1·38–1·81; $P < 0.001$), as well as of cardiovascular death, new myocardial infarction, stroke, and new congestive heart failure.[25] The risk of death in diabetic women was significantly higher than the risk in diabetic men (RR 1·98 and 1·28 respectively). Diabetic patients without prior cardiovascular disease had the same event rates for all outcomes as non-diabetic patients with previous vascular disease (see Figure 30.3). The impact of depression on prognosis is more and more recognized. In a study of 430 patients with a non-ST-segment elevation ACS, depression predicted the end point of cardiac death or non-fatal MI, with an adjusted odds ratio of 6·73 (95% CI 2·43–18·64; $P < 0.001$) after controlling for other significant prognostic factors that included baseline ECG, left ventricular ejection fraction, and number of diseased coronary vessels.[49]

The 12-lead ECG and the troponin T or I blood levels have become powerful instruments for risk evaluation. They are now part of the entry criteria in clinical trials and of recommended treatment algorithms. Troponin elevation in the blood follows the ischemic insult by 6 hours, as does CK-MB. Myoglobin serum concentration rises earlier, within 2 hours after the onset of pain, and peaks within 4–6 hours. Myoglobin can be useful as an early and sensitive marker of necrosis, but it is non-specific, mandating confirmation of the cardiac origin with the CK-MB or troponin levels. Although failure to detect a rise of myoglobin after 2–4 hours rules out an infarction, the prognostic value with regard to recurrent coronary events in patients with non-ST-segment elevation ACS has been less well characterized.

The presence of ST-segment shifts and/or the elevation in troponin T or I levels confirm the working diagnosis of a non-ST-segment elevation ACS, identify the patient at high risk for an ischemic event, and are useful for immediate patient orientation and management by identifying those who will benefit most from the new treatment strategies that include enoxaparin, the Gp IIb/IIIa antagonists and revascularization procedures. The absence of such changes does not rule out the diagnosis, but places the patient in a more favorable risk category. Patients with an indefinite but possible diagnosis of an ACS need to be observed for the clinical evolution, changes on serial ECGs, and elevation of troponin levels after 8–12 hours.

Prognostic value of troponin levels

In contrast to CK-MB and myoglobin, cardiac troponins T and I are usually not detectable in the peripheral blood and, thus, provide a more distinct and sensitive marker of minute

cardiomyocyte damage. The damage detected is usually of ischemic origin but may be due to non-ischemic myocardial injury, such as myocarditis, severe heart failure, pulmonary embolism, trauma or cardiotoxic agents. Multiple studies since the original publication by Hamm *et al* have validated the prognostic value of an elevation in the blood troponin levels.[50]

Figure 30.6 depicts the results of one trial of patients enrolled in a clinical trial[18] and of one study of patients consulting in the emergency department for acute chest pain;[18] the 30 day rate of death or myocardial infarction was highest in patients with elevated troponin T or troponin I levels, intermediate in patients with ST-segment depression, and lowest in patients with normal troponin levels. The higher the elevation in troponin levels,[51] the worse the prognosis, but even small elevations are associated with a significantly impaired prognosis.[52] In the FRISC study, among patients with a non-ST-segment elevation ACS, the risk of myocardial infarction or cardiac death at 6 months was respectively 4·3%, 10·5%, and 16·1% in patients within the first, second, and third tertile of maximal elevation of troponin during the first 24 hours.[53]

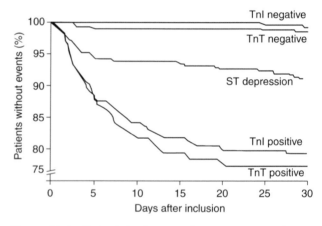

Figure 30.6 Risk of death or non-fatal myocardial infarction during 30 days of follow up by troponin T (TnT) and I (TnI) levels, elevation (positive) or no elevation (negative), and ST-segment depression on the ECG. The risk for myocardial infarction and death increases with increasing serum troponin concentrations and may be 20% in 30 days and 25% within 6 months in patients with the highest troponin levels. Reproduced with permission from Hamm *et al*.[13]

Three meta-analyses were performed and provided results in the same direction. The first, including 12 reports with troponin T and nine with troponin I of patients with unstable angina, demonstrated risk ratios for occurrence of myocardial infarction at 30 days of 4·2 (95% CI 2·7–6·4; $P < 0.001$) for troponin I and of 2·7 (95% CI 2·1–3·4; $P < 0.001$) for troponin T.[54] The second included 18 982 patients with unstable angina from 21 studies and showed odds of death or myocardial infarction at 30 days of 3·44

(95% CI 2·94–4·03; $P < 0.00001$) for the total population of troponin positive patients, 2·86 (95% CI 2·35–3·47; $P < 0.0001$) for patients with ST-segment elevation, 4·93 (95% CI 3·77–6·45; $P < 0.0001$) for patients with non-ST-segment elevation, and 9·39 (95% CI 6·46–13·67; $P < 0.0001$) for patients with unstable angina.[55] The third meta-analysis included seven clinical trials and 19 cohort studies. The odds of mortality among 11 963 patients with positive troponin T or I was 3·1 (5·2% v 1·6%). The discriminative value of elevated troponin levels was greater in cohort studies than in clinical trials, 8·4% v 0·7% (OR 8·5) for troponin I, and 11·6% v 1·7% (OR 5.1) for troponin T.[56]

Determination of troponin levels has many utilities. Beyond providing a highly sensitive and specific test for the diagnosis of myocardial infarction, any elevation provides important prognostic information in acute coronary syndromes. Patients with troponin elevation are also more likely to profit from therapy with a Gp IIb/IIIa antagonist,[57] from a low molecular weight heparin,[58] and from interventional procedures.[59] All evidence converges to relate the elevation of troponin to an ongoing intracoronary thrombotic process, associated with small foci of myocardial necrosis, likely related to distal embolization of thrombotic material originating from the culprit lesion.

Prognostic value of the 12-lead ECG

Current information on the prevalence of ECG abnormalities is difficult to obtain, in part because ECG criteria are often used to define eligibility for clinical studies and the use of heterogeneous inclusion criteria among trials. In a report by Langer *et al* on 135 patients hospitalized with unstable angina without evidence of acute myocardial infarction, ST-segment depression was found in 25% of patients, ST-segment elevation in 16%, both in 4%, and none in 55%.[60] In this study, ST-segment depression and the magnitude of depression were both associated with a higher prevalence of multivessel and left main disease.[60] In the TIMI-3 Registry of 1416 patients enrolled because of unstable angina or non-Q wave MI, ST-segment deviation ≥ 1 mm was present in 14·3% of patients, isolated T wave inversion in 21·9%, and left bundle branch block (LBBB) in 9·0%. By 1 year follow up, death or MI occurred in 11% of patients with ST-segment depression, 6·8% of patients with isolated T wave inversion, and in 8·2% of those with no ECG changes. ST-segment depression 0·5 mm or more and LBBB were significant predictors of death and MI, with rates of 16·3% and 22·9%, respectively.[61] The ECG is not infrequently confounded by LBBB, left ventricular hypertrophy, paced rhythm or other derangements. In the PARAGON-A study, these confounders were associated with near doubling in the 1 year mortality rates (12·6% v 6·5%).[62] Among the 12 142 patients enrolled in the GUSTO-II trial with symptoms at

rest within 12 hours of admission and ischemic ECG changes, 22% had T wave inversion, 28% ST-segment elevation, 35% ST-segment depression, and 15% ST-segment elevation and depression.[26] The 30 day rates of death or myocardial re-infarction were 5·5%, 9·4%, 10·5%, and 12·4% respectively ($P < 0.001$). The cumulative rates of death in this study are shown in Figure 30.4.

There exists therefore a gradient of increasing risk of death or myocardial infarction in hospital and up to 1 year, from non-specific ECGs to T wave inversion to ST-segment depression including confounding ST-T changes. Such a gradient exists from ST-segment depression >0·05 mm, to >1 mm, to >2 mm, to ≥ 2 mm, and to depression in more than two contiguous leads.[62] The prognostic value of ST-segment depression extends to 4 years following hospital discharge.[63] Special attention is required for patients showing deep T wave inversions in leads V1 through V6 and in leads 1 and AVL on the admission or subsequent ECGs; the changes are quite specific for the presence of significant disease in the proximal left anterior coronary artery disease and are predictive of a high risk of progression to an infarction that can be massive.[64]

The importance of recording the 12-lead ECG during chest pain must be emphasized. The detection of ST-segment depression during pain has diagnostic and prognostic value.[65] Occasionally, transient ST-segment elevation will be detected associated with a critical dynamic coronary artery stenosis caused by spasm or thrombus formation. ST-segment shifts during pain occurring on medical management indicate refractory ischemia, an end point commonly used in clinical trials. Refractory ischemia predicts near tripling of adjusted 1 year mortality.[66]

Risk scores

Prognosis can be predicted by various clinical, ECG, and laboratory parameters. Accordingly, predictive models have been derived from various databases by applying multiple regression analyses to identify the independent predictors of prognosis. The results of such analyses are influenced by the characteristics of the test populations and by the baseline data collected. From the population of 9461 patients enrolled in the PURSUIT trial, more than 20 parameters were predictive of mortality and the composite end point of death or MI, the most important being age, heart rate, systolic blood pressure, ST-segment depression, signs of heart failure, and cardiac enzyme elevation.[67]

The TIMI risk score has gained popularity, since it can be readily and simply assessed at admission or shortly thereafter. It was derived from the control cohort of patients in the TIMI-11B study.[68] The seven independent predictors of death, myocardial infarction or recurrent ischemia that were identified are shown in Table 30.4. Their mathematical

Table 30.4 Components of the TIMI risk score

Age 65 yr
At least three risk factors for CAD
Significant coronary stenosis (for example, prior coronary stenosis 50%)
ST-segment deviation
Severe anginal symptoms (for example, two anginal events in last 24 h)
Use of aspirin in last 7 days
Elevated serum cardiac markers

Source: Antman et al[68]

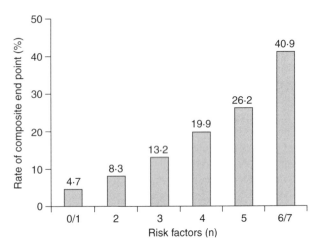

Figure 30.7 Original validation of the TIMI risk score. Rates of all-cause mortality, myocardial infarction, and severe recurrent ischemia prompting urgent revascularization through 14 days by TIMI risk score at admission. The score discriminates a gradient in risk from 5% to 40%. Reproduced with permission from Antman et al.[68]

addition provided a seven-point score that could discriminate a 10-fold difference in risk through 14 days (Figure 30.7). The score was subsequently validated in other populations including PRISM-PLUS[69] and TACTICS.[44] Greater treatment benefit was observed with enoxaparin treatment,[68] Gp IIb/IIIa antagonists[69] and reperfusion procedures[44] in patients with higher scores, ST-segment shifts, and elevated troponin levels.

Inflammation markers

Blood levels of numerous markers of inflammation are elevated in patients with an ACS, including acute phase proteins (C-reactive protein, serum amyloid A protein, fibrinogen), pro-inflammatory cytokines (interleukin-6, TNF-α, interleukin-18), soluble adhesion molecules (sVCAM-1,

sICAM-1, E-selectin, P-selectin), and matrix metalloproteinases. C-reactive protein (CRP) is a non-specific but highly sensitive marker of an inflammatory state. Interleukin-6, which is induced by TNF-α, IL-1, IL-18, platelet derived growth factor, antigens, and endotoxins, is the main stimulus for the production of CRP by the liver. CRP has a half life of 19 hours and can be assessed in the blood by tests with high sensitivity. Many epidemiologic studies in individuals with or without known cardiovascular disease have consistently shown a 3- to 3·5-fold increase in the risk of cardiac events in the highest distribution quartile. The predictive value is additive to that of cholesterol levels.[70] CRP levels are elevated in myocardial infarction. The elevation preceded that of markers of myocardial necrosis in patients who had previous unstable angina, but not in patients who had no preceding angina.[71] Levels are elevated in 40–50% of patients with a non-ST-segment elevation acute coronary syndrome and remain high for months after the acute phase. These elevated levels are associated with high rates of late cardiac events, including death/MI/recurrent ischemia at 12 months,[72] death/MI at 6 months[73,74] and up to 2 years,[75] and death at 36 months.[76] The predictive value for occurrence of early events has been less consistent. In the TIMI-11A study of 630 patients with a non-ST-segment elevation ACS, the risk of death at 14 days was highest with elevated troponin T and CRP, intermediate when either marker was elevated, and lowest when both were normal (CRP < 1·55 mg/l).[77] In the CAPTURE trial of 447 patients, CRP levels >10 mg/l did not predict mortality or myocardial infarction at 72 hours in contrast to elevated troponin T levels, but did predict death or MI at 6 months (18·9% compared to 9·5%), independently of the troponin status (Figure 30.8).[74]

The assessment of CRP levels is not currently part of the recommendations of various guidelines. The cut points that best predict early and late prognosis as well as the ideal timing for blood sampling at admission or hospital discharge remain to be better defined. Moreover, the impact on risk evaluation of treatment with statins, which reduce the CRP levels and the prognostic significance of elevated levels,[78] and of aspirin, which reduces the prognostic value,[79] need additional characterization. Of interest, PCI or CABG appear to have little effect on the 1 year excess of recurrent ischemic events in patients with a non-ST-segment elevation ACS and high CRP levels. Elevated CRP levels are associated with increased risk of restenosis and of acute complications after PCI,[80,81] and with an increased risk of new ischemic events up to 8 years after CABG.[82]

Pathophysiology

This section will focus on the mechanisms of acute coronary syndromes that are the most relevant with respect to management. Interested readers are referred to more exhaustive

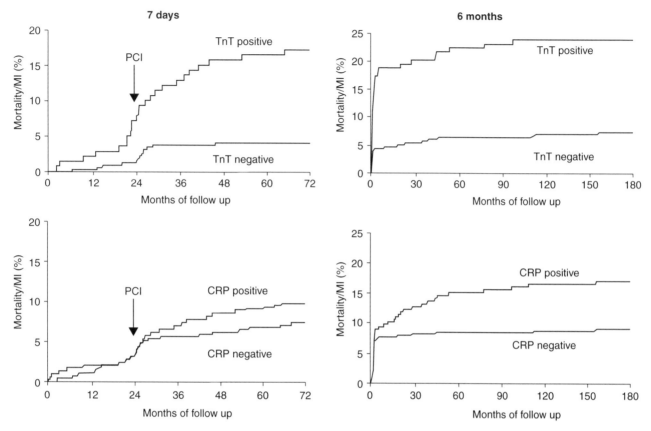

Figure 30.8 Rates of death or MI at 7 days (top left panel) and at 6 months (top right panel) by troponin T (TnT) status (top panels), and C-reactive protein (CRP) status (lower panels) at admission. PCI was performed in all patients 20–24 hours after admission. The risk of death or MI was especially high in TnT positive patients within the first 7 days and increased only slightly thereafter. The event rates were not statistically different for CRP negative patients and CRP positive patients after 7 days (including the coronary intervention) (10·3% v 8%; P = 0·41). During the 6 month follow up period, however, the event rate curves for CRP positive and CRP negative patients continually diverged. There were significant differences both after 30 days (14·1% v 7·6%; P = 0·03) and especially at 6 months (18·9% v 9·5%; P = 0·003). The excess events in CRP-positive patients were related to higher incidence of MI (13·5% v 8·4%; P = 0·16) and of mortality rate (5·4% v 1·1%; P = 0·005). Reproduced with permission from Heeschen *et al.*[74]

reviews.[83–85] Figure 30.9 outlines the cascade of patho physiologic events that build up on an atherosclerotic plaque and eventually result in myocardial infarction and death. The culprit lesion becomes clinically manifest only with the development of an obstruction severe enough to impede coronary blood flow at rest, or when it is the site of a thrombotic occlusion shedding thromboembolic material into the distal circulation. Therefore, the active plaque is clinically detected only at an advanced stage of the underlying disease. Further, the concept of a single active plaque has been challenged. Pathologic studies have shown multiple rupture sites and thrombi at multiple sites often associated with platelet aggregates in small intramyocardial arteries and microscopic foci of necrosis.[7,86–88] An angiographic study in 253 patients with an acute myocardial infarction documented that complex and ruptured plaques could be found in 40% of patients and that these were associated with a 10-fold increase in the risk of a recurrent ACS.[89]

Atherosclerosis is the substrate for ACS. The severity of atherosclerosis in acute coronary syndromes is highly variable, ranging from absence of significant stenoses to the presence of left main disease in 5–10% of patients, and single, double or three vessel disease in respectively 20%, 30%, and 40%.[90] A severely obstructive lesion is most often identified, providing a rationale for coronary revascularization. On inspection and histologic analyses, the culprit lesion is clearly distinct from the stable plaque; it is most often of only moderate severity, with an inner core rich in cholesterol and cholesterol esters and a thin fibrous cap, poor in connective tissue and smooth muscle cells.[83] At microscopy, the culprit lesion is rich in monocyte-macrophages, mast cells, lymphocytes, and neutrophils. Biologically, it is extremely active, with an intense inflammatory reaction marked by heterotypic cell-to-cell interactions and activity of proinflammatory cytokines, matrix-degrading metalloproteinases, and growth factors.[84,85] This culprit lesion is the site of a rupture or

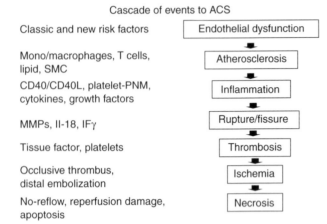

Figure 30.9 Cascade of events leading to ACS. There is a progression of events at the level of an atherosclerotic plaque to excessive inflammation, plaque degeneration, plaque rupture, and intravascular thrombus formation. These events become clinically manifest only when the thrombus becomes obstructive or sheds distal emboli to cause myocardial ischemia and eventually myocardial infarction and death. The cascade of events offers multiple possibilities for intervening at various levels to control and prevent ACS. Il-18, interleukin 18; IFγ, interferon γ.

fissure, occurring most often at the shoulder region of the plaque. The endothelial disruption is occupied by a thrombus extending variably within the lumen of the artery and the vessel wall.[83] The mainstay of immediate therapy in ACS is the control of the thrombotic activity to prevent its rapid progression to occlusion or distal microembolization of thrombotic material. The best results have been achieved with combinations of antiplatelet and anticoagulant therapy consistent with the contributions of both intravascular coagulation and platelet activation and aggregation to arterial thrombosis. Circulating platelets adhere within seconds to the damaged endothelium through receptor–ligand interactions. Gp Ib/IX recognizes von Willebrand factor present in large quantities in the subendothelium, and Gp Ia/IIa recognizes collagen. Platelet adhesion and other local agonists produce intracellular signaling that increases cytosolic Ca^{2+} content and induces shape change, release of potent vasoactive, proaggregant and procoagulant substances, and activation of the Gp IIb/IIIa receptor.[83] The activated Gp IIb/IIIa receptor recognizes and binds the RGD sequence of various moieties, particularly fibrinogen, resulting in platelet cross-bridging and platelet aggregation. The outside translocation of the inner anionic phospholipid layer of platelets early during activation provides a membrane surface well suited for the assembly of coagulation factors and thrombus formation and growth. Tissue factor, expressed by lipid laden macrophages in the core of the atherosclerotic plaque and the diseased endothelium, forms a complex with circulating factor VIIa to activate factors IX and X of the coagulation cascade. Factor IXa is part of the intrinsic tenase complex that

activates factor X. Factor Xa converts prothrombin to thrombin within the prothrombinase complex. Thrombin has multiple pathophysiologic effects. It converts fibrinogen to fibrin, activates factor XIII which cross-links fibrin, amplifies its own generation by activation of factors V, VIII, and XI on the platelet surface, and is a potent platelet agonist. P-selectin expressed on the platelet membrane and on the endothelial cell attracts leukocytes, linking thrombosis and inflammation.

In addition to antithrombotic therapies, other strategies may be employed to control the acute coronary syndromes, as shown in Figure 30.9. The prevention of atherosclerosis is the ultimate goal. Realistic targets in the shorter term are plaque passivation to control the pathophysiologic triggers to plaque rupture and thrombus formation, and cell protection to prevent progression of ischemia to irreversible cell necrosis.[91]

Management

The goals of treatment in ACS are to decrease the substantial risk of myocardial infarction and death, relieve pain, and prevent recurrent ischemia. These objectives can be collectively regrouped under the term plaque passivation, implying the conversion of an unstable plaque into a plaque that will be stable and not prone to complications. During the acute phase, this is best achieved with prompt use of antithrombotic agents, and in selected patients reperfusion procedures. Anti-ischemic therapy is also used to control symptoms. Therapies to control the inflammatory processes within the plaque are effective in secondary prevention and their potential is now being investigated during the more acute phase.

Acute therapy

The therapeutic approaches include general measures, anti-ischemic therapies, antithrombotic therapies, and revascularization procedures. The intensity of treatment is guided by risk as estimated from the clinical presentation, the 12-lead ECG and the troponin levels, as discussed above. Additional patient characteristics associated with an enhanced risk must also be considered. These are listed in Table 30.3 above, along with other predictors of an impaired long-term prognosis. Risk stratification is an ongoing process that must be repeatedly updated during the clinical course and integrated with the results of the various tests performed.

General measures

The patient may present in a non-medical setting or by telephone, in the office, or in the hospital emergency room or ward. Those with the simple new onset of angina or mild exacerbation of previously stable angina, with no angina at rest, ECG changes, or hemodynamic abnormalities should be carefully assessed, initial treatment and educational materials provided, and medical follow up planned, but they may generally be managed as outpatients with initial limitation of activities, providing that necessary investigations can be performed promptly. High-risk patients require admission to the CCU, generally to remain for about 24 hours following the last episode of rest pain. Patients at intermediate risk might go to the CCU, an intermediate care unit, or even to a regular ward depending on the availability of facilities and the specific level of risk.

Whatever the pathophysiology of the acute ischemia in a given patient, there is an imbalance of myocardial oxygen supply and demand, and restricted activities and rest in bed or a recliner chair will be helpful in reducing myocardial oxygen demand. Stool softeners are likely to be helpful. Emotional distress with its attendant increase in myocardial oxygen demand should be minimized by judicious control of environmental noise and light, supportive medical and nursing care, limitation and education of visitors, provision for restful sleep, and control of ischemic pain with intravenous narcotics and nitrates, and other specific anti-ischemic agents as appropriate. Special attention is indicated to detect depressive symptoms that carry an impaired prognosis independently of other predictors.[49] Routine oxygen administration is not recommended unless chest pain is ongoing or respiratory or left heart failure are present. **Grade C** Finger pulse oximetry is then recommended to monitor arterial oxygen saturation. **Grade B**

Anti-ischemic therapies

Nitroglycerin has been a mainstay in the therapy of unstable angina since the prognostic importance was first recognized, and as longer-acting nitrate preparations became available, these were incorporated into treatment regimens without rigorous comparisons to placebo. Studies of the use of IV nitroglycerin among patients with unstable angina have been relatively small, of sequential or case–control design, and the dose regimens have varied considerably.[92] At least partial relief of anginal episodes is usually achieved, occasionally relief is complete, and absence of benefit is an infrequent observation. However, the trials have been of brief duration, generally a few days only, and problems of nitrate tolerance and recurrence of ischemic events emphasize that nitrates are not definitive therapy for unstable angina beyond the acute phase. A trial comparing nitrate therapy and diltiazem[93] indicates that diltiazem is more effective in controlling angina and preventing ischemic events but these studies do not reflect clinical approaches that have employed long acting or intravenous nitroglycerin in combination with a β blocker or a rate limiting calcium antagonist. The widespread use of oral, topical, and IV nitrates in unstable angina is based upon reasonable extrapolation from pathophysiologic observations, case series, evidence of modest reduction of mortality in acute MI,[94–96] and extensive clinical experience using regimens developed in careful clinical studies.[96] **Grade B**

Patients must be monitored for the potential adverse effect of marked arterial hypotension, which must be managed quickly to avoid exacerbating ischemia. The use of sildenafil (Viagra) within the preceding 24 hours is a contraindication to nitrate therapy.[97] **Grade B** Efforts should be made to minimize the development of nitrate tolerance by reducing IV dosage and intermittent dosing by non-IV routes when ischemic pain allows.

The β blockers were introduced in the 1960s and their effectiveness in the treatment of stable angina resulted in rapid acceptance for the management of unstable angina. There was remarkably little objective evidence for the efficacy of β blockers prior to their widespread use.[29] Subsequently, β blockers were evaluated in well-designed studies. In one study, a group of 126 patients hospitalized with unstable angina (characterized by progressive or rest ischemic pain plus ECG changes with pain and documented coronary artery disease) were randomly allocated to the addition to their regular therapy of either nifedipine or the combination of propranolol/isosorbide dinitrate, with appropriate placebos.[98] The principal outcome was absence of recurrent chest pain for at least 48 hours, and the period of evaluation was 14 days. There was no overall difference between the two treatment regimens. However, in a post-hoc analysis of the data amongst the 59 patients not receiving β blocker on admission, the propranolol/isosorbide was more effective than the nifedipine in producing pain relief ($P < 0.001$). Conversely, among the 67% of patients already receiving a β blocker on admission, nifedipine was more effective than augmentation of β blocker accompanied by isosorbide ($P = 0.026$).

The HINT study[99] examined metoprolol and nifedipine in patients hospitalized with prolonged rest pain. The 338 patients who were not receiving β blocker on admission were randomly allocated to nifedipine, metoprolol, both, or neither in a double-blind placebo-controlled fashion. The outcome of AMI or recurrent angina with ST change within 48 hours occurred with the following frequencies: placebo (37%), nifedipine (47%), metoprolol (28%), nifedipine plus metoprolol (30%). Metoprolol was significantly more effective than nifedipine ($P < 0.05$). The 177 patients already on a β blocker on admission were randomly allocated in double-blind fashion to nifedipine or placebo and treatment failure occurred in 51% of placebo and 30% of nifedipine ($P < 0.05$).

Gottlieb *et al.*[100] studied 81 patients hospitalized with at least 10 minutes of ischemic chest pain at rest. All patients were receiving "optimal" doses of nitrates and nifedipine and were therefore treatment failures on this regimen. They were randomly allocated to the addition of either propranolol or placebo. In the first 4 days, propranolol resulted in a statistically significant reduction of recurrent rest angina episodes, duration of angina, nitroglycerin requirement, and ECG abnormalities. Although recurrences of rest angina remained less among the propranolol treated group over the next 4 weeks, the incidence of aortocoronary bypass, AMI, and sudden death was no different between the two groups.

In another study, patients hospitalized with prolonged pain accompanied by ECG abnormalities, and who had failed maximum treatment with propranolol and long-acting nitrates, were randomized to the addition of nifedipine or placebo;[101] the failure of medical treatment (sudden death, AMI, or bypass surgery) was less frequent with nifedipine than with placebo ($P = 0.03$). The benefit was most marked among patients with ST-segment elevation.

These trials suggest that among patients not receiving a β blocker on hospitalization, the institution of β blockade and the institution or maintenance of nitrates is more effective treatment than the institution of nifedipine. **Grade A** Amongst patients whose pain persists with optimal doses of nitrates and nifedipine, the addition of a β blocker is efficacious in the initial few days, although the incidence of ischemic outcomes (bypass surgery, AMI, sudden death) is not reduced. **Grade A** On the other hand, in patients hospitalized and already receiving a β blocker, then the addition of nifedipine is more effective than simply augmenting the β blocker dose. **Grade B** Recent data suggesting potentially harmful effects of short-acting dihydropyridines[102] indicate that a more prudent choice for the addition to a β blocker would be a long-acting dose preparation or an agent with an intrinsically long half-life such as amlodipine, although rigorous studies have not been conducted. **Grade C**

Diltiazem was compared to propranolol in a randomized single-blind study of patients hospitalized for crescendo rest, or following MI angina accompanied by ECG abnormalities.[103] Chest pain frequency was significantly reduced by both regimens, and there was no difference in efficacy. The 5 month follow up was rather discouraging in both groups, with a high incidence of AMI, death, and bypass surgery, and few patients without bypass surgery were symptom free. In another study, patients with rest angina were randomized to diltiazem or propranolol in maximum tolerated doses.[104] The agents were equally effective in reducing the frequency of daily anginal episodes, but in the subgroup with angina only at rest, diltiazem was efficacious whereas propranolol was not.

There is little rigorous evidence for the value of verapamil in unstable angina. Small placebo-controlled trials[105,106] demonstrated statistically significant reductions in the frequency of ischemia. Long-term follow up in these small trials[107] showed that in general ischemic pain continued to be well controlled but there was a high incidence of AMI and death.

In addition to reducing ischemic episodes, a reduction in MI would be desirable. Yusuf *et al*[108] examined five trials involving about 4700 patients with threatened MI who were placed on intravenous β blocker followed by oral therapy for about a week. There was a modest 13% reduction

in the risk of development of MI in this group. Meta-analysis of studies of calcium antagonists among patients with unstable angina shows no reduction of death or non-fatal MI.[108] Diltiazem and verapamil appear to be effective as initial single agents in the management of unstable angina, and diltiazem appears to be no different in efficacy from propranolol in one direct comparison. However, the meta-analytic data for benefit of β blocker but not calcium antagonists and the evidence for improved long-term outcomes with β blocker therapy among survivors of myocardial infarction,[108] and those with chronic ischemia, support β blockers over rate-limiting calcium antagonists as the first choice therapy in patients with unstable angina. **Grade A** Patients at high risk may have benefit from initial intravenous β blocker, followed by an oral regimen. **Grade C** Diltiazem or verapamil are suitable alternatives for patients with a contraindication to β blocker therapy. **Grade B** Nifedipine should not be the initial single agent for patients with unstable angina.[98] **Grade A** The new dihydropyridines have not been evaluated in patients with an acute coronary syndrome. Nicorandil, an ATP sensitive potassium (K^+) channel opener with arterial and venous vasodilator properties and cardioprotective potential by pharmacologic preconditioning, was shown in one small trial of 188 patients to reduce the number of transient ischemic episodes on continuous Holter monitoring.[109] Nicorandil is not approved for use in North America.

Among patients with variant angina, characterized by recurrent ischemic episodes occurring mainly at rest and in the early morning hours accompanied by transient ST-segment elevation, randomized placebo-controlled, double-blind trials of verapamil,[110–112] diltiazem,[113–116] and nifedipine[117–119] have demonstrated the efficacy of each of these agents in reduction of angina frequency. Several comparisons of calcium antagonists to β blockers have demonstrated greater efficacy with the calcium antagonists.[111,112,116] These agents are regarded along with nitrates as the therapy of choice for variant angina, although there is little direct comparative data with long-acting nitrates. **Grade A**

Antithrombotic therapy

Antithrombotic therapy is cornerstone therapy in ACS. It prevents death or myocardial infarction in patients managed medically and in patients undergoing a reperfusion procedure. Optimal benefit is obtained with combined inhibition of platelets and of the coagulation process. Thrombolytic therapy is beneficial in ST-segment elevation MI but contraindicated in non-ST-segment elevation MI.[120]

Antiplatelet therapy – Whereas aspirin has long been, and is still, the gold standard of antiplatelet therapy, a new armamentarium of agents acting on different platelet functions has been developed. Physicians now have options in drug selection used in mono- or poly-therapy. Antiplatelet agents evaluated in ACS have been aspirin, dipyridamole, prostacyclin, sulfinpyrazone, inhibitors of thromboxane synthase and/or its receptor, ticlopidine, clopidogrel, and the intravenous and oral Gp IIb/IIIa antagonists. The various drugs can be classified first by their site of action on the main steps of platelet function from adhesion to activation and aggregation, and secondarily by their specific effects at each step (Figure 30.10). Adhesion can be inhibited by agents under development acting mainly on von Willebrand factor and its ligand, Gp 1b/IX. Activation can be inhibited by agents acting on intracellular calcium mobilization such as dypiridamole, which prevents catabolism of cAMP and nitric oxide, which promotes production of cGMP, and by agents inhibiting specific activation pathways. Aspirin blocks the thromboxane pathway and ADP-receptor antagonists block purinergic receptors on platelets. Gp IIb/IIIa antagonists occupy the receptor to prevent fibrinogen binding and platelet aggregation.

Aspirin – Four conclusive trials have shown consistent benefit with aspirin in patients with non-ST-segment elevation ACS, despite different study designs and different doses. The Veterans Administration Study, performed between 1974 and 1981, included 1338 men with unstable angina randomly allocated within 72 hours of admission to ASA 324 mg or placebo.[121] The rate of death or myocardial infarction was reduced from 10·1% to 5·0% (RR 49%, $P = 0.0005$) over a 12 week treatment period.

In the Canadian Multicenter Trial conducted between 1979 and 1984, 555 patients (73% men) with unstable angina were randomized before hospital discharge to aspirin (325 mg four times daily), sulfinpyrazone (200 mg four times daily), placebo, or both drugs.[122] The outcome of death or myocardial infarction at 2 years was reduced from 17% to 8·6% (RR 49·2%; $P = 0.008$) by efficacy analysis and by 30% ($P = 0.072$) by intention-to-treat analysis, and the outcome of death was reduced by 71% ($P = 0.004$) and 43·4% ($P = 0.035$) respectively. Sulfinpyrazone had no

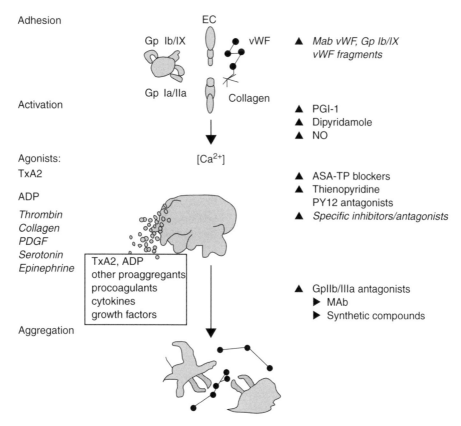

Figure 30.10 Mechanisms of platelet adhesion, secretion and aggregation, and sites of action of various antiplatelet drugs. The drugs approved for clinical use are in bold and the drugs under development in italics. Adhesion to the damaged endothelium and other agonists triggers intracellular signaling with an increase in cytosolic free calcium content (Ca^{2+}), shape change, and release of numerous proaggregants, procoagulants, growth factors, and inflammatory mediators. The GP IIb/IIIa receptors undergo conformational changes making them competent to cross-link fibrinogen to form platelet aggregates and the platelet thrombus. ADP, adenosine diphosphate; ASA, aspirin; Mab, monoclonal antibody; PDGF, platelet derived growth factor; PGI_1, prostacyclin; TP, thromboxane receptor; TxA2, thromboxane A2; vWF, von Willebrand factor. Reproduced with permission from Theroux P. Thrombosis in coronary artery disease: its pathophysiology and control. *Dialogues Cardiovas Med* 2002;**7**:3–18.

significant effect or interaction with aspirin. In the Montreal study, 479 patients were randomized during the acute phase of disease to aspirin (325 mg bid), heparin, both or neither in a 2×2 factorial design.[32] Aspirin reduced the risk of death or myocardial infarction at 6 days from 6·3% to 2·6%, a 63% risk reduction ($P = 0·04$). The RISC study randomized 945 patients to aspirin (80 mg daily), intravenous heparin, both or placebos.[31] End points were assessed in 796 patients meeting the entry criteria. Aspirin, compared to no aspirin, reduced the rate of death or MI at 5 days from 5·8% to 2·6% ($P = 0·033$), at 7 days from 13·4% to 4·3% ($P = 0·0001$), and at 30 days from 17·1% to 6·5% ($P = 0·0001$).

The Antiplatelet Trialists' Collaboration updated their initial meta-analysis by including 287 studies involving 135 000 patients administered antiplatelet therapy versus control and 77 000 patients randomized to different antiplatelet regimens.[123] Overall, among high-risk patients, allocation to antiplatelet therapy reduced the outcome of any serious vascular event by 25%, non-fatal MI by 33%, non-fatal stroke by 25%, and vascular mortality by 16%. Aspirin was the most widely studied antiplatelet drug. The absolute benefit of aspirin increases with the inherent risk of the condition for which it is prescribed, and is substantial in patients with a non-ST-segment elevation ACS, as illustrated in Figure 30.11.[124] Aspirin has numerous physiologic effects on platelets and the inflammatory process, many of which are only partly characterized. The mechanism accounting for the benefit in ACS is believed to be the irreversible inhibition of cyclo-oxygenase-1 (COX-1) in platelets, blocking formation of thromboxane A2; the doses of 75–160 mg daily that have been shown to be at least as clinically effective as higher doses are quite specific for this effect.[123] This inhibition is dose-related, cumulative and irreversible. A loading dose of 160–365 mg is recommended followed by doses of 80–160 mg daily. **Grade A** Higher doses have anti-inflammatory effects and inhibit cyclo-oxygenase-2 (COX-2). COX-2 is not constitutive and is expressed in endothelial cells and white cells in response to an inflammatory stimulus. It is inhibited selectively by the coxibs and less selectively by the non-steroidal anti-inflammatory drugs (NSAIDs). The term aspirin resistance is increasingly used to describe failure of aspirin to prevent events in some patients. Laboratory data suggest that there is a non-optimal biologic response in about 30% of patients.[125,126] Practical reasons for the failure of aspirin are non-compliance to therapy and intake of NSAIDs prior to aspirin. NSAIDS, and typically ibuprofen, flurbiprofen, indomethacin, and suprofen, bind COX-1 on the same serine residue as aspirin to mask the active site; the biologic actions of aspirin are therefore prevented when these NSAIDS are present in blood, an effect that is favored by the short plasma half life of aspirin.[127] Other reasons for aspirin failure could be individual variations in metabolism

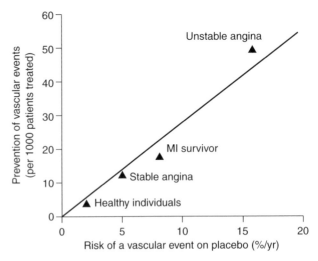

Figure 30.11 Benefits of aspirin by risk groups. The absolute risk of vascular complications is the major determinant of the absolute benefit of antiplatelet prophylaxis. Data are plotted from placebo-controlled aspirin trials in different clinical settings. For each category of patients, the abscissa denotes the absolute risk of experiencing a major vascular event as recorded in the placebo arms of the trials. The absolute benefit of antiplatelet treatment is reported on the ordinate axis as the number of subjects in whom an important vascular event (that is, non-fatal MI, non-fatal stroke, or vascular death) is actually prevented by treating 1000 subjects with aspirin for 1 year. Reproduced with permission from Patrono *et al.*[124]

of low doses of aspirin possibly influenced by genetic polymorphism, thromboxane A2 independent pathways of thrombus formation, generation of thromboxane A2 by COX-2, and agonists of thromboxane receptors other than thromboxane A2, such as the isoprostanes which are non-enzymatically derived products of arachidonic acid.[128] The diagnosis of aspirin resistance is based on clinical suspicion as no single test has so far been prospectively and reproducibly validated. Since an alternative therapy to aspirin exists with drugs that have been shown to be at least as useful as aspirin, aspirin monotherapy should be questioned in patients clinically suspected of aspirin resistance because of recurrent ischemic events occurring on aspirin therapy. **Grade B**

Other agents acting on the cyclo-oxygenase pathway – The inhibition of prostacyclin (PGI_2) generation by aspirin does not appear to limit its protective effects significantly. Nevertheless, it was shown that an infusion of prostacyclin in unstable angina patients resulted in no benefit.[129] Analogs of PGI_1 that are more stable and that have less hemodynamic effects are now being investigated in various situations. The thromboxane synthase inhibitors and/or receptor antagonists investigated so far were not shown to be superior or inferior to aspirin. S18886 is a new agent under clinical investigation, which blocks the thromboxane (TP) receptor and has favorable pharmacokinetic and pharmaco-dynamic profiles. Experimental data have suggested that the drug could be protective against progression of atherosclerosis.[130]

ADP receptor antagonists

The thienopyridines ticlopidine and clopidogrel are the two ADP receptor antagonists currently approved. Clopidogrel has replaced ticlopidine as it is devoid of the serious life-threatening adverse effects of leukopenia and thrombocyto-penia found with ticlopidine. Clopidogrel is also more potent than ticlopidine and can be safely administered in loading doses to achieve full drug effects approximately 2 hours after the administration of a bolus dose of 300 mg. Clopidogrel effects are dose-related, cumulative, and irre-versible, as are those of aspirin. Placebo-controlled trials with ticlopidine in unstable angina and in the secondary pre-vention of stroke have documented risk reductions in the range of those observed with aspirin.[131] One direct compar-ison trial has shown superiority of ticlopidine over aspirin in the secondary prevention of stroke.[132] Many trials in coro-nary stenting have confirmed the greater efficacy and safety of clopidogrel.[133]

Clopidogrel was evaluated in two large trials, in one as single therapy,[134] and in the other as combined therapy with aspirin versus aspirin alone.[135] In the CAPRIE trial, a total of 19 185 patients with atherosclerotic vascular disease manifested as recent ischemic stroke, recent myocardial infarction, or symptomatic peripheral vascular disease were randomized to aspirin, 325 mg/day, or clopidogrel, 75 mg/day.[134] The annual risk of ischemic stroke, myocardial infarction, or vascular death during a follow up of 1–3 years was reduced by 8·7% from 5·83% to 5·32% by clopidogrel ($P = 0·043$). The risk reductions (RR) were, however, het-erogeneous among the entry groups: 23·8% ($P = 0·00028$) in patients enrolled because of peripheral vascular disease, 7·3% in patients enrolled because of stroke, and an excess of 5·03% ($P = 0·66$) in patients enrolled because of a myocar-dial infarction.

In the CURE trial, 12 562 patients were randomized within 24 hours after the onset of a non-ST-segment elevation ACS to receive clopidogrel (300 mg bolus, 75 mg daily) or placebo in addition to aspirin 160–360 mg daily for 3–12 months. The primary composite outcome of cardiovascular death, non-fatal MI, or stroke occurred in 9·3% of patients in the clopidogrel group and 11·4% of patients in the placebo group (RR 0·80; 95% CI 0·72–0·90; $P < 0·001$) (Figure 30.12).[136] Clopidogrel further reduced the rates of inhospital severe ischemia and of revascularization, the need for thrombolytic therapy or intravenous Gp IIb/IIIa-receptor antagonists, and the occurrence of heart failure. The benefits became

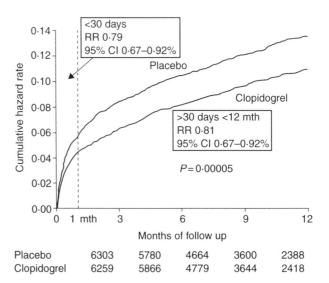

Figure 30.12 Cumulative hazard rates for the outcome of cardiovascular death, non-fatal myocardial infarction, or stroke during the 12 months of the CURE study with the use of clopi-dogrel versus placebo on a background of aspirin in all patients. The results demonstrate sustained benefit of clopidogrel from the time of randomization through to the end of the study. Reproduced with permission from The CURE Investigators.[136]

apparent within a few hours of treatment initiation and increased throughout the follow up period to one year. These benefits were homogeneous among all secondary end points, subgroup analyses, and patients at low, medium, and high risk, enhancing the clinical relevance of the trial. Thus even patients with no ST-segment depression and patients with no elevation of cardiac markers benefit, contrasting with the benefits of enoxaparin and the Gp IIb/IIIa antago-nists which are apparent only in high-risk patients. There were significantly more patients with major bleeding in the clopidogrel group than in the placebo group (3·7% v 2·7%; RR 1·38; $P = 0·001$), but there was no excess in life-threatening bleeding (2·2% v 1·8%; $P = 0·13$) or hemor-rhagic stroke (0·1% v 0·1%). The risk of major bleeding was particularly increased in patients undergoing CABG surgery within the first 5 days of stopping clopidogrel (9·6% v 6·3%, RR 1·53; $P = 0·06$) but not when CABG was performed after 5 days (4·4% v 5·3% with placebo). The CURE trial was mainly aimed at medical management, although revas-cularization was performed during the initial admission in 23% of the patients, among whom there was a benefit of clopidogrel. A benefit of clopidogrel was also noted in patients who received thrombolytic therapy or a Gp IIb/IIIa antagonist, but these drugs were administered in only 1·1% and 5·9% of patients respectively.

Gp IIb/IIIA-receptor blockers – Three Gp IIb/IIIa antago-nists are approved for clinical use: abciximab, eptifibatide, and tirofiban. Clinical trials failed to show a benefit of lamifiban, a synthetic Gp IIb/IIIa antagonist with properties similar to those of eptifibatide and tirofiban.[37,137] Abciximab is a Fab fragment of a chimeric monoclonal antibody that binds the RGD and dodecapeptide recognition sequences of the receptor. The plasma half life of the drug is approximately 10 minutes but the biologic half life extends to 6–12 hours. Abciximab has strong affinity for the receptor and receptor occupancy persists weeks after drug exposure, although platelet aggregation progressively returns to normal within 12–24 hours. Abciximab is not specific for the Gp IIb/IIIa integrin, also inhibiting the vitronectin receptor (αvβ3) on the endothelium and smooth muscle cell and the MAC-1 (αmβ2) integrin on neutrophils and monocytes. The clinical relevance of occupancy of these receptors involved in cell proliferation and leukocyte activation respectively remains ill defined. Eptifibatide is a cyclic heptapeptide derived from the structure of barbourin in the venom of the pigmy rattlesnake possessing a KGD sequence recognized by the receptor. Tirofiban is a non-peptide mimetic of the RGD sequence. The half life of the two small molecules is approximately 2 hours. After drug discontinuation, there is 50% recovery of receptor occupancy and platelet aggregation within 4 hours and nearly 100% within 8 hours. These drugs have no special affinity for the receptor and receptor occupancy parallels blood levels. Many trials have documented the efficacy of abciximab in reducing periprocedural MI and the need for urgent revascularization when it is administered in the cardiac catheterization laboratory before a revascularization procedure and continued for 12 hours thereafter.[138,139] In the c7E3 Fab Antiplatelet Therapy in Unstable Refractory angina (CAPTURE)[140] trial involving 1265 patients with refractory unstable angina, abciximab was administered after a first angiogram identifying a culprit lesion suitable for coronary angioplasty. The procedures were performed 20–24 hours later and abciximab was continued for one hour after the procedure.[140] Abciximab, compared with placebo, reduced the rate of death and myocardial infarction by 30 days from 15·9% to 11·3% ($P = 0.012$). In a comparison trial, abciximab was shown to be significantly superior to tirofiban in preventing complications associated with urgent or elective stent placement.[141] The doses of tirofiban used in this study had previously been shown to be ineffective.[142] Contrasting with the benefits observed in percutaneous intervention and in stent implantation trials, the GUSTO-IV trial failed to show a benefit of abciximab in the medical management of patients with a non-ST-segment elevation ACS. In this trial, 7800 patients with chest pain and either ST-segment depression or raised troponin T or I concentrations were randomly assigned placebo, an abciximab bolus and 24 h infusion, or an abciximab bolus and 48 h infusion.[42] The primary outcome of death or myocardial infarction 30 days after randomization occurred in 8·0% of patients on placebo, 8·2% of patients on 24 h abciximab, and 9·1% of

patients on 48 h abciximab (OR 1·0 between placebo and 24 h abciximab, and 1·1 (95% CI 0·94–1·39) for difference between placebo and 48 h abciximab). The lack of benefit with abciximab was consistent in most subgroups investigated including, remarkably, patients with elevated troponin T or I, although they were at a high risk of subsequent events.

Tirofiban was investigated in two ACS trials. In one, tirofiban alone with placebo heparin versus heparin with placebo tirofiban was associated with an early benefit at 72 hours, a benefit that was not, however, sustained after 30 days.[35] The second trial compared the combination of tirofiban with heparin to heparin alone. The combination reduced the occurrence of the primary end point of death, myocardial infarction, or refractory ischemia at 7 days by 32% ($P= 0.004$) and of death or myocardial infarction by 43% ($P= 0.006$).[36] The gain appeared early and was sustained after 6 months.

Many trials were performed with eptifibatide. In the PURSUIT trial, 9461 patients with a non-ST-segment elevation ACS were randomized to eptifibatide or placebo; the rate of death or myocardial infarction after 30 days was reduced by 10% with eptifibatide (14·2% v 15·7%, $P = 0.042$).[39] In the placebo-controlled ESPRIT trial, eptifibatide used at higher doses and with a double bolus injection significantly reduced the event rate associated with coronary stenting to an extent similar to that observed with abciximab.[143]

Altogether, these trials show efficacy of abciximab and eptifibatide in reducing event rates in percutaneous coronary interventions and of tirofiban and eptifibatide in non-ST-segment elevation ACS. The benefits were additive to those of aspirin and of heparin. **Grade A**

Several meta-analyses demonstrated a benefit of intravenous Gp IIb/IIIa antagonist therapy in patients with an ACS. One meta-analysis published in 1999, before the confounding results of GUSTO-IV were known and including the data from the CAPTURE, PURSUIT, and PRISM-PLUS trials, showed event rates of 2·5% with treatment and 3·8% with placebo during the period of medical management and of 4·9% and 8·0% respectively in the 48 hours that followed PCI in the subgroups of patients who underwent a procedure (RR reduction 34%, $P< 0.001$). An early benefit of Gp IIb/IIIa inhibitors during medical treatment was documented, and a larger benefit when PCI was performed on drug therapy.[144] A second meta-analysis with data on individual patients included trials, which enrolled at least 1000 patients and did not recommend early coronary revascularization (this criterion did not apply in PRISM-PLUS).[36,145] Among 31 402 patients from six trials, including GUSTO-IV, the Gp IIb/IIIa antagonists reduced the odds of death or MI at 30 days by 9% (10·8% v 11·8%; OR 0·91; 95% CI 0·84–0·98; $P= 0.015$). The relative treatment benefit was largest in high-risk patients. Benefit was present in both males and females when the baseline troponin levels were elevated but only in males when normal.

A third meta-analysis examined more specifically the 6458 diabetic patients enrolled in the six trials. In these patients, the Gp IIb/IIIa inhibitors reduced the mortality at 30 days from 6·2% to 4·6% (OR 0·74; 95% CI 0·59–0·92; *P* < 0·007) with a statistically significant interaction between treatment and diabetic status (*P* = 0·036). Mortality at 30 days among the 1279 who underwent PCI was reduced from 4·0% to 1·2% (OR 0·30; 95% CI 0·14–0·69; *P* < 0·002).[146]

Puzzling observations with the use of Gp IIb/IIIa antagonists include the absence of benefit in patients with prolonged use of abciximab not referred for invasive management, the failure of lamifiban to show a significant benefit, and, as will be seen below, the excess mortality observed with the prolonged use of orally active agents.

Oral Gp IIb/IIIa antagonists – In an attempt to extend the benefit of intravenous Gp IIb/IIIa antagonists to the subacute and chronic phases of the disease, orally active inhibitors were developed. Four different agents – xemilofiban, orbofiban, sibrafiban and latrofiban – were investigated in five large trials. These agents have rapid on and off binding to the receptor. No single trial showed a benefit in reducing ischemic events and two were prematurely interrupted because of excess mortality. A meta-analysis of four of these trials totaling 33 326 patients showed a statistically significant increase in mortality with therapy (OR 1·37; *P* = 0·001) and trends to more MI. There was a twofold increase in the rate of major bleeding and a high rate of less severe bleeding leading to study drug discontinuation.[147]

Anticoagulants

Anticoagulants evaluated during the acute phase of non-ST-segment elevation ACS have been unfractionated heparin, direct thrombin inhibitors including recombinant hirudin and small molecules, and the low molecular weight heparins. New and promising agents such as r-tissue factor pathway inhibitor, r-protein C, and pentasaccharide and other specific inhibitors of factor Xa are under investigation (Figure 30.13). Documentation of reactivation of the disease

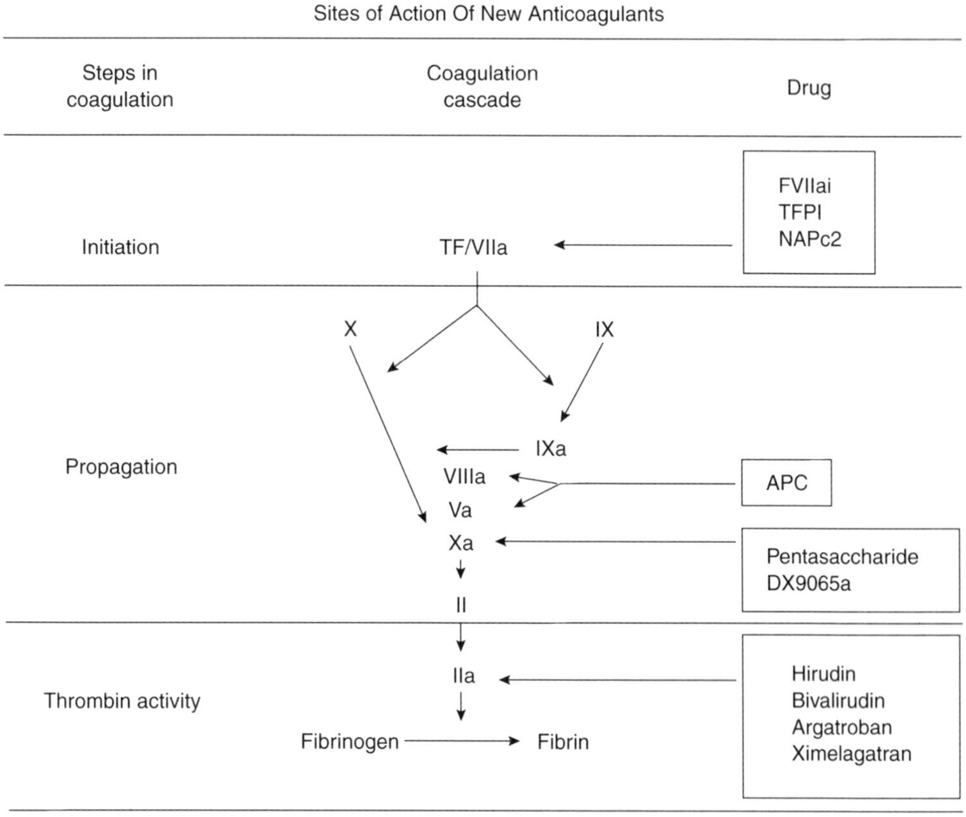

Figure 30.13 The coagulation cascade and sites of action of new anticoagulants. Initiation of coagulation is triggered by the tissue factor/factor VIIa complex (TF/VIIa), which activates factor IX (IX) and factor X (X). Activated factor IX (IXa) propagates coagulation by activating factor X in a reaction that utilizes activated factor VIII (VIIIa) as a cofactor. Activated factor X (Xa), with activated factor V (Va) as a cofactor, converts prothrombin (II) to thrombin (IIa). Thrombin then converts fibrinogen to fibrin. Active site-blocked VIIa (VIIai) competes with VIIa for TF, whereas tissue factor pathway inhibitor (TFPI) and nematode anticoagulant peptide (NAPc2) target VIIa bound to TF. Synthetic pentasaccharide and DX-9065a inactivate Xa, activated protein C (APC) inactivates Va and VIIIa, and hirudin, bivalirudin, argatroban, and ximelagatran target thrombin. Reproduced with permission from Weitz and Buller.[154]

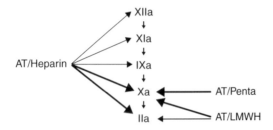

Figure 30.14 Antithrombin (AT)-mediated inhibition of coagulation factors. The complex heparin/AT inhibits especially factor Xa and thrombin (IIa) and also factor XIIa, factor XIa, and factor IXa. The shorter saccharide chains contained in the low molecular weight heparins (LMWH) allow more selective inhibition of factor Xa than factor IIa. The unique pentasaccharide chain of fondaparinux allows highly specific inhibition of factor Xa. Adapted with permission from Hirsh *et al.*[149]

following the discontinuation of heparin[148] and persisting prothrombotic activity past the acute phase have led to the evaluation of long-term therapy with coumadin and the low molecular weight heparins.

Unfractionated and low molecular weight heparins – Unfractionated heparin, low molecular weight heparins, and the heparin pentasaccharide inhibit coagulation factors by greatly enhancing the physiologic properties of circulating antithrombin, with differential effects on factor Xa and thrombin related to the molecular weight of the various heparins (Figure 30.14).[149] In the study by Theroux *et al* of 479 patients, the incidence of fatal and non-fatal myocardial infarction was reduced from 7·5% to 1·2% (RR 85%; $P= 0·007$) with unfractionated heparin compared with placebo, and of recurrent refractory ischemia from 19·7% to 9·6% (RR 51%; $P= 0·02$).[32] In the RISC study, which enrolled 945 men, the combination of aspirin and heparin resulted in a significant risk reduction in death and myocardial infarction at 5 days.[31] In the FRISC study, 1506 patients were randomized to subcutaneous dalteparin twice daily for 6 days followed by once a day for 35–45 days or placebo.[150] During the first 6 days the rate of death or MI was reduced with dalteparin (1·8% *v* 4·8%; RR = 0·37; 95% CI 0·20–0·68). Survival analysis showed a risk of reactivation and re-infarction when the dose was decreased; the benefit persisted at 40 days but not at 4–5 months.[150] A meta-analysis of 12 trials that compared unfractionated heparin or a low molecular weight heparin to placebo in a total of 17 157 patients showed an odds ratio for myocardial infarction or death during the short term (up to 7 days) of 0·53 (95% CI 0·38–0·73; $P= 0·0001$) in favor of the anticoagulant. These results validate the use of unfractionated heparin or of a low molecular weight heparin in combination with aspirin in patients with a non-ST-segment elevation ACS. **Grade A**

Low molecular weight heparins present distinct advantages over unfractionated heparin. They can be administered subcutaneously once or twice a day. They bind plasma proteins and endothelial cells less avidly than unfractionated heparin resulting in more predictable anticoagulation, with no need for monitoring. The ratio of inhibition factor Xa/thrombin is greater. Low molecular weight heparins also stimulate platelets less and are less often associated with heparin-induced thrombocytopenia.

Four trials have directly compared a low molecular weight heparin with unfractionated heparin. No advantages were observed with dalteparin in a trial involving 1482 patients[151] and with nadroparin in a trial of 3468 patients.[152] Enoxaparin was shown to be superior to unfractionated heparin in the two trials that evaluated the drug. In the ESSENCE trial, enoxaparin, 1 mg/kg administered twice daily for 48 hours to 8 days (median 2·6 days) in 3171 patients, reduced the composite outcome of death, MI or recurrent angina by 16·2% at 14 days (16·6% *v* 19·8%; $P= 0·019$), and by 19% at 30 days (19·8% *v* 23·3%; $P= 0·017$) compared to unfractionated heparin. The rate of death was unaffected, but the rate of myocardial infarction was reduced by 29% (3·2% *v* 4·5%; $P= 0·06$) at 14 days, and by 26% (3·9% *v* 5·2%) at 30 days ($P= 0·08$).[34] The TIMI-11B trial showed in 3910 patients a reduction in the composite outcome of death, myocardial infarction or refractory ischemia requiring an urgent revascularization from 16·6% to 14·2% at 14 days ($P= 0·04$) and from 19·6% to 17·3% at 43 days ($P= 0·06$).[41] A meta-analysis of trials that directly compared any low molecular weight heparin to unfractionated heparin showed no statistically significant difference in the odds of death or MI (OR 0·88; 95% CI 0·69–1·12; $P= 0·34$). On the other hand, a combined analysis of the data from ESSENCE and TIMI-11B showed a statistically significant reduction in the rate of death or myocardial infarction in favor of enoxaparin.[153]

The pentasaccharide binds antithrombin to inhibit factor Xa with high specificity. It does not produce thrombocytopenia. The drug is now approved for the prevention of deep vein thrombosis in orthopedic surgery and is under investigation in ST-segment elevation and non-ST-segment elevation acute coronary syndromes.

Direct thrombin inhibitors – These drugs are potent anticoagulants that specifically inhibit thrombin (Figure 30.13); they require a cofactor for their effects and have a highly predictable response. Hirudin, now produced by recombinant technology, is the prototype of these agents. Various other inhibitors have been synthesized with different binding properties to the active site and substrate-binding site of thrombin that affect their relative potency and bleeding risk.[154]

Hirudin tightly binds the active and substrate-binding sites of thrombin. The drug has been investigated in four major trials. The dose regimen of 0·6 mg/kg bolus followed

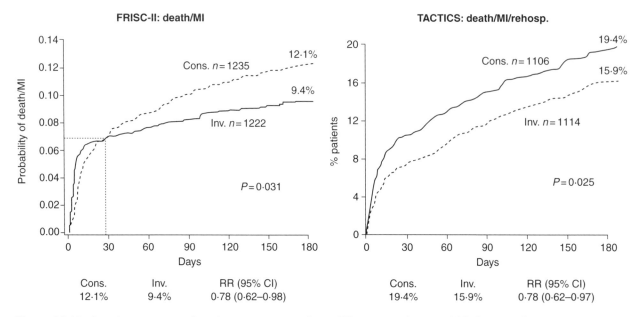

Figure 30.15 Invasive versus non-invasive management of non-ST-segment elevation ACS. Results of the two most recent trials that have compared an early routine invasive management strategy to an early routine medical management strategy. The intervention was performed relatively late in the FRISC-II study after a course of treatment with aspirin and dalteparin and relatively early after a median of 22 hours in TACTICS on treatment with aspirin, heparin, and tirofiban. The two trials show a definitive gain with the early invasive approach in patients with high-risk features as documented by ST-segment shifts and/or an elevation of cardiac markers. Adapted with permission from the FRISC-II Investigators[43] and Cannon *et al*.[44]

by 0·2 mg/kg/hour infusion initially evaluated had to be dropped because of excess bleeding.[155] A dose of 0·2 mg/kg bolus with infusion of 0·1 mg/kg/hour was used in the GUSTO-IIb, which enrolled 12 142 patients, two thirds of them with a non-ST-segment elevation ACS and one third with ST-segment elevation MI,[33] and in the TIMI-9B trial, which enrolled 3002 patients with ST-segment elevation MI.[156] Among patients with no ST-segment elevation in GUSTO-IIb, the composite end point of death or MI at 30 days occurred in 8·3% of the patients on hirudin and in 9·1% of patients on heparin (OR 0·90; 95% CI 0·78–1·06; *P* = 0·22); at 24 h, the risk of death or MI was significantly lower in the patients who received hirudin (2·1% *v* 1·3%; *P* = 0·001). The OASIS pilot study suggested a greater benefit with an intermediate dose of 0·4 mg/kg bolus and 0·15 mg/kg/hour infusion.[157] This dose was used in the large OASIS-2 trial, which randomized 10 141 patients to UFH (5000 IU bolus plus 15 U/kg/h) or recombinant hirudin for 72 h.[40] The primary end point of cardiovascular death or new MI at 7 days was reduced with hirudin from 4·2% to 3·6% (*P* = 0·064); there was an excess of major bleeds requiring transfusions (1·2% *v* 0·7%; *P* = 0·014). A meta-analysis of the GUSTO-IIb, TIMI-9B, OASIS pilot and OASIS-2 showed that the risk of death or MI at 35 days was significantly reduced with hirudin compared with heparin (RR 0·90; *P* = 0·015).[40]

Bivalirudin, argatroban, efegatran, and inogatran have been evaluated in smaller trials in acute coronary syndromes and in

coronary angioplasty. A meta-analysis of 35 970 patients in 11 trials, including the hirudin trials, showed an overall reduction in the risk of death or MI at the end of the treatment period with the direct antithrombin (4·3% *v* 5·1%; OR 0·85; 95% CI 0·77–0·94; *P* = 0·001) and after 30 days (7·4% *v* 8·2%; OR 0·91; 95% CI 0·84–0·99; *P* = 0·02).[158] The benefit was, however, restricted to hirudin and bivalirudin, the two agents inhibiting the two active sites of thrombin, and was not present with agents inhibiting only the catalytic or exosite binding site of thrombin. Hirudin increased the risk of major bleeding compared with heparin but bivalirudin reduced it.[158] Hirudin, bivalirudin, and argatroban are approved for use in patients with heparin-induced thrombocytopenia. Hirudin is also approved for the prevention of deep vein thrombosis in patients undergoing orthopedic surgery and bivalirudin for use in percutaneous interventions.

Long-term anticoagulation – Prolonged administration of low molecular weight heparins and of warfarin has been evaluated to prolong the benefit of anticoagulants past the acute phase and prevent reactivation of the disease. In the ATACS trial, 214 patients were randomized to ASA alone or the combination of ASA plus UFH followed by warfarin. At 14 days, there was a reduction in the composite outcome of death, MI, and recurrent ischemia with the combination therapy (27·0% *v* 10·5%; *P* = 0·004). In a small randomized pilot study of 57 patients allocated to warfarin or placebo in addition to ASA, there was less progression and more regression in the severity of the culprit lesion after a few weeks of treatment with warfarin. The OASIS pilot study[157] compared a fixed dosage of 3 mg of warfarin with a moderate dose titrated to an international normalized ratio (INR) of 2 to 2·5 administered for 7 months. Low-intensity warfarin had no benefit, whereas the moderate-intensity regimen reduced the risk of death, MI, or refractory angina by 58% and the need for rehospitalization for unstable angina by 58%. These results were not reproduced in the larger OASIS-2 trial[40] which randomized 3712 patients to the moderate-intensity regimen. The rate of cardiovascular death, MI, or stroke after 5 months was 7·65% with the anticoagulant and 8·4% without ($P = 0·37$). The authors suggested that poor compliance with treatment in some countries could have explained the negative results. A meta-analysis of 30 randomized studies published between 1960 and July 1999 among patients with CAD showed that high-intensity and moderate-intensity anticoagulation were effective in reducing MI and stroke but increased the risk of bleeding. In the presence of aspirin, low-intensity anticoagulation was not superior to aspirin alone, while moderate- to high-intensity anticoagulation and aspirin versus aspirin alone appeared promising with a modest increase in bleeding risk.[159]

A meta-analysis of prolonged use of low molecular weight heparin for up to 3 months after hospital discharge showed no consistent benefit (OR 0·98; 95% CI 0·81–1·17; $P = 0·80$) but an excess risk of major bleeding (OR 2·26; 95% CI 1·63–3·14; $P < 0·0001$).[160] In FRISC-II, dalteparin was administrated double-blind for 3 months following 5 days of open label administration. A significant reduction in rates of death, MI, and revascularization was observed after 30 days (3·1% v 5·9%; RR 0·53; $P = 0·02$) and 3 months (29·1% v 33·4%; $P = 0·03$), which was not sustained at 6 months.[161]

Coronary reperfusion procedures

Reperfusion therapy is increasingly successful as expertise, adjunctive pharmacotherapies, and technology are improving. It is a common clinical experience that reperfusion is the only effective means to control the unstable patient. It has also been long recognized that interventions are associated with a higher risk of complications when performed early during an unstable coronary condition and which are attenuated when interventions can be delayed past a period of medical stabilization. This early hazard can now be minimized with the use of coronary stenting and of ticlopidine or clopidogrel, and of the Gp IIb/IIIa antagonists. Modern trials are comparing treatment strategies randomizing patients to an early invasive or an early conservative management strategy. In the early invasive approach, coronary angiography is routinely performed followed by revascularization with either PCI or CABG; the choice of procedures is

governed by expert judgment. In the early non-invasive approach, coronary angiography is performed only when there is evidence of recurrent spontaneous ischemia or when the ischemia can be induced by a provocative test, the criteria for evaluation being more or less stringent. Earlier trials that had compared CABG to medical therapy failed to show a difference in mortality with the two treatment strategies but succeeded in identifying subgroups of patients with depressed ejection fraction and with three vessel disease that benefitted significantly from surgery. Short- and long-term quality of life was also generally improved with reperfusion, and crossovers from medical therapy to CABG were frequent.[162–164]

The results of four major recent trials and of a few smaller trials comparing early invasive management to early conservative management were reported. The TIMI-3b randomized 1473 patients. The primary outcome of death, MI or an unsatisfactory symptom-limited exercise stress test performed at 6 weeks occurred in 18·1% of patients assigned to the early conservative strategy and 16·2% of patients assigned to the early invasive strategy (NS). The average length of initial hospitalization, the incidence of rehospitalization within 6 weeks, and days of rehospitalization were all decreased in the early invasive group.[165]

In the VANQWISH trial, 920 patients with a NSTEMI on the basis of CK-MB elevation were randomized within 72 hours of admission. More patients in the early invasive group experienced inhospital death (21 v 6; $P = 0·007$) or a composite of death or MI (36 v 15; $P = 0·004$); statistically significant differences persisted at 1 year and a trend towards higher mortality was still observed at 2 years.[166] The results of this study were questioned on the basis of the high mortality associated with CABG; no mortality was seen with PCI.

The MATE trial assigned 201 ACS patients ineligible for thrombolytic therapy to triage angiography within 24 hours, or early conservative strategy. Follow up at a median of 21 months showed no significant difference in the cumulative incidence of death, MI, rehospitalization, or revascularization between the two groups.[167] In the VINO study, 131 patients were randomized to first day angiography/angioplasty or conservative strategy. Death by 6 months occurred in 3·1% of invasive patients versus 13·4% of conservative patients ($P < 0·03$) and non-fatal MI in 3·1% and 14·9% ($P < 0·02$) respectively.[168]

More recently, the FRISC-II study enrolled 2457 patients with chest pain within the previous 48 hours and ST or T wave changes or elevated troponin T or CK-MB.[43] All patients received dalteparin in addition to aspirin in the first 5 days and were thereafter randomized to placebo or continued dalteparin administration for 3 months. Coronary angiography was done within the first 7 days in 96% of patients in the invasive arm and in 10% in the non-invasive arm, and revascularization was performed within the first

10 days in 71% and 9% of patients respectively. After 6 months there was a decrease in the composite end point of death or MI in the invasive group (9·4% v 12·1%; RR 0·78; 95% CI 0·62–0·98; $P<0·031$) (Figure 30.15). At 1 year the mortality rate in the invasive strategy group was 2·2% compared with 3·9% in the non-invasive strategy group ($P= 0·016$).[169] There was a heterogeneous effect of the invasive strategies, which provided greater advantages at older age, in men, and with longer duration of angina, chest pain at rest, and ST-segment depression or Troponin-T elevation. The frequencies of symptomatic angina and readmission were halved by the invasive strategy. It was concluded that patients who first received an average of 6 days of treatment with LMWH, ASA, nitrates, and β blockers have a better outcome at 6 months.

The TACTICS trial enrolled 2220 patients with non-ST-segment elevation ACS characterized by ST-T changes suggestive of ischemia or elevated levels of cardiac markers or a history of coronary artery disease.[44] All patients received aspirin, heparin, and tirofiban. In the invasive arm, routine coronary angiography was performed within 4 to 48 hours and revascularization as appropriate. The primary outcome of death, non-fatal MI, or rehospitalization for an acute coronary syndrome at 6 months was 15·9% with use of the early invasive strategy and 19·4% with use of the conservative strategy (OR 0·78; 95% CI 0·62–0·97; $P= 0·025$). The rate of death or non-fatal MI at 6 months was similarly reduced (7·3% v 9·5%; OR 0·74; 95% CI 0·54–1·00; $P<0·05$) (Figure 30.15). As in the FRISC-II trial, the patients who benefitted were those at medium or high risk, as defined by an elevation of TnT greater than 0·01 ng/ml, the presence of ST-segment deviation, or a TIMI risk score of greater than 3. In the absence of these high-risk features, outcomes in patients assigned to the two strategies were similar. Women in the FRISC-II trial derived no benefit from invasive management.[48] They were older, yet had less severe CAD and a better prognosis compared with men. Such a gender difference was not present in the TACTICS trial,[48] suggesting that the differences were related to baseline risk. Rates of major bleeding were similar, and lengths of hospital stay were reduced in patients assigned to the invasive strategy.

Thus, the two most recent trials comparing invasive versus conservative strategies in patients with non-ST-segment elevation ACS showed a benefit in patients assigned to the invasive strategy using state-of-the-art pharmacologic therapy and stenting in the majority of cases. In FRISC-II, the invasive strategy involved treatment for an average of 6 days in the hospital with ASA and dalteparin. In TACTICS–TIMI-18, treatment included ASA, unfractionated heparin, and tirofiban and interventions were performed earlier (mean 22 h). A routine invasive management strategy is therefore recommended in patients with a non-ST-segment elevation ACS with high-risk features characterized by

elevation of troponin levels, ST-segment ischemic changes or a high risk score determined by the global clinical evaluation. **Grade A** These patients also require aggressive antithrombotic therapy. **Grade A** Drugs that have been shown to be useful in randomized placebo-controlled studies include aspirin, clopidogrel, heparin, dalteparin, bivaluridin, and the Gp IIb/IIa antagonists eptifibatide and tirofiban in medical management and abciximab and eptifibatide in patients undergoing percutaneous intervention. **Grade A** Direct comparisons of the various drugs have shown superiority of enoxaparin over unfractionated heparin,[34,44] and over tinzaparin,[170] and of abciximab over tirofiban when administered in the cardiac catheterization laboratory before procedures. The combination of enoxaparin with eptifibatide[171] and with tirofiban[172] has been shown to be at least as effective and safe as the combination with unfractionated heparin. No direct comparisons, however, have been conducted between the various regimens that have been shown to be useful in non-ST-segment elevation ACS. Thus, the relative benefits of the combination of aspirin and clopidogrel (CURE regimen) versus the combination of aspirin and a Gp IIb/IIa antagonist (PURSUIT and PRISM-PLUS regimen), versus the combination of enoxaparin and ASA (ESSENCE regimen), are unknown. Further, the potential benefits of various drug combinations, such as for example ASA and enoxaparin with clopidogrel or with a Gp IIb/IIIa antagonist, have not been studied. Also, uncertainties exist as to the optimal timing for performing interventions. FRISC-II employed a delayed intervention strategy and TACTICS an accelerated strategy. Many centers used an immediate intervention strategy. On the other hand, no early routine invasive procedure was used in the CURE trial. The PCI–CURE study was designed to characterize prospectively the event rates in patients who underwent PCI in the trial. A total of 1313 patients, 21·2% of the total population, had such an intervention a median of 10 days after randomization; in 65% of patients, it was performed during the initial hospitalization, a median of 6 days after randomization. Open labeled ticlopidine or clopidogrel was administered during PCI and for 4 weeks thereafter. The primary end point of cardiovascular death, MI, or urgent target vessel revascularization within 30 days of PCI occurred in 4·5% of patients in the clopidogrel group compared with 6·4% in the placebo group (RR 0·70; 95% CI 0·50–0·97; $P= 0·03$). There was also less use of Gp IIb/IIIa inhibitor in the clopidogrel group ($P= 0·001$).[173] These results may suggest that more prolonged administration of clopidogrel before percutaneous interventions could amplify the benefit, possibly by more complete plaque passivation. Thus, much evidence remains to be acquired to define the optimal modalities for medical and invasive management of patients with non-ST-segment elevation ACS. In the mean time, the best current evidence dictates the use of a combination of ASA and clopidogrel, **Grade A** plus unfractionated heparin or low molecular weight heparin, **Grade A** plus a Gp IIb/IIIa antagonist in the patients remaining unstable and referred for an interventional procedure. **Grade A** An early invasive management approach is recommended for patients with ST-segment shifts or an elevation of troponin T or I. **Grade A** Enoxaparin is preferred over unfractionated heparin when the primary emphasis is placed on medical management with no immediate intervention planned, **Grade A** and caution is advised in the use of clopidogrel in patients with immediate PCI and a possibility of rapid CABG. **Grade A** In the low-risk patients with no ischemic changes, no troponin elevation and no recurrent ischemia, risk stratification with a treadmill or another provocative test is recommended. **Grade A**

Case series support the use of the intra-aortic balloon pump as a bridge to PCI or CABG to stabilize hemodynamically unstable patients and patients with severe recurrent ischemia on treatment. **Grade B**

Cell protection

Cell necrosis is a significant problem in patients with a non-ST-segment elevation acute coronary syndrome, as close to 50% of patients have some degree of necrosis at admission and 5–15% develop a new myocardial infarction within a few weeks (Figure 30.5). Reperfusion procedures are frequently associated with myocardial infarction and there is a correlation between subsequent mortality and elevation of blood markers of necrosis, even within the range of only one and three times normal.[174] Measures that could prevent or halt the progression of myocardial cell ischemia to necrosis could therefore optimize the benefit of current treatment strategies (see Figure 30.9).[91] These have been investigated mainly in evolving ST-segment elevation MI, with the goal of reducing infarct size. A number of interventions have been shown to be protective in experimental models of ischemia reperfusion. None of these interventions, however, have translated into relevant benefit in humans. Beta blockers were shown in a meta-analysis to be of moderate benefit to prevent myocardial infarction in patients with threatened myocardial infarction.[108] A recent trial with cariporide, an inhibitor of the Na^+/H^+ exchanger that prevents the accumulation of anions within the ischemic cell, failed to prevent myocardial infarction in patients with a non-ST-segment elevation ACS and in patients undergoing high-risk percutaneous interventions.[175] Pilot studies with antibodies against leukocyte integrins and against the cytokine tissue necrosis factor α (TNF-α) suggested no reductions of infarct size.[176]

Plaque passivation

An attractive treatment strategy for acute coronary syndromes is control of inflammatory processes associated with plaque degradation that result in plaque rupture and thrombus formation (see Figure 30.9). In principle, these therapies could be applied before, during or after the rupture. Since there are no means to easily and reliably identify vulnerable plaques, administration of these therapies before the clinical manifestations of acute coronary syndromes is not practicable. On the other hand, secondary preventive measures applied past the very acute phase, as will be discussed in the next section, are rewarding, particularly statin therapy and control of risk factors. Percutaneous interventions including stent implantation are very effective during the acute process, possibly by interrupting some of the processes implicated in the disease. A 48 hour course of methylprednisone in a small pilot study in patients with unstable angina was ineffective to prevent ischemic events and even accelerated their manifestations.[177] Statins and ACE inhibitors can promote plaque stabilization by their anti-inflammatory, antioxidant, anti-cell proliferative and anticoagulant properties.[178]

Many trials and registries have shown that statins started 2–10 days after an ACS are well tolerated and associated with reductions in total and low density lipoprotein cholesterol. In pooled observational data of 20 809 ACS patients enrolled in clinical trials, the presence of lipid lowering therapy at hospital discharge was associated with a 56% reduction in risk of mortality at 1 month ($P = 0.001$).[179] A Swedish registry of 5528 AMI survivors reported a 1 year mortality of 9.3% in the 14 071 patients who had no statin at hospital discharge and of 4.0% in the 5528 patients with a statin.[180]

In a small randomized trial, the initiation of pravastatin 6 days after the acute phase was associated with a significant reduction in the incidence of major cardiovascular events at 2 years ($P < 0.03$).[181] The MIRACL study was the first large-scale clinical trial to investigate early treatment with a statin in patients with an ACS.[182] A total of 3086 patients with no interventions anticipated were randomized within 24–96 hours of hospital admission to high-dose atorvastatin or placebo. The primary outcome of death, non-fatal MI, resuscitated cardiac arrest or worsening angina requiring urgent rehospitalization occurred at 16 weeks in 14.8% of treated patients and 17.4% of placebo patients (RR 0.84; $P = 0.048$). The benefit was limited to the reduction of the outcome of worsening angina and there were no significant differences in the risk of death, non-fatal MI, or cardiac arrest. The survival curves diverged after a few weeks. The MIRACL trial showed no definitive evidence of an early benefit for statins. Nevertheless, until the results of ongoing trials are known, it is recommended to initiate statin therapy in hospital, before hospital discharge. **Grade B** This approach increases the likelihood that patients will continue to comply with statin therapy and results in a greater percentage of patients using a statin after one year.[183] Numerous large-scale trials have documented marked benefits of statins used in primary and secondary prevention.

Subacute therapy

Those patients who respond quickly to optimal medical therapy in hospital, and who are found to be at relatively low risk based upon a variety of prognostic factors and non-invasive testing, require long-term follow up. Once they have stabilized for about 24–48 hours in hospital, with no ischemic pain recurrence, intravenous nitrate therapy is generally tapered with the substitution of oral or topical nitrates. The early efficacy of β blockers, and evidence for long-term benefits in patients following MI[184] and with stable ischemia, suggest that the therapy should be continued indefinitely. Similar analogies appear reasonable if a rate-limiting calcium antagonist was chosen because of contraindications to a β blocker, although there is no good evidence for long-term benefit in terms of major cardiovascular outcomes. If large doses of β blocker or calcium antagonists, or combined therapy, were required for control of the ischemic episodes, judicious decrements of intensity are likely to be appropriate once the patient is fully mobilized and non-invasive testing has indicated that revascularization is not obligatory. **Grade A**

The evidence from the initial trials of aspirin for unstable angina[121] demonstrated ongoing benefit for up to 2 years, consistent with evidence in survivors of MI and patients with stable angina.[123] Accordingly, aspirin should be continued indefinitely. Clopidogrel, 75 mg daily should be started on admission, and continued for at least 9–12 months, in conjunction with aspirin. **Grade A1b** For those patients intolerant of aspirin, clopidogrel alone is likely to be efficacious. **Grade A** Heparin should be sustained for at least 48 hours following the resolution of acute ischemic episodes.[148] Low molecular weight heparins appear to be at least as efficacious as unfractionated heparin and may be preferable in terms of ease of use and cost–benefit considerations. They have generally been used in clinical trials for longer periods of time than unfractionated heparin and can therefore be administered until hospital discharge. **Grade C** Clinical trials of oral Gp IIb/IIIa receptor antagonists have demonstrated no benefit and potential harm from these agents. **Grade A**

Early attention to optimal management of coronary risk factors is mandatory as their control is definitively of benefit. **Grade A** It is recommended to initiate a statin in hospital. **Grade A1c** The HPS study showed benefit independently of initial cholesterol levels.[185]

Recent evidence indicates that tight control of glucose in patients with type 2 diabetes reduces the risk of death following MI and among patients with newly detected type 2 diabetes.[186–188] The recurrence of an unstable phase of coronary artery disease or poor symptomatic control in patients being managed on medical therapy generally mandates reconsideration of the option of revascularization **Grade A** and, if not feasible, alternative medical therapy and the consideration

of possible aspirin failure. **Grade B** Risk factor management is of great importance in those patients who have undergone revascularization and is focused on limiting progression of disease in non-revascularized vessels and in areas of percutaneous intervention and bypass conduits. The long-term use of an ACE inhibitor is likely to be beneficial in all but the lowest-risk patients who have experienced non-ST-segment elevation acute coronary syndromes.[189] **Grade A**

References

1. Fowler NO. "Preinfarctional" angina: a need for an objective definition and for a controlled clinical trial of its management. *Circulation* 1971;**44**:755–8.
2. Wood P. Therapeutic application of anticoagulants. *Trans Med Soc Lond* 1948;**66**:80.
3. Fuster V, Steele PM, Chesebro JH. Role of platelets and thrombosis in coronary atherosclerotic disease and sudden death. *J Am Coll Cardiol* 1985;**5**:175B–184B.
4. Davies MJ and Thomas A. Thrombosis and acute coronary artery lesions in sudden cardiac ischemic death. *N Engl J Med* 1984;**310**:1137–40.
5. Davies M, Thomas A, Knapman P, Hangartner R. Intramyocardial platelet aggregation in patients with unstable angina suffering sudden ischaemic cardiac death. *Circulation* 1986;**73**:418–27.
6. Falk E. Unstable angina with fatal outcome: dynamic coronary thrombosis leading to infarction and/or sudden death: autopsy evidence of recurrent mural thrombosis with peripheral embolization culminating in total coronary occlusion. *Circulation* 1985;**71**:699–708.
7. Falk E. Plaque rupture with severe pre-existing stenosis precipitating coronary thrombosis. Characteristics of coronary atherosclerotic plaque underlying fatal occlusive thrombi. *Br Heart J* 1983;**50**:127–34.
8. DeWood MA, Spores J, Notske R *et al.* Prevalence of total coronary occlusion during the early hours of transmural myocardial infarction. *N Engl J Med* 1980;**303**:897–902.
9. Braunwald E, Antman EM, Beasley JW *et al.* ACC/AHA guidelines for the management of patients with unstable angina-non-ST-segment elevation myocardial infarction: a report of the American College of Cardiology/American Heart Association Task Force on Practice Guidelines (Committee on the Management of Patients With Unstable Angina). 2002. Available at: http://www.acc.org/clinical/guidelines/unstable/unstable.pdf
10. Braunwald E. Unstable angina. A classification. *Circulation* 1989;**80**:410–14.
11. Antman EM, Braunwald E. Acute myocardial infarction. In: Braunwald E, Zipes DP, Libby P, eds. *Heart disease: a textbook of cardiovascular medicine*. Philadelphia: WB Saunders, 2001.
12. The Joint European Society of Cardiology/American College of Cardiology Committee. Myocardial infarction redefined – a consensus document of the Joint European Society of Cardiology/American College of Cardiology Committee for the

redefinition of myocardial infarction. *J Am Coll Cardiol* 2000;**36**:959–69.

13. Hamm CW, Braunwald E. A classification of unstable angina revisited. *Circulation* 2000;**102**:118–22.

14. Nourjah P. National Hospital Ambulatory Medical Care Survey: 1997 emergency department summary. Advance data from Vital and Health Statistics. Hyattsville, MD: National Center for Health Statistics, 1999;**304**.

15. National Center for Health Statistics. Detailed diagnoses and procedures. National Hospital Discharge Survey, 1996.

16. Data from Vital and Health Statistics. Hyattsville, MD: National Center for Health Statistics, 1998;**13**.

17. Bata IR, Gregor RD, Eastwood BJ, Wolf HK. Trends in the incidence of acute myocardial infarction between 1984 and 1993 – The Halifax County MONICA Project. *Can J Cardiol* 2000;**16**:589–95.

18. Volmink JA, Newton JN, Hicks NR, Sleight P, Fowler GH, Neil HA. Coronary event and case fatality rates in an English population: results of the Oxford myocardial infarction incidence study. The Oxford Myocardial Infarction Incidence Study Group. *Heart* 1998;**80**:40–4.

19. Madsen M, Rasmussen S, Juel K. [Acute myocardial infarction in Denmark. Incidence development and prognosis during a 20-year period]. *Ugeskr Laeger* 2000;**162**:5918–23.

20. van der Pal-de Bruin KM, Verkleij H, Jansen J, Bartelds A, Kromhout D. The incidence of suspected myocardial infarction in Dutch general practice in the period 1978–1994. *Eur Heart J* 1998;**19**:429–34.

21. Fox KA, Cokkinos DV, Deckers J, Keil U, Maggioni A, Steg G. The ENACT study: a pan-European survey of acute coronary syndromes. European Network for Acute Coronary Treatment. *Eur Heart J* 2000;**21**:1440–9.

22. Goldberg RJ, Steg PG, Sadiq I *et al.* Extent of, and factors associated with, delay to hospital presentation in patients with acute coronary disease (the GRACE registry). *Am J Cardiol* 2002;**89**:791–6.

23. Furman MI, Dauerman HL, Goldberg RJ, Yarzebski J, Lessard D, Gore JM. Twenty-two year (1975 to 1997) trends in the incidence, in-hospital and long-term case fatality rates from initial Q-wave and non-Q-wave myocardial infarction: a multi-hospital, community-wide perspective. *J Am Coll Cardiol* 2001; **37**:1571–80.

24. Braunwald E, Mark DB, Jones RH *et al.* Unstable angina: diagnosis and management. Clinical practice guideline, no. 10 (Agency for Health Care Policy and Research Publications No. 94: 6–2). Rockville, MD: US Department of Health and Human Services, 1994.

25. Malmberg K, Yusuf S, Gerstein HC *et al.* Impact of diabetes on long-term prognosis in patients with unstable angina and non-Q-wave myocardial infarction: results of the OASIS (Organization to Assess Strategies for Ischemic Syndromes) Registry. *Circulation* 2000;**102**:1014–19.

26. Savonitto S, Ardissino D, Granger CB *et al.* Prognostic value of the admission electrocardiogram in acute coronary syndromes. *JAMA* 1999;**281**:707–13.

27. Bogaty P, Poirier P, Simard S, Boyer L, Solymoss S, Dagenais GR. Biological profiles in subjects with recurrent acute coronary events compared with subjects with long-standing stable angina. *Circulation* 2001;**103**:3062–8.

28. Bahit MC, Granger CB, Wallentin L. Persistence of the prothrombotic state after acute coronary syndromes: implications for treatment. *Am Heart J* 2002;**143**:205–16.

29. Cairns JA, Fantus IG, Klassen GA. Unstable angina pectoris. *Am Heart J* 1976;**92**:373–86.

30. Cairns J, Singer J, Gent M *et al.* One-year mortality outcomes of all coronary and intensive care units with acute myocardial infarction, unstable angina or other chest pain in Hamilton, Canada, a city of 375 000 people. *Can J Cardiol* 1989;**5**: 239–46.

31. The RISC Group. Risk of myocardial infarction and death during treatment with low-dose aspirin and intravenous heparin in men with unstable coronary artery disease. *Lancet* 1990;**226**:827–30.

32. Theroux P, Waters D, Qiu S *et al.* Aspirin versus heparin to prevent myocardial infarction during the acute phase of unstable angina. *Circulation* 1993;**88**:2045–8.

33. The Global Use of Strategies to Open Occluded Coronary Arteries (GUSTO) IIb Investigators. A comparison of recombinant hirudin with heparin for the treatment of acute coronary syndromes. *N Engl J Med* 1996;**335**:775–82.

34. Cohen M, Demers C, Gurfinkel EP *et al.* A comparison of low molecular-weight heparin with unfractionated heparin for unstable coronary artery disease. Efficacy and Safety of Subcutaneous Enoxaparin in Non-Q-Wave Coronary Events Study Group. *N Engl J Med* 1997;**337**:447–52.

35. Platelet Receptor Inhibition for Ischemic Syndrome Management in Patients Limited by Unstable Signs and Symptoms (PRISM) Study Investigators. A comparison of aspirin plus tirofiban versus aspirin plus heparin for unstable angina. *N Engl J Med* 1998;**338**:1498–505.

36. Platelet Receptor Inhibition in Ischemic Syndrome Management in Patients Limited by Unstable Signs and Symptoms (PRISM-PLUS) Study Investigators. Inhibition of the platelet glycoprotein IIb/IIIa receptor with tirofiban in unstable angina and non-Q-wave myocardial infarction. *N Engl J Med* 1998;**338**:1488–97.

37. The PARAGON Investigators. International, randomized, controlled trial of lamifiban (a platelet glycoprotein IIb/IIIa inhibitor), heparin, or both in unstable angina. Platelet IIb/IIIa Antagonism for the Reduction of Acute Coronary Syndrome Events in a Global Organization Network. *Circulation* 1998;**97**:2386–95.

38. Mahaffey KW, Roe MT, Dyke CK *et al.* Misreporting of myocardial infarction end points: results of adjudication by a central clinical events committee in the PARAGON-B trial. Second Platelet IIb/IIIa Antagonist for the Reduction of Acute Coronary Syndrome Events in a Global Organization Network Trial. *Am Heart J* 2002;**143**:242–8.

39. PURSUIT Investigators. Inhibition of platelet glycoprotein IIb/IIIa with eptifibatide in patients with acute coronary syndromes. Platelet Glycoprotein IIb/IIIa in Unstable Angina: Receptor Suppression Using Integrilin Therapy. *N Engl J Med* 1998;**339**:436–43.

40. Organisation to Assess Strategies for Ischemic Syndromes (OASIS-2) Investigators. Effects of recombinant hirudin (lepirudin) compared with heparin on death, myocardial infarction, refractory angina, and revascularisation procedures in patients with acute myocardial ischaemia without ST elevation: a randomized trial. *Lancet* 1999;**353**:429–38.

41. Antman EM, McCabe CH, Gurfinkel EP *et al.* Enoxaparin prevents death and cardiac ischemic events in unstable angina/non-Q-wave myocardial infarction: results of the thrombolysis in myocardial infarction (TIMI) 11B trial. *Circulation* 1999;**100**:1593–601.

42. The GUSTO IV-ACS Investigators. Effect of glycoprotein IIb/IIIa receptor blocker abciximab on outcome in patients with acute coronary syndromes without early coronary revascularisation: the GUSTO IV-ACS randomized trial. *Lancet* 2001;**357**:1915–24.

43. FRISC II Investigators. Invasive compared with non-invasive treatment in unstable coronary-artery disease: FRISC II prospective randomized multicenter study. *Lancet* 1999; **354**:708–15.

44. Cannon CP, Weintraub WS, Demopoulos LA *et al.* Comparison of early invasive and conservative strategies in patients with unstable coronary syndromes treated with the glycoprotein IIb/IIIa inhibitor tirofiban. *N Engl J Med* 2001; **344**: 1879–87.

45. Jayes RL Jr, Beshansky JR, D'Agostino RB, Selker HP. Do patients' coronary risk factor reports predict acute cardiac ischemia in the emergency department? A multicenter study. *J Clin Epidemiol* 1992;**45**:621–6.

46. Sheifer SE, Manolio TA, Gersh BJ. Unrecognized myocardial infarction. *Ann Intern Med* 2001;**135**:801–11.

47. Hochman JS, Tamis JE, Thompson TD *et al.* Sex, clinical presentation, and outcome in patients with acute coronary syndromes. Global Use of Strategies to Open Occluded Coronary Arteries in Acute Coronary Syndromes IIb Investigators. *N Engl J Med* 1999;**341**:226–32.

48. Lagerqvist B, Safstrom K, Stahle E, Wallentin L, Swahn E. Is early invasive treatment of unstable coronary artery disease equally effective for both women and men? FRISC II Study Group Investigators. *J Am Coll Cardiol* 2001;**38**:41–8.

49. Lesperance F, Frasure-Smith N, Juneau M, Theroux P. Depression and 1-year prognosis in unstable angina. *Arch Intern Med* 2000;**160**:1354–60.

50. Hamm CW, Ravkilde J, Gerhardt W *et al.* The prognostic value of serum troponin T in unstable angina. *N Engl J Med* 1992;**327**:146–50.

51. Antman EM, Tanasijevic MJ, Thompson B *et al.* Cardiac-specific troponin I levels to predict the risk of mortality in patients with acute coronary syndromes. *N Engl J Med* 1996;**335**:1342–9.

52. Lindahl B, Venge P, Armstrong P *et al.* Troponin-T 0·03 μg/l is the most appropriate cut-off level between high and low risk acute coronary syndrome patients: prospective verification in a large cohort of placebo patients from the GUSTO-IV ACS study. *J Am Coll Cardiol* 2001;**37**(Suppl. A):326A.

53. Lindahl B, Venge P, Wallentin L. Relation between troponin T and the risk of subsequent cardiac events in unstable coronary artery disease. The FRISC study group. *Circulation* 1996; **93**:1651–7.

54. Olatidoye AG, Wu AH, Feng YJ, Waters D. Prognostic role of troponin T versus troponin I in unstable angina pectoris for cardiac events with meta-analysis comparing published studies. *Am J Cardiol* 1998;**81**:1405–10.

55. Ottani F, Galvani M, Nicolini FA *et al.* Elevated cardiac troponin levels predict the risk of adverse outcome in patients with acute coronary syndromes. *Am Heart J* 2000;**140**: 917–27.

56. Heidenreich PA, Alloggiamento T, Melsop K, McDonald KM, Go AS, Hlatky MA. The prognostic value of troponin in patients with non-ST elevation acute coronary syndromes: a meta-analysis. *J Am Coll Cardiol* 2001;**38**:478–85.

57. Hamm CW, Heeschen C, Goldmann B *et al.* Benefit of abciximab in patients with refractory unstable angina in relation to serum troponin T levels. c7E3 Fab Antiplatelet Therapy in Unstable Refractory Angina (CAPTURE) Study Investigators. *N Engl J Med* 1999;**340**:1623–9.

58. Morrow DA, Antman EM, Tanasijevic M *et al.* Cardiac troponin I for stratification of early outcomes and the efficacy of enoxaparin in unstable angina: a TIMI-11B substudy. *J Am Coll Cardiol* 2000;**36**:1812–17.

59. Morrow DA, Cannon CP, Rifai N *et al.* The TACTICS-TIMI 18 Investigators. Ability of minor elevations of troponins I and T to predict benefit from an early invasive strategy in patients with unstable angina and non-ST elevation myocardial infarction: results from a randomized trial. *JAMA* 2001;**286**: 2405–12.

60. Langer A, Freeman MR, Armstrong PW. ST segment shift in unstable angina: pathophysiology and association with coronary anatomy and hospital outcome. *J Am Coll Cardiol* 1989;**13**:1495–502.

61. Cannon CP, McCabe CH, Stone PH *et al.* The electrocardiogram predicts one-year outcome of patients with unstable angina and non-Q wave myocardial infarction: results of the TIMI III Registry ECG Ancillary Study. Thrombolysis in Myocardial Ischemia. *J Am Coll Cardiol* 1997;**30**:133–40.

62. Kaul P, Fu Y, Chang WC *et al.* Prognostic value of ST-segment depression in acute coronary syndromes: insights from PARAGON-A applied to GUSTO-IIb. *J Am Coll Cardiol* 2001; **38**:64–71.

63. Hyde TA, French JK, Wong CK *et al.* Four-year survival of patients with acute coronary syndromes without ST segment elevation and prognostic significance of 0·5-mm ST segment depression. *Am J Cardiol* 1999;**84**:379–85.

64. de Zwaan C, Bär FW, Janssen JHA *et al.* Angiographic and clinical characteristics of patients with unstable angina showing an ECG pattern indicating critical narrowing of the proximal LAD coronary artery. *Am Heart J* 1989;**117**:657–65.

65. Cohen M, Hawkins L, Greenberg S, Fuster V. Usefulness of ST-segment changes in >2 leads on the emergency room electrocardiogram in either unstable angina pectoris or non-Q-wave myocardial infarction in predicting outcome. *Am J Cardiol* 1991;**67**:1368–73.

66. Armstrong PW, Fu Y, Chang WC *et al.* Acute coronary syndromes in the GUSTO-IIb trial. Prognostic insights and impact of recurrent ischemia. *Circulation* 1998;**98**:1860–8.

67. Boersma E, Pieper KS, Steyerberg EW *et al.* Predictors of outcome in patients with acute coronary syndromes without persistent ST-segment elevation. Results from an international trial of 9461 patients. The PURSUIT Investigators. *Circulation* 2000;**101**:2557–67.

68. Antman EM, Cohen M, Bernink PJ *et al.* The TIMI risk score for unstable angina/non-ST elevation MI: a method for prognostication and therapeutic decision-making. *JAMA* 2000; **284**:835–42.

69. Morrow DA, Antman EM, Snapinn S *et al.* An integrated clinical approach to predicting the benefit of tirofiban in non-ST elevation acute coronary syndromes: application of the TIMI

risk score for UA/NSTEMI in PRISM-PLUS. *Eur Heart J* 2002;**23**:223–9.

70. Ridker PM, Glynn RJ, Hennekens CH. C-reactive protein adds to the predictive value of total and HDL cholesterol in determining risk of first myocardial infarction. *Circulation* 1998;**97**:2007–11.

71. Liuzzo G, Biasucci LM, Gallimore JR *et al.* Enhanced inflammatory response in patients with pre-infarction unstable angina. *J Am Coll Cardiol* 1999;**34**:1696–703.

72. Biasucci LM, Liuzzo G, Grillo RL *et al.* Elevated levels of C-reactive protein at discharge in patients with unstable angina predict recurrent instability. *Circulation* 1999;**99**: 855–60.

73. Toss H, Lindahl B, Siegbahn A *et al.* Prognostic influence of increased fibrinogen and C-reactive protein levels in unstable coronary artery disease. FRISC Study Group. Fragmin during Instability in Coronary Artery Disease. *Circulation* 1997; **96**:4204–10.

74. Heeschen C, Hamm CW, Bruemmer J *et al.* Predictive value of C-reactive protein and troponin T in patients with unstable angina: a comparative analysis. CAPTURE Investigators. Chimeric c7E3 AntiPlatelet Therapy in Unstable angina REfractory to standard treatment trial. *J Am Coll Cardiol* 2000;**35**:1535–42.

75. Haverkate F, Thompson SG, Pyke SD *et al.* Production of C-reactive protein and risk of coronary events in stable and unstable angina. European Concerted Action on Thrombosis and Disabilities Angina Pectoris Study Group. *Lancet* 1997;**349**:462–6.

76. Lindahl B, Toss H, Siegbahn A *et al.* Markers of myocardial damage and inflammation in relation to long-term mortality in unstable coronary artery disease. FRISC Study Group. Fragmin during Instability in Coronary Artery Disease. *N Engl J Med* 2000;**343**:1139–47.

77. Morrow DA, Rifai N, Antman EM *et al.* C-reactive protein is a potent predictor of mortality independently of and in combination with troponin T in acute coronary syndromes: a TIMI 11A substudy. Thrombolysis in Myocardial Infarction. *J Am Coll Cardiol* 1998;**31**:1460–5.

78. Ridker PM, Rifai N, Clearfield M *et al.* Measurement of C-reactive protein for the targeting of statin therapy in the primary prevention of acute coronary events. *N Engl J Med* 2001;**344**:1959–65.

79. Ridker PM, Cushman M, Stampfer MJ *et al.* Inflammation, aspirin, and the risk of cardiovascular disease in apparently healthy men. *N Engl J Med* 1997;**336**:973–9.

80. Buffon A, Liuzzo G, Biasucci LM *et al.* Preprocedural serum levels of C-reactive protein predict early complications and late restenosis after coronary angioplasty. *J Am Coll Cardiol* 1999;**34**:1512–21.

81. Chew DP, Bhatt DL, Robbins MA *et al.* Incremental prognostic value of elevated baseline C-reactive protein among established markers of risk in percutaneous coronary intervention. *Circulation* 2001;**104**:992–7.

82. Milazzo D, Biasucci LM, Luciani N *et al.* Elevated levels of C-reactive protein before coronary artery bypass grafting predict recurrence of ischemic events. *Am J Cardiol* 1999;**84**:459–61.

83. Theroux P, Fuster V. Acute coronary syndromes: unstable angina and non-Q-wave myocardial infarction. *Circulation* 1998;**97**:1195–206.

84. Libby P, Ridker PM, Maseri A. Inflammation and atherosclerosis. *Circulation* 2002;**105**:1135–43.

85. Libby P. Current concepts of the pathogenesis of the acute coronary syndromes. *Circulation* 2001;**104**:365–72.

86. Arbustini E, Bello BD, Morbini P *et al.* Plaque erosion is a major substrate for coronary thrombosis in acute myocardial infarction. *Heart* 1999;**82**:269–72.

87. Frink RJ. Chronic ulcerated plaques: new insights into the pathogenesis of acute coronary disease. *J Invas Cardiol* 1994;**6**:173–85.

88. Tracy RE, Devaney K, Kissling G. Characteristics of the plaque under a coronary thrombus. *Virchows Arch A Pathol Anat Histopathol* 1985;**405**:411–27.

89. Goldstein JA, Demetriou D, Grines CL, Pica M, Shoukfeh M, O'Neill WW. Multiple complex coronary plaques in patients with acute myocardial infarction. *N Engl J Med* 2000; **343**:915–22.

90. The TIMI IIIA Investigators. Early effects of tissue-type plasminogen activator added to conventional therapy on the culprit coronary lesion in patients with ischemic cardiac pain at rest. Results of the Thrombolysis in Myocardial Ischemia (TIMI IIIA) Trial. *Circulation* 1993;**87**:38–52.

91. Theroux P. Myocardial cell protection: a challenging time for action and a challenging time for clinical research. *Circulation* 2000;**101**:2874–6.

92. Orlander R. Use of nitrates in the treatment of unstable and variant angina. *Drugs* 1987;**33**:131–9.

93. Gobel EJAM, Hautvast RWH, van Gilst WH *et al.* Randomized, double-blind trial of intravenous diltiazem versus glyceral tinitrate for unstable angina pectoris. *Lancet* 1995;**346**:1653–7.

94. Jugdutt BL, Warnica JW. Intravenous nitroglycerin therapy to limit myocardial infarction size, expansions and complications. Effective timing, dosage and infarct location. *Circulation* 1988;**78**:906–20.

95. ISIS-4. A randomized factorial trial assessing early oral captopril, oral mononitrate, and intravenous magnesium sulphate in 58 050 patients with suspected myocardial infarction. *Lancet* 1995;**345**:669–85.

96. Gruppo Italiano per lo Studio della Sopravvivenze nell'Infarto Miocardico. GISSI-3: effects of lisinopril and tranidermal glyceryl trinitrate single and together on 6-week mortality and ventricular function after acute myocardial infarction. *Lancet* 1994;**343**:1115–22.

97. Cheitlin MD, Hutter AMJ, Brindis RG *et al.* ACC/AHA expert consensus document use of sildenafil (Viagra) in patients with cardiovascular disease: American College of Cardiology/American Heart Association. *J Am Coll Cardiol* 1999;**33**:273–82.

98. Muller JE, Turi ZG, Pearle DL *et al.* Nifedipine and conventional therapy for unstable angina pectoris: a randomized, double-blind comparison. *Circulation* 1984;**69**:728–39.

99. The Netherlands Interuniversity Nifedipine/Metropolol Trial (HINT) Research Group. Early treatment of unstable angina in the coronary care unit: a randomized, double-blind, placebo controlled comparison of recurrent ischemia in patients treated with nifedipine or metropolol or both. *Br Heart J* 1986;**73**:331–7.

100. Gottlieb So, Weisfeldt M, Ouyang P *et al.* Effect of the addition of propranolol to therapy with nifedipine for unstable

angina pectoris. A randomized, double-blind, placebo-controlled trial. *Circulation* 1986;**73**:331–7.

100.Gerstenblith G, Ouyang P, Achuff SC *et al.* Nifedipine in unstable angina: a double-blind, randomized trial. *N Engl J Med* 1982;**306**:885–9.

102.Furberg CD, Psaty BM, Meye JV. Nifedipine. Dose-related increase in mortality in patients with coronary heart disease. *Circulation* 1995;**92**:1326–31.

103.Theroux P, Taeymans Y, Morrissette D, Bosch Y, Pelletier GB, Waters DD. A randomized study comparing propranolol and diltiazem in the treatment of unstable angina. *J Am Coll Cardiol* 1985;**5**:717–22.

104.Andre-Fouet X, Usdin JP, Gayet CH *et al.* Comparison of short-term efficacy of diltiazem and propranolol in unstable angina at rest. A randomized trial in 70 patients. *Eur Heart J* 1983;**4**:691–8.

105.Parodi O, Maseri A, Simonetti I. Management of unstable angina by verapamil. A double-blind crossover study in CCU. *Br Heart J* 1979;**41**:167–74.

106.Mehta J, Pepine CJ, Day M, Guerrero JR, Conti CR. Short-term efficacy of oral verapamil in rest angina. A double-blind controlled trial in CCU patients. *Am J Med* 1981;**71**:977–82.

107.Scheidt S, Frishman WH, Packer M, Parodi O, Subramanian VB. Long-term effectiveness of verapamil in stable and unstable angina pectoris. One-year follow-up of patients treated in placebo-controlled double-blind randomized clinical trials. *Am J Cardiol* 1982;**50**:1185–90.

108.Yusuf S, Wittes J, Friedman L. Overview of results of randomized clinical trials in heart disease. II. Unstable angina, heart failure, primary prevention with aspirin, and risk factor modification. *JAMA* 1988;**260**:2259–63.

109.Patel DJ, Purcell HJ, Fox KM. Cardioprotection by opening of the K(ATP) channel in unstable angina. Is this a clinical manifestation of myocardial preconditioning? Results of a randomized study with nicorandil. CESAR 2 investigation. Clinical European studies in angina and revascularization. *Eur Heart J* 1999;**20**:51–7.

110.Johnson SM, Mauritson DR, Willerson JT, Hillis LD. A controlled trial of verapamil for Prinzmetal's variant angina. *N Engl J Med* 1981;**304**:862–66.

111.Capucci A, Bracchetti D, Carini GC, DiCio G, Maresta A, Magnani B. Propranolol versus verapamil in patients with unstable angina. In: Zanchetti A, Krikler DM, eds. *Calcium antagonism in cardiovascular therapy. Experience with verapamil.* Amsterdam: Excerpta Medica, 1981.

112.Parodi O, Simoneti I, Michelassi C *et al.* Comparison of verapamil and propranolol therapy for angina pectoris at rest. A randomized, multiple-crossover, controlled trial in the coronary care unit. *Am J Cardiol* 1986;**57**:899–906.

113.Rosenthal SJ, Ginsburg R, Lamb IH, Baim DS, Schroeder JS. Efficacy of diltiazem for control of symptoms of coronary artery spasm. *Am J Cardiol* 1980;**46**:1027–32.

114.Pepine CJ, Feldman RL, Whittle J, Curry RC, Conti GR. Effect of diltiazem in patients with variant angina. A randomized double-blind trial. *Am Heart J* 1981;**101**:719–25.

115.Schroeder JS, Feldman RL, Giles TD *et al.* Multiclinic controlled trial of diltiazem for Prinzmetal's variant angina. *JAMA* 1982;**72**:227–32.

116.Tilmant PY, LaBlanche JM, Thieuleux FA, Dupuis BA, Bertrand ME. Detrimental effect of propranolol in patients with coronary arterial spasm countered by combination with diltiazem. *Am J Cardiol* 1983;**52**:230–3.

117.Previtali M, Salerno J, Tavazzi L *et al.* Treatment of angina at rest with nifedipine: a short-term controlled study. *Am J Cardiol* 1980;**45**:825–30.

118.Ginsburg R, Lab IH, Schroeder JS, Hu M, Harrison DC. Randomized double-blind comparison of nifedipine and isosorbide dinitrate therapy in variant angina pectoris due to coronary artery spasm. *Am Heart J* 1982;**103**:44–8.

119.Hill JA, Feldman RI, Pepine CJ, Conti CR. Randomized double-blind comparison of nifedipine and isosorbide dinitrate in patients with coronary arterial spasm. *Am J Cardiol* 1982;**49**:431–8.

120.Rizik DG, Healy S, Margulis A *et al.* A new clinical classification for hospital prognosis of unstable angina pectoris. *Am J Cardiol* 1995;**75**:993–7.

121.Lewis HD, Davis JW, Archibald DG *et al.* Protective effects of aspirin against myocardial infarction and death in men with unstable angina. *N Engl J Med* 1983;**313**:396–403.

122.Cairns JA, Gent M, Singer J *et al.* Aspirin, sulfinpyrazone, or both in unstable angina. *N Engl J Med* 1985;**313**:1369–75.

123.Collaborative meta-analysis of randomized trials of antiplatelet therapy for prevention of death, myocardial infarction, and stroke in high-risk patients. *BMJ* 2002;**324**:71–86.

124.Patrono C, Coller B, Dalen JE *et al.* Platelet-active drugs. The relationships among dose, effectiveness, and side effects. *Chest* 2001;**119**:39S–63S.

125.Gum PA, Kottke-Marchant K, Poggio ED *et al.* Profile and prevalence of aspirin resistance in patients with cardiovascular disease. *Am J Cardiol* 2001;**88**:230–5.

126.Eikelboom JW, Hirsh J, Weitz JI, Johnston M, Yi Q, Yusuf S. Aspirin-resistant thromboxane biosynthesis and the risk of myocardial infarction, stroke, or cardiovascular death in patients at high risk for cardiovascular events. *Circulation* 2002;**105**:1650–5.

127.Catella-Lawson F, Reilly MP, Kapoor SC *et al.* Cyclooxygenase inhibitors and the antiplatelet effects of aspirin. *N Engl J Med* 2001;**345**:1809–17.

128.Cipollone F, Ciabattoni G, Patrignani P *et al.* Oxidant stress and aspirin-insensitive thromboxane biosynthesis in severe unstable angina. *Circulation* 2000;**102**:1007–13.

129.Theroux P, Latour JG, Diodati J *et al.* Hemodynamic, platelet, and clinical response to prostacycline in unstable angina pectoris. *Am J Cardiol* 1990;**65**:1084–9.

130.Cayatte AJ, Du Y, Oliver-Krasinski J, Lavielle G, Verbeuren TJ, Cohen RA. The thromboxane receptor antagonist S18886 but not aspirin inhibits atherogenesis in apo E-deficient mice. Evidence that eicosanoids other than thromboxane contribute to atherosclerosis. *Arterioscler Thromb Vasc Biol* 2000;**20**:1724–8.

131.Balsano F, Rizzon P, Violi F *et al.* Antiplatelet treatment with ticlopidine in unstable angina. *Circulation* 1990;**82**:17–26.

132.Gent M, Blakely JA, Easton JD *et al.* The Canadian American Ticlopidine Study (CATS) in thromboembolic stroke. *Lancet* 1989;**1**:1215–20.

133. Bhatt DL, Chew DP, Hirsch AT, Ringleb PA, Hacke W, Topol EJ. Superiority of clopidogrel versus aspirin in patients with prior cardiac surgery. *Circulation* 2001;**103**:363–8.

134. CAPRIE Steering Committee. A randomized, blinded, trial of clopidogrel versus aspirin in patients at risk of ischaemic events (CAPRIE). *Lancet* 1996;**348**:1329–39.

135. Yusuf S, Zhao F, Mehta SR, Chrolavicius S, Tognoni G, Fox KK. Effects of clopidogrel in addition to aspirin in patients with acute coronary syndromes without ST-segment elevation. *N Engl J Med* 2001;**345**:494–502.

136. The CURE Trial Investigators. Effects of clopidogrel in addition to aspirin in patients with acute coronary syndromes without ST-segment elevation. *N Engl J Med* 2001; **345**: 494–502.

137. The Platelet IIb/IIIa Antagonist for the Reduction of Acute Coronary Syndrome Events in a Global Organization Network (PARAGON)-B Investigators. Randomized, placebo- controlled trial of titrated intravenous lamifiban for acute coronary syndromes. *Circulation* 2002;**105**:316–21.

138. EPIC Investigators. Use of a monoclonal antibody directed against the platelet glycoprotein IIb/IIIa receptor in high-risk coronary angioplasty. *N Engl J Med* 1997;**336**: 1689–96.

139. The EPISTENT Investigators. Randomized placebo-controlled and balloon-angioplasty-controlled trial to assess safety of coronary stenting with use of platelet glycoprotein-IIb/IIIa blockade. Evaluation of Platelet IIb/IIIa Inhibitor for Stenting. *Lancet* 1998;**352**:87–92.

140. The CAPTURE Investigators. Randomized placebo-controlled trial of abciximab before and during coronary intervention in refractory unstable angina: the CAPTURE trial. *Lancet* 1997;**349**:1429–35.

141. Topol EJ, Moliterno DJ, Herrmann HC *et al.* Comparison of two platelet glycoprotein IIb/IIIa inhibitors, tirofiban and abciximab, for the prevention of ischemic events with percutaneous coronary revascularization. *N Engl J Med* 2001;**344**:1888–94.

142. The RESTORE Investigators. Randomized Efficacy Study of Tirofiban for Outcomes and REstenosis. Effects of platelet glycoprotein IIb/IIIa blockade with tirofiban on adverse cardiac events in patients with unstable angina or acute myocardial infarction undergoing coronary angioplasty. *Circulation* 1997;**96**:1445–53.

143. O'Shea JC, Hafley GE, Greenberg S *et al.* Platelet glycoprotein IIb/IIIa integrin blockade with eptifibatide in coronary stent intervention: the ESPRIT trial: a randomized controlled trial. *JAMA* 2001;**285**:2468–73.

144. Boersma E, Akkerhuis KM, Theroux P, Califf RM, Topol EJ, Simoons ML. Platelet glycoprotein IIb/IIIa receptor inhibition in non-ST-elevation acute coronary syndromes early benefit during medical treatment only, with additional protection during percutaneous coronary intervention. *Circulation* 1999;**100**:2045–8.

145. Boersma E, Harrington RA, Moliterno DJ *et al.* Platelet glycoprotein IIb/IIIa inhibitors in acute coronary syndromes: a meta-analysis of all major randomized clinical trials. *Lancet* 2002;**359**:189–98.

146. Roffi M, Chew DP, Mukherjee D *et al.* Platelet glycoprotein IIb/IIIa inhibitors reduce mortality in diabetic patients with non-ST-segment-elevation acute coronary syndromes. *Circulation* 2001;**104**:2767–71.

147. Chew DP, Bhatt DL, Sapp S, Topol EJ. Increased mortality with oral platelet glycoprotein IIb/IIIa antagonists. A meta-analysis of phase III multicenter randomized trials. *Circulation* 2001;**103**:201–6.

148. Theroux P, Waters D, Lam J, Juneau M, McCans J. Reactivation of unstable angina after the discontinuation of heparin [see comments]. *N Engl J Med* 1992;**327**: 141–5.

149. Hirsh J, Anand SS, Halperin JL, Fuster V. Guide to anticoagulant therapy. Heparin: a statement for healthcare professionals from the American Heart Association. *Circulation* 2001;**103**: 2994–3018.

150. Fragmin during Instability in Coronary Artery Disease (FRISC) study group. Low-molecular-weight heparin during instability in coronary artery disease. *Lancet* 1996;**347**: 561–8.

151. Klein W, Buchwald A, Hillis SE *et al.* Fragmin in unstable coronary artery disease study: comparison of low- molecular weight- heparin with unfractionated heparin acutely and with placebo for 6 weeks in the management of unstable coronary artery disease. *Circulation* 1997;**96**:61–8.

152. The FRAXIS Study Group. Comparison of two treatment durations (6 days and 14 days) of a low molecular weight heparin with a 6-day treatment of unfractionated heparin in the initial management of unstable angina or non-Q-wave myocardial infarction: FRAXIS (FRAXiparine in Ischaemic Syndrome). *Eur Heart J* 1999;**20**:1553–62.

153. Antman EM, Cohen M, Radley D *et al.* Assessment of the treatment effect of enoxaparin for unstable angina/non-Q-wave myocardial infarction. TIMI 11B-ESSENCE meta-analysis. *Circulation* 1999;**100**:1602–8.

154. Weitz JI, Buller HR. Direct thrombin inhibitors in acute coronary syndromes. Present and future. *Circulation* 2002;**105**: 1004–11.

155. The Global Use of Strategies to Open Occluded Coronary Arteries (GUSTO) IIa Investigators. Randomized trial of intravenous heparin versus recombinant hirudin for acute coronary syndromes. *Circulation* 1994;**90**:1631–7.

156. Antman EM. Hirudin in acute myocardial infarction. Thrombolysis and Thrombin Inhibition in Myocardial Infarction (TIMI) 9B trial. *Circulation* 1996;**94**:911–21.

157. Organization to Assess Strategies for Ischemic Syndromes (OASIS) Investigators. Comparison of the effects of two doses of recombinant hirudin compared with heparin in patients with acute myocardial ischemia without ST elevation: a pilot study. *Circulation* 1997;**96**:769–77.

158. The Direct Thrombin Inhibitor Trialists' Collaborative Group. Direct thrombin inhibitors in acute coronary syndromes: principal results of a meta-analysis based on individual patients' data. *Lancet* 2002;**359**:294–302.

159. Anand SS, Yusuf S. Oral anticoagulant therapy in patients with coronary artery disease: a meta-analysis. *JAMA* 1999; **282**: 2058–67.

160. Eikelboom JW, Anand SS, Malmberg K, Weitz JI, Ginsberg JS, Yusuf S. Unfractionated heparin and low- molecular weight-heparin in acute coronary syndrome without ST elevation: a meta-analysis. *Lancet* 2000;**355**:1936–42.

161. Fragmin and Revascularization during InStability in Coronary artery disease (FRISC II) Investigators. *Lancet* 1999;**353**: 701–7.

162. Luchi RJ, Scott SM, Deupree RH *et al.* Comparison of medical and surgical treatment for unstable angina pectoris. Results of a Veterans Administration Cooperative Study. *N Engl J Med* 1987;**316**:977–84.

163. Parisi AF, Khuri S, Deupree RH, Sharma GV, Scott SM, Luchi RJ. Medical compared with surgical management of unstable angina: 5-year mortality and morbidity in the Veterans Administration Study. *Circulation* 1989;**80**: 1176–89.

164. Booth DC, Deupree RH, Hultgren HN *et al.* Quality of life after bypass surgery for unstable angina. *Circulation* 1991;**83**: 87–95.

165. Effects of tissue plasminogen activator and a comparison of early invasive and conservative strategies in unstable angina and non-Q-wave myocardial infarction. Results of the TIMI IIIB Trial. Thrombolysis in Myocardial Ischemia. *Circulation* 1994;**89**:1545–56.

166. Boden WE, O'Rourke RA, Crawford MH *et al.* Outcomes in patients with acute non-Q-wave myocardial infarction randomly assigned to an invasive as compared with a conservative management strategy. Veterans Affairs Non-Q-Wave Infarction Strategies in Hospital (VANQWISH) Trial Investigators. *N Engl J Med* 1998;**338**:1785–92.

167. McCullough PA, O'Neill WW, Graham M *et al.* A prospective randomized trial of triage angiography in acute coronary syndromes ineligible for thrombolytic therapy. Results of the medicine versus angiography in thrombolytic exclusion (MATE) trial. *J Am Coll Cardiol* 1998;**32**: 596–605.

168. Spacek R, Straka SE, Polasek JD *et al.* Value of first day angiography/angioplasty in evolving non-ST-segment elevation myocardial infarction: an open multicenter trial. The VINO Study. *Eur Heart J* 2002;**23**: 230–8.

169. Wallentin L, Lagerqvist B, Husted S *et al.* Outcome at one year after an invasive compared with a non-invasive strategy in unstable coronary artery disease: the FRISC II invasive randomized trial. *Lancet* 2000;**356**:9–16.

170. Michalis LK, Papamichail N, Katsouras C *et al.* Enoxaparin versus tinzaparin in the management of unstable coronary artery disease (EVET Study) (Abstract). *J Am Coll Cardiol* 2001;**37**:365a.

171. Goodman S. The INTERACT trial. Presented at the ACC Scientific Sessions, Atlanta, GA, March 2002.

172. Cohen M, Theroux P, Frey MJ *et al.* Anti-thrombotic combination using tirofiban and enoxaparin: the ACUTE II Study (Abstract). *Circulation* 2000;**102**(Suppl. II):II-826.

173. Mehta SR, Yusuf S, Peters RJ *et al.* Effects of pretreatment with clopidogrel and aspirin followed by long-term therapy in patients undergoing percutaneous coronary intervention: the PCI-CURE study. *Lancet* 2001;**358**:527–33.

174. Tardiff BE, Califf RM, Tcheng JE *et al.* Clinical outcomes after detection of elevated cardiac enzymes in patients undergoing percutaneous intervention. IMPACT-II Investigators. Integrilin (eptifibatide) to Minimize Platelet Aggregation and Coronary Thrombosis-II. *J Am Coll Cardiol* 1999; **33**:88–96.

175. Theroux P, Chaitman BR, Danchin N *et al.* Inhibition of the sodium-hydrogen exchanger with cariporide to prevent myocardial infarction in high-risk ischemic situations. Main results of the GUARDIAN trial. Guard During Ischemia Against Necrosis (GUARDIAN) Investigators. *Circulation* 2000;**102**:3032–8.

176. Baran KW, Nguyen M, McKendall GR *et al.* Double-blind, randomized trial of an anti-CD18 antibody in conjunction with recombinant tissue plasminogen activator for acute myocardial infarction: limitation of myocardial infarction following thrombolysis in acute myocardial infarction (LIMIT AMI) study. *Circulation* 2001;**104**: 2778–83.

177. Azar RR, Rinfret S, Theroux P *et al.* A randomized placebo-controlled trial to assess the efficacy of anti-inflammatory therapy with methylprednisolone in unstable angina (MUNA trial). *Eur Heart J* 2000;**21**:2026–32.

178. Davignon J, Mabile L. Mechanisms of action of statins and their pleiotropic effects. *Ann Endocrinol (Paris)* 2001; **62**: 101–12.

179. Aronow HD, Topol EJ, Roe MT *et al.* Effect of lipid-lowering therapy on early mortality after acute coronary syndromes: an observational study. *Lancet* 2001;**357**:1063–8.

180. Stenestrand U, Wallentin L. Early statin treatment following acute myocardial infarction and 1-year survival. *JAMA* 2001;**285**:430–6.

181. Arntz HR, Wunderlich W, Schnitzer L. The decisive importance of cholesterol lowering therapy for coronary lesions and clinical course immediately after an acute coronary event: short and long-term results of a controlled study. *Circulation* 1998;**98**(Suppl. 1):I-45.

182. Schwartz GG, Olsson AG, Ezekowitz MD *et al.* Myocardial Ischemia Reduction with Aggressive Cholesterol Lowering (MIRACL) Study Investigators. Effects of atorvastatin on early recurrent ischemic events in acute coronary syndromes: the MIRACL study: a randomized controlled trial. *JAMA* 2001;**285**:1711–18.

183. Fonarow GC, Gawlinski A, Moughrabi S, Tillisch JH. Improved treatment of coronary heart disease by implementation of a Cardiac Hospitalization Atherosclerosis Management Program (CHAMP). *Am J Cardiol* 2001;**87**:819–22.

184. Yusuf S, Peto R, Lewis J, Collins R, Sleight P. Beta blockade during and after myocardial infarction: an overview of the randomized trials. *Progr Cardiovasc Dis* 1985;**27**:335–71.

185. Heart Protection Study Collaborative Group. MRC/BHF Heart Protection Study of cholesterol lowering with simvastatin in 20/536 high-risk individuals: a randomised placebo-controlled trial. *Lancet* 2002;**360**:7–22.

186. Malmberg K, Ryden L, Efendic S *et al.* Randomized trial of insulin-glucose infusion followed by subcutaneous insulin treatment in diabetic patients with acute myocardial infarction (DIGA-MI study): effects on mortality at 1 year. *J Am Coll Cardiol* 1995;**26**:57–65.

187. American Diabetes Association. Standards of medical care for patients with diabetes mellitus (position statement). *Diabetes Care* 1999;**22**(Suppl. 1):S32–41.

188. UK Prospective Diabetes Study Group. Tight blood pressure control and risk of macrovascular and microvascular complications in type 2 diabetes: UKPDS 38. *BMJ* 1998;**317**: 703–13.

189. Yusuf S, Sleight P, Pogue J, Bosch J, Davies R, Dagenais G. Effects of an angiotensin-converting-enzyme inhibitor, ramipril, on cardiovascular events in high-risk patients. The Heart Outcomes Prevention Evaluation Study Investigators. *N Engl J Med* 2000;**342**:145–53.

31 Fibrinolytic therapy

James S Zebrack, Jeffrey L Anderson

Impact, pathophysiology, and rationale

Over 5 million people visit US emergency departments each year for evaluation of chest pain and related symptoms, and almost 1·5 million are hospitalized for an acute coronary syndrome.[1–3] Acute myocardial infarction (AMI) is the primary discharge diagnosis in the US in 750 000 annually,[4,5] and over 225 000 deaths are attributed to AMI each year.[4] At least one half of AMI-related deaths occur within one hour of onset of symptoms and before reaching a hospital emergency department.[6] In addition, the majority of sudden cardiac deaths (300 000 annually in the US) are believed to have an ischemic basis.[7–9]

Acute reperfusion (achieved by fibrinolysis or coronary angioplasty) represents the greatest of global conceptual and practical advance for therapy ST-segment elevation (STE) AMI.[10] STE-AMI currently represents approximately one third of AMI presentations.[5,11] With broad application of reperfusion therapy, 30 day mortality rates from STE-AMI have progressively declined (from 20–30% to 5–10%).[11–14]

Herrick in the US and Obraztsov in Russia postulated almost a century ago that thrombosis-related coronary occlusion precipitates AMI.[15,16] However, controversy about the role of thrombosis continued[17–19] until 1980 when DeWood *et al*[20] demonstrated coronary occlusion in 87% of STE-AMI patients studied within 4 hours of symptom onset. The occlusion was proved to be thrombotic by observations during emergent bypass surgery or intracoronary fibrinolysis. Renewed focus on acute coronary thrombosis and reperfusion therapy ensued.

Erosion or sudden rupture of an atherosclerotic cap, weakened by internal metalloproteinase activity, has been determined to be the precipitant of coronary thrombosis.[21] Exposure of blood to collagen, other matrix elements, and the lipid core with its macrophage-derived tissue factor stimulates platelet adhesion, activation, and aggregation; thrombin generation; and fibrin formation. Vasospasm and initiation of a platelet-rich clot ensue. When these processes lead to reduction or interruption of coronary blood flow, myocardial infarction may occur. In canine models,[22,23] myocardial cell death begins within 15 minutes of coronary occlusion and proceeds rapidly in a wavefront from endocardium to epicardium. Timely reperfusion (within about 3 hours) achieves partial myocardial salvage. The rate and extent of necrosis (and salvage) is modified by metabolic demands and collateral blood supply.

The benefits of therapy depend on the rate and extent to which myocardial perfusion is effectively achieved.[24–26] Reperfusion is scored by the Thrombolysis In Myocardial Infarction (TIMI) visual[24] or frame-counts[27] supplemented, recently, by a TIMI myocardial perfusion (TMP) score.[28] Restoration of TIMI grade 3 (normal) epicardial flow is associated with lower mortality rates than TIMI grades 0–2 (3·7% *v* 7·0%).[25,28] Among those with TIMI 3 flow, lower mortality is associated with TMP grade 3 (0·7%) than with TMP grades 2 (2·9%) or 0–1 (5·4%).[28] The factors differentiating epicardial and myocardial reperfusion are incompletely understood. Platelet and platelet-leukocyte aggregates and secreted vasoactive and thrombogenic factors have received recent attention, and combinations of fibrinolytic therapy with potent platelet inhibitors to further improve myocardial perfusion are being actively studied.[29]

Early observational and controlled studies

In 1933, Tillet and Garner published their discovery of a streptococcal fibrinolysin.[30,31] Clinical application of streptokinase to AMI was first reported in 1958.[32] From then until 1979, at least 17 studies were published, but AMI pathophysiology was not well understood, and results were inconclusive and poorly accepted.[33–35] With the establishment of the thrombotic nature of coronary occlusion[20] several groups demonstrated the feasibility of clinical fibrinolysis to achieve early reperfusion under angiographic monitoring ($\cong$75% success with intracoronary [IC] SK) in the period 1976–83.[36–39]

Randomized studies in AMI followed. Anderson *et al.* reported in 1983[40] a benefit of early (<4 h) IC SK on clinical, ECG, enzymatic, and imaging end points. Later therapy (at >6 hours) relieved ischemic pain but did not benefit regional myocardial function in another study.[41] The potential for mortality benefit of IC SK was suggested by subsequent Western Washington and Dutch studies in a few hundred patients.[42–44] The logistic difficulties with intracoronary administration stimulated the re-evaluation of IV SK (Schröder *et al*[45]). By the mid-1980s, favorable comparisons with IC SK[46–48] and a larger outcomes study of

IV SK (ISAM)[49] established the intravenous route for subsequent clinical trials.

Fibrinolytic agents

General mechanisms of action and pharmacological properties

Fibrinolysis is mediated by plasmin, a non-specific serine protease that degrades clot-associated fibrin and fibrinogen, disrupting a forming thrombus, facilitating reperfusion. The fibrinolytic (or "thrombolytic") agents are all plasminogen activators, directly or indirectly converting the proenzyme plasminogen to plasmin by cleaving the arginine 560–valine 561 bond (Figure 31.1). Plasmin degrades several proteins, including fibrin, fibrinogen, prothrombin, and factors V and VII. The fibrinolytic agents differ in several properties, as summarized in the text and Table 31.1.

Approved fibrinolytic agents

Streptokinase

Streptokinase (SK) is a 415 amino acid bacterial protein sharing homology with serine proteases.[35,53] Upon

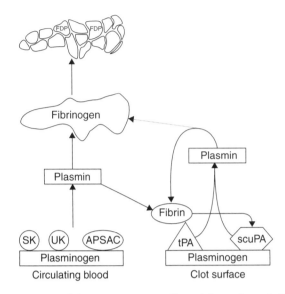

Figure 31.1 Schematic representation of the action of fibrinolytic enzymes. Streptokinase (SK), urokinase (UK), and anisoylated plasminogen streptokinase activator complex (APSAC) work predominantly on circulating plasminogen, whereas tissue type plasminogen activator (tPA) and single chain urokinase-type plasminogen activator (scuPA) are relatively clot-selective. (From Topol EJ. Clinical use of streptokinase and urokinase to treat acute myocardial infarction. *Heart Lung* 1987;**16**:760.)

Table 31.1 Comparison of fibrinolytic agents approved by the US FDA for intravenous use

	SK (Streptokinase)	APSAC (anistreplase)	tPA (alteplase)	rPA (reteplase)	TNK (tenecteplase)
Dose	1·5 million units (MU) in 30–60 min	30 U in 5 min	100 mg in 90 min[a]	10 U+10 U, 30 min apart	30–50 mg[b] over 5 seconds
Circulating half life (min)	≅20	≅100	≅6	≅18	≅20
Antigenic	Yes	Yes	No	No	No
Allergic reactions	Yes	Yes	No	No	No
Systemic fibrinogen depletion	Severe	Severe	Mild–moderate	Moderate	Minimal
Intracerebral hemorrhage	≅0·4%	≅0·6%	≅0·7%	≅0·8%	≅0·7%
Patency (TIMI-2/3) rate, 90 min[c]	≅51%	≅70%	≅73–84%	≅83%	≅77–88%
Lives saved per 100 treated	≅3[c]	≅3[d]	≅4[e]	≅4	≅4
Cost per dose (approx US dollars)	290	1700	2750	2750	2750

[a] Accelerated tPA given as follows: 15 mg bolus, then 0·75 mg/kg over 30 min (maximum, 50 mg), then 0·50 mg/kg over 60 min (maximum 35 mg).
[b] TNK is dosed by weight (supplied in 5 mg/ml vials): <60 kg = 6 ml; 61–70 kg = 7 ml; 71–80 kg = 8 ml; 81–90 kg = 9 ml; >90 kg = 10 ml.
[c] Based on Granger *et al*[50] and Bode *et al*[51]
[d] Patients with ST elevation or BBB, treated in <6 h.
[e] Based on the finding from the GUSTO trial[52] that tPA saves 1 more additional life per 100 treated than does SK.

injection, SK forms a 1:1 stoichiometric complex with plasminogen or plasmin, activating a catalytic site that cleaves plasminogen to plasmin. The half life of the SK complex is about 23 minutes. SK is antigenic, has little fibrin specificity, and causes substantial systemic lytic effects in clinical doses. Least expensive of fibrinolytics and still widely used globally, SK is administered by short-term (≤ 1 h) infusions.

Urokinase

Urokinase (UK) is a native, 2-polypeptide protein derived from human urine or renal cell cultures.[54] UK directly converts plasminogen to plasmin. It is non-antigenic and is cleared from the circulation predominantly by the liver with a half life of 16 minutes. Clinically used doses produce moderately extensive systemic fibrinolysis. Its principal use in North America has been for intra-arterial (including intra-coronary) fibrinolysis. It has not been approved for and currently is not available for IV use in AMI.

Anistreplase

Anisoylated plasminogen streptokinase activator complex (APSAC or anistreplase) was the first "designer" fibrinolytic, synthesized by complexing streptokinase with lysplasminogen and reversibly inactivating it by reacting it with the anisoyl group of a special reversible acylating agent.[55] It was tailored to allow simple injection ("bolus") delivery, more rapid onset and prolonged duration of action than SK (half life 90–105 min), with improved plasma stability and fibrin binding compared with SK. Like SK, it is antigenic and produces extensive systemic fibrinolysis. Its greater expense and bleeding risk than SK, coupled with little evidence for added benefit, has limited its clinical acceptance.

Tissue-type plasminogen activator (tPA)

Tissue-type plasminogen activator (tPA), a 526 amino acid single polypeptide chain, is the major intrinsic (physiological) plasminogen activator.[56] The marketed form (alteplase) is manufactured by recombinant DNA technology (rtPA). tPA is converted by plasmin to a double-chain form with equivalent fibrinolytic activity.[57] tPA has greater activity in the locale of the thrombus and causes less systemic plasminemia, fibrinogenolysis, and proteolysis than SK. tPA is non-antigenic, is inhibited by a circulating plasminogen activator inhibitor (PAI-1), and is rapidly cleared (half life about 5 minutes). This short half life has necessitated bolus/infusion regimens (over 1–3 hours); bolus-only tPA regimens have been tested but abandoned in favor of longer-acting mutant forms of tPA (see below).

Reteplase

Reteplase (rPA) was the first variant (mutant) of tPA to be developed and marketed.[58] It is a non-glycosylated, single-chain deletion variant consisting only of the kringle 2 and proteinase (plasmin cleavage site) domains of human tPA. Fibrin specificity is lower and half life longer (14–18 minutes) than tPA, allowing more convenient, double-bolus administration.

Tenecteplase

Tenecteplase (TNK-tPA) is a triple-site substitution variant of tPA: at amino acid 103, threonine (T) is replaced by asparagine, adding a glycosylation site; at site 117, asparagine (N) is replaced by glutamine, removing a glycosylation site; at a third site, four amino acids (lysine [K], histidine, arginine and arginine) are replaced by four alanines.[59] The first two changes decrease clearance rate (half life 20 minutes), allowing for single bolus dosing. The third change confers greater fibrin specificity and resistance to PAI-1.

Selected investigational fibrinolytics

Prourokinase or single chain urokinase-type plasminogen activator (scuPA)

In the early 1980s, a glycosylated, single chain form of urokinase (scuPA) was isolated from human urine and cell culture media and characterized biochemically as a proenzyme form of the active two-chain urokinase (tcuPA).[10] Prourokinase was of interest in part because it appeared to be more fibrin-specific than urokinase. This effect is believed to be mediated by the preferential conversion of scuPA to active tcuPA at the fibrin surface. The circulating half life of natural and recombinant scuPA is 4 and 8 minutes respectively, with predominant hepatic clearance.[60] A Phase II study of glycosylated prourokinase produced in mouse hybridoma cells suggested promising coronary patency rates,[61] but further development for AMI has not been undertaken.

Saruplase

Saruplase is a recombinant non-glycosylated form of human prourokinase which has less fibrin specificity and stability than glycosylated prourokinase.[10] Elimination is biphasic, with an initial half life of 6–9 minutes. Administration has been by bolus (20 mg) plus infusion (60 mg/60 min). Saruplase has undergone comparative clinical studies with SK and tPA.[62–64] Saruplase achieves early (60–90 minute) coronary patency rates greater than SK and similar to 3 hour tPA infusions. Mortality rates were at least equivalent to SK, but intracranial hemorrhage rates were greater.

An application for clinical use was rejected by the European Medical Evaluation Agency (EMEA).

Lanoteplase

Lanoteplase (nPA) is a tPA mutant with deletions of the epidermal growth factor, the fibronectin finger domain, and the amino acid 117-glycosylation site.[10] The result is slower clearance (half life 37 minutes), allowing for bolus injection, but decreased fibrin specificity. In comparative studies with tPA, nPA achieved equivalent patency rates[65] and similar 30 day mortality rates,[66] but an increase in intracranial hemorrhage was seen (1·13% v 0·62%). It is believed that the dosing strategy of both nPA and heparin may have contributed, but further development of nPA is uncertain.

Staphylokinase

Staphylokinase (SAK) is a single chain, 136 amino acid protein secreted by strains of *Staphylococcus aureus* and manufactured for clinical use by recombinant DNA technology.[67,68] The SAK-plasmin complex is fibrin selective, efficiently activating plasminogen while bound to fibrin at the thrombus surface. SAK has shown at least equivalent reperfusion potential and greater fibrin-specificity than accelerated-dose tPA in Phase II studies. Staphylokinase is antigenic, inducing neutralizing antibodies within 1 week. A pegylated form has been generated to increase half life and allow for bolus dosing.

Efficacy of intravenous fibrinolytic therapy

Effects on coronary arterial patency

Because myocardial reperfusion is the postulated mechanism of benefit of fibrinolysis for AMI, many angiographic studies have been undertaken to assess patency profiles of the infarct-related coronary artery after fibrinolytic therapy.[24] Granger *et al* summarized 14 124 angiographic observations from 58 studies (Figure 31.2).[50] Because the extent of myocardial salvage is time-dependent, early (60–90 min) patency has generally formed the primary end point in these studies. Without fibrinolytic therapy, spontaneous perfusion early after ST elevation AMI occurs in only 15% and 21% at 60 and 90 minutes after study entry, respectively, remains unchanged at 1 day, then gradually increases to about 60% by 3 weeks. All fibrinolytic regimens improve early patency rates. At 60 and 90 minutes, streptokinase had the lowest rates (48%, 51%), APSAC and standard (3 hour) tPA infusions intermediate rates (about 60%, 70%), and accelerated (90 minute) tPA infusions the highest rates (74%, 84%). However, patency rates at ≥3 hours were similar for all regimens, and reocclusion rates were higher after tPA than non-fibrin-specific (systemically active) agents (13% v 8%) (P = 0·002). The GUSTO angiographic

study,[69] embedded within a larger comparative mortality study,[52] directly demonstrated that early but not late patency rates accurately predict mortality differences among AMI therapies (see below), providing direct support for the open artery hypothesis of fibrinolytic benefit.

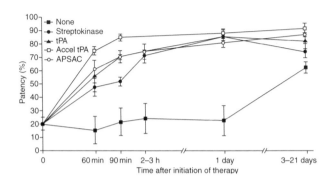

Figure 31.2 Pooled angiographic patency rates with 95% confidence intervals over time after no fibrinolytic agent, streptokinase, conventional dose tPA, accelerated dose tPA, and APSAC from 14 124 angiographic observations. (From Granger CB, White HD, Bates ER, Ohman EM, Califf RM. A pooled analysis of coronary arterial patency and left ventricular function after intravenous thrombolysis for acute myocardial infarction. *Am J Cardiol* 1994;**74**:1220–8.[50])

Effects on mortality

Selected randomized trials with non-fibrinolysis controls

By the late 1980s, accumulating clinical trials data provided support for a survival benefit of IV fibrinolysis.[70–72] The most important survival trials, comparing fibrinolysis to placebo or standard non-fibrinolytic care, are summarized in Figure 31.3.

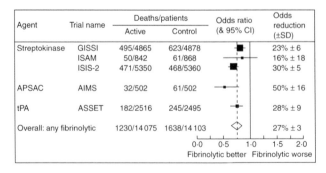

Figure 31.3 Reduction in the odds of early death among ST elevation AMI patients treated within 6 hours; overview from five largest randomized control trials of fibrinolytic therapy versus placebo. (From Granger CB, Califf RM, Topol EJ. Thrombolytic therapy for acute myocardial infarction. *Drugs* 1992;**44**:293.)

The *Gruppo Italiano per lo Studio della Streptochinasi nell'Infarto Miocardico (GISSI)* – This study[73] was the first "definitive" mortality trial. Eleven thousand eight hundred and six AMI patients with ST elevation were randomized to receive 1·5 million units (MU) of IV SK over 1 hour or standard therapy. Aspirin was not routinely given. Inhospital mortality was 10·7% in the SK group and 13·0% in the control group, a 17·6% risk reduction (*P* = 0·0002; RR [relative risk]; 0·81). Survival differences remained at 1–2 years.[74] Benefit was time-dependent and particularly large for treatment within 1 hour of symptom onset (47% mortality reduction, RR 0·49) but was not significant after 6 hours.

The *second International Study of Infarct Survival (ISIS-2)* – This study[75] randomized 17 187 patients with *suspected* AMI within 24 hours to IV SK (1·5 MU), aspirin (162·5 mg), both, or neither (placebos) in a 2 × 2 factorial design. The 35 day vascular mortality rate (13·2% for the double placebo group) was reduced 23% by aspirin alone, 25% by SK alone, and 42% by combined aspirin and SK (all *P* < 0·00001). When both were given early (within 4 hours of symptom onset), a 53% odds reduction was achieved.

The *APSAC Intervention Mortality Study (AIMS)* – This[76,77] was a randomized, double-blind, placebo-controlled trial of APSAC (30 U) in 1258 AMI patients under age 70 with ST elevation and symptoms of <6 hours' duration. Adjunctive therapy included heparin, begun 6 hours after APSAC, followed by warfarin for at least 3 months. APSAC reduced 30 day mortality from 12·2% to 6·4% (odds reduction (OR) 51%, *P* = 0·0006) and 1 year mortality from 17·8% to 11·1% (OR 43%, *P* = 0·0007). Virtually all patient subgroups benefitted.

The *Anglo-Scandinavian Study of Early Thrombolysis (ASSET)* – This Study[78] evaluated tPA (alteplase) with heparin versus heparin alone within a randomized, double-blind, placebo-controlled design. ASSET enrolled 5013 patients within 5 hours of *suspected* AMI. Therapies were IV tPA (100 mg over 3 hours) plus heparin (5000 U IV bolus, then 1000 U/h), or placebo plus heparin. The 30 day mortality was lower in the tPA than the placebo group (7·2% *v* 9·8%, *P* = 0·0011). Hemorrhagic risk was acceptable.

The *Fibrinolytic Therapy Trialists' (FTT) Collaborative Group* – This group[79] pooled data from nine controlled trials that randomized 1000 or more patients with suspected AMI. The database consisted of 58 600 patients of whom 6177 (10·7%) died, 564 (1·0%) had strokes, and 436 had major non-cerebral bleeds. The 45 000 patients who presented with ST elevation or bundle branch block (BBB) had an absolute mortality reduction of 30 per 1000 for treatment within the first 6 hours, 20 per 1000 for hours 7–12, and a statistically uncertain reduction of 13 per 1000 beyond 12 hours.

Given its large size, FTT also performed subgroup analysis. Analysis by presenting electrocardiogram (ECG) (Figure 31.4) showed mortality reductions for those with ST elevation (21%, *P* < 0·000001) and bundle branch block (BBB) (25%, *P* < 0·01). Benefit was greater for those with anterior (37 lives saved per 1000 treated) compared with inferior (8 per 1000) or other (27 per 1000) AMI sites. The absolute benefit was greater in those with greater risk, for example, BBB (49 lives saved per 1000 treated) and anterior ST elevation (37 per 1000). Those with normal ECGs or with ST depression alone showed no benefit and adverse trends (7 and 14 more deaths per 1000, respectively).

The FTT study[79] suggested that proportional mortality reduction was little influenced by systolic blood pressure or heart rate. Benefits also were confirmed for other high-risk groups, including those with prior MI and diabetes.

Benefits of very early (<1 hour) therapy

The magnitude of mortality reductions in FTT was dependent on time to therapy from symptom onset. For those with ST elevation or BBB, the absolute benefit was 39 (at 0–1 h), 30 (>1–3 h), 27 (>3–6 h), 21 (>6–12 h), and 7 (>12–24 h) lives saved per 1000 treated (Figure 31.5).

Others also studied the benefits of therapy within 1 hour.[80,81] Boersma *et al*[81] reappraised very early therapy

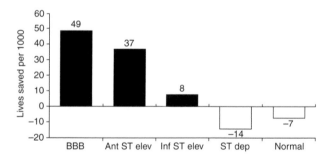

Figure 31.4 The effect of fibrinolytic therapy on mortality (lives saved per 1000 treated) in various patient subsets classified according to admission ECG. Patients presenting with bundle branch block and anterior ST segment elevations derived most benefit from fibrinolytic therapy. Patients with inferior ST segment elevation derived much less benefit, while those with ST depression or normal ECG did not benefit. (Based on data from FTT Collaborative Group[79]). The FTT found that for elderly patients (over age 75), proportional mortality reduction was less and the trend to benefit was not significant. Absolute mortality reduction was interpreted to be still worthwhile (Figure 31.5). Fibrinolytic therapy in the very elderly continues to be debated (see later).

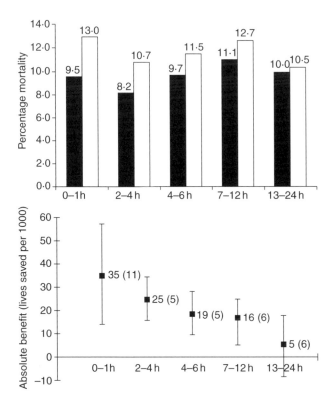

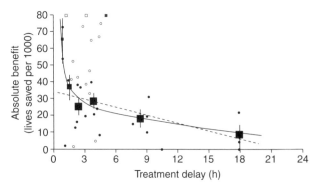

Figure 31.6 Absolute 35 day mortality reduction *v* treatment delay: small closed dots, information from trials included in FTT analysis; open dots, information from additional trials; small squares, data beyond scale of X/Y cross. The linear $(34{\cdot}7 - 0{\cdot}6X)$ and non-linear $(19{\cdot}4 - 0{\cdot}6X + 29{\cdot}3X^{-1})$ closed regression lines are fitted within these data, weighted by the inverse of the variance of the absolute benefit at each data point. The black squares denote the average effects in six time-to-treatment groups (areas of squares inversely proportional to the variance of absolute benefits described). (From Boersma E, Maas ACP, Deckers JW *et al.* Early thrombolytic treatment in acute myocardial infarction: reappraisal of the golden hour. *Lancet* 1996;**348**:771–5.[81])

Figure 31.5 The effect of fibrinolytic therapy on mortality in various patient subsets classified according to duration of symptoms before treatment: (*above*) mortality in each subgroup of fibrinolytic treated (black bars) versus placebo treated (white bars) patients; (*below*) absolute benefit (lives saved per 1000 treated, standard deviation in parentheses) with confidence intervals. (Based on data from FTT Collaborative Group.[79])

based on a larger database (50 246 patients, derived from all randomized trials of ≥100 patients). The absolute mortality reduction for treatment within 1 hour of symptom onset was 65 per 1000. The delay/benefit relation (Figure 31.6) was non-linear.

Benefit of delayed (≥6 hour) therapy

In contrast to earlier therapy, the benefit of fibrinolysis after 6 hours is less certain. The Late Assessment of Thrombolytic Efficacy (LATE) study[82] enrolled 5711 patients with evidence of AMI between 6 and 24 hours from symptom onset and randomized them to tPA (100 mg over 3 h) or placebo. A 26% relative mortality reduction (8·9% *v* 11·9%, *P* = 0·02) was observed for those treated within 12 hours. The 12–24 hour subgroup showed a non-significant trend to benefit (8·7% *v* 9·2% mortality rate). The South American EMERAS collaborative group[83] treated 4534 patients with IV SK or placebo within 24 hours after onset of suspected AMI and found a non-significant trend towards a mortality benefit between hours 7 and 12 (SK 11·7%, placebo 13·2%). These with

other late treatment trials[79] have provided the rationale for recommending fibrinolysis for hours 7–12 after the onset of AMI in patients with persistent symptoms and ECG changes.[5]

Risks of thrombolytic therapy

Bleeding

Bleeding is the primary risk of fibrinolytic therapy. Intracranial (or intracerebral) hemorrhage (ICH) is the most important bleeding risk, occurring in about 0·5–1·0%, with substantial risk of fatality (44–75%) or disability.[84–88] Non-cerebral but not cerebral bleeding risk has benefitted by increased fibrin selectivity. The absolute and relative contraindications to fibrinolytic therapy are summarized in Box 31.1 (after[5]).

> **Box 31.1   Absolute and relative contraindications to fibrinolytic therapy**
> *Contraindications, absolute*
>   Active bleeding; bleeding diathesis
>   Prior hemorrhagic stroke; intracranial pathology
>   Aortic dissection
> *Contraindications, relative*
>   Severe, uncontrolled hypertension (>180/110 mmHg)
>   Oral anticoagulation with INR >1·5
>   Major recent trauma/surgery
>   Pregnancy
>   Recent non-hemorrhagic stroke

Non-compressible recent vascular punctures
Recent retinal laser therapy
Cardiogenic shock when revascularization available

The risk of ICH varies with patient characteristics, the fibrinolytic agent, and adjunctive antithrombotic therapy.[84–88] Simoons et al[87] identified four independent predictors of increased ICH risk: age > 65 years (OR 2·2; 95% CI 1·4–3·5), weight <70 kg (OR 2·1; 95% CI 1·3–3·2), hypertension on admission (OR 2·0; 95% CI 1·2–3·2), and use of tPA (alteplase) (OR 1·6; 95% CI 1·0–2·5) versus SK. The GUSTO-1 group[88] identified seven predictors of ICH: advanced age, lower weight, history of cerebrovascular disease, history of hypertension, higher systolic or diastolic pressure on presentation, and randomization to tPA (v SK). In contrast, the incidence of non-cerebral bleeding is higher with SK.[89]

The safety of bolus compared with infusion administration of fibrinolysis for ICH was questioned by a meta-analysis of several different agents.[90] However, problems with the meta-analysis have been raised,[91,92] and large, well-controlled trials of the two bolus agents in general use, rPA[93] and TNK-PA,[94] have not shown excess ICH rates compared with front-loaded rt-PA.

The critical importance of dose and adjunctive therapies to ICH risk is now realized. Excessive ICH was observed with tPA doses >100 mg.[24] Excessive adjunctive therapy (for example, heparin, hirudin, glycoprotein IIb/IIIa receptor inhibition) with fibrinolytics also has resulted in unacceptable rates of bleeding including ICH.[95–97] In the GUSTO-I trial, the risk of ICH increased with aPTT levels beyond 70 seconds.[98] Three concurrent trials[95–97] were stopped prematurely and reconfigured because of excessive hemorrhage. With lower doses of antithrombins, hemorrhage rates subsequently decreased. Recommendations for adjuvant heparin therapy have been adjusted downward to 60 U/kg bolus (maximum 4000 units) and 12 units/kg/hour (maximum 1000 units), adjusted after 3 hours to maintain aPTT at 50–70 seconds for 48 hours.[5] Further reductions in heparin dosing have been required with combined fibrinolytic and glycoprotein IIb/IIIa receptor inhibitor therapy (see below).

Previously, prolonged cardiopulmonary resuscitation (CPR) has been considered a contraindication to fibrinolytic therapy. Recently, Bottiger et al observed 90 patients with AMI who had out-of-hospital cardiac arrest.[99] Patients treated with heparin and tPA more frequently had return of spontaneous circulation (68% v 44%, P< 0·03), admission to the ICU (P< 0·01), and survival to discharge (15% v 8%). Bleeding complications were not problematic.

Allergy, hypotension, and fever

SK and APSAC are antigenic and may be allergenic although serious anaphylaxis or bronchoconstriction are rare

(<0·2–0·5%).[75] In ISIS-3,[86] any allergic-type reaction was reported after SK in 3·6%, APSAC in 5·1%, and tPA (duteplase) in 0·8%; only 0·3%, 0·5%, and 0·1%, respectively, required treatment. Angioneurotic and periorbital edema, hypersensitivity vasculitis, serum sickness or renal failure due to interstitial nephritis, and purpuric rashes have been rarely reported, especially after repeat administration.[35,75,77,86]

SK and APSAC may acutely release bradykinin, a vasodilator. The incidence of clinical hypotension was similar after SK (11·8%) and APSAC (12·5%) but lower after tPA (7·1%);[86] only half of episodes required treatment.

Fever occurs in 5–30% of SK and 5–10% of APSAC treated patients. Delayed-type hypersensitivity may provoke fever and may respond to acetaminophen. The role of fibrinolytics in reports of splenic rupture, aortic dissection, and cholesterol embolization is uncertain.

Comparative fibrinolytic trials

After establishing the general utility of fibrinolysis in STE-AMI, clinical trials focused on comparisons with new drug regimens. Salient features of major early comparative outcomes trials are presented in Table 31.2; bolus fibrinolytic trials are summarized in Table 31.3; and recent combination therapy trials are shown in Table 31.4.

The GISSI-2/International Study Group trial[100,101] randomized 20 891 patients with STE-AMI <6 h old to tPA (alteplase, 100 mg/3 h) or SK (1·5 MU/1 h) and to subcutaneous (SC) heparin (12 500 U twice daily) beginning 12 hours later or no heparin. Aspirin and atenolol were given as standard therapies. Inhospital mortality was: SK 8·5% and tPA 8·9% (P= NS). ICH rates were 0·5% and 0·8%, respectively; other major bleeds were most frequent with SK plus heparin. At 35 days, death or severe left ventricular dysfunction did not differ by fibrinolytic. Delayed, SC heparin added little benefit (RR 0·95; 95% CI 0·86–1·04).

The third ISIS study (ISIS-3)[86] randomized 41 299 patients with suspected AMI <24 h old to receive SK (1·5 MU/1 h), tPA (duteplase 0·6 MU/kg/4 h) or APSAC (30 U/3 min) and to SC heparin (12 500 U, 4 hours after beginning thrombolytics and bid) or no heparin. Aspirin (162 mg/day) was given to all patients. The median time to treatment was 4 hours; 88% presented within 6 hours and had ST elevation. Mortality rates at 35 days were: SK 10·6%, APSAC 10·5%, and tPA 10·3% overall, and 10·0%, 9·9%, and 9·6%, respectively, in those with clear indications (P= NS). Similar outcomes also were observed after 6 months. SC heparin tended to improve 1 week mortality (7·4% v 7·9%, P= 0·06) at the expense of increased bleeding, but mortality rates at 35 days were similar (10·3% v 10·6%, P= NS).

In comparing fibrinolytic regimens, GISSI-2 and ISIS-3 were limited by the suboptimal use of heparin for short-acting,

Table 31.2 Clinical end points in early comparative fibrinolytic outcomes trials

End points	GISSI-2/ International[100]		ISIS-3[86]			GUSTO-1[69]		
	SK (10 396)	tPA (10 372)	SK (13 607)	tPA (13 569)	APSAC (13 599)	SK (20 173)	tPA[a] (10 344)	SK+tPA (10 328)
Death (%)	8·5	8·9	10·6	10·3	10·5	7·3	6·3[b]	7·0
Re-infarction (%)	3·0	2·6	3·5	2·9[b]	3·6	3·7	4·0	4·0
Any stroke (%)	0·9	1·3[b]	1·0	1·4[b]	1·3	1·3	1·6	1·7
Hemorrhagic stroke (%)	0·3	0·4	0·2	0·7[b]	0·6	0·5	0·7[b]	0·9
Non-CNS bleeds (%)	0·9	0·6[b]	4·5	5·2[b]	5·4	6·0	5·4[b]	6·1

[a] Accelerated dose tPA.
[b] Statistically significant; statistical comparisons are only listed for SK *v* tPA.

Table 31.3 Comparative trials of bolus agents with accelerated tPA

End points	ASSENT-II[94]		GUSTO-III[93]		In-TIME-II[66]	
	tPA (*n* = 8488)	TNK (8461)	tPA (4921)	rPA (10 138)	tPA (5022)	nPA (10 038)
Death (%) at 30 days	6·15	6·18	7·24	7·47	6·61	6·75
Re-infarction (%)	3·8	4·1	4·2	4·2	5·5	5·0
Any stroke (%)	1·66	1·78	1·79	1·64	1·53	1·87
Hemorrhagic stroke (%)	0·94	0·93	0·87	0·91	0·64*	1·12*
Major bleed (%)	5·94*	4·66*	1·2	0·95	0·6	0·5

* *P* < 0·001 for comparisons.

Table 31.4 Comparative outcomes trials with combined fibrinolytic and GP IIb/IIIa inhibitor therapy

End points	GUSTO-V AMI1[25]		ASSENT-3[14]		
	rPA (*n* = 8260)	1/2 rPA + abciximab (8328)	TNK-tPA with heparin (2038)	TNK-tPA with enoxaparin (2040)	1/2 dose TNK-tPA + abciximab (2017)
30 day death (%)	6·2	5·9	6·0	5·4	6·6
Re-infarction (%)	3·5	2·3*	4·2[d]	2·7[d]	2·2[d]
Combined death, Re-AMI, UA (or urgent revasc) (%)	20·6	16·2*	15·4[e]	11·4[e]	11·1[e]
Any stroke (%)	0·9	1·0	1·52	1·62	1·49
ICH (%)	0·6[a]	0·6[b]	0·93	0·88	0·94
Major bleed (%)	2·3[c]	4·6[c]	2·2[f]	3·0[f]	4·3[f]

[a] ICH rates for patients >75 = 1·1%.
[b] ICH rates for patients >75 = 2·1%.
[c] Severe and moderate bleeding combined.
[d] Inhospital events, *P* = 0·0009 among groups.
[e] *P* < 0·0001 among groups for 30 day death, inhospital re-infarction, or inhospital refractory ischemia.
[f] Major inhospital bleeding (other than ICH), *P* = 0·0005 among groups.
* *P* < 0·0001 between groups.

fibrin-selective tPA (SC dosing after a delay of 4–12 hours), treatment was relatively late (mean times >4 hours) and did not require ST elevation (ISIS-3), and tPA was not front-loaded.[102–104]

These concerns led to the Global Use of Streptokinase and tPA for Occluded Coronary Arteries (GUSTO) study.[52] GUSTO randomized 41 021 patients with STE-AMI <6 h old to:

1. SK 1·5 MU/1 h with SC heparin 12 500 U every 12 h starting 4 h after SK;
2. IV SK with IV heparin, 5000 U bolus then 1000 U/h, titrating aPTT to 60–85 seconds;
3. front-loaded tPA (15 mg bolus, 0·75 mg/kg – maximum 50 mg – over 30 minutes, then 0·50 mg/kg – maximum 35 mg – over 60 minutes, for a maximum of 100 mg over 90 minutes) and IV heparin as per the SK regimen;
4. a combination of tPA 1·0 mg/kg and SK 1·0 MU, administered concurrently over 60 minutes, plus IV heparin.

The primary end point, 30 day mortality, was lowest with accelerated tPA with IV heparin (6·3%), representing a 14% risk reduction ($P = 0·001$) compared to the two SK strategies (7·3%), which did not differ. Combined tPA and SK gave an intermediate outcome. The risk of hemorrhagic stroke was higher with tPA (0·7%) than SK (0·5%), but the combined end point of death or disabling stroke favored tPA (6·9% v 7·8%, $P = 0·006$). Implications of GUSTO for selection of fibrinolytic regimens have been debated.

Three additional angiographic studies compared APSAC and tPA.[105–107] Early patency profiles, convalescent ejection fraction, and unsatisfactory clinical outcomes end points tended to favor tPA.

Comparative trials with bolus fibrinolytics

INJECT (The International Joint Efficacy Comparison of Thrombolytics)[58] compared reteplase (rPA) and SK in a 6010 patient double-blind, randomized trial. Mortality rates at 35 days were: rPA 9·0% and SK 9·5% (0·5% absolute reduction; 95% CI 1·9–0·96). On this basis "equivalence" (non-inferiority) of rPA to standard, SK therapy, was established and rPA approved. Outcomes trials of bolus agents subsequent to INJECT used accelerated tPA as comparator (Table 31.3).

Reteplase

Reteplase was next favorably compared to tPA in an angiographic study, leading to a large mortality study. In RAPID 2 (Reteplase v Alteplase Patency Investigation During acute myocardial infarction)[51] 90 minute TIMI grade 2 or 3 patency rates among 324 patients were 83% v 73% (rPA v tPA, $P = 0·03$), with TIMI-3 flow rates of 60% v 45%, $P = 0·01$. On this basis, a comparative mortality trial,

GUSTO-3,[93] was undertaken and randomized 15 059 patients 2:1 to rPA (two 10 mg IV injections 30 minutes apart), or accelerated tPA (alteplase). A postulated survival advantage for rPA was not demonstrated (30 day mortality: rPA 7·5%, tPA 7·2%).

Lanoteplase

Lanoteplase (nPA), a longer-acting tPA variant, was studied in doses of 15–120 kU/kg in the Phase II angiographic trial Intravenous n-PA for Treating Infarcting Myocardium Early (InTIME).[65] A dose response in 60 minute TIMI-3 patency was observed over the 3 lowest doses but not between 60 and 120 kU/kg, and neither of these doses was superior to rt-PA. A subsequent double-blind mortality equivalence trial, InTIME-2[66] selected the 120 kU/kg dose and randomized 15 078 STE-AMI patients within 6 hours to nPA or tPA (2 : 1). Although 30 day mortality rates were similar (nPA = 6·77%, tPA = 6·60%), a significantly higher ICH rate occurred in the nPA group (1·13% v 0·62%). As concerns developed about excessive ICH rates during InTIME-2, heparin down-titration was undertaken earlier (at 3 hours) if PTT exceeded 70 seconds. Reductions in ICH with both nPA and tPA ensued. In an extension study (InTIME-2b, $n = 1491$), the heparin bolus was omitted and heparin initiated with an infusion of 15 U/kg/h (1000 U/h maximum). ICH rates declined further for nPA to 0·87%. These observations have impacted heparin recommendations generally (see below).

Tenecteplase

Tenecteplase (TNK-tPA), a fibrin-selective, single bolus fibrinolytic, was evaluated in the TIMI 10 dose finding trials.[108,109] In Phase II studies, a clear dose-response was observed[109] both for coronary patency and hemorrhage (including ICH for the 50 mg dose). With limitation and weight-adjustment of TNK-tPA dose and reduction and earlier down-titration of heparin dosing, satisfactory bleeding rates and comparable TIMI-3 patency rates were demonstrated at 90 minutes compared to accelerated rt-PA.[110] The double-blind Phase III Assessment of the Safety and Efficacy of a New Thrombolytic-2 (ASSENT-2) mortality equivalence trial[94] compared weight adjusted TNK (as a 30–50 mg bolus over 5–10 seconds) and accelerated rt-PA. All patients received aspirin and heparin. Thirty day mortality rates were virtually identical for TNK-tPA (6·18%) and rt-PA (6·15%) and met statistical criteria for equivalence. ICH rates also were identical (at 0·93% and 0·94%, respectively). However, major non-cerebral bleeding was lower with the more fibrin-selective TNK (4·66% v 5·94%, $P = 0·0002$) as was need for blood transfusion (4·25% v 5·49%, $P = 0·0002$). A lower mortality rate with TNK-tPA was observed among patients presenting >4 hours after symptom onset (7·0% v 9·2%), which may be due to either greater activity of the more fibrin-specific TNK-tPA against older, fibrin-rich clots or chance.

Thus, none of the newer fibrinolytic regimens has surpassed accelerated tPA. However, the ease of administration of TNK-tPA, together with its reduced transfusion requirements, is likely to lead to rapid acceptance of its clinical use. Lower rates of dosing errors with bolus fibrinolytics such as TNK-tPA also may contribute to superior clinical outcomes.[111]

Combinations of fibrinolytic therapy and glycoprotein IIb/IIIa receptor inhibitors or low molecular weight heparins

With the failure of new fibrinolytic monotherapies to improve early coronary patency and clinical outcomes compared to rt-PA, interest has shifted toward combination pharmacotherapies. A strong theoretical argument can be made for combined fibrinolytic and augmented antiplatelet therapy.[29] The platelet membrane glycoprotein (GP) IIb/IIIa receptor, a specific fibrinogen receptor, is the final common pathway in platelet activation and an attractive therapeutic target. Antibodies, peptides, and small molecules have been developed that block the platelet GP IIb/IIIa receptor. These have potent platelet anti-aggregatory effects and have demonstrated efficacy in the setting of non-STE acute coronary syndromes and coronary angioplasty.[112–115] In STE-AMI, their utility as adjunctive therapy for patients undergoing direct PTCA with stenting has been recently shown.[116] Given the critical role of platelets in coronary arterial thrombosis, the combination of fibrinolytic with GPIIb/IIIa inhibitor (GPI) therapy has substantial appeal as an approach to improving pharmacologic reperfusion.

Abciximab, a monoclonal chimeric antibody against GP IIb/IIIa, was tested as conjunctive therapy with lower doses of tPA in the TIMI-14 dose-ranging angiographic trial.[117] The combination of half dose rt-PA and full dose abciximab (with reduced doses of heparin) produced impressive increments in TIMI-3 flow rates at 60 minutes (72% *v* 43%, *P* < 0·001) and 90 minutes (77% *v* 62%, *P* = 0·02) with acceptable bleeding rates.

Another angiographic study, Strategies for Patency Enhancement in the Emergency Department (SPEED)[118] tested reteplase with abciximab (versus rPA alone) in two phases. The best combination in phase A (half dose reteplase −5 U + 5 U 30 minutes apart − with full dose abciximab) was re-evaluated in phase B with two heparin bolus doses (40 or 60 U/kg). Improved TIMI-3 flow rates were observed with combination therapy, 54% *v* 47%, although differences were not significant. Higher rates of bleeding (9·8% *v* 3·7%) were observed with combination therapy. SPEED piloted the GUSTO-V AMI outcomes trial (Table 31.4).

An argument also has been made for substituting an antithrombin more effective than heparin in combination with a fibrinolytic. Low molecular weight heparins (LMWHs) have theoretical advantages over unfractionated heparin. Unlike unfractionated heparin, LMWHs do not bind extensively to plasma proteins, do not activate platelets, have more predictable kinetics, are effective inhibitors of thrombin activity (anti factor Xa activity) as well as thrombin activity (anti-IIa activity), and are given in fixed doses without the requirement for monitoring.[119] LMWHs are effective in the non-STE acute coronary syndromes,[120] and some LMWH trials also have shown clinical superiority to unfractionated heparin.[121,122] Combinations of fibrinolytics with LMWH have been less extensively tested but have shown promise, with improved late patency and reduced re-infarction/reocclusion compared to intravenous heparin.[123,124]

GUSTO-V AMI[125] was an unblinded mortality study in 16 588 patients with STE-AMI enrolled within 6 hours and randomized to standard rPA (10 U + 10 U) or half dose rPA (5 U + 5 U) plus full dose abciximab. The primary hypothesis, that 30 day mortality rates with combination therapy would be less than with standard fibrinolytic therapy, was disproved (5·6% *v* 5·9%, respectively, *P* = 0·43) although the criterion for non-inferiority was reached. However, of 16 prespecified inhospital adverse AMI-related outcomes, 14 occurred less frequently with combination therapy. Combined death or non-fatal re-infarction (relative risk, 0·83, *P* = 0·001), non-fatal MI alone (*P* < 0·0001), recurrent ischemia (*P* = 0·004), urgent coronary intervention (relative risk, 0·64, *P* < 0·0001), ventricular tachycardia or fibrillation, and high-grade AV block, and total complications (28·5% *v* 31·7%, *P* < 0·0001) were significantly reduced. On the other hand, spontaneous bleeding rates and transfusion requirements were increased up to twofold with combination therapy (*P* < 0·0001). Moreover, there was a significant (*P* = 0·03) adverse treatment interaction by age for ICH: 2·1% *v* 1·1% for combined versus standard therapy for age >75; ICH 0·4% *v* 0·5%, respectively, for age ≤75. GUSTO-V AMI was interpreted as validating an alternative reperfusion strategy for patients ≤75 years old, although the lack of incremental mortality benefit and the increased bleeding risks were disappointing. Younger patients at higher AMI risk (anterior AMI) arguably now might be considered for the GUSTO-V AMI combination regimen although ASSENT-3 suggests another alternative (below).

ASSENT-3[14] was a randomized but unblinded trial in 6095 patients with STE-AMI enrolled within 6 hours of symptom onset and assigned to one of three regimens:

- TNK-tPA and unfractionated heparin (both weight adjusted)
- TNK-tPA with the low molecular weight heparin enoxaparin
- half dose TNK-tPA with heparin and full dose abciximab.

Enoxaparin was given as a 30 mg IV bolus and 1 mg/kg SC repeated every 12 hours until hospital discharge or for

7 days except that the first two SC doses could not exceed 100 mg. Unfractionated heparin was dosed according to recent ACC/AHA guidelines: 60 U/kg bolus (maximum, 4000 U) and 12 U/kg per hour initial infusion (maximum, 1000 U/h), adjusted after 3 hours to an aPTT of 50–70 sec. With abciximab co-therapy, the heparin dose was further reduced to 40 mg/kg bolus (maximum 3000 U) followed by 7 U/kg per h initial infusion (maximum, 800 U/h).

The primary efficacy end point of ASSENT-3 was the composite of 30 day mortality and inhospital re-infarction or refractory ischemia. The primary efficacy plus safety end point was the efficacy end point plus inhospital ICH or other major bleeding. The efficacy end point was significantly lower in both the enoxaparin (11·4%, $P = 0·0002$) and the abciximab co-therapy groups (11·1%, $P < 0·0001$) than the TNK-tPA/heparin group (15·4%). The efficacy plus safety end point also was significantly lower with adjunctive enoxaparin (13·7%, $P < 0·004$) and conjunctive abciximab (14·2%, $P = 0·014$) than with unfractionated heparin (17·0%) (Figure 31.7). A lesser need for urgent coronary interventions was observed with the two experimental therapies. Despite the positive overall results with combination abciximab, there was no mortality benefit (6·6%, v 6·0% for TNK-tPA/heparin control). Moreover, a significant adverse interaction of treatment with age (RR 1·30 for >75 years v 0·74 for ≤75, $P = 0·001$) (Figure 31.7) and diabetes (RR = 1·35 with v 0·74 without diabetes, $P = 0·0007$) was observed for the efficacy plus safety end point. More major bleeding complications, transfusions, and thrombocytopenia occurred in the abciximab group (all $P < 0·001$), and the rates were three times higher in those older than 75 years. Bleeding was only slightly increased with enoxaparin and

no treatment interactions were seen. Taking into account efficacy and safety, TNK-tPA with adjunctive enoxaparin therapy emerged as the best overall therapy. Ease of administration and lack of need for monitoring advantaged enoxaparin over heparin, and greater safety in the elderly and diabetics distinguished it from the abciximab combination.

A combination of half dose fibrinolytic, GP IIb/IIIa inhibition and enoxaparin was studied in ENTIRE-TIMI 23 (Enoxaparin and TNK-tPA with or without GP IIb/IIIa Inhibitor as Reperfusion strategy in ST Elevation MI), and results were recently presented.[126] A total of 461 patients were enrolled. Patients tended to have higher rates of ST segment resolution with enoxaparin versus heparin and with combination therapy versus TNK-tPA alone. Rates of major hemorrhage were higher with TNK-tPA combinations, as expected. However, bleeding rates tended to be lower if enoxaparin was used instead of heparin (5·6% v 7·8%). Although the study was not powered to detect efficacy, the 30 day rates of death or MI were reduced in the enoxaparin groups (15·9% with TNK-tPA/heparin v 4·4% with TNK-tPA/enoxaparin, and 6·5% with half TNK-tPA/abciximab/heparin v 5·5% with half TNK-tPA/abciximab/enoxaparin).

Based on these two recent trials (Table 31.4), combined enoxaparin and TNK-tPA appears to be the most attractive current alternative pharmacological reperfusion strategy and deserves further study. The role of combined GP IIb/IIIa and fibrinolytic therapy, in contrast, is less certain after GUSTO-V and ASSENT-3. Further studies should be limited to younger patients at lower risk of bleed and high risk of AMI-related complications and might include those likely to undergo early percutaneous coronary interventions or include combination therapy with enoxaparin. Whether shorter-acting GPI's (such as eptifibatide or tirofiban) or further changes in adjunctive heparin dosing can improve the benefit/risk ratio of combination regimens with fibrinolytics must await ongoing and future studies.

Combinations of fibrinolytic therapy and direct antithrombins

Initial testing of antithrombins as adjuncts to fibrinolytics was complicated by excessive bleeding.[95–97] Recently, the results of HERO-2, which used adjusted doses, were reported.[127] HERO-2 randomized 17 073 AMI patients to unfractionated heparin or bivalirudin, given 3 minutes before streptokinase administration. All patients received aspirin. Thirty day mortality, the primary end point, did not differ between the bivalirudin and heparin groups (10·8% v 10·9%). However, adjudicated 30 day re-infarction was reduced (2·8% v 3·6%, $P = 0·004$) at the expense of increased moderate to severe bleeding (2·1% v 1·5%, $P < 0·05$) and increased ICH (0·55% v 0·37%, $P = 0·09$). Thus, bivalirudin could lead to 8 fewer AMI's at a cost of 3 more transfusions for every

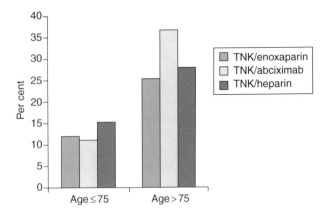

Figure 31.7 Efficacy plus Safety End point (death at 30 days, inhospital re-infarction, refractory ischemia, ICH or major bleeding) from ASSENT-3 trial, by age and treatment group. Patients over age 75 years had poorer outcomes with abciximab, those 75 or younger had poorer outcomes with heparin as adjunc-tive therapy ($P = 0·0010$ for interaction or age, therapy). TNK, TNK-tPA.

1000 patients treated. The value of hirudin analogs as adjuncts to fibrinolytics, instead of heparin, continues to be uncertain.

Indications for fibrinolytic therapy in AMI

In the 1999 guidelines of the American College of Cardiology (ACC) and American Heart Association (AHA),[5] fibrinolytic therapy is strongly recommended **Grade A1a** within 12 hours of the onset of suggestive clinical features (ischemic chest discomfort or equivalent) and ST elevation (>0·1 mV, ≥2 contiguous ECG leads) or BBB (obscuring ST segment analysis), and age ≤75 years. Fibrinolytic therapy also is generally recommended **Grade A1c** for these same features and age >75 years (in the absence of contraindications). Therapy is considered possibly effective – that is, consider selected use **Grade B/C** for these ECG findings but time 12–24 hours or blood pressure on presentation >180 mmHg systolic and/or >110 mmHg diastolic and

associated with a high risk AMI. Fibrinolysis is not indicated for those with ST elevation (or BBB) but time to therapy >24 hours and ischemic pain resolved and those with ST depression (at any time). These recent ACC/AHA guidelines are summarized in Table 31.5.

Fibrinolysis in the elderly

The appropriate use of fibrinolytics in the elderly continues to be debated. In a recent analysis of over 37 000 Medicare patients with AMI age 65 or older who were eligible for fibrinolytic therapy,[128] 38% received fibrinolytic therapy and 4·2% received primary angioplasty. After multivariate adjustments, fibrinolytic therapy was not associated with improved 30 day survival (OR 1·01; 95% CI [0·94–1·09]), whereas primary angioplasty was (OR 0·79; 95% CI [0·66–0·94]). However, at 1 year, both fibrinolytic therapy (OR 0·84 ; 95% CI [0·79–0·89]) and primary angioplasty (OR 0·71 ; 95% CI [0·61–0·83]) were associated with lower

Table 31.5   ACC/AHA guidelines for management of acute myocardial infarction (1999)

Prerequisites for considering fibrinolytic therapy	Choice/time of fibrinolytic agent	Adjuvant therapy
Class I: **Grade A1a**	No specific recommendations	Aspirin 162–325 mg/d
1. ST elevation, time to therapy less than 12 h and age <75 years	In patients with large area of infarction, early after symptom onset, and at low risk for ICH may consider the use of tPA.	β Blockers unless contraindicated or CHF
2. BBB with history suggestive of MI	In smaller infants with smaller potential of survival benefit and if a greater risk of ICH exists, SK may be the choice	ACE inhibitors for anterior MI, CHF or ejection fraction <40% (alternatively: all patients, reassess need for continued therapy at 6 weeks).
Class IIa: **Grade A1c**		IV heparin with tPA, rPA, TNK-tPA, and non-STE-AMI
1. Age >75 years with ST elevation or BBB, suggestive history, time <12 hours		SC heparin with SK or APSAC unless at high risk for thromboembolism, when IV heparin is preferred
Class IIb: **Grade B/C**	Door to needle time less than 30 min	
1. ST elevation, time to therapy 12–24 h 2. Systolic BP >180 mmHg, or diastolic BP >110 mmHg with high-risk MI No evidence for benefit, possibly harmful **Grade A1a** against therapy 1. ST elevation, time to therapy >24 h, pain resolved 2. ST segment depression		

mortality rates. Another Medicare analysis[129] suggested that fibrinolytic therapy even might be harmful in those over 75 years. In contrast, a large Swedish registry found a 12% risk reduction in the composite end point of cerebral bleeding and 1 year mortality.[130] Similarly, the Fibrinolytic Therapy Trialists' overview of randomized trials data in patients over 75 years reported 35 day mortality to be reduced (trend) from 29·4% to 26·0% with fibrinolytic therapy.[79] Analyses restricted to elderly patients with clear indications for fibrinolytic therapy, suggested similar greater *absolute* benefit from fibrinolytic therapy than in younger patients. Fibrinolytic regimens should be chosen to minimize the risk of ICH, which increases in the elderly. Weight adjusting treatment regimens and avoidance of excessive heparin and other adjunctive antithrombotics (for example GP IIb/IIIa inhibitors) is important. When safety concerns predominate, SK, which carries a lower risk of ICH, or primary angioplasty should be considered as preferred reperfusion strategies in the elderly.

LBBB and fibrinolysis

In patients with left BBB *not known to be new*, diagnosis of AMI may be obscured and fibrinolytics withheld. In order to define a prediction rule for evaluating left BBB, the GUSTO-1 investigators[131] found three ECG criteria to have independent value in the diagnosis of AMI:

- ST elevation of 1 mm or more in leads with a positive QRS complex
- ST depression of 1 mm or more in leads V1, V2 or V3
- ST elevation of 5 mm or more with a negative QRS complex. Using an index score, a sensitivity of 36% and a specificity of 96% for AMI were found in a validation group.

Current use of fibrinolytics

The National Registry of Myocardial Infarction (NRMI) tracks the use of reperfusion therapies in the United States, which is accomplished through surveys of 1432 hospitals. Over three phases, from 1990 to 1999, information on 1 514 292 patients with AMI were accumulated.[11] During this decade, the percentage of AMIs eligible for fibrinolytic therapy (ST elevation or LBBB presenting within 12 hours) fell from 36% to 27%, but the percentage of eligible patients who received reperfusion therapy remained constant (69% v 70%). Among patients eligible for reperfusion therapy, the relative use of fibrinolytic therapy fell, from 59% to 48%, whereas use of primary coronary angioplasty increased, from 12% to 24%. Of those receiving fibrinolytic therapy, the mean time from hospital arrival to drug delivery decreased, from 62 minutes to 38 minutes.

Selection of a fibrinolytic regimen

The selection of a fibrinolytic regimen is based on the risk of the AMI, a benefit versus risk analysis of therapy, and consideration of economic constraints. Using these factors, tPA-related fibrinolytics have become dominant in the United States, whereas in Europe and elsewhere, less costly SK is still widely used. These same factors undoubtedly will influence the rate of incorporation of new fibrinolytics and adjunctive therapies into practice. A number of algorithms for selecting the reperfusion regimen (that is, a specific fibrinolytic or primary PTCA) have been proposed,[132,133] but none has been prospectively validated and universally accepted.

The authors view primary percutaneous coronary intervention (PCI) as preferred therapy when readily available (time to PCI <90±30 min).[5] In other circumstances, fibrinolytic therapy is standard of care. TNK-tPA, accelerated dose rt-PA, or rPA may be recommended for high risk patients who have the potential for a large therapeutic benefit, for example, anterior AMI, BBB-related AMI, or poor-prognosis inferior AMI (that is, with right ventricular involvement, anterior reciprocal ST depression, or lateral and posterior extension), time <6 hours, and age <75 years. (Older patients have greater mortality risk but also greater bleeding risk and derive less proportionate benefit.) TNK-tPA offers the advantage of single bolus dosing and lower transfusion requirement, yet maintains efficacy equivalent to rt-PA. For other patients, efficacy advantages are less clear, and physician preference, patient safety, cost issues, and availability can guide choice. SK is preferred when the risk of ICH is high (for example, the elderly) and when cost is an important consideration. A non-immunogenic fibrinolytic is preferred in patients with a history of prior SK or APSAC use (neutralizing antibodies may persist for several years).

Despite two large outcomes trials,[14,125] the role of combination therapies with GP IIb/IIIa inhibitors remains unclear and recommendations on use cannot be given. Clearly, the combinations tested in GUSTO-V and ASSENT-3 should be avoided in the elderly (>75 years old).

Adjunctive therapy with the LMWH enoxaparin presents another co-therapy option. Based on ASSENT-3,[14] enoxaparin appears to be an attractive alternative to unfractionated heparin as an adjunctive antithrombin with standard dose TNK-tPA. Further testing and assimilation of enoxaparin into official guidelines is anticipated in the near future.

Adjunctive therapy

Adjunctive medical and antithrombotic therapy will be covered more completely in related chapters. Current guidelines strongly recommend **Grade A1a** aspirin on admission in a dose of 162–325 mg, preferably chewed. Aspirin is then continued in the same dose, once daily, indefinitely (enteric coated forms are popular).[5] For aspirin allergy, clopidogrel (preferred) or ticlopidine may be used.

Intravenous heparin is recommended **Grade A1c** with tPA-related fibrinolytics,[5] beginning concurrently and given for 48 hours, with a target aPTT at $\geq$12 hours after thrombolytics of 50–70 seconds (1·5 to 2 times control).[98] Currently recommended dosing includes a 60 U/kg bolus (maximum 4000 U) followed initially with a 12 U/kg per hour infusion (maximum 1000 U/hour) with adjustment after *3* hours based on aPTT.[5]

IV heparin is not routinely recommended with systemically active (non-fibrin-selective) agents such as SK and APSAC, especially within 6 hours of fibrinolysis. **Grade A1c** [5] Rather, subcutaneous heparin (7500–12 500 U twice daily until ambulatory) or low molecular weight heparin may be given. IV heparin is "probably effective" after 6 hours in patients at high risk for further thrombosis or thromboembolism (for example, those with large or anterior MI, atrial fibrillation, previous embolus, or known left ventricular thrombus) **Grade B** .[5]

It is likely that the LMWH enoxaparin may be included as an antithrombin option or preference in future guidelines, based on ASSENT-3 **Grade A1d** . Direct antithrombins (hirudin derivatives) also have been tested as adjunctive therapies (for example, HERO-2), but their role has not yet been clearly established.

References

1. Braunwald E, Antman EM, Beasley JW *et al*. ACC/AHA guidelines for the management of patients with unstable angina and non-ST-segment elevation myocardial infarction. A report of the American College of Cardiology/American Heart Association Task Force on Practice Guidelines (Committee on the Management of Patients With Unstable Angina). *J Am Coll Cardiol* 2000;**36**:970–1062.

2. Nourjah P. National Hospital Ambulatory Medical Care Survey: 1997 emergency department summary. *National Center for Health Statistics; advance data from vital and health statistics*. Hyattsville, MD: National Institutes of Health, 1999.

3. Statistics NCfH. *Detailed diagnoses and procedures: National Hospital Discharge Survey, 1996*. Hyattsville, MD: National Center for Health Statistics, 1998.

4. National Heart Lung, and Blood Institute. *Morbidity and mortality: 1996 chartbook on cardiovascular, lung, and blood diseases*. Bethesda, MD: US Department of Health and Human Services, Public Health Service, National Institutes of Health, 1996.

5. Ryan TJ, Antman EM, Brooks NH *et al*. 1999 update: ACC/AHA guidelines for the management of patients with acute myocardial infarction. A report of the American College of Cardiology/American Heart Association Task Force on Practice Guidelines (Committee on Management of Acute Myocardial Infarction). *J Am Coll Cardiol* 1999;**34**:890–911.

6. Herlitz J, Blohm M, Hartford M, Hjalmarsson A, Holmberg S, Karlson BW. Delay time in suspected acute myocardial infarction

and the importance of its modification. *Clin Cardiol* 1989; **12**:370–4.

7. Priori SG, Aliot E, Blomstrom-Lundqvist C *et al*. Task force on sudden cardiac death of the European Society of Cardiology. *Eur Heart J* 2001;**22**:1374–450.

8. Myerburg RJ, Kessler KM, Castellanos A. Sudden cardiac death. Structure, function, and time-dependence of risk. *Circulation* 1992;**85**(Suppl. 1):I2–10.

9. Farb A, Tang AL, Burke AP, Sessums L, Liang Y, Virmani R. Sudden coronary death. Frequency of active coronary lesions, inactive coronary lesions, and myocardial infarction. *Circulation* 1995;**92**:1701–9.

10. Armstrong PW, Collen D. Fibrinolysis for acute myocardial infarction: current status and new horizons for pharmacological reperfusion, part 1. *Circulation* 2001;**103**:2862–6.

11. Rogers WJ, Canto JG, Lambrew CT, *et al*. Temporal trends in the treatment of over 1·5 million patients with myocardial infarction in the US from 1990 through 1999: the National Registry of Myocardial Infarction 1, 2 and 3. *J Am Coll Cardiol* 2000;**36**:2056–63.

12. Hunink MG, Goldman L, Tosteson AN *et al*. The recent decline in mortality from coronary heart disease, 1980–1990. The effect of secular trends in risk factors and treatment. *JAMA* 1997;**277**:535–42.

13. Rogers WJ, Canto JG, Barron HV, Boscarino JA, Shoultz DA, Every NR. Treatment and outcome of myocardial infarction in hospitals with and without invasive capability. Investigators in the National Registry of Myocardial Infarction. *J Am Coll Cardiol* 2000;**35**:371–9.

14. Efficacy and safety of tenecteplase in combination with enoxaparin, abciximab, or unfractionated heparin: the ASSENT-3 randomised trial in acute myocardial infarction. *Lancet* 2001;**358**:605–13.

15. Herrick JB. Clinical features of sudden obstruction of the coronary arteries. *JAMA* 1912;**59**:220–8.

16. Obraztsov VP, Strazhesko ND. On the symptomatology and diagnosis of coronary thrombosis. In: Vorobeva VA, Konchalovski MP, eds. *Works of the First Congress of Russian Therapists*: Comradeship typography of A E Mamontov, 1910.

17. Blumgart HL, Schlesinger MJ, Davis D. Studies on the relation of the clinical manifestations of angina pectoris, coronary thrombosis and myocardial infarction to the pathologic findings with particular reference to the significance of the collateral circulation. *Am Heart J* 1940;**19**:1–91.

18. Roberts WC. Coronary arteries in fatal acute myocardial infarction. *Circulation* 1972;**45**:215–30.

19. Davies MJ, Woolf N, Robertson WB. Pathology of acute myocardial infarction with particular reference to occlusive coronary thrombi. *Br Heart J* 1976;**38**:659–64.

20. DeWood MA, Spores J, Notske R *et al*. Prevalence of total coronary occlusion during the early hours of transmural myocardial infarction. *N Engl J Med* 1980;**303**:897–902.

21. Shah PK, Falk E, Badimon JJ *et al*. Human monocyte-derived macrophages induce collagen breakdown in fibrous caps of atherosclerotic plaques. Potential role of matrix-degrading metalloproteinases and implications for plaque rupture. *Circulation* 1995;**92**:1565–9.

22. Reimer KA, Lowe JE, Rasmussen MM, Jennings RB. The wavefront phenomenon of ischemic cell death. 1. Myocardial infarct

size vs duration of coronary occlusion in dogs. *Circulation* 1977;**56**:786–94.

23. Reimer KA, Jennings RB. The "wavefront phenomenon" of myocardial ischemic cell death. II. Transmural progression of necrosis within the framework of ischemic bed size (myocardium at risk) and collateral flow. *Lab Invest* 1979; **40**:633–44.

24. Chesebro JH, Knatterud G, Roberts R *et al.* Thrombolysis in Myocardial Infarction (TIMI) Trial, Phase I: A comparison between intravenous tissue plasminogen activator and intravenous streptokinase. Clinical findings through hospital discharge. *Circulation* 1987;**76**:142–54.

25. Anderson JL, Karagounis LA, Califf RM. Meta-analysis of five reported studies on the relation of early coronary patency grades with mortality and outcomes after acute myocardial infarction. *Am J Cardiol* 1996;**78**:1–8.

26. Ito H, Okamura A, Iwakura K *et al.* Myocardial perfusion patterns related to thrombolysis in myocardial infarction perfusion grades after coronary angioplasty in patients with acute anterior wall myocardial infarction. *Circulation* 1996;**93**:1993–9.

27. Gibson CM, Murphy SA, Rizzo MJ *et al.* Relationship between TIMI frame count and clinical outcomes after thrombolytic administration. Thrombolysis In Myocardial Infarction (TIMI) Study Group. *Circulation* 1999;**99**:1945–50.

28. Gibson CM, Cannon CP, Murphy SA *et al.* Relationship of TIMI myocardial perfusion grade to mortality after administration of thrombolytic drugs. *Circulation* 2000;**101**:125–30.

29. Topol EJ. Toward a new frontier in myocardial reperfusion therapy: emerging platelet preeminence. *Circulation* 1998; **97**:211–18.

30. Tillet WS, Garner RL. The fibrinolytic activity of hemolytic streptococci. *J Exp Med* 1933;**58**:485–502.

31. Sherry S. The origin of thrombolytic therapy. *J Am Coll Cardiol* 1989;**14**:1085–92.

32. Fletcher AP, Alkjaersig N, Smyrniotis FE *et al.* Treatment of patients suffering from early acute myocardial infarction with massive and prolonged streptokinase therapy. *Trans Assoc Am Phys* 1958;**71**:287–97.

33. Streptokinase in acute myocardial infarction. European Cooperative Study Group for Streptokinase Treatment in Acute Myocardial Infarction. *N Engl J Med* 1979;**301**:797–802.

34. Sharma GV, Cella G, Parisi AF, Sasahara AA. Thrombolytic therapy. *N Engl J Med* 1982;**306**:1268–76.

35. Anderson JL, Smith BR. Streptokinase in acute myocardial infarction. In: Anderson JL, ed. *Modern management of acute myocardial infarction in the community hospital.* New York: Marcel Dekker, 1991.

36. Chazov EI, Matveeva LS, Mazaev AV *et al.* Intracoronary administration of fibrinolysin in acute myocardial infarction (in Russian). *Ter Arkh* 1976;**48**:8–19.

37. Rentrop KP, Blanke H, Karsch KR *et al.* Acute myocardial infarction: intracoronary application of nitroglycerin and streptokinase. *Clin Cardiol* 1979;**2**:354–63.

38. Rentrop P, Blanke H, Karsch KR, Kaiser H, Kostering H, Leitz K. Selective intracoronary thrombolysis in acute myocardial infarction and unstable angina pectoris. *Circulation* 1981; **63**:307–17.

39. Ganz W, Ninomiya K, Hashida J *et al.* Intracoronary thrombolysis in acute myocardial infarction: experimental background and clinical experience. *Am Heart J* 1981; **102**:1145–9.

40. Anderson JL, Marshall HW, Bray BE *et al.* A randomized trial of intracoronary streptokinase in the treatment of acute myocardial infarction. *N Engl J Med* 1983;**308**:1312–18.

41. Khaja F, Walton JA, Jr., Brymer JF, *et al.* Intracoronary fibrinolytic therapy in acute myocardial infarction. Report of a prospective randomized trial. *N Engl J Med* 1983;**308**:1305–11.

42. Kennedy JW, Ritchie JL, Davis KB, Fritz JK. Western Washington randomized trial of intracoronary streptokinase in acute myocardial infarction. *N Engl J Med* 1983;**309**: 1477–82.

43. Kennedy JW, Ritchie JL, Davis KB, Stadius ML, Maynard C, Fritz JK. The western Washington randomized trial of intracoronary streptokinase in acute myocardial infarction. A 12-month follow-up report. *N Engl J Med* 1985;**312**:1073–8.

44. Simoons ML, Serruys PW, vd Brand M, Bar F, de Zwaan C, Res J *et al.* Improved survival after early thrombolysis in acute myocardial infarction. A randomized trial by the Interuniversity Cardiology Institute in The Netherlands. *Lancet* 1985; **2**:578–82.

45. Schröder R, Biamino G, von Leitner ER *et al.* Intravenous short-term infusion of streptokinase in acute myocardial infarction. *Circulation* 1983;**67**:536–48.

46. Rogers WJ, Mantle JA, Hood WP, Jr. *et al.* Prospective randomized trial of intravenous and intracoronary streptokinase in acute myocardial infarction. *Circulation* 1983;**68**:1051–61.

47. Anderson JL, Marshall HW, Askins JC *et al.* A randomized trial of intravenous and intracoronary streptokinase in patients with acute myocardial infarction. *Circulation* 1984;**70**:606–18.

48. Alderman EL, Jutzy KR, Berte LE *et al.* Randomized comparison of intravenous versus intracoronary streptokinase for myocardial infarction. *Am J Cardiol* 1984;**54**:14–9.

49. A prospective trial of intravenous streptokinase in acute myocardial infarction (I.S.A.M.). Mortality, morbidity, and infarct size at 21 days. The I.S.A.M. Study Group. *N Engl J Med* 1986;**314**:1465–71.

50. Granger CB, White HD, Bates ER, Ohman EM, Califf RM. A pooled analysis of coronary arterial patency and left ventricular function after intravenous thrombolysis for acute myocardial infarction. *Am J Cardiol* 1994;**74**:1220–8.

51. Bode C, Smalling RW, Berg G *et al.* Randomized comparison of coronary thrombolysis achieved with double-bolus reteplase (recombinant plasminogen activator) and front-loaded, accelerated alteplase (recombinant tissue plasminogen activator) in patients with acute myocardial infarction. The RAPID II Investigators. *Circulation* 1996;**94**:891–8.

52. An international randomized trial comparing four thrombolytic strategies for acute myocardial infarction. The GUSTO investigators. *N Engl J Med* 1993;**329**:673–82.

53. Sherry S, Marder MJ. Streptokinase. In: Messerli FH, ed. *Cardiovascular drug therapy, 2nd edn.* Philadelphia: W B Saunders, 1996.

54. Rutherford RB, Comerota AJ. Urokinase. In: Messerli FH, ed. *Cardiovascular Drug Therapy, 2nd edn.* Philadelphia: W B Saunders, 1990.

55. Anderson JL, Califf RM. Anisoylated plasminogen-streptokinase activator complex (APSAC). In: Messerli FH, ed. *Cardiovascular drug therapy*. Philadelphia: W B Saunders, 1996.

56. Tiefenbrunn AJ. Tissue-type plasminogen activator. In: Messerli FH, ed. *Cardiovascular drug therapy.* Philadelphia: W B Saunders, 1996.

57. Rijken DC, Hoylaerts M, Collen D. Fibrinolytic properties of one-chain and two-chain human extrinsic (tissue-type) plasminogen activator. *J Biol Chem* 1982;**257**:2920–5.

58. Randomized, double-blind comparison of reteplase double-bolus administration with streptokinase in acute myocardial infarction (INJECT): trial to investigate equivalence. International Joint Efficacy Comparison of Thrombolytics. *Lancet* 1995;**346**:329–36.

59. Keyt BA, Paoni NF, Refino CJ *et al.* A faster-acting and more potent form of tissue plasminogen activator. *Proc Natl Acad Sci USA* 1994;**91**:3670–4.

60. Van de Werf F, Vanhaecke J, de Geest H, Verstraete M, Collen D. Coronary thrombolysis with recombinant single-chain urokinase-type plasminogen activator in patients with acute myocardial infarction. *Circulation* 1986;**74**:1066–70.

61. Weaver WD, Hartmann JR, Anderson JL, Reddy PS, Sobolski JC, Sasahara AA. New recombinant glycosylated prourokinase for treatment of patients with acute myocardial infarction. Prourokinase Study Group. *J Am Coll Cardiol* 1994;**24**:1242–8.

62. Randomized double-blind trial of recombinant pro-urokinase against streptokinase in acute myocardial infarction. PRIMI Trial Study Group. *Lancet* 1989;**1**:863–8.

63. Bar FW, Meyer J, Vermeer F *et al.* Comparison of saruplase and alteplase in acute myocardial infarction. SESAM Study Group. The Study in Europe with Saruplase and Alteplase in Myocardial Infarction. *Am J Cardiol* 1997;**79**:727–32.

64. Tebbe U, Michels R, Adgey J *et al.* Randomized, double-blind study comparing saruplase with streptokinase therapy in acute myocardial infarction: the COMPASS Equivalence Trial. Comparison Trial of Saruplase and Streptokinase (COMASS) Investigators. *J Am Coll Cardiol* 1998;**31**:487–93.

65. den Heijer P, Vermeer F, Ambrosioni E *et al.* Evaluation of a weight-adjusted single-bolus plasminogen activator in patients with myocardial infarction: a double-blind, randomized angiographic trial of lanoteplase versus alteplase. *Circulation* 1998;**98**:2117–25.

66. Intravenous NPA for the treatment of infarcting myocardium early; InTIME-II, a double-blind comparison of single-bolus lanoteplase vs accelerated alteplase for the treatment of patients with acute myocardial infarction. *Eur Heart J* 2000;**21**:2005–13.

67. Collen D, Lijnen HR. Staphylokinase, a fibrin-specific plasminogen activator with therapeutic potential? *Blood* 1994; **84**:680–6.

68. Vanderschueren S, Barrios L, Kerdsinchai P *et al.* A randomized trial of recombinant staphylokinase versus alteplase for coronary artery patency in acute myocardial infarction. The STAR Trial Group. *Circulation* 1995;**92**:2044–9.

69. The effects of tissue plasminogen activator, streptokinase, or both on coronary-artery patency, ventricular function, and survival after acute myocardial infarction. The GUSTO Angiographic Investigators. *N Engl J Med* 1993;**329**: 1615–22.

70. Yusuf S, Collins R, Peto R *et al.* Intravenous and intracoronary fibrinolytic therapy in acute myocardial infarction: overview of results on mortality, re-infarction and side-effects from 33 randomized controlled trials. *Eur Heart J* 1985;**6**: 556–85.

71. Yusuf S, Wittes J, Friedman L. Overview of results of randomized clinical trials in heart disease. I. Treatments following myocardial infarction. *JAMA* 1988;**260**:2088–93.

72. Yusuf S, Sleight P, Held P, McMahon S. Routine medical management of acute myocardial infarction. Lessons from overviews of recent randomized controlled trials. *Circulation* 1990;**82**:II117–34.

73. Effectiveness of intravenous thrombolytic treatment in acute myocardial infarction. Gruppo Italiano per lo Studio della Streptochinasi nell'Infarto Miocardico (GISSI). *Lancet* 1986;**1**:397–402.

74. Long-term effects of intravenous thrombolysis in acute myocardial infarction: final report of the GISSI study. Gruppo Italiano per lo Studio della Streptochinasi nell'Infarto Miocardico (GISSI). *Lancet* 1987;**2**:871–4.

75. Randomised trial of intravenous streptokinase, oral aspirin, both, or neither among 17 187 cases of suspected acute myocardial infarction: ISIS-2. ISIS-2 (Second International Study of Infarct Survival) Collaborative Group. *Lancet* 1988;**2**:349–60.

76. Effect of intravenous APSAC on mortality after acute myocardial infarction: preliminary report of a placebo-controlled clinical trial. AIMS Trial Study Group. *Lancet* 1988;**1**:545–9.

77. Long-term effects of intravenous anistreplase in acute myocardial infarction: final report of the AIMS study. AIMS Trial Study Group. *Lancet* 1990;**335**:427–31.

78. Wilcox RG, von der Lippe G, Olsson CG, Jensen G, Skene AM, Hampton JR. Trial of tissue plasminogen activator for mortality reduction in acute myocardial infarction. Anglo-Scandinavian Study of Early Thrombolysis (ASSET). *Lancet* 1988;**2**:525–30.

79. Indications for fibrinolytic therapy in suspected acute myocardial infarction: collaborative overview of early mortality and major morbidity results from all randomized trials of more than 1000 patients. Fibrinolytic Therapy Trialists' (FTT) Collaborative Group. *Lancet* 1994;**343**:311–22.

80. Gersh BJ, Anderson JL. Thrombolysis and myocardial salvage. Results of clinical trials and the animal paradigm–paradoxic or predictable? *Circulation* 1993;**88**:296–306.

81. Boersma E, Maas AC, Deckers JW, Simoons ML. Early thrombolytic treatment in acute myocardial infarction: reappraisal of the golden hour. *Lancet* 1996;**348**:771–5.

82. Late Assessment of Thrombolytic Efficacy (LATE) study with alteplase 6–24 hours after onset of acute myocardial infarction. *Lancet* 1993;**342**:759–66.

83. Randomised trial of late thrombolysis in patients with suspected acute myocardial infarction. EMERAS (Estudio Multicentrico Estreptoquinasa Republicas de America del Sur) Collaborative Group. *Lancet* 1993;**342**:767–72.

84. Anderson JL, Karagounis L, Allen A, Bradford MJ, Menlove RL, Pryor TA. Older age and elevated blood pressure are risk factors for intracerebral hemorrhage after thrombolysis. *Am J Cardiol* 1991;**68**:166–70.

85. Maggioni AP, Franzosi MG, Santoro E, White H, Van de Werf F, Tognoni G. The risk of stroke in patients with acute myocardial infarction after thrombolytic and antithrombotic

treatment. Gruppo Italiano per lo Studio della Sopravvivenza nell'Infarto Miocardico II (GISSI-2), and The International Study Group. *N Engl J Med* 1992;**327**:1–6.

86.ISIS-3: a randomised comparison of streptokinase vs tissue plasminogen activator vs anistreplase and of aspirin plus heparin vs aspirin alone among 41299 cases of suspected acute myocardial infarction. ISIS-3 (Third International Study of Infarct Survival) Collaborative Group. *Lancet* 1992;**339**:753–70.

87.Simoons ML, Maggioni AP, Knatterud G, *et al.* Individual risk assessment for intracranial haemorrhage during thrombolytic therapy. *Lancet* 1993;**342**:1523–8.

88.Gore JM, Granger CB, Simoons ML *et al.* Stroke after thrombolysis. Mortality and functional outcomes in the GUSTO-I trial. Global Use of Strategies to Open Occluded Coronary Arteries. *Circulation* 1995;**92**:2811–18.

89.Berkowitz SD, Granger CB, Pieper KS *et al.* Incidence and predictors of bleeding after contemporary thrombolytic therapy for myocardial infarction. The Global Utilization of Streptokinase and Tissue Plasminogen activator for Occluded coronary arteries (GUSTO) I Investigators. *Circulation* 1997;**95**:2508–16.

90.Mehta SR, Eikelboom JW, Yusuf S. Risk of intracranial haemorrhage with bolus versus infusion thrombolytic therapy: a meta-analysis. *Lancet* 2000;**356**:449–54.

91.Armstrong PW, Granger C, Van de Werf F. Bolus fibrinolysis: risk, benefit, and opportunities. *Circulation* 2001;**103**:1171–3.

92.Anderson JL. Bolus thrombolytic treatment is associated with an increased risk of intracranial hemorrhage in patients with ST segment elevation infarction. A Commentary. *Evidence-based Cardiovasc Med* 2000;**4**:110–111.

93.A comparison of reteplase with alteplase for acute myocardial infarction. The Global Use of Strategies to Open Occluded Coronary Arteries (GUSTO III) Investigators. *N Engl J Med* 1997;**337**:1118–23.

94.Single-bolus tenecteplase compared with front-loaded alteplase in acute myocardial infarction: the ASSENT-2 double-blind randomised trial. Assessment of the Safety and Efficacy of a New Thrombolytic Investigators. *Lancet* 1999;**354**:716–22.

95.Randomized trial of intravenous heparin versus recombinant hirudin for acute coronary syndromes. The Global Use of Strategies to Open Occluded Coronary Arteries (GUSTO) IIa Investigators. *Circulation* 1994;**90**:1631–7.

96.Antman EM. Hirudin in acute myocardial infarction. Safety report from the Thrombolysis and Thrombin Inhibition in Myocardial Infarction (TIMI) 9A Trial. *Circulation* 1994; **90**:1624–30.

97.Neuhaus KL, von Essen R, Tebbe U *et al.* Safety observations from the pilot phase of the randomized r-Hirudin for Improvement of Thrombolysis (HIT-III) study. A study of the Arbeitsgemeinschaft Leitender Kardiologischer Krankenhausarzte (ALKK). *Circulation* 1994;**90**:1638–42.

98.Granger CB, Hirsch J, Califf RM *et al.* Activated partial thromboplastin time and outcome after thrombolytic therapy for acute myocardial infarction: results from the GUSTO-I trial. *Circulation* 1996;**93**:870–8.

99.Bottiger BW, Bode C, Kern S *et al.* Efficacy and safety of thrombolytic therapy after initially unsuccessful cardiopulmonary resuscitation: a prospective clinical trial. *Lancet* 2001;**357**:1583–5.

100.GISSI-2: a factorial randomised trial of alteplase versus streptokinase and heparin versus no heparin among 12490 patients with acute myocardial infarction. Gruppo Italiano per lo Studio della Sopravvivenza nell'Infarto Miocardico. *Lancet* 1990;**336**:65–71.

101.In-hospital mortality and clinical course of 20891 patients with suspected acute myocardial infarction randomised between alteplase and streptokinase with or without heparin. The International Study Group. *Lancet* 1990;**336**:71–5.

102.de Bono DP, Simoons ML, Tijssen J *et al.* Effect of early intravenous heparin on coronary patency, infarct size, and bleeding complications after alteplase thrombolysis: results of a randomised double blind European Cooperative Study Group trial. *Br Heart J* 1992;**67**:122–8.

103.Hsia J, Hamilton WP, Kleiman N, Roberts R, Chaitman BR, Ross AM. A comparison between heparin and low-dose aspirin as adjunctive therapy with tissue plasminogen activator for acute myocardial infarction. Heparin-Aspirin Reperfusion Trial (HART) Investigators. *N Engl J Med* 1990;**323**:1433–7.

104.Anderson JL, Karagounis LA. Does intravenous heparin or time-to-treatment/reperfusion explain differences between GUSTO and ISIS-3 results? *Am J Cardiol* 1994;**74**:1057–60.

105.Anderson JL, Becker LC, Sorensen SG *et al.* Anistreplase versus alteplase in acute myocardial infarction: comparative effects on left ventricular function, morbidity and 1-day coronary artery patency. The TEAM-3 Investigators. *J Am Coll Cardiol* 1992;**20**:753–66.

106.Neuhaus KL, von Essen R, Tebbe U *et al.* Improved thrombolysis in acute myocardial infarction with front-loaded administration of alteplase: results of the rt-PA-APSAC patency study (TAPS). *J Am Coll Cardiol* 1992;**19**:885–91.

107.Cannon CP, McCabe CH, Diver DJ *et al.* Comparison of front-loaded recombinant tissue-type plasminogen activator, anistreplase and combination thrombolytic therapy for acute myocardial infarction: results of the Thrombolysis in Myocardial Infarction (TIMI) 4 trial. *J Am Coll Cardiol* 1994;**24**:1602–10.

108.Cannon CP, McCabe CH, Gibson CM *et al.* TNK-tissue plasminogen activator in acute myocardial infarction. Results of the Thrombolysis in Myocardial Infarction (TIMI) 10A dose-ranging trial. *Circulation* 1997;**95**:351–6.

109.Cannon CP, Gibson CM, McCabe CH *et al.* TNK-tissue plasminogen activator compared with front-loaded alteplase in acute myocardial infarction: results of the TIMI 10B trial. Thrombolysis in Myocardial Infarction (TIMI) 10B Investigators. *Circulation* 1998;**98**:2805–14.

110.Van de Werf F, Cannon CP, Luyten A *et al.* Safety assessment of single-bolus administration of TNK tissue-plasminogen activator in acute myocardial infarction: the ASSENT-1 trial. The ASSENT-1 Investigators. *Am Heart J* 1999; **137**:786–91.

111.Cannon CP. Thrombolysis medication errors: benefits of bolus thrombolytic agents. *Am J Cardiol* 2000;**85**:17C–22C.

112.Randomised placebo-controlled trial of abciximab before and during coronary intervention in refractory unstable angina: the CAPTURE Study. *Lancet* 1997;**349**:1429–35.

113.Inhibition of platelet glycoprotein IIb/IIIa with eptifibatide in patients with acute coronary syndromes. The PURSUIT Trial Investigators. Platelet Glycoprotein IIb/IIIa in Unstable

Angina: Receptor Suppression Using Integrilin Therapy. *N Engl J Med* 1998;**339**:436–43.

114. Inhibition of the platelet glycoprotein IIb/IIIa receptor with tirofiban in unstable angina and non-Q-wave myocardial infarction. Platelet Receptor Inhibition in Ischemic Syndrome Management in Patients Limited by Unstable Signs and Symptoms (PRISM-PLUS) Study Investigators. *N Engl J Med* 1998;**338**:1488–97.

115. Novel dosing regimen of eptifibatide in planned coronary stent implantation (ESPRIT): a randomized, placebo-controlled trial. *Lancet* 2000;**356**:2037–44.

116. Montalescot G, Barragan P, Wittenberg O *et al.* Platelet glycoprotein IIb/IIIa inhibition with coronary stenting for acute myocardial infarction. *N Engl J Med* 2001;**344**:1895–903.

117. Antman EM, Giugliano RP, Gibson CM *et al.* Abciximab facilitates the rate and extent of thrombolysis: results of the thrombolysis in myocardial infarction (TIMI) 14 trial. The TIMI 14 Investigators. *Circulation* 1999;**99**:2720–32.

118. Trial of abciximab with and without low-dose reteplase for acute myocardial infarction. Strategies for Patency Enhancement in the Emergency Department (SPEED) Group. *Circulation* 2000;**101**:2788–94.

119. Hirsh J, Anand SS, Halperin JL, Fuster V. Guide to anticoagulant therapy: Heparin : a statement for healthcare professionals from the American Heart Association. *Circulation* 2001;**103**:2994–3018.

120. Turpie AG, Antman EM. Low molecular weight heparins in the treatment of acute coronary syndromes. *Arch Intern Med* 2001;**161**:1484–90.

121. Cohen M, Blaber R, Demers C *et al.* The Essence Trial: Efficacy and Safety of Subcutaneous Enoxaparin in unstable angina and non-Q-wave MI: a double-blind, randomized, parallel-group, multicenter study comparing enoxaparin and intravenous unfractionated heparin: methods and design. *J Thromb Thrombolysis* 1997;**4**:271–4.

122. Antman EM, Cohen M, Radley D *et al.* Assessment of the treatment effect of enoxaparin for unstable angina/non-Q-wave myocardial infarction. TIMI 11B-ESSENCE meta-analysis. *Circulation* 1999;**100**:1602–8.

123. Ross AM, Molhoek P, Lundergan C *et al.* Randomized comparison of enoxaparin, a low molecular-weight heparin, with unfractionated heparin adjunctive to recombinant tissue plasminogen activator thrombolysis and aspirin: second trial of Heparin and Aspirin Reperfusion Therapy (HART II). *Circulation* 2001;**104**:648–52.

124. Wallentin L, Dellborg DM, Lindahl B *et al.* The low molecular weight heparin dalteparin as adjuvant therapy in acute myocardial infarction: the ASSENT Plus study. *Clin Cardiol* 2001;**24**:I12–14.

125. Topol EJ. Reperfusion therapy for acute myocardial infarction with fibrinolytic therapy or combination reduced fibrinolytic therapy and platelet glycoprotein IIb/IIIa inhibition: the GUSTO V randomised trial. *Lancet* 2001;**357**:1905–14.

126. Antman EM, Louwerenburg HW, Baars HF *et al.* Enoxaparin as adjunctive antithrombin therapy for ST-elevation myocardial infarction: results of the ENTIRE-Thrombolysis in Myocardial Infarction (TIMI) 23 Trial. *Circulation* 2002;**105**:1642–9. (Erratum in *Circulation* 2002;**105**:2799).

127. White H and the The Hirulog and Early Reperfusion or Occlusion (HERO)-2 Trial Investigators. Thrombin-specific anticoagulation with bivalirudin versus heparin in patients receiving fibrinolytic therapy for acute myocardial infarction: the HERO-2 randomised trial. *Lancet* 2001;**358**:1855–63.

128. Berger AK, Radford MJ, Wang Y, Krumholz HM. Thrombolytic therapy in older patients. *J Am Coll Cardiol* 2000;**36**:366–74.

129. Thiemann DR, Coresh J, Schulman SP, Gerstenblith G, Oetgen WJ, Powe NR. Lack of benefit for intravenous thrombolysis in patients with myocardial infarction who are older than 75 years. *Circulation* 2000;**101**:2239–46.

130. Stenestrand U, Wallentin L. Thrombolysis is beneficial in elderly acute myocardial infarctin patients. *J Am Coll Cardiol* 2002:in press.

131. Sgarbossa EB, Pinski SL, Barbagelata A *et al.* Electrocardiographic diagnosis of evolving acute myocardial infarction in the presence of left bundle-branch block. GUSTO-1 (Global Utilization of Streptokinase and Tissue Plasminogen Activator for Occluded Coronary Arteries) Investigators. *N Engl J Med* 1996;**334**:481–7.

132. Simoons ML, Arnold AE. Tailored thrombolytic therapy. A perspective. *Circulation* 1993;**88**:2556–64.

133. Cairns JA, Fuster V, Gore J, Kennedy JW. Coronary thrombolysis. *Chest* 1995;**108**:401S–23S.

32 Mechanical reperfusion strategies in patients presenting with acute myocardial infarction

Sanjaya Khanal, W Douglas Weaver

Introduction

Mechanical reperfusion of the coronary artery is well established as an effective modality of treatment in patients presenting with an acute myocardial infarction. As the pathophysiology of an acute myocardial infarction most commonly involves thrombosis in an area of coronary artery with atherosclerotic narrowing with plaque rupture, advances in treating the thrombus and the underlying stenosis have significantly improved the therapy of this group of patients. Most patients with non-ST-segment elevation myocardial infarction (NSTEMI) have a non-occlusive or partially occlusive thrombus in an atherosclerotic coronary artery with the exception of true posterior myocardial infarction. The pathophysiology and the initial 30 day course of the group of patients with NSTEMI is similar to those who have unstable angina. These patients are initially managed with anticoagulants and antiplatelet agents and then risk stratified. Recently it has been shown that invasive risk stratification and appropriate revascularization in these patients improve outcomes compared to continued medical management.[1] **Grade A**

Patients with ST-segment elevation MI (STEMI) usually have a total thrombotic occlusion of the infarct artery and therefore it is critical to re-establish flow to the distal myocardium as rapidly as possible to reduce the ongoing damage to the cardiac tissue. Antiplatelet and fibrinolytic therapy has been shown to improve outcome and reduce mortality in multiple randomized studies in these patients.[2–4] **Grade A** At the same time, catheter-based percutaneous coronary interventions (PCI) have also been shown to re-establish flow in the infarct artery quite effectively, improving outcome in these patients.[5] **Grade A** Surgical revascularization is required only in a very small percentage of patients with acute STEMI. As the technology has advanced, besides balloon angioplasty, current mechanical reperfusion strategies involve stenting, various thrombectomy devices, distal protection devices, and adjunctive medications. Therefore the terminology percutaneous coronary interventions (PCI) is more appropriate than

balloon angioplasty. The focus of this chapter is to explore therapies for STEMI.

Patients who present with STEMI should be treated with either fibrinolytics or percutaneous coronary intervention (PCI) as the initial modality of reperfusion if they are otherwise eligible and have potential to benefit from therapy. **Grade A** The clear advantage of fibrinolytic therapy remains its rapidity and ease of use. It can be used in medical facilities without dedicated cardiac catheterization laboratories and the outcome does not depend on the volume of patients treated by the institution as opposed to PCI. Despite multiple randomized studies showing improved outcome with fibrinolytic therapy as compared to placebo, it is still underused in appropriate patients, most often due to perceived risk of bleeding or cerebral complications. Appropriate contraindications are infrequent. Even with the newer fibrinolytic agents, a small but significant risk (<1%) of intracranial hemorrhage remains and results in death or disability in two thirds of these patients.[7,8,25] **Grade A** The fibrinolytics establish normal TIMI grade 3 flow in only 50–60% of the patients (Figure 32.1).[9,10] **Grade A** Only a third of treated patients have complete resolution of ST-segment elevation and only about 50% have >70% resolution of ST-segment elevation 24–36 hours after fibrinolytic administration – a marker of lower mortality.[11] Since there are no absolutely reliable clinical symptoms or signs that indicate success of fibrinolytic therapy, it is difficult to evaluate whether the infarct artery is open with the treatment in

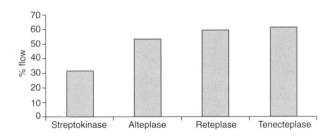

Figure 32.1 Percent TIMI-3 flow at 90 minutes with different fibrinolytic agents

an individual patient. Even in those patients who have successful fibrinolysis, many go on to have reocclusion and re-infarction due to the ongoing vulnerability of the underlying atherosclerotic plaque (Figure 32.2).[9,12,13] **Grade A**

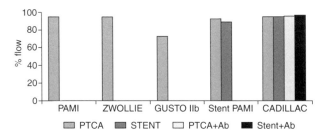

Figure 32.2 Percent TIMI-3 flow in the infarct artery after direct PCI. (Ab, abciximab; PTCA, balloon angioplasty.)

Mechanical reperfusion can overcome many of these limitations. Direct (or primary) PCI, intervention of the infarct artery without prior fibrinolysis, can be done in many patients with contraindications for fibrinolytic therapy. The overall risk of intracranial bleeding is significantly lower with direct PCI.[5] **Grade A** With the strategy of direct PCI, there is an opportunity to evaluate coronary anatomy, ventricular function, and intracardiac pressures essentially at the time of admission and possibly to detect anatomic features or mechanical complications that would require earlier treatment with surgery. The cardiac catheterization laboratory also gives an opportunity to observe directly the effects of medications and mechanical devices like intra-aortic balloon counterpulsation. The other benefit of direct PCI is the availability of highly trained staff in the cardiac catheterization laboratory if circulatory resuscitation is needed. In most randomized studies of direct PCI, the success rate is quite high and the rate of TIMI-3 flow in the infarct artery is substantially higher than is achieved with fibrinolytic therapy (Figure 32.3).[5,14,15] **Grade A** Rapid assessment and treatment also results in shorter lengths of

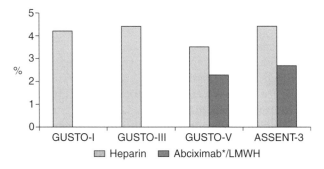

Figure 32.3 Re-infarction rates (per cent) after successful fibrinolytic therapy. (*GUSTO-V: half dose reteplase and abciximab; †ASSENT-3: half dose tenecteplase and enoxaparin; LMWH, low molecular weight heparin.)

hospital stay for patients, potentially reducing the cost of care.[16] **Grade B** The primary limitation of direct PCI in acute MI is logistical. Access to a tertiary care center with a cardiac catheterization laboratory facility and highly trained personnel is required. The majority of the patients with acute MI present to hospitals with neither of these. Even in facilities able to do PCI, the time to treatment is usually longer compared to administering fibrinolytic therapy. Transfer to these tertiary centers is often impractical because it would further delay therapy.[17] One study has suggested that the initial advantage of primary PCI over fibrinolytics is lost when the delay in doing primary PCI is more than 90 minutes from the time of presentation.[17] **Grade B** Despite these limitations, direct PCI for STEMI and elective PCI for NSTEMI are done in a significant proportion of patients with acute MI. Better understanding of the cardiovascular hemodynamics, advances in catheter technology and stents, and use of adjunctive pharmacologic therapies in the cardiac catheterization laboratory have improved results and outcomes in patients with acute MI. This has resulted from improvement in procedure safety, procedural success, and decreased need for repeat revascularization.

Randomized controlled trials: direct PTCA *v* fibrinolytic therapy

Randomized controlled trials have compared various regimens of fibrinolytic therapy with balloon angioplasty (Table 32.1). **Grade A** These studies were small in size compared to the studies of fibrinolytics versus placebo and the results may not be as generalizable. The studies are limited in that third generation fibrinolytics such as tenecteplase and reteplase along with modern regimens of heparin were not used; nor do they include the use of stents and glycoprotein (Gp) IIb/IIIa receptor inhibitors in those patients treated by direct PCI. Overall, direct balloon angioplasty seems to result in better outcomes than fibrinolysis in certain settings (Table 32.2). **Grade A** The first reported studies to compare the strategies in a randomized setting used 3 hour infusion of tPA and 1·5 MU of streptokinase.[14,15] These were done in specialized centers dedicated to direct PCI. Grines *et al* reported a trend towards improved hospital mortality and a significant decrease in the end point of death and re-infarction in patients treated with direct balloon angioplasty (OR 0·40; 95% CI 0·16–0·89). Zijlstra *et al* also reported significant mortality benefit for direct angioplasty (OR 0·25; 95% CI 0·04–0·99). **Grade A** Among the three other smaller randomized studies comparing streptokinase to direct angioplasty, two of them favored angioplasty and one streptokinase.[15,18,19] Among the smaller studies using 3–4 hour tPA regimens there were no differences in survival.[20,21] Two small studies and one large study compared the optimum accelerated tPA regimen with direct angioplasty.[22–24] The smaller studies showed a trend

Table 32.1 Trials comparing direct balloon angioplasty and fibrinolytics

Study (first author)	Lytic agent	Patient population description	Duration of symptoms (h)	Primary follow up period	Patients PTCA (n)	Patients FTX (n)	Time to Rx (min) PTCA	Time to Rx (min) FTx
DeWood[21]	Duteplase 4 h	ST ↑ <76 yr	<12	30 days	46	44	294	258
Grines[14]	tPA 3 h	ST ↑	<12	Discharge	195	200	60	32
Zijlstra[15]	1·5 mU SK ×1 h	ST ↑ <76 yr	<6	Discharge	152	149	62	30
Gibbons[20]	Duteplase 4 h	ST ↑ <80 yr	<12	Discharge	47	56	45	20
Ribeiro[18]	1·2 mU SK ×1 h	ST ↑ <75 yr	<6	Discharge	50	50	238	179
Zijlstra[15]	1·5 mU SK ×1 h	ST ↑ Low risk	<6	30 days	45	50	68	30
Ribichini[22]	tPA 90 min	Inf. MI Ant. ST ↓ <80 yr	<6	Discharge	41	42	40[a]	33[a]
Grinfeld[19]	1·5 mU SK ×1 h	ST ↑	<12	30 days	54	58	63[a]	18[a]
GUSTO-II[24]	tPA 90 min	ST ↑ LBBB	<12	30 days	565	573	72[a]	114[a]
Garcia[23]	tPA 90 min	Ant. MI	5	30 days	95	94	69	84
Total					1290	1316		

[a] From randomization.
Arrow indicates ST-segment elevated or depressed; FTx, fibrinolysis; LBBB, left bundle branch block; PTCA, percutaneous trans-luminal coronary angioplasty

Table 32.2 Mortality at end of study period: direct PTCA *v* fibrinolysis

Study	PTCA	Fibrinolysis	Odds ratio (95% CI)
Zijlstra[15]	3/152 (2·0%)	11/149 (7·4%)	0·25 (0·04–0·99)
Ribeiro[18]	3/50 (6·0%)	1/50 (2·0%)	3·13 (0·24–1·67)
Grinfeld[19]	5/54 (9·3%)	6/58 (10·3%)	0·88 (0·20–3·73)
Zijlstra[15]	1/45 (2·2%)	0/50 (0·0%)	
DeWood[21a]	3/46 (6·5%)	2/44 (4·6%)	1·47 (0·16–18·3)
Grines[14]	5/195 (2·6%)	13/200 (6·5%)	0·38 (0·11–1·16)
Gibbons[20a]	2/47 (4·3%)	2/56 (3·6%)	1·20 (0·08–17·1)
Ribichini[22]	0/41 (0%)	1/42 (2·4%)	0·00 (0·0–19·6)
Garcia[23]	3/95 (3·2%)	10/94 (10·6%)	0·27 (0·04–1·12)
GUSTO-II[24]	32/565 (5·7%)	40/573 (7·0%)	0·80 (0·48–1·32)
Total	57/1290(4·4%)[b]	86/1316 (6·5%)[b]	0·66 (0·46–0·94)

[a] Duteplase.
[b] Percentages are pooled results and odds ratio calculated by exact method using all trials.

that favored angioplasty, but the difference was not statistically significant. **Grade A**

The largest study to date that compared accelerated tPA and direct angioplasty is the GUSTO-IIb.[24] This was a multicenter study that was a substudy of the larger GUSTO-II study comparing hirudin and heparin in the treatment of acute MI. It represented more of community practice for treating MI, with 57 hospitals participating rather than a few specialized centers. In this study, the incidence of the primary end point (death, non-fatal re-infarction and stroke at 30 days) was 9·6% in the angioplasty group and 13·7% in the tPA group (*P* = 0·03). However, there was no difference in the incidence

of the composite end point (14·1% *v* 16·1% *P* = NS) at 6 months. **Grade A** Of note, this study reported only 73% of patients undergoing direct angioplasty achieved TIMI-3 flow when analyzed by a core laboratory. Most of other direct PCI studies have reported achieving TIMI-3 flow rates of over 90%. Subgroup analysis of the GUSTO-IIb study seems to suggest more benefit of direct angioplasty in elderly patients and patients who present after 4 hours of symptoms. **Grade B** When the results of GUSTO-IIb are combined with all others, it appears that there is a significant reduction in the composite mortality and re-infarction (approximately 70% net reduction at 30 days that is maintained to at least 6 months).

A meta-analysis of the studies described above by Weaver *et al* found that patients treated with direct angioplasty had 30 day or less mortality of 4·4% compared with 6·5% in patients treated with fibrinolytic therapy (OR 0·66; 95% CI 0·46–0·94).[5] The rates of death or non-fatal re-infarction were 7·2% for angioplasty and 11·9% for fibrinolytics (OR 0·58; 95% CI 0·44–0·76). Furthermore, the risk of stroke was also significantly reduced (0·7% *v* 2·0%; *P* = 0·007). **Grade A** Intracranial hemorrhage is a significant limitation of intravenous fibrinolytic therapy. Major fibrinolytic studies have consistently reported a small but significant risk of intracranial hemorrhage.[9,25] **Grade A** This risk is lower with direct angioplasty compared to fibrinolytics in the randomized trials.[5] Patients at higher risk of intracranial bleeding (for example, age >75 years or systemic hypertension) may derive more benefit from direct PCI as opposed to fibrinolytic therapy.[24] **Grade A** The risk of bleeding increases with more aggressive fibrinolytic therapy. Pilot studies suggested better TIMI-3 flow rates in the infarct artery when a reduced dose fibrinolytic was combined with a GP IIb/IIIa inhibitor.[26–28] However, there was no mortality benefit seen with the use of half-dose fibrinolytic therapy plus a GP IIb/IIIa inhibitor compared to full-dose fibrinolytic in the GUSTO-V study.[29] There was a reduction in re-infarction rate but a higher bleeding rate with the combination therapy. **Grade A** In the ASSENT-3 study, the combination of low molecular weight heparin had greater efficacy (30 day mortality, re-infarction or refractory ischemia) and safety (intracranial hemorrhage or major bleeding) than tenecteplase plus unfractionated heparin or half-dose tenecteplase plus abciximab.[30] **Grade A** Therefore, it appears that adjusting fibrinolytic dose or combining it with IIb/IIIa inhibitors has not reduced overall mortality in AMI without compromising safety.

Observational studies: direct angioplasty *v* fibrinolytic therapy

Randomized controlled trials have demonstrated that direct angioplasty results in superior outcomes if done in a controlled setting. Whether this superiority is maintained in the community is not clear. Observational studies of large registries provide insight into this.[31,32] Randomized trials of direct angioplasty are usually carried out in tertiary hospitals with the facility and personnel dedicated to PCI. Therefore, a community hospital may not be able to replicate the results of the randomized trial for various reasons. The Myocardial Infarction Triage and Intervention Investigation registry compared mortality in 1050 patients undergoing direct angioplasty with 2095 patients treated with fibrinolytics for AMI.[32] The primary angioplasty patients were treated in three high volume and seven low volume centers, reflecting community practice. There was no difference of inhospital

mortality or long-term mortality between the groups (5·6% *v* 5·5%, *P* = 0·93; long-term adjusted hazard ratio 0·95; 95% CI 0·8–1·2) (Figure 32.4). **Grade B** Procedure use and costs were lower in patients in the fibrinolytic group by the time of hospital discharge and at 3 years (33% fewer coronary angiograms, 20% fewer PCIs, and 14% lower costs). **Grade B** However, this study did not include the use of stents, which have been shown to significantly reduce target vessel revascularization. Currently, 40–60% of patients who are treated with fibrinolytics undergo further revascularization, and it is now likely that cost–benefit analysis will favor PCI. **Grade B/C**

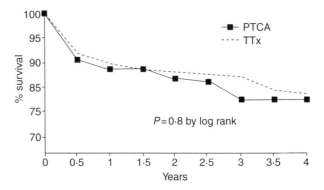

Figure 32.4 Cumulative survival among 1050 patients in the primary-angioplasty group and 2095 patients in the fibrinolytic group

Tierfenbrunn *et al* reported a similar comparison between 4939 patients undergoing direct angioplasty and 24 705 patients undergoing fibrinolysis for AMI.[33] The time to treatment with fibrinolytic was shorter than direct angioplasty (42 min *v* 111 min, *P* < 0·0001). Inhospital mortality in the two groups was the same (5·2% *v* 5·4%). The stroke rate was higher in the fibrinolytic group (1·6% *v* 0·7%, *P* < 0·001). The inhospital mortality was higher in patients with shock treated with fibrinolytics than direct angioplasty (52% *v* 32%). The results were maintained after adjustments for baseline risk by multivariate analysis. **Grade B**

Observational studies therefore suggest that the mortality advantage of direct PCI may not be maintained in the community setting, although the results are probably no worse than with fibrinolytic therapy. There are various explanations for this, but the delay in doing direct PCI as compared to administering fibrinolytic in the community setting is likely a major factor. Since the experience of the institution and the operator doing the PCI influences outcome, results of direct PCI in the community may not be as good as those from specialized tertiary centers.[34] **Grade B** Cannon *et al*, using a retrospective analysis, have demonstrated that an increase in the door-to-balloon time increases mortality significantly in patients undergoing direct angioplasty for AMI (121–150 min, OR 1·41; 151–180 min OR 1·62; >180 min, OR 1·61).[17] **Grade B** Canto *et al*, reporting from the same registry, noted that inhospital mortality was 28% lower among patients who underwent direct angioplasty in hospitals with the highest volume compared with those who were treated at hospitals with the lowest volume (adjusted RR 0·72; 95% CI 0·60–0·87).[31] At the same time there was no significant relation between inhospital mortality and volume of patients when fibrinolytic therapy was used. **Grade B** Another possible factor explaining this finding may be the bias of treating sicker patients with direct angioplasty in a non-randomized setting. Although baseline risk adjustments were done to exclude this, it is possible that the risk adjustments may have been incomplete.

There has been continuous improvement in the outcomes following both fibrinolytic therapy and direct angioplasty over time. However, direct angioplasty may have had more incremental improvement than fibrinolytic therapy over time. Rogers *et al* reported that the temporal trend in 1·5 million patients with MI in the USA from 1990 through 1999 revealed that patients are being administered fibrinolysis more rapidly, there is increasing use of direct PCI, and more frequent use of adjunctive therapies.[35] **Grade B** These factors may be contributing to shorter hospital stays (median duration from 8·3 days *v* 4·3 days) and lower inhospital mortality (11·2% *v* 9·4%). Zahn *et al* reported data from two large German registries of 10 118 fibrinolytic eligible patients.[36] There were 1385 patients treated with direct angioplasty and 8733 who received fibrinolysis. The proportion of an inhospital delay of more than 90 minutes significantly decreased inpatients treated with direct angioplasty between 1994 and 1998 (multivariate OR 0·84; 95% CI 0·73–0·96) but did not change significantly for patients treated with fibrinolysis. Hospital mortality decreased significantly in the direct angioplasty group (multivariate OR 0·73; 95% CI 0·58–0·93), but there was no significant improvement in mortality over time in patients treated with fibrinolysis. **Grade B**

Fibrinolytic therapy *v* stenting

Use of stents in elective percutaneous coronary interventions has been shown to have superior results in the form of lower restenosis and better target vessel revascularization rates in many coronary lesion subsets. **Grade A** Stent implantation in the setting of MI has been studied in comparison to fibrinolytic therapy and balloon angioplasty alone with and without concomitant Gp IIb/IIIa inhibitor therapy. Schomig *et al* randomized 140 AMI patients to receive either accelerated intravenous tPA or direct coronary stenting plus abciximab.[37] The median size of the infarct as measured by Tc[99m] sestamibi scan was smaller in the stent plus abciximab group compared to the tPA group (14·3% *v* 19·4%, *P* = 0·002). The combined end point of death, re-infarction, or stroke was also lower in the stent

plus abciximab group (8·5% *v* 23·2%, *P* = 0·02). **Grade A** Le May *et al*, in a smaller study of 123 AMI patients, reported that compared to accelerated tPA, stenting reduced the combined end point of death, re-infarction, stroke or repeat target vessel revascularization in a 6 month follow up (24·2% *v* 55·7%, *P* < 0·001).[38] The median length of hospital stay was significantly reduced in the stented patients (4 days *v* 7 days, *P* < 0·001). **Grade A** Kastrati *et al* compared the administration of alteplase plus abciximab with stenting plus abciximab in 162 AMI patients.[39] Stenting was associated with greater myocardial salvage than alteplase (median 13·6% *v* 8·0%, *P* = 0·007). Stenting therefore results in superior outcome to fibrinolytic therapy if done in appropriate settings. **Grade A**

Fibrinolytics, transport or direct PCI without on-site cardiac surgery

One major limitation of direct PCI is the excessive time it takes to mobilize the patient and do the procedure. The advantage of direct PCI is decreased in the community setting primarily because of major difference in treatment times as compared to randomized studies.[32,33] Ideally, if door-to-balloon time could be substantially reduced, direct PCI would probably have a significant advantage over fibrinolytic therapy. The Air PAMI study randomized patients to on-site fibrinolysis versus transfer to tertiary facility for direct PCI.[40] There was a non-statistically significant 38% reduction in the end point of death, re-infarction or disabling stroke (8·4% *v* 13·6%) in patients treated with direct PCI. **Grade A** Widimsky *et al* have shown that patients transported from presenting hospitals to tertiary hospitals for direct PCI have lower incidence of the combined end point of death, re-infarction, and stroke at 30 days than patients treated with fibrinolytic therapy in the community hospital or fibrinolytic therapy during transportation to PCI (8% *v* 23% *v* 15%, *P* < 0·02).[41] **Grade A** Anderson *et al* presented data in a randomized study reporting that patients treated with direct PCI with or without transfer had a lower incidence of the combined end point of death, re-infarction or disabling stroke at 30 days than patients treated with fibrinolytic therapy (9·8% *v* 13·7%, *P* = 0·0003).[42] **Grade A** The delay in door-to-balloon time with the transport in both these studies averaged only 10 minutes, which is hard to achieve in most settings.

The other limitation of direct PCI is the accessibility of patients to centers that can perform the procedure safely. Whether direct PCI can or should be done in facilities without surgical backup has been debated. Aversano *et al* compared fibrinolytic therapy versus primary PCI in patients presenting to hospitals without on-site cardiac surgery.[43] After extensive formal PCI programs were developed at the treating facilities, 451 patients were randomly assigned to either direct PCI or fibrinolytic therapy with accelerated tPA. The composite end point of death, re-infarction or stroke was reduced in patients treated with direct PCI at 6 weeks (10·7% *v* 17·7%, *P*= 0·03) and 6 months (12·4% *v* 19·9%, *P*= 0·03). The median length of hospital stay was also reduced in the PCI group (4·5 days *v* 6·0 days, *P*= 0·02). **Grade A**

Therefore, the choice of whether to treat AMI patients with direct PCI or fibrinolytic therapy should be made depending on each institution's preparedness to do direct PCI and its success rate. If conditions close to those in the randomized studies prevail the choice should clearly be direct PCI. In less optimal conditions, the choice depends on the likelihood of good outcomes in individual and groups of patients. **Grade A** Finally, as advances in pharmacologic therapy and PCI continue, there may be a role in doing both approaches in the form of facilitated PCI. **Grade B/C**

Balloon angioplasty *v* stenting

Grines *et al* compared balloon angioplasty to implantation of a heparin coated stent in a randomized study of 900 patients with AMI undergoing direct PCI.[44] The combined primary end point of death, re-infarction, disabling stroke or target vessel revascularization was lower in the stent group (12·6% *v* 20·1%, *P*< 0·001). The benefit resulted primarily from a reduction in target vessel revascularization, with a larger minimal luminal diameter achieved after stenting (2·56 + 0·44 mm *v* 2·12 + 0·45 mm, *P*< 0·001) resulting in a lower restenosis rate (20·3% *v* 33·5%, *P*< 0·001) than the angioplasty group. **Grade A** This study was done without significant use of Gp IIb/IIIa inhibitors and reported a marginally higher death rate in the stent group than the angioplasty group (3·5% *v* 1·8%, *P*= 0·15). Although this was not statistically significant, there was a question as to whether the lower TIMI-3 flow rate achieved with stenting in this study (89·4% *v* 92·7%, *P*= 0·10) contributed to this. Subsequent studies have not reproduced this. Maillard *et al* reported a study which randomized 211 AMI patients to direct angioplasty versus stenting and found that the primary end point of restenosis at 6 months was lower in the stent group (25% *v* 40%, *P*= 0·04).[45] There was no acute difference in angiographic success rates between the two groups (86% for stent and 82% for angioplasty, *P*= NS). **Grade A** Stone *et al* demonstrated that implantation of stents to treat lesions causing an acute MI had the best overall results when compared to balloon angioplasty with or without the Gp IIb/IIIa inhibitor abciximab.[46] In this study 2082 patients with acute MI undergoing direct PCI were randomly assigned four different treatment groups: angioplasty alone, angioplasty with abciximab, stent alone, and stent with abciximab. The stent group had the lowest

incidence of major cardiovascular events at 6 months (20·0% PTCA, 16·5% PTCA plus abciximab, 11·5% stenting and 10·2% stenting plus abciximab, *P*< 0·001). **Grade A** This benefit was primarily driven by target vessel revascularization. There was no deterioration of flow or possible early hazard seen with the stent in this study. It therefore appears safe and desirable in patient undergoing direct PCI in the setting of an acute MI to treat the coronary lesions with stents if feasible. **Grade A**

PCI with or without Gp IIb/IIIa inhibitors

There are several studies evaluating the use of Gp IIb/IIIa inhibitors during direct PCI for AMI. Brener *et al* randomized 483 patients to receive abciximab or placebo during direct AMI angioplasty. When the results were analyzed by intention to treat, there was no difference in the incidence of the combined end point of death, re-infarction, and target vessel revascularization (TVR) at 6 months (28·1% *v* 28·2%, *P*= 0·97).[45] There was a trend toward a lower rate of death or re-infarction with abciximab in an actual treatment analysis (6·9% *v* 12·0%, *P* = 0·07) but this was achieved with more frequent major bleeding in the abciximab group (16·6% *v* 9·5%, *P*= 0·02). **Grade A** Montalescot *et al* randomly assigned 300 patients to abciximab and stenting or placebo and stenting. The composite end point of death, re-infarction or urgent TVR was lower in the abciximab group at 30 days (6·0% *v* 14·6%, *P*= 0·01) and at 6 months (7·4% *v* 15·9%, *P*= 0·02).[48] The TIMI-3 flow was better in the abciximab group immediately prior to the procedure (16·8% *v* 5·4%, *P*= 0·01), immediately after the stenting procedure (95·1% *v* 86·7%, *P*= 0·04) and at 6 month angiographic follow up (94·3% *v* 82·8%, *P*= 0·04). There was significantly more minor bleeding (12·1% *v* 3·3%, *P*= 0·004) but only one major bleed was reported in the abciximab group. The better results with abciximab in this study may be influenced by the better TIMI-3 flow rate achieved prior to PCI in the patients who received abciximab well ahead of the PCI. **Grade A** In the 2082 patient randomized study reported by Stone *et al*, patients treated with abciximab and stent did not have statistically significantly better outcome than those treated with stent alone.[46] In this study, the abciximab was used after angiography and randomization with no difference in the TIMI-3 flow between the groups treated with stent alone or stent plus abciximab either before (21·3% *v* 24%) or after (94·5% *v* 96·9%) the PCI. The combined end point of death, re-infarction, disabling stroke or TVR was also not statistically different between the groups (11·5% *v* 10·2%). **Grade A** We have to therefore conclude that use of the Gp IIb/IIIa inhibitor abciximab during direct PCI has either marginal or no advantage over stenting alone. There are no randomized data with the other Gp IIb/IIIa inhibitors in this setting.

Facilitated PCI

Earlier achievement of normal perfusion of the infarct artery results in better myocardial salvage and clinical outcome.[49] **Grade A** Facilitated PCI is the term used to designate the use of pharmacologic therapy to aid reperfusion of the infarct artery while preparing for direct PCI. This may be achieved with either full-dose fibrinolytics or reduced dose fibrinolytics combined with platelet inhibitors. Earlier studies showed that routinely undertaking PCI after full-dose fibrinolytic administration results in worse outcomes and therefore is not recommended unless there is clinical evidence of failure of fibrinolytic therapy.[50,51] **Grade A** However, with advancements in catheter technology, better hemostatic techniques, and safer pharmacologic regimens, it may be feasible to combine various doses of fibrinolytics and direct PCI. Since fibrinolytics can be administered much more quickly than PCI can be performed, whether this approach results in better patient outcome needs to be studied. The potential advantage of this approach would be that more patients would have open infarct arteries prior to doing PCI resulting in better myocardial salvage. Ross *et al.* reported a pilot study of 606 AMI patients randomly assigned to half-dose rtPA or placebo before undergoing angiography.[52] PCI was carried out only if there was less than TIMI-3 flow in the infarct artery. More patients with half-dose rtPA had TIMI-3 flow at first angiography (33% *v* 15%, $P < 0.001$) but there was no difference in bleeding rates, stroke or 30 day mortality between the groups. **Grade B** Herrman *et al* reported the result of a subanalysis of the GUSTO-IV Pilot in which 323 patients underwent PCI at the time of initial angiography.[53] In this analysis PCI was done safely and efficaciously in patients receiving half-dose rtPA and full-dose abciximab. **Grade B**

Facilitated PCI may also address the delay in reperfusion in patients undergoing direct PCI. If PCI in patients who have received a combination of reduced dose fibrinolytic and platelet inhibitors can be demonstrated to be safe, this strategy may reduce time to reperfusion and maintain the benefit of direct PCI. **Grade B/C** Whether transferring patients after administration of combination therapy from community medical centers to tertiary centers to perform facilitated PCI results in better outcome requires further study.

The other potential advantage of facilitated PCI may be the opportunity to improve distal myocardial perfusion. Distal myocardial perfusion is normal only in the one third of patients who undergo direct PCI and achieve TIMI-3 flow in the culprit artery. Poor distal myocardial perfusion in spite of TIMI-3 flow in the epicardial artery predicts a worse outcome in patients with AMI.[54] **Grade B** Thrombectomy devices or distal protection devices may decrease the chance of worsening distal myocardial flow during PCI. **Grade B/C** Systemic or intracoronary administration of agents such as Gp IIb/IIIa inhibitors and adenosine may improve distal myocardial perfusion.[53,55] **Grade A/B** A variety of other pharmacologic agents is being tested in combination with fibrinolysis or PCI to see if infarct size can be reduced. Invasive assessments of the coronaries and myocardium currently allow accurate assessment. Facilitated PCI is in its early stages of investigation and no definite recommendations can be made with the current evidence.

Resource use and cost effectiveness of direct PCI

As clinical outcomes vary between randomized trials and observational studies of direct PCI and fibrinolysis, so too does cost analysis between individual randomized studies and observational studies. In general, randomized studies report cost advantages of direct angioplasty because of reduced length of stay, repeat hospitalizations, and need for subsequent revascularization. **Grade A** Whether these factors overcome the higher upfront costs of an invasive procedure requires systematic analysis. Zijlstra *et al* have reported a 5 year follow up of 395 patients randomly treated with intravenous streptokinase or direct angioplasty.[56] The direct angioplasty group had higher survival (mortality 13% *v* 24%, RR 0·54; 95% CI 0·15–0·52%) less non-fatal re-infarctions, and fewer readmissions for heart failure and ischemia. The total medical charges were also lower in the angioplasty group ($16 090 *v* 16 813, $P = 0.05$). **Grade A** In the randomized PAMI study, Stone *et al* reported direct angioplasty achieved better clinical outcomes with no significant difference in cost ($27 653 for angioplasty *v* $30 227 for fibrinolysis, $P = 0.21$).[57] **Grade A**

Analysis of the MITI registry, however, shows that patients treated with angioplasty for AMI were more likely to undergo further catheterization and revascularization procedures and incurred 13% higher costs than patients treated with fibrinolysis.[32] **Grade B** This is in contrast with the results of most of the randomized studies of direct PCI and fibrinolysis. When patients are randomly assigned in a carefully conducted study, the physician preference or bias is controlled. But in an observational study, it may be that sicker patients are referred for direct PCI and the additional invasive assessment after the primary PCI may be driven by the physician preference for invasive assessment.

Therefore the cost of direct PCI probably is lower or equal to the cost of fibrinolysis in the long term if it is done in centers practicing methods used in the randomized control trials, but the comparison of the costs in the community setting is not as favorable. Estimates of cost effectiveness using randomized data and assuming a large (40–50%) mortality benefit from direct PCI favor direct PCI.[58] But if the more modest reduction in events noted in the GUSTO-IIb or the observational studies are used, the estimate of benefit may be much less.[24,32] **Grade B** Because therapeutic strategies for both fibrinolysis and direct PCI are evolving, it is hard to compare the cost or calculate the cost effectiveness of either therapy.[59] Upfront costs of direct PCI have increased with the more frequent use of Gp IIb/IIIa inhibitors and stents during the procedures, but the shorter hospital stay and improving clinical outcomes may offset the initial costs. Grines *et al* have demonstrated that omission of intensive care and discharge at day 3 of hospital stay after direct PCI for AMI is safe in some lower-risk patients and has the potential for cost savings.[16] **Grade B** The cost of fibrinolysis is in flux, with newer agents, adjunctive therapies, and increasing use of invasive risk stratification after fibrinolytic administration. Because of this, and the wide variation of cost of procedures in patients with AMI, formal cost effective analysis is difficult and inaccurate to extrapolate to all settings.

The use of bypass surgery in the setting of AMI

With the advent of stents for acute vessel closures, the percentage of patients requiring emergency bypass surgery for acute myocardial infarction has fallen below 1% in contemporary randomized studies of direct PCI.[37,44] **Grade A** However, earlier studies of direct PCI and observational registries reported this rate as 4–6%.[14,15,60] **Grade B** Bypass surgery may be required owing to anatomical considerations, such as left main disease or coronary disease not suitable for immediate PCI, or mechanical complications from the MI such as acute severe mitral regurgitation, ventricular septal defect or a failed PCI. Observational studies report that stable patients with acute MI can undergo bypass surgery with good results. But, the complexity of performing cardiac surgery in patients with acute MI and potentially other manifestations like failed PCI or cardiogenic shock is definitely greater. Randomized studies comparing surgery to medical therapy or PCI in this situation are lacking.

When bypass surgery was the only available therapy for acute coronary reperfusion in the 1970s, there were some studies that reported surprisingly good results. DeWood *et al* reported on their experience with 187 patients treated with early coronary bypass surgery.[61] In this observational study, all patients under 65 years of age who presented with ST-segment elevation underwent cardiac catheterization. After exclusion of 28 patients (comorbidity, diffuse or no coronary disease), 187 patients were treated with bypass surgery and 200 were treated medically. Although treatment was not randomly assigned, the groups were well balanced in terms of age, prior history, and presenting signs and symptoms. Hospital and long-term mortality was lower in the bypass patients (5·8% *v* 11·5%, *P* = 0·08 in hospital; 11·7% *v* 20·5%, *P* < 0·03 at 56 months). In surgical patients placed on cardiopulmonary bypass within 6 hours

of symptoms, hospital mortality was 2%. **Grade B** Similar results have been reported in 261 patients treated with acute bypass surgery at the Iowa Heart Center (hospital mortality 5·7%).[62] **Grade B** These findings, however, are limited by the fact that the comparisons between surgical and medical therapy were not randomized. Patients were excluded from the surgical cohort due to coronary anatomy, comorbidity or shock. Thus, these excellent results are probably not generalizable to the larger population of acute infarct patients.

In the PAMI-2 study of AMI patients treated with direct angioplasty, 10·9% underwent cardiac surgery before hospital discharge, 57% of whom underwent the surgery urgently.[55] The inhospital mortality was 6·4% in those who underwent surgery urgently versus 2·0% in the elective surgery group. **Grade B** The mortality associated with bypass surgery after AMI increases with the instability of the patient. Lee *et al* reported on 316 patients undergoing bypass surgery after AMI, among whom the mortality was 1·2% in stable patients and 26% in patients with cardiogenic shock.[63] Hochman *et al* reported the results a randomized study comparing medical therapy versus revasularization therapy in 304 patients with acute MI and cardiogenic shock.[64] In the revascularization group 64% were treated with angioplasty and 36% by surgery. At 30 days the mortality was 46·7% in the revascularization group versus 56% in the medical therapy group (*P* = 0·11) but at 6 months the mortality was statistically lower in the revascularization group (50·3% *v* 63·1%, *P* = 0·027). There was no difference in mortality between the angioplasty group (45·3%) and the surgery group (42%). Although patients have a high mortality when they present with acute MI and cardiogenic shock, revascularization strategy may improve the outcome in selected patients. **Grade A** As a subgroup, patients ≥75 years of age had higher mortality with the revascularization strategy (RR 1·41; 95% CI 0·97–2·03) than medical therapy. **Grade B** Therefore, it is unclear at this time whether elderly patients in cardiogenic shock should undergo revascularization therapy in the setting of an acute MI.

The American College of Cardiology/American Heart Association practice guidelines for the treatment of AMI recommend acute bypass surgery only in the case where catheter-based intervention has failed or is not feasible.[65] Class I recommendations for urgent/emergent bypass in the setting of AMI include those patients with failed PTCA with persistent pain or hemodynamic instability, persistent or recurrent ischemia refractory to medical therapy in candidates not eligible/suitable for catheter-based intervention, or in the setting of a surgical repair for ventricular septal defect or mitral valve insufficiency. Class II indications include cardiogenic shock or failed angioplasty in patients with a small amount of myocardium at risk.

Conclusions and recommendations

Although a small subset of patients will require emergent surgery, in the current environment, mechanical reperfusion in the setting of an acute MI is mostly limited to percutaneous coronary intervention. The majority of patients with STEMI present to hospitals without dedicated PCI facilities or personnel and will be treated pharmacologically with fibrinolytics, antithrombotics, and platelet inhibitors. In centers with dedicated PCI facilities, the choice of therapy should be direct PCI in all patients presenting with STEMI unless contraindicated. **Grade A** This is especially so if it can be done in an expeditious manner, by an experienced operator in a high volume center. **Grade B** Although there are no randomized study data to substantiate the numbers associated with the time to therapy, operator volume or institution PCI volume, the American College of Cardiology and American Heart Association recommends a door-to-balloon time of <90 minutes, operator PCI volume of >75 per year, and institution volume of >200 per year.[65] Whether surgical backup is necessary to do direct AMI PCI is debatable, but a small number of patients continue to require emergency surgical therapy because of coronary anatomy or failed PCI, and surgical backup close at hand is recommended. **Grade B** Younger patients (<75 years) with cardiogenic shock, patients with contraindications to fibrinolytic therapy with high risk of bleeding, and patients who have failed fibrinolytic therapy should also be considered for PCI.[64] **Grade A**

Myocardial salvage and therefore prognosis depends on the time delay to opening the blocked infarct artery. Everything possible should be done to expedite the re-establishment of flow into the distal myocardium. **Grade A** Whether the benefit of direct PCI by transferring patients from community hospitals to tertiary centers outweighs the additional myocardial damage brought on by the delay needs to be studied further. **Grade B** Facilitated PCI by using full or reduced dose fibrinolytics with or without IIb/IIIa inhibitors during the time delay to the catheterization laboratory also shows promise, but again needs further study. **Grade C**

During the actual PCI, there are no clear guidelines about procedural approaches. Many operators minimize the time to open the infarct artery by forgoing the right heart catheterization or the left ventriculography in the majority of patients and using a guiding catheter to do culprit vessel angiography. **Grade C** Gp IIb/IIIa inhibitors, especially abciximab, have been shown to improve periprocedural outcome in some randomized studies if started well in advance to achieve better TIMI-3 flow prior to the PCI.[48] **Grade A** Implantation of a stent to treat the culprit stenosis also reduces combined event rates, especially target vessel revascularization. **Grade A** The possible early hazard observed in the PAMI stent study was not seen in other studies using different stents with or without a GP IIb/IIIa inhibitor.[44,46] Elective use of intra-aortic balloon counterpulsation in stable patients after successful PCI is not beneficial. **Grade B** Distal protection and thrombectomy devices have potential for reducing distal embolization but need systematic study.[66] **Grade B/C**

Although a large majority of patients achieve TIMI-3 flow in the culprit artery after PCI, distal myocardial perfusion is completely normal in only a minority of these patients. The status of myocardial perfusion also directly influences prognosis, with the best outcomes observed in patients with normal myocardial perfusion. Some studies found that vasodilators like adenosine seem to improve the distal myocardial perfusion.[53,54,67] **Grade A/C** Whether these agents and other newer anti-inflammatory agents will result in improved outcomes by improving distal myocardial perfusion needs to be studied further. Other strategies to reduce myocardial damage, such as lowering body temperature and infusing supersaturated oxygen, also need further study.[68,69] **Grade C**

References

1. Cannon CP, Weintraub W, Demopoulos LA *et al*. Comparison of early invasive and conservative strategies in patients with unstable coronary syndromes treated with the glycoprotein IIb/IIIa inhibitor tirofiban. *N Engl J Med* 2001;**344**:1879–87.
2. Second International Study of Infarct Survival (ISIS-2) Collaborative Group. Randomized trial of intravenous streptokinase, oral aspirin, both or neither in 17 187 cases of suspected acute myocardial infarction. *Lancet* 1988;**ii**:349–60.
3. Fibrinolytic Therapy Trialists (FTT) Collaborative Group. Indications for fibrinolytic therapy in suspected acute myocardial infarction: collaborative overview of early mortality and major morbidity results from all randomized trials of more than 1000 patients. *Lancet* 1994;**343**:311–22.
4. The GUSTO Investigators. An international randomized trial comparing four thrombolytic strategies for acute myocardial infarction. *N Engl J Med* 1993;**329**:673–82.
5. Weaver WD, Simes J, Betriu A *et al*. Comparison of primary coronary angioplasty and intravenous thrombolytic therapy for acute myocardial infarction. *JAMA* 1997;**278**:2093–8.
6. Magid DJ, Calonge BN, Rumsfeld JS *et al*. Relation between hospital primary angioplasty volume and mortality for patients treated with acute MI treated with primary angioplasty vs thrombolytic therapy. *JAMA* 2000;**284**:3131–8.
7. Gore JM, Granger CB, Simoons ML *et al*. Stroke after thrombolysis. Mortality and functional outcomes in the GUSTO-I trial. Global Use of Strategies to Open Occluded Coronary Arteries. *Circulation* 1995;**92**:2811–18.
8. The GUSTO-III Investigators. An international, multicenter, randomized comparison of reteplase with alteplase for acute myocardial infarction. *N Engl J Med* 1997;**337**;1118–23.
9. The GUSTO Angiographic Investigators. The effects of tissue plasminogen activator, streptokinase, or both on coronary-artery patency, ventricular function, and survival after acute myocardial infarction. *N Engl J Med* 1993;**329**:1615–22.

10.TIMI Study Group. The Thrombolysis in Myocardial Infarction (TIMI) Trial, Phase 1 findings. *N Engl J Med* 1985; **312**:932–7.

11.Fu Y, Goodman S, Chang WC, Van De Werf F, Granger CB, Armstrong PW. Time to treatment influences the impact of ST-segment resolution on one year prognosis: insights from the assessment of the safety and efficacy of a new thrombolytic (ASSENT-2) trial. *Circulation* 2001;**104**:2653–9.

12.Hudson MP, Granger CB, Topol EJ *et al.* Early reinfarction after fibrinolysis: experience from the global utilization of streptokinase and tissue plasminogen activator (alteplase) for occluded coronary arteries (GUSTO-I) and global use of strategies to open occluded arteries (GUSTO-III) trials. *Circulation* 2001;**104**:1229–35.

13.Gibson CM, Cannon CP, Piana RN *et al.* Angiographic predictors of reocclusion after thrombolysis: results from the Thrombolysis in Myocardial Infarction (TIMI) 4 trial. *J Am Coll Cardiol* 1995;**25**:582–9.

14.Grines CL, Browne KF, Marco J *et al.* A comparison of immediate angioplasty with thrombolytic therapy for acute myocardial infarction. The Primary Angioplasty in Myocardial Infarction Study Group. *N Engl J Med* 1993;**328**:673–9.

15.Zijlstra F, de Boer MJ, Hoornje JC *et al.* A comparison of immediate coronary angioplasty with intravenous streptokinase in acute myocardial infarction. *N Engl J Med* 1993;**328**:680–4.

16.Grines CL, Marsalese DL, Brodie B *et al.* Safety and cost-effectiveness of early discharge after primary angioplasty in low risk patients with acute myocardial infarction. *J Am Coll Cardiol* 1998;**31**:967–72.

17.Cannon CP, Gibson CM, Lambrew CT *et al.* Relationship of symptom-onset-to-balloon time and door-to-balloon time with mortality in patients undergoing angioplasty for acute myocardial infarction. *JAMA* 2000;**283**:2941–7.

18.Ribeiro EE, Silva LA, Carneiro R *et al.* Randomized trial of direct coronary angioplasty versus intravenous streptokinase in acute myocardial infarction. *J Am Coll Cardiol* 1993;**22**:376–80.

19.Grinfeld L, Berrocal D, Belardi J *et al.* Fibrinolytics vs primary angioplasty in acute myocardial infarction (FAP): a randomized trial in a community hospital in Argentina. *J Am Coll Cardiol* 1996;**27**:222A (Abstract).

20.Gibbons RJ, Holmes DR, Reeder GS *et al.*, for the Mayo Coronary Care Unit and Catheterization Laboratory Groups. Immediate angioplasty compared with the administration of a thrombolytic agent followed by conservative treatment for myocardial infarction. *N Engl J Med* 1993;**328**:685–91.

21.DeWood MA. Direct PTCA vs intravenous t-PA in acute myocardial infarction: results from a prospective randomized trial. Thrombolysis and interventional therapy in acute myocardial infarction. George Washington University, VI Symposium, 1990, pp 28–9.

22.Ribichini F, Steffenino G, Dellavalle A *et al.* Primary angioplasty versus thrombolysis in inferior acute myocardial infarction with anterior ST-segment depression: a single-center randomized study. *J Am Coll Cardiol* 1996;**27**:221A (Abstract).

23.Garcia E, Elizaga J, Soriano J *et al.* Hospital Gregorio Maranon, Madrid Spain. Primary angioplasty versus thrombolysis with t-PA in the anterior myocardial infarction: results from a single center trial. *J Am Coll Cardiol* 1997;**389**(Suppl. A) (Abstract).

24.GUSTO-IIb. A clinical trial comparing primary coronary angioplasty with tissue plasminogen activator for acute myocardial infarction. *N Engl J Med* 1997;**336**:1621–8.

25.ASSENT-2 (Assessment of the Safety and Efficacy of a New Thrombolytic) Investigators. The ASSENT-2 double-blind randomized trial. *Lancet* 1999;**354**;716–22.

26.Antman EM, Guigliano RP, Gibson CM *et al.* Abciximab facilitates the rate and extent of thrombolysis: results of the thrombolysis in myocardial infarction-14 (TIMI-14) trial. *Circulation* 1999;**99**:2720–32.

27.SPEED Group. Trial of Abciximab with and without low dose reteplase for acute myocardial infarction. *Circulation* 2000; **101**:2788–94.

28.Brener SJ, Zeymer U, Adgey AA *et al.* Eptifibatide and low-dose tissue plasminaogen activator in acute myocardial infarction: the integrilin and low-dose thrombolysis in acute myocardial infarction (INTRO AMI) trial. *J Am Coll Cardiol* 2002;**39**:377–86.

29.GUSTO-V Investigators. Reperfusion therapy for acute myocardial infarction with fibrinolytic therapy or combination reduced fibrinolytic therapy and platelet glycoprotein IIb/IIIa inhibition: the GUSTO-V randomized trial. *Lancet* 2001; **357**:1905–14.

30.The Assessment of the Safety and Efficacy of a New Thrombolytic Regimen (ASSENT)-3 Investigators. Efficacy and safety of tenecteplase in combination with enoxaparin, abciximab, or unfractionated heparin: the ASSENT-3 randomized trial in acute myocardial infarction. *Lancet* 2001;**358**:605–13.

31.Canto JG, Every NR, Magid DJ *et al.* The volume of primary angioplasty procedures and survival after acute myocardial infarction. *N Engl J Med* 2000;**342**:1573–80.

32.Every NR, Parson LS, Hlatky M *et al.*, for the MITI Investigators. A comparison of thrombolytic therapy with primary coronary angioplasty for acute myocardial infarction. *N Engl J Med* 1996;**335**:1253–60.

33.Tierfenbrunn AJ, Chandra NC, French WJ, Gore JM, Rogers WJ. Clinical experience with primary PTCA compared with alteplase (rtPA) in patients with acute myocardial infarction. A report from the Second National Registry of Myocardial Infarction (NRMI-2). *J Am Coll Cardiol* 1998;**31**:1240–5.

34.Ritchie J, Phillips D, Luft H. Coronary angioplasty. Statewide experience in California. *Circulation* 1993;**88**:2735–43.

35.Rogers WJ, Canto JG, Lambrew CT *et al.* Temporal trends in the treatment of over 1.5 million patients with myocardial infarction in the US from 1990 through 1999: the National Registry of Myocardial Infarction 1, 2 and 3. *J Am Coll Cardiol* 2000;**36**;2056–63.

36.Zahn R, Schiele R, Schneider S *et al.* Decreasing hospital mortality between 1994 and 1998 in patients with acute myocardial infarction treated with primary angioplasty but not in patients treated with intravenous thrombolysis. Results from the pooled data of the Maximal Individual Therapy in Acute Myocardial Infarction (MITRA) registry and the Myocardial Infarction Registry (MIR). *J Am Coll Cardiol* 2000;**36**:2064–71.

37.Schomig A, Kastrati A, Dirschinger J *et al.* Coronary stenting plus platelet glycoprotein IIb/IIIa blockade compared with tissue plasminogen activator in acute myocardial infarction. *N Engl J Med* 2000;**343**:385–91.

38. Le May MR, Labinaz M, Davies RF *et al*. Stenting versus thrombolysis in acute myocardial infarction trial (STAT). *J Am Coll Cardiol* 2001;**37**:985–91.

39. Kastrati A, Mehilli J, Dirshinger J *et al*. Myocardial salvage after coronary stenting plus abciximab versus fibrinolysis plus abciximab in patients with acute myocardial infarction: a randomized trial. *Lancet* 2002;**359**:920–5.

40. Grines CL, Westerhausen DR, Grines LL *et al*. A randomized trial of transfer for primary angioplasty versus on-site thrombolysis in high-risk myocardial infarction (Air PAMI study). *J Am Coll Cardiol* 2002;**39**:1713–19.

41. Widimsky P, Groch L, Zeliko M, Aschermann M, Bednar F, Suryapranata H. Multicenter randomized trial comparing transport to primary angioplasty vs immediate thrombolysis vs combined strategy for patients with acute myocardial infarction presenting to a community hospital without a catheterization laboratory. The PRAGUE study. *Eur Heart J* 2000;**21**:823–31.

42. Danish Trial in Acute Myocardial Infarction-2 (DANAMI-2) Investigators. The Danish multicenter randomized trial on thrombolytic therapy versus acute coronary angioplasty in acute myocardial infarction. Oral presentation ACC 3/20/2002.

43. Aversano T, Aversano LT, Passamani E *et al*., for the Atlantic Cardiovascular Patient Outcomes Research Team (C-PORT). Thrombolytic therapy vs primary percutaneous coronary intervention for myocardial infarction in patients presenting to hospitals without on-site cardiac surgery. A randomized controlled trial. *JAMA* 2002;**287**:1943–51.

44. Grines CL, Cox DA, Stone GW *et al*. Coronary angioplasty with or without stent implantation for acute myocardial infarction. *N Engl J Med* 1999;**341**:1949–56.

45. Maillard L, Hamon M, Khalife K *et al*., for the STENTIM-2 Investigators. A comparison of systematic stenting and conventional balloon angioplasty during primary percutaneous transluminal coronary angioplasty for acute myocardila infarction. *J Am Coll Cardiol* 2000;**35**:1729–36.

46. Stone GW, Grines CL, Cox DA *et al*., for the Controlled Abciximab and Device Investigation to Lower Late Angioplasty Complications (CADILLAC) Investigators. Comparison of angioplasty with stenting, with or without abciximab, in acute myocardial infarction. *N Engl J Med* 2002;**346**:957–66.

47. Brener SJ, Barr LA, Burchenal JE *et al*. Randomized, placebo-controlled trial of platelet glycoprotein IIb/IIIa blockade with primary angioplasty for acute myocardial infarction. ReoPro and primary PTCA organization and randomization trial (RAPPORT) investigators. *Circulation* 1998;**98**:734–41.

48. Montalescot G, Barragan P, Wittenberg O *et al*. Platelet glycoprotein IIb/IIIa inhibition with coronary stenting for acute myocardial infarction. *N Engl J Med* 2001;**344**:1895–903.

49. Gibson CM, Cannon CP, Murphy SA *et al*. Relationship of TIMI myocardial perfusion grade to mortality after administration of thrombolytic drugs. *Circulation* 2002;**101**:125–30.

50. The TIMI Research Group. Immediate vs delayed catheterization and PCI following thrombolytic therapy for acute myocardial infarction: TIMI II A results. *JAMA* 1988;**260**:2849–58.

51. Topol EJ, Califf RM, George BS *et al*. The Thrombolysis and Angioplasty in Myocardial Infarction Study Group. A randomized trial of immediate versus delayed elective PCI after intravenous tissue plasmiogen activator in acute myocardial infarction. *N Engl J Med* 1987;**317**:581–8.

52. Ross AM, Coyne KS, Reiner JA *et al*. A randomized trial comparing primary angioplasty with a strategy of short-acting thrombolysis and immediate planned rescue angioplasty in acute myocardial infarction: the PACT trial. *J Am Coll Cardiol* 1999;**34**:1954–62.

53. Herrmann HC, Moliterno DJ, Ohman EM *et al*. Facilitation of early percutaneous coronary intervention after reteplase with or without abciximab in acute myocardial infarction: results from the SPEED (GUSTO-IV Pilot) trial. *J Am Coll Cardiol* 2000;**36**:1497–9.

54. Stone GW, Peterson MA, Lansky AJ, Dangas G, Mehran R, Leon MB. Impact of normalized myocardial perfusion after successful angioplasty in acute myocardial infarction. *J Am Coll Cardiol* 2002;**39**:591–7.

55. Stone GW, Brodie BR, Griffin JJ *et al*. Role of cardiac surgery in the hospital phase management of patients treated with primary angioplasty for acute myocardial infarction. *Am J Cardiol* 2000;**85**:1292–6.

56. Zijlstra F, Hoorntje JCA, De Boer M *et al*. Long term benefit of primary angioplasty as compared with thrombolytic therapy for acute myocardial infarction. *N Engl J Med* 1999;**341**:1413–19.

57. Stone GW, Grines CL, Rothbaum D *et al*. Analysis of the relative costs and effectiveness of primary angioplasty versus tissue-type plasminogen activator: the Primary Angioplasty in Myocardial Infarction (PAMI) trial. *J Am Coll Cardiol* 1997;**29**:901–7.

58. Parmley WW. Cost-effectiveness of reperfusion strategies. *Am Heart J* 1999;**138**:142–52.

59. Cohen DJ, Taira DA, Berezin R *et al*. Cost-effectiveness of coronary stenting in acute myocardial infarction: results form the Stent Primary Angioplasty in Myocardial Infarction (Stent-PAMI) Trial. *Circulation* 2001;**104**:3039–345.

60. Grassman ED, Johnson SA, Krone RJ. Predictors of success and major complications for primary percutaneous transluminal coronary angioplasty in acute myocardial infarction. An analysis of the 1990 to 1994 Society for Cardiac Angiography and Interventions registries. *J Am Coll Cardiol* 1997;**30**:201–8.

61. DeWood MA, Spores J, Notske RN *et al*. Medical and surgical management of acute myocardial infarction. *Am J Cardiol* 1979;**44**:1356–64.

62. Phillips SJ, Zeff RH, Skinner JR *et al*. Reperfusion protocol and results in 738 patients with evolving myocardial infarction. *Ann Thorac Surg* 1986;**41**:119–25.

63. Lee JH, Murrell HK, Strony J *et al*. Risk analysis of coronary bypass surgery after acute myocardial infarction. *Surgery* 1997;**122**:675–80.

64. Hochman JS, Sleeper LA, Webb JG *et al*. Early revascularization in acute myocardial infarction complicated by cardiogenic shock. *N Engl J Med* 1999;**341**:625–34.

65. Ryan TJ, Anderson JL, Antman EM *et al*. ACC/AHA guidelines for the management of patients with acute myocardial infarction: report of the American College of Cardiology/American Heart Association Task Force on Practice Guidelines (Committee on Management of Acute Myocardial Infarction). *J Am Coll Cardiol* 1996;**28**:1328–428.

66. Silva JA, Ramee SR, Cohen DJ *et al*. Rheolytic thrombectomy during percutaneous revascularization for acute myocardial infarction: experience with the Angiojet catheter. *Am Heart J* 2001;**141**:353–9.

67. Marzilli, M, Orsini E, Marraccini P, Roberto T. Beneficial effects of intracoronary adenosine as an adjunct to primary angioplasty in acute myocardial infarction. *Circulation* 2000; **101**:2154–9.

68. Dixon SR, Bartorelli AL, Marcovitz PA *et al.* Initial experience with hyperoxemic reperfusion after primary angioplasty for acute myocardial infarction: results of a pilot study utilizing intracoronary aqueous oxygen therapy. *J Am Coll Cardiol* 2002;**39**:387–92.

69. The Hypothermia After Cardiac Arrest Study Group. Mild therapeutic hypothermia to improve the neurologic outcome after cardiac arrest. *N Engl J Med* 2002;**346**:549–56.

33 Adjunctive antithrombotic therapy for ST-elevation acute myocardial infarction

John K French, Harvey D White

Introduction

In reperfusion-eligible patients[1] with acute myocardial infarction (MI), the aim of treatment is to restore normal (Thrombolysis in Myocardial Infarction [TIMI] grade 3)[2] epicardial blood flow in the infarct-related coronary artery and microvascular blood flow to the affected myocardium as soon as possible,[3,4] in order to preserve left ventricular function[5] and improve early survival rates.[6] Sustained patency of the infarct artery is associated with enhanced late survival.[7] In reperfusion-eligible patients, high rates of both early and sustained TIMI-3 flow may be achieved by using a combination of fibrinolytic, antiplatelet, and antithrombin agents and/or percutaneous coronary intervention (PCI). Although TIMI-3 flow has been shown to correlate with improved survival,[4] bleeding and intracranial hemorrhage are major adverse effects of the current fibrinolytic regimens, and the balance of benefit and risk needs to be assessed in appropriately designed large clinical trials. This chapter will examine the evidence for the use of adjunctive antithrombin therapies in patients with ST-segment elevation acute MI treated with or without reperfusion therapies.

Indirect antithrombins

Unfractionated heparin

Mechanism of action of heparin

Unfractionated heparin, the clinical prototypical antithrombin agent, is a heterogeneous glycoprotein with a molecular mass that varies between 5000 and 30 000 kilodaltons (mean 15 000 kDa). Upon binding to antithrombin III, heparin forms a complex that inhibits the actions of thrombin (Figure 33.1) and factors IXa, Xa, and XIa. The varying molecular masses of commercial heparin preparations result in only partial (approximately one third) stoichiometric binding to antithrombin III, with unpredictable pharmacokinetics and pharmacodynamics and hence an unpredictable anticoagulant effect.[8] Low molecular weight

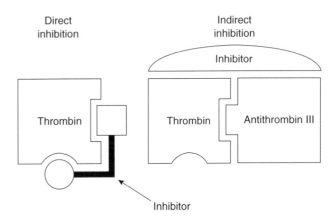

Figure 33.1 Direct thrombin inhibitors such as bivalirudin and hirudin bind to both the catalytic and antithrombin III binding sites of thrombin, directly inhibiting each function. Indirect thrombin inhibitors affect the activation of thrombin indirectly by binding at different sites.

heparins have lower mean molecular masses than unfractionated heparin, and lack the 18 saccharide moieties required for simultaneous binding of thrombin and antithrombin III, thus they effectively inhibit factor Xa without concurrent binding to thrombin and antithrombin. At a heparin concentration that prolongs the activated partial thromboplastin time (APTT) to twice normal, there is only 20–40% inhibition of clot-bound thrombin activity.[9] The heparin–antithrombin III complex is inhibited by fibrin monomer II and is relatively inaccessible to factor Xa in the prothrombinase complex. Heparin binds to several other plasma proteins including platelet factor 4, vitronectin, fibronectin and von Willebrand factor, which inhibits platelet function.

The procoagulant state after administration of fibrinolytic therapy

Administration of fibrinolytic therapy results in a procoagulant state. Plasmin activates platelets either by activating the thrombin receptor[10] or by triggering thrombin generation through activation of factor V (Figure 33.2).[11] The amount of thrombin activity induced by fibrinolytic agents is directly related to the extent of free plasmin activity (Figure 33.3).[12] Administration of streptokinase results in the breakdown of circulating fibrinogen and an increase in fibrin degradation products, which have anticoagulant effects. However, because streptokinase induces extensive plasmin activity, it may be associated with more marked procoagulant effects than fibrin-specific agents such as alteplase, reteplase or tenecteplase, which activate plasminogen to a lesser degree.[12] The exposure of clot-bound thrombin acts as a nidus for further thrombosis, and provides the rationale for adjunctive use of antithrombotic therapies.

Effect on infarct artery patency of unfractionated heparin alone

The effect of a large single bolus of intravenous unfractionated heparin on infarct artery patency in patients not given fibrinolytic therapy was examined in the Heparin in Early Patency (HEAP) trial after the HEAP pilot study showed that a single intravenous heparin bolus of 300 IU/kg produced TIMI-3 flow in 31% of patients.[13] The HEAP trial,[14] which randomized 584 patients, found that 13% of patients given weight adjusted high-dose heparin (20 000–30 000 IU) had TIMI-3 flow at a mean of 79 minutes, compared with 9% of patients given either no heparin or weight adjusted low-dose heparin (0–5000 IU). These rates of TIMI-3 flow are similar to those seen prior to primary angioplasty,[13] and show that heparin on its own does not enhance early infarct artery patency.

Effect on infarct artery patency of adjunctive unfractionated heparin with fibrinolytic therapy

Early angiographic studies evaluated the use of heparin versus aspirin (but not heparin with aspirin) after fibrinolytic therapy. In the Thrombolysis and Angioplasty in Myocardial Infarction (TAMI)-3 study,[15] patients receiving a 3 hour infusion of alteplase were randomized to receive either a 10 000 IU bolus of heparin or a placebo. There was no difference in the rates of TIMI-3 flow at 90 minutes (54% in the heparin group versus 53% in the placebo group). However, three other studies that performed angiography at means of 18,[16] 57,[17] and 81 hours[18] after administering alteplase concluded that heparin did improve patency; in the third study all patients also received 80 mg of aspirin. No trials have found that heparin improved 90 minute patency rates when an aspirin dose of >100 mg was used in conjunction with alteplase.

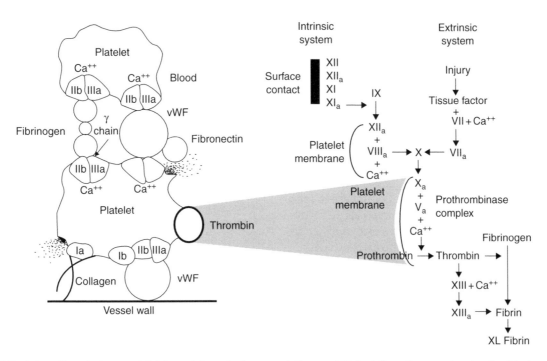

Figure 33.2 Interactions between platelets and thrombotic, coagulation, and fibrinolytic pathways, showing the biochemical interactions between platelet membrane receptors, vessel walls, and adhesive macromolecules during platelet adhesion and aggregation (*left*). Also depicted are the intrinsic and extrinsic systems of the coagulation cascade and their interaction with the platelet membrane (*right*), such as via the prothrombinase complex, which is the activator complex for thrombin. Coronary thrombosis is associated with both platelet and coagulation processes. Ca^{++}, calcium; Ia, glycoprotein Ia; Ib, glycoprotein Ib; IIb/IIIa, glycoprotein IIb/IIIa; vWF, von Willebrand factor; XL, cross-linked. (Modified with permission from Stein B, Fuster V, Halperin JL, Chesebro JH. Antithrombotic therapy in cardiac disease: an emerging approach based on pathogenesis and risk. *Circulation* 1989;**80**:1501–13.)

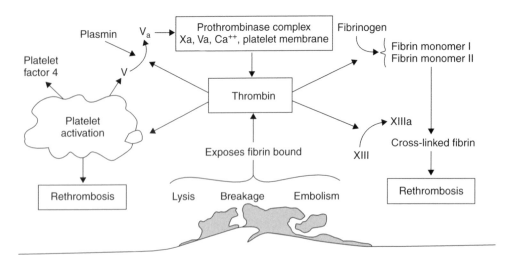

Figure 33.3 Clot lysis and thrombin generation. Disturbance of thrombus by lysis (endogenous or exogenous), mechanical breakage (including PCI), or spontaneous embolism exposes thrombin bound to fibrin. Thrombin activates platelets, activates factor V to Va (which leads to generation of more thrombin via the prothrombinase complex), converts fibrinogen to fibrin I and fibrin II, and activates factor XIII to XIIIa (which cross-links fibrin). These processes combine to produce rethrombosis. Heparin may only partially prevent rethrombosis because factor Xa within the prothrombinase complex is protected from heparin–antithrombin III, platelet factor 4 neutralizes heparin, and fibrin monomer II inhibits heparin–antithrombin III. (Modified with permission from Webster MWI, Chesebro JH, Fuster V. Antithrombotic therapy in acute myocardial infarction: enhancement of thrombolysis, reduction of reocclusion, and prevention of thromboembolism. In: Gersh BJ, Rahimtoola SH, eds. *Current topics in cardiology – acute myocardial infarction.* New York: Elsevier Science, 1990.)

Adjunctive subcutaneous heparin

Subcutaneous heparin is usually administered at either 4 or 12 hours after the start of fibrinolytic therapy. This route of administration results in variable absorption and can take up to 24 hours to achieve significant prolongation of the APTT, hence it may not prevent early reocclusion prior to that time.[19]

In the Studio sulla Calciparina nell-Angina e nella Trombosi Ventricolare nell'Infarto (SCATI) trial,[20] 433 patients were given streptokinase without routine aspirin and randomized to receive either control treatment or a 2000 IU heparin bolus followed 9 hours later by 12 500 IU given subcutaneously twice daily. The inhospital mortality rates were 8·8% in the control group and 4·6% in the heparin group ($P = 0·05$).

Several large trials have tested subcutaneous heparin regimens in conjunction with aspirin and fibrinolytic therapy.[21–23] The Gruppo Italiano per lo Studio della Sopravvivenza nell'Infarto Miocardico (GISSI-2) study[21] randomized 20 891 patients to receive either control treatment or subcutaneous heparin (12 500 IU twice daily throughout hospitalization starting 12 hours after the initiation of either streptokinase or alteplase). The patients also received 160–325 mg of aspirin. Heparin was found to reduce the inhospital mortality rate from 6·0% to 5·4% ($P < 0·05$).

In the Third International Study of Infarct Survival (ISIS-3),[22] 41 299 patients were given 162 mg of crushed enteric coated aspirin and randomized to receive either streptokinase, duteplase or anisoylated plasminogen streptokinase activator complex (APSAC). Four hours after the start of fibrinolytic therapy the patients were randomized to receive either control treatment or 12 500 IU of subcutaneous heparin twice daily. During the scheduled heparin treatment period there was a trend towards a mortality reduction in the patients randomized to receive heparin (7·4% v 7·9% in the control group, $P = 0·06$), which may represent a benefit of 5 lives saved per 1000 patients treated. However, because 12% of the patients randomized to receive heparin were given none and 25% of those randomized to receive no heparin were given intravenous heparin (14%) or high-dose subcutaneous heparin (11%), the true benefit of subcutaneous heparin is estimated to have been nearer 7 lives saved per 1000 patients treated.[22] A meta-analysis of the GISSI-2 and ISIS-3 studies showed that the groups randomized to receive subcutaneous heparin had 2 fewer deaths and 2 fewer non-fatal re-infarctions per 1000 patients treated, at a cost of 3 more transfusions and 0·3 more non-fatal disabling strokes (Table 33.1).[24]

Comparison of intravenous heparin with control treatment

Four trials[18,25–27] have randomized patients treated with aspirin to receive either intravenous heparin or control treatment after fibrinolysis (Table 33.2). There were no significant differences in mortality or re-infarction rates, but these trials lacked the statistical power to evaluate these outcomes, and would have needed to randomize at least five times as many patients in order to detect clinically meaningful differences of 15% in either end point.[28]

Attempts to evaluate the potential benefit of intravenous heparin after fibrinolysis have been confounded in clinical trials because a significant proportion of patients in the control or placebo treatment arms were given intravenous heparin electively by the treating physicians. It is appropriate to conclude that there is a paucity of information comparing intravenous heparin with placebo in patients receiving streptokinase or alteplase.

Meta-analyses of heparin trials

In a meta-analysis of trials that randomized a total of 5459 patients to receive either heparin or no antithrombotic therapy in the absence of routine aspirin therapy (although 14%

received fibrinolytic therapy), heparin was found to reduce mortality by 25% (95% CI 10–37) from 14·9% to 11·4% at a mean of 10 days ($P = 0·002$). The re-infarction rate was not significantly reduced (6·8% v 8·3%, $P = 0·1$), but the rate of stroke was reduced from 2·1% to 1·1% ($P = 0·01$) and the rate of pulmonary embolism was reduced from 3·8% to 2·0% ($P \leqslant 0·001$).[29] In patients with contraindications for aspirin, the use of intravenous heparin is recommended. Although there is no supporting clinical trial evidence, the use of clopidogrel may be appropriate in these circumstances. **Grade A1c**

A total of 68 000 patients treated with aspirin (93% of whom also received fibrinolytic therapy) have been randomized in trials examining various heparin regimens.[24] In patients randomized to receive heparin, 35 day mortality was reduced from 9·1% to 8·6% (95% CI 0–10, $P = 0·03$), inhospital re-infarction from 3·3% to 3·0% ($P = 0·04$), and inhospital pulmonary embolism from 0·4% to 0·3% ($P = 0·01$). There was no significant difference in the rate of stroke (1·2% with heparin v 1·4% with control treatment, $P = $ NS), but major bleeding was more common in patients randomized to receive heparin (1·0% v 0·7%, $P = 0·001$).

Intravenous versus subcutaneous heparin

In the Global Use of Strategies to Open Occluded Coronary Arteries (GUSTO)-I trial, 20 173 patients were randomized to receive streptokinase and either subcutaneous or intravenous heparin.[30] However, 36% of the patients randomized to receive subcutaneous heparin were electively given intravenous heparin (not counting the use of intravenous heparin for cardiac catheterization, which occurred in 54% of patients), and this reduced the power of the study to detect a difference between these two treatment randomizations to 71%. In effect, the heparin comparison in GUSTO-I was actually between intravenous heparin and the ISIS-3 regimen[22] of subcutaneous heparin delayed 4 hours after fibrinolytic therapy with a substantial crossover of patients to intravenous heparin. A "no heparin" strategy was not tested. It is perhaps not surprising, therefore, that there was no difference in

Table 33.1 Benefits and risks associated with adjunctive delayed subcutaneous heparin in patients receiving streptokinase in the ISIS-3[22] and GISSI-2[21] studies

	Events per 1000 patients treated		
	ISIS-3	GISSI-2	Combined
Benefit			
Reduction in mortality	2·8	1·0	2·2[a]
Reduction in non-fatal MI	1·8	1·9	1·8
Risk			
Transfusions	2·6	4·5	3·2
Non-fatal strokes	0·5	0·6	0·6[b]

[a] Figures do not sum up because of rounding.
[b] Half of the patients had fully recovered by the time of discharge.

Table 33.2 Effect of adjunctive intravenous heparin in patients treated with aspirin and fibrinolytic therapy

	Death (%)		Re-infarction (%)		Bleeding (%)	
	Control	Heparin	Control	Heparin	Control	Heparin
ISIS-2 Pilot ($n = 626$)[25]	6	8	5	1	1	0
ECSG ($n = 1296$)[18]	3	2	10	10	NA	NA
OSIRIS ($n = 256$)[26]	11	9	1	2	4	6
DUCCS ($n = 250$)[27]	9	12	4	9	8	15

Abbreviations: DUCCS, Duke University Clinical Cardiology Study; ECSG, European Cooperative Study Group; NA, not available; OSIRIS, Optimization Study of Infarct Reperfusion Investigated by ST Monitoring

clinical end points. However, at 5–7 days, 84% of patients randomized to receive streptokinase and intravenous heparin had TIMI-2 or -3 (that is, slow or normal) flow (the same percentage as in the alteplase group), compared with 72% of those randomized to receive streptokinase and subcutaneous heparin ($P < 0.05$). Given the importance of long-term patency of the infarct-related artery, this may partly explain why those randomized to streptokinase and intravenous heparin had a 5 year survival rate equal to that of those randomized to alteplase, and a 1% higher absolute survival rate than those randomized to streptokinase and subcutaneous heparin.[31] Furthermore, in patients with cardiogenic shock, those randomized to streptokinase and intravenous heparin had the lowest mortality rate (54% *v* 58% in those randomized to streptokinase and subcutaneous heparin, and 63% in those randomized to alteplase and intravenous heparin).[32]

Recent dose adjustments in adjunctive intravenous heparin regimens

Because of concern about the high bleeding rates (including intracranial hemorrhage) seen with alteplase and with modified fibrinolytic regimens including alteplase or other genetically modified plasminogen activators, the dose of adjunctive unfractionated heparin used in conjunction with fibrinolytic therapy has been reduced in recent trials.[33] The current American College of Cardiology (ACC)/American Heart Association (AHA) guidelines[34] recommend an APTT of 1·5–2·0 times control (50–70 seconds) at 12 hours, as this was associated with the lowest mortality rates in GUSTO-I irrespective of the fibrinolytic agent used.[35] In GUSTO-I, heparin was initially administered as a 5000 IU bolus and 1000 IU/hour infusion, but after approximately 10 000 patients had been enrolled the infusion dose was changed to 1200 IU/hour in patients weighing >80 kg. It was observed that the overall rates of moderate bleeding, severe bleeding, and intracranial hemorrhage increased in a linear manner in patients with APTTs above 60–70 seconds at both 12 and 24 hours. The risk factors for these complications included older age, lower body weight, female gender, and African ethnicity. In the GUSTO-I hemostasis substudy, these regimens (which showed good correlation between heparin levels and APTTs) were associated with attenuation of increases in the levels of fibrinopeptide A, but not thrombin generation as measured by prothrombin fragment 1·2.[30]

Unfractionated heparin was compared with hirudin in the TIMI-9A trial[36] and the GUSTO-IIA trial.[37] Both trials were stopped early because of increased rates of intracranial bleeding in both the heparin and the hirudin treatment groups. In patients with ST-segment elevation acute coronary syndromes, the overall intracranial hemorrhage rates were 1·3% in those randomized to receive heparin (a 5000 IU bolus and

1000 IU/hour infusion or a 1300 IU/hour infusion in those weighing >80 kg) and 2·1% in those randomized to receive hirudin (a 0·6 mg/kg bolus and 0·2 mg/kg infusion for 96 hours). TIMI-9 and GUSTO-II were recommenced using lower doses of hirudin (a 0·1 mg bolus and 0·1 mg/kg/hour infusion) and heparin (a 5000 IU bolus and 1000 IU/hour infusion), with the APTT adjusted to 55–85 seconds in TIMI-9B[38] and 60–85 seconds in GUSTO-IIB.[39] These adjustments resulted in lower bleeding rates. The results are discussed below in the section on meta-analysis of direct thrombin inhibitors.

In the TIMI-10B[40] and Assessment of the Safety and Efficacy of a New Thrombolytic Agent (ASSENT)-1[41] trials, the doses of unfractionated heparin used in conjunction with alteplase or tenecteplase were reduced and weight adjusted (a 5000 IU bolus and 1000 IU/hour infusion in patients weighing >67 kg, and a 4000 IU bolus and 800 IU/hour infusion in those weighing <67 kg). The infusion rates were modified according to the APTT at 6 hours, with a target APTT of 50–70 seconds.

The unfractionated heparin dose was also reduced in the TIMI-14 trial[42] and in the Strategies for Patency Enhancement in the Emergency Department (SPEED) trial,[43] which tested the effect on TIMI flow grades of abciximab used in conjunction with reduced doses of alteplase or reteplase. In both trials the patients receiving a full-dose fibrinolytic were given a 70 IU/kg bolus of unfractionated heparin, while those receiving a reduced-dose fibrinolytic were given either a 30 IU/kg bolus of unfractionated heparin plus abciximab or a 60 IU/kg bolus of unfractionated heparin without abciximab. In TIMI-14 the heparin bolus was followed by an infusion of either 7 IU/kg/hour or 4 IU/kg/hour. In SPEED the heparin infusion was adjusted to maintain an APTT of 50–70 seconds if early sheath removal (recommended in the protocol) did not occur. With the reduced heparin regimens, the point estimates for TIMI-3 flow at 60 minutes were 4% lower in the TIMI-14 trial and 10% lower in the SPEED trial, but the confidence intervals were wide (Figure 33.4).

In the ASSENT-2 trial[44] comparing alteplase with tenecteplase and the Intravenous NPA for Treatment of Infarcting Myocardium Early (InTIME)-II study[45] comparing alteplase with lanoteplase (also known as NPA), unfractionated heparin was administered as a 70 IU/kg bolus (maximum 4000 IU) and a 15 IU/kg/hour infusion (maximum 1000 IU/hour). In the ASSENT-3 trial[46] (where patients received either half-dose tenecteplase plus low-dose unfractionated heparin plus abciximab, full-dose tenecteplase plus unfractionated heparin, or full-dose tenecteplase plus enoxaparin), the unfractionated heparin regimen in patients not receiving abciximab was reduced to a 60 IU/kg bolus (maximum 4000 IU) and a 12 IU/kg/hour infusion (maximum 1000 IU/hour). The first adjustment of the heparin infusion took place after measurement of

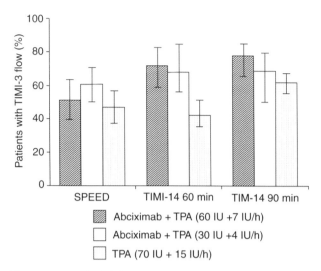

Figure 33.4 TIMI-3 flow rates with different unfractionated heparin regimens in the SPEED[43] and TIMI-14[42] trials

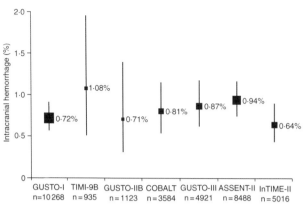

Figure 33.5 Rates of intracranial hemorrhage in the GUSTO-I,[23] TIMI-9B,[38] GUSTO-IIB,[39] COBALT,[94] GUSTO-III,[95] ASSENT-2,[44] and InTIME-II[45] trials using accelerated alteplase and intravenous unfractionated heparin. COBALT, Continuous Infusion Versus Double-Bolus Administration of Alteplase. (Modified with permission from Giugliano RP, McCabe CH, Antman EM *et al.* Lower dose heparin with fibrinolysis is associated with lower rates of intracranial haemorrhage. *Am Heart J* 2001;**141**:742–50.)

the APTT at 3 hours. In the initial phase of InTIME-II, the heparin dose was adjusted according to the APTT at 6 hours, but in the latter part of the trial this was done at 3 hours. Compared with previous trials, these trials had stricter entry criteria for patients at increased risk of intracranial hemorrhage, and excluded those with a documented blood pressure of >180/110 mmHg at any time. Despite these precautions, intracranial hemorrhage occurred in 0·88% of all patients in ASSENT-2 and 0·92% of all patients in ASSENT-3. By comparison, the intracranial hemorrhage rate in patients randomized to receive accelerated alteplase and intravenous heparin in GUSTO-I was 0·72%.[23] The intracranial hemorrhage rates in alteplase-treated patients were 0·94% in ASSENT-2, 0·74% in the initial phase of InTIME-II, and 0·51% in the latter phase of In-TIME-II. The confidence intervals of the point estimates for intracranial hemorrhage in the alteplase groups in these trials overlap (Figure 33.5). The intracranial hemorrhage rate in lanoteplase-treated patients fell from 1·22% to 1·00% when the APTT measurement was brought forward from 6 hours to 3 hours in InTIME-II, and dropped further to 0·50% when the heparin bolus was omitted in InTIME-IIB (χ^2 trend $P = 0·021$).

Comparison of patients with similar baseline characteristics who received tenecteplase in ASSENT-2 and ASSENT-3 showed that the heparin dose reduction and use of the 3 hour APTT measurement in ASSENT-3 was associated with lower rates of major bleeding (2·16 *v* 4·66%) and transfusion (2·31 *v* 4·25%), although the rates of intracranial hemorrhage were the same (0·93%). Randomized trials with clinical end points are required to determine whether lower heparin doses really do improve safety without compromising efficacy.

Table 33.3 and Figure 33.6 show the rates of major, moderate, and minor bleeding, transfusion, stroke, and intracranial hemorrhage in the ASSENT-3 trial,[46] the GUSTO-V trial,[47] which tested abciximab in patients receiving reteplase and unfractionated heparin, and the Hirulog and Early Reperfusion or Occlusion (HERO)-2 trial,[48] which compared bivalirudin with unfractionated heparin in patients receiving streptokinase.

Low molecular weight heparins

Low molecular weight heparins, which block ongoing thrombin generation by inhibiting factor Xa (see Figure 33.1), have recently been evaluated as adjuncts to fibrinolytic therapy. Factor Xa inhibition is dose-dependent, and significant inhibition occurs at a comparatively lower dose of low molecular weight heparin than unfractionated heparin. The ratio of inhibition of factor Xa:thrombin varies from one low molecular weight heparin to another, and is approximately 2:1 with dalteparin and 3:1 with enoxaparin, the two agents most commonly evaluated in clinical trials. Low molecular weight heparins are not inactivated by platelet factor 4, and stimulate the release of tissue factor pathway inhibitor from endothelium.

Dalteparin

Two randomized placebo-controlled trials have compared twice-daily subcutaneous dalteparin with a placebo in patients treated with aspirin and streptokinase. In the Fragmin in Acute Myocardial Infarction (FRAMI) study,[49]

Table 33.3 Bleeding and stroke rates in the ASSENT-3,[46] GUSTO-V[47] and HERO-2[48] trials

	ASSENT-3			GUSTO-V		HERO-2	
	Tenecteplase + UF heparin	Tenecteplase + enoxaparin	Half-dose tenecteplase + UF Heparin + abciximab	Full-dose reteplase	Half-dose reteplase + abciximab	Streptokinase + UF heparin	Streptokinase + bivalirudin
Bleeding							
Severe (%)	2·16	3·04	4·31[a]	0·51	1·08[b]	0·47	0·68
Moderate (%)	–	–	–	1·79	3·47[b]	1·05	1·39[c]
Minor (%)	18·7	22·6	35·3[b]	11·4	20·01[b]	9·0	12·8[b]
Transfusions (%)	2·31	3·43[d]	4·16[b]	3·98	5·71[b]	1·11	1·39
Strokes							
All strokes (%)	1·52	1·62	1·49	0·88	0·97	0·90	1·24
Non-fatal disabling stroke	–	–	–	0·3	0·2	0·3	0·2
Intracranial (%) hemorrhages	0·93	0·88	0·94	0·59	0·62	0·39	0·55

[a] $P = 0.003$.
[b] $P < 0.0001$.
[c] $P = 0.05$.
[d] $P = 0.03$.
Abbreviations: LMW, low molecular weight; UF, unfractionated

which randomized 776 patients, dalteparin (150 IU/kg twice daily during hospitalization) reduced the incidence of left ventricular thrombus or embolism within 9 days from 21·9% to 14·2% ($P = 0.03$). The only significant difference in clinical end points was in the rate of major hemorrhage, which occurred in 2·9% of the dalteparin group versus 0·3% of the placebo group ($P = 0.006$). In the Biochemical Markers in Acute Coronary Syndromes (BIOMACS)-II study of 101 patients,[50] TIMI-3 flow was observed at 20–28 hours in 68% of patients given dalteparin (100 IU/kg initially and 120 IU/kg at 12 hours) versus 51% of those given a placebo ($P = 0.10$). Dalteparin reduced the incidence of recurrent ischemic episodes (recorded by continuous electrocardiography) from 38% to 16% ($P = 0.037$). There were no differences in major bleeding or clinical events.

In the ASSENT PLUS trial,[51] patients were given alteplase ($n = 439$) and randomized to receive either subcutaneous dalteparin (120 IU/kg every 12 hours) for 4–7 days or an intravenous infusion of unfractionated heparin for 48 hours. TIMI-3 flow was achieved in similar proportions of the dalteparin and heparin treatment groups (69·3% v 62·5%, $P = 0.16$), but patients in the dalteparin group were less likely to have TIMI-0 or -1 flow (13·4% v 24·4%, $P = 0.006$) or intraluminal thrombus with or without TIMI 0-1 flow (27·9% v 42·0%, $P = 0.003$). Although there were fewer re-infarctions within 7 days in the dalteparin group (1·4% v 5·4%, $P = 0.01$), there was no significant difference in the re-infarction rates at 30 days (6·5% v 7·0%, $P = $ NS), and no difference in the combined end point of death/

re-infarction at 30 days. Intracranial hemorrhage occurred in 0·9% of the dalteparin group versus 1·9% of the unfractionated heparin group ($P = 0.43$), major bleeding in 7·2% v 9·5% respectively ($P = 0.37$), and minor bleeding in 24·1% v 20% respectively ($P = 0.30$) (Table 33.4).

Enoxaparin

In the Acute Myocardial Infarction–Streptokinase (AMI–SK) trial,[52] 496 patients with MI were given aspirin and streptokinase and randomized to receive either enoxaparin or a placebo for 3–8 days. The primary end point was TIMI-3 flow at 5–10 days, which was observed in 70% of the enoxaparin group and 58% of the placebo group ($P = 0.01$). Major bleeding occurred in 2·5% v 4·8% respectively ($P = 0.13$). ST recovery of ≥70% was more common in the enoxaparin group than in the placebo group ($P = 0.012$ at 90 minutes and $P = 0.004$ at 180 minutes).

In the Heparin and Aspirin Reperfusion Therapy (HART)-II trial,[54] 400 patients were given aspirin and alteplase and randomized to receive either unfractionated heparin or enoxaparin (30 mg intravenously and 1 mg/kg subcutaneously every 12 hours) for at least 3 days. The primary aim of the trial was to show that enoxaparin was not inferior to adjunctive unfractionated heparin for the end point of TIMI-2 or -3 flow at 90 minutes, which was achieved in 80% of the enoxaparin group versus 75% of the unfractionated heparin group ($P = $ NS), while TIMI-3 flow was achieved in 53% v 48% respectively ($P = $ NS). By 5–7 days, reocclusion

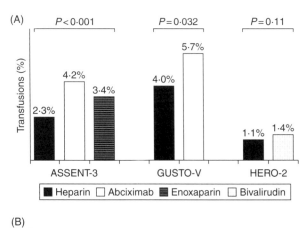

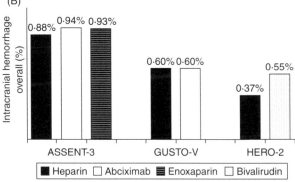

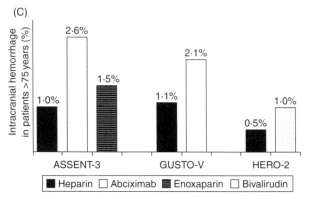

Figure 33.6 Transfusion and intracranial hemorrhage in the ASSENT-3,[46] GUSTO-V,[47] and HERO-2[48] trials: (A) transfusion; (B) intracranial hemorrhage; (C) intracranial hemorrhage in patients >75 years

(TIMI-0 or -1 flow) had occurred in 9·8% of enoxaparin patients and 9·1% of heparin patients who had initially had TIMI-3 flow, and in 5·9% of enoxaparin patients and 3·1% of heparin patients who had initially had TIMI-2 or -3 flow (*P* = 0·26). The rates of major bleeding were similar in both treatment groups (see Table 33.4), and intracranial hemorrhage occurred in 1% of each group.

In the ASSENT-3 trial, 6095 patients were randomized to receive either full-dose tenecteplase plus enoxaparin for a maximum of 7 days, half-dose tenecteplase plus weight

adjusted low-dose unfractionated heparin for 48 hours and a 12 hour infusion of abciximab, or full-dose tenecteplase plus weight-adjusted unfractionated heparin for 48 hours.[46] The trial did not have a prespecified primary hypothesis. The combined rates of 30 day mortality/inhospital investigator-reported re-infarction/inhospital refractory ischemia were significantly lower in the enoxaparin group (11·4%; RR 0·74; 95% CI 0·63–0·87; *P* = 0·0002) and in the abciximab group (11·1%; RR 0·72; 95% CI 0·61–0·84; *P* < 0·0001) than in the unfractionated heparin group (15·4%). The combined rates of 30 day mortality/inhospital investigator-reported re-infarction/inhospital refractory ischemia/inhospital intracranial hemorrhage/inhospital major bleeding were 13·7% in the enoxaparin group (RR 0·81; 95% CI 0·70–0·93; *P* = 0·0037), 14·2% in the abciximab group (RR 0·84; 95% CI 0·72–0·96; *P* = 0·014) and 17·0% in the unfractionated heparin group. In patients with anterior MI, the lowest rates of 30 day mortality/inhospital investigator-reported re-infarction/inhospital refractory ischemia were seen in the abciximab group (13·6% *v* 14·6% in the enoxaparin group and 19·4% in the unfractionated heparin group). Overall, intracranial hemorrhage occurred in 0·88% of the enoxaparin group, 0·94% of the abciximab group and 0·93% of the unfractionated heparin group. Transfusions were less common in the unfractionated heparin group (2·3%) than in the enoxaparin (3·4%) and abciximab groups (4·2%, *P* = 0·003 for the three-way comparison, and *P* = 0·03 for the comparison between unfractionated heparin and enoxaparin) (Figure 33.6 and Table 33.3). In patients over 75 years of age, intracranial hemorrhage occurred in 1·0% of those given unfractionated heparin and 1·5% of those given enoxaparin (*P* = 0·72).

Given the increased transfusion rates with enoxaparin versus unfractionated heparin in ASSENT-3, and the need to define the bleeding risks in high-risk subgroups such as the elderly, women, patients with low body weights and patients with renal dysfunction, further trials will be needed to evaluate low molecular weight heparins in conjunction with new fibrinolytic regimens. The Enoxaparin and Thrombolysis Reperfusion for Acute Myocardial Infarction Treatment (ExTRACT-TIMI-25) trial is currently randomizing 20 000 patients to receive either enoxaparin or unfractionated heparin in a double-blind manner, together with a fibrinolytic agent chosen by the treating physician. The composite primary end point of the trial is death/re-infarction within 30 days. Low molecular weight heparins will also need to be tested with regimens combining modified-dose fibrinolytics and glycoprotein IIb/IIIa inhibitors, and in patients undergoing primary or facilitated PCI. The high rates of bleeding (including intracranial hemorrhage) in patients aged >75 years suggest that specific studies are needed to examine the efficacy and safety of low molecular weight heparins in elderly patients.

Low molecular weight heparin is recommended as an acceptable alternative to intravenous unfractionated heparin for adjunctive use with tenecteplase. **Grade A1c**

Table 33.4 Bleeding rates in angiographic fibrinolytic trials comparing adjunctive low molecular weight heparin with unfractionated heparin

		LMW heparin	UF heparin or placebo*	*P* value
Dalteparin				
FRAMI[49]	Major bleeding (%)	2·9	0·3*	0·006
	Minor bleeding (%)	13·4	2·1*	<0·001
BIOMACS-II[50]	Major bleeding (%)	3·7	0*	0·50
	Minor bleeding (%)	5·5	2·0*	0·62
ASSENT PLUS[51]	Major bleeding (%)	7·4	9·5	0·39
	Minor bleeding (%)	24.0	20.0	0·35
Enoxaparin				
AMI–SK[52]	Major bleeding (%)	4·8	2·5*	0·23
	Major bleeding defined according to TIMI bleeding criteria[53] (%)	1·6	0·8*	–
	Transfusion of ≥2 units (%)	0·8	1·3*	0·68
HART-II[54]	Major bleeding defined according to TIMI bleeding criteria[53] (%)	3·6	3·0	0·79
	Transfusion of ≥2 units (%)	5·6	7·1	0·68
ENTIRE-TIMI-23[55]	Major bleeding with full-dose tenecteplase (%)	2·5	2·5	–
	Major bleeding with half-dose tenecteplase + abciximab (%)	8·5	5·2	–

Abbreviations: LMW, low molecular weight; UF, unfractionated

Direct thrombin inhibitors

A number of direct antithrombins have been shown in animal models to accelerate lysis of platelet-rich thrombi and to limit the size of the infarct.[56–59] The prototypical agent is hirudin, which is a leech-derived protein containing 65 amino acids. Because it is excreted renally, blood levels may be increased in patients with renal impairment. Bivalirudin (previously known as hirulog) is a synthetic 20-amino-acid peptide that directly inhibits free and clot-bound thrombin, and is 20% renally excreted. The univalent direct thrombin inhibitors, argatroban, inogatran and efegatran, are synthetic thrombin inhibitors. The evidence for the adjunctive use of direct thrombin inhibitors has recently been strengthened by the publication of a meta-analysis of direct thrombin inhibitor trials[60] and the 17 073-patient HERO-2 trial.[48]

Hirudin

The TIMI-5 trial[61] randomized patients to receive either adjunctive intravenous heparin or escalating doses of hirudin prior to alteplase. Although there was no significant difference in the proportion of patients achieving TIMI-3 flow by 90 minutes (57% in the heparin group *v* 65% in the hirudin group, *P* = NS), there was a trend towards less reocclusion at 18–36 hours in the hirudin group (1·6% *v* 6·7%, *P* = 0·07) and a lower combined rate of death/re-infarction (6·8% *v* 16·7%, *P* = 0·02). The highest incidence of TIMI-3 flow (73%) was seen with the same dose of hirudin (a 0·1 mg/ kg

bolus and 0·1 mg/kg/hour infusion for 3–5 days to maintain an APTT of 60–85 seconds) that was subsequently tested in the TIMI-9B and GUSTO-IIb trials, where it was given after the start of fibrinolytic therapy. When the data from these two trials were combined, there was no reduction in mortality with hirudin, but the incidence of re-infarction was 14% lower (*P* = 0·024).[62]

In the Hirudin for the Improvement of Thrombolysis (HIT)-4 study,[63] 1200 patients were given streptokinase and randomized to receive either intravenous heparin or intravenous hirudin (a 0·2 mg/kg bolus followed by 0·5 mg/kg subcutaneously twice daily). At 30 days there was no difference in the combined incidence of death/re-infarction/ stroke/rescue angioplasty/refractory angina (22·7% with hirudin *v* 24·3% with heparin, *P* = NS). In an angiographic substudy of 447 patients,[64] TIMI-3 flow was achieved by 90 minutes in 41% of the hirudin group versus 33% of the heparin group (*P* = 0·08). The rates of intracranial hemorrhage (0·2% with hirudin *v* 0·3% with heparin) and major bleeding (3·3% *v* 3·5%) were similar in both treatment groups, and there were no clinical or electrocardiographic differences between the groups.

Bivalirudin

Bivalirudin has a half life of approximately 25 minutes compared with 2–3 hours for hirudin. When used in appropriate regimens as an adjunctive agent with fibrinolytic therapy, bivalirudin may prevent clot formation and extension and facilitate clot lysis.

In the HERO-1 trial,[65] 412 patients presenting within 12 hours of symptom onset were given aspirin and streptokinase (administered over 30–60 minutes) and randomized to receive either heparin, low-dose bivalirudin (a 0·125 mg/kg bolus and 0·25 mg/kg/hour infusion for 12 hours, then 0·125 mg/kg/hour) or high-dose bivalirudin (a 0·25 mg/kg bolus and 0·5 mg/kg/hour infusion for 12 hours, then 0·25 mg/kg/hour). TIMI-3 flow at 90–120 minutes was achieved in 35% of the heparin group, 46% of the low-dose bivalirudin group and 48% of the high-dose bivalirudin group (*P* = 0·024).[65] Continuous ST-segment monitoring showed that the patients given bivalirudin achieved stable ST recovery earlier than those given heparin.[66]

In the HERO-2 trial,[48] 17 073 patients presenting within 6 hours of symptom onset were randomized to receive a bolus and 48 hour infusion of either bivalirudin or heparin immediately prior to beginning streptokinase. By 30 days, 10·8% of the bivalirudin group and 10·9% of the heparin group had died (OR 0·99; 95% CI 0·90–1·09). After adjustment for a gender imbalance (as more women had been randomized to receive bivalirudin than heparin) and for the factors identified in the GUSTO risk model,[67] the mortality rates were 10·5% in the bivalirudin group and 10·9% in the heparin group (OR 0·96; 95% CI 0·86–1·07) (Figure 33.7). At 96 hours the rates of re-infarction (adjudicated by an independent blinded committee) were 1·6% in the bivalirudin group versus 2·3% in the heparin group (OR 0·70; 95% CI 0·56–0·88; *P* = 0·001). Analysis of investigator-reported re-infarctions (as was done in the ASSENT-3 and GUSTO-V trials) showed that the combined rate of death/re-infarction was lower

in the bivalirudin group than in the heparin group (12·9% *v* 14·2%, OR 0·90; 95% CI 0·82–0·99; *P* = 0·023). The overall rates of intracranial bleeding (0·5%) and transfusion (1·2%) were lower than those reported by the ASSENT-3 and GUSTO-V trials (see Figure 33.6), even though the HERO-2 population had greater baseline risk factors for bleeding. The rates of non-fatal disabling stroke, intracerebral bleeding, and severe bleeding were low and similar in both treatment groups, but moderate and minor bleeding were more common with bivalirudin than with heparin (see Table 33.3). This may be partially explained by the fact that the bivalirudin group had more prolonged APTTs at 12 and 24 hours than the heparin group. Statistical adjustment for this factor did not affect the reduction in re-infarction seen with bivalirudin, but did explain 50–100% of the increase in bleeding. In a non-prespecified analysis, the adjusted rates of the composite end point of death/re-infarction/non-fatal disabling stroke were 12·7% in the bivalirudin group versus 13·8% in the heparin group (*P* = 0·049) (Figure 33.7). Based on these data, bivalirudin should be used instead of intravenous heparin as adjunctive therapy with streptokinase to reduce the risk of re-infarction. **Grade A1a**

Univalent direct thrombin inhibitors

The univalent direct thrombin inhibitors include argatroban, inogatran, efegatran, and D-Phe-Pro-Arg-CH$_2$Cl. These anticoagulants inhibit early stages of the coagulation pathway and have been shown experimentally to be effective adjuncts to fibrinolytic therapy.[68–70]

In the Antithrombin-Argatroban in Acute Myocardial Infarction (ARGAMI-2) study,[71] 1001 patients were given either streptokinase or alteplase and randomized to receive

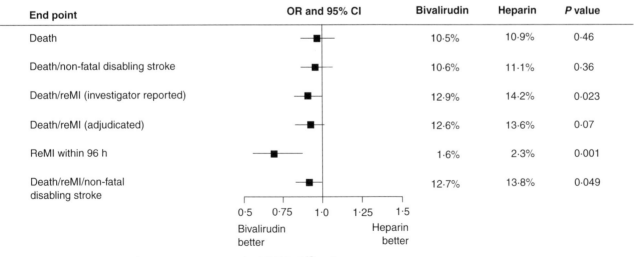

Figure 33.7 Forrest plot of clinical outcomes in the HERO-2[48] trial

either heparin or argatroban (a 120 micrograms bolus and 4 micrograms/kg/minute infusion for 72 hours). A third treatment arm in which patients received half this argatroban regimen was terminated due to lack of efficacy after 609 patients had been enrolled. By 30 days, 5·5% of the argatroban group and 5·7% of the heparin group had died (*P* = NS). There was a trend towards less bleeding in patients randomized to receive argatroban, but there was no difference in other clinical event rates.

Meta-analysis of direct thrombin inhibitor trials

The Direct Thrombin Inhibitor Trialists' Collaborative Group recently published a meta-analysis of 11 randomized trials in which direct thrombin inhibitors (hirudin, bivalirudin, argatroban, efegatran or inogatran) were compared with unfractionated heparin in a total of 35 970 patients with ST-segment elevation or non-ST-segment elevation acute coronary syndromes.[60] There were no significant differences in mortality between the patients given direct thrombin inhibitors and those given unfractionated heparin: 1·9% *v* 2·0% respectively at the cessation of therapy (OR 0·97; 95% CI 0·83–1·13, *P* = 0·69), 2·2% *v* 2·3% at 7 days (OR 1·00; 95% CI 0·87–1·16; *P* = 0·95), and 3·6% *v* 3·7% at 30 days (OR 1·01; 95% CI 0·90–1·12; *P* = 0·90). Likewise, direct thrombin inhibitors did not reduce mortality at 6 months (OR 1·00; 95% CI 0·91–1·09; *P* = 0·92). However, they did reduce the incidence of MI compared with heparin: 2·8% *v* 3·5% at the cessation of therapy (OR 0·80; 95% CI 0·71–0·90; *P* < 0·001), 3·2% *v* 3·9% at 7 days (OR 0·81; 95% CI 0·72–0·91; *P* < 0·001) and 4·7% *v* 5·3% at 30 days (OR 0·87; 95% CI 0·79–0·95; *P* = 0·004). The absolute risk reduction of 7 MIs prevented per 1000 patients treated with direct thrombin inhibitors remained constant at the cessation of therapy, at 7 days and at 30 days. Direct thrombin inhibitors were also shown to reduce the combined incidence of death/MI at the cessation of therapy (4·3% *v* 5·1% with heparin, OR 0·85; 95% CI 0·77–0·94; *P* = 0·001), at 7 days (5·0% *v* 5·8%, OR 0·88; 95% CI 0·80–0·96; *P* = 0·006) and at 30 days (7·4% *v* 8·2%, OR 0·91; 95% CI 0·84–0·99; *P* = 0·02). The 0·8% absolute risk reduction in death/MI remained constant at the cessation of therapy, at 7 days and at 30 days.

Five trials in this meta-analysis[38,39,63,65,71] (not including HERO-2) involved patients with ST-elevation MI. When the HERO-2 data[48] are combined with the data from these five trials (Figure 33.8), the results show that direct thrombin inhibitors have no effect on mortality alone, but do reduce the combined risk of death/re-infarction by 5% at 30 days compared with unfractionated heparin. This is due primarily to a 20% reduction in the rate of re-infarction. When compared with intravenous heparin, direct thrombin inhibitors reduce the risk of re-infarction after fibrinolytic therapy

without altering the rates of ischemic stroke, intracranial hemorrhage or major bleeding. **Grade A1a**

Factor X inhibitors

The newer antithrombotic drugs, vasoflux and pentasaccharide (which also has other effects as detailed below), have been recently evaluated as adjuncts to fibrinolytic therapy in patients with acute MI. These agents inhibit factor Xa, and offer potential advantages over unfractionated and low molecular weight heparin in that they do not interact with platelets or bind to platelet factor 4.

Vasoflux is a derivative of low molecular weight heparin that catalyzes fibrin-bound thrombin inactivation by heparin cofactor II, and inhibits factor IXa activation of factor X independently of antithrombin and heparin cofactor II. In the Vasoflux International Trial for Acute Myocardial Infarction Lysis (VITAL),[72] patients presenting within 6 hours of the onset of acute ST-elevation MI were given aspirin and streptokinase and randomized to receive either intravenous heparin or one of four intravenous doses of vasoflux (1 mg/kg, 4 mg/kg, 8 mg/kg or 16 mg/kg) in a dose-escalating phase II study. The incidence of TIMI-3 flow was similar in all treatment groups (35–42% with the various vasoflux doses *v* 41% with heparin), but major bleeding was more common with the higher doses of vasoflux (13% with 8 mg/kg of vasoflux (*P* = 0·05) and 28% with 16 mg/kg of vasoflux (*P* = 0·01) versus 8% with heparin). The development of this drug has been abandoned.

The Synthetic Pentasaccharide as an Adjunct to Fibrinolysis in ST-Elevation Acute Myocardial Infarction (PENTALYSE) study investigated the efficacy of pentasaccharide (a selective factor Xa inhibitor with a half life of 15–18 hours) in 316 patients presenting within 6 hours of the onset of ST-elevation MI.[73] The patients were given aspirin and alteplase and randomized to receive either unfractionated heparin or weight adjusted low-dose (4–6 mg), medium-dose (6–10 mg) or high-dose (10–12 mg) pentasaccharide administered once daily for 5–7 days. The first dose was given intravenously prior to alteplase, and the subsequent doses were given subcutaneously. The incidence of TIMI-3 flow at 90 minutes was similar in all treatment groups (68% with unfractionated heparin *v* 64% with all three pentasaccharide doses). While there was a trend towards less reocclusion (measured on day 6 ± 1) with pentasaccharide among patients who had achieved TIMI-3 flow by 90 minutes (0·9% *v* 7% with unfractionated heparin, *P* = 0·065), there was no difference in the rate of re-infarction within 30 days (3·8% with pentasaccharide *v* 3·6% with unfractionated heparin, *P* = 1·00). One patient randomized to receive 4 mg of pentasaccharide suffered an intracranial hemorrhage. Transfusions (excluding those related to bypass surgery)

(A)

Trial	N	OR and 95% CI	Death	
			Study drug	Control
TIMI-9B	3002		6·1%	5·0%
GUSTO-IIB	4131		5·9%	6·2%
HERO-1	412		5·1%	6·4%
HERO-2	17 073		10·8%	10·9%
HIT-4	1210		6·8%	6·4%
ARGAMI-2	1200		7·2%	4·5%
Overall	27 028		9·1%	9·0%

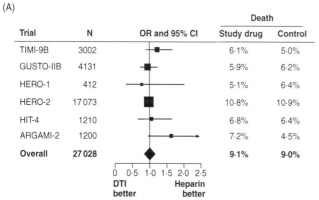

0 0·5 1·0 1·5 2·0 2·5
DTI better   Heparin better

Adjusted summary OR and 95% CI, P=0·6806
Test for homogeneity of ORs: χ²=5·8857, df=4, P=0·3175

(B)

Trial	N	OR and 95% CI	Re-infarction	
			Study drug	Control
TIMI-9B	3002		4·3%	5·0%
GUSTO-IIB	4131		5·0%	6·0%
HERO-1	412		5·1%	8·6%
HERO-2	17 073		3·5%	4·5%
HIT-4	1210		4·5%	4·9%
ARGAMI-2	1200		2·9%	2·8%
Overall	27 028		3·9%	4·8%

0 0·5 1·0 1·5 2·0 2·5
DTI better   Heparin better

Adjusted summary OR and 95% CI, P=0·0002
Test for homogeneity of ORs: χ²=1·7769, df=4, P=0·8791

(C)

Trial	N	OR and 95% CI	Death/re-infarction	
			Study drug	Control
TIMI-9B	3002		9·7%	9·3%
GUSTO-IIB	4131		9·9%	11·3%
HERO-1	412		9·9%	15·0%
HERO-2	17 073		13·0%	13·6%
HIT-4	1210		10·4%	10·9%
ARGAMI-2	1200		9·8%	6·5%
Overall	27 028		11·8%	12·4%

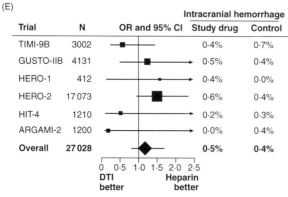

0 0·5 1·0 1·5 2·0 2·5
DTI better   Heparin better

Adjusted summary OR and 95% CI, P=0·1756
Test for homogeneity of ORs: χ²=8·4714, df=4, P=0·1321

(D)

Trial	N	OR and 95% CI	Stroke	
			Study drug	Control
TIMI-9B	3002		1·1%	2·1%
GUSTO-IIB	4131		1·3%	0·8%
HERO-1	412		1·1%	1·4%
HERO-2	17 073		1·2%	1·0%
HIT-4	1210		1·0%	1·0%
ARGAMI-2	1200		0·4%	0·4%
Overall	27 028		1·2%	1·0%

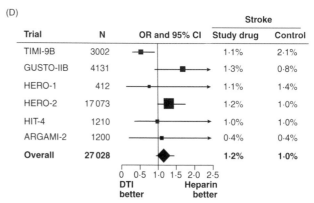

0 0·5 1·0 1·5 2·0 2·5
DTI better   Heparin better

Adjusted summary OR and 95% CI, P=0·2545
Test for homogeneity of ORs: χ²=9·8726, df=4, P=0·0789

(E)

Trial	N	OR and 95% CI	Intracranial hemorrhage	
			Study drug	Control
TIMI-9B	3002		0·4%	0·7%
GUSTO-IIB	4131		0·5%	0·4%
HERO-1	412		0·4%	0·0%
HERO-2	17 073		0·6%	0·4%
HIT-4	1210		0·2%	0·3%
ARGAMI-2	1200		0·0%	0·4%
Overall	27 028		0·5%	0·4%

0 0·5 1·0 1·5 2·0 2·5
DTI better   Heparin better

Adjusted summary OR and 95% CI, P=0·3908
Test for homogeneity of ORs: χ²=7·674, df=4, P=0·1751

(F)

Trial	N	OR and 95% CI	Major bleeding	
			Study drug	Control
TIMI-9B	3002		3·4%	3·8%
GUSTO-IIB	4131		1·1%	1·5%
HERO-1	412		16·5%	27·1%
HERO-2	17 073		0·7%	0·5%
HIT-4	1210		3·8%	3·6%
ARGAMI-2	1200		1·3%	1·8%
Overall	27 028		1·5%	1·5%

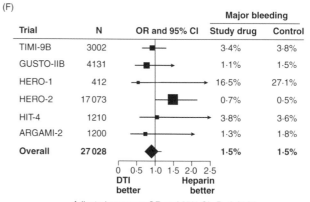

0 0·5 1·0 1·5 2·0 2·5
DTI better   Heparin better

Adjusted summary OR and 95% CI, P=0·3535
Test for homogeneity of ORs: χ²=11·11, df=4, P=0·0492

Figure 33.8 30 day event rates in patients with ST-elevation MI randomized to receive direct thrombin inhibitors (DTI) or unfractionated heparin in the HERO-1,[65] HERO-2,[48] TIMI-9B,[38] GUSTO-IIB,[39] HIT-4,[63] and ARGAMI-2[71] trials: (A) death; (B) re-infarction; (C) death/re-infarction; (D) stroke; (E) intracranial hemorrhage; (F) major bleeding. HIT=Hirudin for Improvement of Thrombolysis

were given to 3·3% of the pentasaccharide patients and 7·1% of the unfractionated heparin patients ($P = 0.21$).

Antiplatelet agents

Aspirin

Aspirin inhibits the cyclo-oxygenase-1 pathway of platelet activation (Figure 33.9).[74] The major support for its use in conjunction with fibrinolytic therapy comes from the ISIS-2 study, which was designed as a double-blind placebo-controlled 2×2 factorial trial.[75] Over 17 000 patients presenting within 24 hours of the onset of suspected acute MI were randomized to receive either streptokinase (1·5 million IU over 1 hour) or aspirin (162·5 mg daily for 1 month), or both, or neither. Aspirin on its own was found to reduce vascular mortality by 23% at 1 month, and when combined with streptokinase the reduction in this end point was 42%. The rates of non-fatal re-infarction (OR 0·51) and non-fatal stroke (OR 0·49) were also reduced by aspirin.

Aspirin should be given to all patients with ST-elevation MI and without contraindications in a dose of $\geqslant 150$ mg.
Grade A1a

The results of a 1992 meta-analysis suggested that aspirin reduced reocclusion in the first 2 weeks after MI,[76] but there has been no convincing evidence that aspirin prevents late reocclusion.[77,78]

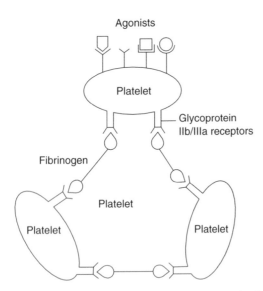

Agonists

Platelet

Glycoprotein IIb/IIIa receptors

Fibrinogen

Platelet

Platelet

Platelet

Figure 33.9 Glycoprotein IIb/IIIa receptors and platelet aggregation. Platelets are activated to aggregate by several mechanisms including high shear stress. The most common mechanism is the binding of an agonist to an external receptor, which activates signal transduction pathways. This causes the glycoprotein IIb/IIIa receptor to bind to fibrinogen, which binds to other platelets.

Glycoprotein IIb/IIIa inhibitors

Inhibition of the glycoprotein IIb/IIIa receptor blocks the final common site of several signal transduction pathways that lead to platelet aggregation (see Figure 33.9). There are two main types of drug in this class: (1) abciximab, which is a composite (human–murine) monoclonal antibody to the IIb/IIIa receptor; and (2) "small molecule" non-competitive IIb/IIIa inhibitors.

Abciximab used alone

Abciximab has been shown to enhance the likelihood of achieving TIMI-3 flow, but its effect is time-dependent. Figure 33.10 shows the percentages of patients achieving TIMI-2 and TIMI-3 flow after ST-elevation MI in five studies[45,79–82] where abciximab was administered prior to angiography.

Abciximab with percutaneous coronary interventions (PCI)

In the Abciximab Before Direct Angioplasty and Stenting in Myocardial Infarction Regarding Acute and Long-Term Follow-Up (ADMIRAL) study, 300 patients with acute MI were randomized in a double-blind manner to receive either abciximab or a placebo prior to primary angioplasty with stenting.[81] Some patients received the study drugs in the ambulance en route to hospital. Death/re-infarction/urgent target vessel revascularization occurred in 6·0% of the abciximab group versus 14·6% of the placebo group within 30 days ($P = 0.01$), and in 7·4% versus 15·9% respectively

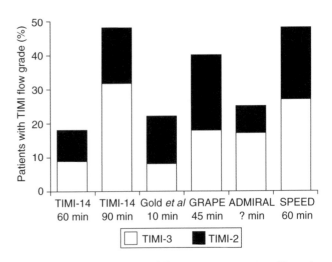

Figure 33.10 TIMI-2 and -3 flow rates in patients with acute MI treated with abciximab prior to angiography in the TIMI-14,[42] Gold *et al*,[79] GRAPE,[80] ADMIRAL,[81] and SPEED[82] trials. The time intervals between administration of the abciximab bolus and angiography are shown. GRAPE, Glycoprotein Receptor Antagonist Patency Evaluation.

within 6 months ($P= 0.02$). Patients in the abciximab group had a higher incidence of TIMI-3 flow prior to the procedure (16·8% v 5·4%; $P= 0.01$), immediately afterwards (95·1% v 86·7%; $P= 0.04$) and at 6 months (94·3% v 82·8%; $P= 0.04$). There was one major bleeding event in the abciximab group (0·7%) and none in the placebo group.

In the larger Controlled Abciximab and Device Investigation to Lower Late Angioplasty Complications (CADILLAC) trial,[83] 2082 patients presenting within 12 hours of the onset of ST elevation MI without cardiogenic shock were randomized in a 2×2 manner to receive either abciximab or a placebo, and either stenting or balloon angioplasty. Abciximab was not administered prior to angiography. TIMI-3 flow was achieved in 94·5% of the angioplasty group, 96·1% of the angioplasty plus abciximab group, 92·9% of the stenting group, and 96·4% of the stenting plus abciximab group. The mortality rates at 6 months were 5·3%, 2·9%, 3·2%, and 5·0% respectively, and reocclusion occurred in 12·9%, 9·7%, 5·4%, and 6·9% respectively. At 12 months the incidence of major adverse cardiac events was reduced (mainly due to a reduction in target vessel revascularization) from 15·9% in both balloon angioplasty groups to 9·3% and 6·6% in the stenting and stenting plus abciximab groups respectively ($P< 0.01$ for the four-way comparison between the groups).

The Stent Versus Thrombolysis for Occluded Coronary Arteries in Patients With Acute Myocardial Infarction (STOPAMI)-1 and -2 trials evaluated the effects of abciximab in conjunction with stenting or alteplase on myocardial salvage indices, measured by technetium-99m sestamibi on paired scintigrams at presentation (area at risk) and at 10 days (final infarct size). In the STOPAMI-1 trial,[84] 140 patients were randomized to receive either stenting plus abciximab, or alteplase. The salvage indices were 0·57 (interquartile range (IQR) 0·35–0·69) in the stenting plus abciximab group versus 0·26 (IQR 0·09–0·61; $P< 0.001$) in the alteplase group. In the STOPAMI-2 trial,[85] 162 patients were randomized to receive either half-dose alteplase plus abciximab or stenting plus abciximab. The salvage indices were 0·41 (IQR 0·13–0·58) in the alteplase plus abciximab group versus 0·60 (IQR 0·37–0·82) in the stenting plus abciximab group ($P= 0.001$). At 6 months 5% of the stenting plus abciximab group versus 9% of the alteplase plus abciximab group had died (RR 0·56; 95% CI 0·17–1·88; $P= 0.35$), while 0% v 4·9% respectively had suffered reinfarction ($P= 0.12$). There were no differences in the rates of stroke (1·2% in both groups) or major bleeding (also 1·2% in both groups).

Glycoprotein IIb/IIIa inhibitors and full-dose fibrinolytics

In the Combined Accelerated Tissue-Plasminogen Activator and Platelet Glycoprotein IIb/IIIa Integrin Receptor Blockade

With Integrilin in Acute Myocardial Infarction (IMPACT-AMI) dose-escalation study, 180 patients were given alteplase, aspirin, intravenous unfractionated heparin, and either a placebo or one of six doses of eptifibatide (previously known as integrilin).[86] TIMI-3 flow was achieved in 66% of patients given the highest dose of eptifibatide (a 180 micrograms/kg bolus and 0·75 micrograms/kg/minute infusion) versus 39% of those not given eptifibatide ($P= 0.007$). The major bleeding rates in these two groups were 3·9% and 5·4% respectively. However, this study involved small patient numbers, and so the results need to be confirmed in a larger study.

A pilot study[87] tested three doses of eptifibatide in conjunction with full-dose streptokinase in 181 patients who were randomized to receive a 180 micrograms/kg bolus of eptifibatide (or a placebo) followed by an infusion of 0·75, 1·33 or 2 micrograms/kg/minute. TIMI-3 flow at 90 minutes was achieved in 44–53% of patients in the various eptifibatide groups versus 38% of the group given streptokinase alone ($P=$ NS). Bleeding requiring transfusion (mainly angiography-related) occurred in 17% of patients given the highest dose of eptifibatide, 11% of those given the two lower doses, and none of those given the placebo ($P= 0.007$).

Glycoprotein IIb/IIIa inhibitors and modified-dose fibrinolytics

A number of angiographic and clinical trials have tested full-dose IIb/IIIa inhibitors in conjunction with reduced doses of fibrinolytic agents.

Angiographic studies

In the TIMI-14 trial,[42] patients were randomized to one of four treatment strategies: accelerated alteplase (a 100 mg infusion); full-dose abciximab with 20, 35 or 50 mg of alteplase; full-dose abciximab with 0·5, 0·75 or 1·25 million IU of streptokinase; or full-dose abciximab alone. All patients received a bolus of either 40 IU/kg or 60 IU/kg of unfractionated heparin. The highest incidence of TIMI-3 flow (77% at 90 minutes) was achieved with 50 mg of alteplase plus full-dose abciximab and 40 IU/kg of heparin. Overall, 3 of the 181 patients (1·7%) who received abciximab suffered intracranial hemorrhage. A high bleeding rate led to discontinuation of the treatment limbs that included streptokinase.

The SPEED trial[82] randomized patients to receive either abciximab alone (a 0·25 microgram/kg bolus and 0·125 microgram/kg/minute infusion for 12 hours), reteplase alone (two 10 mg boluses), or abciximab plus one of six double-bolus doses of reteplase (2·5–15 mg). Abciximab alone achieved TIMI-3 flow in 23% of patients by 60 minutes, while the highest incidence of TIMI-3 flow (62%) was achieved with 60 IU/kg of heparin plus two 5 mg boluses of reteplase and full-dose abciximab. Major bleeding occurred in 9·8% of the patients who received two 5 mg boluses of reteplase plus abciximab versus 3·7% of those who received reteplase alone ($P = 0·11$).

In the dose-finding phase of the Integrilin and Low-Dose Thrombolytics in Acute Myocardial Infarction (INTRO AMI) study,[88] eptifibatide was administered as a single 180 micrograms/kg bolus or as double boluses (30 minutes apart) of $180+90$ micrograms/kg or $180+180$ micrograms/kg, followed by an infusion of 1·33 or 2·0 micrograms/kg/minute for 72 hours after 25 or 50 mg of alteplase. In the dose-confirmation phase, the highest rates of TIMI-3 flow (65% at 60 minutes and 78% at 90 minutes) were achieved with 50 mg of alteplase plus a $180+90$ micrograms/kg double bolus and 1·33 micrograms/kg/minute infusion of eptifibatide. The $180+90$ micrograms/kg double bolus (given 10 minutes apart) and 2·0 micrograms/kg/minute infusion of eptifibatide achieved TIMI-3 flow in 54% of patients by 60 minutes, but major bleeding occurred in 11%, intracranial hemorrhage in 3%, and death in 5% of patients treated with this dose. For reasons that are not fully understood, the rates of intracranial hemorrhage have been higher in angiographic studies than in large clinical trials.

Glycoprotein IIb/IIIa inhibitors and low molecular weight heparin

In the Enoxaparin and TNK-t-PA With or Without Glycoprotein IIb/IIIa Inhibitor as Reperfusion Strategy in ST-Elevation Myocardial Infarction (ENTIRE-TIMI-23) trial,[55] patients were randomized to one of three treatment regimens: tenecteplase (0·53 mg/kg) plus either enoxaparin or unfractionated heparin, or half this dose of tenecteplase plus abciximab. The TIMI-3 flow rates at 60 minutes ranged from 47% to 58% with the various treatment regimens, but did not differ significantly between the groups. Major bleeding was less common with enoxaparin than with unfractionated heparin (1·9% v 2·4%, $P < 0·05$).

In the Integrilin and Tenecteplase in Acute Myocardial Infarction (INTEGRITI) trial,[89] patients received either tenecteplase alone (0·375 mg) or reduced-dose tenecteplase (0·25 mg) plus eptifibatide (two boluses of 180 and 90 mg/kg given 10 minutes apart followed by a 2 mg/kg infusion). TIMI-3 flow was achieved by 60 minutes in 49% of patients receiving tenecteplase alone versus 59% of those receiving tenecteplase and eptifibatide ($P = NS$).

The Fibrinolytic and Aggrastat ST-Elevation Resolution (FASTER) trial[90] tested various bolus doses of tirofiban (between 10 and 15 micrograms/kg followed by 0·15 micrograms/kg/minute for 24 hours) in combination with half or two thirds doses of tenecteplase (0.27 or 0.36 mg/kg, respectively). A control group received full-dose tenecteplase alone (0.53 mg/kg). The patients receiving the half and two thirds doses of tenecteplase were given a 40 IU/kg heparin bolus

(maximum 3000 IU) and a 7 IU/kg/hour infusion (maximum 800 IU/hour) to maintain an APTT of 50–70 seconds, while those receiving full-dose tenecteplase (the control group) were given a 60 IU/kg heparin bolus (maximum 4000 IU) and a 12 IU/kg/hour infusion (maximum 1000 IU). The end points of the trial were TIMI-3 flow in the infarct artery at 60 minutes, the corrected TIMI frame count at 60 minutes and ST-segment resolution at 60 and 180 minutes. TIMI-3 flow was achieved by 60 minutes in 59% of the tirofiban groups overall versus 58% of the control group, and there were no differences in their corrected TIMI frame counts. Complete ST-segment resolution was achieved by 60 minutes in 41% of the tirofiban groups overall versus 29% of the control group ($P = 0.07$), and by 180 minutes in 76 versus 65%, respectively ($P = 0.10$). TIMI major bleeding[53] occurred within the first 48 hours in 2.3% of the tirofiban groups overall versus 4·7% of the control group. There were no episodes of intracranial hemorrhage (personal communication from Dr EM Ohman).

Trials with clinical end points

The ASSENT-3 trial[46] randomized patients to receive either full-dose tenecteplase plus enoxaparin (30 mg intravenously plus 1 mg/kg subcutaneously every 12 hours) for a maximum of 7 days, half-dose tenecteplase plus weight adjusted low-dose unfractionated heparin and a 12 hour infusion of abciximab, or full-dose tenecteplase plus weight adjusted unfractionated heparin for 48 hours. A summary of the clinical outcomes, including a reduction in investigator-reported re-infarction, is shown in Figure 33.11.

In the GUSTO-V trial,[47] 16 588 patients presenting within 6 hours of the onset of acute ST-segment elevation MI were randomized to receive either half-dose reteplase plus a modified dose of heparin and abciximab, or full-dose reteplase and heparin without abciximab. By 30 days, 5·6% of the abciximab group versus 5·9% of the no-abciximab group had died (OR 0·95; 95% CI 0·83–1·08; $P = 0·43$). The abciximab group had a lower rate of investigator-reported re-infarction (Figure 33.11), but higher rates of severe bleeding (1·1% v 0·5%; OR 2·14; 95% CI 1·48–3·09; $P < 0·001$) and transfusion (5·7% v 4·0%; OR 1·46; 95% CI 1·26–1·69; $P < 0·001$). Intracranial hemorrhage occurred in 0·6% of both groups. In a prespecified analysis, the regimen including abciximab was shown not to be inferior to the regimen excluding abciximab. Subgroup analysis showed that the abciximab group had a lower point estimate for mortality in patients presenting after 4 hours (7·1% v 8·1%; $P = 0·33$) and in patients with anterior MI (7·6% v 8·5%, $P = 0·17$).

In ASSENT-3[46] and GUSTO-V[47] the risk of bleeding in patients aged >75 years (including intracranial hemorrhage) (see Figure 33.6) was higher with regimens involving half-dose fibrinolytic therapy plus full-dose abciximab than in those involving full-dose fibrinolytic therapy without abciximab.

-tion
144

(A)

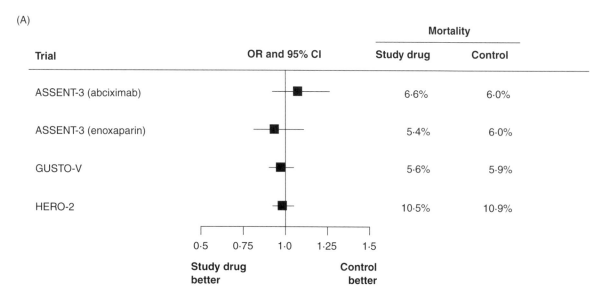

(B)

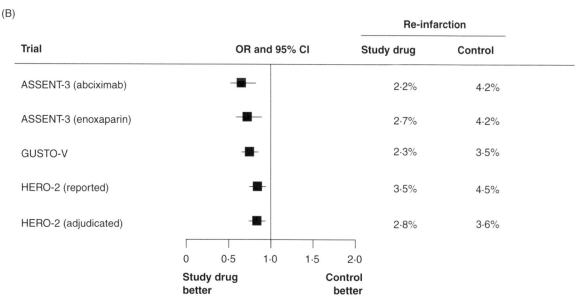

Figure 33.11 Clinical outcomes in the ASSENT-3,[46] GUSTO-V,[47] and HERO-2[48] trials: (A) mortality; (B) re-infarction

In ASSENT-3, bleeding occurred in 13·3% of elderly patients given tenecteplase plus abciximab versus 4·1% of those given tenecteplase plus unfractionated heparin ($P= 0·0002$). In GUSTO-V, bleeding occurred in 1·9% of elderly patients given reteplase plus abciximab versus 1·2% of those given reteplase plus unfractionated heparin ($P= 0·17$). These findings suggest that the combination of abciximab with half-dose reteplase or tenecteplase reduces the risk of re-infarction compared with full doses of these fibrinolytic agents combined with intravenous unfractionated heparin although in GUSTO-V this did not translate into a mortality benefit at 12 months, including in prespecified subgroups.[96] Based on the data currently available, no firm recommendations can be made for the use of glycoprotein IIb/IIIa inhibitors as adjuncts to either fibrinolytic therapy or percutaneous intervention. **Grade A1b**

Recommendations for use of adjunctive antithrombotic therapies

The 1999 ACC/AHA guidelines[34] and the 2000 American College of Chest Physicians (ACCP)[91] guidelines recommend that patients receiving a fibrin-specific fibrinolytic agent for acute MI should be given a 60 IU/kg bolus (maximum 4000 IU) and a 12 IU/kg/hour infusion (maximum 1000 IU/hour) of unfractionated heparin (Table 33.5). **Grade A1c** This dose is lower than that recommended in

Table 33.5 Recommendations for the use of adjunctive unfractionated heparin with fibrinolytic therapy from two consensus conferences

Fibrinolytic agent	ACC/AHA 1999[34]	ACCP 2000[91]
Fibrin-specific agents	Intravenous unfractionated heparin should be used in patients undergoing reperfusion therapy with alteplase. The recommended regimen is 60 IU/kg as a bolus at initiation of the alteplase infusion, then an initial maintenance dose of approximately 12 IU/kg/hour (maximum 4000 IU bolus and maximum 1000 IU/hour infusion for patients weighing >70 kg), adjusted to maintain the APTT at 1·5–2·0 times control (50–70 seconds) for 48 hours. Continuation of the heparin infusion beyond 48 hours should be considered in patients at high risk of systemic or venous thromboembolism	Patients receiving alteplase, reteplase or tenecteplase should be given intravenous unfractionated heparin for 48 hours. Either standard dosing (a 5000 IU bolus and 1000 IU/hour infusion) or weight adjusted dosing (a 60 IU/kg bolus (maximum 4000 IU) and 12 IU/kg/hour infusion (maximum 1000 IU/hour) may be used, both adjusted to maintain an APTT of 50–70 seconds
Streptokinase	Intravenous unfractionated heparin should be used in patients at high risk of systemic emboli (large or anterior MI, atrial fibrillation, previous embolus or known left ventricular thrombus). It is recommended that heparin be withheld for 6 hours and that APTT testing begin at that time. Heparin should be started when the APTT returns to <2 times control (approximately 70 seconds), then infused to keep the APTT at 1.5–2.0 times control (initial infusion rate approximately 1000 IU/hour). After 48 hours, a change to subcutaneous heparin, warfarin or aspirin alone should be considered	Patients at high risk of systemic or venous thromboembolism (that is, those with Q wave anterior MI, severe left ventricular dysfunction, congestive heart failure, a history of systemic or pulmonary embolism, evidence of left ventricular thrombus, or atrial fibrillation) should receive intravenous unfractionated heparin, starting not less than 4 hours after the commencement of streptokinase and when the APTT is <70 seconds. The target APTT should be 50–70 seconds, and the infusion should continue for ≥48 hours Patients who are not at high risk of systemic or venous thromboembolism should receive subcutaneous unfractionated heparin (12 500 IU) every 12 hours for 48 hours

the 1996 guidelines. The time for the first APTT measurement is not specified. Although the recent reduction in the unfractionated heparin regimen is aimed at lowering the rates of major bleeding and intracranial hemorrhage while maintaining efficacy as assessed by TIMI-3 flow rates, this is only supported by Grade C evidence.

The ACC/AHA and ACCP guidelines recommend the use of intravenous heparin in patients treated with streptokinase if they have high-risk features (Table 33.5). **Grade A1c** Our personal approach is to use intravenous heparin (commencing with a weight adjusted bolus) to achieve a high level of thrombin inhibition in patients receiving streptokinase, and to measure the APTT at 3 hours. This is based on the results of the overview (which indicated a possible saving with unfractionated heparin of 2·2 lives and 1·8 infarctions prevented per 1000 patients treated, at a cost of 3·2 transfusions and 0·3 non-fatal disabling strokes compared with a placebo or control treatment),[29] angiographic data from GUSTO-I (showing significantly better patency at 5–7 days with intravenous versus subcutaneous heparin),[6] and follow up data from GUSTO-I (showing that the 5 year survival rate of patients given streptokinase and intravenous heparin was equal to that of patients given alteplase, and higher than those given streptokinase plus subcutaneous heparin).[31]

If a fibrin-specific fibrinolytic agent is being used, the patient should receive a weight adjusted bolus of intravenous heparin followed by an infusion to maintain the APTT at 50–70 seconds for 48 hours if the patient is not undergoing PCI (see Table 33.5). The APTT should be measured at 3 hours. Further trials of adjunctive intravenous low molecular weight heparins with fibrinolytic therapy will need to be performed before recommendations can be made regarding combinations of these agents.

Future directions

Despite greater understanding of the mechanism of benefit of adjunctive antithrombin therapies, and recent large clinical trials in patients with ST-segment elevation MI, many questions remain unanswered. It has not yet been resolved whether combinations of newer fibrinolytic agents with newer antithrombin agents and/or glycoprotein IIb/IIIa inhibitors improve clinical outcomes with acceptable bleeding risks. These regimens, along with agents such as P-selectin inhibitors[92] and tissue factor pathway inhibitors,[93] will need to be tested in combination with clopidogrel and with facilitated PCI.

Key points

- There is ongoing thrombin generation in patients with ST-segment elevation acute coronary syndromes.
- Fibrinolytic therapy results in a procoagulant state.
- Unfractionated heparin has proven efficacy in the absence of aspirin and a modest effect in the presence of aspirin.
- Unfractionated heparin has several limitations as an antithrombin agent, including variable pharmacokinetics and pharmacodynamics and relative inefficacy against clot-bound thrombin.
- Reduction of the unfractionated heparin dose may reduce the risk of major bleeding, but does not alter the risk of intracranial hemorrhage.
- Low molecular weight heparins are easier to administer than unfractionated heparin, and have been shown to reduce the risk of re-infarction when used as adjuncts to fibrinolytic therapy. However, they may increase the need for transfusion compared with unfractionated heparin.
- Bivalirudin has no effect on mortality when used as adjunctive therapy with streptokinase, but does reduce the incidence of re-infarction compared with unfractionated heparin increases the risks of minor and moderate bleeding.
- When combined with reteplase or tenecteplase, abciximab reduces the risk of re-infarction compared with unfractionated heparin, but increases the risk of major bleeding, particularly in elderly patients.

References

1. French JK, Williams BF, Hart HH *et al.* Prospective evaluation of eligibility for thrombolytic therapy in acute myocardial infarction. *BMJ* 1996;**312**:1637–41.
2. Chesebro JH, Knatterud G, Roberts R *et al.* Thrombolysis in Myocardial Infarction (TIMI) trial, Phase I: a comparison between intravenous tissue plasminogen activator and intravenous streptokinase: clinical findings through hospital discharge. *Circulation* 1987;**76**:142–54.
3. TIMI Study Group. The Thrombolysis in Myocardial Infarction (TIMI) trial: Phase I findings. *N Engl J Med* 1985; **312**:932–6.
4. Simes RJ, Topol EJ, Holmes DR Jr *et al.* Link between the angiographic substudy and mortality outcomes in a large randomized trial of myocardial reperfusion: importance of early

and complete infarct artery reperfusion. *Circulation* 1995; **91**:1923–8.
5. White HD, Norris RM, Brown MA *et al.* Effect of intravenous streptokinase on left ventricular function and early survival after acute myocardial infarction. *N Engl J Med* 1987; **317**:850–5.
6. The GUSTO Angiographic Investigators. The effects of tissue plasminogen activator, streptokinase, or both on coronary-artery patency, ventricular function, and survival after acute myocardial infarction. *N Engl J Med* 1993;**329**:1615–22 [published erratum appears in *N Engl J Med* 1994;**330**:516].
7. White HD, Cross DB, Elliott JM, Norris RM, Yee TW. Long-term prognostic importance of patency of the infarct-related coronary artery after thrombolytic therapy for acute myocardial infarction. *Circulation* 1994;**89**:61–7.
8. Hirsh J, Raschke R, Warkentin TE *et al.* Heparin: mechanism of action, pharmacokinetics, dosing considerations, monitoring, efficacy, and safety. *Chest* 1995;**108**:258S–75S.
9. Weitz JI, Hudoba M, Massel D, Maraganore J, Hirsh J. Clot-bound thrombin is protected from inhibition by heparin–antithrombin III but is susceptible to inactivation by antithrombin III-independent inhibitors. *J Clin Invest* 1990;**86**:385–91.
10. Eisenberg PR, Miletich JP. Induction of marked thrombin activity by pharmacologic concentrations of plasminogen activators in nonanticoagulated whole blood. *Thromb Res* 1989; **55**:635–43.
11. Lee CD, Mann KG. Activation/inactivation of human coagulation factor V by plasmin. *Blood* 1989;**73**:185–90.
12. Eisenberg PR. Role of heparin in coronary thrombolysis. *Chest* 1992;**101**(Suppl. 4):131S–9S.
13. Verheugt FW, Liem A, Zijlstra F *et al.* High dose bolus heparin as initial therapy before primary angioplasty for acute myocardial infarction: results of the Heparin in Early Patency (HEAP) pilot study. *J Am Coll Cardiol* 1998;**31**:289–93.
14. Liem A, Zijlstra F, Ottervanger JP *et al.* High dose heparin as pretreatment for primary angioplasty in acute myocardial infarction: the Heparin in Early Patency (HEAP) randomized trial. *J Am Coll Cardiol* 2000;**35**:600–4.
15. Topol EJ, George BS, Kereiakes DJ *et al.* A randomized controlled trial of intravenous tissue plasminogen activator and early intravenous heparin in acute myocardial infarction. *Circulation* 1989;**79**:281–6.
16. Hsia J, Hamilton WP, Kleiman N *et al.* A comparison between heparin and low-dose aspirin as adjunctive therapy with tissue plasminogen activator for acute myocardial infarction. *N Engl J Med* 1990;**323**:1433–7.
17. Bleich SD, Nichols TC, Schumacher RR *et al.* Effect of heparin on coronary arterial patency after thrombolysis with tissue plasminogen activator in acute myocardial infarction. *Am J Cardiol* 1990;**66**:1412–17.
18. de Bono DP, Simoons ML, Tijssen J *et al.* Effect of early intravenous heparin on coronary patency, infarct size, and bleeding complications after alteplase thrombolysis: results of a randomized double blind European Cooperative Study Group trial. *Br Heart J* 1992;**67**:122–8.
19. Turpie AGG, Robinson JG, Doyle DJ *et al.* Comparison of high-dose subcutaneous heparin to prevent left ventricular mural thrombosis in patients with acute transmural anterior myocardial infarction. *N Engl J Med* 1989;**320**:352–8.

20. The SCATI (Studio sulla Calciparina nell-Angina e nella Trombosi Ventricolare nell'Infarto) Group. Randomized controlled trial of subcutaneous calcium-heparin in acute myocardial infarction. *Lancet* 1989;**ii**:182–6.

21. Gruppo Italiano per lo Studio della Sopravvivenza nell'Infarto Miocardico (GISSI). GISSI-2: a factorial randomized trial of alteplase versus streptokinase and heparin versus no heparin among 12 490 patients with acute myocardial infarction. *Lancet* 1990;**336**:65–71.

22. ISIS-3 (Third International Study of Infarct Survival) Collaborative Group. ISIS-3: a randomized comparison of streptokinase vs tissue plasminogen activator vs anistreplase and of aspirin plus heparin vs aspirin alone among 41 299 cases of suspected acute myocardial infarction. *Lancet* 1992; **339**: 753–70.

23. The GUSTO Investigators. An international randomized trial comparing four thrombolytic strategies for acute myocardial infarction. *N Engl J Med* 1993;**329**:673–82.

24. Collins R, Peto R, Baigent C, Sleight P. Aspirin, heparin, and fibrinolytic therapy in suspected acute myocardial infarction. *N Engl J Med* 1997;**336**:847–60.

25. Collins R, Conway M, Alexopoulos D *et al*, for the ISIS Pilot Study Investigators. Randomized factorial trial of high-dose intravenous streptokinase, of oral aspirin and of intravenous heparin in acute myocardial infarction. *Eur Heart J* 1987; **8**:634–42.

26. Col J, Decoster O, Hanique G *et al*. Infusion of heparin conjunct to streptokinase accelerates reperfusion of acute myocardial infarction: results of a double blind randomized study (OSIRIS) [abstract]. *Circulation* 1992;**86**(Suppl. I):I-259.

27. O'Connor CM, Meese R, Carney R *et al*, for the DUCCS Group. A randomized trial of heparin in conjunction with anistreplase (anisoylated plasminogen streptokinase activator complex) in acute myocardial infarction: the Duke University Clinical Cardiology Study (DUCCS). *J Am Coll Cardiol* 1994;**23**:11–18.

28. Topol EJ, Califf RM, Van de Werf F *et al*. Perspectives on large-scale cardiovascular clinical trials for the new millenium. *Circulation* 1997;**95**:1072–82.

29. Collins R, MacMahon S, Flather M *et al*. Clinical effects of anticoagulant therapy in suspected acute myocardial infarction: systematic overview of randomized trials. *BMJ* 1996; **313**:652–9.

30. Granger CB, Becker R, Tracy RP *et al*. Thrombin generation, inhibition and clinical outcomes in patients with actue myocardial infarction treated with thrombolytic therapy and heparin: results from the GUSTO-1 trial. *J Am Coll Cardiol* 1998;**31**:497–505.

31. Tardiff BE, McCants B, Hellkamp AS *et al*. Long term results from the Global Utilization of Streptokinase and TPA for Occluded Coronary Arteries (GUSTO-I) trial: sustained benefit of fibrin-specific therapy [abstract]. *Circulation* 1999; **100**(Suppl. I):I-498-9.

32. Holmes DR Jr, Califf RM, Van de Werf F *et al*. Difference in countries' use of resources and clinical outcome for patients with cardiogenic shock after myocardial infarction: results from the GUSTO trial. *Lancet* 1997;**349**:75–8.

33. Giugliano RP, McCabe CH, Antman EM *et al*. Lower-dose heparin with fibrinolysis is associated with lower rates of intracranial hemorrhage. *Am Heart J* 2001;**141**:742–50.

34. Ryan TJ, Antman EM, Brooks NH *et al*. 1999 update: ACC/AHA guidelines for the management of patients with acute myocardial infarction: a report of the American College of Cardiology/American Heart Association Task Force on Practice Guidelines (Committee on Management of Acute Myocardial Infarction). *J Am Coll Cardiol* 1999;**34**: 890–911.

35. Granger CB, Hirsh J, Califf RM *et al*. Activated partial thromboplastin time and outcome after thrombolytic therapy for acute myocardial infarction: results from the GUSTO-I trial. *Circulation* 1996;**93**:870–8.

36. Antman EM, for the TIMI-9A Investigators. Hirudin in acute myocardial infarction: safety report from the Thrombolysis and Thrombin Inhibition in Myocardial Infarction (TIMI) 9A trial. *Circulation* 1994;**90**:1624–30.

37. The Global Use of Strategies to Open Occluded Coronary Arteries (GUSTO) IIa Investigators. Randomized trial of intravenous heparin versus recombinant hirudin for acute coronary syndromes. *Circulation* 1994;**90**:1631–7.

38. Antman EM, for the TIMI-9B Investigators. Hirudin in acute myocardial infarction: Thrombolysis and Thrombin Inhibition in Myocardial Infarction (TIMI) 9B trial. *Circulation* 1996; **94**:911–21.

39. The Global Use of Strategies to Open Occluded Coronary Arteries (GUSTO) IIB Investigators. A comparison of recombinant hirudin with heparin for the treatment of acute coronary syndromes. *N Engl J Med* 1996;**335**:775–82.

40. Cannon CP, Gibson CM, McCabe CH *et al*. TNK-tissue plasminogen activator compared with front-loaded alteplase in acute myocardial infarction: results of the TIMI-10B trial. *Circulation* 1998;**98**:2805–14.

41. Van de Werf F, Cannon CP, Luyten A *et al*. Safety assessment of single-bolus administration of TNK tissue-plasminogen activator in acute myocardial infarction: the ASSENT-1 trial. *Am Heart J* 1999;**137**:786–91.

42. Antman EM, Giugliano RP, Gibson CM *et al*. Abciximab facilitates the rate and extent of thrombolysis: results of the Thrombolysis in Myocardial Infarction (TIMI) 14 trial. *Circulation* 1999;**99**:2720–32.

43. Strategies for Patency Enhancement in the Emergency Department (SPEED) Group. Trial of abciximab with and without low-dose reteplase for acute myocardial infarction. *Circulation* 2000;**101**:2788–94.

44. Assessment of the Safety and Efficacy of a New Thrombolytic (ASSENT-2) Investigators. Single-bolus tenecteplase compared with front-loaded alteplase in acute myocardial infarction: the ASSENT-2 double-blind randomized trial. *Lancet* 1999; **354**:716–22.

45. The InTIME-II Investigators. Intravenous NPA for the treatment of infarcting myocardium early: InTIME-II, a double-blind comparison of single-bolus lanoteplase vs accelerated alteplase for the treatment of patients with acute myocardial infarction. *Eur Heart J* 2000;**21**:2005–13.

46. The Assessment of the Safety and Efficacy of a New Thrombolytic Regimen (ASSENT)-3 Investigators. Efficacy and safety of tenecteplase in combination with enoxaparin, abciximab, or unfractionated heparin: the ASSENT-3 randomized trial in acute myocardial infarction. *Lancet* 2001;**358**: 605–13.

47. The GUSTO V Investigators. Reperfusion therapy for acute myocardial infarction with fibrinolytic therapy or combination

reduced fibrinolytic therapy and platelet glycoprotein IIb/IIIa inhibition: the GUSTO V randomized trial. *Lancet* 2001; **357**:1905–14.

48. The Hirulog and Early Reperfusion or Occlusion (HERO)-2 Trial Investigators. Thrombin-specific anticoagulation with bivalirudin versus heparin in patients receiving fibrinolytic therapy for acute myocardial infarction: the HERO-2 randomized trial. *Lancet* 2001;**358**:1855–63.

49. Kontny F, Dale J, Abildgaard U, Pedersen TR, on behalf of the FRAMI Study Group. Randomized trial of low molecular weight heparin (dalteparin) in prevention of left ventricular thrombus formation and arterial embolism after acute anterior myocardial infarction: the Fragmin in Acute Myocardial Infarction (FRAMI) study. *J Am Coll Cardiol* 1997;**30**:962–9.

50. Frostfeldt G, Ahlberg G, Gustafsson G *et al.* Low molecular weight heparin (dalteparin) as adjuvant treatment to thrombolysis in acute myocardial infarction – a pilot study: Biochemical Markers in Acute Coronary Syndromes (BIOMACS II). *J Am Coll Cardiol* 1999;**33**:627–33.

51. Wallentin L, Dellborg DM, Lindahl B *et al.* The low-molecular-weight heparin dalteparin as adjuvant therapy in acute myocardial infarction: the ASSENT PLUS study. *Clin Cardiol* 2001;**24**:I-12–14.

52. Simoons ML, Krzeminska-Pakula M, Alonso A *et al.* Improved reperfusion and clinical outcome with enoxaparin as an adjunct to streptokinase thrombolysis in acute myocardial infarction: the AMI-SK study. *Eur Heart J.* In press 2002.

53. Rao AK, Pratt C, Berke A *et al.* Thrombolysis in Myocardial Infarction (TIMI) trial – phase I: hemorrhagic manifestations and changes in plasma fibrinogen and the fibrinolytic system in patients treated with recombinant tissue plasminogen activator and streptokinase. *J Am Coll Cardiol* 1988;**11**:1–11.

54. Ross AM, Molhoek P, Lundergan C *et al.* Randomized comparison of enoxaparin, a low molecular weight heparin, with unfractionated heparin adjunctive to recombinant tissue plasminogen activator thrombolysis and aspirin: second trial of Heparin and Aspirin Reperfusion Therapy (HART II). *Circulation* 2001;**104**:648–52.

55. Antman EM, Louwerenburg HW, Baars HF *et al.* Enoxaparin as adjunctive antithrombin therapy for ST-elevation myocardial infarction: results of the ENTIRE-Thrombolysis in Myocardial Infarction (TIMI) 23 trial. *Circulation* 2002;**105**:1642–9.

56. Maraganore JM, Bourdon P, Jablonski I, Ramachandran KL, Fenton JW II. Design and characterization of hirulogs: a novel class of bivalent peptide inhibitors of thrombin. *Biochem J* 1990;**29**:7095–101.

57. Collen D, Matsuo O, Stassen JM, Kettner C, Shaw E. *In vivo* studies of a synthetic inhibitor of thrombin. *J Lab Clin Med* 1982;**99**:76–83.

58. Yasuda T, Gold HK, Yaoita H *et al.* Comparative effects of aspirin, a synthetic thrombin inhibitor and a monoclonal antiplatelet glycoprotein IIb/IIIa antibody on coronary artery reperfusion, reocclusion and bleeding with recombinant tissue-type plasminogen activator in a canine preparation. *J Am Coll Cardiol* 1990;**16**:714–22.

59. Haskel EJ, Prager NA, Sobel BE, Abendschein DR. Relative efficacy of antithrombin compared with antiplatelet agents in accelerating coronary thrombolysis and preventing early reocclusion. *Circulation* 1991;**83**:1048–56.

60. The Direct Thrombin Inhibitor Trialists' Collaborative Group. Direct thrombin inhibitors in acute coronary syndromes: principal results of a meta-analysis based on individual patients' data. *Lancet* 2002;**359**:294–302.

61. Cannon CP, McCabe CH, Henry TD *et al.* A pilot trial of recombinant desulfatohirudin compared with heparin in conjunction with tissue-type plasminogen activator and aspirin for acute myocardial infarction: results of the Thrombolysis in Myocardial Infarction (TIMI) 5 trial. *J Am Coll Cardiol* 1994; **23**:993–1003.

62. Simes RJ, Granger CB, Antman EM *et al.* Impact of hirudin versus heparin on mortality and (re)infarction in patients with acute coronary syndromes: a prospective meta-analysis of the GUSTO-IIb and TIMI 9b trials [abstract]. *Circulation* 1996; **94**(Suppl. I):I-430.

63. Neuhaus K-L, Molhoek GP, Zeymer U *et al.* Recombinant hirudin (lepirudin) for the improvement of thrombolysis with streptokinase in patients with acute myocardial infarction: results of the HIT-4 trial. *J Am Coll Cardiol* 1999;**34**: 966–73.

64. Zeymer U, Schroder R, Tebbe U *et al.* Non-invasive detection of early infarct vessel patency by resolution of ST-segment elevation in patients with thrombolysis for acute myocardial infarction; results of the angiographic substudy of the Hirudin for Improvement of Thrombolysis (HIT)-4 trial. *Eur Heart J* 2001;**22**:769–75.

65. White HD, Aylward PE, Frey MJ *et al.* Randomized, double-blind comparison of hirulog versus heparin in patients receiving streptokinase and aspirin for acute myocardial infarction (HERO). *Circulation* 1997;**96**:2155–61.

66. Andrews J, Straznicky IT, French JK *et al.* Hirulog reduces re-ischaemic episodes as assessed by continuous ST segment monitoring following acute myocardial infarction treated with streptokinase [abstract]. *J Am Coll Cardiol* 1999; **33**(Suppl. A):375A.

67. Lee KL, Woodlief LH, Topol EJ *et al.* Predictors of 30-day mortality in the era of reperfusion for acute myocardial infarction: results from an international trial of 41 021 patients. *Circulation* 1995;**91**:1659–68.

68. Abendschein DR, Meng YY, Torr-Brown S, Sobel BE. Maintenance of coronary patency after fibrinolysis with tissue factor pathway inhibitor. *Circulation* 1995;**92**:944–9.

69. Sitko GR, Ramjit DR, Stabilito II *et al.* Conjunctive enhancement of enzymatic thrombolysis and prevention of thrombotic reocclusion with the selective factor Xa inhibitor, tick anticoagulant peptide. *Circulation* 1992;**85**:805–15.

70. Gruber A, Harker LA, Hanson SR, Kelly AB, Griffin JH. Antithrombotic effects of combining activated protein C and urokinase in nonhuman primates. *Circulation* 1991;**84**: 2454–62.

71. Kaplinsky E. Direct antithrombin-argatroban in acute myocardial infarction (ARGAMI-2). Proceedings of the Late-Breaking Clinical Trials III Session, 47th Scientific Sessions of the American College of Cardiology; Atlanta, Georgia, USA; March 1998.

72. Peters RJG, Spickler W, Théroux P *et al.* Randomized comparison of a novel anticoagulant, vasoflux, and heparin as adjunctive therapy to streptokinase for acute myocardial infarction: results of the VITAL study (Vasoflux International Trial for

Acute Myocardial Infarction Lysis). *Am Heart J* 2001;**142**:237–43.

73. Coussement PK, Bassand JP, Convens C *et al.* A synthetic factor-Xa inhibitor (ORG31540/SR9017A) as an adjunct to fibrinolysis in acute myocardial infarction: the PENTALYSE study. *Eur Heart J* 2001;**22**:1716–24.

74. Antiplatelet Trialists' Collaboration. Collaborative overview of randomized trials of antiplatelet therapy – I: prevention of death, myocardial infarction, and stroke by prolonged antiplatelet therapy in various categories of patients. *BMJ* 1994;**308**:81–106.

75. ISIS-2 (Second International Study of Infarct Survival) Collaborative Group. Randomized trial of intravenous streptokinase, oral aspirin, both, or neither among 17 187 cases of suspected acute myocardial infarction: ISIS-2. *Lancet* 1988;**ii**:349–60.

76. Roux S, Christeller S, Ludin E. Effects of aspirin on coronary reocclusion and recurrent ischemia after thrombolysis: a meta-analysis. *J Am Coll Cardiol* 1992;**19**:671–7.

77. Meijer A, Verheugt FWA, Werter CJPJ *et al.* Aspirin versus coumadin in the prevention of reocclusion and recurrent ischemia after successful thrombolysis: a prospective placebo-controlled angiographic study: results of the APRICOT study. *Circulation* 1993;**87**:1524–30.

78. White HD, French JK, Hamer AW *et al.* Frequent reocclusion of patent infarct-related arteries between 4 weeks and 1 year: effects of antiplatelet therapy. *J Am Coll Cardiol* 1995;**25**: 218–23.

79. Gold HK, Garabedian HD, Dinsmore RE *et al.* Restoration of coronary flow in myocardial infarction by intravenous chimeric 7E3 antibody without exogenous plasminogen activators: observations in animals and humans. *Circulation* 1997;**95**:1755–9.

80. van den Merkhof LFM, Zijlstra F, Olsson H *et al.* Abciximab in the treatment of acute myocardial infarction eligible for primary percutaneous transluminal coronary angioplasty: results of the Glycoprotein Receptor Antagonist Patency Evaluation (GRAPE) pilot study. *J Am Coll Cardiol* 1999;**33**:1528–32.

81. Montalescot G, Barragan P, Wittenberg O *et al.* Platelet glycoprotein IIb/IIIa inhibition with coronary stenting for acute myocardial infarction. *N Engl J Med* 2001;**344**:1895–903.

82. Herrmann HC, Moliterno DJ, Ohman EM *et al.* Facilitation of early percutaneous coronary intervention after reteplase with or without abciximab in acute myocardial infarction: results from the SPEED (GUSTO-4 Pilot) trial. *J Am Coll Cardiol* 2000;**36**:1489–96.

83. Stone GW, Grines CL, Cox DA *et al.* Comparison of angioplasty with stenting, with or without abciximab, in acute myocardial infarction. *N Engl J Med* 2002;**346**:957–66.

84. Schömig A, Kastrati A, Dirschinger J *et al.* Coronary stenting plus platelet glycoprotein IIb/IIIa blockade compared with tissue plasminogen activator in acute myocardial infarction. *N Engl J Med* 2000;**343**:385–91.

85. Kastrati A, Mehilli J, Dirschinger J *et al.* Myocardial salvage after coronary stenting plus abciximab versus fibrinolysis plus abciximab in patients with acute myocardial infarction: a randomized trial. *Lancet* 2002;**359**:920–5.

86. Ohman EM, Kleiman NS, Gacioch G *et al.* Combined accelerated tissue-plasminogen activator and platelet glycoprotein IIb/IIIa integrin receptor blockade with integrilin in acute myocardial infarction: results of a randomized, placebo-controlled, dose-ranging trial. *Circulation* 1997;**95**:846–54.

87. Ronner E, van Kesteren HA, Zijnen P *et al.* Safety and efficacy of eptifibatide vs placebo in patients receiving thrombolytic therapy with streptokinase for acute myocardial infarction; a phase II dose escalation, randomized, double-blind study. *Eur Heart J* 2000;**21**:1530–6.

88. Brener SJ, Zeymer U, Adgey AA *et al.* Eptifibatide and low-dose tissue plasminogen activator in acute myocardial infarction: the Integrilin and Low-Dose Thrombolysis in Acute Myocardial Infarction (INTRO AMI) trial. *J Am Coll Cardiol* 2002;**39**:377–86.

89. Giugliano RP, Roe MT, Zeymer U *et al.* Restoration of epicardial and myocardial perfusion in acute ST-elevation myocardial infarction with combination eptifibatide + reduced-dose tenecteplase: results from the INTEGRITI trial [abstract]. *Circulation* 2001;**104**(Suppl. II):II-538.

90. The Fibrinolytic and Aggrastat ST-Elevation Resolution (FASTER) trial. Proceedings of the American College of Cardiology 51st Annual Scientific Session, Atlanta, GA, March 2002.

91. Ohman EM, Harrington RA, Cannon CP *et al.* Intravenous thrombolysis in acute myocardial infarction. *Chest* 2001;**119**(Suppl.):253S–77S.

92. Lefer AM, Campbell B, Scalia R, Lefer DJ. Synergism between platelets and neutrophils in provoking cardiac dysfunction after ischemia and reperfusion: role of selectins. *Circulation* 1998;**98**:1322–8.

93. Ott I, Malcouvier V, Schomig A, Neumann FJ. Proteolysis of tissue factor pathway inhibitor-1 by thrombolysis in acute myocardial infarction. *Circulation* 2002;**105**:279–81.

94. The Continuous Infusion Versus Double-Bolus Administration of Alteplase (COBALT) Investigators. A comparison of continuous infusion of alteplase with double-bolus administration for acute myocardial infarction. *N Engl J Med* 1997;**337**:1124–30.

95. The Global Use of Strategies to Open Occluded Coronary Arteries (GUSTO III) Investigators. A comparison of reteplase with alteplase for acute myocardial infarction. *N Engl J Med* 1997;**337**:1118–23.

96. Lincoff AM. One-year follow-up of the GUSTO-V trial. Proceedings of the Late Breaking Clinical Trials Session, XIVth World Congress of Cardiology. Sydney, Australia; May 2002.

34 Pain relief, general management, and other adjunctive treatments

Aldo P Maggioni, Roberto Latini, Gianni Tognoni, Peter Sleight

The prognosis of patients admitted to hospital with acute myocardial infarction (AMI) has improved greatly since the introduction of reperfusion therapies into clinical practice. Several trials testing different fibrinolytic agents, aspirin, and more recently, primary PTCA, have shown that mortality can be reduced by 20–30% when these therapies are begun in the first few hours after the onset of symptoms of AMI. The favorable effects were proportional to the patency rates obtained. Although there is no objective evidence for mortality reduction, pain relief, oxygen, bed rest, and adjunctive therapies should be considered to reduce clinical symptoms and possibly improve prognosis.

Pain relief

The relief of pain is a priority in patients with AMI, not only for humane reasons, but also because pain activates the sympathetic nervous system increasing cardiac work and myocardial oxygen consumption **Grade A1b**. Two approaches are used:

- reduction of ischemia
- direct analgesia.

Nitroglycerin by the sublingual route or by IV infusion is the most commonly used drug to reduce pain due to ischemia (see the section on Nitrates below). A double-blind randomized trial on 69 patients[1] showed that inhaled nitrous oxide can decrease pain in the absence of hemodynamic changes or other major adverse events. Few controlled data are available, so the recommendations are based mainly on empiricism and personal expertise **Grade C**.

Among direct analgesics, morphine is the drug of choice, while meperidine and pentazocine can be substituted in patients with documented hypersensitivity to morphine. Morphine, besides its analgesic effect, has useful hemodynamic actions, including peripheral vasodilation without a decrease of left ventricular (LV) filling pressure. This action, together with central reduction of tachypnea, can be particularly useful in patients with pulmonary edema.[2–5]

Effective analgesia should not be delayed because of the fear of masking the effects of anti-ischemic therapy with recommended agents – fibrinolytic agents, β blockers, aspirin, nitrates. Morphine is given at doses of 4–8 mg IV and repeated every 5–15 minutes in doses of 2–8 mg until pain is relieved. Morphine also reduces anxiety, thereby decreasing metabolic demands of the heart during the early critical phase. The decrease in heart rate resulting from the reduction of sympathetic tone and the vagomimetic action of morphine contributes to the reduction of anxiety. Usually opioids are sufficient and tranquillizers are not needed.

Adverse reactions to morphine such as severe vomiting, hypotension, and respiratory depression may limit its administration. Hypotension (systolic blood pressure <100 mmHg) can be minimized by keeping the patient supine with elevated lower extremities. In the case of excessive bradycardia, atropine may be administered IV (0·5–1·5 mg). Depression of respiration seldom occurs and can be treated with intravenous naloxone (0·1–0·2 mg, repeated after 15 minutes if necessary). Nausea and vomiting, if severe or recurrent, may be treated with a phenothiazine.

The widespread use of reperfusion therapy early after AMI has decreased the intensity and duration of pain, which is largely due to ongoing cardiac ischemia. The additional use of IV β blockers[6,7] further decreases the severity of pain by reducing cardiac work.

New approaches to analgesia after AMI include synthetic and semisynthetic narcotics like fentanyl and sufentanyl and thoracic epidural anesthesia, but clinical experience is too limited to recommend regimens and modalities.

General management

Oxygen

Grade B Experimental studies have shown that breathing oxygen can decrease myocardial injury;[8] moreover, in patients with AMI the administration of oxygen reduced ST segment elevation.[9] It is assumed that oxygen breathing might improve the ventilation/perfusion mismatch which may be seen in AMI patients. Arterial Po_2 is reduced for about 48 hours in many uncomplicated cases of AMI.[10]

There are no objective randomized trials on the benefit of oxygen breathing after AMI. However, in the presence of severe hypoxemia oxygen is recommended, while in uncomplicated cases its use should probably be limited to the first day or less. **Grade C**

Oxygen therapy is indicated if monitored oxygen saturation is lower than 90%. In complicated AMI, with severe heart failure, pulmonary edema or mechanical complications, supplemental oxygen is not sufficient and continuous positive pressure breathing or tracheal intubation with mechanical ventilation are sometimes required.[11] **Grade C**

Excessive oxygen can cause systemic vasoconstriction with a consequent increase in cardiac workload, an important consideration in uncomplicated patients.

Bed rest

Bed rest has been traditionally advised for patients with AMI on the assumption that it would decrease cardiac workload. However, it is now recognized that the intensive use of

recommended treatments – fibrinolysis, IV β blockade, aspirin – allows a much shorter stay in bed for AMI patients. **Grade B** This may decrease the risk of thromboembolism and help to prevent the adverse effects of deconditioning.[12]

Prophylactic use of lidocaine (lignocaine)

Grade A The observation that life-threatening arrhythmias occur within the first 24–48 hours of onset of AMI in a substantial proportion of patients led to the hypothesis that the prophylactic administration of lidocaine could prevent or reduce the incidence of ventricular fibrillation and resulting early mortality.[13]

However, an overview of 14 controlled trials testing the effects of prophylactic lidocaine (administered by the IM or IV route) on a total of 9155 patients confirmed a significant reduction of 35% in the rate of ventricular fibrillation, but a strong trend to an increase of 38% in early mortality (OR 1·38, 95% CI 0·98–1·95).[14] The increase in mortality appeared to be caused by bradyarrhythmias, advanced atrioventricular

Table 34.1   Other adjunctive therapies: summary of evidence

Therapies	Study	*n*	Follow up duration	Mortality (%) Treated	Control	*P* value	NNT
β blockers							
ISIS-1[19]	LSRCT	16027	7 days	3·9	4·6	0·04	143
Sleight *et al.*[18]	OV	27536	7 days	3·7	4·3	0·03	167
CAPRICORN[23]	LSRCT	1959	1.3 years	12	15	0·03	34
ACE inhibitors							
Early unselected strategy							
GISSI-3[34]	LSRCT	19394	42 days	6·4	7·2	0·03	125
ISIS-4[35]	LSRCT	58050	35 days	7·2	7·7	0·02	200
ACE-i MICG[37]	OV	98469	30 days	7·1	7·6	0·004	200
Late selected strategy							
SAVE[38]	LSRCT	2231	42 months (mean)	20·4	24·6	0·019	24
AIRE[39]	LSRCT	2006	15 months (mean)	17·0	23·0	0·002	17
TRACE[40]	LSRCT	1749		34·7	62·3	0·001	13
Nitrates							
Yusuf *et al.*[55]	OV	3041	Inhospital	13·3	18·9	0·002	18
GISSI-3[34]	LSRCT	19394	42 days	6·5	6·9	NS	–
ISIS-4[35]	LSRCT	58050	35 days	7·3	7·5	NS	–
Overview[35]	OV	81908	35 days	7·4	7·7	0·03	333
Calcium antagonists							
Teo *et al.*[62]	OV	20342	–	9·6	9·3	NS	–
Magnesium							
Teo *et al.*[67]	OV	1301	Inhospital	3·8	8·2	0·001	23
LIMIT-2[68]	LSRCT	2316	28 days	7·8	10·4	0·04	42
ISIS-4[35]	LSRCT	58050	35 days	7·6	7·2	NS	–
Overview[35]	OV	61860	35 days	7·6	7·5	NS	–

Abbreviations: LSRCT, large-scale randomized clinical trials; NNT, number of patients needed to treat to save one life; NS, non-significant; OV, overview

block, and asystole. In view of these findings, prophylactic lidocaine is no longer considered as a standard treatment in patients with AMI, but is reserved for those patients who have already experienced ventricular fibrillation. **Grade A**

Other adjunctive treatments (Table 34.1)

We will now discuss adjunctive drug therapy with β blockers, ACE inhibitors, nitrates, magnesium, and calcium-antagonists. The results of published randomized trials which were of adequate size to show reliable data in terms of mortality, together with overviews of the data, will be summarized. We will also indicate areas of doubt.

Specific therapy

β Blockers

Rationale

Early after AMI, activation of the sympathetic nervous system occurs. β Blockers reduce oxygen demand by lowering heart rate and blood pressure, and decreasing myocardial wall stress, thereby limiting infarct size, the incidence of cardiac rupture, and improving ventricular function and mortality.[15] By their β adrenergic antagonist properties, they can also prevent the life-threatening ventricular arrhythmias related to the increased adrenergic activity occurring in the first hours after the onset of AMI.[16]

Evidence from trials and overviews of early IV β blockade

Studies testing the effects of early IV β blockade on the mortality of patients with AMI show consistent results.[17] Available data on more than 27 000 patients from 27 trials show that the mortality rate of the patients allocated to the active treatment was significantly reduced by about 14% in comparison with placebo-allocated patients (from 4·3% to 3·7%; in absolute terms, six lives saved per 1000 patients treated with β blockers).[18] The largest study testing this treatment, the ISIS-1 trial, showed that the mortality reduction by atenolol treatment in patients with AMI was concentrated in the first day or two from the onset of AMI symptoms.[19] Further, this study suggested that reduction in cardiac rupture and cardiac arrest were the most notable changes in early death associated with β blocker therapy.[20] These observations may be considered as the rationale for the combined use of β blockers and fibrinolytics, which are both known to reduce mortality. In particular, in the first few days from the onset of AMI, β blockers may reduce cardiac rupture, the incidence of which may be increased by fibrinolytic induced hemorrhage of infarcted myocardium.[21,22] However, β blocker trials in AMI were

conducted mostly during the 1970s and 1980s, when no fibrinolysis or primary angioplasty was performed, and adjunctive therapy was characterized by much less use of aspirin and no ACE inhibitors. Further, study populations were mostly at lower risk and patients with heart failure were usually excluded. For these reasons, the CAPRICORN trial was planned with the aim to evaluate whether long-term treatment with carvedilol (titrated up to 25 mg ×2/day) could reduce all-cause mortality in postinfarction patients (from 3 to 21 days from symptom onset) with an LV ejection fraction ≤ 40% and who were receiving an ACE inhibitor for ≥48 hours.[23] All-cause mortality was reduced from 15% in the placebo group and to 12% in the carvedilol group (23% relative reduction), while the combined end point of all-cause deaths plus CV hospitalizations was not modified by the active treatment.

Recommendations

All patients with AMI, in the absence of specific contraindications, should be treated with a β blocker within 24 hours from the onset of symptoms and treatment should be continued for at least 2 years. **Grade A** Clear contraindications are pulmonary edema, asthma, hypotension, bradycardia, or advanced atrioventricular block. Even in the absence of trials of adequate size testing specifically the effects of the combination of a β blocker and a fibrinolytic, pathophysiologic premises, observational data, and the few controlled studies suggest that this treatment should be considered in association with reperfusion treatment with fibrinolysis. In the GISSI-2 trial, IV atenolol was used in conjunction with fibrinolytics in 48% of the patients.

Lack of randomized trials of early β blockade in the era of reperfusion

With the exception of the recently published CAPRICORN trial that included patients with LV dysfunction some days after AMI, the trials testing the early effects on mortality of β blockers in all-comers with AMI were conducted in the early 1980s, before the widespread use of reperfusion therapy. Trials formally testing the effects of the combination of a β blocker and a fibrinolytic are few and underpowered to provide reliable data in terms of mortality reduction. The only data available are from the TIMI-2B trial, in which 1434 patients, all treated with tPA and aspirin, were randomized to receive immediate or delayed (6–8 days) oral metoprolol.[24] Total mortality rate at 6 and 42 days was not significantly decreased by the immediate treatment, but the number of deaths was fewer, and the rate of non-fatal re-infarction was reduced in the group receiving immediate metoprolol.

More recently, data from the National Registry of Myocardial Infarction 2 showed that immediate β blocker administration in patients with AMI treated with tPA reduces the occurrence of intracranial hemorrhage. Among patients receiving tPA, the incidence of intracranial hemorrhage was 0·7% (158/23 749) in patients receiving β blockers and 1·0% (384/3658) in patients not receiving β blockers (*P* < 0·001).[25] Multivariate analysis showed that immediate β blocker use was associated with a 31% reduction in the rate of intracranial hemorrhage. No other drugs given within the first 24 hours were associated with a reduction in the rate of intracranial hemorrhage.

Long-term use

The effects of β blocker therapy started after the acute phase of MI (5–28 days from the onset of symptoms) have been tested among more than 35 000 patients not receiving a reperfusion therapy in several placebo-controlled trials.[26] Overall, the long-term composite outcome of mortality and non-fatal infarction was reduced by 20–25%. **Grade A**

Timolol, metoprolol, and propranolol were the most extensively studied drugs.[27–29] In the Norwegian Multicenter Study,[27] patients allocated to timolol showed a 39% mortality reduction and a 28% reduction of re-infarction. The initial benefit persisted for at least 72 months in the patients who continued timolol treatment after trial termination. Similar results have been obtained by the Beta-Blocker Heart Attack Trial (BHAT),[28] in which 3837 patients were allocated to propranolol or placebo. After 25 months of treatment overall mortality was reduced by 28%. Subgroup analysis showed that the beneficial effects of β blockers were apparent among the various subgroups, but the magnitude of the benefit was greater in high-risk patients (those with large or anterior AMI or with signs or symptoms of moderate left ventricular dysfunction). This subgroup analysis of the BHAT trial has been recently confirmed by the results of the CAPRICORN trial, which showed a significant mortality reduction in post-AMI patients with LV dysfunction treated with carvedilol.[23]

Definite contraindications to β blocker therapy are pulmonary edema, asthma, severe hypotension, bradycardia, or advanced atrioventricular block. Evidence from trials and overviews suggests that all patients with AMI who do not have clear contraindications should be treated with intravenous β blockers within 24 hours from the onset of symptoms. If tolerated, the treatment should be continued for at least 2–3 years, and perhaps longer. **Grade A** A debate is still open about whether β blockers should be prescribed to all patients without contraindications or whether they should be given only to the patients at moderate to high risk who have the most to gain from a long-term treatment.

Despite the clear evidence of benefit, observational studies showed that in clinical practice β blockers are generally underused, only 36–42% of patients receiving a β blocker at discharge.[30]

ACE inhibitors

Rationale

The rationale behind this strategy is based mainly on the fact that activation of the renin–angiotensin system occurs during the very early phase of MI, with deleterious consequences, including an increase of peripheral resistance and heart rate, decrease of coronary perfusion, and alteration in endogenous fibrinolytic activity.[31,32]

Evidence from trials and overviews

After the disappointing results of the CONSENSUS-2 trial,[33] which did not show a benefit from enalapril treatment, the results of GISSI-3 and ISIS-4 studies were published.[34,35] In the GISSI-3 trial, 6 week total mortality was significantly lower in the patients treated with lisinopril: 6 week lisinopril treatment significantly reduced mortality from 7·2% to 6·4% (in absolute terms eight lives saved per 1000 treated patients).[34]

The favorable results on mortality shown by the GISSI-3 study have been confirmed by the larger ISIS-4 trial. During the first 5 weeks there were 2088 (7·19%) deaths recorded among 29 028 captopril-allocated patients compared with 2231 (7·69%) among 29 022 patients allocated placebo.[35] This 7% relative reduction in total mortality was statistically significant (*P* = 0·02) and corresponded in absolute terms to five fewer deaths per 1000 patients treated with captopril for 1 month. The reduction in total mortality shown by CCS-1[36] was similar to that demonstrated by the larger GISSI-3 and ISIS-4 trials, but statistical significance was not achieved, presumably because of inadequate sample size.

An overview of the trials testing an early unselected approach with ACE inhibitors in 98 496 patients with AMI showed that immediate treatment is safe, well tolerated and that it produces a small, but significant reduction of 30 day mortality.[37] This benefit is quantifiable as about five extra lives saved for every 1000 patients treated with ACE inhibitors early after the onset of AMI.

With respect to the safety profile, persistent hypotension and renal dysfunction were (as expected) reported significantly more often in the patients treated with ACE inhibitors than in corresponding controls.

The overview also confirmed the important benefit achievable with early ACE inhibitor treatment. Of the total 239 lives saved by early ACE inhibitor treatment, 200 were saved in the first week after AMI.

The "selective" strategy of starting ACE inhibitors some days after AMI only in patients with clinical heart failure and/or objective evidence of LV dysfunction was tested in three trials (SAVE, AIRE, TRACE), involving about 6000 patients overall.[38–40] These trials consistently showed that long-term ACE inhibitor treatment in this selected population of patients was associated with a significant reduction of mortality. **Grade A**

Controversy: aspirin and ACE inhibitors

It has been proven that part of the hypotensive/unloading effect of ACE inhibitors is attributable to increased synthesis of vasodilatory prostaglandins such as PGE_2.[41] It has been shown that the concomitant administration of salicylate reduces the effectiveness of ACE inhibitors in patients with congestive heart failure.[42,43] However, the appropriateness of extrapolating these data to post-AMI patients in clinical practice is questionable since other studies have yielded conflicting results on the interaction between ACE inhibitor and aspirin.[44,45] In relatively unselected AMI patients enrolled in the GISSI-3 trial there was a beneficial effect from ACE inhibitors irrespective of aspirin use.[46] The GISSI-3 findings have been confirmed by the overview of the individual data of 98 496 patients enrolled in trials involving more than 1000 patients randomly allocated to receive ACE inhibitors or control starting in the acute phase of AMI. ACE inhibitor treatment was associated with a similar proportional reduction in 30 day mortality among the 86 484 patients who were taking aspirin (6%) and among the 10 228 patients who were not (10%).[47] The lack of negative interaction between aspirin and ACE inhibitors has also been reported in the overview of 12 763 AMI patients with LV dysfunction or heart failure.[48]

In conclusion, it seems that the pharmacologic interaction between salicylates and ACE inhibitors is devoid of major clinical relevance in the setting of AMI, both in terms of reduction of the unloading effect of ACE inhibitors and in terms of adverse effects on renal function. Therefore in the absence of adequate data from randomized controlled trials (RCTs), both ACE inhibitors and aspirin may be safely administered in the early phase of AMI. Since patients with left ventricular (LV) dysfunction have a mortality rate of about 50% if they experience a new infarction, prevention with aspirin should not be abandoned on the basis of inadequate data. The lack of negative interaction between aspirin and ramipril in the prevention of cardiovascular events, recently shown by the HOPE trial,[49] further supports this conclusion.

Recommendations

ACE inhibitor treatment should be started during the first day following AMI in most patients after timely and careful observation of the patient's hemodynamic and clinical status, and after administration of routinely recommended treatments (fibrinolysis, aspirin, and β blockers). **Grade A** If echocardiography shortly before discharge shows LV dysfunction, the treatment should be continued for a long period of time. In the patients showing neither clinical symptoms nor objective evidence of LV dysfunction, the treatment can be stopped and ventricular function re-evaluated after an appropriate time interval. **Grade A** These recommendations

derive from the results of trials testing ACE inhibitors in patients with a recent AMI. More recently, the results of the HOPE trial have been published.[49] The HOPE trial tested the effects of ramipril versus placebo in nearly 9000 patients at increased risk of cardiovascular disease, defined as a history of MI, angina, cerebrovascular or peripheral arterial disease. People with diabetes were also included, even in the absence of a previous cardiovascular event. The trial showed a significant 22% reduction of a composite measure of MI, stroke, and death from cardiovascular causes. The HOPE findings indicate that virtually all patients with a history of cardiovascular disease should be treated with ACE inhibitors, and not just those who after an AMI have signs or symptoms of heart failure. **Grade A** The PEACE and EUROPA trials, still ongoing, will provide further data from such patients.[50]

The main contraindications to early ACE inhibitor treatment are hypotension, bilateral renal artery stenosis, severe renal failure, or a history of cough or angioedema attributed to previous treatment with ACE inhibitors. Caution is needed in patients previously receiving high-dose diuretic (>50 mg furosemide/day) therapy.

Nitrates

Rationale

Experimental and clinical studies showed that nitrates can reduce oxygen demand and myocardial wall stress during AMI by reducing pre- and afterload.[51] Further, nitrates can increase coronary blood supply to the ischemic muscle by reducing coronary vasospasm.[52] These favorable effects of reduced infarct size and improved LV function have been demonstrated in both animals and humans.[53,54]

Evidence from trials and overviews

Controlled clinical trials and overviews provide conflicting results. Yusuf *et al* carried out a meta-analysis of seven small trials testing IV nitroglycerin and three trials testing IV nitroprusside. Overall, the results on 2041 patients showed that nitrate treatment reduced mortality by about 35%.[55]

More recently, the effects of different nitrate treatments in patients with AMI has been tested in two large-scale mortality trials enrolling more than 80 000 patients, receiving currently recommended concomitant therapies (90% received aspirin and about 70% fibrinolysis).[35] Both trials showed that routine nitrate use does not produce an improvement in survival, either in the total population of patients with AMI or in the subgroups with different risks of death. A large number of patients allocated to the control groups in these trials received out-of-protocol nitrate treatment because of a specific indication (pain, angina, heart failure, hypertension), possibly obscuring a true benefit in terms of mortality reduction. Accordingly, the ISIS-4 investigators analyzed the effects of nitrates in the subgroup of patients not receiving out-of-protocol nitrate treatment. The results of this subanalysis confirmed the main results of the study.[35]

A further trial, ESPRIM, of the nitric oxide donor molsidomine also failed to show any mortality benefit in AMI patients.[56] The overview of all existing data (the first 10 small trials plus the two recent large scale studies) confirms the negative results in terms of mortality reduction.[35]

Recommendations

Grade A Nitrates are not a recommended treatment for all patients with AMI. However, nitrates are confirmed to be well tolerated even in the context of the other treatments (β blockers, aspirin, fibrinolysis, ACE inhibitors), suggesting that their use, limited to the patients with specific indications such as angina or pump failure, is safe and likely to be beneficial in the treatment of ischemic chest pain and pump failure. **Grade A** Definite data on the short-term mortality benefit of IV nitroglycerin started in the first 24 hours after the beginning of AMI symptoms are not available.

Unclear interaction with ACE inhibitors

The results of the GISSI-3 trial suggest that nitrates can produce some additive beneficial effect when used in combination with ACE inhibitors but this was not seen in ISIS-4. Additional trials should be conducted to confirm or reject this hypothesis.[34,35]

Calcium-channel blockers

Rationale

Calcium-channel blockers can reduce oxygen demand by lowering blood pressure and reducing contractility;[57] verapamil and diltiazem also reduce heart rate.[58] These mechanisms could be beneficial in patients during AMI.

Evidence from trials and overviews

Trials testing nifedipine at different dosages either in the acute phase of MI or after discharge showed a non-significant increase of mortality.[59] Controlled clinical trials testing calcium-channel blockers other than dihydropyridines, such as diltiazem or verapamil, have also found no significant reduction of mortality. However, the DAVIT-2 trial did show a 20% reduction of the combined end point of cardiovascular mortality and re-infarction.[60] Similarly, the largest trial testing diltiazem showed a 23% reduction of deaths from cardiac causes and re-infarction in the subgroup of patients without signs of pulmonary congestion, while in the

subgroup of patients with pulmonary congestion a 41% increase of these events was observed.[61] An overview of the 24 trials testing any kind of calcium-channel blocker in patients with AMI showed a non-significant increase of mortality of about 4%.[62]

Recommendations

Grade A Since individual trials and overviews revealed no statistically significant evidence of harm or benefit in terms of mortality reduction, these drugs are not recommended as standard therapy in patients in the acute phase of MI. Verapamil or diltiazem may be useful after AMI in patients intolerant of β blockade. Despite the consistent negative results of trials and overviews, the rate of use of calcium-channel blockers remains high.[30,63]

Newer drugs

Few data are available concerning the effects either of long-acting nifedipine or of newer, more selective dihydropyridines, such as felodipine or amlodipine. New trials of these drugs are planned or under way.

Magnesium

Rationale

In experimental models of AMI, high plasma levels of magnesium can prevent extensive myocardial damage, possibly through inhibition of the inward current of calcium in ischemic cardiac cells, and the reduction of coronary tone.[64,65] Infusion of magnesium in experimental models of AMI can increase the threshold for malignant arrhythmias, reducing the occurrence of ventricular fibrillation.[66] In humans, high plasma levels of magnesium reduce peripheral vascular resistance and increase cardiac output without affecting myocardial oxygen consumption. Thus, infusions of magnesium started early during AMI could theoretically reduce infarct size, prevent life-threatening arrhythmias and improve survival.

Evidence from trials and overviews

Conflicting results have been provided by the trials in which IV infusion of magnesium has been tested. A first overview by Teo *et al* of seven trials among about 1300 patients showed that mortality was reduced by 58% (from 8·2% to 3·8%) by an early intravenous infusion of magnesium.[67] The greatest part of the benefit was due to the reduction of life-threatening ventricular arrhythmias. These favorable data received further support from a large single center study, LIMIT-2, in which 2316 patients were randomized to receive IV magnesium or placebo.[68] This study showed that the 28 day mortality rate was significantly reduced by 24% ($P = 0.04$) (but with a lower confidence interval near zero). No difference was observed in terms of ventricular arrhythmias, but surprisingly a reduction in clinical heart failure was observed. More recently the results of the ISIS-4 trial on more than 58 000 patients did not confirm that IV magnesium can reduce mortality.[35] As expected, the current overview of all the existing data is dominated by the results of ISIS-4.[35]

Recommendations

Intravenous magnesium cannot be recommended for routine use for patients with AMI. **Grade A** Its use should be limited to the patients with specific indications (that is, patients with ventricular arrhythmias and prolonged QT interval, or those with high blood pressure not controlled by usual therapy).

A new trial

Experimental studies suggested in animal models that magnesium is effective only if administered before fibrinolysis, thereby preventing reperfusion injury.[69,70] This hypothesis is supported by animal models of AMI and by the LIMIT-2 trial, which showed a reduction of the cases of heart failure after magnesium infusion.

Even though the ISIS-4 trial showed that magnesium treatment was not effective in any of the studied subgroups of patients, including those treated with fibrinolysis within 6 hours from the onset of symptoms, the possibility that magnesium treatment can limit reperfusion injury after recanalization therapy has not been formally tested. Because of this disparity between ISIS-4 and LIMIT-2, a further trial (MAGIC) is ongoing in selected patients.

Other adjunctive therapies in search of evidence

Adenosine

The excess of mortality in the day after fibrinolytic therapy may be, at least in part, attributed to reperfusion injury. Adenosine has been shown to exert a cardioprotective action in animal studies and in small-scale clinical trials. In particular, adenosine reduced infarct size and improved LV function in animal models of reperfusion injury.

In the Acute Myocardial Infarction Study of Adenosine (AMISTAD) trial, among patients receiving IV fibrinolytic therapy within 6 hours from symptom onset, an IV infusion of adenosine reduced infarct size by 33% compared to placebo ($P = 0.085$). Infarct size was significantly reduced by 67% ($P = 0.014$) in patients with anterior MI, while it had no effect in those with non-anterior MI. The effect of adenosine on final infarct size appeared to be independent of the

fibrinolytic (alteplase or streptokinase) and of lidocaine use.[71] Based on these promising results obtained in 236 patients, a large-scale trial, AMISTAD II, was conducted to assess the effect of two doses of adenosine versus placebo on mortality and heart failure over 6 months after MI. Although the overall analysis did not show significant improvement with adenosine versus placebo, the higher dose group showed a significant reduction in infarct size and a trend in event reduction (American College of Cardiology, 2002).

Inhibition of leukocyte adhesion

Inflammation plays a role in determining the extent of myocardial damage after ischemia and reperfusion. Anti-inflammatory treatments have yielded contrasting results in animal models of MI, but have never been proven beneficial in humans. Specific inhibition of leukocyte adhesion reduced cardiac ischemia-reperfusion injury in animals. In the Limitation of Myocardial Injury following Thrombolysis in Acute Myocardial Infarction (LIMIT AMI), 394 patients with signs and symptoms of AMI were randomized within 12 hours of symptom onset to two doses of IV bolus of a monoclonal antibody to the CD18 subunit of the β2 integrin adhesion receptors (rhu MAB CD18) or placebo. The MAB CD18 was well tolerated, but ineffective either in increasing 90 minute TIMI grade 3 flow or in decreasing MI size.[72]

Along the same line, 420 patients with TIMI flow 0 or 1 after MI were randomized to two doses of LeukArrest or placebo in the HALT-MI trial. LeukArrest is a human monoclonal antibody which binds all four integrin receptors on leukocytes. LeukArrest did not reduce infarct size or clinical and adverse event rates. The agent appeared well tolerated, except for a significant increase in the rate of major infections.[73]

Metabolic interventions

The old concept of metabolic protection of the ischemic myocardium has been tested in a randomized open trial on 407 patients with suspected MI, the ECLA Glucose-Insulin-Potassium (GIK) trial.[74] Patients were randomized to two doses of GIK or to control within 24 hours from symptom onset. Overall mortality and morbidity reduction by GIK did not reach statistical significance. However, the reduction in mortality was significant in patients who received reperfusion therapy. GIK appeared to be well tolerated even if volumes of the order of 2–3 liters had to be infused over 24 hours. A mortality trial is being conducted to verify the benefit of this cheap intervention in AMI.

Ischemia/reperfusion damage is due partly to the Na^+/H^+ exchange system. Animal experiments and a pilot study in patients suggested that inhibitors of Na^+/H^+ exchanger, amiloride derivatives (cariporide, eniporide) exerted cardioprotective effects. Two recent placebo-controlled trial have shown neutral results of NHE inhibitors versus placebo.[75,76]

In the GUARd During Ischemia Against Necrosis (GUARDIAN) trial 11 590 patients with unstable angina or non-ST-elevation MI were randomized to cariporide or placebo and followed for 36 days. No difference between cariporide and placebo was documented on the primary end point of death or MI.[75] In the Evaluation of the Safety and Cardioprotective Effects of Eniporide in AMI (ESCAMI) trial, 1389 patients with ST-elevation MI undergoing reperfusion treatments were studied. Eniporide administered before reperfusion neither reduced infarct size (the primary end point), nor improved clinical outcome.[76]

Nicorandil, has been proposed for several years with indications ranging from stable effort angina to MI. In an open study, 81 patients with a first anterior MI were randomized to control or nicorandil started IV before PTCA. Nicorandil plus PTCA improved clinical outcome and left-ventricular functional recovery in respect to PTCA alone.[77] However, the number of patients in the study was too small, even for a pilot trial, to draw any conclusion.

Conclusions

The therapeutic approaches discussed in the chapter can provide benefits only to patients who survive long enough to reach a monitored bed. The potential reduction of mortality obtainable with the use of evidence-based therapies is applicable to only about half of the population of patients suffering an AMI.[78]

Besides research efforts aimed at designing new strategies to further improve survival, the challenges are several:

- to broaden the correct use of evidence-based treatments for the patients reaching the hospital;
- to apply these or new treatments to the subgroup of patients generally excluded from randomized clinical trials (elderly patients, patients with comorbidities, etc.);
- to reduce the number of patients who die before reaching the hospital.

Appendix: long-term use of aspirin after the acute phase of myocardial infarction

Grade A Besides the favorable effects in terms of mortality reduction when used in the first 24 hours from the onset of symptoms of AMI,[79] long-term use of aspirin in the postinfarction period also results in a significant reduction of morbidity and mortality.

The Antiplatelet Trialists' Collaborative Group reviewed all the long-term trials of antiplatelet agents in secondary prevention.[80] Six randomized, placebo-controlled trials tested the effects of aspirin started between 1 week and 7 years after the initial infarct. Vascular mortality, non-fatal re-infarction and non-fatal stroke rates were significantly reduced respectively by 13%, 31%, and 42% among the patients allocated to aspirin in comparison with the placebo-allocated patients. The beneficial effects on major vascular events were apparent in all subgroups examined.

The overview also shows that, although other antiplatelet agents, such as dipyridamole or sulfinpyrazone, have been used in postinfarct patients, there is no evidence that they can be more efficacious than aspirin alone.

The benefits of aspirin were seen to be similar in the trials which evaluated doses from 160 mg to 1500 mg daily. These observations suggest that it is reasonable to recommend aspirin at 160–325 mg/day, starting early after the onset of symptoms of AMI and continuing for a long period of time (probably lifelong). **Grade A** A trial in patients with stable angina recently showed that lower doses of aspirin (75 mg/day) were associated with a significant reduction (34%) of non-fatal MI and sudden death.[81] These data suggest that lower doses of aspirin can be effective with fewer adverse effects.

References

1. Thompson PL, Lown B. Nitrous oxide as an analgesic in acute myocardial infarction. *JAMA* 1976;**235**:924–7.
2. Roth A, Keren G, Gluck A, Braun S, Laniado S. Comparison of nalbuphine hydrochloride versus morphine sulfate for acute myocardial infarction with elevated pulmonary artery wedge pressure. *Am J Cardiol* 1988;**62**:551–5.
3. Semenkovich CF, Jaffe AS. Adverse effects due to morphine sulfate. Challenge to previous clinical doctrine. *Am J Med* 1985;**79**:325–30.
4. Timmis AD, Rothman MT, Henderson MA, Geal PW, Chamberlain DA. Haemodynamic effects of intravenous morphine in patients with acute myocardial infarction complicated by severe left ventricular failure. *BMJ* 1980;**280**: 980–2.
5. Nielsen JR, Pedersen KE, Dahlstrom CG *et al.* Analgesic treatment in acute myocardial infarction. A controlled clinical comparison of morphine, nicomorphine and pethidine. *Acta Med Scand* 1984;**215**:349–54.
6. Waagstein F, Hjalmarson A. Double blind study of the effect of cardioselective beta-blockade on chest pain in acute myocardial infarction. *Acta Med Scand* 1975;**587**:201–8.
7. Ramsdale DR, Faragher EB, Bennett DH *et al.* Ischemic pain relief in patients with acute myocardial infarction by intravenous atenolol. *Am Heart J* 1982;**103**:459–67.
8. Maroko PR, Radvany P, Braunwald E, Hale SL. Reduction of infarct size by oxygen inhalation following acute coronary occlusion. *Circulation* 1975;**52**:360–8.
9. Madias JE, Hood WB Jr. Reduction of precordial ST-segment elevation in patients with anterior myocardial infarction by oxygen breathing. *Circulation* 1976;**53**(Suppl. I):I-198–200.
10. Fillmore SJ, Shapiro M, Killip T. Arterial oxygen tension in acute myocardial infarction: serial analysis of clinical state and blood gas changes. *Am Heart J* 1970;**79**:620–9.

11. Aubier M, Trippenbach T, Roussos C. Respiratory muscle fatigue during cardiogenic shock. *J Appl Physiol* 1981;**51**: 499–508.

12. Coats AJS, Adamopoulos S, Meyer TE, Conway J, Sleight P. Effects of physical training of chronic heart failure. *Lancet* 1990;**335**:63–6.

13. Lie KI, Wellens HJJ, Downar E, Durrer D. Observations on patients with primary ventricular fibrillation complicating acute myocardial infarction. *Circulation* 1975;**52**:755–9.

14. MacMahon S, Collins R, Peto R, Koster RW, Yusuf S. Effects of prophylactic lidocaine in suspected acute myocardial infarction: an overview of results from the randomized, controlled trials. *JAMA* 1988;**260**:1910–16.

15. Yusuf S, Sleight P, Rossi PRF *et al.* Reduction in infarct size, arrhythmias, chest pain and morbidity by early intravenous beta-blockade in suspected acute myocardial infarction. *Circulation* 1983;**67**:32–41.

16. Rossi PRF, Yusuf S, Ramsdale D *et al.* Reduction of ventricular arrhythmias by early intravenous atenolol in suspected acute myocardial infarction. *BMJ* 1983;**286**:506–10.

17. Yusuf S, Peto R, Lewis J, Collins R, Sleight P. Beta-blockade during and after myocardial infarction: an overview of the randomized trials. *Prog Cardiovasc Dis* 1985;**27**:335–43.

18. Sleight P (for ISIS Study Group). Beta blockade early in acute myocardial infarction. *Am J Cardiol* 1987;**60**:6A–12A.

19. ISIS-1 (First International Study of Infarct Survival) Collaborative Group. Randomised trial of intravenous atenolol among 16 027 cases of suspected acute myocardial infarction. ISIS-1. *Lancet* 1986;**ii**:57–66.

20. ISIS-1 (First International Study of Infarct Survival) Collaborative Group. Mechanisms for the early mortality reduction produced by beta-blockade started early in acute myocardial infarction: ISIS-1. *Lancet* 1988;**i**:921–7.

21. Mauri F, DeBiase AM, Franzosi MD *et al.* GISSI: analisi delle cause di morte intraospedaliera. *G Ital Cardiol* 1987;**17**:37–44.

22. Honan MB, Harrell FE, Reimer KA *et al.* Cardiac rupture, mortality and the timing of thrombolytic therapy: a meta-analysis. *J Am Coll Cardiol* 1990;**16**:359–67.

23. Dargie HJ. Effect of carvedilol on outcome after myocardial infarction in patients with left-ventricular dysfunction: the CAPRICORN randomised trial. *Lancet* 2001;**357**:1385–90.

24. Roberts R, Rogers WJ, Mueller HS *et al.* Immediate versus deferred beta-blockade following thrombolytic therapy in patients with acute myocardial infarction: results of the Thrombolysis in Myocardial Infarction (TIMI) II-B Study. *Circulation* 1991;**83**:422–37.

25. Barron HV, Rundle AC, Gore JM, Gurwitz JH, Penney J, for the participants in the National Registry of Myocardial Infarction-2. Intracranial hemorrhage rates and effect of immediate beta-blocker use in patients with acute myocardial infarction treated with tissue plasminogen activator. *Am J Cardiol* 2000;**85**:294–8.

26. Yusuf S, Lessem J, Jha P, Lonn E. Primary and secondary prevention of myocardial infarction and strokes: an update of randomly allocated controlled trials. *J Hypertens* 1993;**11** (Suppl. 4):S61–73.

27. The Norwegian Multicenter Study Group. Timolol-induced reduction in mortality and reinfarction in patients surviving acute myocardial infarction. *N Engl J Med* 1981;**304**:801–7.

28. Beta-Blocker Heart Attack Trial Research Group. A randomized trial of propranolol in patients with acute myocardial infarction. I. Mortality results. *JAMA* 1982;**247**:1707–14.

29. Hjalmarson A, Elmfeldt D, Herlitz J *et al.* Effect on mortality of metoprolol in acute myocardial infarction: a double-blind randomised trial. *Lancet* 1981;**ii**:823–7.

30. Rogers WJ, Bowlby LJ, Chandra NC *et al.* Treatment of myocardial infarction in the United States (1990 to 1993): observations from the National Registry of Myocardial Infarction. *Circulation* 1994;**90**:2103–14.

31. Liang CS, Gavras H, Black J, Sherman LG, Hood WB Jr. Renin-angiotensin system inhibition in acute myocardial infarction in dogs. Effects on systemic hemodynamics, myocardial blood flow, segmental myocardial function and infarct size. *Circulation* 1982;**66**:1249–55.

32. Ertl G, Kloner RA, Alexander RW, Braunwald E. Limitation of experimental infarct size by an angiotensin-converting enzyme inhibitor. *Circulation* 1982;**65**:40–8.

33. Swedberg K, Held P, Kjekshus J *et al.* CONSENSUS II Study Group. Effects of the early administration of enalapril on mortality in patients with acute myocardial infarction. *N Engl J Med* 1992;**327**:678–84.

34. Gruppo Italiano per lo Studio della Sopravvivenza nell'Infarto Miocardico. GISSI-3: effects of lisinopril and transdermal glyceryl trinitrate singly and together on 6-week mortality and ventricular function after acute myocardial infarction. *Lancet* 1994;**343**:1115–22.

35. ISIS-4 Collaborative Group. ISIS-4: A randomised factorial trial assessing early oral captopril, oral mononitrate, and intravenous magnesium sulphate in 58 050 patients with suspected acute myocardial infarction. *Lancet* 1995;**345**: 669–85.

36. Chinese Cardiac Study Collaborative Group. Oral captopril versus placebo among 13 634 patients with suspected acute myocardial infarction: interim report from the Chinese Cardiac Study (CCS-1). *Lancet* 1995;**345**:686–7.

37. ACE Inhibitor Myocardial Infarction Collaborative Group. Indications for ACE inhibitors in the early treatment of acute myocardial infarction: systematic overview of individual data from 100 000 patients in randomized trials. *Circulation* 1998; **97**:2202–12.

38. Pfeffer MA, Braunwald E, Moyé LA *et al.* Effect of captopril on mortality and morbidity in patients with left ventricular dysfunction after myocardial infarction. Results of the survival and ventricular enlargement trial (SAVE). *N Engl J Med* 1992; **327**:669–77.

39. The Acute Infarction Ramipril Efficacy (AIRE) Study Investigators. Effect of ramipril on mortality and morbidity of survivors of acute myocardial infarction with clinical evidence of heart failure. *Lancet* 1993;**342**:821–8.

40. The Trandolapril Cardiac Evaluation (TRACE) Study Group. A clinical trial of the angiotensin-converting-enzyme inhibitor trandolapril in patients with left ventricular dysfunction after myocardial infarction. *N Engl J Med* 1995;**333**: 1670–6.

41. Swartz SL, Williams GH, Hollenberg NK *et al.* Captopril-induced changes in prostaglandin production. Relationship to vascular responses in normal man. *J Clin Invest* 1980;**65**: 1257–64.

42. Hall D, Zeitler H, Rudolph W. Counteraction of the vasodilator effect of enalapril by aspirin in severe heart failure. *J Am Coll Cardiol* 1992;**20**:1549–55.

43. Pitt B, Yusuf S, for the SOLVD Investigators, University of Michigan Medical Center. Studies of left ventricular dysfunction (SOLVD): subgroup results (abstract). *J Am Coll Cardiol* 1992;**19**:215A.

44. Baur LHB, Schipperheyn JJ, van der Laarse A *et al.* Combining salicylate and enalapril in patients with coronary artery disease and heart failure. *Br Heart J* 1995; **73**:227–36.

45. Nguyen KN, Aursnes I, Kjeskshus J. Interaction between enalapril and aspirin on mortality after acute myocardial infarction: subgroup analysis of the Cooperative New Scandinavian Enalapril Survival Study II (CONSENSUS II). *Am J Cardiol* 1997;**79**:115–19.

46. Latini R, Santoro E, Masson S *et al.*, for the GISSI-3 investigators. Aspirin does not interact with ACE inhibitors when both are given early after acute myocardial infarction. Results of the GISSI-3 Trial. *Heart Dis* 2000;**2**:185–90.

47. Latini R, Tognoni G, Maggioni AP *et al.*, on behalf of the Angiotensin-converting Enzyme Inhibitor Myocardial Infaction Collaborative Group. Clinical effects of early angiotensin-converting enzyme inhibitor treatment for acute myocardial infarction are similar in the presence and absence of aspirin. Systematic overview of individual data from 96712 randomized patients. *J Am Coll Cardiol* 2000;**35**:1801–7.

48. Flather MD, Yusuf S, Køber L *et al.*, for the ACE-Inhibitor Myocardial Infarction Collaborative Group. Long-term ACE-inhibitor therapy in patients with heart failure or left-ventricular dysfunction: a systematic overview of data from individual patients. *Lancet* 2000;**355**:1575–81.

49. The Heart Outcomes Prevention Evaluation Study Investigators. Effects of an angiotensin-converting-enzyme inhibitor, ramipril, on cardiovascular events in high-risk patients. *N Engl J Med* 2000;**342**:145–53.

50. Maggioni AP. Secondary prevention: improving outcomes following myocardial infarction. *Heart* 2000;**84**(Suppl.1):5–7.

51. Jugdutt BI, Becker LC, Hutchins GM *et al.* Effect of intravenous nitroglycerin on collateral blood flow and infarct size in the conscious dog. *Circulation* 1981;**63**:17–28.

52. Hackett D, Davies G, Chierchia S, Maseri A. Intermittent coronary occlusion in acute myocardial infarction: value of combined thrombolytic and vasodilator therapy. *N Engl J Med* 1987;**317**:1055–9.

53. Jugdutt BI, Warnica JW. Intravenous nitroglycerin therapy to limit myocardial infarction size, expansion, and complications: effect of timing, dosage and infarct location. *Circulation* 1988;**78**:906–19.

54. Mahmarian JJ, Moye LA, Chinoy DA *et al.* Transdermal nitroglycerin patch therapy improves left ventricular function and prevents remodeling after acute myocardial infarction: results of a multicenter prospective randomized, double-blind, placebo-controlled trial. *Circulation* 1998;**97**:2017–24.

55. Yusuf S, Collins R, MacMahon S, Peto R. Effect of intravenous nitrates on mortality in acute myocardial infarction: an overview of the randomised trials. *Lancet* 1988;**i**:1088–92.

56. The European Study of Prevention of Infarction with molsidomine (ESPRIM) Group. The ESPRIM trial: short-term treatment of acute myocardial infarction with molsidomine. *Lancet* 1994;**344**:91–7.

57. Kloner RA, Braunwald E. Effects of calcium antagonists on infarcting myocardium. *Am J Cardiol* 1987;**59**:84–94B.

58. Opie LE, Buhler FR, Fleckenstein A *et al.* Working group on classification of calcium antagonists for cardiovascular disease. *Am J Cardiol* 1987;**60**:630–2.

59. Yusuf S, Furberg CD. Effects of calcium-channel blockers on survival after myocardial infarction. *Cardiovasc Drugs Ther* 1987;**1**:343–4.

60. The Danish Study Group on Verapamil in Myocardial Infarction. Effect of verapamil on mortality and major events after acute myocardial infarction (the Danish Verapamil Infarction Trial II – DAVIT II). *Am J Cardiol* 1990;**66**:779–85.

61. The Multicenter Diltiazem Postinfarction Trial Research Group. The effect of diltiazem on mortality and reinfarction after myocardial infarction. *N Engl J Med* 1988;**319**:385–92.

62. Teo KK, Yusuf S, Furberg CD. Effects of prophylactic antiarrhythmic drug therapy in acute myocardial infarction: an overview of results from randomized controlled trials. *JAMA* 1993;**270**:1589–95.

63. Zuanetti G, Latini R, Avanzini F *et al.*, on behalf of the GISSI Investigators. Trends and determinants of calcium antagonist usage after acute myocardial infarction (the GISSI experience). *Am J Cardiol* 1996;**78**:153–7.

64. Vormann J, Fischer G, Classen HG, Thoni H. Influence of decreased and increased magnesium supply on the cardiotoxic effects of epinephrine in rats. *Arzneimittelforschung* 1983;**33**:205–10.

65. Turlapaty PDMV, Altura BM. Magnesium deficiency produces spasms of coronary arteries: relationship to etiology of sudden death ischemic heart disease. *Science* 1980;**208**:198–200.

66. Watanabe Y, Dreifus LS. Electrophysiological effects of magnesium and its interactions with potassium. *Cardiovasc Res* 1972;**6**:79–88.

67. Teo KK, Yusuf S, Collins R, Held PH, Peto R. Effect of intravenous magnesium in suspected acute myocardial infarction: overview of randomized trials. *BMJ* 1991;**303**:1499–503.

68. Woods KL, Fletcher S, Roffe C, Haider Y. Intravenous magnesium sulphate in suspected acute myocardial infarction: results of the second Leicester Intravenous Magnesium Intervention Trial (LIMIT-2). *Lancet* 1992;**339**:1553–8.

69. Herzog WR, Schlossberg ML, MacMurdy KS *et al.* Timing of magnesium therapy affects experimental infarct size. *Circulation* 1995;**92**:2622–6.

70. Christensen CA, Rieder MA, Silvestein EL, Gencheff NE. Magnesium sulfate reduces myocardial infarct size when administered before but not after coronary reperfusion in a canine model. *Circulation* 1995;**92**:2617–21.

71. Mahaffey KW, Puma JA, Barbagelata NA *et al.*, for the AMISTAD Investigators. Adenosine as an adjunct to thrombolytic therapy for acute myocardial infarction. Results of a multicenter, randomized, placebo-controlled trial: the Acute Myocardial Infarction Study of Adenosine (AMISTAD) Trial. *J Am Coll Cardiol* 1999;**34**:1711–20.

72. Baran KW, Nguyen M, McKendall GR *et al.*, for the LIMIT AMI Investigators. Double-blind, randomized trial of an anti-CD18 antibody in conjunction with recombinant tissue plasminogen activator for acute myocardial infarction.

Limitation of Myocardial Infarction Following Thrombolysis in Acute Myocardial Infarction (LIMIT AMI) Study. *Circulation* 2001;**104**:2778–83.

73. Rother K. HALTing myocardial injury didn't work. *Heart Wire News* 1999; Nov.11.

74. Diaz R, Paolasso EA, Piegas LS *et al.*, on behalf of the ECLA (Estudios Cardiológicos Latinoamérica) Collaborative Group. Metabolic modulation of acute myocardial infarction. The ECLA Glucose-Insulin-Potassium Pilot Trial. *Circulation* 1998; **98**:2227–34.

75. Théroux P, Chaitman BR, Danchin N *et al.*, for the GUARd During Ischemia Against Necrosis (GUARDIAN) Investigators. *Circulation* 2000;**102**:3032–8.

76. Zeymer U, Suryapranata H, Monassier JP *et al.*, for the ESCAMI Investigators. The Na$^+$/H$^+$ exchange inhibitor eniporide as an adjunct to early reperfusion therapy for acute myocardial infarction. *J Am Coll Cardiol* 2001;**38**:1644–50.

77. Ito H, Taniyama Y, Iwakura K *et al.* Intravenous nicorandil can preserve microvascular integrity and myocardial viability in patients with reperfused anterior wall myocardial infarction. *J Am Coll Cardiol* 1999;**33**:654–60.

78. Tunstall-Pedoe H, Morrison C, Woodward M, Fitzpatrick B, Watt G. Sex difference in myocardial infarction and coronary deaths in the Scottish MONICA population of Glasgow 1985 to 1991. Presentation, diagnosis, treatment and 28-day case fatality of 3991 events in men and 1551 events in women. *Circulation* 1996;**93**:1981–92.

79. ISIS-2 (Second International Study of Infarct Survival) Collaborative Group. Randomized trial of intravenous streptokinase, oral aspirin, both, or neither among 17 187 cases of suspected acute myocardial infarction: ISIS-2. *Lancet* 1988;**2**: 349–60.

80. Antiplatelet Trialists' Collaboration. Secondary prevention of vascular disease by prolonged antiplatelet treatment. *BMJ* 1988;**296**:320–31.

81. Becker RC. Antiplatelet therapy in coronary heart disease: emerging strategies for the treatment and prevention of acute myocardial infarction. *Arch Pathol Lab Med* 1993;**117**:89–96.

35 Complications after myocardial infarction

Peter L Thompson, Barry McKeown

Introduction

Despite major changes in treatment and prevention, myocardial infarction (MI) remains a common and lethal condition. Recent statistical updates estimate that there are 7·3 million persons in the United States who have suffered a myocardial infarction, and each year there are 1·1 million new or recurrent coronary attacks, of whom 40% die.[1] Mechanical complications of myocardial infarction include acute and chronic heart failure, cardiogenic shock, ventricular aneurysm, right ventricular infarction and failure, mitral regurgitation due to papillary muscle dysfunction or rupture, rupture of the interventricular septum and rupture of the free wall of the left ventricle. Electrical complications include ventricular fibrillation, ventricular tachycardia, atrial fibrillation, and atrioventricular block. A common and important category of complication that is frequently neglected is the psychosocial and socioeconomic complications of MI.

Other chapters in this book cover the topics of left ventricular dysfunction and heart failure (Chapter 46) ventricular arrhythmias (Chapter 42) bradyarrhythmias (Chapter 74) and atrial fibrillation (Chapter 38–40). The major complications of MI, such as left ventricular (LV) dysfunction, heart failure or ventricular and atrial arrhythmias lend themselves to study with controlled clinical trials. However, for many of the acute complications of MI, clinical trials have not been performed, and clinical decision making must rely on evidence from other sources including uncontrolled trials, observational studies and inference from pathophysiologic data. The evidence base for managing the complications of MI will be discussed under the headings of clinical features and prognosis, and management.

Left ventricular dysfunction and failure

Clinical features and prognosis

Pathophysiology

Acute coronary occlusion with ST segment elevation (STEMI) affects the function of the left ventricle within seconds, even before irreversible myocardial damage has occurred.[2] Adverse remodeling of the ventricle can occur early in the course of myocardial infarction, and continues over the ensuing months and years, leading to an increase in end-diastolic and end-systolic volumes, an increase in the sphericity of the ventricle, and systolic bulging and thinning of the infarct zone, without necessarily any extension of the infarcted zone.[3] Results from autopsy studies suggested that MIs that involved greater than 40% of the left ventricle were usually fatal.[4] However, a more recent prospective study conducted in the reperfusion era showed that out of 16 patients with residual infarcts of >40%, and followed for 13 months, only one had persistent heart failure and subsequently died.[5] The likely explanation for this discrepancy lies in the inherent bias of autopsy studies and the improved management of post-MI patients in the reperfusion era. Extensive damage can occur as a consequence of one large infarction or multiple smaller ones. Non-ST elevation MI may also cause left ventricular dysfunction if there has been prior cumulative myocardial damage. Echocardiographic evidence from infarct survivors shows that up to 60–80% of the left ventricle may be akinetic or severely hypokinetic in those with a history of multiple infarctions.[6]

Prognostic markers based on left ventricular dysfunction

The extent of LV dysfunction is a strong predictor of short- and long-term prognosis after MI. The Killip and Kimball[7] classification stratifies MI patients from low to very high risk based upon clinical signs of heart failure. It remains a reasonably accurate indicator of short term survival. In patients undergoing primary PTCA, the inhospital mortality was 2·4%, 7% and 19% for class I, II and III, respectively and 6 month mortality was 4%, 10% and 28% for class I, II, and III, respectively.[8] The presence of left ventricular dysfunction as determined by Killip class may be a predictor of response to invasive coronary procedures in acute myocardial infarction.[9] The Forrester classification comprising four categories defined according to the presence or absence of pulmonary congestion and peripheral hypoperfusion requires measurement of the pulmonary artery pressure using a balloon flotation catheter.[10] Although this is safe in experienced hands, it has a recognized risk of adverse events, including ventricular tachyarrhythmias and pulmonary hemorrhage or infarction.[11]

In both postinfarction patients[12] and in a wider range of critically ill patients in intensive care units,[13] hemodynamic variables determined from right heart catheterization correlate strongly with a higher mortality even after adjusting for other prognostic variables. This association may be spurious, due to a failure to identify and adjust for all relevant variables. However, recent guidelines recommend the use of balloon flotation catheters only in severe or progressive CHF or pulmonary edema, cardiogenic shock or progressive hypotension or suspected mechanical complications of acute infarction – that is, ventricular septal defect (VSD), papillary muscle rupture, or pericardial tamponade.[11] The mechanism whereby right heart catheterization might increase mortality is uncertain.[14]

Late postinfarction mortality is also affected by the extent of left ventricular dysfunction. The presence of clinical signs of left ventricular failure is a strong indicator of a poor long-term prognosis.[15] In some patients, more detailed assessment is necessary, and the use of echocardiography or radionuclide assessment may provide information which cannot be obtained clinically.[16] Late postinfarction mortality was 3% in patients with an EF above 0·40, 12% when the EF was between 0·20 and 0·40, and 47% when it was below 0·20.[17] The measurement of left ventricular function adds incremental value to the clinical detection of left ventricular failure. Approximately two thirds of patients with an EF low enough to indicate a poor long-term prognosis for example, <0·40, have no radiological evidence of left ventricular failure.[18] The choice of modality for assessment of left ventricular function depends on local availability and expertise. The information obtained from assessing left ventricular function by echocardiography, radionuclide imaging or cardiac catheterization has been found to be of equivalent value in predicting 1 year prognosis.[19]

Biochemical markers

Biochemical markers of necrosis provide an index of the extent of left ventricular infarction which in turn is correlated with the extent of left ventricular dysfunction. Creatine kinase was shown in the prereperfusion era to predict short- and long-term prognosis.[20] The introduction of reperfusion into routine clinical practice has reduced the utility of CK or CK-MB to reflect the extent of left ventricular dysfunction because of early, direct release of the myocardial enzymes into the plasma during reperfusion and high, early peaking of the serum levels. The use of newer markers such as troponin is now widespread, and both troponin-I[21] and troponin-T[22] correlate well with prognosis, although their value in estimating infarct size is limited. Multivariate analysis of data from large clinical trials has provided sound evidence that prognosis can be predicted with accuracy using clinical information which is readily available during the assessment of the patient. Demographics

(advanced age, lower weight), more extensive infarction (higher Killip class, lower blood pressure, faster heart rate, longer QRS duration), higher cardiac risk (smoking, hypertension, prior cerebrovascular disease), and arrhythmia were important predictors of death between 30 days and 1 year in 41 021 patients enrolled in the Global Utilization of Streptokinase and TPA for Occluded Coronary Arteries (GUSTO) trial,[23] and in the GISSI trial.[24]

Management

Pharmacologic therapy

Since left ventricular function is a critical determinant of prognosis, there have been many attempts to limit the extent of left ventricular dysfunction during myocardial infarction. Pharmacologic attempts to achieve this after myocardial necrosis is well established have achieved limited success. Improvements in hemodynamic status have not translated to better outcomes. For example, furosemide has been shown to reduce elevated LV filling pressures without adversely affecting cardiac output,[25] but there is no evidence of improvement in outcomes with diuretic therapy in AMI. Nitrates have been shown to improve the hemodynamic status in and adverse remodeling post-AMI,[26] and nitroglycerin may increase collateral blood flow to the infarct zone and thus limit infarct size, particularly if heart rate is controlled.[27] The fact that remodeling begins soon after the onset of infarction is a justification for beginning intravenous nitroglycerin or an ACE inhibitor early, even when these drugs are not required to correct a hemodynamic abnormality. While preliminary meta-analysis of small trials of intravenous nitrates showed an apparent benefit on outcomes,[28] larger clinical trials have shown no benefit of nitrates in improving prognosis.[29,30]

In contrast to the neutral effects of nitrate vasodilators, the beneficial effects of angiotensin converting enzyme (ACE) inhibitors in the treatment of patients with left ventricular function complicating myocardial infarction have been striking. Eight large randomized, placebo-controlled trials have assessed the effect of an ACE inhibitor on mortality after MI.

ACE inhibitors unequivocally reduce mortality overall, and the benefit appears to be the greatest among patients with depressed LV function, overt heart failure, or anterior infarction.[31–38] **Grade A1a**

In a meta-analysis of data from all randomized trials involving more than 1000 patients in which ACE inhibitor treatment was started within 36 hours of onset of myocardial infarction, there were results available on 98 496 patients from four eligible trials.[39] Among patients allocated to ACE inhibitors there was a 7% (95% CI 2–11; $2P < 0.004$) proportional reduction in early mortality, an absolute reduction of 5 (SD 2) deaths per 1000 patients. While the relative benefit was similar in patients at different underlying risks, the absolute benefit was greatest in those patients with evidence of left ventricular dysfunction (that is, Killip class II to III, heart rate ≥100 bpm at entry) and in anterior MI. ACE inhibitor therapy also reduced the incidence of non-fatal manifestations of left ventricular dysfunction. During longer term follow up of patients enrolled in randomized controlled trials, ACE inhibitors have also been shown to be effective. In three long-term follow up trials involving 5966 postinfarction patients, mortality was significantly lower with ACE inhibitors than with placebo, odds ratio 0·74 (95% CI 0·66–0·83).[40] Whether low-risk postinfarction patients with normal EFs derive benefit from ACE inhibitors is still controversial. The AHA/ACC guidelines for acute myocardial infarction conclude that ACE inhibitors are supported by a class 1 recommendation for all patients with MI and LV ejection fraction less than 40%, or patients with clinical heart failure on the basis of systolic pump dysfunction during and after convalescence from AMI.[11] The optimum timing of initiation of ACE inhibitor therapy has been studied in only a small number of direct comparative trials. In a meta-analysis of 845 patients receiving thrombolysis, ACE inhibitor treatment within 6 to 9 h after MI was compared with other usual therapy.[41] ACE inhibition could not be demonstrated to attenuate LV dilation on 3 month echocardiographic follow up. Three hundred and fifty-two patients with acute anterior myocardial infarction were randomized to early (1 to 14 days) or late (14 to 19 days) post-MI treatment with the angiotensin converting enzyme (ACE) inhibitor ramipril and were followed by echocardiography. Those receiving early ramipril had a greater improvement in ejection fraction, suggesting that such patients should be commenced on ACE inhibitor therapy early in their course of infarction.[42] In considering treatment for left ventricular dysfunction, the hemodynamic benefits need to be balanced against the possible adverse effect of extending the infarct size. In the only ACE inhibitor trial that did not show a mortality benefit, CONSENSUS-II, treatment was begun early with an intravenous ACE inhibitor.[31]

Inotropic agents

Inotropic agents are used widely in cardiogenic shock complicating myocardial infarction.

The choice of inotropic agents is dependent on the known pathophysiologic effects of the drugs rather than clinical trial evidence.[43] **Grade C5**

Digitalis may help the acute postinfarction patient with heart failure when the left ventricle is dilated and damaged, but use of this drug carries more risk than benefit when heart failure complicates a large infarction in a previously healthy ventricle.[44] Digoxin reduced the rate of hospitalization for heart failure, but did not alter total mortality, in a large randomized trial of patients with chronic heart failure, 70% of whom had ischemic heart disease as the primary cause.[45]

Reperfusion therapy

Attempts to prevent myocardial necrosis and subsequent left ventricular dysfunction, and the disappointing results of efforts to limit infarct size when myocardial necrosis is well advanced, have driven the so-called reperfusion era of treatment in myocardial infarction. However, the relationship between improvements in left ventricular function and prognosis after reperfusion therapy has been surprisingly difficult to demonstrate. Although some of the early studies demonstrated clear benefits on left ventricular function from coronary thrombolysis,[46,47] the evidence since then has been conflicting, with some groups showing a worse left ventricular function despite an improved prognosis. In a meta-analysis of ten studies enrolling 4088 patients treated with thrombolytic therapy versus control, only a modest improvement in left ventricular function was demonstrated after thrombolytic therapy.[48] By 4 days, mean LV ejection fraction was 53% versus 47% (thrombolytic *v* control therapy, $P < 0·01$); by 10 to 28 days it was 54·1% and 51·5%, respectively. The reason for the discrepancy in the marked improvement in survival and the limited benefit on left ventricular function is not clear. Patients who have had coronary reperfusion after MI may have myocardium that is stunned[49] or even hibernating,[50] phenomena that may affect the assessment of ventricular function. Stunned myocardium has been successfully reperfused but has not regained its normal contractile function.

A study of 352 patients with anterior MI found that out of the 252 patients with abnormal LV function on day 1, 22% had complete and 36% had partial recovery of function by day 90.[51] This result highlights the potential for improvement in LV function over time due to recovery of stunned myocardium. Hibernating myocardium is underperfused and non-contractile, but is not infarcted and may gradually improve its function with revascularization. The degree of success in achieving coronary patency with thrombolysis is an obvious confounding factor.[52] The most recent analysis demonstrates that left ventricular function is improved by successful coronary reperfusion and that the previous inability to demonstrate this has been due to confounding by the following factors: the variable relationship between left ventricular function and prognosis (irrespective of reperfusion status), variable methods of measuring left ventricular function, the effects of hibernation and stunning on interpretation of left ventricular functional recovery, and the variable success in achieving coronary patency in the coronary reperfusion trials.[53]

Overall reperfusion therapy results in a modest improvement in systolic LV function. **Grade A1c**

Cardiogenic shock

Clinical features and prognosis

Cardiogenic shock is a syndrome characterized by hypotension and peripheral hypoperfusion, usually accompanied by high LV filling pressures. The common clinical manifestations of these hemodynamic derangements include mental obtundation or confusion, cold and clammy skin, and oliguria or anuria.[11] Cardiogenic shock is the commonest cause of inhospital mortality after MI.[54] When cardiogenic shock is not secondary to a correctable cause, such as arrhythmia, bradycardia, hypovolemia or a mechanical defect, short-term mortality is 80% or higher, depending upon the strictness of the definition. Despite the major improvements in treatment in the past two decades, the inhospital mortality in a recent international registry for patients with cardiogenic shock treated with modern therapy in the late 1990s was 66%.[55] Old age, diabetes, previous infarction and extensive infarction as assessed either by enzymatic or electrocardiographic criteria are factors commonly associated with cardiogenic shock.[54] A recent analysis of predictors of cardiogenic shock in patients treated with thrombolytic therapy showed that each decade increase in age increased the risk of cardiogenic shock by 47%.[56]

Management

Inotropic drugs have been subjected to detailed study and widespread use in cardiogenic shock, but no clearcut effect on mortality has been demonstrated.[57] Intra-aortic balloon pumping has been used to stabilize patients with cardiogenic shock; clearcut benefits on hemodynamic status and coronary blood flow have been shown, but benefits on survival, have not been shown; inhospital mortality remained at 83% despite the use of balloon pumping in a cooperative clinical trial.[58] Nevertheless, intra-aortic balloon pumping has a clear place in stabilizing the unstable cardiogenic shock patient for more definitive treatment such as coronary angioplasty or bypass surgery,[59] as has been demonstrated in a randomized trial in the setting of rescue angioplasty.[60] Newer methods of circulatory support have shown highly encouraging results,[61,62] but benefits on survival remain to be established.

Although the outcome of cardiogenic shock has been shown to be dependent on the patency of the infarct related artery, clinical trials of thrombolytic therapy have not shown a benefit in patients with established cardiogenic shock.[63] Alternative antithrombotic strategies may improve outcomes, but data is limited to observational studies.[64] There has been increased interest in alternative approaches to reperfusion in patients with cardiogenic shock. Observational studies and clinical trials suggest that an aggressive approach with early revascularization reduces the mortality of patients with cardiogenic shock after MI. For example, the 30 day mortality was 38% in 406 patients who underwent early angiography and were usually revascularized, most often with angioplasty, compared to 62% in the 1794 patients without early angiography in the GUSTO-1 trial.[65] A registry report has suggested that an aggressive approach with reperfusion therapy and intra-aortic balloon pulsation treatment of patients in cardiogenic shock due to predominant LV failure is associated with lower inhospital mortality rates than standard medical therapy.[66] This benefit persisted after adjustment for baseline differences (odds ratio 0·43; 95% CI 0·34–0·54; $P = 0·0001$). The use of early catheterization may influence the outcome by helping to direct therapy.[55] In a controlled clinical trial of an aggressive approach involving early catheterization with revascularization and intra-aortic balloon pumping, in cardiogenic shock patients (the SHOCK trial),[67] 87% of patients in the invasive arm underwent revascularization (surgical or percutaneous). There was a clear trend at 30 days towards reduced mortality in the invasive group compared with the medical therapy group (46·7% v 56·0%), however this difference did not reach statistical significance. There was an early hazard in the first 5 days after assignment to the invasive approach, which was possibly associated with procedure-related complications. However, after the first 5 days there was a survival benefit in favor of the revascularization group, which persisted at one year, when survival in the early revascularization group was 46·7% compared with 33·6% in those treated with early medical stabilization (relative risk for death: 0·7; 95% CI 0·54–0·95).[68]

Evidence from clinical trials supports invasive intervention in patients with cardiogenic shock post-MI. These patients should undergo coronary angiography with a view to coronary angioplasty, or in selected patients, coronary bypass surgery. **Grade A1d**

Right ventricular infarction and failure

Clinical features and prognosis

Right ventricular (RV) infarction typically occurs in association with inferior or posterior MI, as a consequence of total occlusion of the right coronary artery proximal to its marginal branches,[69] or of the proximal circumflex in patients with a dominant left coronary system. RV infarction was present in 54% of patients with inferior MI in one series, although clinical manifestations are usually evident in only 10–15%.[70] RV involvement is much less common in anterior infarction, with 13% being the highest incidence reported.[71] Right ventricular involvement in inferior infarction has been reported to increase the mortality by fivefold. In one series of 200 consecutive cases,[72] the inhospital mortality in inferior MI complicated by RV infarction was 31%, compared to 6% when RV involvement was absent. RV dysfunction almost always resolves in survivors during the first few weeks. Some studies have shown that RV infarction is an independent predictor of long-term prognosis, while others have not demonstrated a difference in long-term mortality between patients with and without this complication.[69]

The clinical features of RV infarction complicating inferior MI include hypotension, an elevated jugular venous pressure and clear lung fields; however, the sensitivity of this combination of findings for the diagnosis of right ventricular infarction is less than 25%.[69] Jugular venous distension on inspiration (Kussmaul's sign) has been reported to be a sensitive and specific sign of RV infarction.[73] The hemodynamic features of RV infarction may disappear with volume depletion or may emerge only after volume loading, making the clinical diagnosis elusive in some cases.

ST segment elevation in a right precordial lead (V_{4R}) has been reported to have a sensitivity of 70% and a specificity of nearly 100% for the diagnosis of RV infarction when the electrocardiogram is recorded within the first hours after the onset of symptoms.[74] Echocardiography commonly reveals wall motion abnormalities of the right ventricle and interventricular septum. Bowing of the interatrial septum toward the left atrium indicates that the right atrial pressure exceeds the left atrial pressure,[75] and bowing of the interventricular septum into the right ventricle, compounding the dysfunction of the right ventricle;[76] both indicate a poor prognosis. Detection of a low RVEF and a segmental wall motion abnormality by radionuclide right ventriculography had a sensitivity of 92% and a specificity of 82% for identifying hemodynamically significant RV infarction in one study.[73]

Management

Volume loading can normalize blood pressure and increase cardiac output.[77] Earlier trials of RV infarction demonstrated a marked response to volume loading.[78] Many of these patients were volume depleted secondary to aggressive diuresis in response to a raised venous pressure.

Although this therapy remains very important, these trials may have exaggerated the importance of volume loading. Grade B4

Inotropic agents are often used in the treatment of right ventricular infarction when volume loading fails to improve cardiac output, but the effect of this on prognosis is unclear. The maintenance of atrioventricular synchrony is often critical to the maintenance of a satisfactory cardiac output; atrioventricular pacing has been shown to improve hemodynamics.[79] Successful thrombolysis appears to reduce the

incidence of RV infarction.[80] Patients with inferior MI in the TIMI-II study were less likely to have RV involvement when the culprit artery was patent as compared to patients with persistent occlusion.[81] In patients with hemodynamically significant right ventricular infarction, right coronary artery reperfusion with angioplasty was associated with dramatic recovery of right ventricular function and reduced mortality.[82] In contrast, unsuccessful right coronary artery reperfusion was associated with a high mortality.

In summary, reperfusion therapy in right ventricular infarction has not been studied in randomized trials but appears to be effective. Grade B4

Left ventricular aneurysm

Clinical features and prognosis

Left ventricular aneurysms develop most commonly after large transmural anterior MIs, although in 5–15% of cases the site is inferior or posterior.[83] The coronary anatomy is an important determinant of the development of left ventricular aneurysm. Total occlusion of the left anterior descending artery in association with poor collateral blood supply is a significant determinant of aneurysm formation in anterior MI. Multivessel disease with either good collateral circulation or a patent left anterior descending artery is uncommonly associated with the development of left ventricular aneurysm.[84] Coronary patency also determines the likelihood of developing an aneurysm.[85] A ventricular aneurysm can often be palpated as a dyskinetic region adjacent to the apical impulse. A third heart sound and signs of heart failure may also be detected. A non-specific marker of an aneurysm is ST segment elevation that persists weeks after the acute phase of infarction. Echocardiography can delineate LV aneurysms as well as left ventriculography and has a higher sensitivity in the detection of thrombus.[86] A left ventricular aneurysm may cause no problems, but may be associated with heart failure because the left ventricle functions at a mechanical disadvantage. Ventricular tachycardia late after infarction is commonly associated with an aneurysm, but its incidence may be reduced in patients receiving thrombolysis. In a non-randomized study of patients who developed a ventricular aneurysm after myocardial infarction, inducible ventricular tachycardia was less likely in patients who received thrombolytic therapy than those who did not (8% *v* 88%; $P = 0.0008$) and there was a reduced incidence of sudden death on subsequent follow up (0% *v* 50%; $P = 0.002$).[87]

A ventricular aneurysm also provides a nidus for the development of an intracavitary thrombus. The risk of a clinical embolic event, based on four observational studies, is approximately 5%.[88] The risk of thromboembolism after infarction is greatest within the first few weeks.

Management

Surgical removal of a left ventricular aneurysm is indicated in patients with heart failure that is difficult to control medically, in patients with recurrent ventricular tachycardia not controlled by other means, and in patients with embolic episodes in spite of adequate anticoagulation.[89] Grade B4

Aneurysmectomy is often performed at the time of coronary bypass surgery, and coronary bypass of severe lesions almost always accompanies aneurysmectomy.

Pseudoaneurysm

A pseudoaneurysm is a rare complication of MI that develops when a myocardial rupture is sealed off by surrounding adherent pericardium. The aneurysmal sac may progressively enlarge but maintains a narrow neck, in contrast to a true ventricular aneurysm. In a series of 290 patients with LV pseudoaneurysms; congestive heart failure, chest pain and dyspnea were the most frequently reported symptoms, but >10% of patients were asymptomatic.[90] Physical examination revealed a murmur in 70% of patients. Almost all patients had electrocardiographic abnormalities, but only 20% of patients had ST segment elevation. Radiographic findings were frequently non-specific, however a mass was detected, in more than one half of patients. Differentiation of left ventricular pseudoaneurysms from true aneurysms may be difficult,[91] and can be assisted with echocardiography. The ratio of the maximum diameter of the orifice to the maximum internal diameter of the cavity has been recommended as a useful index to differentiate the two conditions. In one series, the ratio of the orifice of the aneurysm to the cavity was 0·25 to 0·50 for pseudoaneurysms, while the range for true aneurysms was 0·90 to 1·0.[92] Regardless of treatment, patients with LV pseudoaneurysms have a high mortality rate, but especially those who are managed non-surgically.[93]

Therefore urgent surgery should be considered in all patients with LV pseudoaneurysms. Grade B4

Cardiac thromboembolism

Clinical features and prognosis

Left ventricular thrombi develop in up to 40% of patients with large anterior transmural MIs.[94–96] If left untreated, up to 15% of thrombi will dislodge and result in a symptomatic embolic event.[97,98] Overall, 1·5–3·6% of patients with MIs suffer a complicating stroke, most often from a dislodged mural thrombus. This risk is higher in patients with large anterior infarctions.[99,100] Emboli are more common within the first few months after infarction than later, and with large, irregular shaped thrombi, particularly those with frond-like appendages.[97] When a thrombus is visualized by echocardiography, the risk ratio for embolization is 5·45 (95% CI 3·0–9·8) according to a meta-analysis.[101]

Management

Anticoagulation with heparin followed by warfarin for 6 months has been shown to reduce the incidence of thromboembolism in patients with documented intracavitary thrombi (OR 0·14; 95% CI 0·04–0·52).[102] The benefits in terms of reduction of embolic potential outweigh the risks of hemorrhage with anticoagulation. Meta-analysis of trials of anticoagulant therapy to prevent thrombus formation confirmed a benefit (OR 0·32; 95% CI 0·20–0·52), but no effect for antiplatelet drugs.[102] It is important to consider this evidence in the light of whether the anticoagulants are given in the presence or absence of aspirin, and the relationship to thrombolytic therapy. In a meta-analysis of all trials involving heparin administration in over 70 000 patients with acute myocardial infarction,[103] in the *absence* of aspirin, anticoagulant therapy reduced the risk of stroke to 1·1% from 2·1% ($2P = 0·01$), equivalent to 10 fewer strokes per 1000 ($2P = 0·01$). In the *presence* of aspirin, however, heparin was associated with a small non-significant excess of stroke and a definite excess of three major bleeds per 1000 ($2P < 0·0001$). The use of heparin after thrombolytic therapy was studied in a meta-analysis of six trials involving 1735 patients in which intravenous heparin was compared with placebo after thrombolysis.[104] Mortality before hospital discharge was 5·1% for patients allocated to intravenous heparin compared with 5·6% for controls (relative risk reduction of 9%, OR 0·91; 95% CI 0·59–1·39). The rates of total stroke, intracranial hemorrhage, and severe bleeding were similar in patients allocated to heparin; however, the risk of any severity of bleeding was significantly higher (22·7% *v* 16·2%; OR 1·55; 95% CI 1·21–1·98). Thrombolytic therapy may be associated with a reduced risk of intraventricular thrombus and thromboembolic events, but the analysis is confounded by the potential for thrombolytic therapy to cause hemorrhagic stroke. Thrombolytic therapy is associated with an excess of stroke of four extra strokes on day 1 compared with placebo.[105] This risk is reduced if angioplasty is used instead of thrombolytic therapy. In a meta-analysis comparing the effects of angioplasty with thrombolysis, angioplasty was associated with a significant reduction in total stroke (0·7% *v* 2·0%; $P = 0·007$) primarily due to a reduction in hemorrhagic stroke (0·1% *v* 1·1%; $P < 0·001$).[106]

Acute mitral regurgitation

Clinical features and prognosis

Mitral regurgitation complicating acute myocardial infarction is usually due to dysfunction of the papillary muscles.[107,108] The milder form of mitral regurgitation is a relatively common complication of myocardial infarction, found in 19% of postinfarction patients who undergo left ventriculography[109] and 39% of those who undergo Doppler echocardiography.[110] Mitral regurgitation is an independent predictor of cardiovascular mortality in postinfarction patients. In the SAVE trial, the relative risk was 2·00 (95% CI 1·28–3·04) in patients who had mitral regurgitation detected on catheterization early after MI. In a recent series studied with Doppler echocardiography, the hazard ratio for 1 year mortality after adjustment for other prognostic variables was 2·31 (95% CI 1·03–5·20) for mild MR and 2·85 (95% CI 0·95–8·51) for moderate or severe MR.[111] The most severe form of mitral regurgitation results from complete rupture of the head of a papillary muscle and usually leads quickly to severe heart failure or cardiogenic shock. In the SHOCK trial registry, cardiogenic shock was associated with severe mitral regurgitation in 98 of 1190 patients.[112] The mitral regurgitation patients were more likely to be female and to have non-ST elevation MI at the time of presentation, and to have inferior or posterior rather than anterior infarction. In fact one should suspect acute MR or another mechanical complication in any patient with a first inferior MI who develops heart failure or cardiogenic shock.

Early diagnosis of mitral regurgitation complicating MI is important because mitral valve surgery can be life saving. Usually the diagnosis is evident clinically with a loud pansystolic murmur maximal at the apex, and radiation to the axilla; however, if LV function is severely impaired or if left atrial pressure is very high, the murmur may be of low intensity or entirely absent. Echocardiography Doppler examination is invaluable in confirming the diagnosis.[113] However, in some cases transthoracic echocardiography is non-diagnostic and transesophageal echocardiography is required to assess the extent of the regurgitation. Transesophageal echocardiography has been demonstrated to be safe and produce a high diagnostic yield in hemodynamically unstable, critically ill patients who are suspected of having an underlying cardiovascular disorder.[114] The presence of cardiogenic shock or severe failure with preserved LV function usually indicates that an important mechanical complication is present, and further investigation should be urgently pursued. If the mitral regurgitation is acute in its onset, the left atrium may not be greatly enlarged, and the pulmonary capillary wedge pressure tracing should exhibit large v waves. Large v waves are neither highly sensitive nor highly specific for severe chronic mitral regurgitation,[115] but the correlation between giant v waves and severe acute mitral regurgitation is stronger.[116]

Management

Treatment with arterial dilators such as nitroprusside may improve hemodynamic status temporarily, by reducing afterload and the regurgitant fraction.[117]

Observational data suggest that surgery for acute mitral regurgitation should be performed acutely, even in patients who appear to stabilize with medical therapy, because subsequent deterioration is usual, abrupt, and unpredictable. Grade B4

The perioperative mortality associated with mitral valve surgery for postinfarction papillary muscle rupture is high, 27% in one series, but two thirds of the survivors were still alive at 7 years.[118] Patients with a low preoperative EF had the highest short-term and long-term mortality. The use of mitral valve repair in this situation can give excellent long-term results.[119] There is evidence from the SHOCK trial registry that transfer to a center skilled in mitral valve surgery for early operation may be helpful.[112] Early reperfusion with thrombolytic therapy[120] has been shown to reduce the frequency of mitral regurgitation after myocardial infarction. There is some evidence that angioplasty may be superior in achieving this, although this is based on an indirect comparison of clinical trial results.[121] There have been reports of striking improvement in mitral regurgitation after emergency coronary angioplasty in patients with acute myocardial infarction.[122]

Ventricular septal rupture

Clinical features and prognosis

Rupture of the interventricular septum occurs in approximately 2% of patients with acute myocardial infarction.[123] The pathology of septal rupture is determined by the location of the associated myocardial infarction and has implications for surgical repair. Septal rupture complicating anterior infarction is usually apical and involves one direct perforation; septal rupture complicating inferior infarction often involves the posterior or basal septum with complex, serpiginous defects.[124] The median time of onset of rupture was at 2·5 days in one study[123] and 7 days in another.[124] In the SHOCK trial registry of cardiogenic shock patients,[125] ventricular septal rupture occurred a median of 16 h after infarction. The patients tended to be older ($P = 0·053$), were more often female ($P = 0·002$) and less often had previous infarction ($P < 0·001$), diabetes mellitus ($P = 0·015$) or smoking history ($P = 0·033$). The inhospital mortality was higher in the shock patients with septal rupture 87% v 61%, $P < 0·001$. Even when most patients undergo surgical repair, inhospital or 30 day mortality remains high: 43% to 59%.[125–127] Early diagnosis may offer some hope of early repair. Most patients with septal rupture develop signs of acute right and left sided heart failure and a loud pansystolic murmur at the left sternal border. This may be difficult to distinguish from the murmur of acute mitral regurgitation. The murmur may be unimpressive or even absent when cardiac contractility is depressed. A large proportion of patients have a systolic thrill at the left sternal border. Echocardiography with Doppler color flow mapping is very sensitive and specific in the diagnosis of this condition; this technique also localizes the defect accurately and provides important prognostic information.[128]

Management

Early closure is now recognized to yield better results than attempting to wait for days or weeks until the conditions for surgery improve. Although early surgical intervention may increase operative mortality there is reduced patient mortality overall.

This practice is based on observational data, as there have not been any controlled trials of early versus late intervention. Grade B4

In the SHOCK trial register, surgical repair was performed in 31 patients with rupture, of whom six (19%) survived. Of the 24 patients managed medically, only one survived.[125] Technical improvements in repair have resulted in improvements in outcome, but mortality remains high.[129] Transcatheter closure has been described, but with a high mortality in early reports.[130]

Free wall rupture

Clinical features and prognosis

Rupture of the free wall of the left ventricle is an almost uniformly fatal complication of MI that now probably accounts for 10–20% of inhospital deaths.[131] Older patients are at far greater risk than younger patients. In the GISSI trial, cardiac rupture was the cause of 19% of the deaths among patients 60 years old or younger and 86% of deaths among those more than 70 years old.[132] Rupture occurs most frequently in elderly women.[133] Anterior infarctions, hypertension on admission and marked or persistent ST elevation are also risk factors for rupture.[134] The usual presentation is sudden collapse, associated electrical-mechanical dissociation, and failure to respond to cardiopulmonary resuscitation. However, in some patients ventricular rupture is subacute, allowing time for ante-mortem diagnosis,[135] this clinical entity is probably underrecognized. Premonitory symptoms of chest discomfort, a sense of impending doom and intermittent bradycardia signal impending myocardial rupture in many cases,[136] and if recognized, can lead to life saving surgery.[137] There has been some evidence that thrombolytic therapy can increase the risk of cardiac rupture[138] and that the timing of rupture is accelerated to within 24 to 48 hours of treatment.[139] A meta-analysis of 58 cases of rupture involving 1638 patients from four trials showed that the odds ratio (treated/control) of cardiac rupture was directly correlated with time to treatment ($P = 0.01$); late administration of thrombolytic therapy may increase the risk of cardiac rupture.[140]

Management

Urgent surgical repair is mandatory for acute rupture, but for subacute rupture, medical management may be effective but on balance all patients should be treated surgically if possible. Grade B4

In one recent report[141] of 81 consecutive patients presenting with acute hypotension with electrical mechanical dissociation, 19 survived with medical management alone.

Pericarditis

Clinical features and prognosis

Pericarditis occurs in approximately 25% of patients with Q wave infarctions and 9% of patients with non-Q wave infarctions,[142] and usually occurs within the first week.[143] A pericardial friction rub may be present but is not found in half of patients with typical symptoms and is not required for diagnosis or treatment.[143] On the other hand, the only evidence of pericarditis in many patients is a transient pericardial rub, with no symptoms. Pericarditis following myocardial infarction is associated with a higher risk of death in the year post-infarction, possibly due to the associated large infarction.[142]

Management

High dose aspirin and non-steroidal anti-inflammatory drugs are recommended to treat the symptoms of postinfarction pericarditis, although no randomized studies have been done to document their efficacy.

A single dose of a non-steroidal agent may be very effective, avoiding the need for long-term therapy. Grade C5

A serial echocardiographic study of patients with postinfarction pericarditis showed that patients treated with indomethacin or ibuprofen showed a greater tendency for infarct expansion, but it was not clear if the infarct expansion was due to the non-steroidal anti-inflammatory drugs or to the selection for treatment of those with larger infarctions.[144] Thrombolytic therapy reduces the incidence of pericarditis by approximately half.[143]

Pericardial effusion and tamponade

A pericardial effusion can be detected by echocardiography in one quarter of patients with acute Q wave MI.[145,146] This finding correlates with the presence of heart failure and a poor prognosis. Cardiac tamponade is a rare complication of thrombolytic therapy for acute MI, being reported in four of 392 consecutively treated patients in one series.[147]

Dressler's syndrome

A form of postinfarction pericarditis occurring 2–11 weeks after the acute event was described in 1956 by Dressler.[148] The full syndrome includes prolonged or recurrent pleuritic chest pain, a pericardial friction rub, fever, pulmonary infiltrates or a small pulmonary effusion, and an increased sedimentation rate. There has been a striking reduction in the incidence of this postinfarction complication.[149]

Non-steroidal anti-inflammatory drugs may be required for control of Dressler's syndrome, but there are no randomized trials to confirm their efficacy. Grade C5

Ventricular fibrillation and sustained ventricular tachycardia

Clinical features and prognosis

Sustained monomorphic ventricular tachycardia is not common in the early postinfarction period but it is a marker of adverse prognosis. Results of the GISSI-3 database showed that sustained ventricular tachycardia occuring after the first 24 hours of MI was a strong independent predictor of 6-week mortality (hazard ratio 6·13; 95% CI 4·56–8·25).[150] Risk factors for this arrhythmia included: older age, a history of hypertension, diabetes, and myocardial infarction and non-administration of lytic therapy.

The frequency of ventricular fibrillation (VF) has declined over the past 20 years as noted by Antman *et al*, who demonstrated from the randomized trials of prevention of ventricular fibrillation that the frequency in the 1970s was 5 to 10%, dropping through the 1980s to less than 2%.[151] The reasons for this may include the admission of lower risk patients to coronary care units, wider use of beta blocking drugs and more effective treatment of ventricular dysfunction and electrolyte imbalances in the coronary care unit. The prognosis of ventricular fibrillation depends on the associated clinical state. VF occurring in the presence of hemodynamic compromise has a high hospital mortality of 80%.[152] VF occurring in the absence of cardiogenic shock, severe heart failure or hypotension (primary VF) has a good short-term prognosis[153] although one major study of primary VF showed higher hospital mortality.[154] Patients surviving early inhospital VF complicating myocardial infarction, experience no adverse effect on long-term survival following hospital discharge.[155,156]

Management of VF

Results of individual trials of prophylactic lidocaine were conflicting. Meta-analyses of the clinical trials[157,158] have shown that prophylactic lidocaine was effective in reducing the frequency of ventricular fibrillation, but paradoxically did not improve mortality and was associated with a possible adverse effect. For this reason the use of intravenous lidocaine as prophylaxis against ventricular fibrillation has been virtually abandoned.[11]

Intravenous β blockers have been shown to reduce mortality, particularly in high-risk patients, with an apparent benefit in reduction of ventricular fibrillation.[159] Grade A1d

Low serum potassium is associated with a higher risk of VF[160] especially in patients on diuretic therapy prior to their infarction.[161]

The potential of intravenous magnesium to reduce the risk of ventricular fibrillation early in acute myocardial infarction has been studied in several trials. A meta-analysis of nine small trials showed an apparent improvement in survival.[162] A clinical trial involving 2316 patients randomized to early magnesium or placebo showed a significant 24% reduction in mortality[163] but wider use in non-selected patients in the much larger ISIS-4 trial was disappointing, with no significant effect on short-term mortality.[164] A meta-analysis included in the ISIS-4 publication which included all of the previous magnesium trials failed to show a mortality benefit. Overall there is insufficient evidence for the routine use of intravenous magnesium early in the post-MI period.

Postinfarction ventricular premature beats and non-sustained ventricular tachycardia

Clinical features and prognosis

While frequent ventricular premature beats (more than 10 per hour) in the postinfarction patient are an independent risk factor for subsequent mortality (both total mortality and sudden death), the significance of non-sustained ventricular tachycardia in this setting is controversial.[165] The suppression of these ventricular arrhythmias has consistently failed to improve survival.

Management

Antiarrhythmic drugs

A meta-analysis of 138 randomized trials of prophylactic antiarrhythmic drug therapy involving 98 000 postinfarction patients, reported by Teo *et al* in 1993,[166] showed that the mortality of patients randomized to receive Class I agents was increased (OR 1·14; 95% CI 1·01–1·28, *P*= 0·03). The most convincing evidence of the deleterious effects of antiarrhythmic drugs for suppression of ventricular extrasystoles came from the Cardiac Arrhythmia Suppression Trial (CAST).[167] In patients randomized to Class IC drugs, mortality was significantly higher even though these drugs effectively suppressed ventricular extrasystoles. Subsequently, the SWORD study was stopped after enrollment of only 3400 of the planned 6400 high-risk survivors of MI because of an excess mortality (4·6% v 2·7%, P = 0·005) in patients randomized to D-sotalol.[168]

Clinical trials have shown some support for the use of the predominantly Class III drug amiodarone. Two randomized clinical trials, each with more than 1000 postinfarction patients with either frequent or repetitive ventricular extrasystoles (CAMIAT)[169] or an EF of 0·40 or less (EMIAT),[170] have compared amiodarone to placebo. EMIAT reported no difference in mortality between treatment groups but CAMIAT reported a decrease in the primary end point, a composite of resuscitated ventricular fibrillation or arrhythmic death (3·3% v 6·0%, RR 48%; 95% CI 4–72), and a trend toward decreased all-cause mortality. A subsequent analysis indicated that a beneficial interaction between amiodarone and beta adrenergic blocker drugs may have contributed to the benefit of amiodarone in these trials.[171] A limitation of amiodarone therapy is the high incidence of serious adverse effects seen with long-term therapy. The clinical trial evidence that is now available does not appear to be strong enough to recommend amiodarone therapy to MI survivors with asymptomatic ventricular extrasystoles or a depressed EF. However, patients with symptomatic ventricular tachycardia as a long-term complication of MI often benefit from amiodarone therapy.

Implantable defibrillator

The implanted defibrillator reduced total mortality over 27 months in MADIT, a small randomized clinical trial in a specific high-risk subgroup of postinfarction patients.[172] Eligible patients had an EF of 0·35 or less, a documented episode of unsustained ventricular tachycardia, and inducible, non-suppressible ventricular tachyarrhythmia during electrophysiologic study. The risk ratio for total mortality was 0·46 (95% CI 0·26–0·82). The AVID (Antiarrhythmics Versus Implantable Defibrillators) study included a group of patients with ventricular fibrillation or ventricular tachycardia associated with a low EF or hemodynamic compromise.[173] The effect of an implanted cardiac defibrillator was compared to therapy with amiodarone or sotalol, the treatment decision guided by Holter or electrophysiologic study. There was a statistically significant benefit of defibrillator therapy compared to drug therapy. Similar results have been reported in two smaller randomized trials, the Canadian Implantable Defibrillator Study[174] and the Cardiac Arrest Study Hamburg.[175] In a subgroup analysis of the AVID database, in patients with better-preserved left ventricular function with ejection fractions in the range of 35 to 40%, cardioverter-defibrillator therapy had no advantage over drug therapy.[176] In a meta-analysis of the defibrillator

secondary prevention trials (AVID, CASH and SIDS), there was a 28% reduction in the relative risk of death in favor of defibrillator therapy over amiodarone therapy.[177] The MADIT II trial of 1200 post-MI patients with impaired left ventricular function was terminated early after observing a 30% reduction in mortality in patients randomized to receive an implantable defibrillator device compared to those receiving conventional treatment.[178]

Overall, the evidence indicates that Class I antiarrhythmic drugs should not be used to treat ventricular extrasystoles or unsustained ventricular tachycardia postinfarction. Amiodarone may be effective in some high-risk patients, but with a risk of side effects with long term use. β Blockers reduce total mortality and the incidence of re-infarction by one quarter in postinfarction patients.

Although no trial has specifically addressed the use of an implanted defibrillator in the early postinfarction period, it appears to be the treatment of choice in specific subgroups who have a history of MI and impaired LV systolic function. Grade A1a

Atrial fibrillation

Clinical features and prognosis

Atrial fibrillation is a relatively common complication of myocardial infarction. In patients with MI treated with thrombolytic therapy in the GUSTO 1 trial, atrial fibrillation was present on admission in 2·5% and developed during hospitalization in an additional 7·9% of cases.[179] Patients with atrial fibrillation more often had underlying three-vessel disease and an incompletely patent infarct-related artery. Inhospital stroke developed more often (3·1%) in patients with atrial fibrillation compared to those without atrial fibrillation (1·3%) (P = 0·0001). Atrial fibrillation was more likely to complicate the inhospital course of older patients with larger infarctions, worse Killip class and higher heart rates. The unadjusted mortality was higher at 30 days (14·3% v 6·2%, P = 0·0001) and at 1 year (21·5% v 8·6%, P = 0·0001) in patients with atrial fibrillation. The adjusted 30 day mortality ratio was 1·3 (95% CI 1·2–1·4). In a study from the GISSI trial, the incidence of inhospital atrial fibrillation or flutter was 7·8%, and was associated with a worse prognosis.[180] After adjustment for other prognostic factors, atrial fibrillation remained an independent predictor of increased inhospital mortality, adjusted relative risk (RR) 1·98 (95% CI 1·67–2·34). Four years after acute myocardial infarction the negative influence of atrial fibrillation persisted (RR 1·78; 95% CI 1·60–1·99).

The onset of atrial fibrillation is usually after the first hospital day, and the usual underlying causes are heart failure, pericarditis, and atrial ischemia, with heart failure being by far the most common.[181] In a study based on 106 780 US

Medicare beneficiaries 65 years of age or over, patients were categorized on the basis of the presence of AF, and those with AF were further subdivided by timing of AF (present on arrival *v* developing during hospitalization);[182] 11 510 presented with AF and 12 055 developed AF during hospitalization. Patients developing AF during hospitalization had a worse prognosis than patients who presented with AF. In another study, detailed analysis of the prognosis of AF in AMI showed that AF was an independent predictor of cardiac death when it developed within 24 hours (OR 2·5; 95% CI 1·2–5·0; *P* = 0·0012) and later (OR 3·7; 95% CI 1·8–7·5; *P* = 0·0005), but not when it preceded the onset of AMI.[183]

Management

Amiodarone has been shown to be more effective than digoxin in achieving reversion to sinus rhythm.[184] In a prospective but not randomized study, the combination of amiodarone and digoxin was superior to amiodarone alone in restoring sinus rhythm faster, maintaining sinus rhythm longer, and allowing the use of a lower cumulative amount of amiodarone.[185]

Heart block and conduction disturbances

Clinical features and prognosis

Complete atrioventricular block occurred in 7·7% of patients with inferior MI in one large series.[186] In one study patients with inferior infarction complicated by complete heart block had higher inhospital mortality rates than did those without this complication: 42% *v* 14% (*P* < 0·01), adjusted odds ratio of 2·7 (95% CI 1·6–4·6).[186] In another series the inhospital mortality rate was also higher (24·2% *v* 6·3%, *P* < 0·001), but at hospital discharge the survivors had similar clinical characteristics to patients without complete atrioventricular block, and a similar mortality rate during the next year.[187] In a study of elderly patients who had suffered an acute MI, heart block was associated with increased inhospital mortality but had no effect on prognosis at 1 year among hospital survivors.[188] There is some evidence that the widespread adoption of reperfusion therapy may have reduced the incidence of this complication of MI.[189] But even in the "reperfusion era", among patients with inferior MI treated with thrombolytic therapy, the development of complete atrioventricular block is associated with a relative risk of 4·5 for 21 day mortality.[190]

Management

In patients with inferior infarction pacing is indicated if there is persistent high-grade atrioventricular block.[191] In anterior infarction, the prognostic significance of atrioventricular block is even greater than for inferior MI. Patients with anterior MI and complete atrioventricular block had a 63% inhospital mortality rate, compared with a 19% mortality rate in those without complete heart block.[186] When right bundle branch block and left anterior hemiblock develop within the first few hours of infarction prophylactic pacing may be considered; however this practice remains controversial. If the patient survives, this type of heart block usually regresses, but there is a risk of complete heart block causing death after hospital discharge.[192] A small randomized trial showed no benefit of prophylactic placement of a permanent pacemaker.[193]

Transvenous pacing is required urgently for atrioventricular block complicating anterior infarction because the escape rhythm originates below the level of the atrioventricular node and is therefore unstable and usually very slow (20–40 bpm). Grade C5

The development of left or right bundle branch block, as a complication of MI is a marker of a larger infarct size and a higher mortality after hospital discharge,[194] but is not an indication for pacing. A randomized trial of pacing for bundle branch block complicating MI showed no advantage.[195] Left anterior hemiblock denotes neither a larger infarct size nor a worse prognosis.[196]

Postinfarction angina and myocardial ischemia

Clinical features and prognosis

Approximately 20% of patients develop angina during hospitalization after MI. Patients with early postinfarction angina are 10 times more likely to develop infarct extension during hospitalization, have a worse long-term prognosis and have more extensive coronary disease at arteriography.[197]

Management

Coronary angioplasty can be performed with a low risk in patients with postinfarction angina.[198] In trials of angioplasty performed after thrombolytic therapy there was no important difference in early mortality, but an apparent reduction in mortality between 6 and 52 weeks.[199] A study of the effect of coronary interventional procedures on improved postinfarction outcomes could not attribute the improvement to increased procedural management because most of the procedures were directed to the lowest risk patients.[200] Early intervention with coronary bypass surgery can relieve symptoms in almost all patients with postinfarction angina, with low complication rates.[201] The timing of surgery after infarction has not been shown to be a risk factor except when surgery is performed within the first 2 to 3 days postinfarction.[202] Early surgery is not an important risk factor in patients with normal left ventricular function but when the LV function is significantly depressed, delayed surgery is safer than early surgery.[203] The outcome of surgery performed after thrombolytic therapy depends on the hemodynamic stability of the patient at the time of surgery. When CABG was performed within 8 hours of thrombolytic therapy in the TIMI II trial, operative mortality was higher (13% to 17%) and there was an increased use of blood products when the patient was hemodynamically unstable compared with hemodynamically stable patients, who had a relatively low (2·8%) mortality.[204] Operative survivors in this group had a low 1 year mortality.

The Danish Trial in Acute MI (DANAMI) randomized 503 patients with inducible ischemia after thrombolytic therapy for MI to an invasive strategy, with coronary bypass surgery or angioplasty done in 82% of cases, or to a conservative strategy.[205] After 2·4 years of follow up, there was no difference in mortality (3·6% in the invasive group and 4·4% in the conservative group (*P* = NS)). But there was a reduction in re-infarction in the invasive group (5·6%) compared with the conservative group (10·5%) (*P* = 0·038), and far fewer hospitalizations for unstable angina in the invasive group (17·9% *v* 29·5%, *P* < 0·00001).

Overall invasive intervention is indicated in patients with postinfarction myocardial ischemia.
Grade A1c

Psychosocial complications

Clinical features and prognosis

An estimated 20–50% of postinfarction patients have high levels of psychosocial stress, including anxiety, depression, denial, hostility, and social isolation.[206] A major depressive disorder may occur in as many as 15–20% of patients hospitalized with myocardial infarction,[207] and depression has been shown to have a significantly adverse effect on outcome.[208] The effects of depression are compounded by lifestyle factors, including isolation, which themselves have been shown to have an adverse effect.[209] Poor adherence to postinfarction therapies has been shown to be a possible mechanism for the adverse outcome of depressed postinfarction patients.[210] Other postulated mechanisms are an increased risk of postinfarction ventricular arrhythmias[211] and abnormalities in platelet function[212] associated with depression. The possible association between depression and ventricular arrhythmias may be explained by the finding of reduced heart rate variability (HRV) in depressed post-MI patients.[213]

Management

Cardiac rehabilitation programs provide psychological and social support to patients after MI, in addition to education about risk factors and their modification. Randomized clinical trials of formal exercise programs post infarction have shown benefits on quality of life, but have not yielded definitive results individually on prognosis. An overview that included 36 trials involving 4554 patients was suggestive of benefit. After an average follow up of 3 years, the odds ratio was 0·80 for total mortality (95% CI 0·66–0·96) but the rate of non-fatal re-infarction was not reduced.[214]

An overview of randomized trials of disease management programs in patients with known coronary disease (including myocardial infarction) showed improvements in processes of care, quality of life and functional status, and admissions to hospital (RR 0·84 (95% CI 0·76–0·94), but no reductions in all-cause mortality (RR 0·91 (95% CI 0·79–1·04)) or recurrent myocardial infarction (RR 0·94 (95% CI 0·80–1·10)).[215] The effect of a specific nursing intervention designed to improve the psychological and social status of postinfarction patients was assessed in the Montreal Heart Attack Readjustment Trial (M-HART). The 1376 patients were randomized to usual care or to a treatment plan consisting of nurse visits and telephone calls to patients exhibiting high levels of psychological stress. The intervention had no effect on mortality in men, and was associated with an increased mortality in women that was of borderline statistical significance (*P* = 0·069).[216] Berkman *et al* recently compared the use of psychosocial intervention to usual care in 2481 post-MI patients who were depressed and with a low level of social support.[217] The intervention included cognitive behavioral therapy and pharmacotherapy for non-responders with severe depression. There was no significant difference between the two groups with regard to the primary end point of death and MI over a period of 48 months. A preliminary clinical trial of sertraline did however show benefits, not only on mood, but on ventricular ectopic activity.[218]

Overall, trials of psychosocial interventions have yielded inconsistent results with regard to hard cardiovascular end points such as death and MI; there is some evidence however, that these interventions improve functional status and quality of life.

References

1. American Heart Association. *2001 Heart and stroke statistical update*. Dallas, Texas: American Heart Association, 2000.
2. Braunwald E, Rutherford JD. Reversible ischemic left ventricular dysfunction: evidence for the "hibernating myocardium". *J Am Coll Cardiol* 1986;**8**:1467–70.
3. Pfeffer MA, Braunwald E. Ventricular remodeling after myocardial infarction. Experimental observations and clinical implications. *Circulation* 1990;**81**:1161–72.
4. Page DL, Caulfield JB, Kastor JA, DeSanctis RW, Saunders CA. Myocardial changes associated with cardiogenic shock. *N Engl J Med* 1971;**285**:133–7.
5. McCallister BD Jr, Christian TF, Gersh BJ, Gibbon RJ. Prognosis of myocardial infarctions involving more than 40% of the left

ventricle after acute reperfusion therapy. *Circulation* 1993;**88**:1470–5.

6. Fisher JP, Picard MH, Mikan JS *et al.* Quantitation of myocardial dysfunction in ischemic heart disease by echocardiographic endocardial surface mapping: correlation with hemodynamic status. *Am Heart J* 1995;**129**:1114–21.

7. Killip T, Kimball JT. Treatment of myocardial infarction in a coronary care unit: a two year experience with 250 patients. *Am J Cardiol* 1967;**20**:457–64.

8. DeGeare VS, Boura JA, Grines LL, O'Neill WW, Grines CL. Predictive value of the Killip classification in patients undergoing primary percutaneous coronary intervention for acute myocardial infarction. *Am J Cardiol* 2001;**87**:1035–8.

9. Rott D, Behar S, Leor J *et al*, Working Group on Intensive Cardiac Care, Israel Heart Society. Effect on survival of acute myocardial infarction in Killip classes II or III patients undergoing invasive coronary procedures. *Am J Cardiol* 2001;**88**:618–23.

10. Forrester JS, Diamond G, Chatterjee K, Swan HJC. Medical therapy of acute myocardial infarction by application of hemodynamic subsets. *N Engl J Med* 1976;**295**:1356–62,1404–14.

11. Ryan TJ, Antman EM, Brooks NH *et al.* 1999 update: ACC/AHA guidelines for the management of patients with acute myocardial infarction: executive summary and recommendations: a report of the American College of Cardiology/American Heart Association Task Force on Practice Guidelines (Committee on Management of Acute Myocardial Infarction). *Circulation* 1999;**100**:1016–30.

12. Zion MM, Balkin J, Rosenmann D *et al.* Use of pulmonary artery catheters in patients with acute myocardial infarction: analysis of experience in 5841 patients in the SPRINT Registry. *Chest* 1990;**98**:1331–5.

13. Connors AF, Speroff T, Dawson N *et al.* The effectiveness of right heart catheterization in the initial care of critically ill patients. *JAMA* 1996;**276**:889–97.

14. Dalen JE, Bone RC. Is it time to pull the pulmonary artery catheter? *JAMA* 1996;**276**:916–18.

15. Stevenson R, Ranjadayalan K, Wilkinson P, Roberts R, Timmis AD. Short and long term prognosis of acute myocardial infarction since introduction of thrombolysis. *BMJ* 1993;**307**:349–53.

16. Villanueva FS, Sabia PJ, Afrookteh A, Pollock SG, Hwang LJ, Kaul S. Value and limitations of current methods of evaluating patients presenting to the emergency room with cardiac-related symptoms for determining long-term prognosis. *Am J Cardiol* 1992;**69**:746–50.

17. The Multicenter Postinfarction Research Group. Risk stratification and survival after myocardial infarction. *N Engl J Med* 1983;**309**:331–6.

18. Gottlieb S, Moss AJ, McDermott M, Eberly S. Interrelation of left ventricular ejection fraction, pulmonary congestion and outcome in acute myocardial infarction. *Am J Cardiol* 1992;**69**:977–84.

19. Candell-Riera J, Permanyer-Miralda G, Castell J, *et al.* Uncomplicated first myocardial infarction: strategy for comprehensive prognostic studies. *J Am Coll Cardiol* 1991;**18**:1207–19.

20. Thompson PL, Fletcher EE, Katavatis V. Enzymatic indices of myocardial necrosis: influence on short-and long-term prog-

nosis after myocardial infarction. *Circulation* 1979;**59**:113–19.

21. Antman EM, Tanasijevic MJ, Thompson B *et al.* Cardiac-specific troponin I levels to predict the risk of mortality in patients with acute coronary syndromes. *N Engl J Med* 1996;**335**:1342–9.

22. Ohman EM, Armstrong PW, White HD *et al.* Risk stratification with a point-of-care cardiac troponin T test in acute myocardial infarction. GUSTO III investigators. Global Use of Strategies to Open Occluded Coronary Arteries. *Am J Cardiol* 1999;**84**:1281–6.

23. Califf RM, Pieper KS, Lee KL *et al.* Prediction of 1-year survival after thrombolysis for acute myocardial infarction in the global utilization of streptokinase and TPA for occluded coronary arteries trial. *Circulation* 2000;**101**:2231–8.

24. Marchioli R, Avanzini F *et al.*, on behalf of GISSI-Prevenzione Investigators. Assessment of absolute risk of death after myocardial infarction by use of multiple-risk-factor assessment equations; GISSI-Prevenzione mortality risk chart. *Eur Heart J* 2001;**22**:2085–103.

25. Dikshit K, Vyden JK, Forrester JS *et al.* Renal and extrarenal hemodynamic effects of furosemide in congestive heart failure after myocardial infarction. *N Engl J Med* 1973;**288**:1087–90.

26. Jugdutt BI. Effect of nitrates on myocardial remodeling after acute myocardial infarction. *Am J Cardiol* 1996;**77**:17C–23C.

27. Armstrong PW, Walker DC, Burton JR, Parker JO. Vasodilator therapy in acute myocardial infarction. A comparison of sodium nitroprusside and nitroglycerin. *Circulation* 1975;**52**:1118–22.

28. Yusuf S, Collins R, MacMahon S, Peto R. Effect of intravenous nitrates on mortality in acute myocardial infarction: an overview of the randomised trials. *Lancet* 1988;**1**:1088–92.

29. GISSI-3: effects of lisinopril and transdermal glyceryl trinitrate singly and together on 6-week mortality and ventricular function after acute myocardial infarction. Gruppo Italiano per lo Studio della Sopravvivenza nell'infarto Miocardico. *Lancet* 1994;**343**:1115–22.

30. ISIS-4: a randomised factorial trial assessing early oral captopril, oral mononitrate, and intravenous magnesium sulphate in 58050 patients with suspected acute myocardial infarction. ISIS-4 (Fourth International Study of Infarct Survival) Collaborative Group. *Lancet* 1995;**345**:669–85.

31. Swedberg K, Held P, Kjekshus J *et al.* Effects of the early administration of enalapril on mortality in patients with acute myocardial infarction. *N Engl J Med* 1992;**327**:678–84.

32. Pfeffer MA, Braunwald E, Moye LA *et al.* Effect of captopril on mortality and morbidity in patients with left ventricular dysfunction after myocardial infarction. Results of the Survival and Ventricular Enlargement Trial. *N Engl J Med* 1992;**327**:669–77.

33. Gruppo Italiano per lo Studio della Sopravvivenza nell'Infarto Miocardico. GISSI-3: effects of lisinopril and transdermal glyceryl trinitrate singly and together on 6-week mortality and ventricular function after acute myocardial infarction. *Lancet* 1994;**343**:1115–22.

34. The Acute Infarction Ramipril Efficacy (AIRE) Study Investigators. Effect of ramipril on mortality and morbidity of survivors of acute myocardial infarction with clinical evidence of heart failure. *Lancet* 1993;**342**:821–8.

35.Ambrosioni E, Borghi C, Magnani B. The effect of angiotensin-converting-enzyme inhibitor zofenopril on mortality and morbidity after anterior myocardial infarction. *N Engl J Med* 1995;**332**:80–5.

36.ISIS-IV Collaborative Group. A randomized factorial trial assessing early oral captopril, oral mononitrate and intravenous magnesium sulphate in 58050 patients with suspected acute myocardial infarction. *Lancet* 1995;**345**:669–85.

37.Kober L, Torp-Pedersen C, Carlsen JE *et al.* A clinical trial of the angiotensin-converting-enzyme inhibitor trandolapril in patients with left ventricular dysfunction after myocardial infarction. *N Engl J Med* 1995;**333**:1670–6.

38.Chinese Cardiac Study Collaborative Group. Oral captopril vs placebo among 13634 patients with suspected acute myocardial infarction: interim report from the Chinese Cardiac Study (CCS-1). *Lancet* 1995;**345**:686–7.

39.Indications for ACE inhibitors in the early treatment of acute myocardial infarction: systematic overview of individual data from 100000 patients in randomized trials. ACE Inhibitor Myocardial Infarction Collaborative Group. *Circulation* 1998;**97**:2202–12.

40.Flather MD, Yusuf S, Kober L *et al.* Long-term ACE-inhibitor therapy in patients with heart failure or left-ventricular dysfunction: a systematic overview of data from individual patients. ACE-Inhibitor Myocardial Infarction Collaborative Group. *Lancet* 2000;**355**:1575–81.

41.de Kam PJ, Voors AA, van den Berg MP *et al.* Effect of very early angiotensin-converting enzyme inhibition on left ventricular dilation after myocardial infarction in patients receiving thrombolysis: results of a meta-analysis of 845 patients. FAMIS, CAPTIN and CATS Investigators. *J Am Coll Cardiol* 2000;**36**:2047–53.

42.Pfeffer MA, Greaves SC, Arnold JM *et al.* Early versus delayed angiotensin-converting enzyme inhibition therapy in acute myocardial infarction. The healing and early afterload reducing therapy trial. *Circulation* 1997;**95**:2643–51.

43.McGhie AI, Golstein RA. Pathogenesis and management of acute heart failure and cardiogenic shock: role of inotropic therapy. *Chest* 1992;**102**(Suppl. 2):626S–32S.

44.Van Veldhuisen DJ, de Graeff PA, Remme WJ. Value of digoxin in heart failure and sinus rhythm: new features of an old drug? *J Am Coll Cardiol* 1996;**28**:813–19.

45.The Digitalis Investigation Group. The effect of digoxin on mortality and morbidity in patients with heart failure. *N Engl J Med* 1997;**336**:525–33.

46.White HD, Norris RM, Brown MA *et al.* Effect of intravenous streptokinase on left ventricular function and early survival after acute myocardial infarction. *N Engl J Med* 1987; **317**:850–5.

47.Coronary thrombolysis and myocardial salvage by tissue plasminogen activator given up to 4 hours after onset of myocardial infarction. National Heart Foundation of Australia Coronary Thrombolysis Group. *Lancet* 1988;**1**:203–7.

48.Granger CB, White HD, Bates ER, Ohman EM, Califf RM. A pooled analysis of coronary arterial patency and left ventricular function after intravenous thrombolysis for acute myocardial infarction. *Am J Cardiol* 1994;**74**:1220–8.

49.Bolli R. Myocardial "stunning" in man. *Circulation* 1992; **86**:1671–91.

50.Braunwald E, Rutherford JD. Reversible ischemic left ventricular dysfunction: evidence for the "hibernating myocardium". *J Am Coll Cardiol* 1986;**8**:1467–70.

51.Solomon SD, Glynn RJ, Greaves S *et al.* Recovery of ventricular function after myocardial infarction in the reperfusion era: the healing and early afterload reducing therapy study. *Ann Intern Med* 2001;**134**:451–8.

52.Marroquin OC, Lamas GA. Beneficial effects of an open artery on left ventricular remodeling after myocardial infarction. *Prog Cardiovasc Dis* 2000;**42**:471–83.

53.Lundergan CF, Ross AM, McCarthy WF *et al.* Predictors of left ventricular function after acute myocardial infarction: effects of time to treatment, patency, and body mass index: the GUSTO-I angiographic experience. *Am Heart J* 2001; **142**: 43–50.

54.Goldberg RJ, Gore JM, Alpert JS *et al.* Cardiogenic shock after acute myocardial infarction. Incidence and mortality from a community wide perspective, 1975–1988. *N Engl J Med* 1991;**325**:1117–22.

55.Hochman JS, Boland J, Sleeper LA *et al.* Current spectrum of cardiogenic shock and effect of early revascularization on mortality. Results of an international registry. *Circulation* 1995;**91**:873–81.

56.Hasdai D, Califf RM, Thompson TD *et al.* Predictors of cardiogenic shock after thrombolytic therapy for acute myocardial infarction. *J Am Coll Cardiol* 2000;**35**:136–43.

57.Richard C, Ricome JL, Rimailho A, Bottineau G, Auzepy P. Combined hemodynamic effects of dopamine and dobutamine in cardiogenic shock. *Circulation* 1983;**67**:620–6.

58.Scheidt S, Wilner G, Mueller H *et al.* Intra-aortic balloon counterpulsion in cardiogenic shock. Report of a co-operative clinical trial. *N Engl J Med* 1973;**288**:979–84.

59.Bengtson JR, Kaplan AJ, Pieper KS *et al.* Prognosis in cardiogenic shock after acute myocardial infarction in the interventional era. *J Am Coll Cardiol* 1992;**20**:1482–9.

60.Ohman EM, George BS, White CJ *et al.*, the Randomized IABP Study Group. Use of aortic counterpulsation to improve sustained coronary artery patency during acute myocardial infarction: results of a randomized trial. *Circulation* 1994; **90**: 792–9.

61.Park SJ, Nguyen DQ, Bank AJ, Ormaza S, Bolman RM 3rd. Left ventricular assist device bridge therapy for acute myocardial infarction. *Ann Thorac Surg* 2000;**69**:1146–51.

62.Thiele H, Lauer B, Hambrecht R, Boudriot E, Cohen HA, Schuler G. Reversal of cardiogenic shock by percutaneous left atrial-to-femoral arterial bypass assistance. *Circulation* 2001; **104**:2917–22.

63.Bates ER, Topol EJ. Limitations of thrombolytic therapy for acute myocardial infarction complicated by congestive heart failure and cardiogenic shock. *J Am Coll Cardiol* 1991;**18**: 1077–84.

64.Hasdai D, Harrington RA, Hochman JS *et al.* Platelet glycoprotein IIb/IIIa blockade and outcome of cardiogenic shock complicating acute coronary syndromes without persistent ST-segment elevation. *J Am Coll Cardiol* 2000;**36**:685–92.

65.Berger PB, Holmes DR, Stebbins AL *et al.* for the GUSTO-1 Investigators. Impact of an aggressive invasive catheterization and revascularization strategy on mortality in patients with cardiogenic shock in the Global Utilization of Streptokinase and

Tissue Plasminogen Activator for Occluded Coronary Arteries (GUSTO-1) Trial. *Circulation* 1997;**96**:122–7.

66. Sanborn TA, Sleeper LA, Bates ER *et al.* Impact of thrombolysis, intra-aortic balloon pump counterpulsation, and their combination in cardiogenic shock complicating acute myocardial infarction: a report from the SHOCK Trial Registry. SHould we emergently revascularize Occluded Coronaries for cardiogenic shocK? *J Am Coll Cardiol* 2000;**36**(Suppl. A): 1123–9.

67. Hochman JS, Sleeper LA, Webb JG *et al.* Early revascularization in acute myocardial infarction complicated by cardiogenic shock. SHOCK Investigators. SHould we emergently revascularize Occluded Coronaries for cardiogenic shocK. *N Engl J Med* 1999;**341**:625–34.

68. Hochman JS, Sleeper LA, White HD *et al.* One-year survival following early revascularization for cardiogenic shock. *JAMA* 2001;**28**:190–2.

69. Kinch JW, Ryan TJ. Right ventricular infarction. *N Engl J Med* 1993;**330**:1211–17.

70. Zehender M, Kasper W, Kauder E *et al.* Eligibility for and benefit of thrombolytic therapy in inferior myocardial infarction: focus on the prognostic importance of right ventricular infarction. *J Am Coll Cardiol* 1994;**24**:362–9.

71. Cabin HS, Clubb KS, Wackers FJT, Zaret BL. Right ventricular myocardial infarction with anterior wall left ventricular infarction: an autopsy study. *Am Heart J* 1987;**113**:16–23.

72. Zehender M, Kasper W, Kauder E *et al.* Right ventricular infarction as an independent predictor of prognosis after acute inferior myocardial infarction. *N Engl J Med* 1993;**328**: 981–8.

73. Dell'Italia LJ, Starling MR, Crawford MH *et al.* Right ventricular infarction: identification by hemodynamic measurements before and after volume loading and correlation with noninvasive techniques. *J Am Coll Cardiol* 1984;**4**:931–9.

74. Erhardt IR, Sjogren A, Wahlberg I. Single right sided precordial lead in the diagnosis of right ventricular involvement in inferior myocardial infarction. *Am Heart J* 1976;**91**:571–6.

75. López-Sendón J, López de Sá E, Roldán I *et al.* Inversion of the normal interatrial septum convexity in acute myocardial infarction: incidence, clinical relevance and prognostic significance. *J Am Coll Cardiol* 1990;**15**:801–5.

76. Goldstein JA, Barzilai B, Rosamond TL, Eisenberg PR, Jaffe AS. Determinants of hemodynamic compromise with severe right ventricular infarction. *Circulation* 1990;**82**:359–68.

77. Goldstein JA, Vlahakes GJ, Verrier ED *et al.* Volume loading improves low cardiac output in experimental myocardial infarction. *J Am Coll Cardiol* 1993;**2**:270–8.

78. Lloyd EA, Gersh BJ, Kennelly BM. Hemodynamic spectrum of "dominant" right ventricular infarction in 19 patients. *Am J Cardiol* 1981;**48**:1016–22.

79. Love JC, Haffajee CI, Gore JM, Alpert JS. Reversibility of hypotension and shock by atrial or atrioventricular sequential pacing in patients with right ventricular infarction. *Am Heart J* 1984;**108**:5–13.

80. Schuler G, Hofmann M, Schwarz F *et al.* Effect of successful thrombolytic therapy on right ventricular function in acute inferior wall myocardial infarction. *Am J Cardiol* 1984;**54**: 951–7.

81. Berger PB, Ruocco NA, Ryan TJ *et al.* Frequency and significance of right ventricular dysfunction during inferior wall left ventricular myocardial infarction treated with thrombolytic therapy (results from the Thrombolysis in Myocardial Infarction [TIMI] II trial). *Am J Cardiol* 1993;**71**:1148–52.

82. Bowers TR, O'Neill WW, Grines C, Pica MC, Safian RD, Goldstein JA. Effect of reperfusion on biventricular function and survival after right ventricular infarction. *N Engl J Med* 1998;**338**:933–40.

83. Ba'albaki HA, Clements SD. Left ventricular aneurysm: a review. *Clin Cardiol* 1989;**12**:5–13.

84. Forman MB, Collins HW, Kopelman HA *et al.* Determinants of left ventricular aneurysm formation after anterior myocardial infarction: a clinical and angiographic study. *J Am Coll Cardiol* 1986;**8**:1256–62.

85. Popovic AD, Neskovic AN, Babic R *et al.* Independent impact of thrombolytic therapy and vessel patency on left ventricular dilation after myocardial infarction. Serial echocardiographic follow-up. *Circulation* 1994;**90**:800–7.

86. Sechtem U, Theissen P, Heindel W *et al.* Diagnosis of left ventricular thrombi by magnetic resonance imaging and comparison with angiocardiography, computed tomography and echocardiography. *Am J Cardiol* 1989;**64**:1195–9.

87. Sager PT, Perlmutter RA, Rosenfeld LE, McPherson CA, Wackers FJ, Batsford WP. Electrophysiologic effects of thrombolytic therapy in patients with a transmural anterior myocardial infarction complicated by left ventricular aneurysm formation. *J Am Coll Cardiol* 1988;**12**:19–24.

88. Ba'albaki HA, Clements SD. Left ventricular aneurysm: a review. *Clin Cardiol* 1989;**12**:5–13.

89. Cohen M, Packer M, Gorlin R. Indications for left ventricular aneurysmectomy. *Circulation* 1983;**67**:717–22.

90. Roberts WC, Morrow AG. Pseudoaneurysm of the left ventricle: an unusual sequel of myocardial infarction and rupture of the heart. *Am J Med* 1967;**43**:639–54.

91. Brown SL, Gropler RJ, Harris KM. Distinguishing left ventricular aneurysm from pseudoaneurysm. A review of the literature. *Chest* 1997;**111**:1403–9.

92. Gatewood RP, Nanda NC. Differentiation of left ventricular pseudoaneurysm from true aneurysm with two-dimensional echocardiography. *Am J Cardiol* 1980;**46**:869–78.

93. Frances C, Romero A, Grady D. Left ventricular pseudoaneurysm. *J Am Coll Cardiol* 1998;**32**:557–61.

94. Vecchio C, Chiarella F, Lupi G, Bellotti P, Domenicucci S. Left ventricular thrombus in anterior acute myocardial infarction after thrombolysis. A GISSI-2 connected study. *Circulation* 1991;**84**:512–19.

95. Nihoyannopoulos P, Smith GC, Maseri A, Foale RA. The natural history of left ventricular thrombus in myocardial infarction: a rationale in support of masterly inactivity. *J Am Coll Cardiol* 1989;**14**:903–11.

96. Funke Küpper AJ, Verheugt FWA, Peels CH, Galema TW, Roos JP. Left ventricular thrombus incidence and behavior studied by serial two-dimensional echocardiography in acute anterior myocardial infarction: left ventricular wall motion, systemic embolism and oral anticoagulation. *J Am Coll Cardiol* 1989;**13**:1514–20.

97. Stratton JR, Resnick AD. Increased embolic risk in patients with left ventricular thrombi. *Circulation* 1987;**75**:1004–11.

98. Keren A, Goldberg S, Gottlieb S *et al.* Natural history of left ventricular thrombi: their appearance and resolution in the post-hospital period of acute myocardial infarction. *J Am Coll Cardiol* 1990;**15**:790–800.

99. Thompson PL, Robinson JS. Stroke after acute myocardial infarction: relation to infarct size. *BMJ* 1978;**2**:457.

100. Konrad MS, Coffey CE, Coffey KS *et al.* Myocardial infarction and stroke. *Neurology* 1984;**34**:1403–9.

101. Vaitkus PT, Barnathan ES. Embolic potential, prevention and management of mural thrombus complicating anterior myocardial infarction: a meta-analysis. *J Am Coll Cardiol* 1993;**22**:1004–9.

102. Vaitkus PT, Berlin JA, Schwartz JS, Barnathan ES. Stroke complicating acute myocardial infarction: a meta-analysis of risk modification by anticoagulation and thrombolytic therapy. *Arch Intern Med* 1992;**152**:2020–4.

103. Collins R, MacMahon S, Flather M *et al.* Clinical effects of anticoagulant therapy in suspected acute myocardial infarction: systematic overview of randomised trials. *BMJ* 1996; **313**:652–9.

104. Mahaffey KW, Granger CB, Collins R *et al.* Overview of randomized trials of intravenous heparin in patients with acute myocardial infarction treated with thrombolytic therapy. *Am J Cardiol* 1996;**77**:551–6.

105. Fibrinolytic Therapy Trialists' (FTT) Collaborative Group. Indications for fibrinolytic therapy in suspected acute myocardial infarction: collaborative overview of early mortality and major morbidity results from all randomised trials of more than 1000 patients. *Lancet* 1994;**343**:311–22.

106. Weaver WD, Simes RJ, Betriu A *et al.* Comparison of primary coronary angioplasty and intravenous thrombolytic therapy for acute myocardial infarction: a quantitative review. *JAMA* 1997;**278**:2093–8.

107. Shelburne JC, Rubinstein D, Gorlin R. A reappraisal of papillary muscle dysfunction: correlative clinical and angiographic study. *Am J Med* 1969;**46**:862–71.

108. Izumi S, Miyatake K, Beppu S *et al.* Mechanism of mitral regurgitation in patients with myocardial infarction: a study using real-time two-dimensional Doppler flow imaging and echocardiography. *Circulation* 1987;**76**:777–85.

109. Lamas GA, Mitchell GF, Flaker GC *et al.* Clinical significance of mitral regurgitation after acute myocardial infarction. *Circulation* 1997;**96**:827–33.

110. Barzilai B, Gessler C, Pérez JE, Schaab C, Jaffe AS. Significance of Doppler-detected mitral regurgitation in acute myocardial infarction. *Am J Cardiol* 1988;**61**:220–3.

111. Feinberg MS, Schwammenthal E, Shlizerman L, *et al.* Prognostic significance of mild mitral regurgitation by color Doppler echocardiography in acute myocardial infarction. *Am J Cardiol* 2000;**86**:903–7.

112. Thompson CR, Buller CE, Sleeper LA *et al.* Cardiogenic shock due to acute severe mitral regurgitation complicating acute myocardial infarction: a report from the SHOCK Trial Registry. SHould we use emergently revascularize Occluded Coronaries in cardiogenic shocK? *J Am Coll Cardiol* 2000; **36**(Suppl. A):1104–9.

113. Patel AR, Mochizuki Y, Yao J, Pandian NG. Mitral regurgitation: comprehensive assessment by echocardiography. *Echocardiography* 2000;**17**:275–83.

114. Sohn DW, Shin GJ, Oh JK *et al.* Role of transesophageal echocardiography in hemodynamically unstable patients. *Mayo Clin Proc* 1995;**70**:925–31.

115. Fuchs RM, Heuser RR, Yin FCP, Brinker JA. Limitations of pulmonary wedge v waves in diagnosing mitral regurgitation. *Am J Cardiol* 1982;**49**:849–54.

116. Baxley W, Kennedy JW, Field B, Dodge HT. Hemodynamics in ruptured chordae tendinae and chronic rheumatic mitral regurgitation. *Circulation* 1973;**48**:1288–94.

117. Chatterjee K, Parmley WW, Swan HJC *et al.* Beneficial effects of vasodilator agents in severe mitral regurgitation due to dysfunction of subvalvular apparatus. *Circulation* 1973;**47**: 684–90.

118. Kishon Y, Oh JK, Schaff HV *et al.* Mitral valve operation in postinfarction rupture of a papillary muscle: immediate results and long-term follow-up of 22 patients. *Mayo Clin Proc* 1992;**67**:1023–30.

119. Yamanishi H, Izumoto H, Kitahara H, Kamata J, Tasai K, Kawazoe K. Clinical experiences of surgical repair for mitral regurgitation secondary to papillary muscle rupture complicating acute myocardial infarction. *Ann Thorac Cardiovasc Surg* 1998;**4**:83–6.

120. Leor J, Feinberg MS, Vered Z *et al.* Effect of thrombolytic therapy on the evolution of significant mitral regurgitation in patients with a first inferior myocardial infarction. *J Am Coll Cardiol* 1993;**21**:1661–6.

121. Kinn JW, O'Neill WW, Benzuly KH, Jones DE, Grines CL. Primary angioplasty reduces risk of myocardial rupture compared to thrombolysis for acute myocardial infarction. *Cathet Cardiovasc Diagn* 1997;**42**:151–7.

122. Shawl FA, Forman MB, Punja S, Goldbaum TS. Emergent coronary angioplasty in the treatment of acute ischemic mitral regurgitation: long-term results in five cases. *J Am Coll Cardiol* 1989;**14**:986–91.

123. Moore CA, Nygaard TW, Kaiser DL, Cooper AA, Gibson RS. Postinfarction ventricular septal rupture: the importance of location of infarction and right ventricular function in determining survival. *Circulation* 1986;**74**:45–55.

124. Edwards BS, Edwards WD, Edwards JE. Ventricular septal rupture complicating acute myocardial infarction: identification of simple and complex types in 53 autopsied hearts. *Am J Cardiol* 1984;**54**:1201–5.

125. Menon V, Webb JG, Hillis LD, Sleeper LA, *et al.* Outcome and profile of ventricular septal rupture with cardiogenic shock after myocardial infarction: a report from the SHOCK Trial Registry. SHould we emergently revascularize Occluded Coronaries in cardiogenic shocK. *J Am Coll Cardiol* 2000;**36**(Suppl. A):1110–6.

126. Lemery R, Smith HC, Giuliani ER, Gersh BJ. Prognosis in rupture of the ventricular septum after acute myocardial infarction and role of early surgical intervention. *Am J Cardiol* 1992;**70**:147–51.

127. Hill JD, Stiles QR. Acute ischemic ventricular septal defect. *Circulation* 1989;**79**(Suppl. I):I-112–15.

128. Helmcke F, Mahan EF, Nanda NC *et al.* Two-dimensional echocardiography and Doppler color flow mapping in the diagnosis and prognosis of ventricular septal rupture. *Circulation* 1990;**81**:1775–83.

129. Alvarez JM, Brady PW, Ross AM. Technical improvements in the repair of acute post infarction ventricular septal rupture. *J Cardiovasc Surg* 1992;**3**:198.

130. Landzberg MJ, Lock JE. Transcatheter management of ventricular septal rupture after myocardial infarction. *Semin Thorac Cardiovasc Surg* 1998;**10**:128–32.

131. Reddy SG, Roberts WC. Frequency of rupture of the left ventricular free wall or ventricular septum among necroscopy cases of fatal acute myocardial infarction since introduction of coronary care units. *Am J Cardiol* 1989;**63**:906–11.

132. Maggioni AP, Maseri A, Fresco C *et al.* Age-related increase in mortality among patients with first myocardial infarctions treated with thrombolysis. The Investigators of the Gruppo Italiano per lo Studio della Sopravvivenza nell'Infarto Miocardico (GISSI-2). *N Engl J Med* 1993;**329**:1442–8.

133. Shapira I, Isakov A, Burke M, Almog C. Cardiac rupture in patients with acute myocardial infarction. *Chest* 1987; **92**:219–23.

134. Figueras J, Curos A, Cortadellas J, Sans M, Soler-Soler J. Relevance of electrocardiographic findings, heart failure, and infarct site in assessing risk and timing of left ventricular free wall rupture during acute myocardial infarction. *Am J Cardiol* 1995;**76**:543–7.

135. López-Sendón J, Gonzalez A, López de Sá E *et al.* Diagnosis of subacute left ventricular wall rupture after acute myocardial infarction: sensitivity and specificity of clinical, hemodynamic and echocardiographic criteria. *J Am Coll Cardiol* 1992;**19**:1145–53.

136. Oliva PB, Hammill SC, Edwards WD. Cardiac rupture: a clinically predictable complication of acute myocardial infarction: a report of 70 cases with clinical-pathological correlations. *J Am Coll Cardiol* 1993;**22**:720–6.

137. Bashour T, Kabbani SS, Ellertson DG, Crew J, Hanna ES. Surgical salvage of heart rupture: report of two cases and review of the literature. *Ann Thorac Surg* 1983;**36**:209–13.

138. Pollak H, Nobis H, Miczoch J. Frequency of left ventricular free wall rupture complicating acute myocardial infarction since the advent of thrombolysis. *Am J Cardiol* 1994;**74**:184–6.

139. Becker RC, Hochman JS, Cannon CP *et al.* Fatal cardiac rupture among patients treated with thrombolytic agents and adjunctive thrombin antagonists: observations from the Thrombolysis and Thrombin in Myocardial Infarction 9 Study. *J Am Coll Cardiol* 1999;**33**:479–87.

140. Honan MB, Harrell FE Jr, Reimer KA *et al.* Cardiac rupture, mortality and the timing of thrombolytic therapy: a meta-analysis. *J Am Coll Cardiol* 1990;**16**:359–67.

141. Figueras J, Cortadellas J, Evangelista A, Soler-Soler J. Medical management of selected patients with left ventricular free wall rupture during acute myocardial infarction. *J Am Coll Cardiol* 1997;**29**:512–18.

142. Tofler GH, Muller JE, Stone PH *et al.* Pericarditis in acute myocardial infarction: characterization and clinical significance. *Am Heart J* 1989;**117**:86–92.

143. Oliva PB, Hammill SC, Talano JV. Effect of definition on incidence of postinfarction pericarditis. Is it time to redefine postinfarction pericarditis? *Circulation* 1994;**90**:1537–41.

144. Jugdutt BI, Basualdo CA. Myocardial infarct expansion during indomethacin or ibuprofen therapy for symptomatic post infarction pericarditis. Influence of other pharmacologic agents during early remodelling. *Can J Cardiol* 1989;**5**: 211–21.

145. Pierard LA, Albert A, Henrard L *et al.* Incidence and significance of pericardial effusion in acute myocardial infarction as determined by two-dimensional echocardiography. *J Am Coll Cardiol* 1986;**8**:517–20.

146. Sugiura T, Iwasaka T, Takayama Y *et al.* Factors associated with pericardial effusion in acute Q wave myocardial infarction. *Circulation* 1990;**81**:477–81.

147. Renkin J, De Bruyne B, Benit E *et al.* Cardiac tamponade early after thrombolysis for acute myocardial infarction: a rare but not reported hemorrhagic complication. *J Am Coll Cardiol* 1991;**17**:280–5.

148. Dressler W. A post-myocardial-infarction syndrome: preliminary report of a complication resembling idiopathic, recurrent, benign pericarditis. *JAMA* 1956;**160**:1379–83.

149. Northcote RJ, Hutchison SJ, McGuinness JB. Evidence for the continued existence of the postmyocardial infarction (Dressler's) syndrome. *Am J Cardiol* 1984;**53**:1201–2.

150. Volpi A, Cavalli A, Turato R, Barlera S, Santoro E, Negri E. Incidence and short-term prognosis of late sustained ventricular tachycardia after myocardial infarction: results of the Gruppo Italiano per lo Studio della Sopravvivenza nell'Infarcto Miocardio (GISSI-3) Data Base. *Am Heart J* 2001;**142**:87–92.

151. Antman EM, Berlin JA. Declining incidence of ventricular fibrillation in myocardial infarction. Implications for the prophylactic use of lidocaine. *Circulation* 1992;**86**:764–73.

152. Bigger JT, Dresdale RJ, Heissenbutter RH, Weld FM, Wit AL. Ventricular arrhythmias in ischemic heart disease: mechanism, prevalence, significance and management. *Prog Cardiovasc Dis* 1977;**19**:255–300.

153. Tofler GH, Stone PH, Muller JE *et al* and the MILIS study group. Prognosis after cardiac arrest due to ventricular tachycardia or ventricular fibrillation associated with acute myocardial infarction. *Am J Cardiol* 1987;**60**:755–61.

154. Volpi A, Maggioni A, Franzosi MG, Pampallona S, Mauri F, Tognoni G. In-hospital prognosis of patients with acute myocardial infarction complicated by primary ventricular fibrillation. *N Engl J Med* 1987;**317**:257–61.

155. Nicod P, Gilpin E, Dittrich H *et al.* Late clinical outcome in patients with early ventricular fibrillation after myocardial infarction. *J Am Coll Cardiol* 1988;**11**:464–70.

156. Volpi A, Cavalli A, Franzosi MG *et al* and the GISSI Investigators. One-year prognosis of primary ventricular fibrillation complicating acute myocardial infarction *Am J Cardiol* 1989;**63**:1174–8.

157. MacMahon S, Collins R, Peto R, Koster RW, Yusuf S. Effects of prophylactic lignocaine in suspected acute myocardial infarction. An overview of results from the randomized, controlled trials. *JAMA* 1988;**260**:1910–6.

158. Da Silva RA, Hennekens CH, Lown B, Cascells W. Lignocaine prophylaxis in acute myocardial infarction: an evaluation of the randomised trials. *Lancet* 1981;**2**:855–8.

159. Norris RM, Barnaby PF, Brown MA *et al.* Prevention of ventricular fibrillation during acute myocardial infarction with intravenous propranolol. *Lancet* 1984;**2**:883–6.

160. Nordrehaug JE, Lippe GVD. Hypokalaemia and ventricular fibrillation in acute myocardial infarction. *Br Heart J* 1983; **50**:525–9.

161. Stewart DE, Ikram H, Espiner EA, Nicholls MG. Arrhythmogenic potential of diuretic induced hypokalaemia in patients with mild hypertension and ischaemic heart disease. *Br Heart J* 1985;**54**:290–7.

162. Teo KK, Yusuf S, Collins R, Held PH, Peto R. Effects of intravenous magnesium in suspected acute myocardial infarction: overview of randomised trials. *BMJ* 1991;**303**:1499–503.

163. Baxter GF, Sumeray MS, Walker JM. Infarct size and magnesium: insights into LIMIT-2 and ISIS-4 from experimental studies. *Lancet* 1996;**348**:1424–6.

164. ISIS Collaboration Group. ISIS-4: a randomized factorial trial assessing oral captopril, oral mononitrate and intravenous magnesium sulphate in 58 080 patients with suspected acute myocardial infarction. *Lancet* 1995;**345**:669–85.

165. Maggioni AP, Zuanetti G, Franzosi MG et al. Prevalence and prognostic significance of ventricular arrhythmias after myocardial infarction in the fibrinolytic era. GISSI-2 Results. *Circulation* 1993;**87**:312–22.

166. Teo K, Yusuf S, Furberg CD. Effects of prophylactic antiarrhythmic drug therapy in acute myocardial infarction: an overview of results from randomized controlled trials. *JAMA* 1993;**270**:1589–95.

167. Echt DS, Liebson PR, Mitchell B et al. Mortality and morbidity in patients receiving encainide, flecainide, or placebo. The Cardiac Arrhythmia Suppression Trial. *N Engl J Med* 1991;**324**:781–8.

168. Domanski MJ, Zipes DP, Schron E. Treatment of sudden cardiac death. Current understandings from randomized trials and future research directions. *Circulation* 1997;**95**:2694–9.

169. Cairns JA, Connolly SJ, Roberts R, Gent M. Randomised trial of outcome after myocardial infarction in patients with frequent or repetitive ventricular premature depolarisations: Canadian Amiodarone Myocardial Infarction Arrhythmia Trial (CAMIAT). *Lancet* 1997;**349**:675–82.

170. Julian DG, Camm AJ, Frangin G et al. Randomised trial of the effect of amiodarone on mortality in patients with left-ventricular dysfunction after recent myocardial infarction: European Myocardial Infarction Amiodarone Trial (EMIAT). *Lancet* 1997;**349**:667–74.

171. Boutitie F, Boissel JP, Connolly SJ et al. Amiodarone interaction with beta-blockers: analysis of the merged EMIAT (European Myocardial Infarct Amiodarone Trial) and CAMIAT (Canadian Amiodarone Myocardial Infarction Trial) databases. *Circulation* 1999;**99**:2268–75.

172. Moss AJ, Hall J, Cannom DS et al. Improved survival with an implanted defibrillator in patients with coronary disease at high risk for ventricular arrhythmia. Multicenter Automatic Defibrillation Implantation Trial (MADIT). *N Engl J Med* 1996;**335**:1933–40.

173. The Antiarrhythmics versus Implantable Defibrillators (AVID) Investigators. A comparison of antiarrhythmic-drug therapy with implantable defibrillators in patients resuscitated from near-fatal ventricular arrhythmias. *N Engl J Med* 1997;**337**:1576–83.

174. Connolly SJ, Gent M, Roberts RS et al. Canadian Implantable Defibrillator Study (CIDS): a randomized trial of the implantable cardioverter defibrillator against amiodarone. *Circulation* 2000;**101**:1287–302.

175. Kuck KH, Cappato R, Siebels J, Ruppel R. Randomized comparison of antiarrhythmic drug therapy with implantable defibrillators in patients resuscitated from cardiac arrest: the Cardiac Arrest Study Hamburg (CASH). *Circulation* 2000;**102**:748–54.

176. Domanski MJ, Sakseena S, Epstein AE et al. Relative effectiveness of the implantable cardioverter-defibrillator and antiarrhythmic drugs in patients with varying degrees of left ventricular dysfunction who have survived malignant ventricular arrhythmias. *J Am Coll Cardiol* 1999;**34**:1090–5.

177. Connolly SJ, Hallstrom AP, Cappato R et al. Meta-analysis of the implantable cardioverter defibrillator secondary prevention trials. AVID, CASH and CIDS studies; Antiarrythmics vs Implantable Defibrillator Study, Cardiac Arrest Study Hamburg, Canadian Implantable Defibrillator Study. *Eur Heart J* 2000;**21**:2071–8.

178. Editorial MADIT II, the Multi-center Autonomic Defibrillation Implantation Trial II stopped early for mortality reduction, has ICD therapy earned its evidence-based credentials? *Int J Cardiol* 2002;**82**:1–5.

179. Crenshaw BS, Ward SR, Granger CB et al. for the GUSTO-1 Trial Investigators. Atrial fibrillation in the setting of acute myocardial infarction: the GUSTO-1 experience. *J Am Coll Cardiol* 1997;**30**:406–13.

180. Pizzetti F, Turazza FM, Franzosi MG et al. GISSI-3 Investigators. Incidence and prognostic significance of atrial fibrillation in acute myocardial infarction: the GISSI-3 data. *Heart* 2001;**86**:527–32.

181. Sugiura T, Iwasaka T, Takahashi N et al. Factors associated with atrial fibrillation in Q wave anterior myocardial infarction. *Am Heart J* 1991;**121**:1409–12.

182. Rathore SS, Berger AK, Weinfurt KP et al. Acute myocardial infarction complicated by atrial fibrillation in the elderly: prevalence and outcomes. *Circulation* 2000;**101**:969–74.

183. Sakata K, Kurihara H, Iwamori K et al. Clinical and prognostic significance of atrial fibrillation in acute myocardial infarction. *Am J Cardiol* 1997;**80**:1522–7.

184. Cowan JC, Gardiner P, Reid DS, Newell DJ, Campbell RW. A comparison of amiodarone and digoxin in the treatment of atrial fibrillation complicating suspected acute myocardial infarction. *J Cardiovasc Pharmacol* 1986;**8**:252–6.

185. Kontoyannis DA, Anastasiou-Nana MI, Kontoyannis SA, Zaga AK, Nanas JN. Intravenous amiodarone decreases the duration of atrial fibrillation associated with acute myocardial infarction. *Cardiovasc Drugs Ther* 2001;**15**:155–60.

186. Goldberg RJ, Zevallos JC, Yarzebski J et al. Prognosis of acute myocardial infarction complicated by complete heart block (the Worcester Heart Attack Study). *Am J Cardiol* 1992;**69**:1135–41.

187. Nicod P, Gilpin E, Dittrich H et al. Long-term outcome in patients with inferior myocardial infarction and complete atrioventricular block. *J Am Coll Cardiol* 1988;**12**:589–94.

188. Rathore SS, Gersh BJ, Berger PB, Oetgen WJ, Schulman KA, Solomon AJ: Acute myocardial infarction complicated by heart block in the elderly: prevalence and outcomes: *Am Heart J* 2001;**141**:47–54.

189. Harpaz D, Behar S, Gottlieb S, Boyko V, Kishon Y, Eldar M. Complete atrioventricular block complicating acute myocardial infarction in the thrombolytic era. SPRINT Study Group and the Israeli Thrombolytic Survey Group. Secondary Prevention Reinfarction Israeli Nifedipine Trial. *J Am Coll Cardiol* 1999;**34**:1721–8.

190. Berger PB, Ruocco NA Jr, Ryan TJ, Frederick MM, Jacobs AK, Faxon DP. Incidence and prognostic implications of heart block complicating inferior myocardial infarction treated with thrombolytic therapy: results from TIMI II. *J Am Coll Cardiol* 1992;**20**:533–40.

191. Ritter WS, Atkins JM, Blomqvist CG, Mullins CB. Permanent pacing in patients with transient trifascicular block during acute myocardial infarction. *Am J Cardiol* 1976;**38**:205–8.

192. Atkins JM, Leshin SJ, Blomqvist G, Mullins CB. Ventricular conduction blocks and sudden death in acute myocardial infarction. Potential indications for pacing. *N Engl J Med* 1973;**288**:281–4.

193. Grigg L, Kertes P, Hunt D *et al.* The role of permanent pacing after anterior myocardial infarction complicated by transient complete atrioventricular block. *Aust N Z J Med* 1988;**18**:685–8.

194. Ricou F, Nicod P, Gilpin E, Henning H, Ross J. Influence of right bundle branch block on short- and long-term survival after acute anterior myocardial infarction. *J Am Coll Cardiol* 1991;**17**:858–63.

195. Watson RD, Glover DR, Page AJ *et al.* The Birmingham Trial of permanent pacing in patients with intraventricular conduction disorders after acute myocardial infarction. *Am Heart J* 1984;**108**:496–501.

196. Bosch X, Theroux P, Roy D, Moise A, Waters DD. Coronary angiographic significance of left anterior fascicular block. *J Am Coll Cardiol* 1985;**5**:9–15.

197. Bosch X, Theroux P, Waters DD, Pelletier GB, Roy D. Early postinfarction ischemia: clinical, angiographic, and prognostic significance. *Circulation* 1987;**75**:988–95.

198. De Feyter PJ, Serruys PW, Soward A *et al.* Coronary angioplasty for early postinfarction unstable angina. *Circulation* 1986;**74**:1365–70.

199. Michels KB, Yusuf S. Does PTCA in acute myocardial infarction affect mortality and reinfarction rates? A quantitative overview (meta-analysis) of the randomized clinical trials. *Circulation* 1995;**91**:476–85.

200. Blanton C, Thompson PL. Role of coronary interventional procedures in improved postinfarction survival in the 1990s. *Am J Cardiol* 2001;**87**:832–7.

201. Levine FH, Gold HK, Leinbach RC *et al.* Safe early revascularization for continuing ischemia after acute myocardial infarction. *Circulation* 1979;**60**:I-5–I-9.

202. Kaul TK, Fields BL, Riggins SL, Dacumos GC, Wyatt DA, Jones CR. Coronary artery bypass grafting within 30 days of an acute myocardial infarction. *Ann Thorac Surg* 1995;**59**: 1169–76.

203. Hochberg MS, Parsonnet V, Gielinschky I *et al.* Timing of coronary revascularization after acute myocardial infarction. Early and late results in patients revascularized within seven weeks. *J Thorac Cardiovasc Surg* 1984;**88**:914–21.

204. Gersh BJ, Chesebro JH, Braunwald E *et al.* Coronary artery bypass graft surgery after thrombolytic therapy in the Thrombolysis in Myocardial Infarction Trial, Phase II (TIMI II). *J Am Coll Cardiol* 1995;**25**:395–402.

205. Madsen JK, Grande P, Saunamäki K *et al.* Danish multicenter randomized study of invasive vs conservative treatment in patients with inducible ischemia after thrombolysis in acute myocardial infarction (DANAMI). *Circulation* 1997;**96**: 748–55.

206. Balady G, Fletcher BJ, Froelicher ES *et al.* Cardiac rehabilitation programs. A statement for healthcare professionals from the American Heart Association. *Circulation* 1994;**90**: 1602–10.

207. Frasure-Smith N, Lesperance F, Talajic M. Depression following myocardial infarction. *JAMA* 1993;**270**:1819–25.

208. Frasure-Smith N, Lesperance F, Talajic M. Depression and 18-month prognosis after myocardial infarction. *Circulation* 1995;**91**:999–1005.

209. Ruberman W, Weinblatt E, Goldberg JD *et al.* Psychosocial influences on mortality after myocardial infarction. *N Engl J Med* 1984;**311**:552–9.

210. Ziegelstein RC, Fauerbach JA, Stevens SS *et al.* Patients with depression are less likely to follow recommendations to reduce cardiac risk during recovery from a myocardial infarction. *Arch Intern Med* 2000;**160**:1818–23.

211. Follick MJ, Gorkin L, Capone RJ *et al.* Psychological distress as a predictor of ventricular arrhythmias in a post-myocardial infarction population. *Am Heart J* 1988; **116**:32–6.

212. Nair GV, Gurbel PA, O'Connor CM *et al.* Depression, coronary events, platelet inhibition, and serotonin reuptake inhibitors. *Am J Cardiol* 1999;**84**:321–3.

213. Carney RM, Blumenthal JA, Stein PK *et al.* Depression, heart rate variability, and acute myocardial infarction. *Circulation* 2001;**104**:2024–8.

214. O'Connor GT, Buring JE, Yusuf S *et al.* An overview of randomized trials of rehabilitation with exercise after myocardial infarction. *Circulation* 1989;**80**:234–44.

215. McAlister FA, Lawson FM, Teo KK, Armstrong PW. Randomised trials of secondary prevention programmes in coronary heart disease: systematic review. *BMJ* 2001;**323**: 957–62.

216. Frasure-Smith N, Lesperance F, Prince RH *et al.* Randomised trial of home-based psychosocial nursing intervention for patients recovering from myocardial infarction. *Lancet* 1997; **350**:473–9.

217. Berkman LF, Jaffe AS. Enhancing Recovery In Coronary Heart Disease (ENRICHD) – Treatment of Depression and Social Isolation Post MI. Plenary Session VII. Late Breaking Trials. American Heart Association Scientific Sessions 2001.

218. Shapiro PA, Lesperance F, Frasure-Smith N *et al.* An open-label preliminary trial of sertraline for treatment of major depression after acute myocardial infarction (the SADHAT Trial). Sertraline Anti-Depressant Heart Attack Trial. *Am Heart J* 1999;**137**:1100–6.

36 An integrated approach to the management of patients after the early phase of the acute coronary syndromes

Desmond G Julian

Changing definitions of myocardial infarction and unstable angina

The recent changes in the diagnostic criteria for myocardial infarction (MI) and unstable angina[1] make it difficult to compare contemporary trials with those undertaken many years ago. It is now appreciated that there is a spectrum of acute coronary syndromes and many cases that would previously have been classified as unstable angina would now be designated MI. It is, therefore, no longer appropriate to treat the different syndromes entirely separately. Nonetheless, there are important differences in management depending on whether or not the event is accompanied by, for example, elevation of the ST segment or raised troponin levels.

Management of the postinfarction patient

Treatment of the postinfarction patient can be divided into two categories – secondary prevention and the management of specific complications. Secondary prevention has been studied in many large and well-conducted trials and it is possible to arrive at some firm conclusions as to the optimal program. By contrast, the management of complications has seldom been submitted to randomized controlled trials, mainly for the reason that it may not be ethical to use placebo when seriously ill patients are being treated. Even in this context, however, two or more active treatments can be compared, but this has not often been undertaken.

Secondary prevention trials

Diet and dietary supplements

Although it is usual practice to advise patients after MI to adhere to a lipid lowering diet, no trials to date have shown this to be effective. Nonetheless, as drug trials have demonstrated the beneficial effect of lipid lowering on morbidity and mortality, it seems prudent to advise a diet that would

have a similar effect. It has been found that, if 60% of saturated fats are replaced by other fats and if 60% of the dietary cholesterol is avoided, this would reduce blood total cholesterol level by about 0·8 mmol/l (10–15%),[2] sufficient to achieve a level below 5 mmol/l in many of those with "average" cholesterol levels.

Encouraging data have been provided from four studies in which an increase in the use of omega-3 fatty acids was tested. One study[3] suggested that advising the consumption of fatty fish at least twice a week reduced the risk of re-infarction and death. In a study from India,[4] it was claimed that patients taking a diet high in fiber, omega-3 fatty acids, antioxidants and vitamins had a 42% reduction in cardiac death, and a 45% reduction in total mortality at 1 year compared with a control group on a standard "low fat" diet. In the prematurely terminated Lyon Heart Study,[5] there was reported to be a 70% reduction in MI, coronary mortality, and total mortality after 2 years. In the fourth study, GISSI-Prevenzione,[6] 11 374 patients were randomized to omega-3 or vitamin E after hospital discharge or within 3 months of MI, according to a factorial design. Fish oil, but not vitamin E, showed significant benefit at a median time of 42 months.

Each of the first three trials is open to criticism but, in the absence of any evidence of harm, it is not unreasonable to recommend increased consumption of fatty fish, nuts, vegetables, and fruit.

Smoking

It has not been possible to conduct randomized studies of smoking cessation after MI, but observational studies show that those who quit smoking have a mortality in the succeeding years less than half that of those who continue to do so.[7] This is, therefore, potentially the most effective of all secondary prevention measures. Unfortunately, resumption of smoking is common after return home, and it is important to establish methods to prevent this. A randomized study has demonstrated the effectiveness of a program in which specially trained nurses maintained contact with patients over several months.[8]

Cardiac rehabilitation

Two systematic reviews of exercise-based rehabilitation trials concluded that these reduced mortality after infarction by 20–25%.[9,10] A recent Cochrane review of exercise-based rehabilitation for coronary heart disease (CHD) has been published.[11] This review included not only patients who had experienced MI but also those with angina pectoris or who had undergone revascularization interventions. The outcomes in 8440 patients were reported (7683 contributing to the mortality outcome). For exercise-only interventions, there was a 31% reduction in mortality; the corresponding figure for comprehensive cardiac rehabilitation was 26%.

These claims must be viewed with caution as no single trial has shown a significant benefit, and there has been no evidence of a reduction in re-infarction. Furthermore, it is known that several negative trials of rehabilitation have gone unreported, and the studies showing large reductions in mortality were mainly undertaken before the widespread use of aspirin, β blockers, and ACE inhibitors in postinfarction patients. Nonetheless, there is no doubt that such programs improve exercise performance and a sense of wellbeing, and can be justified on that basis.

Antiplatelet and anticoagulant treatment

The effectiveness of antiplatelet drugs in unstable angina has been demonstrated in many trials, but it must be borne in mind that many patients included in these trials would now be regarded as having sustained an MI. In the US Veterans Administration Study trial of aspirin reported by Lewis *et al*,[12] the intention-to-treat analysis at 12 weeks demonstrated a risk reduction in the primary end point of death and myocardial infarction of 41%. At longer term follow up, mortality was 5·5% in the aspirin group compared with 9·6% in the control group. In the Canadian Multicenter Trial,[13] cardiac death was reduced by aspirin from 9·7% to 4·3%. No benefit was observed with sulfinpyrazone. In the Antithrombotic Trialists' Collaboration report on 12 unstable angina trials of antiplatelet therapy published up to 1997,[14] the number of vascular events was reduced by 46% from 13·3% to 8·0%.

The value of antiplatelet treatment with aspirin in the acute phase of myocardial infarction was shown clearly by the ISIS-2 trial,[15] and this has been further confirmed by the Antithrombotic Trialists' Collaboration.[14] In the latter survey of 19 288 patients included in trials up to 1997, 1 month of antiplatelet treatment was associated with 38 fewer events per 1000 patients, with non-fatal MI being reduced by 13 events per 1000, vascular deaths by 23 per 1000, and non-fatal stroke by two per 1000. Against this

was an increase of one to two extracranial bleeds per 1000. In the trials analyzed, aspirin dosages ranged from 75 to 1500 mg daily. There is some evidence that the lower dosages were effective and produced fewer adverse effects.

In this report,[14] it was also observed that there were 36 fewer serious vascular events in 18 788 patients with a prior history of MI followed for a mean duration of 27 months. There were 18 fewer non-fatal infarctions, 14 fewer vascular deaths, and five fewer non-fatal strokes per 1000 patients treated. On the other hand, there were three additional major extracranial bleeds. Because few patients have contraindications to aspirin therapy, it is appropriate for most postinfarction patients.

Clopidogrel was studied as an alternative to aspirin in the CAPRIE trial of 11 630 survivors of MI.[16] This failed to show any difference between this drug and aspirin in terms of death or re-infarction. It had few side effects and can be considered an alternative for those who cannot be prescribed aspirin.

Subsequently, the CURE trial[17] has demonstrated the value of adding clopidogrel to aspirin in patients with unstable angina, many of whom would now be classified as having sustained an MI because of their enzyme/troponin levels. This combination reduced the primary end point of cardiovascular death, myocardial infarction, and stroke by 20% when administered over a mean period of 9 months. Further trials will be necessary to establish how long it is cost effective to maintain the combination.

The role of antithrombins after myocardial infarction is less clear. In the Antithrombotic Therapy in Acute Coronary Syndromes (ATACS) study,[18] aspirin alone was compared with aspirin with intravenous heparin for 3–4 days, followed by warfarin. The primary outcome of death, MI, and recurrent angina was observed in 27% of the aspirin group compared with 10% in the anticoagulant group ($P = 0·004$). However, the difference was no longer significant at 12 weeks.

In the Fragmin during Instability in Coronary Artery Disease (FRISC) study,[19] aspirin alone was compared with aspirin combined with low molecular weight heparin. While at 6 days, the rate of death and myocardial infarction was 4·8% and 1·8% respectively ($P = 0·001$), the difference at 10·7% and 8·0% respectively was no longer significant at 40 days ($P = 0·07$).

In the Thrombolysis in Myocardial Infarction (TIMI) 11B trial,[20] low molecular weight enoxaparin was compared with intravenous unfractionated heparin during the acute phase, followed by placebo subcutaneous injection for 35 days. At the specified primary outcome time of 43 days, there was a significant reduction in the composite end point of death, re-infarction, and severe recurrent ischemia.

In FRISC II,[21] patients were randomized to the low molecular weight heparin, dalteparin, or placebo. The primary end point of death or MI at 3 months occurred in

6·7% of the dalteparin patients and 8% of those on placebo ($P = 0.17$).

The use of long-term heparin therapy after MI has not been firmly established.

In a meta-analysis of oral anticoagulant trials in patients with coronary artery disease (CAD) performed between 1960 and 1999, Anand and Yusuf[22] concluded that high or moderate intensity oral anticoagulation is effective in reducing MI and stroke but at the expense of an increased risk of bleeding. Low intensity anticoagulation together with aspirin does not seem superior to aspirin alone.

Since this review, two anticoagulant trials have been presented but not yet published. In the Combination Hemotherapy And Mortality Prevention (CHAMP) study,[23] 5059 patients were randomized after an MI to aspirin 160 mg/day or a combination of aspirin 81 mg/day and warfarin titrated to an INR of 1·5–2·5 IU. There was no difference in the end points of overall mortality, cardiovascular mortality, or non-fatal MI.

In the WARIS II trial of antithrombotic therapy after MI,[24] 3630 patients were randomized to one of three regimens: aspirin alone in a dosage of 160 mg/day, warfarin alone to reach a target INR of 2·8–4, or a combination of aspirin 75 mg and warfarin with a target INR of 2·0–2·5. The primary composite end point of death, non-fatal re-infarction, or thromboembolic stroke occurred in 20% of the patients on aspirin, 16·7% of those on warfarin, and 15% of those on a combination of these drugs. The superiority of the combination over aspirin was highly significant at $P = 0.0005$, but there was no significant difference between the two warfarin groups. Major bleeding occurred at a rate of 0·15% per year in the aspirin alone group, 0·58% per year in the warfarin alone group, and 0·52%/year in the combined group. It may be concluded that the beneficial effect of aspirin after MI may be augmented by the addition of warfarin.

Whilst it is clear that adding clopidogrel to aspirin is beneficial in those who have experienced unstable angina, it is still unresolved whether adding this drug to those who have had an ST elevation MI is cost effective.

Whether antithrombins should be routinely used is uncertain. It is likely that the beneficial results of WARIS II reflect the use of a more effective anticoagulant regimen.

β Blockers

Several trials and meta-analyses undertaken in the pre-fibrinolytic era have demonstrated that β adrenoceptor blocking drugs reduce mortality and re-infarction by 20–25% in those who have recovered from acute MI.[25,26] Recently, the CAPRICORN trial of carvedilol involved 1959 postinfarction patients with a left ventricular ejection fraction of 40% or less:[27] 46% of the patients had been treated with fibrinolysis or primary angioplasty, and nearly all patients were also being treated with ACE inhibitors and

aspirin. All-cause mortality was reduced from 15% to 12% ($P = 0.03$). This study confirms that β blockers add to the benefit of ACE inhibitors and are of value in patients with impaired left ventricular function, many of whom have experienced heart failure. It is not possible to say whether carvedilol is superior to the other β blockers (propranolol, metoprolol, timolol, and acebutolol), which have been shown to be effective in the postinfarction patient.

Physicians have been, in the past, reluctant to administer β blockers to patients who are or have been in cardiac failure. This has been partly responsible for the relatively low usage of β blockers in the postinfarction patient. Recent trials in heart failure (see below) have shown that patients with heart failure benefit from β blockers, provided the heart failure is stable and the dosage carefully uptitrated.

About one quarter of postinfarction patients have contraindications to β blockade because of uncontrolled heart failure, respiratory disease, or other conditions. Of the remainder, perhaps half can be defined as of low risk,[26,28] in whom β blockade exerts only a marginal benefit, bearing in mind the minor though sometimes troublesome side effects. β Blockers are most clearly indicated in the higher risk patient without contraindications.

Calcium antagonists

Trials with dihydropyridine calcium antagonists[29] have failed to show a benefit in terms of improved prognosis after MI.

One trial with verapamil[30] (DAVIT-II) suggested that it prevented re-infarction and death. Trials with diltiazem[31] have failed to show a reduction in mortality; indeed, it was increased in those with impaired left ventricular function. A review of heart rate-lowering antagonists in hypertensive postinfarction patients[32] showed a decrease in mortality and recurrent infarction in hypertensive postinfarction patients without heart failure, but an increase in those with this complication. The INTERCEPT trial[33] compared once daily diltiazem with placebo in 874 patients with acute MI, not complicated by heart failure, who had been treated with fibrinolysis. There was no significant reduction in the primary end point of a composite of cardiac death, non-fatal re-infarction, or refractory ischemia, but there was a reduction in non-fatal cardiac events and in the need for revascularization.

Nitrates

Oral or transdermal nitrates did not improve prognosis in the first few weeks after MI in the ISIS-4[34] and GISSI-3[35] trials. There have been no long-term trials of nitrates after MI.

Angiotensin converting enzyme (ACE) inhibitors

Several trials have established that ACE inhibitors reduce mortality after acute MI.[36–40] In the SAVE trial,[36] patients who survived the acute phase of infarction were recruited to receive captopril or placebo if they had an ejection fraction less than 40% on nuclear imaging, and if they were free of manifest ischemia on an exercise test. No mortality benefit was seen in the first year, but there was a 19% mortality reduction in 3–5 years of follow up (from 24·6 to 20·4%) (*P* = 0·019). Fewer re-infarctions and less heart failure were, however, seen even within the first year. In the AIRE trial[37] postinfarction patients were randomized to ramipril or placebo after an MI that had been complicated by the clinical or radiological features of heart failure. At an average of 15 months later, the mortality was reduced from 22·6% to 16·9% (a 27% reduction) (*P* = 0·002). In the TRACE study,[38] patients were randomized to trandolapril or placebo if they had left ventricular dysfunction as demonstrated by a wall motion index of 1·2 or less. At an average follow up of 108 weeks, the mortality was 34·7% in the treated group and 42·3% in the placebo group (*P* = 0·001).

A systematic review of these trials[39] found that at a mean treatment duration of 31 months, there were 702 deaths (23·4%) of 2995 patients randomized to receive ACE inhibitor and 866 (29·1%) of 2971 randomized to control (*P* < 0·0001). Comparable figures for re-infarction were 10·8% and 13·2% (*P* < 0·0057).

In the SMILE (Survival of Myocardial Infarction Long-Term Evaluation) study,[40] 1556 patients with anterior MI were randomized to zofenopril or placebo within 24 hours of onset, the treatment being continued for 6 weeks. At 1 year, the mortality rate was significantly lower in the zofenopril group (10·0%) than in the placebo group (14·1%) (*P* = 0·011). These studies provide powerful evidence of the effectiveness of ACE inhibitors in patients who have experienced heart failure in the acute event, even if no features of this persist, who have an ejection fraction of less than 40%, or a wall motion index of 1·2 or less, provided there are no contraindications. Analysis of the results of these studies indicate that ACE inhibitors are beneficial not only in patients with poor left ventricular function even if they have not experienced heart failure, but also in those who have suffered from heart failure even if their left ventricular function is relatively good. The SMILE study suggests that ACE inhibitor therapy may be appropriate for anterior infarction even in the absence of poor ventricular function. As discussed in chapter 34, there is a case for administering ACE inhibitors to all patients with acute infarction from admission, provided there are no contraindications. Against such a policy is the increased incidence of hypotension and renal failure in those receiving ACE inhibitors in the acute stage, and the small benefit in those at relatively low risk, such as patients with small inferior infarctions.

The indications for ACE inhibitors after infarction have been radically altered following the results of the Heart Outcomes Prevention Evaluation Study (HOPE).[41] This study of ramipril versus placebo included a wide range of patients at high risk of serious cardiovascular events, but 52% of the patients had had a prior MI and 25% unstable angina. Patients with a history of clinical heart failure or a ejection fraction known to be less than 0·40 were excluded. There seemed little difference in the relative benefit observed in the different categories of patients included in the trial, and the overall results may be taken to apply to postinfarction patients. There was a very clear reduction in the primary end point of a composite of cardiovascular death, heart attack, and stroke in the ramipril arm (placebo 17·8%, ramipril 14·0% *P* < 0·001). The incidence of MI was reduced from 12·3% to 9·9%, and stroke from 4·9% to 3·4%. There were comparable reductions in overall mortality, need for hospitalization, and revascularization. It is not yet known whether similar results would be seen with other ACE inhibitors, but this question should be answered by the ongoing EUROPA trial with perindopril[42] and the PEACE trial with trandolapril.[43]

Antiarrhythmic drugs

Trials of antiarrhythmic drugs after MI have proved disappointing. A meta-analysis of 18 trials of Class I drugs showed a significant 21% increase in mortality.[44] The SWORD trial[45] of the Class III drug *d*-sotalol was stopped because of an increased mortality. The Class III agent dofetilide was studied in the DIAMOND trial of 1510 patients with recent MI and left ventricular dysfunction.[46] There was no difference between dofetilide and placebo with regard to overall mortality, cardiac mortality, or arrhythmic death. Similar results have been reported with azimilide in the Azimilide post-Infarct Survival Evaluation trial (ALIVE).[47]

Amiodarone has been studied in four trials. Two small trials were favorable, but the two larger trials – EMIAT[48] and CAMIAT[49] – failed to demonstrate a reduction in total mortality. However, there was a reduction in arrhythmic death in these studies, and a pooling of results from amiodarone trials following MI shows a significant reduction in arrhythmic death (2·6% *v* 4·2% per year) and a non-significant trend towards lower total mortality (10·9% *v* 12·3%).[50] Unlike the other Class I and III antiarrhythmic drugs, amiodarone does not appear to have an important pro-arrhythmic effect, but its use is limited by its significant side effects.

Lipid lowering agents

The Scandinavian Simvastatin Survival Study (4S)[51] clearly demonstrated the benefits of lipid lowering in a population of 4444 anginal and/or postinfarction patients with serum cholesterol levels of 5·5–8·0 mmol/l (212–308 mg/dl) after dietary measures had been tried. Overall mortality at a median of 5·4 years was reduced by 30% (from 12 to 8%) (*P* = 0·0001). This represented 33 lives saved per 1000 patients treated over this period. There were substantial reductions in coronary mortality and in the need for coronary bypass surgery. Older patients appeared to benefit as much as younger patients. Relatively few women were recruited, perhaps accounting for the failure to show a significant reduction in mortality, but coronary events were reduced as they were in men.

In the Cholesterol and Recurrent Events (CARE) trial,[52] 4159 post-MI infarction patients with "average" cholesterol levels were randomized to pravastatin or placebo at least 3 months after the acute event: 13·2% of the placebo group and 10·2% of the treatment group ($P = 0.003$) experienced a primary end point (fatal coronary event or non-fatal MI) in the trial which lasted 5 years. There was also a reduction in stroke and in the need for coronary artery bypass surgery and angioplasty. The effects appeared to be greater in women than in men, and in those with higher low density lipoprotein (LDL) levels. Indeed, no benefit was shown in patients with LDL levels below 125 mg/dl (3·25 mmol/l).

In the Long-term Intervention with pravastatin in ischemic heart disease (LIPID) study,[53] 9014 patients with a history of MI or unstable angina, and with cholesterol 4·0–7·0 mmol/l were randomized to pravastatin or placebo. After a mean follow up of 6·1 years, overall death rate was 14·1% in the placebo group and 11·0% in the pravastatin group ($P < 0.001$) – coronary death rates were 8·3% and 6·4% respectively. There were corresponding reductions in MI and need for revascularization.

The Heart Protection Study (HPS)[54] has provided further information about certain categories of patient, such as women and the elderly, poorly represented in the earlier trials. It has shown that these groups are also benefitted to a similar degree.

The trials cited above were started in postinfarction patients some months or years after the acute event. To determine whether patients would benefit from an earlier administration of lipid lowering, the MIRACL trial[55] of atorvastatin versus placebo was started within days of the onset of unstable angina in 3086 patients not scheduled for early intervention. The primary end point of death, non-fatal MI, resuscitated cardiac arrest, and recurrent symptomatic myocardial ischemia occurred in 14·8% of the atorvastatin patients and 17·4% of the placebo patients ($P = 0.048$). The benefit was essentially confined to the prevention of recurrent myocardial ischemia.

In the FLORIDA study,[56] patients with a recent MI and a cholesterol value less than 6·5 mmol/l on admission were started on fluvastatin or placebo immediately on discharge. The primary end point was that of myocardial ischemia on Holter monitoring; this was observed in 17% of both groups, but at 1 year 2·6% of the fluvastatin group and 4·0% of the placebo group had died. It is difficult to draw confident conclusions from these studies, but it would seem that it is safe to start lipid lowering therapy soon after the acute event,

and it may be wise to do so if the patient is known to be hyperlipidemic in spite of dietary measures.

In the VA-HIT trial,[57] 2531 men with documented CHD, with HDL cholesterol at or less than 40 mg/dl (1 mmol/l), LDL cholesterol at or less than 140 mg/dl (3·6 mmol/l), and triglycerides at or less than 300 mg/dl were randomized to gemfibrozil or placebo. There was a significant reduction in the combined end point of coronary death and MI in the treatment arm, with events occurring in 21·6% of the placebo group and 17·3% of the gemfibrozil group ($P = 0.006$). There were non-significant reductions in death due to CHD, total death, and stroke, but there was a significant reduction in non-fatal MI (from 14·5% to 11·6%, $P = 0.02$).

The Bezafibrate Infarction Prevention (BIP) trial[58] randomized 3090 patients with previous MI or stable angina to bezafibrate or placebo. The primary end point of MI or sudden death occurred in 13·6% of those on bezafibrate and 15·0% in those on placebo ($P = 0.26$).

These trials have firmly established the use of statins in post-MI patients with "average" or high lipid levels. Furthermore, patients with lipid abnormalities other those studied in these trials (for example, hypertriglyceridemia) might benefit from other lipid lowering regimens.

Hormone replacement therapy (HRT)

Many epidemiologic trials have suggested that HRT might reduce cardiovascular risk substantially, but the only large-scale trial in patients with CHD – the Heart and Estrogen/progestin trial (HERS)[59] – showed a significant (52%) increase in the primary combined end point of non-fatal MI and coronary death in the first year of treatment (42·5/1000 person-years compared with 28·0 in the placebo group). There was a trend towards fewer events in the treated group in the ensuing years and, at an average of 4·1 years, there was no longer a significant difference between the two groups. The ongoing Estrogen in the Prevention of Reinfarction Trial (ESPRIT) is studying the effect of estrogen alone in a postinfarction population.

Percutaneous coronary interventions (PCI) and coronary artery bypass graft surgery (CABG)

The role of coronary interventions in preventing recurrent infarction and death when performed in the days after MI remains uncertain. The SWIFT (Should We Intervene Following Thrombolysis?),[58] TIMI-II,[61] and TIMI IIIB trials[61] failed to show any benefit from intervention in terms of recurrent infarction and death in patients after fibrinolysis.

In the Veterans Affairs Non-Q wave Infarction Strategies in-Hospital (VANQWISH) trial,[63] patients with non-Q wave MI were randomized to an invasive or a conservative strategy. In the former, cardiac catheterization was carried out within 3 to 7 days, and, subsequently, PTCA or CABG was carried out according to the coronary anatomy; a total of 920 patients were randomized. Death and MI occurred in 7·8% of the invasive arm and 5·7% of the conservative arm at hospital discharge ($P = 0.012$).

In the Danish Acute Myocardial Infarction (DANAMI) study,[64] however, 1008 survivors of a first acute infarction in whom ischemia could be induced were randomized to catheterization and revascularization, or standard medical therapy. There were significantly fewer non-fatal infarctions in the 2·5 year follow up period in those who underwent revascularization ($P = 0.0038$), as well as a reduction in hospitalization and in medical costs.

In the FRISC II trial,[65] there was a significant reduction in death and/or MI in those randomized to coronary angiography, followed, if appropriate, by angioplasty or CABG in patients with unstable CAD. At 6 months, there was a reduction in the composite end point of death and MI from 12·1% in the non-invasive group to 9·4% in the invasive group ($P = 0.031$). At 1 year, the comparable figures were 14·1% versus 10·4% ($P = 0.005$).[66] The benefit was predominantly in those with raised troponin levels and/or ST depression at entry. There was no evidence of a benefit in women.[67]

In TACTICS-TIMI-18,[68] 2220 patients with an acute coronary syndrome without ST elevation were all administered tirofiban, and randomized to a conservative or invasive strategy. The primary end point of death, MI, or rehospitalization at 6 months occurred in 19·4% of the conservative group, and 15·9% in the invasive group ($P = 0.025$). Death and/or MI occurred in 9·5% and 7·3% respectively ($P < 0.05$). The benefit seemed to be largely confined to those with elevation in troponin or creatine kinase, and in those without prior aspirin treatment.

It seems probable that an invasive approach is appropriate for acute coronary syndromes if there are raised cardiac markers or active ischemia and when there has not been an intervention during the acute event. The place of such a strategy in women, or in those who have not shown these features, remains uncertain.

Management of the complications of MI

Cardiac failure

On the basis of the trials with ACE inhibitors described above and the results of the Consensus[69] and SOLVD[70] trials, ACE inhibitors should be given to patients in heart failure without contraindications, in addition to diuretics and, perhaps, digitalis. The use of diuretics and digitalis is largely based on observational studies.

Several trials have established the value of β blockers in the treatment of heart failure, which, in the majority of cases, was due to ischemic heart disease. The Cardiac Insufficiency Bisoprolol Study II (CIBIS II)[71] of patients with NYHA (New York Heart Association) classes III and IV was

stopped prematurely, after it was found that the bisoprolol-treated group had a highly significantly better survival rate than the placebo group. At an average of 1·4 years, there was a 17·3% mortality rate in the placebo group compared with 11·8% in the bisoprolol group. The Metoprolol CR/XL Randomized Intervention Trial in Congestive Heart Failure (MERIT-HF)[72] was similar, except that the active agent was metoprolol and it included patients with NYHA class II heart failure. All-cause mortality was lower in the metoprolol CR/XL group than in the placebo group (7·2%, per patient-year of follow up v 11·0%, $P = 0.00009$). In the COPERNICUS trial (Carvedilol Prospective Randomized Cumulative Survival),[73] 2289 patients with severe chronic heart failure were randomized to carvedilol or placebo. There were 190 deaths in the placebo group and 135 in the carvedilol group – a 35% reduction in the risk of death ($P = 0.0014$). By contrast, no overall benefit was seen in the BEST (Beta-blocker Evaluation Survival trial)[74] in which 2708 patients with severe chronic heart failure were randomized to receive either bucindolol or placebo. A subgroup analysis suggested that there was a benefit in non-black patients. Whether the different results in BEST were due to chance, the drug being tested, or a different population is uncertain. It would seem that β blockade is effective in patients with heart failure without contraindications.

The Randomized Aldactone Evaluation Study (RALES) study[75] concerned patients with a history of NYHA class IV heart failure and an ejection fraction of less than 40%, who had already received ACE inhibitor therapy. Patients were randomized to receive spironolactone or placebo. The trial was stopped when patients had been followed for a minimum of 18 months. Mortality was reduced by a quarter from 40% to 27% ($P = 0.001$).

It seems reasonable to suggest that patients with NYHA class II–III should receive both β blockers and ACE inhibitors, and that spironolactone should be added in the more severe cases.

Angina pectoris

There have been few randomized studies of the therapy of angina after infarction. The DANAMI[64] study referred to above suggests that PTCA and CABG have an important role in controlling symptoms and improving prognosis.

Life-threatening arrhythmias

As mentioned above, the use of antiarrhythmic drugs is potentially hazardous in the postinfarction patient. However, the findings of the EMIAT[47] and CAMIAT[48] studies have shown that amiodarone is relatively free of arrhythmogenesis, and is effective in preventing sudden death in high-risk patients without life-threatening arrhythmias. It seems an appropriate therapy for those with such arrhythmias.

The place of implantable defibrillators (ICD) in the post-infarction patient with arrhythmias remains uncertain, although recent trials have been encouraging. In the Multicenter Automatic Defibrillator Implantation Trial (MADIT),[76] 202 patients with prior MI, together with an ejection fraction of 0·35 or less, unsustained ventricular tachycardia, and non-suppressible ventricular tachycardia on electrophysiologic study, were randomly assigned to an implantable defibrillator or conventional medical therapy. At an average follow up of 27 months, there were 15 deaths in the defibrillator group and 39 deaths in the conventionally treated group ($P = 0·009$).

In the Antiarrhythmics versus Implantable Defibrillators (AVID) Trial,[77] in which many of the patients were post-infarction, half of those included had experienced ventricular fibrillation and the other half serious ventricular tachycardia. After three years, 25% of the patients in the defibrillator group had died compared with 36% of patients treated with antiarrhythmic drugs ($P < 0·02$).

In the Multicenter Automatic Defibrillator Implantation Trial II (MADIT II)[78] postinfarction patients with an ejection fraction of 0·30 or less were randomized to an implantable defibrillator or conventional medical therapy. At an average follow up of 20 months, 19·8% of the conventional group had died compared with 14.2% of the defibrillator group ($P = 0·016$).

It is evident that an implantable defibrillator is highly effective in the types of patient included in these studies, but its eventual place in the prevention of sudden death following MI remains to be determined.

Limitations of the evidence available

While randomized clinical trials provide the most reliable evidence of efficacy, their findings may not readily be applied to a wide spectrum of patients with the given condition, particularly if the entry criteria are very rigidly defined. Furthermore, even though the internal validity may be beyond question, few trials are sufficiently powered to permit reliable estimates of effect in subgroups, such as women or the elderly, or in relation to concomitant therapy. The latter problem is compounded by the fact that there may be interactions between effective agents.

Subgroup analysis is rightly suspect, although it is important to differentiate between "proper subgroups" (based on baseline characteristics) and "improper subgroups" based on findings after entry into the trial.[79] Analysis of proper subgroups may be of great importance, particularly when there are marked differences in risk in various baseline characteristics so that, even if the effect of therapy is relatively the same whatever the risk, the absolute effect will be very different. In postinfarction and postunstable angina patients, it is possible to define high-, medium-, and low-risk patients on quite simple clinical and investigational criteria, and the

probable effect of the secondary preventive treatment can then be estimated. Thus, one can anticipate little benefit from β blockers or ACE inhibitors in a patient with a small inferior first infarction who has had no complications in the acute phase, whereas the patient, who has had heart failure brought under control, remains at high risk and would benefit from both these therapies.

A further problem with applying trial results to practice is that of adherence to therapy. There is abundant evidence that compliance falls off if therapies have to be taken more than twice a day and when more than three types of drug are prescribed. It is now commonplace for patients to be given five or more drug therapies, and several widely recommended drugs (for example, captopril) have to be taken three or more times a day.

Increasingly, the cost of therapies is being critically scrutinized. An outstanding example is that of the statins, which are now being recommended for most patients with manifest coronary disease. As pointed out by Yusuf and Anand,[80] based on the 4S study, the cost effectiveness of this therapy in high-risk individuals is very favorable. Pedersen *et al*[81] have concluded that the drug costs of treatment are largely offset by savings that result from fewer hospitalizations and less need for revascularization.

These estimates were made on assumptions from the United States. They will be very different in countries with substantially lower hospitalization costs but are also very sensitive to the cost of the drug.

Both compliance issues and health economic considerations argue for economy in the prescription of drugs, and this will influence the integrated approach to management.

An integrated approach to post-MI and unstable angina patients

As far as secondary prevention is concerned, it is possible to base therapy on the results of well-conducted randomized clinical trials. However, one must bear in mind that it may not be feasible to undertake randomized trials with regard to certain lifestyle factors, such as smoking and diet, nor can patients with major remediable symptoms be subjected to placebo-controlled trials. One can, however, advise the cessation of smoking based on strong observational data, and recommend a "Mediterranean" diet, knowing that it is probably beneficial and unlikely to have any harmful effects. The same is true of exercise-based rehabilitation programs.

Aspirin should be administered to all patients with these diagnoses, unless contraindicated. Clopidogrel should be added, at least in the short term, to patients who have had an acute coronary syndrome without ST elevation; it is still not possible to conclude for how long it should be given, or whether it should be given to patients who have sustained an ST elevation MI.

β Blockers should be considered in all patients but the risks and benefits should be carefully weighed up in those at low risk. Calcium antagonists and nitrates should be prescribed for symptomatic reasons only, the former should probably be avoided in those with heart failure or poor left ventricular function.

ACE inhibitors should be prescribed for all patients (except those with contraindications) who have been or are in heart failure, as well as those who have poor left ventricular function. There is also a strong case for giving ramipril to patients who fulfill the criteria of the HOPE trial.

Patients with average or raised lipid levels should first be treated by dietary means, but appropriate lipid modifying therapy should be given if an adequate fall in LDL is not achieved.

PTCA and CABG should be considered in patients with recurrent angina or easily provoked ischemia. Such patients should have coronary angiography and the choice of treatment determined by the anatomical and functional findings.

Evidence-based secondary prevention therapies for postinfarction patients

- Smoking cessation **Grade B**
- Lipid lowering diet **Grade C**
- Lipid lowering drugs if diet fails **Grade A**
- Aspirin for all patients without contraindications. **Grade A** Other antiplatelet agents (for example, clopidogrel) if aspirin contraindicated. **Grade A** Clopidogrel added to aspirin in patients who have experienced non-ST segment elevation MI or unstable angina. **Grade A**
- β Blockers, particularly for high-risk patients, in the absence of contraindications. **Grade A**
- ACE inhibitors for all patients with severely impaired left ventricular function or heart failure. **Grade A**
- In the absence of heart failure, ramipril for those who fulfill the criteria for the HOPE trial. **Grade A**
- Percutaneous transluminal angioplasty or CABG for patients with persistent readily induced ischemia or angina, **Grade A** or for patients with non-ST segment elevation MI or unstable angina with raised troponin levels. **Grade A**

References

1. The Joint European Society of Cardiology/American College of Cardiology Committee. Myocardial infarction redefined. *J Am Coll Cardiol* 2000;**36**:959–69.

2. Clarke R, Frost C, Collins R, Appleby P, Peto R. Dietary lipids and blood cholesterol: quantitative meta-analysis of metabolic ward studies. *BMJ* 1997;**314**:112–17.

3. Burr ML, Fehily AM, Gilbert JF *et al.* The effects of changes in fat, fish and fibre intakes on death and myocardial infarction: diet and reinfarction trial. *Lancet.* 1989;**ii**:757–81.

4. Singh RB, Rastogi SS, Verma T *et al.* Randomised controlled trial of cardioprotective diet in patients with acute myocardial infarction: results of one year follow-up. *BMJ* 1992;**304**:1015–19.

5. de Lorgeril M, Renaud S, Mamelle N *et al.* Mediterranean alpha-linolenic acid-rich diet in secondary prevention of coronary heart disease. *Lancet* 1994;**343**:1454–9.

6. GISSI-Prevenzione Investigators (Gruppo Italiano per lo Studio della Sopravvivenza nell'Infarto miocardico). Dietary supplementation with n-3 polyunsaturated fatty acids and vitamin E after myocardial infarction: results of the GISSI-Prevenzione trial. *Lancet* 1999;**354**:447–55.

7. Åberg A, Bergstrand R, Johansson S *et al.* Cessation of smoking after myocardial infarction. Effects on mortality after 10 years. *Br Heart J* 1983;**49**:416–22.

8. Taylor CB, Houston-Miller N, Killen JD, De Busk RF. Smoking cessation after acute myocardial infarction: effect of a nurse-managed intervention. *Ann Intern Med* 1990;**113**:118–32.

9. O'Connor GT, Buring JE, Yusuf S *et al.* An overview of randomized trials of rehabilitation with exercise after myocardial infarction. *Circulation* 1989;**80**:234–44.

10. Oldridge NB, Guyatt GH, Fischer MD, Rimm AA. Cardiac rehabilitation after myocardial infarction: combined experience of randomized trials. *JAMA* 1988;**260**:945–50.

11. Jolliffe JA, Rees K, Taylor RS, Thompson D, Oldridge N, Ebrahim S. Exercise-based rehabilitation for coronary heart disease (Cochrane Review). *Cochrane Database Syst Rev* 2001;**1**:CD001800.

12. Lewis HD, Davis J, Archibald D *et al.* Protective effects of aspirin against acute myocardial infarction and death in men with unstable angina. *N Engl J Med* 1983;**309**:396–403.

13. Cairns J, Gent M, Singer J *et al.* Aspirin, sulfinpyrazone or both in unstable angina: results of a Canadian Multicenter trial. *N Engl J Med* 1985;**313**:1369–75.

14. Antiplatelet Trialists' Collaboration. Collaborative meta-analysis of randomised trials of antiplatelet therapy for prevention of death, myocardial infarction, and stroke in high-risk patients. *BMJ* 2002;**324**:71–80.

15. ISIS-2 (Second International Study of Infarct Survival Collaborative Group). Randomised trial of intravenous streptokinase, oral aspirin, both or neither among 17 187 cases of suspected myocardial infarction. ISIS-2. *Lancet* 1988;**ii**:349–60.

16. CAPRIE Steering Committee. A randomised, blinded, trial of clopidogrel versus aspirin in patients at risk of ischaemic events (CAPRIE). *Lancet* 1996;**348**:1329–39.

17. The Clopidogrel in Unstable Angina to Prevent Events Trial Investigators. Effects of clopidogrel in addition to aspirin in patients with acute coronary syndromes without ST-segment elevation. *N Engl J Med* 2001;**345**:494–502.

18. Cohen M, Adams P, Parry G *et al.* on behalf of the Antithrombotic Therapy in Acute Coronary Syndromes Research Group. Combination antithrombotic therapy in unstable angina and non-Q wave infarction in non-prior aspirin users: primary end-points from the ATACS trial. *Circulation* 1994;**89**:81–8.

19. Fragmin during Instability in Coronary Artery Disease (FRISC) Study Group. Low molecular weight heparin during instability in coronary artery disease. *Lancet* 1996;**347**:561–8.

20. Antman EM, McCabe CH, Gurfinkel EP *et al.* Enoxaparin prevents death and cardiac ischemic events in unstable

angina/non-Q wave myocardial infarction. *Circulation* 1999; **100**:1593–1601.

21. Fragmin and Fast Revascularisation during InStability in Coronary artery disease (FRISC II) investigators. Low molecular-mass heparin in unstable coronary artery disease: FRISC II prospective randomised multicenter study. *Lancet* 1999;**354**:701–7.

22. Anand SS, Yusuf S. Oral anticoagulant therapy in patients with coronary artery disease: a meta-analysis. *JAMA* 1999; **282**:2058–67.

23. CHAMP. Presented at American Heart Association 1999.

24. WARIS II. Presented at the European Society of Cardiology. Stockholm. September 2001.

25. Yusuf S, Lessem J, Jha P, Lonn E. Primary and secondary prevention of myocardial infarction and strokes: An update of randomly allocated controlled trials. *J Hypertens* 1993;**11** (Suppl. 4):S61–S73.

26. The Beta-Blocker Pooling Project Research Group. The Beta-Blocker Pooling Project (BBPP): subgroup findings from randomized trials in post infarction patients. *Eur Heart J* 1988; **9**:8–16.

27. The CAPRICORN Investigators. Effect of carvedilol on outcome after myocardial infarction in patients with left-ventricular dysfunction: the CAPRICORN randomised trial. *Lancet* 2001;**357**:1385–90.

28. Furberg CD, Hawkins CM, Lichstein F. Effect of propranolol in postinfarction patients with mechanical and electrical complications. *Circulation* 1983;**69**:761–5.

29. Yusuf S, Held P, Furberg C. Update of effects of calcium antagonists in myocardial infarction or angina in light of the second Danish Verapamil Infarction Trial (DAVIT-II) and other recent studies. *Am J Cardiol* 1991;**67**:1295–7.

30. The Danish Study Group on Verapamil in Myocardial Infarction. Effect of verapamil on mortality and major events after myocardial infarction (the Danish Verapamil Infarction Trial II-DAVIT II). *Am J Cardiol* 1990;**66**:779–85.

31. The Multicenter Diltiazem Postinfarction Trial Research Group. The effect of diltiazem on mortality and reinfarction after myocardial infarction. *N Engl J Med* 1988;**319**:385–92.

32. Messerli FH, Hansen JF, Gibson RS, Schechtman KB, Boden WE. Heart-rate lowering calcium antagonists in hypertensive post-myocardial infarction patients. *J Hypertens* 2001; **19**:977–82.

33. Boden WE, Wiek H van G, Scheldewaert RG *et al*. Diltiazem in acute myocardial infarction treated with thrombolytic agents: a randomised placebo controlled trial. *Lancet* 2000; **355**:1751–6.

34. ISIS-4 (Fourth International Study on Infarct Survival) Collaborative group. ISIS-4: A randomised factorial trial assessing early oral captopril, oral mononitrate and intravenous magnesium in 58,000 patients with suspected acute myocardial infarction. *Lancet* 1995;**345**:669–85.

35. Gruppo Italiano per lo Studio della Sopravivenza nell'infarto Miocardico. GISSI-3: Effects of lisinopril and transdermal nitrate singly and together on 6-week mortality and ventricular function after acute myocardial infarction. *Lancet* 1994; **343**:1115–22.

36. Pfeffer MA, Braunwald E, Moyé LA *et al*. Effect of captopril on mortality and morbidity in patients with left ventricular dysfunction after myocardial infarction. *N Engl J Med* 1992;**327**:669–77.

37. AIRE (Acute Infarction Ramipril Efficacy) Investigators. Effect of ramipril on mortality and morbidity of survivors of acute myocardial infarction with clinical evidence of heart failure. *Lancet* 1993;**342**:821–8.

38. Køber L, Torp-Pedersen C, Carlsen JE *et al*. A clinical trial of the angiotensin converting enzyme inhibitor trandolapril in patients with left ventricular dysfunction after myocardial infarction. *N Engl J Med* 1995;**333**:1670–6.

39. Flather MD, Yusuf S, Køber L *et al*. Long-term ACE-inhibitor therapy in patients with heart failure or left-ventricular dysfunction: a systematic overview of data from individual patients. *Lancet* 2000;**355**:1575–81.

40. Ambrosioni E, Borghi C, Magnani B. The effect of angiotensin-converting enzyme inhibitor zofenopril on mortality and morbidity after anterior myocardial infarction. The Survival of Myocardial Infarction Long-Term Evaluation (SMILE) Study Investigators. *N Engl J Med* 1995;**332**:80–5.

41. The Heart Outcomes Prevention Evaluation Study Investigators. Effects of an angiotensin converting-enzyme inhibitor, ramipril, on cardiovascular events in high-risk patients. *N Engl J Med* 2000;**342**:145–53.

42. Pfeffer MA, Domanski M, Rosenberg Y *et al*. Prevention of events with angiotensin-converting enzyme inhibition (the PEACE study design). Prevention of Events with Angiotensin-Converting Enzyme Inhibition. *Am J Cardiol* 1998;**82**: 25H–30H.

43. Fox KM, Henderson JR, Bertrand ME, Ferrari R, Remme WJ, Simoons ML. The European trial on reduction of cardiac events with perindopril in stable coronary artery disease (EUROPA). *Eur Heart J* 1998;**19**(Suppl. J):J52–5.

44. Teo KK, Yusuf S, Furberg CD. Effects of prophylactic antiarrhythmic drug therapy in acute myocardial infarction: an overview of results from randomized controlled trials. *JAMA* 1993;**270**:1589–95.

45. Waldo AL, Camm AJ, deRuyter H *et al*. Effect of d-sotalol on mortality in patients with left ventricular dysfunction after recent and remote myocardial infarction. *Lancet* 1996; **348**:7–12.

46. Køber L and others. Effect of dofetilide in patients with recent myocardial infarction and left ventricular dysfunction: a randomised study. *Lancet* 2000;**356**:2052–8.

47. ALIVE, Presented at the American Heart Association. November 2001.

48. Julian DG, Camm AJ, Frangin G *et al*. Randomised trial of effect of amiodarone on mortality in patients with left ventricular dysfunction after recent myocardial infarction: EMIAT. European Myocardial Infarct Amiodarone Trial Investigators. *Lancet* 1997;**349**:667–74.

49. Cairns JA, Connolly SJ, Roberts R, Gent M. Randomised trial of outcome after myocardial infarction in patients with frequent or repetitive ventricular premature depolarisations: CAMIAT. Canadian Amiodarone Myocardial Infarction Arrhythmia Trial Investigators. *Lancet* 1997;**349**:675–82.

50. Connolly SJ. Meta-analysis of antiarrhythmic drug trials. *Am J Cardiol* 1999; **84**(Suppl. 1):90–3.

51. Scandinavian Simvastatin Survival Study Group. Randomised trial of cholesterol lowering in 4444 patients with coronary

heart disease: the Scandinavian Simvastatin Survival Study (4S). *Lancet* 1994;**344**:1383–9.

52. Sacks FM, Pfeffer MA, Moye LA *et al*. The effect of pravastatin on coronary events after myocardial infarction in patients with average cholesterol levels. *N Engl J Med* 1996;**335**: 1001–9.

53. The Long-Term Intervention with Pravastatin in Ischaemic Disease (LIPID) Study Group. Prevention of cardiovascular events and death with pravastatin in patients with coronary heart disease and a broad base of initial cholesterol levels. *N Engl J Med* 1998;**339**:1349–54.

54. Heart Protection Study presented at the American Heart Association, November 2001.

55. Schwartz GG, Olsson AG, Ezekowitz MD *et al*. Effects of atorvastatin on early recurrent ischemic events in acute coronary syndromes: the MIRACL study: a randomized controlled trial. *JAMA* 2001;**285**:1711–18.

56. FLORIDA, Presented at the American Heart Association, 2000.

57. Rubens HB, Robins SJ, Collins D *et al*. Gemfibrozil for the secondary prevention of coronary heart disease in men with low levels of high-density lipoprotein cholesterol. *N Engl J Med* 1999;**341**:410–18.

58. The BIP Study Group. Secondary prevention by raising HDL cholesterol and reducing triglycerides in patients with coronary artery disease. The bezafibrate infarction prevention (BIP) study. *Circulation* 2000;**102**:21–7.

59. Hulley S, Grady D, Bush T *et al*. Randomized trial of estrogen plus progestin for secondary prevention of coronary heart disease in postmenopausal women. *JAMA* 1998;**290**:605–13.

60. SWIFT (Should we intervene following thrombolysis ?) Study Group. SWIFT trial of delayed elective intervention *v* conservative treatment after thrombolysis with anistreplase in acute myocardial infarction. *BMJ* 1991;**302**:555–60.

61. The TIMI Study Group. Comparison of invasive and conservative strategies after treatment with intravenous tissue plasminogen activator in acute myocardial infarction: results of the Thrombolysis in Myocardial Infarction (TIMI) Phase II trial, *N Engl J Med* 1989;**320**:618–27.

62. Anderson HV, Cannon CP, Stone PH *et al*. One-year results of the thrombolysis in myocardial infarction (TIMI) IIIB clinical trial. *J Am Coll Cardiol* 1995;**26**:1643–50.

63. Boden WE, O'Rourke RA, Crawford MH *et al*. Outcomes in patients with acute non-Q-wave myocardial infarction randomly assigned to an invasive as compared with a conservative management strategy. Veterans Affairs Non-Q-Wave Infarction Strategies in Hospital (VANQWISH) Trial Investigators. *N Engl J Med* 1998;**338**:1785–92.

64. Madsen JK, Grande P, Saunamaki K *et al*. Danish multicenter randomized study of invasive versus conservative treatment in patients with inducible ischemia after thrombolysis in Acute Myocardial Infarction (DANAMI). *Circulation* 1997;**96**: 748–55.

65. FRagmin and Fast Revascularisation during InStability in Coronary artery disease Investigators. Invasive compared with non-invasive treatment in unstable coronary-artery disease: FRISC II prospective randomised multicenter study. *Lancet* 1999; **354**:708–15.

66. Wallentin L, Lagerqvist B, Husted S, Kontny F, Stahle E, Swahn E. Outcome at 1 year after an invasive compared with a non-invasive strategy in unstable coronary-artery disease: the FRISC II invasive randomised trial. FRISC II Investigators. Fast Revascularisation during Instability in Coronary artery disease. *Lancet* 2000;**356**:9–16.

67. Lagerqvist B, Safstrom K, Stahle E, Wallentin L, Swahn E, FRISC II Study Group Investigators. Is early invasive treatment of unstable coronary artery disease equally effective for both women and men? FRISC II Study Group Investigators. *J Am Coll Cardiol* 2001;**38**:41–8.

68. Cannon CP, Weintraub WS, Demopoulos LA *et al*. Comparison of early invasive and conservative strategies in patients with unstable coronary syndromes treated with the glycoprotein IIb/IIIa inhibitor tirofiban. *N Engl J Med* 2001; **344**: 1879–87.

69. The CONSENSUS Trial Study Group. Effects of enalapril on mortality in severe congestive failure. *N Engl J Med* 1987; **316**:1429–44.

70. The SOLVD Investigators. Effect of enalapril on survival in patients with reduced left ventricular ejection fractions and congestive heart failure. *N Engl J Med* 1991;**325**:293–302.

71. CIBIS-II Investigators Committees. The Cardiac Insufficiency Bisoprolol Study II (CIBIS II): a randomised trial. *Lancet* 1999;**353**:9–13.

72. MERIT-HF Study Group. Effect of metoprolol CR/XL in chronic heart failure: Metoprolol CR/XL Randomised Intervention Trial in Congestive Heart Failure (MERIT-HF). *Lancet* 1999, **353**:2001–7.

73. Packer M, Coats AJS, Fowler MB *et al*. Effect of carvedilol on survival in severe chronic heart failure. *N Engl J Med* 2001;**344**:1651–8.

74. The beta-blocker evaluation of survival trial investigators. A trial of the beta-blocker bucindolol in patients with advanced chronic heart failure. *N Engl J Med* 2001;**344**:1659–67.

75. Pitt B, Zannad F, Remme WJ *et al*. The effect of spironolactone on morbidity and mortality in patients with severe heart failure. *N Engl J Med* 1999;**341**:709–17.

76. Moss AJ, Hall WJ, Cannom DS *et al*. Improved survival with an implanted defibrillator in patients with coronary disease at high risk for ventricular arrhythmia. *New Engl J Med* 1996; **335**:1933–40.

77. The Antiarrhythmics versus Implantable Defibrillators (AVID) Investigators. A comparison of anti-arrhythmic therapy with implantable defibrillators in patients resuscitated from near-fatal ventricular arrhythmias. *N Engl J Med* 1997;**337**: 1576–83.

78. Moss AJ, Zareba W, Hall JH *et al*. Prophylactic implantation of a defibrillator in patients with myocardial infarction and reduced ejection fraction. *N Engl J Med* 2002;**346**:877–83.

79. Yusuf S, Wittes J, Probstfield J, Tyroler HA. Analysis and interpretation of treatment effects in subgroups of patients in randomized clinical trials. *JAMA* 1991;**266**:93–8.

80. Yusuf S, Anand S. Cost of prevention. The case of lipid-lowering. *Circulation* 1996;**93**:1774–6.

81. Pedersen TR, Kjekshus J, Berg K *et al*. Cholesterol lowering and the use of healthcare resources. *Circulation*; 1996;**93**: 1796–802.

Part IIIc

Specific cardiovascular disorders: Atrial fibrillation and supraventricular tachycardia

A John Camm and John A Cairns, Editors

Grading of recommendations and levels of evidence used in *Evidence-based Cardiology*

GRADE A

Level 1a   Evidence from large randomized clinical trials (RCTs) or systematic reviews (including meta-analyses) of multiple randomized trials which collectively has at least as much data as one single well-defined trial.

Level 1b   Evidence from at least one "All or None" high quality cohort study; in which ALL patients died/failed with conventional therapy and some survived/succeeded with the new therapy (for example, chemotherapy for tuberculosis, meningitis, or defibrillation for ventricular fibrillation); or in which many died/failed with conventional therapy and NONE died/failed with the new therapy (for example, penicillin for pneumococcal infections).

Level 1c   Evidence from at least one moderate-sized RCT or a meta-analysis of small trials which collectively only has a moderate number of patients.

Level 1d   Evidence from at least one RCT.

GRADE B

Level 2   Evidence from at least one high quality study of non-randomized cohorts who did and did not receive the new therapy.

Level 3   Evidence from at least one high quality case–control study.

Level 4   Evidence from at least one high quality case series.

GRADE C

Level 5   Opinions from experts without reference or access to any of the foregoing (for example, argument from physiology, bench research or first principles).

A comprehensive approach would incorporate many different types of evidence (for example, RCTs, non-RCTs, epidemiologic studies, and experimental data), and examine the architecture of the information for consistency, coherence and clarity. Occasionally the evidence does not completely fit into neat compartments. For example, there may not be an RCT that demonstrates a reduction in mortality in individuals with stable angina with the use of β blockers, but there is overwhelming evidence that mortality is reduced following MI. In such cases, some may recommend use of β blockers in angina patients with the expectation that some extrapolation from post-MI trials is warranted. This could be expressed as Grade A/C. In other instances (for example, smoking cessation or a pacemaker for complete heart block), the non-randomized data are so overwhelmingly clear and biologically plausible that it would be reasonable to consider these interventions as Grade A.

Recommendation grades appear either within the text, for example, **Grade A** and **Grade A1a** or within a table in the chapter.

The grading system clearly is only applicable to preventive or therapeutic interventions. It is not applicable to many other types of data such as descriptive, genetic or pathophysiologic.

37 Atrial fibrillation: antiarrhythmic therapy

Harry JGM Crijns, Isabelle C Van Gelder, Irina Savelieva, A John Camm

Definition of the arrhythmia

The clinical classification of atrial fibrillation has caused much controversy, as ideally it would encompass multiple etiologies, risk factors and precipitating agents, various clinical presentations, variable temporal patterns of behavior, all of which might have an important influence on the selection of the therapeutic strategy and ultimately, determine the effect of treatment.[1] Attempts to classify atrial fibrillation according to etiology or underlying heart disease have been instantly marred by the fact that any process in the atrial tissue that causes infiltration, inflammation, scarring or stretch may lead to the development of atrial fibrillation. Furthermore, the primary pathologies underlying or promoting the occurrence of atrial fibrillation vary, probably, more than for any other cardiac arrhythmia, ranging from autonomic imbalance through organic heart disease to metabolic disorders, such as diabetes mellitus and hyperthyroidism.

Recently approved by the ESC/AHA/ACC Task Force on the management of atrial fibrillation, the classification of atrial fibrillation includes two equally important elements: temporal patterns of the evolution of the arrhythmia which may determine further treatment, and the response to medical interventions (Figure 37.1, Table 37.1).[2] First onset atrial fibrillation is the first clinical presentation of the arrhythmia where the patient is still in atrial fibrillation when evaluated and the episode has been present for less than 48 hours. The new onset, or recent onset atrial fibrillation category is included, but not infrequently the duration of atrial fibrillation is uncertain because the patient is often unaware of symptoms. The paroxysmal form of atrial fibrillation is determined by recurrent episodes of the arrhythmia that typically last from minutes to hours, occasionally days, but eventually self-terminate. Persistent atrial fibrillation is present when the arrhythmia is not self-terminating, but sinus rhythm can be restored by pharmacologic

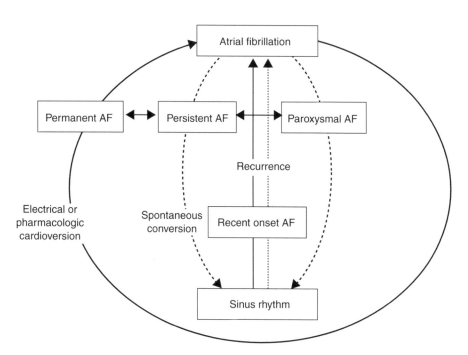

Figure 37.1 Classification of atrial fibrillation, based on the time course of the arrhythmia, and possible transition between the three forms of atrial fibrillation

Table 37.1   Classification of atrial fibrillation

Type	Duration and character	Therapeutic strategy
First detected	Usually <48 hours; usually patient is still in AF when diagnosed	Electrical or pharmacologic cardioversion ± prophylaxis with Class I or III AAD
Paroxysmal	Self-terminating; <2–7 days, frequently <24 hours	Conversion and prevention with Class IC or III AAD and/or
	Spontaneous conversion occurs frequently <2–7 days	Rate control therapy during paroxysm
Persistent	Not self-terminating; usually electrical cardioversion needed to restore sinus rhythm	Electrical cardioversion ± AADs + warfarin pericardioversion
Permanent	Restoration and/or maintenance of sinus rhythm not feasible	Control of the ventricular rate + warfarin or aspirin

Abbreviations: AAD, antiarrhythmic drug; AF, atrial fibrillation

means or, more commonly, by electrical cardioversion. In these patients, atrial fibrillation has usually lasted for weeks or months. Once the arrhythmia is terminated medically, it does not change the designation of the form. Permanent atrial fibrillation is sustained and attempts to restore or maintain sinus rhythm have been abandoned because of frequent recurrence, physician or patient decision, or inability to cardiovert the patient.

Natural history and pathophysiology

Natural history

Atrial fibrillation is the most common cardiac arrhythmia and the incidence increases with age. The Framingham Heart Study showed that the biennial prevalence ranged from 6·2 and 3·8 cases per 1000 in men and women aged 55–64 years, respectively, up to 75·9 and 62·8 per 1000 in men and women aged 85–94 years. Men were 1·5 times more likely to develop atrial fibrillation than women.[3]

Patients with atrial fibrillation are characterized in both sexes by a higher age, the presence of diabetes, hypertension, congestive heart failure, and valve disease. Coronary artery disease is a risk factor for atrial fibrillation only in men.[3] Other predictors are cardiomyopathy and obesity. Echocardiographic predictors include large atria, diminished left ventricular function, and increased left ventricular wall thickness. In the past, rheumatic heart disease was the most common cause of atrial fibrillation, but at present more patients have atrial fibrillation on the basis of coronary artery disease and systemic hypertension.

Mechanisms of atrial fibrillation

Moe and coworkers[4] postulated that atrial fibrillation is maintained by multiple re-entering wavelets circulating randomly in the myocardium and that the stability of the fibrillatory process depends on the average number of wavelets. This hypothesis was confirmed experimentally by Allessie and colleagues,[5] who estimated that the critical number of wavelets to sustain atrial fibrillation was approximately four to six. Atrial fibrillation may also present itself as a focal arrhythmia amenable to ablation. It then occurs in the absence of heart disease in relatively young patients.

Atrial fibrillation has the tendency to become more persistent over time. This is illustrated by the fact that about 30% of patients with paroxysmal atrial fibrillation eventually will develop persistent atrial fibrillation.[6] Also, pharmacologic and electrical cardioversion, and maintenance of sinus rhythm thereafter become more difficult the longer the arrhythmia exists.[7,8] This relates to progression of the underlying disease and possibly also to electrical remodeling of the atria.[9]

Modulating factors

The onset and persistence of atrial fibrillation may be modulated by the autonomic nervous system. Coumel and coworkers distinguished vagal and adrenergic atrial fibrillation.[10] However, the distinction between both mechanisms is not always clear. This implies that it is more appropriate to speak of autonomic imbalance rather than either an increased vagal or an increased sympathetic tone.

Vagally mediated atrial fibrillation

Vagally mediated atrial fibrillation occurs more frequently in men than in women, usually at a younger age (30–50 years). It only rarely progresses to permanent atrial fibrillation and it predominantly occurs in the absence of structural heart disease.[10] Attacks occur at night, end in the morning, and neither emotional stress nor exertion trigger the arrhythmia. On the contrary, when patients feel that atrial fibrillation may start (repeated atrial extrasystoles), some observe that they can prevent an arrhythmia by doing exercise. The arrhythmia frequently starts after exercise or stress. Rest, the postprandial state, and alcohol are other precipitating factors. The pathophysiologic mechanism may relate to vagally induced shortening of the atrial refractory period.

Adrenergic tone in atrial fibrillation

Adrenergic atrial fibrillation is more frequently associated with structural heart disease (ischemic heart disease) than its vagal counterpart.[10] Typically, it occurs during day time and is favored by stress, exercise, tea, coffee or alcohol. Attacks terminate often within a few minutes. It is less frequently observed than vagal atrial fibrillation. The underlying mechanism is unknown.

Familial atrial fibrillation

A hypothesis of genetic predisposition to atrial fibrillation or even specific genetically predetermined forms of the arrhythmia has been confirmed by identification of a gene defect linked to chromosome 10q in three Spanish families, 21 of 49 members of which presented with atrial fibrillation at a relatively young age, ranging from 2 to 46 years.[11] Candidate genes for the familial form of the arrhythmia include genes encoding channel or pore proteins and genes encoding the α- and β adrenergic receptors or signaling proteins. Of interest, since these receptors are involved in normal and abnormal cardiac automaticity, it is tempting to speculate that the basis for familial atrial fibrillation lies in abnormal atrial automaticity or triggering mechanisms.

Recently, a missense mutation in the lamin A/C gene has been found to be a cause of dilated cardiomyopathy associated with progressive conduction system disease, atrioventricular block, atrial fibrillation, congestive heart failure, stroke and sudden death.[12] Similarly, a missense mutation Arg663His in the β-cardiac myosin heavy chain has been identified in patients with specific phenotype of familial hypertrophic cardiomyopathy presenting with moderate left ventricular hypertrophy, predominantly localized in the proximal segment of the interventricular septum, and a 47% prevalence of atrial fibrillation.[13] Although the incidence of familial AF is to be determined, further exploration may reveal a number of possible targets for medical therapy for the prevention or reversal of the arrhythmia.

Clinical impact

Atrial fibrillation causes palpitations, chest pain, dyspnea, and fatigue. Some patients experience presyncope or even drop attacks, especially at arrhythmia onset or termination. All patients with longer lasting atrial fibrillation develop left ventricular dysfunction, even those without underlying heart disease. This is often indicated as tachycardiomyopathy. Conversely, many patients with atrial fibrillation have pre-existent heart failure. Furthermore, atrial fibrillation is associated with excess thromboembolic complications, especially in elderly patients.

However, in at least one third of patients, no obvious symptoms or noticeable degradation of quality of life are observed.[14] In the ALFA (Etude en Activité Liberale sur le Fibrillation Auriculaire) study of 756 patients with atrial fibrillation from general practice in France, of 86 participants who reported no symptoms, 63 (73%) presented with permanent atrial fibrillation, 14 (16%) were diagnosed with recent onset atrial fibrillation, and only 9 (11%) had a paroxysmal form of the arrhythmia.[15] Pharmacologic treatment of the atrial fibrillation has long been known potentially to convert a symptomatic form of the arrhythmia to an entirely asymptomatic variety. In the PAFAC (Prevention of Atrial Fibrillation After Cardioversion) study of more than 1000 patients with atrial fibrillation, antiarrhythmic drug therapy rendered 90% of arrhythmia recurrences completely asymptomatic, as detected in this study by daily transtelephonic ECG monitoring.[16] These observations challenged the validity of symptoms for the reliable detection of recurrence of atrial fibrillation and for the assessment of the efficacy of antiarrhythmic drug therapy.

Hemodynamic consequences and mortality

Atrial fibrillation reduces cardiac output and may lead to heart failure.[17,18] Apart from loss of atrial kick, excessive rate response and rhythm irregularity, two other pathogenetic factors should be mentioned, namely progression of underlying cardiovascular disease and development of tachycardia-related cardiomyopathy.[19] In fact, associated heart disease creates the background hemodynamic derangement which is modulated by the other factors. Tachycardiomyopathy may occur in the absence of heart disease and it may be concealed – that is, heart failure due to tachycardiomyopathy cannot be distinguished from that due to the underlying cardiovascular disease, but may be demonstrable only after restoration of sinus rhythm or adequate rate control.[19,20]

Several cohort and retrospective studies have shown that the relative risk of death in subjects with atrial fibrillation is roughly twice that found in subjects in sinus rhythm.[17,18,21] The reduced survival relates to progression of the underlying cardiovascular disease and stroke. The prognostic impact of atrial fibrillation in patients with heart failure is still uncertain.[22,23]

Progressive increase of atrial size

Atrial enlargement is a cause but also a consequence of atrial fibrillation.[24,25] Atrial enlargement is associated with an increased risk for thromboembolic complications and a high arrhythmia recurrence rate following cardioversion. In addition, drugs used to convert the arrhythmia may be less effective. Restoration of sinus rhythm may reverse the process of atrial enlargement, even in patients with mitral valve disease.[26]

Increased number of thromboembolic complications

Atrial fibrillation is the most common cardiac cause of systemic emboli, usually cerebrovascular.[27] In the presence of atrial fibrillation, the risk of stroke shows an approximately fivefold increase unrelated to age.[27] The proportion of atrial fibrillation-related stroke increases significantly with age from 6·7 for ages 50–59 years to 36·2 for ages 80–89 years. The risk for stroke in lone atrial fibrillation is still uncertain. The cardiac embolus often results in occlusion of a major cerebral artery. The ensuing infarct is often large and may be fatal.[28] Apart from symptomatic strokes, atrial fibrillation has been associated with an increased risk of silent strokes.[28] Risk factors for stroke in atrial fibrillation include rheumatic heart disease, age >65 years, hypertension, previous stroke or transient ischemic attack, diabetes, recent heart failure, and echocardiographic atrial or ventricular enlargement.[27,29,30]

Antiarrhythmic therapy of atrial fibrillation

Essentially, there are three antiarrhythmic strategies: acute pharmacologic termination; drug prevention in paroxysmal atrial fibrillation and persistent atrial fibrillation post cardioversion; and control of the ventricular rate during a paroxysm of atrial fibrillation or during the presence of persistent or permanent atrial fibrillation. Drug treatment to convert or prevent atrial fibrillation aims at prolonging the wavelength or reducing the triggers for atrial fibrillation. The former can be achieved by Class IA or III antiarrhythmic drugs or even the Class IC drugs flecainide and propafenone which prolong refractoriness at short cycle lengths. The latter, for example, through β blockers in the case of adrenergic atrial fibrillation.

Paroxysmal atrial fibrillation

Defining the temporal pattern of atrial fibrillation requires a careful history, an electrocardiogram, and frequently a 24 hour Holter monitor. This implies that the definite pattern cannot always be established on the first consultation. Which strategy will be chosen in the individual patient should depend on the frequency of the paroxysms, the triggers for the arrhythmia, the accompanying symptoms, and the underlying heart disease (Figure 37.2).

The three possible strategies for the pharmacologic treatment of paroxysmal atrial fibrillation will be discussed below.

Acute conversion of paroxysmal atrial fibrillation

If the arrhythmia is not self-limiting, antiarrhythmic drugs can be administered to restore sinus rhythm. Pharmacologic cardioversion is considered to be most effective if initiated within 7 days after the onset of the arrhythmia in which case restoration of sinus rhythm can be achieved in nearly 70% of patients, but the success rate is lower in atrial fibrillation of longer duration.[31] The high rate of spontaneous conversion suggests that a placebo group is required to determine the effects of antiarrhythmic drug therapy.[32] Furthermore, although antiarrhythmic drugs reduce the time to conversion to sinus rhythm, the high rates of spontaneous conversion in recent onset atrial fibrillation may result in an insignificant difference between the intervention and the placebo arms. Figure 37.3 shows conversion rates on placebo and the different antiarrhythmic drugs in recent onset atrial fibrillation. It demonstrates that with time the cumulative conversion rate increases both on placebo and drugs.

Recently published guidelines of ESC Committee and AHA/ACC Task Force members on the management of atrial fibrillation have stated that in atrial fibrillation of less than 7 days' duration, propafenone and flecainide (oral or intravenous), ibutilide or dofetilide should be the first line choice if pharmacologic cardioversion of the arrhythmia is considered.[2] High dose amiodarone (intravenous and in combination with oral administration), and oral quinidine have been shown to be more effective than placebo for converting atrial fibrillation into sinus rhythm and may be used as second choice therapy in selected patients. As the success rate of pharmacologic cardioversion is progressively reduced with increased duration of the arrhythmia, the choice of antiarrhythmic drugs is limited to dofetilide, ibutilide, and possibly, amiodarone. Antiarrhythmic drugs proven to be effective for cardioversion of atrial tachyarrhythmias and recommended by the committee are summarized in Table 37.2.

Conversion rates up to 90% are found 1 hour after intravenous flecainide or propafenone. Both drugs can also be administered orally with success rates reported to be 50–80%.[33–35] The advantage of Class IC antiarrhythmic drugs is their ability to expediently restore sinus rhythm within a short period of time. Thus, cardioversion rates for flecainide and propafenone given as a single dose of 200–300 mg and 450–600 mg respectively were 59% and 51% at 3 hours compared with 18% in the placebo arm, reaching 78% and 72% at 8 hours compared with 39% on placebo.[33] In the third Propafenone in Atrial Fibrillation Italian Trial (PAFIT-3), intravenous infusion of propafenone at a dose of 2 mg/kg restored sinus rhythm within the first hour in nearly half patients with recent onset atrial fibrillation (1–72 hours) compared with 14% on placebo.[36]

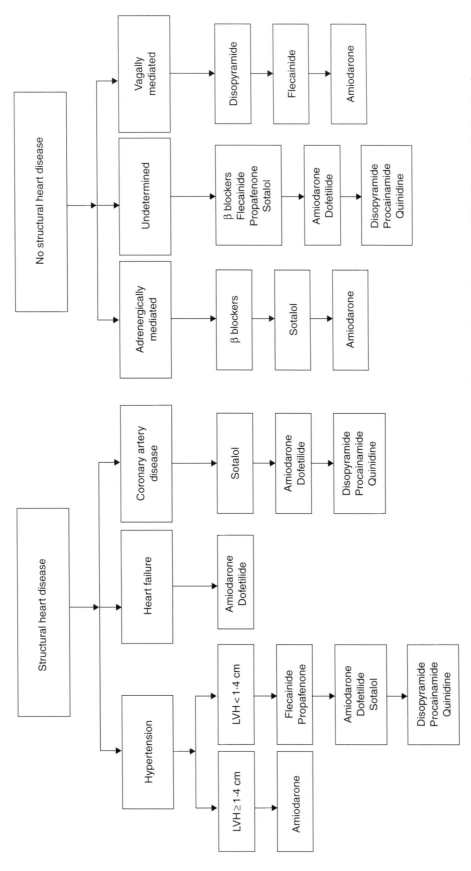

Figure 37.2 Selection of the optimal antiarrhythmic agent to prevent atrial tachyarrhythmias. *No left ventricular dysfunction; LVH, left ventricular hypertrophy

Drug treatment of atrial fibrillation: summary

Type	Strategy	Drugs	Recommendation level
Paroxysmal	(1) Terminate paroxysm	(1) Class IC AAD IV or oral or procainamide IV	Grade A
		Class IA, IC in WPW	Grade B
		Class III drugs (ibutilide, dofetilide)	Grade A
		Amiodarone in hemodynamically compromised patients (cardioversion)	Grade A
	(2) Prevent paroxysm	(2) Class IC	Grade A
		Class III AAD (sotalol, dofetilide, azimilide[a])	Grade A
		Amiodarone (first choice in hemodynamically compromised patients)	Grade A
		Disopyramide/flecainide in vagally induced AF	Grade B
		β blockers in adrenergically induced AF	Grade B
	(3) Rate control during paroxysm	(3) Digitalis	Grade B
		±	
		β blockers	
		±	
		Calcium-channel blockers	
Persistent	Serial cardioversion	DC electrical cardioversion[b]	Grade A
	±	±	
	Serial antiarrhythmic drug therapy	Sotalol (initiate in hospital)	Grade B
	+	Class IC drug (not in patients with significant structural heart disease)	Grade B
	Patient counseling (report to hospital at recurrence)	Amiodarone (first choice in hemodynamically compromised patients)	Grade B
Permanent	Accept AF, rate control therapy:	Digitalis	Grade A
		±	
	if duration AF >36 months	β blockers	
	or	±	
	age >70 years and NYHA III + IV	Calcium-channel blockers	
	or		
	after failure of serial cardioversion therapy		

[a] Investigational agent.
[b] Drugs usually ineffective.
Abbreviation: WPW, Wolff–Parkinson–White syndrome

Ibutilide has been shown to act as much as twice more effectively for conversion of atrial flutter than atrial fibrillation (63% *v* 31%).[37] In 319 patients with persistent atrial tachyarrhythmias (18·5% atrial flutter) of duration up to 45 days, intravenous ibutilide at a dose of 1 mg or 2 mg was more effective than intravenous d,1-sotalol at a dose of 1·5 mg/kg in conversion of atrial fibrillation to sinus rhythm in less than 1 hour (20% with 1 mg, 44% with 2 mg *v* 11%) and was particularly effective in termination of atrial flutter (56% with 1 mg, 70% with 2 mg *v* 19%).[38] In another randomized study in patients with atrial flutter, the comparison also was in favor of ibutilide which was significantly superior

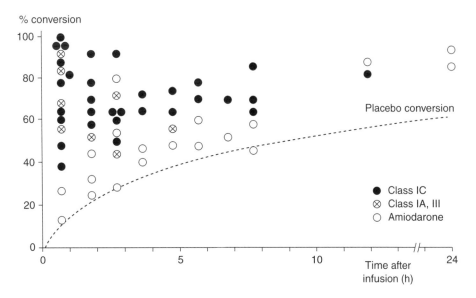

Figure 37.3 Conversion of paroxysmal atrial fibrillation (<3 days). Conversion rates in relation to time after start of the infusion found in studies investigating the efficacy of Class IC (flecainide and propafenone), Class IA and III drugs (procainamide, quinidine, sotalol, ibutilide, dofetilide) and amiodarone are presented. The curve indicating placebo conversion was constructed from placebo conversion rates found in the above studies. Class IC drugs appear most efficacious. Note the late onset of conversion on amiodarone. (Modified after Fresco *et al*.[7])

Table 37.2 Antiarrhythmic drugs for pharmacologic cardioversion of atrial fibrillation of less and more than 7 days duration. Grade A

Drug	Route of administration	Dose
Flecainide	Oral or IV	200–300 mg or 1·5–3·0 mg/kg over 10–20 min
Propafenone	Oral or IV	450–600 mg or 1·5–2·0 mg/kg over 10–20 min
Dofetilide	Oral	125–500 mg twice daily[a]
Ibutilide	IV	1 mg over 10 min; repeat 1 mg if necessary
Amiodarone	Oral or IV	Inpatient: 1200–1800 mg daily in divided doses until 10 g total; then 200–400 mg daily Outpatient: 600–800 mg daily until 10 g total; then 200–400 mg daily 5–7 mg/kg over 30–60 min IV; then 1200–1800 mg daily oral until 10 g total; then 200–400 mg daily
Procainamide	IV	1000 mg over 30 min (33 mg/min) followed by 2 mg/min infusion
Quinidine	Oral	750–1500 mg in divided doses over 6–12 hours + a rate slowing drug

[a] Dose depends on creatinine clearance: >60 ml/min – 500 mg; 40–60 ml/min – 250 mg; 20–40 ml/min – 125 mg twice daily.

to procainamide (76% *v* 14%).[39] However, the efficacy of ibutilide decreased significantly with duration of the arrhythmia more than 7 days: from 71% to 57% for atrial flutter and from 46% to only 18% for atrial fibrillation. Furthermore, as many controlled studies of ibutilide have enrolled patients

with mild or moderate underlying heart disease, these results may not be generalizable to patients with markedly depressed left ventricular function.

Dofetilide has been shown to convert 30·3% of 96 patients with atrial tachyarrhythmias within 3 hours from the start of intravenous infusion of 8 micrograms/kg for 30 minutes compared with a 3·3% conversion rate on placebo.[40] The conversion rates were significantly higher for atrial flutter than for atrial fibrillation (64% *v* 24%). Two large prospective studies, DIAMOND-CHF (Danish Investigations of Arrhythmia and Mortality ON Dofetilide in Congestive Heart Failure) and SAFIRE-D (Symptomatic Atrial Fibrillation Investigative Research on Dofetilide), have recently evaluated effects of oral dofetilide on the conversion rate and maintenance of sinus rhythm in patients with atrial fibrillation. In the DIAMOND study of 1518 patients with symptomatic heart failure and an ejection fraction ≤35%, therapy with dofetilide 1000 micrograms was associated with a greater rate of spontaneous conversion to sinus rhythm (44% *v* 14%).[41] In the SAFIRE-D study of 325 patients with persistent atrial fibrillation and/or atrial flutter, cardioversion rates were 6·1%, 9·8%, and 29·9% for 125, 250, and 500 micrograms of dofetilide twice daily compared with 1·2% of spontaneous conversion in the placebo arm.[42]

However, as far as late conversion has been studied, amiodarone may produce sinus rhythm in over 80% within 24 hours. An advantage of amiodarone is its ability to lower ventricular rates before conversion, whereas Class IC drugs may increase the ventricular rate due to conversion of atrial fibrillation to atrial flutter with 2:1 atrioventricular conduction, and, therefore, should be administered in conjunction with β blockers. Amiodarone is especially recommended in hemodynamically compromised patients since it is less negatively inotropic.[43] A meta-analysis of 12 randomized controlled studies has shown that intravenous amiodarone was moderately effective in converting atrial fibrillation compared with placebo (63% *v* 44%), with the maximum effect at 24 hours (74% *v* 55%).[44] There is evidence from a randomized, controlled study suggesting that higher than usual intravenous dose amiodarone and the combination of intravenous and oral routes of administration may enhance the cardioversion rate.[45]

Quinidine is usually administered in conjunction with rate slowing agents, preferably with β blockers and when given in a cumulative daily dose of up to 1350 mg has been shown to cardiovert 50–77% of patients with recent onset atrial fibrillation.[46,47]

For acute conversion, sotalol must be considered ineffective. This has only become apparent after the drug has been used as an "active" comparator in trials studying new Class III agents.[38,48] The rate of conversion of atrial fibrillation with sotalol did not exceed 19% and was significantly lower for conversion of atrial flutter (11%).[38] On the other hand, sotalol is effective for the *prevention* of atrial fibrillation. This discrepancy relates to its property to prolong the refractory period predominantly at *lower* atrial rates, but not during rapid atrial fibrillation, due to its reverse use dependency.

The availability of studies on the efficacy of procainamide and disopyramide is limited, precluding definite conclusions.

Procainamide has been found to convert at least 65% of the patients with atrial fibrillation within approximately 1 hour. Its lack of efficacy (compared to Class IC drugs) may relate to the rather low dose used in the procainamide studies: up to a maximum of 1 g in 30 minutes, sometimes followed by a low maintenance infusion.

Digitalis, β blockers, and calcium-channel blockers are ineffective for the acute conversion of atrial fibrillation.[7,49,50] The DAAF (Digitalis in Acute Atrial Fibrillation) study has shown that there was no difference in cardioversion rates at 16 hours between intravenous digoxin and placebo (51% *v* 46%).[51] Moreover, the drug has been shown to facilitate AF due to its cholinergic effects which may cause a non-uniform reduction in conduction velocity and effective refractory periods of the atria, and to delay the reversal of remodeling after restoration of sinus rhythm.[52,53]

Self-administered oral drug conversion may be applied if the patient is clinically stable and if the agent has been shown to be safe and effective in that patient.[7]

Prevention of paroxysmal atrial fibrillation

Paroxysmal atrial fibrillation is a chronic disease: the first attack will not be the last in over 90% of patients, despite antiarrhythmic prophylaxis. As a consequence the end point of treatment used in controlled drug studies has been "attack-free rate" or "time to first recurrence". Therefore, when considering drug efficacy, it might be more appropriate to focus on quality of life but firm data concerning this issue are available only for His bundle ablation. In this respect, it is important to note that up to 50% of patients discontinue drug therapy for loss of quality of life due to adverse effects and drug inefficacy. Moreover, too many studies looked at drug effects in mixed populations, including both paroxysmal and persistent atrial fibrillation. Finally, older drugs like procainamide have not been tested extensively in appropriate placebo-controlled studies. Useful data concerning these agents have or will become available only after they have been used as active comparators in studies on Class IC and the new Class III drugs. Therefore, this paragraph contains clinically useful conclusions which, however, are not all evidence-based.

Prophylactic antiarrhythmic drug therapy is usually not recommended after a first episode of the arrhythmia which may self-terminate or require electrical or pharmacologic cardioversion and in patients with infrequent, self-limiting, and well-tolerated paroxysms of the arrhythmia. However, this approach can be appropriate in a small proportion of patients as paroxysmal atrial fibrillation tends to evolve to persistent and eventually to a permanent form. Prophylactic antiarrhythmic drug therapy is, therefore, recommended for a vast majority of patients with paroxysmal tachyarrhythmia when paroxysms occur frequently (1 episode per 3 months) and are associated with significant symptoms or lead to worsening left ventricular function; for patients with persistent atrial fibrillation when the likelihood of maintenance of sinus rhythm is uncertain, especially in the presence of risk factors for recurrence (left atrial enlargement, evidence for depressed atrial function, left ventricular dysfunction, underlying cardiovascular pathology, long duration of the arrhythmia, and advanced age).[54]

The efficacy of propafenone for the prevention of recurrent atrial fibrillation has been assessed in several uncontrolled studies and four placebo-controlled trials.[55–57] In the Propafenone Atrial Fibrillation Trial (PAFT), the likelihood of maintenance of sinus rhythm at 6 months after cardioversion was 67% in the propafenone-treated group compared with 35% with placebo.[56] The UK PSVT (Paroxysmal Supraventricular Tachycardia) study showed that propafenone given at doses of 600 mg and 900 mg daily was effective for suppression of recurrences of the arrhythmia but a dose of 900 mg was associated with a less favorable adverse event profile.[57] Propafenone has proven to be efficacious and safe in patients with supraventricular tachyarrhythmias in meta-analysis involving over 3100 patients.[58] All-cause mortality associated with propafenone was 0·3%. There are now two ongoing studies of the effectiveness of propafenone for the maintenance of sinus rhythm: the North American Recurrence of Atrial Fibrillation Trial (RAFT) and its European equivalent, ERAFT.

Several placebo-controlled and comparative trials of another Class IC antiarrhythmic drug, flecainide, including the Flecainide Multicenter Atrial Fibrillation Study, have found that the efficacy of flecainide in the prevention of first recurrence of AF or flutter and the reduction of the total time spent in the arrhythmia comparable to that of quinidine, with fewer adverse effects.[59–63] In a placebo-controlled, crossover study Anderson and colleagues included 53 patients with two or more attacks of atrial fibrillation within a 4 week baseline period.[61] The median dose of flecainide was 300 mg, which is well above the clinical dose currently instituted (150–200 mg daily). During therapy with flecainide, the median time to the first recurrence was significantly prolonged (15 days v 3 days, $P<0·001$). Similarly, the time interval between subsequent attacks lengthened, from 6 to 27 days during flecainide compared to placebo ($P<0·001$). The efficacy of flecainide was maintained during a mean follow up of 17 months.[62] Naccarelli included 239 patients randomized to flecainide (maximum dose 300 mg) or quinidine (maximum dose 1500 mg/day) and followed them for 12 months. Inadequate response caused 10% and 12% terminations of the drug, respectively. However, 30% of the quinidine patients stopped the drug due to adverse effects, versus only 18% of the flecainide group.[63]

Following the publication of the Cardiac Arrhythmias Suppression Trial (CAST I), and the Stroke Prevention Atrial Fibrillation (SPAF I) study showing a three- to sixfold increase in risk for all-cause and cardiac mortality with Class I antiarrhythmic agents, particularly in patients with structural heart disease,[64,65] a shift has been made to more frequent use of Class III antiarrhythmic drugs, the action of which is based on prolongation of action potential duration. These include amiodarone, sotalol, and dofetilide, a new, investigational agent azimilide, and iodine-free benzofurane derivative dronedarone with affinity for multiple potassium channels. However, the likelihood of remaining free from recurrence of the arrhythmia over the long term is not satisfactory with any of the antiarrhythmic drugs which are presently available but probably, higher for dofetilide (Figure 37.4).

Selected randomized trials of the efficacy of class III antiarrhythmic drugs for conversion of atrial fibrillation and maintenance of sinus rhythm are summarized in Table 37.3.

In randomized comparative and placebo-controlled studies, sotalol has proven to be effective in the prevention of recurrent atrial fibrillation. Sotalol has also been shown to exert additional beneficial effects by suppressing symptoms associated with relapse into atrial fibrillation due to its rate slowing action.[66–69] In 253 patients with atrial fibrillation or flutter, therapy with d,l-sotalol at a dose of 240 mg daily resulted in a significant increase in the median time to first recurrence of symptomatic arrhythmia documented as assessed by transtelephonic monitoring.[69] In the PAFAC study of more than 1000 patients, the recurrence rates during 1 year of daily transtelephonic ECG monitoring were 50% for sotalol, 38% for the combination of quinidine and verapamil, and 77% for placebo.[70] Furthermore, sotalol proved to be inferior to amiodarone in the Canadian Trial of Atrial Fibrillation (CTAF).[71] Sotalol was less effective and had higher rates of withdrawal than dofetilide in the European and Australian Multicenter Evaluative Research on Atrial Fibrillation Dofetilide (EMERALD) study.[72]

In the CTAF study, therapy with amiodarone at a dose of 200 mg/day resulted in a 57% reduction in risk for recurrence of the arrhythmia compared with sotalol and propafenone.[71] However, difficulties with the methodology of the trial, particularly the delay in logging recurrences of the arrhythmia in the amiodarone-treated group, reduce confidence in its results. Data from the CHF-STAT (Congestive Heart Failure Survival Trial of Antiarrhythmic Therapy) substudy showed that amiodarone was effective for the prevention of recurrence of atrial fibrillation in patients with congestive heart failure NYHA Classes II and III.[73] In this study, patients who received amiodarone were twice as less likely to develop new atrial fibrillation compared with placebo (4% v 8%).

Dofetilide has been recently introduced as a safe and effective Class III antiarrhythmic drug for treatment of atrial tachyarrhythmias in patients with underlying heart pathology. In the DIAMOND-CHF study, treatment with dofetilide 500 micrograms twice daily was associated with a significantly greater probability of remaining in sinus rhythm at 1 year

Percentage of patients with sinus rhythm at 6 months

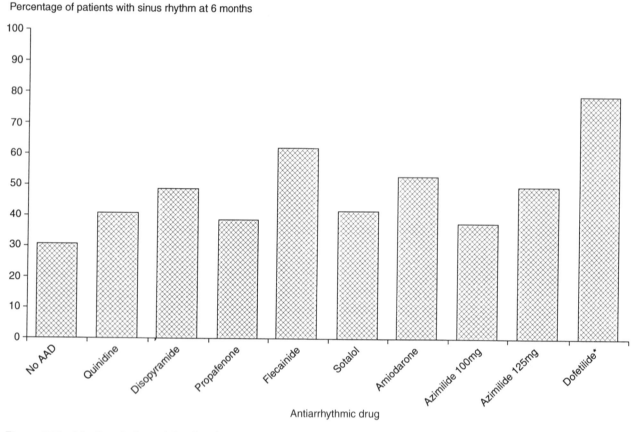

Antiarrhythmic drug

Figure 37.4 Likelihood of remaining free from recurrence of atrial fibrillation or atrial flutter with prophylactic antiarrhythmic drug therapy* at 1 year

Table 37.3 Randomized, controlled studies of efficacy of Class III antiarrhythmic drugs for conversion and/or maintenance of sinus rhythm in patients with atrial fibrillation and flutter

Study	Drug	Patients (n)	Follow up	Cardioverted v control/ placebo	Remained in SR v control	Torsade de pointes
Ibutilide Repeat Dose Study[37]	Ibutilide 1·5 mg or 2 mg IV	266	24 hours	47% v 2%; 63% v 31% flutter v AF	–	8·3% (required cardioversion 1·7%)
Ibutilide/Sotalol Comparator Study (ISCS)[38]	Ibutilide 1 mg or 2 mg IV, d,l-sotalol 1·5 mg/kg IV	319	72 hours	56–70% v 19% on sotalol in atrial flutter; 20–44% v 11% in AF	–	0·9% on ibutilide 2 mg; none on sotalol
Sotalol Multicenter Study Group[48]	d,l-sotalol 160 or 320 mg	49	To first recurrence	–	73% on sotalol 320 mg; 40% on sotalol 160 mg v 29% on placebo	None
D,l-Sotalol Atrial Fibrillation/ Flutter Study Group[69]	d,l-sotalol 160, 240 or 320 mg	253	24 weeks	–	Increased time to first episode: 106–229 days v 27 days on placebo	None

Table 37.3 Continued

Study	Drugs (n)	Patient	Follow up control/ placebo	Cardioverted v control/ placebo	Remained in SR v control	Torsade de pointes
PAFAC	Sotalol quinidine + verapamil	1182	1 year; daily TTE	–	Recurrence rates: 50% on sotalol v 38% on quinidine + verapamil v 77% on placebo	1% (all on sotalol)
Randomized, placebo-controlled study in recent onset AF[45]	Amiodarone IV 125 mg/h for 24 hours; maximum dose 3 g	100	1 month	92% v 64%	88%	Not stated
CTAF[71]	Amiodarone 200 mg	403	16 months	–	65% v 37% on sotalol or propafenone (57% risk reduction)	None
CHF-STAT[73]	Amiodarone 800 mg for 2 weeks; 400 mg for 50 weeks; then 200 mg	667; 103 AF	4–5 years	31·3% v 7·7%	–	–
DDAFF[57]	Dofetilide 8 μg/kg IV	96	3 hours	30·3% v 3·3% 64% flutter v 24% AF	–	3%
DIAMOND[41]	Dofetilide 500 μg	1518	18 months	59% v 34%	79% v 46%	3·3%
SAFIRE-D[42]	Dofetilide 250, 500, 1000 μg	225	1 year	6·1%, 9·8%, 19·9% v 1·2%	40%, 37%, 58% v 25%	0·8%
EMERALD[74]	Dofetilide 250, 500, 1000 μg	671	Phase 1: 72 h; Phase 2: 2 years	6%, 11%, 29% v 5% on sotalol at 72 hours	40%, 52%, 66% v 21% on placebo at 1 year	3 torsades de pointes; 1 sudden death
ASAP[76]	Azimilide 50, 100, 125 mg	384	180 days	–	17%, 38%, 83%[a]	0·99%
Meta-analysis of 4 SVA studies[77]	Azimilide 35, 50, 100, 125 mg	1380	Time to first recurrence	–	1·32–1·34 1·49–1·86[c]	0·9% at 100 and 125 mg v 0% on placebo
ALIVE (unpublished)	Azimilide 100 mg	3381	1 year	26·8% v 10·8% (P = 0·076)	New AF: 0·49% v 1·15% (P = 0·04)	0·3% v 0·1% on placebo

[a] Indicates a reduction in risk of AF recurrence compared with placebo.
[b] Indicates hazards ratios for the time to first recurrence of the arrhythmia compared with placebo.
[c] In patients with structural heart disease.
Abbreviations: AF, atrial fibrillation; AT, atrial tachycardia; DCC, direct current cardioversion; SR, sinus rhythm; SVA, supraventricular arrhythmia

compared with placebo (79% *v* 42%) and a significant reduction in the development of new cases of atrial fibrillation (1·98% *v* 6·55%).[41] In the SAFIRE-D study, 58% of patients treated with the maximal dose of dofetilide (1000 micrograms daily) remained in sinus rhythm at 1 year compared with 25% in the placebo group.[42] The preliminary results of the EMERALD study have shown that therapy with dofetilide at different dose regimens 250, 500, and 1000 micrograms daily was associated with a higher likelihood of maintenance of sinus rhythm compared with placebo (40%, 52%, and 66% *v* 21%, respectively).[74] In the EMERALD study, dofetilide was effective for maintenance of sinus rhythm in the subgroups of patients with high risk of recurrence of the arrhythmia, including those with significantly dilated left atrium, left ventricular dysfunction, and atrial fibrillation of more than 30 days' duration.[75]

Finally, azimilide, a new antiarrhythmic agent which blocks both fast and slow components of the delayed potassium rectifier current, has been shown to significantly prolong the time to first symptomatic arrhythmia episode compared with placebo (the hazard ratio 1·58) in 384 patients with atrial fibrillation.[76] Meta-analysis of four randomized controlled studies of the effectiveness of a range of azimilide doses in 1380 patients with atrial tachyarrhythmias has shown that each of the two highest doses (100 and 125 mg/day) significantly prolonged the time to first recurrence.[77] Patients with a history of coronary artery disease or congestive heart failure derive significantly greater benefit from azimilide than those with other underlying cardiovascular pathologies. In the ALIVE (AzimiLide post Infarct survival Evaluation Trial) of over 3000 post myocardial infarction patients with left ventricular dysfunction, fewer patients who started the trial in sinus rhythm developed atrial fibrillation on azimilide compared with placebo (0·49% *v* 1·15%), and there was a clear tendency to higher pharmacologic conversion rates in the azimilide arm than in the placebo arm (26·8% *v* 10·8%).

In patients suffering from vagally induced atrial fibrillation, β blockers and digitalis should be avoided as these drugs may provoke attacks. Quinidine, disopyramide, and flecainide may be effective due to their vagolytic effect. Propafenone is also considered ineffective due to its β blocking properties.

In patients with adrenergic-dependent atrial fibrillation, underlying cardiac disorders should be treated. After that, patients usually benefit from a β blocker. Class IA and IC drugs are generally ineffective, although some patients may respond to propafenone. At this point it should be stressed that firm data concerning this issue are missing since unequivocal identification of vagal or adrenergic atrial fibrillation may be impossible. This has precluded large, controlled studies on drug efficacy in predominantly vagally or adrenergically induced atrial fibrillation.

Finally, although β blockers have been predominantly used for rate control, recent data suggest that therapy with β blockers appears to be effective in the prevention of recurrence of persistent atrial fibrillation after cardioversion, especially in the presence of hypertension as underlying pathology.[78,79] In a randomized, crossover study, the efficacy of atenolol at a dose of 50 mg daily was comparable to that of low-dose sotalol (160 mg daily) and better than placebo for suppression of recurrent atrial fibrillation, reduction in duration of episodes of the arrhythmia and associated symptoms.[80] Bisoprolol at a dose of 5 mg daily has been shown to maintain sinus rhythm during 1 year after electrical cardioversion in 58% of patients with persistent atrial fibrillation, an effect comparable to that of sotalol (59%).[81]

Control of the ventricular rate during paroxysmal atrial fibrillation

Digitalis, β blockers or calcium-channel blockers may be necessary to control the ventricular rate when a relapse occurs. This holds especially in hemodynamically compromised patients who may decompensate during the attack. These agents may also prevent rate-dependent proarrhythmias (rapid atrioventricular conduction, excessive QRS widening, and ventricular tachycardia) of Class IA and IC drugs during a recurrence of atrial fibrillation, but conclusive data on this issue are lacking.[82] If amiodarone or sotalol are used to prevent atrial fibrillation, addition of conventional rate control drugs is not necessary. Controlling the ventricular rate in patients with paroxysmal atrial fibrillation in the setting of a sick sinus syndrome may be impossible

Table 37.4 Review of controlled studies on maintenance of sinus rhythm after cardioversion of persistent atrial fibrillation with Class I antiarrhythmic drugs

Study (1st author)	Year	Patients (*n*)	Duration AF (mth; mean)	Age (yr; mean)	Underlying heart disease (%)			Lone AF
					CAD	VHD	SH	
Quinidine *v* no treatment								
1 Södermark	1975	176	<36	58	35	27	9	8
2 Byrne-Q	1970	92	<120	54	16[b]	56	—[b]	20
3 Hillestad	1971	100	?	54	10	70	?	8
4 Lloyd	1984	53	<36	46	11	70	5	6

Table 37.4 Continued

Study (first author)	Year	Patients (n)	Duration AF (mth; mean)	Age (yr; mean)	Underlying heart disease (%)			Lone AF
					CAD	VHD	SH	
5 Boissel	1981	212	?	?	1	70	4	20
6 Hartel	1970	175	?	?	18	30	2	11
Disopyramide 450–500 mg *v* no treatment								
7 Karlson	1988	90	4[a]	60	16	13	13	40
Procainamide 3000 mg *v* propranolol 60 mg								
8 Szekely	1970	166-23	NA	NA	8	78	NA	5
Flecainide 150–300 mg *v* no treatment								
9 Van Gelder	1989	73	6–11[a]	58	27	37	10	18
Propafenone 900 mg *v* disopyramide 750 mg								
10 Crijns	1996	56	5[a]	60	12	28	16	40
Quinidine sulfate 1200 mg *v* sotalol 160–320 mg								
11 Juul-Möller	1990	183	5	59	16	6	26	52
Propafenone 450–900 mg (mean 737±177) *v* sotalol 320–950 mg (mean 335±18)								
12 Reimold	1993	53[c]	55	61	16	30	19	19
Quinidine 1200 mg *v* amiodarone 2000 mg/week								
13 Vitolo	1981	54	79%<6	53	56	44	0	0

Study	Follow up (mth)	Patients in SR at 1 mth (%)		Patients in SR at 6 mth (%)		Stat. sig.	Death on (n/n)		Drug-related death
		AA	Ctrl	AA	Ctrl		AA	Ctrl	
1	12	90	50	51	28	Yes	5/91	2/75	0
2	12	NA	NA	54	16	Yes	1/45	0/43	1
3	12	60	46	40	21	Yes	1/48	0/52	0
4	6	70	82	48	39	No	2/26	0/25	1
5	3	NA	NA	75[d]	56[d]	Yes	2/103	1/104	1
6	3	NA	NA	69[d]	41[d]	Yes	1/88	0/87	1
7	12	70	39	54	30	Yes	2/44	0/46	0
8	12	66	61[e]	25	13	No	NA	NA	NA
9	12	70	54	49	36	No	0/36	0/37	0
10	6	76	71[f]	55	67	No	0	0	0
11	6	80	70[g]	49	42[g]	No	1/97	1/86[g]	0[i]
12	12	61	59[h]	37	30[h]	No	2/28	0/25	2[j]
13	6	NA	NA	83	43[g]	Yes	0/28	0/26[g]	0

Abbreviations: AA, antiarrhythmic drug; AF, atrial fibrillation; CAD, coronary artery disease; CTR, control group; lone AF, atrial fibrillation without underlying heart disease; SH, systemic hypertension; SR, sinus rhythm; Stat. sig., statistically significant; VHD, valvular heart disease
[a] Median value.
[b] Ischemic and/or hypertensive heart disease.
[c] For persistent atrial fibrillation only.
[d] Follow up 3 months.
[e] Control drug: propranolol.
[f] Control drug: disopyramide.
[g] Long acting quinidine.
[h] Control drug: propafenone.
[i] Two severe proarrhythmias on each drug early after start of the drug.
[j] Sudden deaths (one documented torsade de pointes) after recent dosage increase.
Modified from Crijns *et al*,[84] where details of the studies are given.

without implanting an artificial pacemaker. This relates to possible sinus node or atrioventricular conduction disturbances caused by negative chronotropic drugs. In Wolff–Parkinson–White syndrome complicated by atrial fibrillation acute rate control (as well as conversion to sinus rhythm) may be achieved by procainamide or flecainide.[83]

Prevention of recurrences of persistent atrial fibrillation

Persistent atrial fibrillation does not disappear spontaneously and is difficult to terminate with drugs. First choice therapy for restoration of sinus rhythm is DC electrical cardioversion. However, the Achilles' heel of cardioversion is that atrial fibrillation frequently relapses if left untreated. Recurrences happen predominantly during the first month after cardioversion (Table 37.4, Figure 37.5).[84] Preliminary data from our institution indicate that there is a vulnerable period which is confined to the first week after the shock.

The notion that about 50% of patients will maintain sinus rhythm for over 1 year after cardioversion should be taken with caution since most studies show a progressive pattern of relapses but do not give information beyond 1 year. After a single shock (without prophylactic drugs) the 4 year arrhythmia-free survival rate presumably does not exceed 10%.[8] This means that most patients need prophylactic therapy after cardioversion. However, even when using a serial

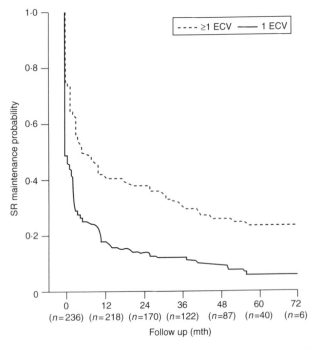

Figure 37.5 Kaplan–Meier plots depicting the probability of maintenance of sinus rhythm (SR) after serial electrical conversions (≥1 ECV) compared to a single cardioversion without drug prescription (1 ECV). *n*, number of patients at risk during serial cardioversion therapy. (From Van Gelder *et al*[8] with permission.)

antiarrhythmic approach only around 30% of patients maintain sinus rhythm for 4 years (Figure 37.5).[8]

Most prophylactic drugs are equally effective, except for amiodarone which appears to be more efficacious. Quinidine has been studied most frequently. A meta-analysis of six controlled trials showed that quinidine was superior to no treatment (50% *v* 25% of the patients remained in sinus rhythm during one year, respectively). However, the total mortality was significantly higher in the quinidine group: 12 of 413 patients (2·9%) *v* 3 of 387 patients (0·8%) respectively ($P < 0·05$).[85] Also, a recent registry demonstrated a relatively high incidence of sudden death with quinidine.[86] Of 570 patients aged younger than 65 years, 6 patients died suddenly, all shortly after restoration of sinus rhythm. These findings make it questionable whether there is still a role for quinidine in the prophylaxis of atrial fibrillation.

Only a few controlled trials evaluated the Class IC drugs flecainide and propafenone and the Class III drug sotalol, showing that they are comparable to Class IA drugs (Table 37.4). However, differences may be observed in the adverse event profile which may guide the choice for one particular drug (see below). In general, Class IC drugs and sotalol are better tolerated than Class IA drugs and amiodarone. On the other hand, all except amiodarone cause significant proarrhythmia. Limited prospective comparative data of amiodarone are available but a favorable outcome has been reported when amiodarone is instituted as a last resort agent. The drug is particularly useful in atrial fibrillation complicated by heart failure. Unfortunately, its use is limited by potentially severe non-cardiac adverse effects. However, low dose amiodarone (200 mg daily) is effective and gives only few adverse events.[87] Gosselink *et al* included 89 patients with chronic atrial fibrillation who had failed previous treatment aimed at maintenance of sinus rhythm. These patients were treated with a mean dose of amiodarone of 204±66 mg. Actuarially, 53% of these patients were still in sinus rhythm after a follow up of 3 years. Adverse events occurred in three patients and were a reason for discontinuation in only one patient.[87] β Blockers are only effective in preventing early but not late recurrences,[88] presumably by suppressing adrenergic-dependent premature beats in the early phase after cardioversion. It is uncertain when to start β blockade and which patients benefit. Obviously, these issues warrant further evaluation.

Rate control in atrial fibrillation

Although increased morbidity and mortality conveyed by atrial fibrillation provide a clear impetus to rhythm control as the first line strategy, there is no direct evidence that rhythm control confers additional benefit over rate control with regard to improved survival or reduced risk for stroke. Furthermore, rate control appears to be more appropriate as a primary strategy in a substantial proportion of patients with atrial fibrillation, including those with a permanent form of the arrhythmia, patients with heart failure and mildly symptomatic, longstanding atrial fibrillation, patients with persistent arrhythmia and failed repeat cardioversions and serial prophylactic antiarrhythmic drug therapy, and those in whom risk/benefit ratio from using specific antiarrhythmic agents is shifted towards increased risk.

To date, there are four studies which have addressed the issue of rate versus rhythm control in a systematic fashion (Table 37.5).

The PIAF (Pharmacological Intervention in Atrial Fibrillation) trial[89] and the pilot STAF (Strategies of Treatment of Atrial Fibrillation) study[90] in patients with persistent atrial fibrillation were not powered to determine survival benefit but showed that both strategies yielded similar results with regard to symptoms, functional status and quality of life improvement. Despite repeat cardioversions and serial antiarrhythmic drug therapy, 56% PIAF patients and 40% STAF patients, who were assigned to rhythm control, maintained sinus rhythm at 1 year. Of note, although there was no difference in the incidence of composite primary end point events (death, cardiovascular event or systemic embolism) in the rhythm

control and the rate control groups (9 and 10 events, respectively) in the STAF population, 18 of these occurred while patients were in atrial fibrillation, providing indirect evidence that maintenance of sinus rhythm is protective.

The preliminary results of the RACE (RAte Control versus Electrical cardioversion) study of 522 patients with persistent AF have also shown no difference in the primary composite end point of cardiovascular death, hospital admissions for heart failure, thromboembolic events, major bleedings, pacemaker implantation, and adverse effects of antiarrhythmic drug therapy between the two strategies (22·6% v 17·2%) (unpublished results at the time of this chapter going to press). This study was designed to prove non-inferiority of rate control, and indeed, a −5·4% absolute difference with 90% confidence intervals ranging from −11·0% to 0·4% showed a non-significant trend in favor of the rate control strategy. After 3 years of follow up, sinus rhythm was maintained in less than half the patients randomized to rhythm control, implying that the strategies appear equal not because atrial fibrillation and sinus rhythm were associated with the equivalent risk for prespecified end points, but due

Table 37.5 Randomized studies of rhythm and rate control strategies in atrial fibrillation

Study	Patients (n)	Follow up	Rhythm control	Rate control	Patients in SR[a]	Primary end point
PIAF[89]	252	1 yr	n = 127 Amiodarone, repeat DCC	n = 125 Diltiazem	56% v 10%	Symptomatic improvement 55% v 61% (n.s.)
STAF[90]	200	2 yr	n = 200 Amiodarone, repeat DCC	n = 200 Digoxin β blockers Calcium blockers	40% v 12% at 1 yr, 26% v 11% at 2 yr; 23% v 0% at 3 yr	Composite end point (all-cause mortality, cardiovascular events, CPR, TE) 9 v 10; 18/19 events occurred during AF
RACE[b]	522	2·3 yr	n = 266 Serial DCC + sotalol, propafenone or flecainide, amiodarone	n = 256 Digoxin β blockers Calcium blockers	40% v 10%	Composite end point (cardiovascular death, admissions for CHF, TE, bleeding, pacemaker implantation, adverse effects of AAD) 22·6% v 17·2%; in HTN 30·8% v 17·3%
AFFIRM[b]	4060	3·5 yr	n = 2033 Amiodarone, sotalol, propafenone, procainamide, quinidine, flecainide	n = 2027 Digoxin, β blockers Calcium blockers	60% v 38% at 5 yr	All-cause mortality 27% v 26% (n.s.)

[a]Rhythm v rate control.
[b]Preliminary results.
Abbreviations: AAD, antiarrhythmic drugs; AF, atrial fibrillation; CHF, congestive heart failure; CPR, cardiopulmonary resuscitation; DCC, direct current cardioversion; HTN, hypertension; SR, sinus rhythm; TE, thromboembolism

to the fact that that it was not possible to achieve rhythm control in a significant proportion of patients assigned to this strategy. This is in consistency with the inclusion criteria for the RACE study, allowing participation of patients with persistent atrial fibrillation who may have had the arrhythmia as long as 12 months' duration and who had undergone one or two electrical cardioversions in the past 2 years. Despite an aggressive rhythm control strategy, including three antiarrhythmic drugs (sotalol, propafenone or flecainide, and amiodarone) and serial cardioversions, the likelihood of maintenance of sinus rhythm in this selected group of patients is expected to be low, thus favoring the rate control strategy. Likewise in the STAF study, atrial fibrillation was an underlying rhythm in more than two thirds of the RACE patients at the time of the primary end point events.

The largest to date AFFIRM (Atrial Fibrillation Follow up Investigation of Rhythm Management) study of 4060 patients over 65 years or under 65 years but with at least one risk factor for stroke, which was designed to assess mortality benefit of different strategies in atrial fibrillation, has shown no difference in the primary end point of all-cause mortality as well as quality of life and functional status between the two strategies (unpublished results at the time of this chapter going to press). However, likewise the results of the RACE study, the conclusions drawn from the AFFIRM trial, which pertained to older patients in whom rate control is generally considered to be preferential, can only be applied to selected groups of patients with atrial fibrillation and cannot be extrapolated on younger patients who are more likely to be symptomatic and to have impaired quality of life associated with the arrhythmia, even if good rate control has been achieved.

The aim of rate control in atrial fibrillation is to improve symptoms, functional status and quality of life and to prevent the progression of left ventricular dysfunction and heart failure. There is no accepted definition for adequate rate control at rest or exercise. To compensate for loss of atrial contribution, the ventricular rate during AF should probably be about 10–20% higher than a corresponding rate during sinus rhythm. The rate is generally considered controlled if the ventricular rate response is between 60 and 80 beats/min at rest and between 90 and 115 beats/min during moderate exercise.[2]

Rate control therapy in atrial tachyarrhythmias is based mainly on depression of conduction through the atrioventricular node. This is achieved by digitalis, calcium-channel blockers and β blockers. The evidence in favor of sotalol or amiodarone as rate slowing agents is poor. In permanent atrial fibrillation, digoxin usually provides rate control at rest by prolongation of atrioventricular nodal conduction and refractoriness through vagal stimulation, by direct effects on the atrioventricular node, and by increasing the amount of concealed conduction in the atrioventricular node due to the increased rate at which atria discharge. Due to

sympathetic overdrive it does not prevent an excessive heart rate increase during daily life exercise, especially in younger, active patients, in which case concomitant use of multiple drugs may be necessary to provide an adequate ventricular rate response, such as β blockers and non-dihydropyridine calcium antagonists. On the other hand, β blockers but also verapamil and diltiazem may reduce peak heart rate too much, thereby limiting the exercise tolerability and quality of life. These agents should be titrated to provide control of both resting and daily life exercise heart rate. In active patients it is necessary to monitor peak exercise heart rate which should not be blunted too much by drugs. Digoxin is accepted as primary rate control treatment in atrial fibrillation complicated by heart failure, but this advice lacks a solid scientific basis. In the light of the positive studies on β blockers in heart failure it seems worthwhile to evaluate their rate controlling effects in this setting. Finally, there is a delay of 30–60 minutes before onset of the therapeutic effect of digoxin, and a peak effect develops after 4–6 hours which limits the use of digoxin in emergency settings.

β blockers, including propranolol, atenolol, metoprolol or esmolol, may be particularly useful in the presence of high adrenergic tone. In the recent crossover, open label study of five drug regimens, the combination of digoxin and atenolol has been shown to be superior to digoxin, atenolol, and diltiazem alone, and the combination of digoxin with diltiazem for rate control, especially during exercise.[91] In randomized, placebo-controlled studies, non-dihydropyridine calcium antagonists, verapamil and diltiazem, have proven effective for rate control in acute atrial fibrillation as they have a rapid onset of action and slow heart rate by 25% within 3–7 minutes of administration but their effects are transient, and repeat doses or a continuous intravenous infusion may be required to maintain adequate rate control.[92,93]

Finally, there are data suggesting that amiodarone may provide adequate rate control during atrial fibrillation if it fails to restore and/or maintain sinus rhythm. In the CHF-STAT study, amiodarone produced a sustained and significant slowing of the mean and maximal ventricular rate responses in the range of 16–20% and 14–22%, respectively.[73] However, the efficacy and safety of amiodarone purely for rate control have not been tested prospectively. Agents that may be administered for control of the ventricular rate response in atrial fibrillation are listed in below.

Atrial fibrillation after cardiac surgery

The incidence of atrial fibrillation after cardiac surgery is 27–37% following coronary bypass surgery and exceeds 50% after valvular surgery.[94–97] Postoperative AF occurs predominantly during the first 4 days and is associated with increased morbidity and mortality, largely due to stroke and circulatory failure, and longer hospital stay. More than 90%

Agents for rate control in atrial fibrillation		
Drug	Dose	Level of evidence
Digoxin	Loading dose: 250 micrograms every 2 hours; up to 1500 micrograms; maintenance dose 125–250 micrograms daily	Grade A
Diltiazem	120–360 mg daily	Grade A
Verapamil	120–360 mg daily	
Metoprolol	50–200 mg daily	Grade A
Atenolol	50–100 mg daily	
Propranolol	80–240 mg daily	
Amiodarone	800 mg daily for 1 week; then 600 mg daily for 1 week; then 400 mg daily for 4–6 weeks; maintenance dose 200 mg daily	Grade C

patients present with a paroxysmal or first onset form of the arrhythmia.[96] Atrial flutter and atrial tachycardias, including multifocal atrial tachycardia, are also not uncommon.

Clinical factors that convey a higher risk for the development of postoperative atrial tachyarrhythmias include advanced age, male sex, a previous history of atrial fibrillation, hypertension, congestive heart failure, valvular heart disease, chronic obstructive pulmonary disease, chronic renal failure, previous cardiac surgery, left atrial enlargement, inadequate cardioprotection and hypothermia, right coronary artery grafting, and a longer bypass time.[98] Recent observations suggest that the incidence of postoperative atrial tachyarrhythmias is lower with minimally invasive techniques, especially for valvular surgery. The pathophysiology of atrial fibrillation after cardiac surgery relates to perioperative changes in atrial electrophysiology, including increased dispersion of atrial refractoriness, decreased atrial conduction velocity, and changes in atrial transmembrane potential. A rhythm control strategy, including electrical or pharmacologic restoration of sinus rhythm with subsequent prophylactic antiarrhythmic therapy should be considered in hemodynamically unstable or highly symptomatic patients with postoperative atrial fibrillation. Low energy internal atrial defibrillation using temporary implanted epicardial coils may be particularly effective in high-risk patients with contraindications to pharmacologic therapy.[99]

Rate control may be preferable in the absence of hemodynamic compromise or poorly tolerated symptoms as atrial fibrillation after coronary bypass surgery appears to be self-limited and there is a high likelihood of spontaneous conversion to sinus rhythm within 6 weeks after discharge.[100] Although digoxin and non-dihydropyridine calcium antagonists (verapamil, diltiazem) are effective in slowing atrioventricular conduction, β blockers should be considered the first line choice because of their beneficial effects on

hyperadrenergic postoperative state and a high probability of restoring sinus rhythm (see below).

Short-acting β blocking agents for intravenous administration, such as esmolol, may be preferable in the presence of increased risk for bradyarrhythmias, hypotension, and bronchospasm. In a small series of patients, intravenous infusion of esmolol was associated with a significantly higher rates of conversion to sinus rhythm compared with intravenous diltiazem (66·6% v 13·3% at 6 hours and 80% v 66·6% at 24 hours).[101] However, diltiazem produced a more rapid rate slowing effect than digoxin (median time to 20% or more decrease in ventricular rates were 2 min and 228 min, respectively).[102] At 2 and 6 hours, the proportion of patients who achieved adequate rate control was significantly higher in the diltiazem-treated group compared with the digoxin-treated group (75% v 35% and 85% v 45%). This difference disappeared only after 12–14 hours of treatment. There is evidence from a retrospective study of 38 hemodynamically unstable patients with atrial tachyarrhythmias suggesting that intravenous amiodarone may provide adequate rate control resulting in a significant hemodynamic improvement and may also potentiate reversion to sinus rhythm.[103]

The role of β blocker therapy in controlling atrial tachyarrhythmias after cardiac surgery is well established. Two meta-analyses of randomized controlled studies have shown that treatment with β blockers may reduce the incidence of atrial fibrillation by approximately 50%.[104,105] β blockade should always be started or continued as soon as possible after cardiac surgery. There is indirect evidence that adding digoxin may further reduce the occurrence of atrial arrhythmias or increased the success rate of pharmacologic cardioversion.[104,106,107]

Class IA and IC antiarrhythmic drugs have been proven to be moderately effective in the prevention of atrial tachyarrhythmias after cardiac surgery. The preliminary results from the Clinical Outcomes from the Prevention of Postoperative Arrhythmia (COPPA) II study of 293 patients who had undergone coronary bypass have shown that treatment with propafenone 675 mg daily reduced the incidence of postoperative atrial fibrillation to 12·4% compared with 22·7% on placebo.[108] However, there was no difference in the prevalence of atrial fibrillation between patients treated with propafenone at a lower dose of 450 mg daily and the placebo group. Of note, in addition to the study drug or placebo, 93% of patients received digoxin and 84% received β blockers.

Propafenone administered intravenously at a dose of 2 mg/kg produced a more rapid effect on restoration of sinus rhythm compared with intravenous procainamide given at a dose of 20 mg/kg to maximum of 1000 mg (59% v 18% at 15 minutes) but there was no significant difference in the conversion rates at 1 hour (76% v 61%).[109] However, procainamide was associated with a significantly higher

Principles of management of atrial tachyarrhythmias after cardiac surgery			
Strategy	**Therapy**	**Effectiveness**	**Level of evidence**
Prophylaxis (before and/or after surgery)	β blockers	Effectiveness proven	**Grade A**
	Class III antiarrhythmic drugs (sotalol, amiodarone)	Effectiveness mainly proven	**Grade A**
	Class IA and IC antiarrhythmic drugs (procainamide, propafenone)	Possibly effective	**Grade A**
	Digoxin	Ineffective alone, possibly increases the effectiveness of the above	**Grade A**
	Calcium-channel blockers	Ineffective	**Grade B**
Pharmacologic cardioversion	Ibutilide	Effectiveness proven, especially for atrial flutter	**Grade A**
	Amiodarone Class IA and IC antiarrhythmic drugs (procainamide, propafenone)	Possibly effective	**Grade A**
Electrical cardioversion	Low energy internal cardioversion	Effective and preferable in high-risk patients	**Grade B**
Rate control	β blockers	Effectiveness proven	**Grade A**
	Calcium antagonists	Effectiveness proven	**Grade A**
	Digoxin	Effectiveness proven	**Grade A**
	Amiodarone	Possibly effective	**Grade B**
Anticoagulation	Warfarin or LMWH	Effective, required if AF persists more than 24–48 h	**Grade B**
Atrial pacing	Single, dual site or biatrial	Possibly effective but controversy exists	**Grade B**

Abbreviations: AF, atrial fibrillation; LMWH, low molecular weight heparin

incidence of hypotension than propafenone (27% *v* 7%) which was clinically relevant and required discontinuation of the drug in 9% cases. Procainamide does not appear to be more effective than placebo in the prevention of atrial fibrillation but it has not been studied systematically.[110,111] Finally, quinidine has been shown to reduce recurrence of atrial fibrillation in patients who developed the arrhythmia after coronary bypass surgery as assessed by serial 24 hour Holter monitoring and regular physical examination during a 3 month period of follow up, but it was associated with a 16·6% rate of adverse effects.[112]

Sotalol has been reported to reduce the incidence of postoperative atrial fibrillation by 20% to 67% compared with placebo and to have a relatively safe profile in randomized, controlled studies.[113–117] Sotalol may be more effective in the prevention of atrial fibrillation as compared with β blockers because of its potential incremental benefit due to Class III antiarrhythmic drug properties. However, in a randomized study of 429 patients who had undergone cardiac surgery, both low- and high-dose propranolol (40 or 80 mg daily) and

low- and high-dose sotalol (120 or 240 mg daily) were comparably effective in reducing the incidence of atrial fibrillation to 14 and 19% or to 11% and 14% respectively.[118] In another series of patients, sotalol proved to be superior to metoprolol resulting in a twofold decrease in atrial fibrillation.[119]

There is compelling evidence from randomized, controlled studies that treatment with amiodarone may reduce the incidence and duration of postoperative atrial fibrillation, and is also effective for control of the ventricular rate.[120–128] Although in some studies amiodarone did not statistically alter the occurrence of atrial tachyarrhythmias, favorable trends were noted for selected groups of patients. The Amiodarone Reduction in Coronary Heart (ARCH) study of 300 patients who had undergone coronary bypass surgery has shown a significant reduction in the incidence of postoperative atrial fibrillation with intravenous amiodarone compared with placebo (35% *v* 47%) without significant risk from the active agent.[126] In the Atrial Fibrillation Suppression Trial (AFIST), there was a significant difference in favor of amiodarone for symptomatic atrial fibrillation

(4·2% *v* 18%).[127] However, adverse events, especially brady-cardia necessitating chronotropic support or pacing, may limit its feasibility. Thus, temporary atrial pacing was required due to bradycardia in 40–48% patients who received prophylactic amiodarone compared with 28% patients in the placebo group.[128] Recent meta-analysis of 42 randomized trials of amiodarone, sotalol and β blockers has shown that each of the three drug treatments prevented postoperative atrial fibrillation with odds ratios of 0·48, 0·35, and 0·39, respectively.[129]

Magnesium sulphate (administered intravenously during the first 4–5 days) has been reported to significantly reduce the incidence and the number of episodes of atrial fibrilla-tion.[130,131] In the recent randomized, controlled study of 200 patients who had undergone elective coronary bypass surgery, infusion of 6 mmol of magnesium sulphate the day before, immediately after and for 4 consecutive days after the inter-vention was associated with a 2% incidence of postoperative atrial fibrillation compared with 21% in the placebo arm.[130] The favorable effects of magnesium may relate to restoration of electrolyte balance after surgery. Alternatively, the stimulat-ing effects of magnesium on the sodium/potassium pump may act beneficially by inducing a calcium-channel blocking effect. However, magnesium infusion did not confer additional bene-fit in patients already treated with propranolol (22·4% com-pared with 19·5% on propranolol alone)[132] and was less effective than intravenous amiodarone (the cumulative rates of atrial fibrillation were 23% and 14% respectively).[126] Finally, glucose–insulin–potassium infusion started at anes-thetic induction and continued for 12 hours postoperatively significantly decreased the incidence of atrial fibrillation com-pared with placebo (15% *v* 60%) in diabetic patients.[133]

Several new Class III antiarrhythmic drugs, ibutilide and dofetilide, have recently proven effective for pharmacologic cardioversion of atrial tachyarrhythmias after cardiac sur-gery. In 302 patients, 101 of whom presented with atrial flutter, intravenous ibutilide given at three dose regimens (0·25, 0·5, or 1 mg) was associated with significantly higher conversion rates (40%, 47%, and 57%, respectively) com-pared with placebo (15%).[112] Conversion rates at all doses were higher for atrial flutter than for atrial fibrillation, reach-ing 78% versus 44% with a dose of 1 mg. Pretreatment with ibutilide was associated with a trend towards lower energy levels required for external defibrillation. Of note, there was a suggestion of a benefit of concomitant therapy with digoxin: 65% patients treated with digoxin were success-fully cardioverted with 1 mg of ibutilide compared with 31% patients who did not receive digoxin. Dofetilide adminis-tered intravenously at a dose of 4 or 8 micrograms/kg was associated with a non-significant trend towards higher inci-dence of restoration of sinus rhythm compared with placebo (36% and 44% *v* 24%).

However, in virtually all randomized studies antiar-rhythmic drug therapy, probably except for amiodarone,

accomplished no reduction in the length of hospital stay. Selected randomized, controlled trials of prophylactic antiar-rhythmic drug therapy for postoperative atrial fibrillation are listed in Table 37.6.

The potential role of preventative atrial pacing for post-operative atrial fibrillation has been investigated in a number of randomized studies, but the efficacy of this therapeutic modality has not yet been proven. This issue will be discussed in more details in the following sections.

Persistent and permanent atrial fibrillation in the setting of heart failure – evidence base for "upstream" therapy

In patients with atrial fibrillation in the setting of heart fail-ure, management should be aimed initially at adequate ther-apy of heart failure. Thereafter, electrical cardioversion may be considered in younger patients with a short arrhythmia duration who have been successfully re-compensated. In case of an early relapse (<6 months after the last shock) re-cardioversion should be performed after pretreatment with amiodarone.[87] Repeat cardioversions with intervals longer than 6 months between each shock is an appropriate man-ner to prevent progression of heart failure.

Effective conventional treatment of congestive heart failure delays progression of left ventricular dysfunction and reduces mitral regurgitation and consequently, may prevent left atrial dilation and stretch which are considered to be important constituents of the substrate for atrial tachyarrhythmias by creating "a critical mass" necessary for multiple wavelet re-entry and stretch-related abnormal automaticity in the atria. Experimental evidence suggests that angiotensin enzyme converting (ACE) inhibitors may provide additional "antiarrhythmic" benefit by reducing adverse electrophysiolo-gic effects of angiotensin II due to lessening the extent of fibrosis within the atrial myocardium.[135,136]

The beneficial effect of an ACE inhibitor on the frequency of atrial fibrillation was first shown in the TRACE (Trandolapril Cardiac Evaluation) study of 1749 post myocar-dial infarction patients with left ventricular dysfunction.[137] In the trandolapril group, significantly fewer patients devel-oped atrial fibrillation during follow up compared with the placebo group (2·8% *v* 5·3%), reflecting a 55% risk reduction. Pretreatment with an ACE inhibitor before electrical cardioversion in patients with congestive heart failure and persistent atrial fibrillation increased a likelihood of restora-tion of sinus rhythm (33% in the ACE inhibitor-treated group *v* 7% in the untreated group) and exhibited a trend towards fewer recurrences of the arrhythmia.[138] Furthermore, angiotensin II AT_1-receptor blocker irbersartan has been shown to promote pharmacologic cardioversion of persistent atrial fibrillation by oral amiodarone (32% compared with 23% on amiodarone alone) and to reduce the recurrence rate

Table 37.6 Clinical evidence of the efficacy of antiarrhythmic therapy with Class I and III antiarrhythmic drugs for conversion and/or prophylaxis of atrial tachyarrhythmias after cardiac surgery

Study (first author)	Patients (n)	Treatment arm	Control arm	Incidence of AF v placebo	Adverse effects
Laub[110]	46	Procainamide IV 12 mg/kg, then 2 mg/min started within 1 h after surgery	Placebo	3·9/day at risk v 10·6 day at risk	–
Gold[111]	100	Oral procainamide (weight adjusted dose) for 4 days after surgery	Placebo	38% v 26% but reduced duration of AF (16 v 28 patient-days)	Hypotension
COPPA II[108]	293	Oral propafenone 675 mg Oral propafenone 400 mg started within 24 h for 15 days or until discharge	Placebo	12·4% v 22·5% v 22·7%	–
Geelen[109]	62	Propafenone IV 2 mg/kg in 10 min	Procainamide IV 20 mg/kg (maximum 1000 mg)	Conversion rates: 59% v 18% at 15 min (P<0·001); 76% v 61% at 1 h (difference n.s.)	Hypotension in 7% in the propafenone arm 27% in the procainamide arm (9% severe)
Nystrom[120]	101	Oral sotalol	β blocker	10% v 29% (P= 0·028)	Sotalol stopped or dose reduced in 10% v none in the control arm
Suttorp[117]	300	Sotalol 240 mg started from the 4th h for 6 days after surgery	Placebo	16% v 33%	Sotalol stopped in 1%; placebo stopped in 3%
Suttorp[118]	429	Sotalol 120 mg or Sotalol 240 mg started from the 4th h for 6 days after surgery	Propranolol 40 mg Propranolol 80 mg	13·9% v 18·8% 10·9% v 13·7% (difference n.s.)	Either low-dose drug stopped in 2·9%; either high-dose drug stopped in 10·7%
Evrard[113]	206	Oral sotalol 160 mg from the 1st day after surgery	Matched control patients; no β blockers	16% v 48% (P< 0·0001); 20% reduction	Sotalol stopped in 7·8% v none in the control arm
Pfisterer[114]	255	Oral sotalol 160 mg started 2 h before until discharge	Placebo	26% v 46% (P= 0·0012); 43% reduction	Sotalol stopped in 5·6%; placebo stopped in 3·9% (difference n.s.)
Matsuura[115]	80	Oral sotalol 80 mg for 14 days after surgery	Matched control patients	15% v 37·5% (P= 0·05)	Hypotension on sotalol in 7·5%
Gomes[116]	85	Oral sotalol 80–120 mg 24–48 h before and 4 days after surgery	Placebo	12·5% v 38% (P= 0·008); 67% reduction	Sotalol stopped (bradycardia, hypotension) in 5% v none in the control arm

Table 37.6 Continued

Study (first author)	Patients (n)	Treatment arm	Control arm	Incidence of AF v placebo	Adverse effects
Parikka[119]	191	Oral sotalol 120 mg after surgery	Oral metoprolol 75 mg	16% v 30% (P< 0·01)	–
Daoud[121]	124	Oral amiodarone 600 mg started for a minimum of 7 days before surgery, then 200 mg until discharge	Placebo	25% v 53% (P= 0·04)	Major morbidity and mortality events occurred in 12% and 5% in the amiodarone arm v 10% and 3% in the placebo arm
Lee[122]	140	Amiodarone 150 mg IV, then 400 mg/kg/h for 3 days before and 5 days after surgery	Placebo	12% v 34% (P< 0·01); longer stay in intensive care in the placebo arm	–
Reddle[123]	143	Oral amiodarone 2000 mg 1–4 days before surgery and 400 mg for 7 days after surgery	Placebo	24·7% v 32·8% (difference n.s.) Amiodarone + β blockers: 16·7% v 32·8% in the remaining patients	–
Solomon[124]	102	Amiodarone IV 1000 mg/day for 48 h, then 400 mg/day	Propranolol IV 1 mg every 6 h for 48 h, then 80 mg/day until discharge	16% v 32·7% (P= 0·05)	–
Treggiari-Venzi[125]	155	Amiodarone IV 900 mg/d for 72 h	Magnesium sulphate 4000 mg/d for 72 h Placebo	14% v 23% v 27% (difference n.s.)	–
ARCH[126]	300	Amiodarone IV 100 mg/d for 2 days	Placebo	35% v 47% (P= 0·01)	Major morbidity and mortality events occurred in 2·5% and 0% in the amiodarone arm v 4·9% and 1·4% in the placebo arm
AFIST[127]	220	Oral amiodarone 600 mg for 5 days or 1600 mg for 1 day before surgery, then 800–1200 mg on the day of surgery and 800 mg for 1–4 days after surgery	Placebo	22·5% v 38·0%; 4·2% v 18·0% for symptomatic AF	Bradycardia and hypotension on amiodarone in 7·5% and 14·2% v 7·5% and 10·0% in the placebo arm

Table 37.6 Continued

Study (first author)	Patients (n)	Treatment arm	Control arm	Incidence of AF v placebo	Adverse effects
VaderLugt[107]	302 (101 with flutter)	Ibutilide IV 0.25 mg, 0.5 mg, 1 mg	Placebo	Conversion rates: 40%, 47%, 57% v 15% in the placebo arm; at 1 mg 44% for AF, 78% for flutter	All ibutilide v placebo: hypotension 2.8% v 1.3%; ventricular arrhythmias 8.3% v 1.2%, torsade de pointes 1.8% v 1.2%
Frost[134]	98 with AF/flutter	Dofetilide IV 8 microgram/kg Dofetilide IV 4 microgram/kg	Placebo	Conversion rates: 44% v 33% v 24% (difference n.s.)	Ventricular tachycardia in 9.3% on high-dose dofetilide

Abbreviaiton: AF, atrial fibrillation

at 2 months of follow up (14% v 30%).[139] Finally, in a series of 750 patients with advanced heart failure who were evaluated for heart transplantation, an increase in use of ACE inhibitors and amiodarone between 1985 and 1993 was associated with an improvement in the 2 year survival rate from 39% to 66% in those with atrial fibrillation.[140]

Although β blockers are usually ineffective for long term maintenance of sinus rhythm, except for adrenergically mediated atrial fibrillation, therapy with β blockers in patients with heart failure may confer benefit in terms of prevention or delay in the development of the arrhythmia likely due to an overall beneficial effect in heart failure. In the CAPRICORN (Carvedilol Post-Infarct Survival Control in Left Ventricular Dysfunction) study of 1959 patients with myocardial infarction and left ventricular dysfunction, therapy with carvedilol reduced risk of the development of atrial fibrillation or flutter by nearly two thirds.[141] However, it is unclear whether it translates into survival benefit. Although the subgroup analysis of CIBIS (Cardiac Insufficiency Bisoprolol Study) II data has shown that bisoprolol reduced all-cause mortality in patients with sinus rhythm (relative risk 0.58) but not in patients presenting with atrial fibrillation (relative risk 1.16),[142] the preliminary data from the COPERNICUS (Carvedilol Prospective Randomized Cumulative Survival) study have suggested that in the subgroup of patients with atrial fibrillation carvedilol was associated with a better survival compared with placebo, but this effect was less pronounced than in patients with sinus rhythm.

These observations open the possibility of exploitation of ACE inhibitors and angiotensin II AT$_1$-receptor blockers to prevent or delay atrial remodeling in atrial fibrillation and introduce the concept of "upstream" therapy targeting the underlying disease process, such as heart failure or hypertension, that may favor the atrial arrhythmia by disorganized hemodynamics or the development of atrial pathology.

Tolerability and safety of antiarrhythmic drugs

The most important adverse effects of drugs used in atrial fibrillation are ventricular proarrhythmia, heart failure, enhanced atrioventricular nodal conduction, and exacerbation of sick sinus syndrome (or atrioventricular conduction disturbances). The latter may be the basis for atrial fibrillation and can be unmasked by all antiarrhythmic drugs, including digitalis.

Class IA and III drugs predominantly cause polymorphic ventricular tachycardia or torsade de pointes,[143,144] and Class IC drugs, incessant monomorphic ventricular tachycardias and ventricular fibrillation.[145,146] In contrast to the quinidine-like drugs, ventricular proarrhythmia or sudden death due to Class IC drugs is virtually absent in patients *without* overt heart disease. Patients treated with quinidine or sotalol may experience sudden death especially *early* after onset of therapy or after dosage increases.[86] Amiodarone shows a low incidence of torsade de pointes and may even be instituted after proarrhythmic events on Class IA drugs. Class III agent, dofetilide, has been shown to exhibit reverse use-dependence, that is, a decline in its ability to prolong action potential duration and effective refractory period at higher heart rates, a property which is associated with potentially proarrhythmic QT prolongation during bradycardia. The incidence of torsade de pointes in the DIAMOND study was 3.3%, the majority of which occurred within the first 3 days.[147]

Proarrhythmic effects of ibutilide are also likely to be due to marked prolongation of ventricular repolarization, favoring the occurrence of early after-depolarizations. The incidence of sustained torsade de pointes associated with ibutilide infusion for conversion of atrial fibrillation or flutter was reported to be 1·7%, with the majority of episodes occurring within 1 hour of drug administration, although patients with a high risk of the development of proarrhythmia, that is, with a history of torsade de pointes and baseline QT interval prolongation, were excluded.[148] Torsade de pointes occurred in 0·9% of patients receiving azimilide at doses of 100 mg and 125 mg.[149]

Electrocardiographic signs, potentially useful in the prediction of proarrhythmia with Class IA and III drugs, include acute and excessive QT prolongation, pause-related TU wave changes, and increased QT dispersion. Torsade de pointes may occur, especially if there is a pre-existing QT prolongation, and is enhanced by bradycardia (for example, occurring after sudden conversion of "rapid" atrial fibrillation to "slow" sinus rhythm). Late proarrhythmia may occur after addition of drugs, like diuretics or during intercurrent bradycardia. Recently, it was demonstrated that women are more susceptible than men.[150] Ventricular proarrhythmia with Class IC drugs should be expected in patients with previous sustained ventricular tachycardia and in those with structural heart disease receiving a high dose. It occurs predominantly late after institution of the drug, and especially during higher heart rates. In this respect, it is considered useful to perform an exercise test after institution of the drug. During higher heart rates conduction slowing may become more prominent. Excessive broadening of the QRS complex during high heart rates may be a marker of future ventricular proarrhythmia necessitating dose reduction or termination of the drug.

Patients using Class IA and IC drugs may experience high ventricular rates during breakthrough atrial fibrillation or flutter. These agents do not suppress and may even augment atrioventricular conduction by anticholinergic stimulation. AV conduction is further reinforced by exercise and anxiety. Therefore patients using these drugs prophylactically must be cautioned to avoid exercise during a recurrence of atrial fibrillation. Digoxin, a β blockers or a calcium-channel blocker may be added but there are no clinical data to support this approach.

Depending on dose and duration of therapy, Class IA and IC drugs especially may cause heart failure, mainly through cardiodepression. Disopyramide allegedly has the largest negative inotropic effects and may cause heart failure early but also late (months) after initiation, especially in patients with a history of cardiac insufficiency. The other Class IA drugs, as well as β blockers (including sotalol) and calcium-channel blockers, rarely cause heart failure in patients with atrial fibrillation. Heart failure induced by amiodarone has not been described.

Where to initiate antiarrhythmic drug therapy

The issue of the proper site for initiation of antiarrhythmic drug therapy for atrial tachyarrhythmias revolves around considerations of risk and practicality.[151] Inhospital initiation under monitored conditions conveys benefits of accurate assessment of the efficacy and prompt recognition of adverse effects, such as bradycardia, conduction abnormalities, excessive QT interval prolongation, proarrhythmias, and intolerance or idiosyncrasy. It should, therefore, be considered in patients in atrial fibrillation in whom sinus node function or QT interval duration during sinus rhythm are unknown and patients at anticipated high risk of developing adverse effects, irrespective of the underlying rhythm. For some antiarrhythmic agents, for example, dofetilide, there is formal mandate for inhospital initiation.

In the absence of proarrhythmic concerns and formal labeling, convenience and cost effectiveness favor out-of-hospital initiation, for example, oral propafenone and flecainide in patients with lone atrial fibrillation or atrial fibrillation associated with hypertension without significant left ventricular hypertrophy. The same approach is valid for amiodarone, given its long elimination half life period and low probability of developing torsade de pointes, especially if transtelephonic monitoring is used to provide the surveillance of heart rate, PR and QT interval durations, QRS width, and the assessment of the efficacy of treatment. Table 37.7 summarizes current recommendations on inhospital or out-of-hospital initiation of antiarrhythmic drug treatment.

Table 37.7 Inhospital versus out-of-hospital initiation of antiarrhythmic drug therapy

Drug	Underlying rhythm	
	Atrial fibrillation/flutter	Sinus rhythm
Quinidine	Inpatient	Inpatient
Procainamide	Inpatient	Inpatient
Flecainide	Outpatient[a]	Outpatient
Propafenone	Outpatient[a]	Outpatient
Sotalol	Inpatient	Outpatient[c]
Dofetilide	Inpatient	Inpatient
Azimilide[b]	Inpatient	Inpatient
Amiodarone	Outpatient[c]	Outpatient[c]

[a] No sinus node dysfunction.
[b] An investigational drug.
[c] With transtelephonic monitoring.

As a general rule, antiarrhythmic drugs should be started at a lower dose with upward titration, reassessing the ECG as each dose change is made or concomitant drug therapies are introduced.[2] Of note, even with inhospital initiation, antiarrhythmic agents impose risk of developing proarrhythmia later in the course of therapy, which may be facilitated by progression of underlying heart disease, electrolyte abnormalities, drug interactions, and changes in absorption, metabolism or clearance.

Conclusion

Rational antiarrhythmic treatment of atrial fibrillation starts with establishing whether one is dealing with the paroxysmal, persistent or permanent subtype. Only then the goal of treatment can be identified: to restore sinus rhythm with the option of prophylactic drug treatment or to adopt atrial fibrillation as the dominant rhythm. Antiarrhythmic treatment is further guided by the duration of the arrhythmia, the tendency for recurrence after conversion, and the potential adverse effects of drugs. At some stage during treatment, rate control is useful in all three subtypes of atrial fibrillation but especially in the *permanent* form. The termination of *paroxysmal* atrial fibrillation is enhanced by intravenous drugs. For fibrillation Class IC drugs are first choice whereas Class III drugs may effectively terminate atrial flutter. Restoration of sinus rhythm in *persistent* atrial fibrillation is most effectively achieved by electrical cardioversion but to reduce post-shock recurrence usually antiarrhythmics are indispensable. Despite drugs, the latter approach will at best postpone progression from persistent to permanent atrial fibrillation.

Most patients cannot be cured from atrial fibrillation: almost all will experience recurrence of the arrhythmia earlier or later after the first attack despite drug treatment. Therefore the primary goal of treatment is to reduce morbidity (and possibly also mortality) rather than simply mending the rhythm at any price. Currently, rhythm and rate control strategies are being evaluated concerning their effect on morbidity and mortality. These studies may help to better define the role of the different antiarrhythmic treatments.

Upstream therapy aimed at the underlying pathology and better identification and modification of risk factors is likely to make possible intervention early in the course of the disease when preventative or corrective strategies are most efficient.

Acknowledgments

Isabelle C Van Gelder is supported by the Dutch Heart Foundation, grant 94·014. John Camm is a British Heart Foundation Professor of Cardiology.

References

1. Lévy S. Classification system of atrial fibrillation. *Curr Opin Cardiol* 2000;**15**:54–57.
2. Fuster V, Rydén LE, Asinger RV *et al*. Task Force Report: ACC/AHA/ESC guidelines for the management of patients with atrial fibrillation. *Eur Heart J* 2001:1852–923.
3. Benjamin EJ, Levy D, Vaziri SM *et al*. Independent risk factors for atrial fibrillation in a population-based cohort. The Framingham study. *JAMA* 1994;**271**:840–4.
4. Moe GK. On the multiple wavelet hypothesis of atrial fibrillation. *Arch Int Pharmacodyn Ther* 1962;**140**:183–8.
5. Allessie MA, Lamers WJEP, Bonke FIM, Hollen SJ. Experimental evaluation of Moe's multiple wavelet hypothesis of atrial fibrillation. In: Zipes DP, Jalife J, eds. *Cardiac electrophysiology and arrhythmias*. New York: Grune and Stratton, 1985.
6. Godtfredsen J. Atrial fibrillation. Etiology, course and prognosis. A follow up study of 1212 cases. Thesis, University of Copenhagen, 1975.
7. Fresco C, Proclemer A, on behalf of the PAFIT-2 Investigators. Management of recent onset atrial fibrillation. *Eur Heart J* 1996;**17**(Suppl. C):C41–7.
8. Van Gelder IC, Crijns HJGM, Tieleman RG *et al*. Value and limitation of electrical cardioversion in patients with chronic atrial fibrillation – importance of arrhythmia risk factors and oral anticoagulation. *Arch Intern Med* 1996;**156**:2585–92.
9. Wijffels MCEF, Kirchhof CJHJ, Dorland R, Allessie MA. Atrial fibrillation begets atrial fibrillation. A study in awake chronically instrumented goats. *Circulation* 1995;**92**:1954–68.
10. Coumel P. Neural aspects of paroxysmal atrial fibrillation. In Falk RH, Podrid PJ, eds. *Atrial fibrillation: mechanisms and management*. New York: Raven Press, 1992.
11. Brugada R, Tapscott T, Czernuszewicz GZ *et al*. Identification of a genetic locus for familial atrial fibrillation. *N Engl J Med* 1997;**336**:905–11.
12. Bharati S, Sasaki D, Siedman S, Vidaillet H. Sudden death among patients with a hereditary cardiomyopathy due to a missense mutation in the rad domain of the lamin a/c gene. *J Am Coll Cardiol* 2001;**37**:174A (Abstract).
13. Gruver EJ, Fatkin D, Dodds GA *et al*. Familial hypertrophic cardiomyopathy and atrial fibrillation caused by Arg663His beta–cardiac myosin heavy chain mutation. *Am J Cardiol* 1999;**83**:13H–18H.
14. Savelieva I, Camm AJ. Clinical relevance of silent atrial fibrillation: prevalence, prognosis, quality of life, and management. *J Intervent Cardiac Electrophysiol* 2000;**4**:369–82.
15. Levy S, Maarek M, Coumel P *et al.*, on behalf of the College of French Cardiologists. Characterization of different subsets of atrial fibrillation in general practice in France: the ALFA Study. *Circulation* 1999;**99**:3028–35.
16. Fetsch T, Breithardt G, Engberding R *et al*. Can we believe in symptoms for detection of atrial fibrillation in clinical routine? The results of the PAFAC study. *Circulation* 2001;**104**:II–699 (Abstract).
17. Krahn AD, Manfreda J, Tate RB, Mathewson FAL, Cuddy TE. The natural history of atrial fibrillation: incidence, risk factors, and prognosis in the Manitoba follow up study. *Am J Med* 1995;**98**:476–84.
18. Önundarson PT, Thorgeirsson G, Jonmundsson E, Sigfusson N, Hardarson Th. Chronic atrial fibrillation – epidemiologic features and 14 years follow-up: a case control study. *Eur Heart J* 1987;**8**:521–7.
19. Crijns HJGM, Van den Berg MP, Van Gelder IC, Van Veldhuisen DJ. Management of atrial fibrillation in the setting of heart failure. *Eur Heart J* 1997;**18**(Suppl. C):C45–9.

20.Van Gelder IC, Crijns HJGM, Blanksma PK *et al.* Time course of hemodynamic changes and improvement of exercise tolerance after cardioversion of chronic atrial fibrillation unassociated with cardiac valve disease. *Am J Cardiol* 1993; **72**: 560–6.

21.Kannel WB, Abbott RD, Savage DD, McNamara PM. Epidemiologic features of chronic atrial fibrillation. *N Engl J Med* 1982;**306**:1018–22.

22.Carson PE, Johnson GR, Dunkman WB *et al.* The influence of atrial fibrillation on prognosis in mild to moderate heart failure: the V–HeFT studies. *Circulation* 1993;**87**(Suppl. VI): VI-102–10.

23.Stevenson WG, Stevenson LW, Middlekauff HR *et al.* Improving survival for patients with atrial fibrillation and advanced heart failure. *J Am Coll Cardiol* 1996;**28**:1458–63.

24.Keren G, Etzion T, Sherez J *et al.* Atrial fibrillation and atrial enlargement in patients with mitral stenosis. *Am Heart J* 1987;**114**:1146–55.

25.Sanfilippo AJ, Abascal VM, Sheehan M *et al.* Atrial enlargement as a consequence of atrial fibrillation. *Circulation* 1990; **82**:792–7.

26.Gosselink ATM, Crijns HJGM, Hamer JPM, Hillege H, Lie KI. Changes in atrial dimensions after cardioversion: role of mitral valve disease. *J Am Coll Cardiol* 1993;**22**:1666–72.

27.Wolf PA, Abbott RD, Kannel WB. Atrial fibrillation: a major contributor to stroke in the elderly. *Arch Intern Med* 1987;**147**:1561–4.

28.Petersen P. Thromboembolic complications of atrial fibrillation and their prevention: a review. *Am J Cardiol* 1990; **65**: 24C–8C.

29.The Stroke Prevention in Atrial Fibrillation investigators. Predictors of thromboembolism in atrial fibrillation: I. Clinical features of patients at risk. *Ann Intern Med* 1992;**116**:1–5.

30.The Stroke Prevention in Atrial Fibrillation investigators. Predictors of thromboembolism in atrial fibrillation: II. Echocardiographic features of patients at risk. *Ann Intern Med* 1992;**116**:6–12.

31.Costeas C, Kassotis J, Blitzer M, Reiffel JA. Rhythm management in atrial fibrillation – with a primary emphasis on pharmacological therapy: part 2. *PACE* 1998;**21**:742–52.

32.Slavik RS, Tisdale JE, Borzak S. Pharmacologic conversion of atrial fibrillation: a systematic review of available evidence. *Prog Cardiovasc Dis* 2001;**44**:121–52.

33.Capucci A, Villani GQ, Piepoli MF, Aschieri D. The role of oral IC antiarrhythmic drugs in terminating atrial fibrillation. *Curr Opin Cardiol* 1999;**14**:4–8.

34.Azpitarte J, Alvarez M, Baun O *et al.* Value of single oral loading dose of propafenone in converting recent-onset atrial fibrillation: results of a randomized double-blind, controlled study. *Eur Heart J* 1997;**18**:1649–54.

35.Boriani G, Biffi M, Capucci A *et al.* Conversion of recent-onset atrial fibrillation to sinus rhythm. Effects of different drug protocols. *PACE* 1998;**21**:2470–4.

36.Bianconi L, Mennuni M, and PAFIT-3 Investigators. Comparison between propafenone and digoxin administered intravenously to patients with acute atrial fibrillation. *Am J Cardiol* 1998;**82**:584–8.

37.Stambler BS, Wood MA, Ellenbogen KA *et al.*, and the Ibutilide Repeat Dose Investigators. Efficacy and safety of repeated intravenous doses of ibutilide for rapid conversion of atrial flutter or fibrillation. *Circulation* 1996;**94**:1613–21.

38.Vos MA, Golitsyn SR, Stangl K *et al.*, for the Ibutilide/Sotalol Comparator Study Group. Superiority of ibutilide (a new class III agent) over d, l–sotalol in converting atrial flutter and atrial fibrillation. *Heart* 1998;**79**:568–75.

39.Volgman AS, Carberry PA, Stambler B *et al.* Conversion efficacy and safety of intravenous ibutilide compared with intravenous procainamide in patients with atrial flutter or fibrillation. *J Am Coll Cardiol* 1998;**31**:1414–19.

40.Norgaard BL, Wachtell K, Christensen PD *et al.* Efficacy and safety of intravenously administered dofetilide in acute termination of atrial fibrillation and flutter: a multicenter, randomized, double blind, placebo–controlled study. *Am Heart J* 1999;**137**:1062–9.

41.Pedersen OD, Bagger H, Keller N *et al.*, for the Danish Investigations of Arrhythmia and Mortality on Dofetilide Study Group. Efficacy of dofetilide in the treatment of atrial fibrillation–flutter in patients with reduced left ventricular function: a Danish Investigations of Arrhythmia and Mortality on Dofetilide (DIAMOND) Substudy. *Circulation* 2001; **104**:292–6.

42.Singh S, Zoble RG, Yellen L *et al.*, for the Dofetilide Atrial Fibrillation Investigators. Efficacy and safety of oral dofetilide in converting to and maintaining sinus rhythm in patients with chronic atrial fibrillation or atrial flutter: the Symptomatic Atrial Fibrillation Investigative Research on Dofetilide (SAFIRE–D) Study. *Circulation* 2000;**102**:2385–90.

43.Hou Z-Y, Chang M-S, Chen C-Y *et al.* Acute treatment of recent-onset atrial fibrillation and flutter with a tailored dosing regimen of intravenous amiodarone. A randomized, digoxin-controlled study. *Eur Heart J* 1995;**16**:521–8.

44.Pinski SL, Labadet C, Villamil A. Is intravenous amiodarone effective in converting atrial fibrillation: a meta-analysis. *Circulation* 2001;**104**:II-700 (Abstract).

45.Vardas PE, Kochiadakis GE, Igomenidis NE *et al.* Amiodarone as a first-choice drug for restoring sinus rhythm in patients with atrial fibrillation. *Chest* 2000;**117**:1538–45.

46.Di Benedetto S. Quinidine versus propafenone for conversion of atrial fibrillation to sinus rhythm. *Am J Cardiol* 1997; **80**:518–19.

47.Hohnloser SH, Van de LA, Baedeker F. Efficacy and proarrhythmic hazards of pharmacologic cardioversion of atrial fibrillation: prospective comparison of sotalol versus quinidine. *J Am Coll Cardiol* 1995;**26**:852–8.

48.Sung RJ, Tan HL, Karagounis L *et al.*, for the Sotalol Multicenter Study Group. Intravenous sotalol for termination of supraventricular tachycardia and atrial fibrillation and flutter: a multicenter, randomized, double-blind, placebocontrolled study. *Am Heart J* 1995;**129**:739–48.

49.Falk RH, Knowlton AA, Bernard SA, Gotlieb NE, Battinelli NJ. Digoxin for converting recent-onset atrial fibrillation to sinus rhythm. *Ann Intern Med* 1987;**106**:503–6.

50.Noc M, Stajer D, Horvat M. Intravenous amiodarone versus verapamil for acute conversion of paroxysmal atrial fibrillation to sinus rhythm. *Am J Cardiol* 1990;**65**:679–80.

51.The Digitalis in Acute Atrial Fibrillation (DAAF) Trial Group. Results of a randomized, placebo-controlled multicenter trial in 239 patients. *Eur Heart J* 1997;**18**:649–54.

52. Sticherling C, Oral H, Horrocks J *et al.* Effects of digoxin on acute, atrial fibrillation-induced changes in atrial refractoriness. *Circulation* 2000;**102**:2503–8.

53. Tieleman RG, Blaau Y, Van Gelder IC *et al.* Digoxin delays recovery from tachycardia-induced electrical remodeling of the atria. *Circulation* 1999;**100**:1836–42.

54. Van Gelder IC, Crijns HJGM, Van Gilst WH *et al.* Prediction of uneventful cardioversion and maintenance of sinus rhythm from direct-current electrical cardioversion of chronic atrial fibrillation and flutter. *Am J Cardiol* 1991;**68**:41–6.

55. Connolly SJ, Hoffest DL. Usefulness of propafenone for recurrent paroxysmal atrial fibrillation. *Am J Cardiol* 1989;**63**:817–19.

56. Stroobandt R, Stiels B, Hoebrechts R, on behalf of the Propafenone Atrial Fibrillation Trial Investigators. Propafenone for conversion and prophylaxis of atrial fibrillation. *Am J Cardiol* 1997;**79**:418–23.

57. UK Propafenone PSVT Study Group. A randomized, placebo-controlled trial of propafenone in the prophylaxis of paroxysmal supraventricular tachycardia and paroxysmal atrial fibrillation. *Circulation* 1995;**92**:2550–7.

58. Reimold SC. Avoiding drug problems. The safety of drugs for supraventricular tachycardia. *Eur Heart J* 1997;**18**:C40–4.

59. Van Gelder IC, Crijns HJ, Van Gilst WH *et al.* Efficacy and safety of flecainide acetate in the maintenance of sinus rhythm after electrical cardioversion of chronic atrial fibrillation or atrial flutter. *Am J Cardiol* 1989;**64**:1317–21.

60. Pietersen AH, Hellemann H, for the Danish–Norwegian Flecainide Multicenter Atrial Fibrillation Study Group. Usefulness of flecainide for prevention of paroxysmal atrial fibrillation and flutter. *Am J Cardiol* 1991;**67**:713–17.

61. Anderson JL, Gilbert EM, Alpert BL *et al.* Prevention of symptomatic recurrences of paroxysmal atrial fibrillation in patients initially tolerating antiarrhythmic therapy. *Circulation* 1989;**80**:1557–70.

62. Anderson JL, Platt ML, Guarnieri T *et al.*, and the Flecainide Supraventricular Tachycardia Study Group. Flecainide acetate for paroxysmal supraventricular arrhythmias. *Am J Cardiol* 1994;**74**:578–84.

63. Naccarelli GV, Dorian P, Hohnloser SH, Coumel P, for the Flecainide Multicenter Atrial Fibrillation Group. Prospective comparison of flecainide versus quinidine for the treatment of paroxysmal atrial fibrillation/flutter. *Am J Cardiol* 1996;**77**:53A–9A.

64. Echt DS, Liebson PR, Mitchell LB *et al.*, and the CAST Investigators. Mortality and morbidity in patients receiving encainide, flecainide, or placebo: the Cardiac Arrhythmia Suppression Trial. *N Engl J Med* 1991;**324**:781–8.

65. Flaker GC, Blackshear JL, McBride R *et al.* Antiarrhythmic drug therapy and cardiac mortality in atrial fibrillation. *J Am Coll Cardiol* 1992;**20**:527–32.

66. Lee SH, Chen SA, Tai CT *et al.* Comparisons of oral propafenone and sotalol as an initial treatment in patients with symptomatic paroxysmal atrial fibrillation. *Am J Cardiol* 1997;**79**:905–8.

67. Bellandi F, Simonetti I, Leoncini M *et al.* Long-term efficacy and safety of propafenone and sotalol for the maintenance of sinus rhythm after conversion of recurrent symptomatic atrial fibrillation. *Am J Cardiol* 2001;**88**:640–5.

68. Wanless RS, Anderson K, Joy M, Joseph SP. Multicenter comparative study of the efficacy and safety of sotalol in the prophylactic treatment of patients with paroxysmal supra-ventricular tachyarrhythmias. *Am Heart J* 1997;**133**:441–6.

69. Benditt DG, Williams JH, Jin J *et al.*, for the D, l-Sotalol Atrial Fibrillation/Flutter Study Group. Maintenance of sinus rhythm with oral d, l-sotalol therapy in patients with symptomatic atrial fibrillation and/or atrial flutter. *Am J Cardiol* 1999;**84**:270–7.

70. Fetsch T, Breithardt G, Engberding R *et al.* Prevention of atrial fibrillation after cardioversion – results of the PAFAC trial. *Circulation* 2001;**104**:II-699 (Abstract).

71. Roy D, Talajic M, Dorian P *et al.*, for the Canadian Trial of Atrial Fibrillation Investigators. Amiodarone to prevent recurrence of atrial fibrillation. *N Engl J Med* 2000;**342**:913–20.

72. Toivonen L, Greenbaum R, Campbell T *et al.* Dofetilide is better tolerated than sotalol for the prevention of recurrence of atrial fibrillation and flutter. *Eur Heart J* 2000;**21**:123 (Abstract).

73. Deedwania PC, Singh BN, Ellenbogen K, for the Department of Veterans Affairs CHF–STAT Investigators. Spontaneous conversion and maintenance of sinus rhythm by amiodarone in patients with heart failure and atrial fibrillation: observations from the Veterans Affairs Congestive Heart Failure Survival Trial of Antiarrhythmic Therapy (CHF–STAT). *Circulation* 1998;**98**:2574–9.

74. European and Australian Multicenter Evaluative Research on Atrial Fibrillation Dofetilide (EMERALD). *Circulation* 1999;**99**:2486–91.

75. Santini M, Greenbaum R, Lehman R *et al.* Oral dofetilide is effective for maintenance of sinus rhythm in patients with atrial fibrillation/flutter independent of patient characteristics. *Eur Heart J* 2000;**21**:327 (Abstract).

76. Pritchett ELC, Page RL, Connolly SJ *et al.* Antiarrhythmic effects of azimilide in atrial fibrillation: efficacy and dose–response. *J Am Coll Cardiol* 2000;**36**:794–802.

77. Connolly SJ, Schnell DJ, Page RL *et al.* Dose–response relations of azimilide in the management of symptomatic, recurrent atrial fibrillation. *Am J Cardiol* 2001;**88**:974–9.

78. Kühlkamp V, Schirdewan A, Stangl K *et al.* Use of metoprolol CR/XL to maintain sinus rhythm after conversion from persistent atrial fibrillation: a randomized, double-blind, placebo-controlled study. *J Am Coll Cardiol* 2000;**36**:139–46.

79. Tieleman RG, Van Noord T, Van Gelder IC *et al.* Beta-blockers prevent subacute recurrences after cardioversion of persistent atrial fibrillation in patients with hypertension but not in lone atrial fibrillation patients. *PACE* 2001;**24**:675 (Abstract).

80. Steeds RP, Birchall AS, Smith M, Channer KS. An open label, randomized, crossover study comparing sotalol and atenolol in the treatment of symptomatic paroxysmal atrial fibrillation. *Heart* 1999;**82**:170–5.

81. Plewan A, Lehmann G, Ndrepepa G *et al.* Maintenance of sinus rhythm after electrical cardioversion of persistent atrial fibrillation: sotalol vs bisoprolol. *Eur Heart J* 2001;**22**:1504–10.

82. Marcus FI. The hazard of using type IC antiarrhythmic drugs for the treatment of paroxysmal atrial fibrillation. *Am J Cardiol* 1990;**66**:366–7.

83.Crozier I. Flecainide in the Wolff–Parkinson–White syndrome. *Am J Cardiol* 1992;**70**:26A–32A.

84.Crijns HJGM, Gosselink ATM, Van Gelder IC *et al.* Drugs after cardioversion to prevent relapses of chronic atrial fibrillation. In: Kingma JH, van Hemel NM, Lie KI, eds. *Atrial fibrillation, a treatable disease?* Dordrecht: Kluwer Academic Publishers, 1992.

85.Coplen SE, Antman EM, Berlin JA, Hewitt P, Chalmers TC. Efficacy and safety of quinidine therapy for maintenance of sinus rhythm after cardioversion. A meta-analysis of randomized control trials. *Circulation* 1990;**82**:1106–16.

86.Carlsson J, Tebbe U, Rox J *et al.*, for the ALKK study group. Cardioversion of atrial fibrillation in the elderly. *Am J Cardiol* 1996;**78**:1380–4.

87.Gosselink ATM, Crijns HJ, Van Gelder IC *et al.* Low-dose amiodarone for maintenance of sinus rhythm after cardioversion of atrial fibrillation or flutter. *JAMA* 1992;**267**:3289–93.

88.Szekely P, Sideris DA, Batson GA. Maintenance of sinus rhythm after atrial defibrillation. *Br Heart J* 1970;**32**:741–6.

89.Hohnloser SH, Kuck KH, Lilienthal J, for the PIAF Investigators. Rhythm or rate control in atrial fibrillation – Pharmacological Intervention in Atrial Fibrillation (PIAF): a randomised trial. *Lancet* 2000;**356**:1789–94.

90.Carlsson J, Tebbe U. Rhythm control versus rate control in atrial fibrillation: results from the STAF Pilot Study (Strategies of Treatment in Atrial Fibrillation). *PACE* 2001;**24**:561 (Abstract).

91.Farshi R, Kistner D, Sarma JSM *et al.* Ventricular rate control in chronic atrial fibrillation during daily activity and programmed exercise: a crossover, open–label study of five drug regimens. *J Am Coll Cardiol* 1998;**22**:304–10.

92.Ellenbogen KA, Dias VC, Plumb VJ *et al.* A placebo-controlled trial of continuous intravenous diltiazem infusion for 24 hour heart rate control during atrial fibrillation and atrial flutter: a multicenter study. *J Am Coll Cardiol* 1991;**18**:891–7.

93.Platia EV, Michelson EL, Porterfield JK, Das G. Esmolol versus verapamil in the acute treatment of atrial fibrillation or atrial flutter. *Am J Cardiol* 1989;**63**:925–9.

94.Mathew JP, Parks R, Savino JS *et al.*, for the Multicenter Study of Perioperative Ischaemia Research Group. Atrial fibrillation following coronary artery bypass graft surgery. *JAMA* 1996;**276**:300–6.

95.Aranki SF, Shaw DP, Adams DH *et al.* Predictors of atrial fibrillation after coronary artery surgery: current trends and impact on hospital resources. *Circulation* 1996;**94**:390–7.

96.Kowey PR, Stebbins D, Igidbashian L *et al.* Clinical outcome of patients who develop PAF after CABG surgery. *PACE* 2001;**24**:191–3.

97.Asher CR, Miller DP, Grimm RA *et al.* Analysis of risk factors for development of atrial fibrillation early after cardiac valvular surgery. *Am J Cardiol* 1998;**82**:892–5.

98.Bharucha DB, Kowey PR. Management and prevention of atrial fibrillation after cardiovascular surgery. *Am J Cardiol* 2000;**85**:20D–4D.

99.Liebold A, Wahba A, Birnbaum DE. Low-energy cardioversion with epicardial wire electrodes: new treatment of atrial fibrillation after open heart surgery. *Circulation* 1998;**98**:883–6.

100.Maisel WH, Rawn JD, Stevenson WG. Atrial fibrillation after cardiac surgery. *Arch Intern Med* 2002;**135**:1061–73.

101.Mooss AN, Wurdeman RL, Mohiuddin SM *et al.* Esmolol versus diltiazem in the treatment of postoperative atrial fibrillation/atrial flutter after open heart surgery. *Am Heart J* 2000;**140**:176–80.

102.Tisdale JE, Padhi ID, Goldberg AD *et al.* A randomized, double blind comparison of intravenous diltiazem and digoxin for atrial fibrillation after coronary bypass surgery. *Am Heart J* 1998;**135**:739–47.

103.Clemo HF, Wood MA, Gilligan DM, Ellenbogen KA. Intravenous amiodarone for acute rate control in the critically ill patient with atrial tachyarrhythmias. *Am J Cardiol* 1998;**81**:594–8.

104.Kowey PR, Taylor JE, Rials SJ, Marinchak RA. Meta-analysis of the effectiveness of prophylactic drug therapy in preventing supraventricular arrhythmia early after coronary artery bypass grafting. *Am J Cardiol* 1992;**69**:963–5.

105.Andrews TC, Reimold SC, Berlin JA, Antman EM. Prevention of supraventricular arrhythmias after coronary artery bypass surgery. A meta-analysis of randomized trials. *Circulation* 1991;**84**(Suppl. III):III-236–44.

106.Kowey PR, Dalessandro DA, Herbertson R *et al.* Effectiveness of digitalis with or without acebutolol in preventing atrial arrhythmias after coronary artery surgery. *Am J Cardiol* 1999:1114–17.

107.VanderLugt JT, Mattioni T, Denker S *et al.*, for the Ibutilide Investigators. Efficacy and safety of ibutilide fumarate for the conversion of atrial arrhythmias after cardiac surgery. *Circulation* 1999;**100**:369–75.

108.SoRelle R. Late-breaking clinical trials at the American Heart Association Scientific Sessions 2001. *Circulation* 2001; **104**:E9046–8.

109.Geelen P, O'Hara GE, Roy N *et al.* Comparison of propafenone versus procainamide for the acute treatment of atrial fibrillation after cardiac surgery. *Am J Cardiol* 1999; **84**:345–7.

110.Laub GW, Janeira L, Muralidharan S *et al.* Prophylactic procainamide for prevention of atrial fibrillation after coronary bypass grafting: a prospective, double-blind, randomized, placebo-controlled pilot study. *Crit Care Med* 1993;**21**: 1474–8.

111.Gold MR, O'Gara PT, Buckley MJ, DeSanctis RW. Efficacy and safety of procainamide in preventing arrhythmias after coronary artery bypass surgery. *Am J Cardiol* 1996;**78**:975–9.

112.Yilmaz AT, Demirkilic U, Arslan M *et al.* Long-term prevention of atrial fibrillation after coronary by-pass surgery: comparison of quinidine, verapamil, and amiodarone in maintaining sinus rhythm. *J Cardiac Surg* 1996;**11**:61–4.

113.Evrard P, Gonzalez M, Jamart J *et al.* Prophylaxis of supraventricular and ventricular arrhythmias after coronary artery grafting with low-dose sotalol. *Ann Thorac Surg* 2000;**70**:151–6.

114.Pfisterer ME, Kloter-Weber UC, Huber M *et al.* Prevention of supraventricular tachyarrhythmias after open heart operation by low-dose sotalol: a prospective, double-blind, randomized, placebo-controlled study. *Ann Thorac Surg* 1997;**64**: 1113–19.

115.Matsuura K, Takahara Y, Sudo Y, Ishida K. Effect of sotalol in the prevention of atrial fibrillation following coronary artery bypass grafting. *Jpn J Thorac Cardiovasc Surg* 2001; **49**:614–17.

116. Gomes JA, Ip J, Santoni-Rugiu F, Mehta D *et al*. Oral d, l sotalol reduces the incidence of postoperative atrial fibrillation in coronary artery bypass surgery patients: a randomized, double-blind, placebo-controlled study. *J Am Coll Cardiol* 1999;**34**:334–9.

117. Suttorp MJ, Kingma JH, Peels HO *et al*. Effectiveness of sotalol in preventing supraventricular tachyarrhythmias shortly after coronary bypass grafting. *Am J Cardiol* 1991;**68**: 1163–9.

118. Suttorp MJ, Kingma JH, Tjon Joe Gin RM *et al*. Efficacy and safety of low and high dose sotalol versus propranolol in the prevention of supraventricular tachyarrhythmias early after coronary artery bypass surgery. *J Thorac Cardiovasc Surg* 1990;**100**:921–6.

119. Parikka H, Toivonen L, Heikkila L *et al*. Comparison of sotalol and metoprolol in the prevention of atrial fibrillation after coronary artery bypass surgery. *J Cardiovasc Pharmacol* 1998;**31**:67–73.

120. Nystrom U, Edvardsson N, Berggren H *et al*. Oral sotalol reduces the incidence of atrial fibrillation after coronary artery bypass. *Thorac Cardiovasc Surg* 1993;**41**:34–7.

121. Daoud EG, Stickberger SA, Man KC *et al*. Preoperative amiodarone as prophylaxis against atrial fibrillation after heart surgery. *N Engl J Med* 1997;**337**:1785–91.

122. Lee SH, Chang CM, Lu MJ *et al*. Intravenous amiodarone for prevention of atrial fibrillation after coronary artery bypass grafting. *Ann Thorac Surg* 2000;**70**:157–61.

123. Reddle JD, Khurama S, Marzan R *et al*. Prophylactic oral amiodarone compared with placebo for prevention of atrial fibrillation after coronary artery bypass surgery. *Am Heart J* 1999;**138**:144–50.

124. Solomon AJ, Greenberg MD, Kilborn MJ, Katz NM. Amiodarone versus a beta-blocker to prevent atrial fibrillation after cardiovascular surgery. *Am Heart J* 2001;**142**: 811–15.

125. Treggiari-Venzi MM, Waeber JL, Perneger TV *et al*. Intravenous amiodarone or magnesium sulphate is not cost–beneficial prophylaxis for atrial fibrillation after coronary artery bypass surgery. *Br J Anaesth* 2000;**85**:690–5.

126. Guarnieri T, Nolan S, Gottlieb SO *et al*. Intravenous amiodarone for the prevention of atrial fibrillation after open heart surgery: the Amiodarone Reduction in Coronary Heart (ARCH) Trial. *J Am Coll Cardiol* 1999; **34**:343–7.

127. Giri S, White CM, Dunn AB *et al*. Oral amiodarone for prevention of atrial fibrillation after open heart surgery, the Atrial Fibrillation Suppression Trial (AFIST): a randomised placebo-controlled trial. *Lancet* 2001;**357**:830–6.

128. Dorge H, Schoendube FA, Schoberer M *et al*. Intraoperative amiodarone as prophylaxis against atrial fibrillation after coronary operations. *Ann Thorac Surg* 2000;**69**:1358–62.

129. Crystal E, Connolly SJ, Sleik K *et al*. Interventions on prevention of postoperative atrial fibrillation in patients undergoing heart surgery: a meta-analysis. *Circulation* 2002;**106**:75–80.

130. Nurozler F, Tokozoglu L, Pasaoglu I *et al*. Atrial fibrillation after coronary bypass surgery: predictors and the role of MgSO$_4$ replacement. *J Cardiac Surg* 1996;**11**:421–7.

131. Toraman F, Karabulut EH, Alhan HC *et al*. Magnesium infusion dramatically decreases the incidence of atrial fibrillation after coronary artery bypass grafting. *Ann Thorac Surg* 2001; **72**:1256–61.

132. Solomon AJ, Berger AK, Trivedi KK, Hannan RL, Katz NM. The combination of propranolol and magnesium does not prevent postoperative atrial fibrillation. *Ann Thorac Surg* 2000; **69**:126–9.

133. Lasar HL, Chipkin S, Philippides G, Bao Y, Apstein C *et al*. Glucose–insulin–potassium solutions improve outcomes in diabetics who have coronary artery operations. *Ann Thorac Surg* 2000;**70**:145–50.

134. Frost L, Mortensen PE, Tingleff J *et al*. Efficacy and safety of dofetilide, a new class III antiarrhythmic agent, in acute termination of atrial fibrillation or flutter after coronary bypass surgery: Dofetilide Post-CABG Study Group. *Int J Cardiol* 1997;**58**:135–40.

135. Goette A, Staack T, Röcken C *et al*. Increased expression of extracellular signal-regulated kinase and angiotensin-converting enzyme in human atria during atrial fibrillation. *J Am Coll Cardiol* 2000;**35**:1669–77.

136. Li D, Shinagawa K, Pang L *et al*. Effects of angiotensin-converting enzyme inhibition on the development of atrial fibrillation substrate in dogs with ventricular tachycardia-induced congestive heart failure. *Circulation* 2001;**104**:2608–14.

137. Pederson OD, Bagger H, Køber L *et al.*, for the TRACE Study Group. Trandolapril reduces the incidence of atrial fibrillation after acute myocardial infarction in patients with left ventricular dysfunction. *Circulation* 1999;**100**:376–80.

138. Van Noord T, Van Gelder IC, Van Den Berg M *et al*. Pretreatment with ACE inhibitors enhances cardioversion outcome in patients with persistent atrial fibrillation. *Circulation* 2001;**104**:II-699 (Abstract).

139. Hernandez-Madrid A, Rebollo JG, Rodriguez A *et al*. A prospective and randomized study on the effect of antiotensin II type 1 receptor blocker irbesartan in maintaining sinus rhythm in patients with persistent atrial fibrillation. *J Am Coll Cardiol* 2002;**39**:103A (Abstract).

140. Stevenson WG, Stevenson LW, Middlekauff HR. Improving survival for patients with atrial fibrillation and advanced heart failure. *J Am Coll Cardiol* 1996;**28**:1458–63.

141. McMurray JJ, Dargie HJ, Ford I *et al*. Carvedilol reduces supraventricular and ventricular arrhythmias after myocardial infarction: evidence form the CAPRICORN study. *Circulation* 2001;**104**:II-700 (Abstract).

142. Lechat P, Hulot JS, Escolano S *et al.*, on behalf of the CIBIS II Investigators. Heart rate and cardiac rhythm relationships with bisoprolol benefit in chronic heart failure in CIBIS II trial. *Circulation* 2001;**103**:1428–35.

143. Hohnloser SH, Van Loo A, Baedeker F. Efficacy and proarrhythmic hazards of pharmacologic cardioversion of atrial fibrillation: prospective comparison of sotalol versus quinidine. *J Am Coll Cardiol* 1995;**26**:852–8.

144. Jackman WM, Friday KJ, Andersen JL *et al*. The long QT syndromes: a critical review, new clinical observations and a unifying hypothesis. *Prog Cardiovasc Dis* 1988;**31**:115–72.

145. Falk RH. Flecainide-induced ventricular tachycardia and fibrillation in patients treated for atrial fibrillation. *Ann Intern Med* 1989;**111**:107–11.

146. Flaker GC, Blackshear JL, McBride R *et al.*, on behalf of the Stroke Prevention in Atrial Fibrillation Investigators. Antiarrhythmic drug therapy and cardiac mortality in atrial fibrillation. *J Am Coll Cardiol* 1992;**20**:527–32.

147.Torp-Pedersen C, Møller M, Bloch-Thomsen PE *et al.*, for the Danish Investigations of Arrhythmia and Mortality on Dofetilide Study Group. Dofetilide in patients with congestive heart failure and left ventricular dysfunction. *N Engl J Med* 1999;**341**:857–65.

148.Kowey PR, Vanderlught JT, Luderer JR. Safety and risk/ benefit analysis of ibutilide for acute conversion of atrial fibrillation/flutter. *Am J Cardiol* 1996;**78**:46A–52A.

149.Pritchett ELC, Page RL, Connolly SJ *et al.* Antiarrhythmic effects of azimilide in atrial fibrillation: efficacy and dose–response. *J Am Coll Cardiol* 2000;**36**:794–802.

150.Lehmann MH, Hardy S, Archibald D, Quart B, MacNeilx DJ. Sex differences in risk of torsade de pointes with d, l-sotalol. *Circulation* 1996;**94**:2534–41.

151.Reiffel JA. Drug choices in the treatment of atrial fibrillation. *Am J Cardiol* 2000;**85**:12D–19D.

38 Atrial fibrillation: antithrombotic therapy

John A Cairns

Definitions, incidence and natural history

Although oral anticoagulant prophylaxis against embolic stroke in rheumatic atrial fibrillation had been in wide use, it remained for the Framingham study[1–5] to demonstrate that the annual incidence of stroke was similar among patients with rheumatic and non-rheumatic atrial fibrillation. These observations, together with evidence of increased safety and maintained efficacy of lower-dose warfarin,[6,7] prompted the initiation of several well designed randomized controlled trials of anticoagulant and antiplatelet therapy for non-rheumatic atrial fibrillation (Table 38.1). Non-rheumatic atrial fibrillation was generally defined by the exclusion of echocardiographic mitral stenosis. The terms non-valvular atrial fibrillation and non-rheumatic atrial fibrillation are not entirely synonymous, although they are often used inter-changeably. The term non-rheumatic atrial fibrillation is generally preferred.

In the Framingham study[4] patients were stratified according to the presence or absence of rheumatic heart disease, and the risk of stroke was adjusted for age and blood pressure. In comparison with patients without atrial fibrillation, the risk ratio for stroke was 17·6 for those with rheumatic atrial fibrillation and 5·6 for those with non-rheumatic atrial

Table 38.1 Non-rheumatic atrial fibrillation: designs of randomized trials

Trial	Sample size	Warfarin	INR	Aspirin
BAATAF[8]	420	Open	1·5–2·7	
CAFA[9]	383	Blind	2·0–3·0	
SPINAF[10]	536	Blind	1·5–2·5	
AFASAK[11,12]	1007	Open	2·8–4·2	75 mg/day
SPAF[13]	1330	Open	2·0–4·5	325 mg/day

Abbreviations: AFASAK, Copenhagen Atrial Fibrillation Aspirin Anticoagulation; BAATAF, Boston Area Anticoagulation Trial for Atrial Fibrillation; CAFA, Canadian Atrial Fibrillation Anticoagulation; INR, international normalized ratio; SPAF, Stroke Prevention in Atrial Fibrillation; SPINAF, Stroke Prevention in Nonrheumatic Atrial Fibrillation

fibrillation. However, the absolute annual rate of stroke was virtually the same in the two groups (4·5% per year for the rheumatic group and 4·2% per year for the non-rheumatic group). The most reliable and current information comes from an analysis of the placebo groups in the recent clinical trials[8–13] where the annual incidence of stroke ranged from 3% to 7% (mean 4·5%) (Table 38.2), and the annual incidence of stroke plus other systemic emboli ranged from 3% to 7·4%. Patients were selected for entry into these trials according to a variety of criteria, including the absence of contraindications to warfarin and in some instances to aspirin, and the willingness to participate in a clinical trial. Hence, generalizations to a wider population must be made cautiously, but it is likely that these rates of stroke and other systemic embolism are reasonably close to those in the general population. In early case series, 50–70% of embolic strokes resulted in either death or severe neurologic deficit,[14] and in the recent randomized trials as many as half the strokes resulted in death or permanent disability.

Several cohort studies[14] have demonstrated a reasonably consistent lower annual stroke risk in patients with paroxysmal or transient atrial fibrillation than in those with chronic atrial fibrillation. On the other hand, the SPAF trial found similar annual rates of ischemic stroke in patients with recurrent (3·2%) and chronic (3·3%) atrial fibrillation,[15] and a meta-analysis of the control groups in five large trials showed no difference.[16] These findings take precedence over earlier perceptions. There is a widespread perception that the risk of stroke is less with atrial flutter than with atrial fibrillation. A large retrospective database analysis confirmed a higher risk with atrial fibrillation, but the risk with atrial flutter was higher than in patients without this arrythmia.[17]

The term "lone atrial fibrillation" is generally used to describe patients who have atrial fibrillation in the absence of other clinically or echocardiographically demonstrable heart disease.[14] The definition is frequently extended to require the exclusion of diabetes mellitus and hypertension, and, in some series, an age younger than 60 years is required to fulfill the criteria. In general, stroke rates are much lower in patients with lone atrial fibrillation, and discrepancies among studies are most likely explained by differences in age, the presence of cardiovascular risk factors and the chronicity of atrial fibrillation.[18,19] Studies suggest

Table 38.2   Non-rheumatic atrial fibrillation: outcomes of randomized trials of warfarin

Trial	Ischemic stroke				Major bleed*
	Control events/ 1000 pt/yr	Warfarin events/ 1000 pt/yr	Relative risk reduction (%)	Absolute risk reduction events/ 1000 pt/yr	Absolute increase events/ 1000 pt/yr
BAATAF[8]	30	4	87	26	2
CAFA[9]	38	26	32	12	15
SPINAF[10]	43	9	79	34	6
AFASAK[11,12]	50	32	36	18	8
SPAF[13]	70	23	67	47	−1
Overview[16]	45	14	68	31	3

*Major bleed defined as intracranial bleeding, a bleeding event requiring 2 U of blood, or an event requiring hospital admission.

that as the study population ages, a decreasing proportion of patients with atrial fibrillation is free of other heart disease.

Antithrombotic management

Anticoagulant therapy

Five randomized controlled trials of warfarin versus control or placebo for the primary prevention of thromboembolism among patients with non-rheumatic (non-valvular) atrial fibrillation have been reported (Tables 38.1, 38.2). The trials generally enrolled patients with chronic atrial fibrillation detected on a routine or screening electrocardiogram (mean age 69 years). AFASAK[11] and SPINAF[10] excluded patients with intermittent atrial fibrillation, whereas the proportion of intermittent atrial fibrillation in CAFA[9] was 7%, in BAATAF[8] 16% and in SPAF[13] 34%. Previous stroke or transient ischemic attack was infrequent. Treatment allocation was randomized in all trials. There was a double-blind comparison of warfarin to placebo in CAFA and SPINAF, and an open label comparison in BAATAF. AFASAK compared warfarin, aspirin and aspirin placebo. SPAF allocated patients as being warfarin eligible (group 1) or warfarin ineligible (group 2). Group 1 patients were randomized to open label warfarin or usual therapy; group 2 patients were randomized to open label warfarin, aspirin or aspirin placebo. The INR range in these trials varied from 1·2–2·5 to 2·8–4·2.

Four of the trials were stopped early by their Data and Safety Monitoring Boards because interim analyses were strongly positive, whereas the fifth[9] was stopped early because of the strongly positive results from two other trials. The primary outcomes varied somewhat among the trials. However, it is possible to determine the rates of ischemic stroke and major bleeding (intracranial, transfusion of 2 or more units, hospitalization) from each trial, to make comparisons and to pool the results. The Atrial Fibrillation Investigators overview[16]

was a collaborative prospective meta-analysis which provides reliable summary data based on individual patient information. The overall risk of ischemic stroke was 4·5% per year, identical to that documented in the Framingham study. This was reduced to 1·4% per year with warfarin, a reduction of 31 strokes for every 1000 patients treated ($P < 0.001$). A major concern with warfarin is hemorrhage, which was carefully documented in each trial. The rate of major hemorrhage with warfarin was 1·3% per year versus 1% per year in controls, an increase of three major hemorrhages per 1000 patients treated, including an excess of intracranial hemorrhage of two per year for every 1000 patients treated. Hence, the overall picture is one of major benefit from warfarin, with only a modest increase in the risk of major hemorrhage and cerebral hemorrhage. **Grade A**

The European Atrial Fibrillation Trial compared warfarin, aspirin and placebo in patients with non-rheumatic atrial fibrillation who had experienced a transient ischemic attack (TIA) or stroke within the preceding 3 months.[20] The risk of recurrence was 12% among the placebo patients, dramatically higher than the 4·5% annual risk in the overall population of patients with non-rheumatic atrial fibrillation. The relative risk reduction on warfarin was 66% ($P < 0.001$), virtually identical to that calculated in the overview of the five major randomized controlled trials, but the absolute reduction of strokes was much greater (80 per year per 1000 versus 31 per year per 1000) because of the high baseline risk of stroke in this population. Major bleeding was more frequent (excess of 21 per year per 1000), but the risk benefit ratio was strongly in favor of warfarin over placebo. **Grade A**

Additional analyses from the five trials have provided useful data on the prognostic stratification of patients as regards the risk of stroke.[16] The Atrial Fibrillation Investigators overview has demonstrated that the statistically significant multivariate predictors of stroke are previous stroke or TIA, increasing age, history of hypertension, congestive heart failure or myocardial infarction, and diabetes. The Stroke Prevention in Atrial Fibrillation investigators have also demonstrated that echocardiographic increased left atrial size and LV dysfunction are important determinants of the risk of stroke.[21] The annual risk of stroke is about 4·5% among the total group of patients with non-rheumatic atrial fibrillation. However, patients under 60 years of age with no risk factors have an annual risk of <1% (there were no strokes among 112 such patients in the Atrial Fibrillation Investigators' overview). Patients of any age with no echocardiographic or clinical risk factors have an annual risk of only 1%, but this rises to 5% with the presence of enlarged left atrium or LV dysfunction, and to 7·2% with the presence of congestive heart failure, previous stroke or hypertension. When two or three clinical risk factors are present, the annual risk of stroke rises to 17·6%[22]. **Grade A**

The short-term risk of stroke appears to be higher in patients with recent-onset atrial fibrillation than in those with atrial fibrillation for more than 1–2 years.[23,24] Among patients with atrial fibrillation who have experienced an embolic event, the risk of recurrence in subsequent months appears to be considerably higher than the overall incidence. The high rate of recurrence, although not observed in every study, suggests that there is some urgency in initiating anticoagulation following the occurrence of embolic stroke in patients with atrial fibrillation. However, such therapy can increase the risk of hemorrhagic transformation of an embolic brain infarction. Based on a review of the literature and the results of the only available randomized clinical trial, the Cerebral Embolism Study Group recommended anticoagulation therapy for patients with small and moderate-sized embolic infarcts if a CT scan performed 24 hours after stroke onset did not show hemorrhage. In patients with a large infarction it was recommended that anticoagulant therapy

be delayed until the CT scan was performed at 7 days to exclude delayed hemorrhage[25]. **Grade B**

The risk of stroke in patients with thyrotoxic atrial fibrillation is substantial, although the mechanism and the relative role of congestive heart failure are uncertain. The risk of stroke is also substantial among patients with hypertrophic cardiomyopathy and atrial fibrillation. Patients with atrial fibrillation and thyrotoxicosis or hypertrophic cardiomyopathy are considered to be at high risk when assigning treatment algorithms[26]. **Grade B**

Aspirin therapy

Comparisons of aspirin and placebo resulted in a somewhat less impressive risk reduction for stroke of about 16% (NS) in AFASAK,[11] 44% ($P = 0.02$) in SPAF[13] and 17% (NS) in the European Atrial Fibrillation Trial (EAFT)[20] (Table 38.3). A meta-analysis of these trials found an overall reduction of 21% ($P = 0.05$) in the rate of ischemic stroke with aspirin compared to placebo.[27] A more recent meta-analysis, including the European Stroke Prevention Study 2 (ESPS-II),[28] the Low Dose Aspirin, Stroke and Atrial Fibrillation pilot study (LASAF)[29] and atrial fibrillation patients from the United Kingdom TIA Study (UK-TIA)[30] confirmed a statistically significant 22% relative risk reduction ($P \leq 0.05$) in the rate of all strokes (ischemic plus hemorrhagic).[31] Hence, aspirin can be expected to reduce the risk of ischemic stroke and all strokes, with a relative risk reduction of about one third that of warfarin and with a somewhat lower risk of major bleeding.

Aspirin v warfarin

The SPAF II trial studied 715 patients aged 75 years or less and 385 patients aged over 75 years, with each group randomly allocated to either warfarin or aspirin.[32] The incidence of

Table 38.3 Non-rheumatic atrial fibrillation trial outcomes: aspirin

Trial	All strokes (ischemic and hemorrhagic)			
	Control events/ 1000 pt/yr	Aspirin events/ 1000 pt/yr	Relative risk reduction (%)	Absolute risk reduction events/ 1000 pt/yr
AFASAK[11]	48	39	17	9
SPAF[13]	60	35	44	25
EAFT[20]	122	103	11	19
ESPF II[28]	207	138	29	69
LASAF[29]	22	27 (125 mg/day)	−17	−5
	6	22 (125 mg/2 days)	67	16
UK-TIA[30]	67	58 (300 mg/day)	17	9
	67	60 (1200 mg/day)	14	7
Overview[31]	80	63	22	17

ischemic stroke was less with warfarin than with aspirin in each group (*P* = NS), but intracranial hemorrhage was more frequent with warfarin and the overall rate of stroke (ischemic plus hemorrhagic) was little different with warfarin than with aspirin. The rate of all strokes with residual deficit was lower with warfarin than with aspirin in the ≤75 year old group (*P* = NS), but slightly higher in the >75 year old group (mean age 80 years) (*P* = NS). When patients with clinical risk factors (congestive heart failure, increased blood pressure, previous stroke) were examined there was a strong trend towards a greater reduction of stroke with warfarin than with aspirin in both groups.

In an attempt to better delineate the relative benefits of warfarin versus aspirin, particularly in patients at high risk of stroke, the SPAF III trial was undertaken.[33] Patients at high risk of embolic stroke because of impaired LV function, systolic hypertension, prior thromboembolism, or female gender and aged over 75 were randomly allocated warfarin, INR 2–3 or warfarin 1–3 mg/day plus aspirin 325 mg/day. This trial was discontinued early after a mean follow up of 1·2 years, because the rate of the composite primary outcome of ischemic stroke or systemic embolus was significantly higher in those given combination therapy than in those given adjusted dose warfarin (7·9% *v* 1·9% per year, risk increase 216%, *P* < 0·0001). Rates of disabling stroke and of the composite of ischemic stroke, systemic embolus or vascular death were also significantly and markedly increased. The rates of major bleeding were similar in the two treatment groups. It is clear that in high-risk patients, targeting INR in the range of 1·2–1·5 does not provide adequate protection against thromboembolism.

Direct comparisons of warfarin and aspirin were undertaken in AFASAK,[11] SPAF-II,[32] EAFT,[20] AFASAK-II[34] and PATAF[35] (Table 38.4). AFASAK-II randomized 339 patients into a primary prevention trial which compared warfarin (INR 2–3) to aspirin (300 ml/day). PATAF randomized 272 patients into a primary prevention trial which compared warfarin (INR 2·5–3·5) to aspirin (150 mg/day). When these five trials are looked at in aggregate,[31] there is a highly statistically significant 36% (95% CI 14–52) relative risk reduction of all strokes (ischemic plus hemorrhagic) with warfarin, equivalent to an absolute risk reduction of approximately 14 events per 1000 patients per year. Major non-cerebral bleeding was somewhat more frequent with warfarin than with aspirin.

Risk of hemorrhage

The efficacy of warfarin for the prevention of ischemic stroke must be balanced against the risk of major hemorrhage, particularly cerebral hemorrhage, which is usually fatal. The risk of major hemorrhage is related to the intensity of anticoagulation, the patient's age, and the fluctuation of INR.[36,37] It is likely to be higher in clinical practice than in the rigorous setting of a clinical trial.[36,37] The 3·1% absolute reduction of ischemic stroke observed in the initial five randomized controlled trials was accompanied by an absolute excess risk of major hemorrhage of only 0·3%. The INR ranged from a low of 1·5 to a high of 4·5. The most widely recommended INR range for patients with NRAF is 2·0–3·0, with a target of 2·5.[26,38] However, the greatest reductions in the rate of ischemic stroke were observed in the two trials with the lowest INR ranges.[8,10] In SPAF II,[32] the greater efficacy of warfarin over aspirin for the prevention of ischemic stroke was outweighed by excess cerebral hemorrhage in the patients over age 75 years (mean 80 years), suggesting that a somewhat lower INR might be preferable. On the other hand, analysis of the INR levels in relation to ischemic stroke and cerebral hemorrhage in EAFT (mean patient age 71 years)[39] found no treatment effect below an INR of 2·0, most major bleeding complications occurred at an INR of 5·0 or above, and the rate of

Table 38.4 Non-rheumatic atrial fibrillation trial outcomes: warfarin *v* aspirin

Trial	All strokes (ischemic and hemorrhagic)			
	Warfarin events/ 1000 pt/yr	Aspirin events/ 1000 pt/yr	Relative risk reduction (%)	Absolute risk reduction events/ 1000 pt/yr
AFASAK[11]	22	39	45	17
SPAF-II[32]				
Age ≤ 75	17	19	10	2
Age ≥ 75	50	55	10	5
EAFT[20]	39	109	67	70
AFASAK-II[34]	31	25	−23	−6
PATAF[35]	7	10	20	3
Overview[31]	26	40	36	14

thromboembolic events was lowest at an INR from 2·0 to 3·9. The authors recommended a target INR of 3·0, with values below 2·0 and above 5·0 to be avoided.

For most patients who are candidates for warfarin an INR range of 2·0–3·0 with a target of 2·5 appears optimal.[26,38] However, those with a previous TIA or minor stroke may benefit from a somewhat higher range of 2·0–3·9 with a target of 3·0,[39] whereas those at higher risk of cerebral hemorrhage, particularly patients over the age of 75, may benefit from a somewhat lower INR range of 1·6–2·5 with a target of 2·0[26]. **Grade A/B**

Cardioversion

The presence of atrial fibrillation increases the risk of systemic embolism, whatever the nature and severity of the underlying heart disease. Accordingly, there is a strong rationale for cardioversion in patients with atrial fibrillation, and maintenance of sinus rhythm to prevent stroke and systemic embolism. Although there is no reliable information in the literature that cardioversion via electrical or pharmacologic means reduces the risk for systemic embolism, this goal remains an expectation, along with a resolution of symptoms related to the atrial fibrillation itself. The strongest predictor of initial and persistent success with cardioversion is short duration of the atrial fibrillation before cardioversion. In general, it may be expected that atrial fibrillation occurring in conjunction with a viral illness, with alcohol or other pharmacologic excess, or in association with thyrotoxicosis or pulmonary embolus, has a high likelihood of reversion with persistence of sinus rhythm if there has been resolution of the precipitating cause. The rate of initial success in restoring sinus rhythm ranges from 76% to 100%, but persistence of sinus rhythm during the next 12 months is noted in 25–81% of patients only.[40–43] Although maintenance of sinus rhythm is more likely with chronic antiarrhythmic drug therapy, a meta-analysis of six randomized placebo-controlled trials of quinidine therapy[41] revealed a statistically significant tripling of mortality during treatment. Other reviews of the use of class I antiarrhythmic therapy in ischemic heart disease indicate a statistically significant excess in mortality.[44] Clinical trials have evaluated class I, II and III drugs for maintenance of sinus rhythm, and individual patient characteristics will influence drug selection.[26] There is no clear evidence yet as to whether antiarrhythmic drug therapy to maintain sinus rhythm reduces the incidence of thromboembolism, congestive failure or death.[45,46]

Although no study has rigorously documented the incidence of systemic embolism following electrical cardioversion, an increased incidence is likely. The best available study,[47] using a prospective cohort design, demonstrated a reduction of postcardioversion systemic embolism from 5·3% to 0·8% among anticoagulated patients. Other studies of less rigorous design have also indicated benefit from

anticoagulation. It is generally believed that a newly formed thrombus will become organized and adherent to the left atrial wall within 2 weeks of formation. Transesophageal echocardiography (TEE) reveals that in the majority of patients thrombus resolves, rather than simply becoming firmly adherent to the wall of the left atrium or left atrial appendage.[48] Accordingly, anticoagulation is usually recommended for about 3 weeks before cardioversion.[26,38] **Grade B** A study that pooled data from 32 studies found that 98% of thromboembolic events occurred within 10 days of cardioversion of atrial fibrillation or flutter.[49] However, evidence exists that even after successful electroversion, atrial contraction may not normalize for some weeks,[50,51] and therefore maintenance of anticoagulation for about 4 weeks following cardioversion seems prudent.[26,38] **Grade B** There is no evidence that the incidence of thromboembolism is less with pharmacologic than with electrical cardioversion, and so accordingly anticoagulant management should not differ.[26] **Grade C**

New-onset atrial fibrillation is generally not thought to warrant anticoagulation if cardioversion is undertaken within 48 hours of its onset. The commencement of intravenous heparin immediately upon diagnosis may be prudent while decisions as to the appropriateness of electrical cardioversion and the preparation for the procedure are undertaken. **Grade B** Emergency cardioversion may be required because of ischemia or hemodynamic compromise in some situations, and if atrial fibrillation has been present for more than 48 hours heparinization may offer some benefit before cardioversion.

The potential role of TEE for the detection of atrial thrombi and the simplification and shortening of the anticoagulation regimen in association with cardioversion was studied in a consecutive series of 230 patients.[52] Atrial thrombi were detected in 15%. Of 196 patients without thrombi, 95% were successfully cardioverted without prolonged anticoagulation, and none had a clinical thromboembolic event. However, a subsequent study[53] and a meta-analysis of several clinical studies[54] indicate that the absence of thrombi on TEE does not mean that a period of 4 weeks of anticoagulation following cardioversion may be safely omitted. **Grade B**

The Assessment of Cardioversion utilizing Echocardiography (ACUTE) pilot study[55] was followed by a multicenter randomized prospective of trial of 1222 patients with atrial fibrillation of more than 2 days' duration.[56] All patients were anticoagulated and assigned to either therapy guided by the findings on TEE or conventional therapy. If TEE showed no thrombus, the patient underwent cardioversion and continued on anticoagulant therapy for 4 weeks. If thrombus was detected, warfarin was given for 3 weeks, TEE was repeated and, if the thrombus had resolved, cardioversion was performed and warfarin continued for 4 weeks. If thrombus was still detected, there was no cardioversion

Table 38.5 Choice of antithrombotic therapies for patients with non-rheumatic atrial fibrillation

Clinical risk factors	Age (yrs)		
	<65	65–75	>75
No	Aspirin definite (A)	Aspirin > warfarin (A) INR target 2·5	Warfarin > aspirin (B) Consider INR target 2·0
Yes	Warfarin definite (A) INR target 2·5	Warfarin definite (A) INR target 2·5	Warfarin definite (A) Consider INR target 2·0

attempted but warfarin was continued for 4 weeks. The patients randomized to no TEE received warfarin for 3 weeks and then underwent cardioversion followed by a further 4 weeks of warfarin. At 8 weeks after the assignment of management strategy there was no significant difference between the two therapeutic groups in the rate of embolic events or in the prevalence of sinus rhythm. The TEE strategy resulted in fewer total hemorrhagic events, most of them minor. Right or left heart thrombi were identified in 13·8% of patients who underwent TEE. Of those patients with thrombi detected, 88·2% had a thrombus in the left atrial appendage. The results of this study indicate that in centers where TEE is readily available and the interpretations reliable, a TEE-guided management strategy can offer a safe, cost effective and convenient alternative to standard anticoagulant regimens. **Grade A** Patients may be anticoagulated and screened by TEE and cardioversion performed immediately if no thrombus is detected, and then receive at least 4 further weeks of anticoagulation. If thrombus is detected, patients should undergo at least 3 weeks of anticoagulation prior to cardioversion, followed by a further 4 weeks of anticoagulation. Among those patients with atrial thrombi detected, the value of repeat TEE after the initial 3 weeks of anticoagulation is uncertain.

Summary recommendations

Patients with persisting atrial fibrillation should generally receive chronic antithrombotic therapy with warfarin or aspirin (Table 38.5). **Grade A** Young patients with atrial fibrillation in the absence of other cardiac abnormality and who are free of a history of hypertension, cerebral vascular disease, congestive heart failure or diabetes mellitus, are at very low risk of thromboembolic events. Aspirin is generally preferable to warfarin, and even no antithrombotic therapy may be acceptable. **Grade A** Warfarin is more effective than aspirin for the prevention of embolic strokes, but the risk of major hemorrhage, including cerebral hemorrhage, is greater. Accordingly, its use should generally be confined to patients who have a substantial risk of embolic stroke. **Grade A** The optimal INR for most patients is 2·0–3·0,

with a target of 2·5. Very elderly patients have a higher risk of cerebral hemorrhage while taking warfarin, and it is possible that the optimal risk–benefit ratio may be achieved with an INR range of 1·6–2·5, with a target of 2·0, although some authorities would recommend a target of 2·5 for all patients. **Grade B**

The most powerful predicator of cerebral embolism is previous TIA or stroke, but substantial increased risk is also associated with a history of congestive heart failure, hypertension or diabetes mellitus and echocardiographic evidence of left atrial enlargement or left ventricular dysfunction. The risk–benefit ratio of warfarin in such patients is increased.

Patients undergoing cardioversion should generally receive oral anticoagulation for about 3 weeks prior to the procedure and for 4 weeks afterwards. **Grade B** If the atrial fibrillation has been present for less than 48 hours, initial heparin therapy before cardioversion, followed by 4 weeks of warfarin therapy after cardioversion, are probably sufficient; in appropriate centers TEE-guided management can offer a safe, cost effective and convenient alternative to standard anticoagulant regimens. **Grade A**

References

1. Kannel WB, Abbott RD, Savage DD *et al.* Coronary heart disease and atrial fibrillation: the Framingham Study. *Am Heart J* 1983;**106**:389–96.
2. Kannel WB, Abbot RD, Savage DD *et al.* Epidemiologic features of chronic atrial fibrillation: the Framingham Study. *N Engl J Med* 1982;**306**:1018–22.
3. Wolf PA, Abbott RD, Kannel WB. Atrial fibrillation: a major contributor to stroke in the elderly. *Arch Intern Med* 1987;**147**:1561–4.
4. Wolf PA, Dawber TR, Thomas E Jr *et al.* Epidemiologic assessment of chronic atrial fibrillation and risk of stroke: the Framingham Study. *Neurology* 1978;**28**:973–7.
5. Wolf PA, Kannel WB, McGee DL *et al.* Duration of atrial fibrillation and eminence of stroke: the Framingham Study. *Stroke* 1983;**14**:664–7.
6. Hull R, Hirsh J, Jay R *et al.* Different intensities of oral anticoagulant therapy in the treatment of proximal-vein thrombosis. *N Engl J Med* 1982;**307**:1676–81.

7. Turpie AGG, Gunstensen J, Hirsh J *et al.* Randomised comparison of two intensities of oral anticoagulant therapy after tissue heart valve replacement. *Lancet* 1988;**i**:1242–5.

8. The Boston Area Anticoagulation Trial of Atrial Fibrillation Investigators. The effect of low-dose warfarin on the risk of stroke in patients with nonrheumatic atrial fibrillation. *N Engl J Med* 1990;**323**:1505–11.

9. Connolly SJ, Laupacis A, Gent M *et al.* for the CAFA Study Coinvestigators. Canadian Atrial Fibrillation Anticoagulation (CAFA) Study. *J Am Coll Cardiol* 1991;18:349–55.

10. Ezekowitz MD, Bridgers SL, James KE *et al.* Warfarin in the prevention of stroke associated with nonrheumatic atrial fibrillation. *N Engl J Med* 1992;**327**:406–12.

11. Petersen P, Boysen G, Godtfredsen J *et al.* Placebo-controlled, randomised trial of warfarin and aspirin for prevention of thromboembolic complications in chronic atrial fibrillation: the Copenhagen AFASAK study. *Lancet* 1989;**i**:175–9.

12. Petersen P, Boysen G. Letter to Editor. *N Engl J Med* 1990; **323**:482.

13. Stroke Prevention in Atrial Fibrillation Investigators. Stroke prevention in atrial fibrillation study: final results. *Circulation* 1991;**84**:527–39.

14. Cairns JA, Connolly SJ. Nonrheumatic atrial fibrillation: risk of stroke and role of antithrombotic therapy. *Circulation* 1991;**84**:469–81.

15. Hart RG, Pearce LA, Rothbart RM, McAnulty JH, Asinger RW, Halperin JL, for the Stroke Prevention in Atrial Fibrillation Investigators. Stroke with intermittent atrial fibrillation: incidence and predictors during aspirin therapy. *J Am Coll Cardiol* 2000;**35**:183–7.

16. Atrial Fibrillation Investigators. Risk factors for stroke and efficiency of antithrombotic therapy in atrial fibrillation analysis of pooled later from five randomized controlled trials. *Arch Intern Med* 1994;**154**:1449–57.

17. Biblo LA, Yuan Z, Quan KJ, Mackall JA, Rimm AA. Risk of stroke in patients with atrial flutter. *Am J Cardiol* 2001;**87**: 346–9, A9.

18. Brand FN, Abbott RD, Kannel WB *et al.* Characteristics and prognosis of lone atrial fibrillation: 30-year follow-up in the Framingham Study. *JAMA* 1985;**254**:3449–53.

19. Kopecky SL, Gersh BJ, McGoon MD *et al.* The natural history of lone atrial fibrillation: a population-based study over three decades. *N Engl J Med* 1987;**317**:669–74.

20. EAFT (European Atrial Fibrillation Trial) Study Group. Secondary prevention in non-rheumatic atrial fibrillation after transient ischemic attack or minor stroke. *Lancet* 1993;**342**: 1255–62.

21. The Stroke Prevention in Atrial Fibrillation Investigation. Prevention of thromboembolism in atrial fibrillation: II Echocardiographic features of patients at risk. *Ann Intern Med* 1992;**116**:6–12.

22. The Stroke Prevention in Atrial Fibrillation Investigation. Prevention of thromboembolism in atrial fibrillation: I Clinical features of patients at risk. *Ann Intern Med* 1992;**116**:1–5.

23. Petersen P, Godtfredsen J. Embolic complications in paroxysmal atrial fibrillation. *Stroke* 1986;**17**:622–6.

24. Wolf PA, Kannel WB, McGee DL *et al.* Duration of atrial fibrillation and eminence of stroke: the Framingham Study. *Stroke* 1983;**14**:664–7.

25. Cerebral Embolism Study Group. Cardioembolic stroke, early anticoagulation, and brain hemorrhage. *Arch Intern Med* 1987;**147**:636–40.

26. Fuster V, Rydén LE, Asinger RW *et al.* ACC/AHA/ESC guidelines for the management of patients with atrial fibrillation: a report of the American College of Cardiology/American Heart Association Task Force on Practice Guidelines and the European Society of Cardiology Committee for Practice Guidelines and Policy Conferences (Committee to Develop Guidelines for the Management of Patients with Atrial Fibrillation). *J Am Coll Cardiol* 2001;**38**:266i–lxx.

27. Atrial Fibrillation Investigators. The efficacy of aspirin in patients with atrial fibrillation: analysis of pooled data from 3 randomized trials. *Arch Intern Med* 1997;**157**:1237–40.

28. Diener HC, Lowenthal A. Antiplatelet therapy to prevent stroke: risk of brain hemorrhage and efficacy in atrial fibrillation. *J Neurol Sci* 1997;**153**:112.

29. Posada IS, Barriales V, for the LASAF Pilot Study Group. Alternate-day dosing of aspirin in atrial fibrillation. *Am Heart J* 1999;**138**:137–43.

30. Benavente O, Hart R, Koudstaal P, Laupacis A, McBride R. Antiplatelet therapy for preventing stroke in patients with non-valvular atrial fibrillation and no previous history of stroke or transient ischemic attacks. In: Warlow C, Van Gijn J, Sandercock P, eds. Stroke Module of the Cochrane Database of Systematic Reviews. Oxford: *The Cochrane Collaboration*, 1999. CD-ROM available from BMJ Publishing Group (London).

31. Hart RG, Benavente O, McBride R, Pearce LA. Antithrombotic therapy to prevent stroke in patients with atrial fibrillation: a meta-analysis. *Ann Intern Med* 1999;**131**:492–501.

32. Stroke Prevention in Atrial Fibrillation Investigators. Warfarin versus aspirin for prevention of thromboembolism in atrial fibrillation. Stroke Prevention in Atrial Fibrillation II Study. *Lancet* 1994;**343**:687–91.

33. Stroke Prevention in Atrial Fibrillation Investigators. Adjusted-dose warfarin versus low-intensity, fixed-dose warfarin plus aspirin for high-risk patients with atrial fibrillation: the Stroke Prevention in Atrial Fibrillation III randomized clinical trial. *Lancet* 1996;**348**:633–8.

34. Gullov AL, Koefoed BG, Petersen P *et al.* Fixed minidose warfarin and aspirin alone and in combination vs adjusted-dose warfarin for stroke prevention in atrial fibrillation. Second Copenhagen Atrial Fibrillation, Aspirit, and Anticoagulation Study. *Arch Intern Med* 1998;**158**:1513–21.

35. Hellemons BS, Langenberg M, Lodder J *et al.* Primary prevention of arterial thromboembolism in patients with non-rheumatic atrial fibrillation in general practice (the PATAF study) [Abstract]. *Cerebrovasc Dis* 1997;**7**(Suppl 4):11.

36. Hylek EM, Singer DE. Risk factors for intracranial hemorrhage in patients taking warfarin. *Ann Intern Med* 1994; **120**:897–902.

37. Fihu SD, Callahan CM, Martin DC *et al.* The risk for and severity of bleeding complications in elderly patients treated with warfarin. *Ann Intern Med* 1996;**124**:970–9.

38. Albers GWM, Dalen JE, Laupacis A *et al.* Antithrombotic therapy in atrial fibrillation. *Chest* 2001;**119**:194S–206S.

39. The European Atrial Fibrillation Trial Study Group. Optimal oral anticoagulant therapy in patients with nonrheumatic atrial

fibrillation and recent cerebral ischemia. *N Engl J Med* 1995; **333**:5–10.

40. Brodsky MA, Allen BJ, Capparelli EV *et al.* Factors determining maintenance of sinus rhythm after chronic atrial fibrillation with left atrial dilatation. *Am J Cardiol* 1989;**63**:1065–8.

41. Coplen SE, Antman EM, Berlin JA *et al.* Prevention of recurrent atrial fibrillation by quinidine: a meta-analysis of randomized trials (abstract). *Circulation* 1989;**80**(Suppl II):II–633.

42. Dittrich HC, Erickson JS, Schneiderman T *et al.* Echocardiographic and clinical predictors for outcome of elective cardioversion of atrial fibrillation. *Am J Cardiol* 1989;**63**: 193–7.

43. Lundstrom T, Ryden L. Chronic atrial fibrillation: long-term results of direct current conversion. *Acta Med Scand* 1988; **223**:53–9.

44. Teo KK, Yusuf S, Furberg CD. Effects of prophylactic antiarrhythmic drug therapy in acute myocardial infarction: an overview of results from the randomized controlled trials. *JAMA* 1993;**270**:1589–95.

45. Planning and Steering Committees of the AFFIRM study for the NHLBI AFFIRM investigators. Atrial fibrillation follow-up investigation of rhythm management: the AFFIRM study design. *Am J Cardiol* 1997;**79**:1198–202.

46. Hohnloser SH, Kuck KH, Lilienthal J. Rhythm or rate control in atrial fibrillation: Pharmacological Intervention in Atrial Fibrillation (PIAF): a randomised trial. *Lancet* 2000;**356**: 1789–94.

47. Bjerkelund CJ, Orning OM. The efficacy of anticoagulant therapy in preventing embolism related to DC electrical conversion of atrial fibrillation. *Am J Cardiol* 1969;**23**:208.

48. Collins LJ, Silverman DI, Douglas PS, Manning WJ. Cardioversion of nonrheumatic atrial fibrillation: reduced thromboembolic complications with 4 weeks of precardioversion anticoagulation are related to atrial thrombus resolution. *Circulation* 1995;**92**:160–3.

49. Berger M, Schweitzer P. Timing of thromboembolic events after electrical cardioversion of atrial fibrillation or flutter: a retrospective analysis. *Am J Cardiol* 1998;**82**:1545–7, A8.

50. Manning WJ, Leeman DE, Gotch PJ *et al.* Pulsed Doppler evaluation of atrial mechanical function after electrical cardioversion of atrial fibrillation. *J Am Coll Cardiol* 1989; **13**:617–23.

51. Padraig GO, Puleo PR, Bolli R *et al.* Return of atrial mechanical function following electrical cardioversion of atrial dysrhythmias. *Am Heart J* 1990;**120**:353–9.

52. Manning WJ, Silverman DI, Keightly CS *et al.* Transesophageal echocardiographically facilitated early cardioversion from atrial fibrillation using short-term anticoagulation – final results of a prospective 4.5 year study. *J Am Coll Cardiol* 1995; **25**:1354–61.

53. Black IW, Fatkin D, Sagar KB *et al.* Exclusion of atrial thrombus by transesophageal echocardiography does not preclude embolism after cardioversion of atrial fibrillation: a multicenter study. *Circulation* 1994;**89**:2509–13.

54. Moreyra E, Finkelhor RS, Debul RD. Limitations of transesophageal echocardiography in the risk assessment of patients before nonanticoagulated cardioversion from atrial fibrillation and flutter: an analysis of pooled trials. *Am Heart J* 1995;**129**:71–5.

55. Klein AL, Grimm RA, Black IW *et al.* Cardioversion guided by transesophageal echocardiography: the ACUTE Pilot Study. *Ann Intern Med* 1997;**126**:200–9.

56. Klein AL, Grimm RA, Murray RD *et al.* Use of transesophageal echocardiography to guide cardioversion in patients with atrial fibrillation. *N Engl J Med* 2001;**344**:1411–20.

39 Atrial fibrillation: non-pharmacologic therapies

Sanjeev Saksena, Andrew J Einstein

The increasing public health burden of atrial fibrillation (AF) is now well recognized and its adverse impact on cardiovascular health and survival for individuals is being fully assessed. Prevalence in the United States has been variously estimated between two and three million, and this has been projected to increase to 5·6 million by 2050. It is the most common arrhythmia, particularly in the elderly. By the age of 80 years, over 9% of the population can suffer from the arrhythmia.[1] In patients with AF, there is a near doubling of cardiovascular mortality in men and a 50% increase in women.[2] While the importance of antithrombotic therapy is now undisputed, the management of this arrhythmia remains controversial. Recent clinical trials and practice guidelines have attempted to provide some insight for clinicians, but major issues remain unclear. Furthermore, epidemiologic data are derived largely from persistent or permanent AF populations, but most rhythm control trials have been conducted primarily in paroxysmal AF patients, from which extrapolation of strategies to other types of AF is problematic. While trials such as RACE,[3] STAF,[4] and AFFIRM[5] have not shown improved morbidity or mortality with rhythm control, it is also clear that effective rhythm control was not often achieved in these studies. In STAF, only 23% of the patients actually achieved freedom from AF on amiodarone therapy.[4] The inability to maintain rhythm control is due to the limited efficacy of antiarrhythmic drugs, which has been repeatedly documented in clinical trials. There is also an absence of good strategies to deal with recurrent AF. This has been limited to cardioversion in an occasional study, and a paucity of options has further compromised development of a sound rhythm control strategy.[6] Recently, an increasing number of non-pharmacologic options have become available and can supplement or even attempt to replace drug therapy in selected patients. In addition, they may be useful strategies in primary prevention approaches. It can be anticipated with some degree of certainty that the current approach of using antiarrhythmic drugs alone is likely to be modified shortly, and refocused on a combined pharmacologic and non-pharmacologic approach, or "hybrid" therapy.

Currently, available non-pharmacologic strategies revolve around implantable device therapy and ablative approaches. Devices available include cardiac pacemakers and pacemaker-defibrillators. Ablation therapy may be classified into catheter-based and intraoperative techniques. Several options now exist for each of these approaches; a classification of current non-pharmacologic strategies is shown in Table 39·1. Several major therapeutic options in current practice will be discussed in this chapter, while those in evaluation will be alluded to. Finally, hybrid therapy is gaining ground, with combinations of non-pharmacologic and pharmacologic methods for longer-term AF management.

Single site atrial pacing

Atrial pacing performed from the high right atrium has been widely reported to reduce the recurrence of AF and progression to permanent AF in observational reports. The Danish Trial of Physiologic Pacing in sick sinus syndrome reported reduction in the incidence of persistent or permanent AF with atrial-based pacing in patients with sick sinus syndrome.[7] **Grade A** This result has been corroborated in the MOST[8] and CTOPP[9] trials. It is particularly effective in patients with sick sinus syndrome alone, reducing the relative risk of AF development by 50%.[8] Clinical investigation of atrial pacing techniques for management of AF in symptomatic or high-risk populations has been the subject of a series of prospective clinical trials.[10–15] Approaches have included high right atrial, septal and dual site atrial pacing. Analysis of the benefit of atrial pacing is complicated by incomplete knowledge of its electrophysiologic effects and interactions with a heterogeneous AF population, by limited knowledge of the natural history of AF, and by the lack of standardized end points for quantifying clinical benefit.[16] Many studies lack a control group without atrial pacing therapy to judge efficacy.[17]

The efficacy of high right atrial pacing alone for prevention of symptomatic paroxysmal AF has been evaluated in clinical studies and remains currently unproven. **Grade A** In a randomized crossover two-phase clinical trial, Gillis and coworkers noted no prolongation in the time to recurrent AF compared to placebo.[10] In patients with refractory AF as the sole arrhythmia, the Jewel AF device experience showed that high right atrial pacing appeared to reduce frequency but not AF burden initially, but more detailed analysis failed to confirm long-term benefit.[11]

Table 39.1   Classification of non-pharmacologic therapies in atrial fibrillation

Therapy	References
Rhythm control strategies	
Device therapy	
Atrial Pacing	
• Single site	
(i) High right atrial	10–15, 20
(ii) Septal	18,19
• Multisite	
(i) Dual site right atrial	23–29
(ii) Biatrial	
Atrial defibrillators	
• Stand alone atrioverter with demand pacing	30
• Atrioventricular pacemaker defibrillator	11, 17
Ablation therapy	
Intraoperative or thoracoscopic	
• His bundle ablation (surgical ligation, mechanical, cryothermia)	33, 34
• Corridor procedure (mechanical)	
• Biatrial maze (mechanical)	35, 36
• Left atrial isolation (mechanical)	
• Pulmonary vein isolation (mechanical or cryothermia)	38
• Epicardial linear ablation (radiofrequency)	37
• Radial incision (mechanical)	39
Transcatheter	
• Trigger ablation	
(i) Focal pulmonary vein (radiofrequency)	22, 40–43
(ii) Pulmonary vein isolation (radiofrequency or ultrasound)	43–46
(iii) Atrial flutter/atrial tachycardia (radiofrequency)	
• Substrate ablation	
(i) Linear ablation (radiofrequency)	
Biatrial	
Right atrial	47, 48
Left atrial	
Rate control strategies	
Catheter AV junctional ablation + pacemaker (DC shock or radiofrequency)	49–51
Catheter AV junctional modification (radiofrequency)	52
Stroke prevention strategy	
Percutaneous left atrial appendage transcatheter occlusion (PLAATO)	53

Thus, in an effort to improve efficacy, several new directions have evolved for single site atrial pacing. These include several new algorithms for ensuring overdrive atrial pacing. The Medtronic AT 500 pacemaker is a DDDRP device which employs two algorithms, atrial preference pacing and atrial rate stabilization, in addition to having antitachycardia pacing capabilities. Atrial preference pacing changes the base pacing rate in response to atrial premature beats, with a programmable increment. Atrial rate stabilization intercedes after premature beats altering the post-ectopic escape interval by reducing it markedly and then slowly easing down to the base pacing rate. Antitachycardia pacing, illustrated in Figure 39·1, can terminate common and non-isthmus-dependent atrial flutter by burst, ramp, or combination rapid pacing sequences. In a non-randomized study, Israel *et al*[12] evaluated 325 patients for efficacy of atrial antitachycardia pacing and device safety, and secondarily, for reliability of atrial tachyarrhythmia detection. Fifty-three per cent of atrial tachycardia episodes were terminated with antitachycardia pacing; there was an 88% complication-free survival at 3 months and 97% reliable detection of atrial tachyarrhythmia episodes. While preventive pacing algorithms were found to increase the median percentage of atrial pacing from 62% to 97%, the frequency and duration of episodes were unchanged. The ATTEST study[13] randomized patients with the AT 500 pacemaker after implantation to all preventive pacing and antitachycardia pacing on or off. Antitachycardia pacing in this study also terminated 53% of

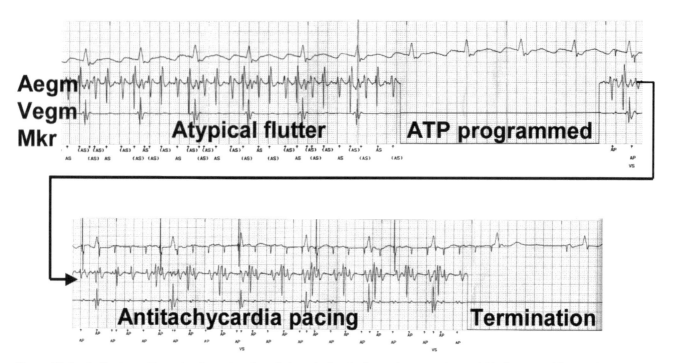

Figure 39.1 Antitachycardia pacing for restoration of sinus rhythm. Left panel represents atrial fibrillation, middle panel represents antitachycardia pacing, right panel represents restored sinus rhythm afterwards

episodes, and positive predictive value for atrial tachycardia detection was 99%. While quality of life improved in both groups, there was no significant difference in frequency or burden of atrial tachyarrhythmia episodes. PROVE, a randomized crossover trial, is evaluating a similar device, the Talent DR 213 pacemaker, combining atrial overdrive pacing with an automatic rest rate function. Preliminary results from 78 patients show 84% prevalence of atrial pacing, a mean 48% shortening of episode duration with overdrive pacing and rest rate, and a slight improvement in quality of life.[14] The ADOPT-A study evaluated a new pacing algorithm, dynamic atrial overdrive, used in St Jude Medical Integrity pacemakers, in patients with AF, and found an approximately 25% decrease in AF burden and some improvement in quality of life.[15] **Grade A**

Alternate site pacing has also been investigated. Single site pacing at a septal location was performed in two prospective randomized studies. Bailin *et al*[18] randomized 120 patients with paroxysmal AF to high septal pacing or right atrial appendage pacing. Patients with high septal pacing had a significantly higher rate of survival free from chronic AF at one year (75% *v* 47%), but no decrease in AF event frequency. A control no treatment arm was absent in this trial. The Atrial Septal Pacing Efficacy Clinical Trial (ASPECT) randomized patients to septal or non-septal RA lead implantation, and pacing prevention using an AT 500 pacemaker. Septal pacing was not associated with a reduction in AF frequency or burden.[19] **Grade B**

Another approach using atrial pacing is high right atrial pacing in combination with other antiarrhythmic therapies, such as drugs. In an early experience from our group, antiarrhythmic drug therapy combined with high right atrial pacing prolonged arrhythmia-free intervals but no long-term data was available on rhythm control.[20] Similarly, we have employed linear ablation with drug therapy and dual site or high right atrial pacing in pilot clinical experience.[21,22] We have noted a decrease in progression to permanent AF (<30% at 3 years) and device datalogs confirm resolution of persistent and permanent AF in a subgroup who underwent right atrial maze procedures.[22] In these refractory patients, early AF recurrence was often observed after intervention, which subsequently resolved after 2–3 months with restoration of rhythm control. **Grade C**

Dualsite right atrial pacing

Current experience with secondary prevention of AF with dual site RA pacing has usually been performed in patients with recurrent, symptomatic, and frequent drug-refractory AF.[23] This method is illustrated in Figures 39.2 and 39.3, which show a representative chest radiograph and electrocardiogram for a patient with dual site right atrial pacing system. The additional atrial pacing lead is inserted just outside the coronary sinus ostium for stability and left atrial synchronization. The ECG shows a biphasic P wave in the

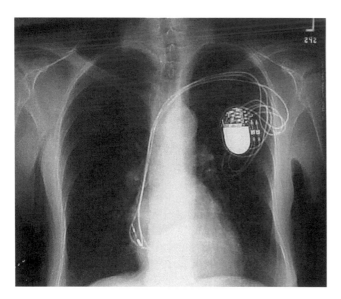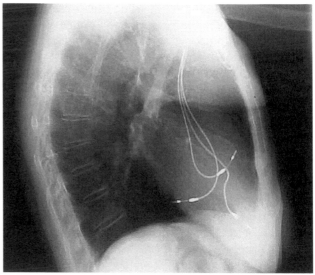

Figure 39.2 Posteroanterior (left) and lateral (right) radiographic views of a dual site right atrial pacemaker system for atrial fibrillation. Two leads are placed in the right atrium, at the high right atrium and outside the ostium of the coronary sinus. A standard right ventricular lead can be placed in patients with AV conduction abnormalities.

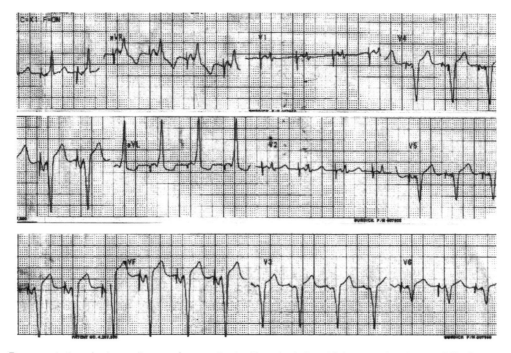

Figure 39.3 Representative electrocardiogram for a patient with a dual site atrial pacemaker for atrial fibrillation treatment. Note that during dual site pacing there is a biphasic P wave in leads II, III, and aVF with abbreviation of total P wave duration.

inferior leads with abbreviation of P wave duration. In our pilot experience, trends to benefit with dual site right atrial pacing were seen in 3 month crossover interim analyses[23] but significant benefit of dual site over high right atrial or septal pacing was only obvious after one year.[20] In our long-term experience, now encompassing over 125 patients with follow up averaging 3 years and ranging to 7 years, the overall patient survival is 80% at 5 years. Freedom from any recurrence of symptomatic AF after institution of pacing was 45% at 5 years and we achieved rhythm control in over 90% of patients at 3 years or more of follow up. The overall stroke incidence is 0·8% per year.[24] Similar efficacy rates can be achieved in paroxysmal, persistent, and permanent AF.

The safety of dual site right atrial pacing can also be assessed. Lead dislodgment rates are well within estimates for any type of atrial pacing and long-term dislodgment concerns have been obviated by the dual right atrial lead technique. The remaining complications have been largely similar to those in any pacemaker implant procedure. Precipitation of angina in a patient with advanced coronary disease and exertional angina occurred in one patient. The major issue has been late intolerance to antiarrhythmic drugs with frequent replacement of class 1 agents with class 3 drugs.

A non-randomized parallel cohort experience from Europe in patients with bradycardias requiring pacing and paroxysmal AF shows similar efficacy.[25] Of 83 patients, 30 had dual site right atrial pacing systems and 53 had single site high right pacemaker implanted. Patients with dual site systems had longer duration of AF (8·1 v 3·8 years for high RA systems, $P < 0.001$) and more failed drug trials (2·4 v 1·6 for high RA systems, $P < 0.05$). During a mean follow up of 18 months, symptomatic paroxysmal AF recurred in 9 patients after dual RA pacing as compared to 24 patients after high RA pacing ($P = 0.03$). Permanent AF supervened in only one patient after dual RA pacing and in 12 patients after high RA pacing ($P < 0.05$). In an observational study, biatrial triggered pacing in patients with intra-atrial conduction delay and recurrent atrial flutter and fibrillation, performed by Revault d'Allonnes and colleagues, resulted in a 64% incidence of rhythm control at a mean follow up of 33 months.[26] A majority of these patients were on antiarrhythmic drug therapy.

Several small, randomized trials have now been reported in addition to several single-center pilot experiences. In a short-term randomized, 12 week comparative study of patients without bradycardia, Lau *et al* reported an increase in mean time to first AF recurrence from 15 to 50 days in patients during dual site pacing as compared to no pacing.[27] In a prospective crossover trial with 6 month treatment periods in patients with recurrent symptomatic AF without structural heart disease, Ramdat Misier and coworkers have shown a significant increase in time to recurrent AF and interventions for symptomatic AF recurrence.[28]

The Dual-Site Atrial Pacing for Prevention of Atrial Fibrillation Trial (DAPPAF) was a longer-term multicenter crossover study with 6 month treatment arms comparing dual site right atrial, high right atrial, and support pacing.[29] It enrolled patients with frequent, symptomatic, and drug-refractory AF with bradyarrhythmias requiring cardiac pacemaker insertion. After dual site right atrial pacing system implant, optimization of drug and pacing therapies was performed. The three modes of pacing were then randomly selected for 6 month periods. Patient tolerance and adherence to the pacing mode was superior in dual RA pacing as compared to support ($P < 0.001$) and high RA pacing ($P = 0.006$). Freedom from any symptomatic AF recurrence

trended to be greater with dual RA (hazard ratio 0·715, $P = 0.07$) but not with high RA pacing ($P = 0.19$) compared to support pacing. Combined symptomatic and asymptomatic AF frequency in patients was significantly reduced during dual RA pacing as compared to high RA pacing ($P < 0.01$). However, in antiarrhythmic drug-treated patients, dual RA pacing increased symptomatic AF-free survival compared to support pacing ($P = 0.011$), and high RA pacing (hazard ratio 0·669, $P = 0.06$). In drug-treated patients with <1 AF event per week, dual RA pacing significantly improved AF suppression compared to support pacing (hazard ratio 0·464, $P = 0.004$) and high RA pacing (hazard ratio 0·623, $P = 0.006$). Lead dislodgment was uncommon (1·7%) with coronary sinus and high RA lead stability being comparable. Thus, the DAPPAF trial showed improved adherence to pacing and rhythm control in the dual site mode, especially when combined with antiarrhythmic drugs, supporting the use of a hybrid approach to rhythm management. **Grade A**

The implantable atrial defibrillator

Catheter-based internal cardioversion of atrial fibrillation was first employed in 1969 and early studies were performed by Mirowski and colleagues. The development of implantable device technology was achieved in the late 1990s and a prototype device was used in pilot studies.[30] Transcatheter atrial defibrillation is often achieved at energies quite similar to ventricular defibrillation. While early enthusiasm suggested that this would be feasible at very low energies (2 J or less) using right atrial and coronary sinus electrodes, more extensive clinical experience suggested significantly higher energy requirements well above the pain threshold.[31] While the initial atrial cardioverter permitted shocks up to 6 J and ventricular pacing, higher energy requirements, risk of ventricular proarrhythmia without ventricular defibrillation and pain related to the therapy limited its adoption. While ventricular proarrhythmia resulting from atrial defibrillation shocks was rare in animal studies, it has been documented in both experimental and clinical studies, particularly in diseased hearts. Initial clinical experience was modest but encouraging and suggested that effective and safe atrial defibrillation was feasible.[30]

The first generation atrial defibrillation device was succeeded by a commercially available dual chamber atrioventricular defibrillator.[11] This device, shown in Figure 39·4, includes atrial and ventricular antitachycardia pacing, cardioversion, and defibrillation. Initial studies have been conducted in patients with atrial fibrillation who may or may not have coexisting lethal ventricular tachyarrhythmias.[11,17] Due to its extensive electrical therapy and monitoring capability, the future of this technology in a hybrid therapy format is quite promising. Dual chamber AV defibrillators

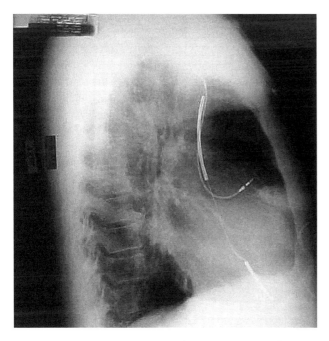

Figure 39.4 Lateral radiograph of atrioventricular defibrillator showing atrial and ventricular defibrillation electrode catheter and an additional atrial pacing lead in the high right atrium

are approved for use in patients with drug-refractory and symptomatic AF and in patients with coexisting symptomatic atrial and ventricular tachyarrhythmias. **Grade B**

In comparison to the widely used ventricular defibrillator, the atrial defibrillator requires insertion of an additional atrial defibrillation electrode used for atrial pacing, AF detection, and atrial shock delivery. Atrial tachyarrhythmia detection is based on two zones, one for monomorphic tachycardias and another for AF events. Antitachycardia pacing is available as well as shock therapy. Burst and ramp pacing is effective in both intra-atrial re-entrant tachycardia and common atrial flutter. Fifty hz pacing trains have been demonstrated to be effective in atypical atrial flutter.[32] Atrial shocks are used if pacing therapies are ineffective. In clinical studies, reliable atrial defibrillation has been obtained with shock energies up to 27 J. A full range of ventricular defibrillation functions is available as in conventional defibrillators.

Newer iterations include prevention algorithms such as continuous atrial pacing for AF prevention. Enhanced monitoring capabilities include atrial and ventricular arrhythmia detection. Device-based testing is available and a handheld patient activator permits delivery of shock therapy on demand by the patient or physician. Combination devices combining atrial defibrillation with the pacing strategies discussed above may offer improvement in AF management. One multicenter crossover study evaluated the use of a dual chamber ICD with both pacing and shock therapies, in

patients otherwise indicated for an implantable ventricular ICD who also had recurrent atrial tachyarrhythmias. The device resulted in a significant reduction in atrial tachyarrhythmia burden.[11] Nevertheless, there have been no controlled trials that compare efficacy, survival, quality of life, or cost in patients treated with implantable atrial defibrillators versus other therapies.

Intraoperative ablation

The first surgical interventions for AF were ligation or cryosurgical ablation of the His bundle followed by implantation of a pacemaker.[33,34] Subsequent efforts included the corridor procedure and left atrial isolation, but definitive treatment awaited the maze procedure, developed by Cox and coworkers.[35] Several refinements of the original technique have been performed. The principle is to compartmentalize both atria so that AF cannot be maintained. Both right and left atrial appendages are resected. The pulmonary vein ostia are isolated, and linear right atrial and left atrial lesions are connected to anatomic structures to form an "electrical maze". Revisions have addressed the problem of sinus node dysfunction, though abnormal hemodynamic function may still exist. Currently, the maze procedure has become an add-on technique during other cardiac surgery procedures including mitral valve replacement and repair,[36] and coronary artery bypass surgery. **Grade B** Furthermore, new techniques described below have limited the extent of the maze. New developments include partial isolation of the pulmonary veins and LA linear ablation[37] or epicardial radiofrequency isolation of the pulmonary veins during thoracoscopy or cardiac surgery.[38] Another recent refinement, introduced to maintain more physiologic atrial transport function, is the radial incision approach, in which incisions radiate from the sinus node to the atrioventricular annular margins and parallel atrial coronary arteries.[39]

Catheter ablation for rhythm control: trigger ablation

Catheter-based approaches to rhythm control in AF utilize focal or linear ablation of the initiating trigger, or introduce linear lesions to modify the substrate maintaining fibrillation. Substantial effort is currently being devoted to trigger ablation, particularly in the pulmonary venous system. Atrial premature beats and monomorphic atrial tachycardias or flutter are the most common triggers for AF. Techniques for isthmus and non-isthmus dependent atrial flutter ablation use linear radiofrequency lesions in critical regions for flutter circuits. Recently, investigative work has focused on ablation of such premature beats or focal tachycardias arising in the pulmonary venous system, as well as mapping of atrial tachycardias and atrial flutter, including non-isthmus dependent atypical forms. Both biatrial contact mapping with multipolar catheters placed in the RA and LA, and also three-dimensional mapping methods have been used.[22,40–43] Three-dimensional mapping can help locate triggers, propagation patterns, zones of slow conduction and re-entry, and refine the focal ablation methodology.[22] An endocardial balloon electrode permits mapping of the atrium obtaining virtual electrogram recordings from up to 3000 endocardial sites which are reconstructed using a Silicon Graphics computer workstation as a three-dimensional image. Specific sites of slow or low amplitude propagation can be defined that could potentially limit efficacy and, in addition, provide insight into the mechanisms of early AF recurrences. These sites can be prophylactically ablated. This can be combined with biatrial catheter mapping and pulmonary vein recordings. Figure 39.5 shows catheter placement in three of the four pulmonary veins in a patient with recurrent refractory AF. The veins can be visualized with angiography and ablation can be performed at the trigger site inside the vein, or partial disconnection of the focus from the left atrium using a spiral electrode configuration for circumferential mapping. Using circumferential electrode arrays on catheters (Lasso or Helix catheters), partial ablation at the site of the connecting muscle bundle can be performed in an effort to avert pulmonary vein stenosis.

Early data from many clinical centers documented elimination of these triggers with modest short-term success ranging from 14% to 63%. In addition, multiple triggers are common, and in some patients ablation within the veins had significant adverse effects including pulmonary vein stenosis. Evolving technology and techniques may address many of these issues. Newer energy sources such as ultrasound are undergoing such clinical trials and early results show modest efficacy and increased safety.[43] Pulmonary vein isolation may have greater success if all four veins are isolated, but remains a demanding and tedious procedure with measurable procedural risk. However, the vast majority of these patients still require adjuvant drug therapy for clinical benefit. Long-term success remains dependent on the number of triggering sites and few data are available in organized clinical trials. The frequency of asymptomatic and symptomatic AF has also not been addressed in a controlled clinical trial with the radiofrequency technique.

Grade C

Pulmonary vein triggers have been directly ablated within the vein, and usually require ablation in multiple or all veins for success. Ablation within the vein has been extensive in early studies but more segmental in recent reports to reduce the risk of pulmonary vein stenosis. Subclinical effects on pulmonary vein flow velocity can occur in many patients (range 25–80%) but clinically significant stenosis occurs in up to 8% of patients. Table 39.2 summarizes efficacy and safety data on this approach in several large reports.[40–46] Another major challenge is the paucity of patients demonstrating spontaneous arrhythmia at the time of study, limiting map-directed targeted ablation. More recently, anatomic approaches to isolate the pulmonary veins by circumferential periostial ablation methods using radiofrequency[44–46] or ultrasound[43] energy have been employed. While there has been demonstrable efficacy, no definite improvement in outcome or safety can be documented at the present time. Furthermore, recurrent AF is common and often has not been systematically monitored in these studies, using advanced or implantable monitoring for asymptomatic as

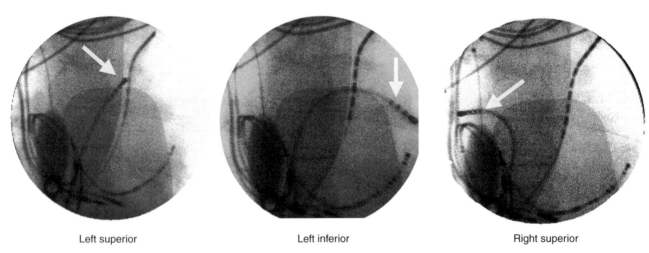

| Left superior | Left inferior | Right superior |

Figure 39.5 Biatrial catheter mapping of refractory atrial fibrillation with three-dimensional mapping of the right atrium. Multielectrode catheters are placed in the right atrium, coronary sinus, left pulmonary artery and transeptally into the pulmonary veins. The arrow points out the individual pulmonary veins in this patient, which are mapped for triggers and then ablated at the focus. There is a pre-existing dual site atrial pacemaker system in this patient with permanent leads in the high right atrium, coronary sinus ostium, and right ventricle.

Table 39.2 Efficacy and safety of pulmonary vein trigger ablation or isolation

Series	Method	Patients (*n*)	Mean follow up (mth)	% AF eliminated	% PV stenosis
Map-directed ablation					
Chen[40]	PVA	79	6	86s	42 (TEE)
Haissaguerre[41]	PVA	225	Not specified	70s	2 (clinical)
Gerstenfeld[42]	PVA	71	6	23s 31c	8 (angiography)
Natale[43]	PVA	293	10	81s 86c	11·5 (CT)
Anatomic ablation					
Pappone[44]	PVI	251	10·4	85pa 68perm	0 (TEE)
Kanagaratnam[45]	PVI	71	29	21s 83c	36 (CT)
Oral[46]	PVI	70	5	70pa 22pers	3 (CT)
Natale[43]	CUVA	30	12	47s 80c	3 (CT)

Abbreviations: c, with drugs; CT, by computed tomography; CUVA, catheter ultrasound vein ablation; pa, paroxysmal; pers, persistent; perm, permanent; PVA, pulmonary vein ablation; PVI, pulmonary vein isolation; s, without drugs; TEE, by transesophageal echocardiography

well as symptomatic AF. These patients require adjuvant drug or device therapy for clinical benefit.

Catheter ablation for rhythm control: substrate ablation

Linear atrial lesions have been employed in the left and right atrium for substrate compartmentalization. In these approaches, contiguous radiofrequency energy lesions are used to create linear ablative lesions, producing lines of block for electrical propagation of triggering or perpetuating arrhythmias in the atrium. During linear ablation, three-dimensional mapping allows assessment of anatomic contiguity of ablation lesions for confluent linear line development. Pacing techniques are used for assessment of the linear lesion's integrity. In addition, new arrhythmias that may develop in compartments can be identified and treated. Left atrial compartmentalization has been modified due to safety concerns and more recent approaches use pulmonary vein ostial or posterior left atrial compartmentalization alone. Again, formal clinical trials of these new approaches are lacking and are awaited.

Right atrial linear compartmentalization has been employed, initially as monotherapy with limited success. Adjuvant drug therapy was often required for modest benefit.[47] Kocheril[48] has reported beneficial effects in paroxysmal AF, and interim results of a large clinical trial have shown benefit in symptomatic AF suppression in over 65% of patients (Cardima Inc., unpublished data). Most patients do require adjuvant antiarrhythmic drug therapy for clinical success but the technique is quite safe in clinical application. Finally, adjuvant pacing therapies such as dual site pacing can be examined. Recently, we have reported successful AF

suppression with atrial pacing after right atrial linear compartmentalization in patients with drug-refractory persistent and permanent AF.[22] In these patients, device datalogs documented elimination of persistent or permanent AF, with the vast majority having non-sustained atrial arrhythmias or brief asymptomatic AF. In summary, ablative AF therapies are in rapid evolution. Early empiric application has been troubled by efficacy and safety concerns. Mapping guided assessment of mechanisms and interventional therapies in the atrium can refine techniques with potential for improving efficacy and safety. **Grade C**

Rate control strategies: catheter ablation and modification of the AV conducting system

As device and ablation therapy advances, permitting restoration of sinus rhythm in more patients, the role of catheter-induced complete AV block to control rapid ventricular response in AF is becoming limited to a smaller population of highly refractory and symptomatic patients. This approach was initially performed operatively with cryoablation. Subsequently, it was performed by catheter using direct current, and ultimately with radiofrequency current. The first prospective, international study of safety and efficacy of the approach was the Catheter Ablation Registry,[49] which evaluated 136 patients treated with direct current energy from 1987 to 1990. The registry reported successful induction of complete heart block in 83% of surviving patients, but an inhospital mortality rate of 5·1%. Patients who died in the hospital were more likely to have had prior sudden cardiac death, congestive heart failure, reduced ejection fraction, and QT prolongation. The Ablate and Pace Trial[50] similarly evaluated radiofrequency ablation. It reported successful ablation of AV conduction in 155 of 156 patients, with no procedural mortality. **Grade B** There was 85·3% 1 year survival, with five sudden cardiac deaths in this period. There were significant improvements in quality of life indices, and slight significant 1 year improvement in New York Heart Association functional class from 2·1 to 1·9. A sustained improvement in left ventricular ejection fraction was only noted in patients with reduced systolic function, indicating that tachycardia-induced cardiomyopathy may be reversed with this approach. Long-term experience with the ablate and pace strategy at the Mayo Clinic, for an average of 3 years, has been reported.[51] Patients were compared with two control groups: age- and sex-matched Minnesota residents, and patients with atrial fibrillation managed with drug therapy. While the observed survival rate was significantly lower than in the Minnesota residents, it was equal when high-risk patients with previous myocardial infarction, congestive heart failure, or drug therapy after ablation were excluded. Survival was equal between the ablation and drug therapy cohorts, suggesting that rate control by AV junctional ablation does not negatively affect long-term survival. Nevertheless, the concern of sudden cardiac death remains, particularly in patients with left ventricular systolic dysfunction.

An alternative to AV junctional ablation and permanent pacemaker placement is modification of AV junctional conduction.[52] This approach typically involves application of radiofrequency energy to the basal portions of Koch's triangle. Experience has been mixed, with results varying widely between series, and the procedure is now employed uncommonly. Progression to complete AV block has been reported as well as loss of efficacy in rate control in a significant proportion of patients. Prospective trial data is lacking for this procedure.

Stroke prevention strategy

While the goal of most device therapy for atrial fibrillation is the restoration of sinus rhythm or rate control, one experimental approach involves implantation of a device to decrease the risk of stroke. Percutaneous left atrial appendage transcatheter occlusion, or PLAATO, involves the insertion of an occlusion device by catheter into the left atrial appendage, the location of over 90% of atrial thrombi, via a transseptal puncture approach. The device is sized for the patient's appendage and anchored in place. It is currently undergoing initial clinical trials in humans in patients deemed not to be candidates for anticoagulation.[53]

Conclusions

An increasingly wide variety of non-pharmacologic approaches now exists for the management of medically refractory AF, spanning devices, surgical approaches, and percutaneous catheter interventions, and with goals including sinus rhythm restoration and maintenance, rate control, and stroke prevention (Table 39.3) Evidence-based application is largely

Table 39.3 Benefits of non-pharmacologic therapy options to treat symptomatic atrial fibrillation

Procedure	Restores sinus rhythm	Restores hemodynamics	Decreases risk of stroke	Need for implantable device (pacemaker/ defibrillator)
Surgical maze procedure	Yes	Yes	Yes	No (usually)
Surgical pulmonary vein isolation/limited maze	Yes	Possibly	Unknown	No
High right atrial pacing/septal pacing	No	No	No	Yes
Dual site atrial pacing	Yes	Improved	Yes	Yes
Implantable atrial/AV defibrillator	Yes	Yes	Unknown	Yes
Catheter-based maze procedure	Yes	Yes	Yes	No
Catheter ablation in pulmonary veins or isolation	Yes	Unknown	Unknown	No
Catheter ablation of AV junction	No	No	No	Yes
Catheter-based modification of AV conduction	No	No	No	No

becoming available for pacing therapies in specific populations, while defibrillation and ablation remain in the technologic evolution and refinement stage with largely observational data. It is becoming clear that non-pharmacologic approaches offer improved efficacy in a rhythm control strategy. They are likely to be implemented in a "hybrid" therapy strategy in a staged or simultaneous manner in the future to achieve effective rhythm control.

Levels of evidence for efficacy and safety of procedures to prevent or manage atrial fibrillation

● Surgical maze procedure	Grade B
● Left atrial isolation	Grade B
● Corridor procedure	Grade B
● Surgical pulmonary vein isolation/ partial maze	Grade B
● High right atrial pacing in sick sinus syndrome	Grade A
● Dual site right atrial pacing	Grade A
● Implantable atrial/AV defibrillator	Grade B
● Catheter-based ablation of AV conduction	Grade A
● Catheter-based modification of AV conduction	Grade B
● Catheter-based maze procedure	Grade C
● Catheter ablation of pulmonary veins or isolation	Grade B

References

1. Go AS, Hylek EM, Phillips KA *et al.* Prevalence of diagnosed atrial fibrillation in adults: national implications for rhythm management and stroke prevention: the anticoagulation and risk factors in atrial fibrillation (ATRIA) study. *JAMA* 2001; **285**:2370–5.
2. Saksena S, Domanski MJ, Benjamin EJ *et al.* Report of the NASPE/NHLBI round table on future research directions in atrial fibrillation. *Pacing Clin Electrophysiol* 2001;**24**: 1435–51.
3. Crijns HJ. Rate control vs. electrical cardioversion for persistent atrial fibrillation. A randomized comparison of two treatment strategies concerning mortality and morbidity: the RACE study. *ACC 2002 late-breaking clinical trials*.
4. Carlsson J. Mortality and stroke rates in a trial of rhythm control versus rate control in atrial fibrillation: results from the STAF pilot phase (strategies of treatment of atrial fibrillation). *ACC 2001 late-breaking clinical trials*.
5. Wyse DG. Survival in patients presenting with atrial fibrillation: the atrial fibrillation follow-up investigation of rhythm management (AFFIRM) study. *ACC 2002 late-breaking clinical trials*.
6. Crijns HJ, van Noord T, van Gelder IC. Recurrence of atrial fibrillation and the need for new definitions. *Eur Heart J* 2001;**22**:1769–71.
7. Andersen HR, Nielsen JC, Thomsen PEB *et al.* Long-term follow-up of patients from a randomized trial of atrial versus ventricular pacing for sick sinus syndrome. *Lancet* 1997; **350**:1210–16.
8. Lamas GA, Lee K, Sweeney M *et al.* Ventricular pacing or dual chamber pacing for sinus node dysfunction. *N Engl J Med* 2002;**346**:1854–62.
9. Connolly SJ, Kerr CR, Gent M *et al.* Effects of physiologic pacing versus ventricular pacing on the risk of stroke and death due to cardiovascular causes. Canadian Trial of Physiologic Pacing Investigators. *N Engl J Med* 2000;**342**:1385–91.
10. Gillis AM, Wyse DG, Connolly SJ *et al.* Atrial pacing periablation for prevention of paroxysmal atrial fibrillation. *Circulation* 1999;**99**:2553–8.
11. Friedman PA, Dijkman B, Warman EN *et al.* Atrial therapies reduce atrial arrhythmia burden in defibrillator patients. *Circulation* 2001;**104**:1023–8.
12. Israel CW, Hügl B, Unterberg C *et al.* on behalf of the AT500 Verification Study Investigators. Pace-termination and pacing for prevention of atrial tachyarrhythmias: results from a multicenter study with an implantable device for atrial therapy. *J Cardiovasc Electrophysiol* 2001;**12**:1121–8.
13. Lee MA, Weachter R, Pollack S *et al.* Can preventive and antitachycardia pacing reduce the frequency and burden of atrial tachyarrhythmias? The ATTEST study results. North American Society of Pacing and Electrophysiology 23rd Annual Scientific Sessions 2002.
14. Funck RC, Adamec R, Lurje L *et al.*, on behalf of the PROVE Study Group. Atrial overdriving is beneficial in patients with atrial arrhythmias: first results of the PROVE study. *PACE* 2000;**23**:1891–3.
15. Carlson MA for the ADOPT-A investigators: the Atrial Dynamic Overdrive Pacing Trial (ADOPT-A): Presented at Late Breaking Clinical Trials Session, North American Society of Pacing and Electrophysiology 22nd Annual Scientific Sessions 2001.
16. Saksena S. Definitions and endpoints for device clinical trials in atrial fibrillation – a pressing need. *J Interv Card Electrophysiol* 1997;**1**:173–4.
17. Saksena S, Sulke N, Manda V *et al.*, on behalf of the Worldwide Jewel AF Investigators. Reduction in frequency of atrial tachyarrhythmia episodes using novel prevention algorithms of an atrial pacemaker defibrillator. *Pacing Clin Electrophysiol* 2000; **23**:581.
18. Bailin SJ, Adler S, Guidici M. Prevention of chronic atrial fibrillation by pacing in the region of Bachmann bundle: results from a multicenter randomized trial. *J Cardiovasc Electrophysiol* 2001;**12**:912–17.
19. Padeletti L, Purerfellner, Adler S *et al.* Atrial septal lead placement and atrial pacing algorithms for prevention of paroxysmal atrial fibrillation: ASPECT study results. North American Society of Pacing and Electrophysiology 23rd Annual Scientific Sessions 2002.
20. Delfaut P, Saksena S, Prakash A, Krol RB. Long-term outcome of patients with drug-refractory atrial flutter and fibrillation after single and dual site right atrial pacing for arrhythmia prevention. *J Am Coll Cardiol* 1998;**32**:1900–8.
21. Prakash A, Saksena S, Krol RB *et al.* Catheter ablation of inducible atrial flutter in combination with atrial pacing and antiarrhythmic drugs (hybrid therapy) improves rhythm control in patients with refractory atrial fibrillation. *J Interv Card Electrophysiol* 2002;**6**:165–74.
22. Filipecki A, Saksena S, Prakash A *et al.* Atrial pacing improves rhythm control after linear right atrial ablation in refractory

permanent and persistent atrial fibrillation. *Pacing Clin Electrophysiol* 2001;**24**:707.

23. Saksena S, Prakash A, Hill M. Prevention of recurrent atrial fibrillation with chronic dual site right atrial pacing. *J Am Coll Cardiol* 1996;**28**:687–94.

24. Saksena S, Lin WH, Prakash A, Filipecki A. Long-term outcome of dual site right atrial pacing in patients with drug-refractory paroxysmal versus persistent or permanent atrial fibrillation. *J Am Coll Cardiol* 2002;**39**:84A.

25. Leclercq JF, DeSisti A, Fiorello P *et al.* Is dual site better than single site atrial pacing in the prevention of atrial fibrillation? *Pacing Clin Electrophysiol* 2000;**23**:2101–7.

26. D'Allonnes GR, Pavin D, Leclercq C *et al.* Long-term effects of biatrial synchronous pacing to prevent drug refractory atrial tachyarrhythmia: a nine-year experience. *J Cardiovasc Electrophysiol* 2000;**11**:1081–91.

27. Lau CP, Tse HF, Yu CM *et al.*, for the New Indication for Preventive Pacing in Atrial Fibrillation (NIPP-AF) Investigators. Dual-site atrial pacing for atrial fibrillation in patients without bradycardia. *Am J Cardiol* 2001;**88**: 371–5.

28. Ramdat Misier AR, Linde C, Beukema WP *et al.* Dual-site right atrial pacing improves quality of life in patients with drug refractory atrial fibrillation. *Pacing Clin Electrophysiol* 2000;**24**:555.

29. Saksena S, Prakash A, Ziegler P *et al.* The Dual Site Atrial Pacing for Permanent Atrial Fibrillation (DAPPAF) trial: improved suppression of drug refractory atrial fibrillation with dual site atrial pacing and antiarrhythmic drug therapy. *J Am Coll Cardiol* 2001;**38**:598–9.

30. Wellens HJ, Lau CP, Luderitz B *et al.* Atrioverter: an implantable device for the treatment of atrial fibrillation. *Circulation* 1998; **98**:1651–6.

31. Saksena S, Prakash A, Mongeon L *et al.* Clinical efficacy and safety of atrial defibrillation using biphasic shocks and current nonthoracotomy endocardial lead configurations. *Am J Cardiol* 1995;**76**:913–21.

32. Giorgberidze I, Saksena S, Mongeon L *et al.* Effects of high-frequency atrial pacing in atypical atrial flutter and atrial fibrillation. *J Interv Card Electrophysiol* 1997;**1**:111–23.

33. Dreifus LS, Nichols H, Morse D. Control of recurrent tachycardia of Wolff–Parkinson–White syndrome by surgical ligature of the AV bundle. *Circulation* 1968;**38**:1030–6.

34. Camm J, Ward DE, Spurrell RA, Rees GM. Cryothermal mapping and cryoablation in the treatment of refractory cardiac arrhythmias. *Circulation* 1980;**62**:67–74.

35. Cox JL, Schuessler RB, D'Agostino HJ Jr *et al.* The surgical treatment of atrial fibrillation. III. Development of a definitive surgical procedure. *J Thorac Cardiovasc Surg* 1991;**101**:569–83.

36. Kosakai Y. Treatment of atrial fibrillation using the Maze procedure: the Japanese experience. *Semin Thorac Cardiovasc Surg* 2000;**12**:44–52.

37. Kottkamp H, Hindricks G, Hammel D *et al.* Intraoperative radiofrequency ablation of chronic atrial fibrillation: a left atrial curative approach by elimination of anatomic "anchor" reentrant circuits. *J Cardiovasc Electrophysiol* 1999;**10**:772–80.

38. Sie HT, Beukema WP, Ramdat Misier AR *et al.* The radiofrequency modified maze procedure. A less invasive surgical approach to atrial fibrillation during open-heart surgery. *Eur J Cardiothorac Surg* 2001;**19**:443–7.

39. Nitta T, Lee R, Schuessler RB, Boineau JP, Cox JL. Radial approach: a new concept in surgical treatment for atrial fibrillation I. Concept, anatomic and physiologic bases and development of a procedure. *Ann Thorac Surg* 1999;**67**:27–35.

40. Chen SA, Hsieh MH, Tai CT *et al.* Initiation of atrial fibrillation by ectopic beats originating from the pulmonary veins: electrophysiological characteristics, pharmacological responses, and effects of radiofrequency ablation. *Circulation* 1999;**100**: 1879–86.

41. Haissaguerre M, Shah DC, Jais P *et al.* Mapping-guided ablation of pulmonary veins to cure atrial fibrillation. *Am J Cardiol* 2000;**86**:K9–19.

42. Gerstenfeld EP, Guerra P, Sparks PB *et al.* Clinical outcome after radiofrequency catheter ablation of focal atrial fibrillation triggers. *J Cardiovasc Electrophysiol* 2001;**12**:900–8.

43. Natale A. Presentation at 16th Annual Course on diagnosis and treatment of cardiac arrhythmias, Milwaukee, 18 April 2002.

44. Pappone C, Oreto G, Rosanio S *et al.* Atrial electroanatomic remodeling after circumferential radiofrequency pulmonary vein ablation: efficacy of an anatomic approach in a large cohort of patients with atrial fibrillation. *Circulation* 2001; **104**:2539–44.

45. Kanagaratnam L, Tomassoni G, Schweikert R *et al.* Empirical pulmonary vein isolation in patients with chronic atrial fibrillation using a three-dimensional nonfluoroscopic mapping system: long-term follow-up. *Pacing Clin Electrophysiol* 2001;**24**:1774–9.

46. Oral H, Knight BP, Tada H *et al.* Pulmonary vein isolation for paroxysmal and persistent atrial fibrillation. *Circulation* 2002;**105**:1077–81.

47. Garg A, Finneran W, Mollerus M *et al.* Right atrial compartmentalization using radiofrequency catheter ablation for management of patients with refractory atrial fibrillation. *J Cardiovasc Electrophysiol* 1999;**10**:763–71.

48. Kocheril AG. Right atrial mapping and linear ablation for paroxysmal atrial fibrillation. *J Intervent Card Electrophysiol* 2001;**5**:505–10.

49. Evans GT, Scheinman MM, Bardy G *et al.* Predictors of in-hospital mortality after DC catheter ablation of atrioventricular junction: results of a prospective, international, multicenter study. *Circulation* 1991;**84**:1924–37.

50. Kay GN, Ellenbogen KA, Giudici M *et al.* The Ablate and Pace Trial: a prospective study of catheter ablation of the AV conduction system and permanent pacemaker implantation for treatment of atrial fibrillation. *J Intervent Card Electrophysiol* 1998;**2**:121–35.

51. Ozcan C, Jahangir A, Friedman PA *et al.* Long-term survival after ablation of the atrioventricular node and implantation of a permanent pacemaker in patients with atrial fibrillation. *N Engl J Med* 2001;**344**:1043–51.

52. Kuck K-H, Kunze K-P, Schluter M *et al.* Transcatheter modulation by radiofrequency current of atrioventricular nodal conduction in patients with atrial fibrillation or flutter. In: Luderitz B, Saksena S, eds. *Interventional electrophysiology*. Mount Kisco, NY: Futura Publishing, 1991.

53. Sievert H, Lesh MD, Trepels T *et al.* Percutaneous left atrial appendage transcatheter occlusion (PLAATO) to prevent stroke in patients with atrial fibrillation: first human experience. *J Am Coll Cardiol* 2002;**39**:6A.

40 Supraventricular tachycardia: drugs *v* ablation

Neil R Grubb, Peter Kowey

"Supraventricular tachycardia", or SVT, is a rather imprecise term used to describe certain types of narrow complex tachycardia. The term is misleading because not all narrow complex tachycardias are "supraventricular" in origin. For example, ventricular tachycardias originating from the His bundle or its environs have a narrow QRS morphology. Also, not all supraventricular tachycardias have narrow complexes. Pre-excited tachycardias (in which the QRS complex is broad because of antegrade conduction through an accessory pathway) and SVTs with aberrant conduction, are cases in point. Furthermore, some "supraventricular" tachycardias involve mechanisms that are not confined to atrial or AV nodal tissue. SVTs involving accessory pathways are absolutely dependent upon conduction through the ventricles for their maintenance.

Ideally, arrhythmias should be described in a manner that reflects the underlying electrophysiological mechanism and the anatomical structures involved. This is not always possible when limited data are available from electrocardiogaphic recordings. In these instances a descriptive term can be applied to the electrocardiogram (for example, "narrow QRS tachycardia") until a more precise mechanism is known. In this way no assumption is made about the arrhythmia mechanism. The term "supraventricular tachycardia" is thus a term used to describe a range of arrhythmias with different mechanisms and involving different components of the cardiac conducting system. The following arrhythmias are encompassed by the term:

- **atrioventricular re-entrant tachycardia [AVRT]** – mediated by re-entry, and involving an accessory pathway and the AV node
- **atrioventricular nodal re-entrant tachycardia [AVNRT]** – mediated by a re-entry circuit involving the atrioventricular (AV) node and its atrial inputs
- **atrial flutter** – involving a re-entry circuit around large scale atrial structure(s), for example, veins, valve orifices
- **atrial tachycardias** – tachycardias involving a smaller scale intra-atrial re-entry circuit or an automatic focus
- **atrial fibrillation** – tachycardias involving multiple complex intra-atrial re-entry circuits.

The use of precise terminology is important. An understanding of the underlying mechanism helps determine whether a pharmacological or non-pharmacological treatment strategy is likely to be helpful. If drug treatment is chosen, the choice of drug used will in part be governed by the underlying arrhythmia mechanism. For radiofrequency ablation to succeed, the arrhythmia mechanism must be understood.

The common SVTs encountered in emergency departments are characterized by sudden onset of palpitation in young and middle-aged adults, with an ECG showing a regular, rapid, narrow complex tachycardia. These tachycardias can be terminated using vagal maneuvers or intravenous adenosine, and mainly involve the first two mechanisms listed above. Management of these tachycardias is the main focus of this chapter.

Issues to consider

Most supraventricular tachycardias are not life-threatening, and are problematic because of the symptoms they cause. For patients with well-tolerated occasional or short-lived episodes of palpitation it is reasonable to adopt a conservative approach and not to recommend drug treatment or ablation. If the arrhythmia does cause significant symptoms, the initial decision between drug treatment or ablation is a matter of patient preference. Patients need to be made aware of the likelihood of achieving symptom control, and of the potential risks of each strategy. For patients with specific occupations (for example, pilots), curative treatment with ablation may be a prerequisite to continuing work. For patients with a history of poor compliance with medication, ablation may also be the favored option. Some patients favor a tiered approach, in which a trial and error approach to drug treatment is used at first, with the option of ablation if symptoms persist or if drugs are poorly tolerated.

Drug treatment for SVTs

There are several categories of drugs that can be used as prophylaxis against SVT. The occurrence of these arrhythmias depends on there being an electrophysiological substrate, and a trigger. The substrate may be fixed, in the case of an accessory pathway mediated tachycardia, or may be dependent on autonomic tone, as in some cases of AV nodal re-entrant tachycardia. Here, the ability of the AV node and its input pathways to maintain tachycardia is dependent on the relative conduction times and refractory periods of the tissues involved. These change dramatically in the presence of sympathetic or vagal stimulation. The trigger for SVT usually takes the form of a critically timed ectopic beat.

Drug treatments may alter substrate, trigger, or both. β Blockers can reduce the frequency of the ectopic beats that potentially trigger tachycardia, as well as altering the conduction properties of the tachycardia circuit to reduce the likelihood of tachycardia being maintained.[1] Some drugs are prescribed because of their effect on the AV nodal component of the re-entry circuit (for example, digoxin, verapamil). Others are used because of a direct effect on the refractory period of conducting tissue (for example, sotalol, dofetilide, amiodarone – potassium-channel blockers)[2] or on excitability and cardiomyocyte depolarization (for example, flecainide, propafenone, quinidine, disopyramide, amiodarone – sodium-channel blockade). Note that amiodarone has mixed properties, including partial beta blockade and calcium-channel blockade. Sodium-channel blockers such as flecainide more potently inhibit conduction through accessory pathways than through the AV node.[3,4] These agents are thus theoretically favorable in the management of atrioventricular re-entrant tachycardia.

How effective are drugs?

There is comparatively little information about the effectiveness of antiarrhythmic drugs for treatment of SVTs. In particular there are few studies that offer information about long-term symptom control, or adverse drug effects, in this setting. Published studies tend to be comparative and with short-term follow up. Other studies are limited in their usefullness because no attempt is made to tailor treatment to the tachycardia mechanism; in most studies all regular SVTs are treated the same. Atrial flutter and atrial fibrillation, which do not share a common mechanism, have been considered together in other trials. The high success rates for radiofrequency ablation have discouraged comparative studies of ablation versus pharmacological management for most SVTs. A summary of drug trials is given in Table 40.1.[5–13]

Both flecainide and propafenone have been shown to be more effective than placebo at preventing paroxysmal SVT.[5,6] In randomized studies, reported mainly in the mid-1990s, success rates for flecainide ranged from 73% to 93%, at the expense of an incidence of adverse effects of up to 53%. The doses used in these trials varied, as did the definitions of success and adverse effects. In some studies success has been defined as a reduction in the incidence or severity of symptom episodes, rather than abolition of the arrhythmia. It is also clear that clinical adverse effects are a significant limiting

Table 40.1 Summary of drug trials

	Patients (n)	Follow up (months)	Drugs	Success rate (%)	Adverse effects (%)
Drugs for "SVT" trial					
Pritchett, 1991[5]	14	1	Flecainide	86	23–53
			Placebo	29	
UK Propafenone PSVT group, 1995[6]	52	3	Propafenone	67–91	2–26
			Placebo	29–41	0–4
Chimienti, 1995[7]	135	12	Flecainide	93	10
			Propafenone	86	8
Hellestrand, 1996[8]	102	48	Flecainide	87	9
Weindling, 1996[9]	106	12	Digoxin ± propranolol	70	0
Dorian, 1996[10]	121	8	Flecainide	86	19
			Verapamil	73	24
Hopson, 1996[11]	67	12	Flecainide	73	64
Drugs for paroxysmal atrial flutter or artial fibrillation					
Pritchett, 1991[5]	28	1	Flecainide	61	23–55
			Placebo	7	31
UK Propafenone PSVT group, 1995[6]	48	3	Propafenone	60–96	3–40
			Placebo	30–32	3–4
Chimienti, 1995[7]	200	12	Flecainide	77	16
			Propafenone	75	14
Hopson, 1996[11]	67	12	Flecainide	56	56
Aliot, 1996[12]	97	12	Flecainide	62	9
			Propafenone	53	17

factor in the use of these drugs. For paroxysmal atrial fibrillation, amiodarone appears to be the most effective prophylactic agent but is not a desirable or realistic treatment option for young patients without structural heart disease, because of its unfavorable adverse effect profile with long-term use.[14] Class IC (flecainide and propafenone) and Class III (d.l sotalol) antiarrhythmic drugs can also be effective at reducing the incidence of symptoms in patients with paroxysmal atrial fibrillation, and are often used as first-line treatment.[5,6,15]

Proarrhythmia

Antiarrhythmic drugs can cause unwanted, sometimes life-threatening arrhythmias. These drugs work by slowing conduction, prolonging repolarization, or by altering automaticity. While these properties can be used to advantage, they can also increase the likelihood of arrhythmia under certain circumstances.[16–18] For example, sodium-channel blockade can have a differential slowing effect on conduction in diseased and healthy tissue, creating an environment in which re-entry is more likely to occur. Furthermore, anisotropy of conduction (that is, different speeds of conduction along the longitudinal and transverse axes between cardiomyocytes) may be exaggerated. These phenomena may explain the increased incidence of sudden death when Class IC drugs (flecainide and encainide) were used in patients with ischemic heart disease in the CAST study.[19] Prolongation of refractoriness through potassium-channel antagonism (for example, with sotalol) also causes proarrhythmia, increasing the risk of polymorphic ventricular tachycardia.[20] This may be caused by exaggerating the differences in refractoriness in diseased and healthy ventricular myocardium, or by a triggering mechanism.

Several risk factors have been identified for occurrence of proarrhythmia. These are: female gender (Class III drugs), history of VT or VF, ischemic heart disease, structural heart disease, and cardiac failure. Most patients with paroxysmal SVT are young and do not have structural heart disease, and are thus not at high risk of proarrhythmia. The incidence of ventricular proarrhythmia in patients treated with flecainide or propafenone for supraventricular arrhythmia is less than 2%, compared with 4–33% when used to treat ventricular arrhythmia.[16,21] Although this risk is small, it is still part of the decision making process when considered in the context of the small risk of serious complication from radiofrequency ablation. Another form of "proarrhythmia" can also occur when Class IC antiarrhythmics are used to treat atrial flutter. These agents slow atrial conduction without significantly affecting the AV nodal refractory period. This causes slowing of atrial flutter, enabling 1:1 atrioventricular conduction to occur.[22] This can paradoxically increase the ventricular rate to well over 200 beats per minute and may lead to hemodynamic compromise.

Ablation for "common" SVTs

For patients with SVTs mediated by atrioventricular nodal re-entry or atrioventricular re-entry via an accessory pathway, it is now accepted that catheter ablation is more effective than drug treatment. Catheter ablation has a more positive impact on quality of life and is more cost effective when assessed for long-term efficacy.[23–25] Catheter ablation is now an accepted first-line treatment for otherwise healthy patients with recurrent, symptomatic tachycardias.

Accessory pathway mediated tachycardias

These tachycardias involve conduction through an accessory atrioventricular connection, usually comprising tissue with electrophysiological properties similar to that of Purkinje tissue. The most common indication here for catheter ablation is *orthodromic* atrioventricular re-entrant tachycardia, during which atrioventricular conduction occurs via the AV node, and ventriculo-atrial re-entry occurs through the accessory pathway. This arrhythmia can occur in patients with manifest electrocardiographic evidence of pre-excitation – Wolf–Parkinson–White syndrome – or in patients with an apparently normal resting electrocardiogram, who may have a concealed accessory pathway. (A less common variant, *antidromic* atrioventricular re-entry, can occur in which the accessory pathway forms the antegrade limb of the circuit, resulting in a broad complex tachycardia.) Initial approaches to curative treatment of this tachycardia involved surgical division of the accessory pathway, and subsequently direct current ablation, but these techniques were rapidly superseded by radiofrequency ablation. Early reports suggested procedural success rates in excess of 95%, with failures and recurrences more frequent when right-sided accessory pathways were treated.[26,27] With refinement of catheter technology, success rates continue to improve and not surprisingly catheter ablation is established as a first-line treatment for this condition in otherwise uncomplicated cases.[28]

Patients with Wolf–Parkinson–White syndrome can also present with pre-excited atrial fibrillation. In some cases the accessory pathway refractory period is very short, allowing rapid, repetitive ventricular stimulation in response to atrial fibrillation. This gives rise to extremely rapid ventricular rates and can precipitate ventricular fibrillation and death. For this reason catheter ablation should be seriously considered in any patient with manifest pre-excitation and palpitation. It is less clear whether asymptomatic patients with pre-excitation should undergo electrophysiological studies.[29] Assessment of accessory pathway refractory period in the EP laboratory is a poor predictor of risk of sudden death because many autonomic variables alter this parameter. It is not clear that the benefit of catheter ablation in asymptomatic patients outweighs the risks of the procedure except in specific circumstances, for example, for competitive athletes or pilots.

AV nodal re-entrant tachycardia

This arrhythmia has a very similar presentation to atrioventricular re-entrant tachycardia. The electrocardiogram typically shows a regular, rapid, narrow complex tachycardia with rate between 160 and 240 beats per minute. For many years the electrophysiology of this arrhythmia was poorly understood. Surgical mapping and autopsy studies have shown that this tachycardia involves atrial as well as AV nodal tissue, and it is sometimes referred to as para AV nodal re-entrant tachycardia.[30,31] Identification that patients with this tachycardia have multiple AV nodal inputs with different electrophysiological properties, and anatomical correlation of a posterior AV nodal extension with the electrophysiological location of a slowly conducting AV nodal input, led to the development of the technique of slow pathway ablation.[32] This technique involves ablation of atrial tissue inferior to the compact AV node, typically at a site anterior to the coronary sinus ostium adjacent to the tricuspid annulus. Initial success rates exceeded 80% at the expense of a 2% risk of development of atrioventricular block requiring permanent pacing.[27,33] With modern catheters and temperature controlled ablation techniques, success rates now exceed 95% and the risk of AV block is approximately 1%.[28]

Atrial flutter

In most cases atrial flutter is mediated by a right atrial macro re-entry circuit with a critical pathway of conduction between the inferior vena cava and the tricuspid annulus. This cavo-tricuspid isthmus zone forms the target for contemporary ablation techniques.[34] Rarer forms of atrial flutter use other anatomic barriers as their substrate (for example, the pulmonary veins, an atrial septal defect, or a surgical scar) and are collectively referred to as atypical atrial flutter. The technique of flutter ablation involves the production of a line of interconnected ablation lesions to create conduction block between two anatomical barriers in a critical part of the flutter circuit. In the case of typical atrial flutter, this line is created in the cavo-tricuspid isthmus. Success rates for catheter ablation of typical atrial flutter were initially limited by an inability to produce full-thickness lesions in patients with pectinate ridges extending into the isthmus region.[35] The use of large tipped catheters or "cooled tip" catheters has allowed delivery of more energy into the atrial myocardium, and has increased success rates over 95%.[36] AV block can complicate flutter ablation, particularly if the line of block is created in the medial (septal) aspect of the cavo-tricuspid isthmus.[28]

Atrial tachycardia

Atrial tachycardias can have an automatic or re-entrant mechanism. Drug treatments have generally proven disappointing,

although flecainide may have a role in their management.[37] Until recently catheter ablation techniques were also of limited use, because of the very large area of potential atrial surface area from which these tachycardias can originate. Furthermore, patients with re-entrant atrial tachycardias often have extensive atrial disease and may have more than one focus for tachycardia. The development of non-fluoroscopic mapping systems, which allow three-dimensional mapping of atrial activation during tachycardia, has proved very helpful in allowing the electrophysiologist to pinpoint the focus or circuit (Figure 40.1).[38] Quoted success rates for treatment of these tachycardias now range from 80–90%.[39]

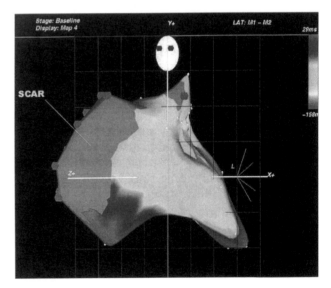

Figure 40.1 Non-fluoroscopic mapping of the right atrium of a patient with suspected right atrial tachycardia. A large zone of atrial infarction is identified by voltage mapping and the patient is subsequently shown to have scar-related atrial flutter.

Atrial fibrillation

Atrial fibrillation is the most common atrial arrhythmia and is the cause of much morbidity because of hemodynamic effects and embolic complications. The arrhythmia itself comprises multiple, interacting, intra-atrial re-entry circuits or wavelets that produce a complex, rapid, irregular atrial rhythm.[40] Atrial fibrillation is most likely to be maintained in enlarged, diseased atria because re-entry is promoted by slow conduction and by long conduction pathways. In these situations atrial fibrillation is likely to be persistent (that is, will not spontaneously terminate) or permanent (that is, will not terminate with pharmacological or electrical cardioversion). Paroxysmal atrial fibrillation can occur in patients with structurally normal hearts and may be initiated by ectopic beats originated from sleeves of atrial tissue extending into the pulmonary veins, or less commonly the superior vena cava.[41,42] Ablation techniques have evolved extremely rapidly in recognition of these mechanisms and can be divided into those directed at ectopic triggers (focal ablation) and at preventing intra-atrial re-entry (linear ablation).

Focal ablation for paroxysmal atrial fibrillation

This technique involves transseptal puncture to pass catheters from the right atrium into the left atrium, and the use of multi-electrode catheters in the ostia of the pulmonary veins to identify the conduction pathways into and out of these veins. The superior pulmonary veins are the most common sources of ectopic triggers and form the targets for ablation.[43] Two approaches may be adopted – electrical isolation of the culprit veins identified from spontaneous ectopic beat activity, or the anatomical approach in which as many pulmonary veins as possible are isolated in an attempt to eliminate all ectopic triggers.[44] Initial techniques involved ablation deep within the veins and were associated with a significant incidence of pulmonary vein stenosis.[45] It is now generally accepted that radiofrequency energy should be applied at or close to the ostia to minimize this risk. Success rates for pulmonary vein ablation are currently around 60% in experienced centers, with success defined as lack of symptomatic recurrence of atrial fibrillation in the medium term (few long-term data are yet available). It is now recognized that pulmonary vein ectopic impulses may be involved in the maintenance of atrial fibrillation as well as its initiation. Ablation of these foci in some patients with persistent atrial fibrillation can acutely terminate the arrhythmia.[46] The

response to antiarrhythmic drugs may be improved by modifying the triggering focus. Recurrences occur because of multiple pulmonary vein triggers, triggers occurring within the atria themselves, or incomplete isolation of veins.

Linear ablation

Linear ablation procedures are designed to compartmentalize atrial tissue to prevent intra-atrial re-entry. These procedures owe much to the early experience with the surgical maze and corridor procedures.[47] Current techniques involve the production of linear lesions around the pulmonary vein ostia, across the superior aspect of the left atrium, and connecting the mitral valve annulus to the pulmonary vein ostial lines. Specially designed compliant, multi-electrode ablation catheters have been developed for this purpose. At present linear ablation is still considered an experimental procedure.[48]

The pace and ablate strategy

For patients with persistent, symptomatic atrial fibrillation, total AV nodal ablation offers a means of controlling heart rate and of regularizing the ventricular rhythm. A physiological (rate responsive) permanent pacemaker is implanted and used to govern heart rate. This technique is effective at improving quality of life in selected patients, especially those with palpitation. Its effectiveness is less clear-cut in patients with non-specific symptoms such as fatigue and dyspnea, in which the underlying cardiac condition may be the main

---

Table 40.2   Potential problems of drugs and ablation for treatment of SVTs

Antiarrhythmic drugs	Ablation

Proarrhythmia
    <2% if otherwise normal heart
    >4% in other patients (that is,
    structural or coronary disease)
	Potentially life-threatening complication
	    (for example, cardiac tamponade, stroke, myocardial
	    infarction) – very rare
	No deaths in 1998 NASPE registry

Non-cardiac side effects
    8 to 60% with Class IC drugs[11]
    24% with verapamil[10]
	AV block requiring pacemaker
	    0·15% (AVRT)
	    to 1% (AVNRT)

Failure to control arrhythmia
    up to 30% with
    short-term follow up
	Inability to ablate target
	    2·6% (AVNRT)
	    6% (AVRT)
	    up to 28% (atrial tachycardia)
	    14% (atrial flutter)[a]

Compliance issues	Pneumothorax (avoided by coronary sinus cannulation via femoral vein route) Tricuspid regurgitation (rare) Vascular complications (rare)

[a] This figure is likely to improve with the use of large tipped catheters and cooled tip catheters that can produce a larger lesion.

cause. Total AV nodal ablation is thus best reserved for patients with atrial fibrillation who have palpitation and for whom AV nodal blocking drugs are ineffective or cause significant adverse effects.

Risks of ablation

In discussing treatment options with patients, the risks of treatment are an important factor (Table 40.2). The risks of antiarrhythmic drugs, especially proarrhythmia, have already been covered. For catheter ablation there are uncommon but important risks. Most patients worry about the risk of a disabling or life-threatening complication. Cardiac tamponade can occur because of transseptal puncture, catheter trauma

Recommendations	Evidence Grade
• Propafenone and flecainide are effective antiarrhythmic drugs for the prophylactic management of paroxysmal supraventricular tachycardia. **Grade A**	
• Sotalol and amiodarone are effective prophylactic therapies for paroxysmal atrial flutter. **Grade B**	
• Potential proarrhythmic complications and other adverse effects of antiarrhythmic therapy should be considered when choosing antiarrhythmic therapy. **Grade C**	
• The choice between ablation and antiarrhythmic drug therapy for the initial treatment of paroxysmal supraventricular tachycardia is dependent on patient preference. **Grade C**	
• Verapamil is a safe first-line treatment for pSVT but has a relatively high rate of failure and side effects. **Grade B**	
• Flecainide and propafenone reduce symptoms from pSVT in most cases and should be considered for individuals who do not have underlying coronary artery disease. **Grade B**	
• RF ablation should be offered as first-line treatment for individuals with pSVT. **Grade B**	
• RF ablation is the treatment of choice in individuals who present with pre-excited atrial fibrillation. **Grade C**	
• RF ablation should be offered as first-line treatment for individuals with paroxysmal or persistent atrial flutter. **Grade B**	
• Pulmonary vein ablation should be considered a second-line treatment for paroxysmal atrial fibrillation in the absence of structural heart disease in selected individuals, where antiarrhythmic drug therapy has failed. **Grade C**	
• The "ablate and pace" strategy should be used to palliate symptoms in patients with atrial fibrillation in whom rate control is not achieved using drugs. **Grade B**	

or ablation in thin-walled tissue. This risk is therefore greatest with left-sided accessory pathways and with ablation of focal atrial arrhythmias, at around 0·7%. For other tachycardias the risk is significantly less. Fatalities were reported particularly during early experience with catheter ablation but in the 1998 NASPE prospective catheter ablation registry there were no deaths reported in more than 3300 procedures. This registry was voluntary and open to reporting bias, but nonetheless death is a very uncommon complication. Other reported complications included myocardial infarction, pneumothorax, pericarditis, tricuspid regurgitation, and femoral artery pseudoaneurysm. AV block requiring pacemaker implantation affected 1 in 100 patients treated for AVNRT, 1 in 650 patients treated for AVRT, and 1 in 150 patients treated for atrial flutter. Complication rates for focal and linear ablation techniques are less well reported but there is concern about the potential for thromoembolic complication when multiple radiofrequency applications are made in the left atrium.

References

1. Frishman WH, Cavusoglu E. Beta-adrenergic blockers and their role in the therapy of arrhythmias. In: Podrid PJ, Kowey PR, eds. *Cardiac arrhythmia: mechanisms, diagnosis and management.* Baltimore, Maryland: Williams and Wilkins, 1995.
2. Gill J, Heel RC, Fitton A. Amiodarone. An overview of its pharmacological properties, and review of its therapeutic use in cardiac arrhythmias. *Drugs* 1992;**43**:69–110.
3. Estes NAM, Garan H, Ruskin JN. Electrophysiologic properties of flecainide acetate. *Am J Cardiol* 1984;**53**(Suppl. B): 26B–9B.
4. Hellestrand KJ, Bexton RS, Nathan AW *et al.* Acute electrophysiological effects of flecainide acetate on cardiac conduction and refractoriness in men. *Br Heart J* 1982;**48**:140–8.
5. Pritchett ELC, Datorre SD, Platt ML *et al.* Flecainide acetate treatment of paroxysmal supraventricular tachycardia and paroxysmal atrial fibrillation – dose response studies. *J Am Coll Cardiol* 1991;**17**:297–303.
6. UK Propafenone PSVT Study Group. A randomized, placebo-controlled trial of propafenone in the prophylaxis of paroxysmal supraventricular tachycardia and paroxysmal atrial fibrillation. *Circulation* 1995;**92**:2550–7.
7. Chimienti M, Cullen Jr MT, Casadei G for the Flecainide and Propafenone Italian Study Investigators. Safety of flecainide versus propafenone for the long-term management of symptomatic paroxysmal supraventricular tachyarrhythmias. Report from the Flecainide and Propafenone Italian Study (FAPIS) Group. *Eur Heart J* 1995;**16**:1943–51.
8. Hellestrand KJ. Efficacy and safety of long-term oral flecainide acetate in patients with responsive supraventricular tachycardia. *Am J Cardiol* 1996;**77**:83A–8A.
9. Weindling SN, Saul JP, Walsh EP. Efficacy and risks of medical therapy for supraventricular tachycardia in neonates and infants. *Am Heart J* 1996;**131**:66–72.
10. Dorian P, Naccarelli GV, Coumel P *et al.* A randomised comparison of flecainide versus verapamil in paroxysmal

supraventricular tachycardia. The Flecainide Multicenter Investigators Group. *Am J Cardiol* 1996;**77**:89A–95A.

11. Hopson JR, Buxton AE, Rinkenberger RL *et al.* Safety and utility of flecainide acetate in the routine care of patients with supraventricular tachyarrhythmias: results of a multicenter trial. The Flecainide Supraventricular Tachycardia Study Group. *Am J Cardiol* 1996;**77**:72A–82A.

12. Aliot E, Denjoy I. Comparison of the safety and efficacy of flecainide and propafenone in hospital out-patients with symptomatic atrial fibrillation/flutter. The Flecainide AF French Study Group. *Am J Cardiol* 1996;**77**:66A–71A.

13. Orejarena LA, Vidaillet H Jr, DeStefano F *et al.* Paroxysmal supraventricular tachycardia in the general population. *J Am Coll Cardiol* 1998;**31**:150–7.

14. Gooselink AT, Crijns HJ, Van Gelder IC *et al.* Low-dose amiodarone for maintenance of sinus rhythm after cardioversion of atrial fibrillation or flutter. *JAMA* 1992;**267**:3289–93.

15. Chung MK, Schweikert RA, Wilkoff BL *et al.* Is hospital admission for initiation of antiarrhythmic therapy with sotalol for atrial arrhythmias required? Yield of in-hospital monitoring and prediction of risk for significant arrhythmia complications. *J Am Coll Cardiol* 1998;**32**:169–76.

16. Stanton MS, Prystowsky EN, Fineberg NS *et al.* Arrhythmogenic effects of antiarrhythmic drugs: a study of 506 patients treated for ventricular tachycardia or fibrillation. *J Am Coll Cardiol* 1989;**14**:209–15.

17. Falk RH. Proarrhythmia in patients treated for atrial fibrillation or flutter. *Ann Intern Med* 1992;**117**:141–50. [Published erratum in *Ann Intern Med* 1992;**117**:446.]

18. Friedman PL, Stevenson WG. Proarrhythmia. *Am J Cardiol* 1998;**82**:50N–8N.

19. Echt DS, Liebson PR, Mitchell LB *et al.* Mortality and morbidity in patients receiving encainide, flecainide or placebo. The Cardiac Arrhythmia Suppression Trial. *N Engl J Med* 1991;**324**:781–8.

20. Reiffel JA. Impact of structural heart disease on the selection of class III antiarrhythmics for the prevention of atrial fibrillation and flutter. *Am Heart J* 1998;**135**:551–6.

21. Pritchett E, Wilkinson WE. Mortality in patients treated with flecainide and encainide for supraventricular arrhythmias. *Am J Cardiol* 1991;**67**:976–80.

22. Nathan AW, Hellestrand KJ, Bexton RS *et al.* Proarrhythmic effects of the new antiarrhythmic agent flecainide acetate. *Am Heart J* 1984;**107**:222–8.

23. Bathina MN, Mickelsen S, Brooks C *et al.* Radiofrequency catheter ablation versus medical therapy for initial treatment of supraventricular tachycardia and its impact on quality of life and healthcare costs. *Am J Cardiol* 1998; **82**:589–93.

24. Weerasooriya HR, Murdock CJ, Harris AH *et al.* The cost- effectiveness of treatment of supraventricular arrhythmias related to an accessory atrioventricular pathway: comparison of catheter ablation, surgical division and medical treatment. *Aust NZ J Med* 1994;**24**:161–7.

25. Ikeda T, Sugi K, Enjoji Y *et al.* Cost effectiveness of radiofrequency catheter ablation versus medical treatment for paroxysmal supraventricular tachycardia in Japan. *J Cardiol* 1994; **24**:461–8.

26. Jackman WM, Beckman KJ, McClelland JH *et al.* Catheter ablation of accessory pathways (Wolff–Parkinson–White syndrome) by radiofrequency current. *N Engl J Med* 1991; **324**:1605–11.

27. Sathe S, Vohra J, Chan W *et al.* Radiofrequency catheter ablation for paroxysmal supraventricular tachycardia: a report of 135 procedures. *Aust NZ J Med* 1993;**23**:317–24.

28. Scheinmann MM, Huang S. The 1998 NASPE prospective catheter ablation registry. *Pacing Clin Electrophysiol* 2000; **23**:1020–8.

29. Fitzsimmons PJ, McWhirter PD, Peterson DW *et al.* The natural history of Wolff–Parkinson–White syndrome in 228 military aviators: a long-term follow-up of 22 years. *Am Heart J* 2001;**142**:530–6.

30. Keim S, Werner P, Jazayeri M *et al.* Localization of the fast and slow pathways in atrioventricular nodal re-entrant tachycardia by intra-operative ice-mapping. *Circulation* 1992; **86**: 919–25.

31. Inoue S, Becker AE. Posterior extensions of the human compact atrioventricular node: a neglected anatomic feature of potential clinical significance. *Circulation* 1998;**97**:188–93.

32. Jackman WM, Beckman KJ, McClelland JH *et al.* Treatment of supraventricular tachycardia due to atrioventricular nodal re-entry by radiofrequency catheter ablation of slow pathway conduction. *N Engl J Med* 1992;**327**:313–18.

33. Kugler JD, Danford DA, Deal BJ *et al.* Radiofrequency catheter ablation for tachyarrhythmias in children and adolescents. The Pediatric Electrophysiology Society. *N Engl J Med* 1994; **330**:1481–7.

34. Cosio FG, Lopez-Gil M, Goicolea A, Arribas F, Barroso JL. Radiofrequency ablation of the inferior vena cava-tricuspid valve isthmus in common atrial flutter. *Am J Cardiol* 1993; **71**:705–9.

35. Chen SA, Chiang CE, Wu TJ *et al.* Radiofrequency catheter ablation of common atrial flutter: comparison of electrophysiologically guided focal ablation and linear ablation technique. *J Am Coll Cardiol* 1996;**27**:860–8.

36. Jaïs P, Hocini M, Gilet T *et al.* Effectiveness of irrigated tip catheter ablation of common atrial flutter. *Am J Cardiol* 2001;**88**:433–5.

37. Anderson JL, Jolivette DM, Fredell PA. Summary of efficacy and safety of flecainide for supraventricular arrhythmias. (Review). *Am J Cardiol* 1988;**62**:62D–6D.

38. Hoffman E, Reithmann C, Nimmermann P *et al.* Clinical experience with electroanatomic mapping of ectopic atrial tachycardia. *Pacing Clin Electrophysiol* 2002;**25**:49–56.

39. Poty H, Saoud N, Haissaguerre M *et al.* Radiofrequency catheter ablation of atrial tachycardias. *Am Heart J* 1996;**131**:481–9.

40. Moe GK. On the multiple wavelet hypothesis of atrial fibrillation. *Arch Int Pharmacodyn* 1962;**140**:183–8.

41. Haïssaguerre M, Jaïs P, Shah DP *et al.* Spontaneous initiation of atrial fibrillation by ectopic beats originating in the pulmonary veins. *N Engl J Med* 1998;**339**:659–66.

42. Tsai CF, Tai CT, Hseih MH *et al.* Initiation of atrial fibrillation by ectopic beats originating from the superior vena cava. Electrophysiological characteristics and results of radiofrequency ablation. *Circulation* 2000;**102**:67–74.

43. Haïssaguerre M, Jaïs P, Shah DC *et al.* Right and left atrial radiofrequency catheter therapy of paroxysmal atrial fibrillation. *J Cardiovasc Electrophysiol* 1996;**7**:1132–44.

44. Hassiguerre M, Jais P, Shah DC *et al.* Electrophysiological end-point for catheter ablation of atrial fibrillation initiated from multiple pulmonary venous foci. *Circulation* 2000;**101**: 1409–17.

45. Robbins IM, Colvin EV, Doyle TP *et al.* Pulmonary vein stenosis after catheter ablation of atrial fibrillation. *Circulation* 1998;**98**:1769–75.

46. Pappone C, Oreto G, Rosanio S *et al.* Atrial electroanatomic remodelling after circumferential radiofrequency pulmonary vein ablation. *Circulation* 2001;**104**:2539–44.

47. Cox JL, Boineau JP, Schuessler RB, Kater KM, Lappas DG. Five year experience with the maze procedure for atrial fibrillation. *Ann Thorac Surg* 1993;**56**:814–24.

48. Maloney JD, Milner L, Barold S, Czerska B, Markel M. Two-staged biatrial linear and focal ablation to restore sinus rhythm in patients with refractory chronic atrial fibrillation: procedure experience and follow-up beyond 1 year. *Pacing Clin Elecrophysiol* 1998;**21**:2527–32.

Part IIId

Specific cardiovascular disorders: Ventricular arrhythmias, bradyarrhythmias and cardiac arrest

A John Camm, Editor

Grading of recommendations and levels of evidence used in *Evidence-based Cardiology*

GRADE A

Level 1a Evidence from large randomized clinical trials (RCTs) or systematic reviews (including meta-analyses) of multiple randomized trials which collectively has at least as much data as one single well-defined trial.

Level 1b Evidence from at least one "All or None" high quality cohort study; in which ALL patients died/failed with conventional therapy and some survived/succeeded with the new therapy (for example, chemotherapy for tuberculosis, meningitis, or defibrillation for ventricular fibrillation); or in which many died/failed with conventional therapy and NONE died/failed with the new therapy (for example, penicillin for pneumococcal infections).

Level 1c Evidence from at least one moderate-sized RCT or a meta-analysis of small trials which collectively only has a moderate number of patients.

Level 1d Evidence from at least one RCT.

GRADE B

Level 2 Evidence from at least one high quality study of non-randomized cohorts who did and did not receive the new therapy.

Level 3 Evidence from at least one high quality case–control study.

Level 4 Evidence from at least one high quality case series.

GRADE C

Level 5 Opinions from experts without reference or access to any of the foregoing (for example, argument from physiology, bench research or first principles).

A comprehensive approach would incorporate many different types of evidence (for example, RCTs, non-RCTs, epidemiologic studies, and experimental data), and examine the architecture of the information for consistency, coherence and clarity. Occasionally the evidence does not completely fit into neat compartments. For example, there may not be an RCT that demonstrates a reduction in mortality in individuals with stable angina with the use of β blockers, but there is overwhelming evidence that mortality is reduced following MI. In such cases, some may recommend use of β blockers in angina patients with the expectation that some extrapolation from post-MI trials is warranted. This could be expressed as Grade A/C. In other instances (for example, smoking cessation or a pacemaker for complete heart block), the non-randomized data are so overwhelmingly clear and biologically plausible that it would be reasonable to consider these interventions as Grade A.

Recommendation grades appear either within the text, for example, **Grade A** and **Grade A1a** or within a table in the chapter.

The grading system clearly is only applicable to preventive or therapeutic interventions. It is not applicable to many other types of data such as descriptive, genetic or pathophysiologic.

41 Prevention and treatment of life-threatening ventricular arrhythmia and sudden death

Eugene Crystal, Stuart J Connolly, Paul Dorian

Introduction

Arrhythmic death and risk stratification

Epidemiologic studies and carefully conducted clinical trials have consistently demonstrated that deaths in patients with severe heart disease are often due to ventricular arrhythmia. The evidence for this comes from several sources, including recordings made by paramedics, Holter monitor studies, and postmortem classification based on suddenness of hemodynamic collapse.[1] Although not all sudden deaths are due to ventricular tachycardia or fibrillation, there is substantial evidence from paramedic monitoring and Holter reports that most are.[2] Although different schemes have been used to classify death according to presumed mechanisms, there is considerable evidence that between one quarter and half of cardiac deaths are sudden and due to arrhythmia. Thus prevention of the sudden death is an important clinical goal.

Over the past two decades methods of risk stratification have been developed and evaluated, in order to target therapy to the subpopulation at greatest risk of sudden death. Techniques have been used in clinical trials of antiarrhythmic agents to select a population at high risk of arrhythmic death. These include some clinical characteristics (decreased left ventricular ejection fraction (LVEF), recent myocardial infarction, New York Heart Association (NYHA) functional class of heart failure), and the use of investigations such as measurement of ventricular ectopy on the 24-hour Holter, programmed ventricular stimulation, signal averaged ECG and heart rate variability. Although all of these techniques identify patients at increased risk of arrhythmic death, and total death as well, there is no evidence that any technique selectively detects increased risk of arrhythmic death.[3] Thus powerful markers of total death, such as poor LVEF, are now used in trials to identify patients at risk of arrhythmic death.

To summarize, risk stratification is necessary to select patients at high enough risk of events to justify intervention; however, left ventricular damage, a powerful risk factor for overall cardiac death risk, may be the most efficient means of selecting patients who are at high risk of arrhythmic death.

Pharmacologic interventions and sudden cardiac death

Classification of antiarrhythmic drugs

There have been a number of attempts to classify antiarrhythmic drugs. The most widely used classification is based on the influence of drugs on different phases of the action potential of myocytes (Table 41.1). This system is relatively simple compared to other classifications, but is limited because of the mixed abilities of most antiarrhythmic drugs.

Table 41.1   Classification of antiarrhythmic drugs*

	Action	Drugs
Class IA	Depression of action potential upstroke, slow conduction, prolong repolarization	Quinidine, procainamide, disopyramide
Class IB	Little effect on upstroke in normal tissue, depression of upstroke in abnormal tissue, shortening of repolarization	Lidocaine, mexiletine
Class IC	Marked depression of upstroke, marked slow conduction, slight effect on repolarization	Flecainide, propafenone, encainade, ajmaline, moricizine
Class II	β Blockers	
Class III	Prolong repolarization	Amiodarone, sotalol, dofetilide, azimilide, ibutilide
Class IV	Calcium-channel blockers	Verapamil, diltiazem

*Many drugs have properties of more than one class, but are classified according to their major effects.

Trials of antiarrhythmic therapy in patients with sustained ventricular arrhythmia

There have been only a few randomized trials of antiarrhythmic therapy in patients with prior sustained ventricular arrhythmia. These have used active controls and the primary outcome has been arrhythmia recurrence or death. Steinbeck *et al*[4] conducted a prospective randomized trial in 170 patients to investigate whether electrophysiologic study (EPS)-guided antiarrhythmic therapy improves the long-term outcome of patients with spontaneous and inducible sustained ventricular arrhythmia compared with metoprolol therapy not guided by EPS. EPS-guided therapy consisted of serial EPS testing of inducibility under different antiarrhythmic agents (in sequence: propafenone → disopyramide → sotalol → amiodarone) to identify one that would suppress an initially inducible sustained arrhythmia. There were 55 patients whose arrhythmia was never inducible during the baseline EPS, thereby precluding further serial drug testing, and these patients were treated with metoprolol. The 2 year incidence of the composite outcome of symptomatic arrhythmia recurrence or sudden death was the same for EPS-guided therapy as for metoprolol (46% *v* 48%).

In the Electrophysiological Study Versus Electrocardiographic Monitoring (ESVEM) study[5,6] patients with inducible VT and any (i) history of cardiac arrest, (ii) sustained VT or (iii) syncope, were randomly assigned to undergo serial testing of the efficacy of the antiarrhythmic drugs either by EPS or by 24 hour Holter monitoring. Patients ($n = 486$) received long-term treatment with the first antiarrhythmic drug that was predicted to be effective on the basis of either repeat EPS or 24 hour Holter. The primary conclusion of ESVEM was that therapy guided by EPS and that guided by Holter monitoring are equally effective.[6] The secondary outcome, related to the efficacy of individual study drug, was very interesting.[5] Sotalol, a β blocking drug with class III activity, was more effective than the class I drugs tested (imipramine, mexiletine, pirmenol, procainamide, propafenone, quinidine). The actuarial probability of a recurrence of arrhythmia after a prediction of drug efficacy by either strategy was significantly lower for patients treated with sotalol than for patients treated with the other drugs (risk ratio (RR) 0·43; 95% CI 0·29, 0·62). With sotalol there were lower risks of death from any cause (RR 0·50; 95% CI 0·30, 0·80), death from cardiac causes (0·50; $P = 0·02$) and death from arrhythmia (0·50; $P = 0·04$). The cumulative percentage of patients in whom a drug was predicted to be effective and in whom it remained effective and tolerated was also higher for sotalol than for the other drugs ($P < 0·001$). Sotalol was more effective than the other six antiarrhythmic drugs in preventing death and recurrences of arrhythmia.

In the Cardiac Arrest in Seattle: Conventional versus Amiodarone Drug Evaluation (CASCADE) study, antiarrhythmic drug therapy was evaluated in survivors of out of hospital VF.[7] Amiodarone without EPS or Holter guidance was compared to class I antiarrhythmic agents (quinidine, procainamide, their combination, or flecainide), selected by serial EPS or Holter monitoring. Most of the 228 randomized patients had coronary artery disease with a prior myocardial infarction, and the mean left ventricular ejection fraction was 35±10%. During a mean follow up of 6 years, amiodarone improved survival compared to the class I agents (53% *v* 40%, $P = 0·007$).

These trials provide evidence that, in survivors of sustained ventricular arrhythmia, amiodarone and sotalol are superior to class I agents.

Recommendation

Grade A Where antiarrhythmic drugs are to be used to prevent the recurrence of ventricular tachyarrhythmia, amiodarone and sotalol are superior to class I antiarrhythmic agents.

Trials of antiarrhythmic therapy in patients with asymptomatic non-sustained ventricular arrhythmia, at risk of sudden death

Asymptomatic non-sustained ventricular arrhythmia on Holter monitor was determined in the 1980s to be a predictor of death in patients surviving myocardial infarction, and these patients were targeted in several trials of antiarrhythmic therapy on the assumption that decreasing asymptomatic ventricular arrhythmia would decrease the occurrence of sudden cardiac death This hypothesis was first tested in the International Mexiletine and Placebo Antiarrhythmic Coronary Trial (IMPACT)[8] and then in the pivotal Cardiac Arrhythmia Suppression Trial (CAST).[9] In IMPACT, 630 patients with recent myocardial infarction were randomly assigned to treatment with mexiletine or placebo.[8] Despite a decrease in the frequency of complex ventricular arrhythmia, after an average follow up of 9 months, the mortality on mexiletine was 7·6% and on placebo was 4·8% ($P = $ NS).

In the Cardiac Arrhythmic Suppression Trial (CAST)[9] 1727 patients with recent onset of myocardial infarction and with asymptomatic, or mildly symptomatic, ventricular arrhythmia (≥ 6 ventricular extrasystoles per hour), suppressible by a class I antiarrhythmic drug (encainide, flecainide or moricizine), were randomized to the active antiarrhythmic drug or placebo and followed for arrhythmic death. The trial was halted early because of an increased incidence of arrhythmic cardiac death and non-fatal cardiac arrests in patients treated with encainide and flecainide (4·5% *v* 1·2%, RR 3·6, 95% CI 1·7, 8·5).

These results led to reappraisal of class I drug therapy for sudden death prophylaxis. In a meta-analysis of the results of 138 trials of antiarrhythmic prophylactic therapy in patients after myocardial infarction,[10] there were 660 deaths among 11 712 patients allocated to receive class I agents and 571 deaths among 11 517 corresponding control patients (51 trials: odds ratio (OR) 1·14; 95% CI 1·01, 1·28; $P = 0·03$). There is therefore considerable evidence that class I antiarrhythmic drugs are harmful when used as prophylactic agents in high-risk patients.

Amiodarone is a class III antiarrhythmic agent which has been extensively studied in patients at risk of sudden arrhythmic death. Amiodarone has several properities other than class III effect, including an antiadrenergic effect. The two largest trials (Canadian Amiodarone Myocardial Infarction Arrhythmia Trial, CAMIAT[11] and European Myocardial Infarction Amiodarone Trial, EMIAT[12]) both showed a reduction in arrhythmic death but no significant reduction in overall death. Meta-analysis of data from all 13 randomized controlled trials of amiodarone (89% of patients, after myocardial infarction) showed a significant reduction in total mortality (OR 0·87, 95% CI 0·78–0·99) and a significant reduction in arrhythmic death (OR 0·71, 95% CI 0·59, 0·85).[13,14] Analysis of the interaction between the treatment and baseline factors suggested an important positive relationship between β blocker use and amiodarone effect,[15] such that patients on β blockers received a significantly greater benefit from amiodarone than those not on β blockers.

D-Sotalol, a pure class III agent, was evaluated for prevention of sudden death in a placebo controlled trial of 3121 patients with recent myocardial infarction and left ventricular ejection fraction <40%, or symptomatic heart failure with a remote myocardial infarction (Survival with Oral d-sotalol, or SWORD trial).[16] Among 1549 patients assigned to d-sotalol there were 78 deaths (5·0%) compared to 48 (3·1%) among the 1572 patients assigned to placebo (RR 1·65, 95% CI 1·15, 2·36). Presumed arrhythmic deaths (RR 1·77, 95% CI 1·15, 2·74) accounted for the excess mortality in the d-sotalol group. This proarrhythmic fatal effect of d-sotalol was greater in patients with a left ventricular ejection fraction of 31–40% than in those with lower ejection fractions (RR 4·0 v 1·2, $P = 0·007$).

Another pure class III compound, dofetilide, was tested in patients with symptomatic heart failure. In the Danish Investigations of Arrhythmia and Mortality on Dofetilide (DIAMOND) 1518 patients were randomized to dofetilide or placebo.[17,18] The study treatment was initiated in hospital and included 3 days of cardiac monitoring and dose adjustment. During a median follow up of 18 months, 311 patients in the dofetilide group (41%) and 317 patients in the placebo group (42%) died (OR, 0·95; 95% CI 0·81, 1·11). Treatment with dofetilide significantly reduced the risk of hospitalization for worsening CHF, rate of conversion and risk of recurrence of atrial fibrillation. There were 25 cases of *torsades de pointes* in the dofetilide group (3·3%), compared to none in the placebo group. Dofetilide has also

been tested in a randomized trial of 1510 patients with severe left ventricular dysfunction (LVEF ≤ 35%) after recent myocardial infarction (DIAMOND MI trial). The primary end point was all-cause mortality. No significant difference was found between the dofetilide and placebo groups in overall mortality (31% v 32%). The cardiac mortality (26% v 28%) and arrhythmic mortality (17% v 18%) were also similar. There were seven cases of *torsades de pointes* ventricular tachycardia, all in the dofetilide group.[19]

In the Azimilide Postinfarct Survival Evaluation (ALIVE) trial the effect of azimilide, another pure class III agent, was evaluated in 3717 patients with recent myocardial infarction, with LVEF < 35% and with low heart rate variability. Azimilide had no effect on mortality (HR = 1·0).[20]

β Blockers in patients at risk of sudden death

β Blockers are the single type of agent most frequently studied in postmyocardial infarction patients for the prevention of death, with more than 12 large trials reported. A meta-analysis of the β blocker trials, reported in 1985, showed a significant reduction in mortality during treatment after myocardial infarction.[21] The data from this meta-analysis also indicated a highly significant 30% reduction in sudden cardiac death with β blockers. The risk of non-sudden death was also decreased by 12%, but this difference was not significant. Recent β blocker trials in CHF patients also show a reduction in both overall and sudden cardiac death.[22–24]

In summary, antiarrhythmic drugs have been extensively evaluated in randomized trials as prophylactic agents against death, but little tested against recurrence of arrhythmia. β Blockers are effective against arrhythmic death (about 20–30% reduction) and non-arrhythmic deaths, and reduce overall mortality significantly. Amiodarone has a moderate effect against sudden death and a neutral effect on other deaths, therefore its overall effect on total mortality is modest. Class I antiarrhythmic drugs are harmful, probably owing to proarrhythmic effects. Pure class III agents are at best neutral, and in the case of one agent, d-sotalol, actually harmful.

β Blocker therapy is indicated in all patients at high risk for sudden death, and amiodarone is the treatment of choice for control of specific arrhythmias where concern about possible proarrhythmic effects is an issue (especially in patients with ischemic heart disease and/or left ventricular dysfunction).

Pure class III antiarrhythmic agents clearly do not reduce mortality when used prophylactically in high-risk patients. The different results of D-sotalol, dofetilide and azimilide trials are probably due to differences in the design of the studies and differences in risk of *torsades de pointes* between the agents.

Recommendations

Grade A β Blockers are indicated in patients with myocardial infarction or congestive heart failure for the prevention of death.

Grade A Amiodarone is the antiarrhythmic drug of choice where there is an above average risk of proarrhythmia.

Grade A Class I antiarrhythmics should be avoided in patients with coronary artery disease or left ventricular dysfunction.

Other pharmacologic interventions decreasing risk of sudden cardiac death

The effect of angiotensin converting enzyme (ACE) inhibitors on the risk of sudden cardiac death (SCD) following myocardial infarction has been demonstrated in randomized trials.[25–27] A recent meta-analysis[28] incorporated data from 15 trials that included 15 104 patients having 900 SCDs. ACE inhibitor therapy resulted in a significant reduction in total mortality (OR 0·83; 95% CI 0·71, 0·97), cardiovascular death (OR 0·82, 95% CI 0·69, 0·97) and SCD (OR 0·80; 95% CI 0·70, 0·92). Also, the meta-analysis suggested that a reduction in SCD risk with ACE inhibitors was an important component of overall survival benefit, the magnitude of effect on SCD being the same as on overall mortality.

Interestingly, in the Heart Outcome Prevention Evaluation Study (HOPE),[29] involving cardiovascular patients without a significant decrease in (LVEF > 40%), the ACE inhibitor, ramipril, significantly decreased the incidence of cardiac arrest (RR 0·62, 95% CI 0·41, 0·94). The mechanism by which ACE inhibitors reduce SCD is poorly understood. In addition to attenuation of remodeling, and thereby reducing the substrate for ventricular tachyarrhythmia, they provide significant neurohumoral modulation and protection from future ischemic events.

In the Randomized Aldactone Evaluation Study (RALES)[30] aldactone was evaluated in patients having NYHA III–IV. After a mean follow up of 24 months the incidence of heart failure symptoms was significantly decreased (RR 0·71, 95% CI 0·54, 0·95). The magnitude of this effect was similar to the effect on total mortality (RR 0·70, 95% CI 0·68, 0·72).

In the GISSI-Prevenzione Trial[31] treatment with *n*-3 polyunsaturated fatty acids in 11 324 postmyocardial infarction patients significantly decreased the incidence of sudden cardiac death (RR 0·74, 95% CI 0·58, 0·93), also significantly decreasing total cardiac mortality and coronary mortality by the same ratio (RR 0·78 and 0·80, respectively, both significant).

Thus, accumulated evidence supports the wide use of the above-mentioned interventions in appropriate patients. However, there is no evidence of a primary antiarrhythmic action and so these agents cannot be recommended as antiarrhythmic agents.

Grade A. ACE inhibitors and spironolactone should be used in patients with congestive heart failure.

ICD treatment trials

ICD therapy

Electrical shock therapy is the most effective acute treatment for life-threatening ventricular arrhythmia. The concept of an implantable device able to diagnose ventricular tachyarrhythmia and to deliver shock therapy automatically was developed in the 1970s. ICD therapy has been the subject of intensive validation since its introduction into clinical practice. The first ICD was implanted in 1980; since then there have been many refinements to the initial technology and improvements continue to occur at a brisk pace. The fundamental therapy is the direct current (DC) shock capable of cardioversion/defibrillation. Overdrive pacing therapy for the termination of VT and bradycardia pacing are available. Therapy can be tiered so that if overdrive pacing fails to convert VT, or transforms it to a more malignant arrhythmia, defibrillation/cardioversion can be deployed subsequently. Detection of VT or VF is achieved by automatic counting of the heart rate. Automatic gain control allows the device to detect VF as well as VT. Major recent refinements are a reduction in size and the addition of atrial electrodes which allow dual chamber pacing, as well as use of the atrial electrogram to improve the specificity of VT and VF detection.

Implantation is generally done under anesthesia in the operating room or the electrophysiology laboratory, with intraoperative testing for pacing and defibrillation thresholds. The operative mortality with modern endocardial systems is <1%.[32,33] The ICD is associated with a number of complications: pneumothorax or vascular complications of implantation; heart perforation; pericarditis; and infectious complications. The rate of infection with non-thoracotomy systems is 0·6–4·1%.[34] A troublesome complication is the painfulness of virtually all cardioversion/defibrillator shocks. The availability of overdrive pacing therapy, which is painless, reduces the frequency of shocks even in fast VT, but many patients still require shocks periodically.[35,36]

ICD therapy has achieved considerable sophistication in the detection and treatment of VT and VF. There is no doubt that it is an effective therapy for the termination of episodes of VT and VF. This has been clear for many years from the fact that VT or VF, artificially induced in hospital, can be reliably terminated by the ICD. Modern ICDs now provide an ECG collection and telemetry ability that allows inspection of the cardiac electrograms immediately before and after discharges of the ICD. It is now possible to directly confirm the success of the ICD against episodes of spontaneously occurring VT and VF. Thus it is safe to conclude that the ICD is very effective for many episodes of VT and VF, preventing their fatal outcomes.

Assessment of ICD effectiveness

Assessment of the overall effectiveness of the ICD is made complex by the fact that in the vast majority of patients VT and VF are not isolated conditions but late complications of ischemic heart disease or cardiomyopathy. In fact, VT and VF only rarely occur in the absence of serious structural heart disease. The typical patient receiving an ICD is at risk of dying not only from recurrence of VT or VF, but also from recurrent myocardial infarction and congestive heart failure. Thus although the ICD is clearly effective against VT and VF, it was not entirely obvious that it would prolong life in the average patient treated. Several trials have addressed this issue.

ICD for survivors of sudden death

There have been four randomized trials which evaluated the ICD as a treatment for patients with previous documented sustained VT or VF. A small (60 patients) Dutch trial randomized patients with inducible sustained cardiac arrhythmia after cardiac arrest to either ICD or conventional therapy (which included antiarrhythmic drugs and VT ablation and VT surgery).[37] During 24 months of follow up patients in the ICD group had non-significantly lower overall, cardiac and sudden cardiac mortality.

Three secondary prevention ICD trials have been conducted. CASH[38] enrolled patients with prior VF, whereas the Canadian Implantable Defibrillator Study (CIDS) and the Antiarrhythmic versus Implantable Defibrillator (AVID) study enrolled both patients with prior VF as well as patients with hemodynamically unstable VT.[39,40] CIDS also enrolled patients with decreased LV function, syncope and inducible VT.

AVID was the first of these three trials to report its results.[40] There were 1016 patients randomized to receive either an ICD or drug therapy, which was specified as either amiodarone or sotalol. In patients eligible for either drug, allocation was random. Forty-five per cent of patients had VF and the rest had VT. Only 13 of 509 patients randomized to drug therapy were actually discharged from hospital on sotalol; the rest received amiodarone. The mean dose of amiodarone at 1 year was 331 mg/day and 87% of patients remained on amiodarone at 1 year. There was a significant imbalance in β blocker use between ICD and amiodarone patients, with 45% of ICD patients receiving this therapy compared to 13% of drug therapy patients. There was a reduction in mortality with the ICD. Over a mean follow up of 18 months, crude death rates were $15·8 \pm 3·2\%$ for the ICD v $24·0 + 3·7\%$ for drug therapy ($P < 0·02$). The relative risk reductions at 1, 2 and 3 years were $39 \pm 20\%$, $27 \pm 21\%$ and $31 \pm 21\%$

($\pm 95\%$ CI). The treatment effect is quite large in terms of relative risk reduction (approximately one third) but the prolongation of life is modest, at only just over 3 months.

CASH was initially planned as a 400 patient study with four treatment arms: ICD, amiodarone, metoprolol and propafenone. The propafenone arm was terminated prematurely owing to excessive mortality compared to the other treatments (61% higher all-cause mortality rate than in ICD patients during a follow up of 11 months). The study continued to recruit patients in the remaining three arms; 99 were assigned to ICDs, 92 to amiodarone and 97 to metoprolol. The primary end point was all-cause mortality. The study was terminated when all patients had concluded a minimum 2 year follow up. Over a mean follow up of 57 ± 34 months, therapy with an ICD was associated with a 23% (non-significant) reduction in all-cause mortality rates compared to treatment with amiodarone/metoprolol.

In CIDS a total of 659 patients were randomly assigned to treatment with the ICD or with amiodarone. The primary outcome measure was all-cause mortality and the secondary outcome was arrhythmic death. At 5 years, 85·4% of patients assigned to amiodarone were still receiving it at a mean dose of 255 mg/day, 28·1% of ICD patients were also receiving amiodarone, and 21·4% of amiodarone patients had received an ICD. A non-significant reduction in the risk of death was observed with the ICD, from 10·2% per year to 8·3% per year (19·7% relative risk reduction; 95% CI $-7·7$ to 40; $P = 0·142$). A non-significant reduction in the risk of arrhythmic death was observed, from 4·5% per year to 3·0% per year (32·8% relative risk reduction; 95% CI $-7·2$ to 57·8; $P = 0·094$).

A meta-analysis of the three trials provides a summary of the benefit of the ICD in the secondary prevention.[41] Individual patient data from AVID, CASH and CIDS were merged into a database. Analysis of the data showed that the estimates of ICD benefit from the three studies were consistent with each other ($P_{\text{heterogeneity}} = 0·306$). It also showed a significant reduction in death from any cause with the ICD, with a summary hazard ratio (ICD v amiodarone) of 0·72 (95% CI 0·60, 0·87; $P = 0·0006$). For the outcome of arrhythmic death the hazard ratio was 0·50 (95% CI 0·37, 0·67; $P < 0·0001$). Survival was extended by a mean of 4·4 months by the ICD over a follow up period of 6 years. Patients with left ventricular ejection fraction $\leq 35\%$ derived significantly more benefit from ICD therapy than those with better left ventricular function (HR 1·2, 95% CI 0·86, 1·76 in patients with LVEF $> 35\%$ v HR 0·66, 95%CI in patients with LVEF $\leq 35\%$, $P_{\text{interaction}} = 0·011$).

At present, when managing a patient with life-threatening sustained VT or VF the balance of evidence now favors ICD therapy over amiodarone. In light of the modest prolongation of life conferred by the ICD and its high cost, where resources are limited, amiodarone may be used as reasonable alternative.

ICD for inducible VT/VF

Two randomized trials have evaluated the ability of the ICD to reduce the risk of death in patients who have not experienced sustained ventricular tachyarrhythmia but who are at high risk of sudden death because they have been shown to have low LVEF, spontaneous non-sustained VT, and inducible sustained ventricular tachyarrhythmia. These are the Multicenter Automatic Defibrillator Implantation Trial (MADIT)[42] and the Multicenter Unsustained Tachycardia Trial (MUSTT).[43,44]

In MADIT, patients with left ventricular ejection fraction <35% and recent myocardial infarction were further screened by programmed ventricular stimulation. Patients found to have inducible VT or VF became eligible for the study if inducibility of the tachycardia could not be suppressed by procainamide.[42] There were 196 patients randomized to either receive an ICD or "conventional" therapy. The choice of conventional therapy was at the discretion of the investigator. Amiodarone and β blockers, the only proven effective drugs against VT and VF, were used predominantly but sporadically (in 45% and 5%, respectively, of "conventional" patients at last contact). The trial was terminated prematurely when about 75% of patients had been enrolled, owing to a benefit of ICD treatment. The hazard ratio was 0·46 (95% CI 0·26, 0·82; $P = 0·009$), indicating a greater than 50% reduction in death with ICD therapy. When the specific causes of death were examined, the ICD not only reduced arrhythmic death (13 *v* 3), but there appeared to be reduction in non-arrhythmic cardiac death (13 *v* 7) and deaths of unknown cause (6 *v* 0), which is not explained and not biologically plausible. There was a marked imbalance in the use of β blocker therapy in favor of the ICD group, but this did not explain the benefit observed with the ICD.

The Multicenter Unsustained Tachycardia Trial (MUSTT) was a randomized trial of electrophysiologically guided antiarrhythmic therapy in patients with coronary artery disease, a left ventricular ejection fraction ≤0·40 and asymptomatic, non-sustained ventricular tachycardia.[43] Seven hundred and four patients who satisfied these criteria, and in whom sustained ventricular tachyarrhythmia was induced by programmed stimulation, were randomly assigned to receive either antiarrhythmic drug tailored by electrophysiological testing, including drugs and ICDs (if drugs failed to suppress inducibility), or no antiarrhythmic therapy at all. The primary end point of cardiac arrest or death from arrhythmia was reached in 25% of those receiving electrophysiologically guided therapy, and in 32% of those assigned to no antiarrhythmic therapy (relative risk 0·73; 95% CI 0·53–0·99), representing a reduction in risk of 27%. Five year total mortality was 42% in patients receiving EPS-guided therapy, versus 48% in controls (RR 0·80, 95% CI 0·64, 1·01). In a non-randomized analysis the primary end point was less frequent among the patients who received ICDs compared to patients discharged without receiving defibrillator treatment (relative risk 0·24; 95% CI, 0·13–0·45; $P < 0·001$). In contrast, the primary end point in those who received antiarrhythmic drugs was not less frequent than in the patients assigned to no antiarrhythmic therapy.

The results of these two trials provide suggestive evidence that the ICD reduces risk of death when used as a prevention therapy in patients with coronary disease, reduced left ventricular function and inducible VT. However, the small size of MADIT and the indirect inference about the role of ICD in MUSTT make it hard to conclude definitely that the ICD benefits these patients.

ICD as a primary prevention of sudden cardiac death

In two other randomized trials, ICDs were tested in patients without spontaneous or inducible life-threatening ventricular arrhythmia: the Coronary Artery Bypass Graft Patch Trial (CABG-Patch)[45] and the Second Multicenter Autonomic Defibrillator Implantation Trial (MADIT II).[46]

The rationale for the CABG-Patch trial was developed at a time when a thoracotomy was required for implantation of an ICD. Patients requiring CABG, who were identified to be at high risk of sudden death, were thought to be good candidates for prophylactic ICD implantation because the detrimental effect of a major surgical procedure to implant the ICD was already accounted for.[45] Thus in the CABG-Patch Trial, patients scheduled for CABG and with LVEF ≤35% were further stratified for risk of arrhythmic death by signal averaged ECG. High-risk patients were randomized either to receive or not to receive an ICD at the time of CABG. The trial randomized 900 patients. Antiarrhythmic drug use was similar between the two groups. There were 52 patients randomized to ICD who either never received a device or who had it removed. There were 196 deaths (101 in the ICD group and 95 in the control group) for a crude mortality rate of 21·8% during an average follow up of 32 ± 16 months. The hazard ratio was 1·07 (95% CI 0·81, 1·42), indicating no benefit from the ICD in this patient population. Secondary analysis showed that the ICD did reduce arrhythmic death, but the benefit was offset by an unexplained increase in non-arrhythmic death.[47]

MADIT II is the second completed trial of ICDs in patients at risk of future sudden death without evidence of sustained VT or VF.[46,48] The target population were patients with LVEF ≤30%, excluding patients with recent (<1 month) myocardial infarction, CABG or PTCA (<2 months); and patients justifying the MADIT I criteria for ICD implantation. There were 1232 patients randomly assigned to receive an ICD (742 patients) or conventional medical therapy (490 patients). During an average follow up of 20 months, the mortality rates were 19·8% in the conventional therapy group and 14·2% in the defibrillator group (HR 0·69, 95% CI 0·51, 0·93).

The discrepancy between the results of the CABG-Patch Trial and MADIT may be explained by differences in severity of left ventricular dysfunction of the target populations (≤30% in MADIT II *v* ≤35% in CABG-Patch). All patients in the CABG-Patch population had CABG performed at the very start of the study. MADIT II enrolled patients who had either been previously revascularized or who were not suitable for revascularization.

There are other ongoing prospective randomized controlled trials evaluating the efficacy of ICD therapy in patients at risk of VT/VF without spontaneous or inducible sustained ventricular arrhythmia. The Sudden Cardiac Death in Heart Failure Trial (SCD-HeFT) is a randomized placebo controlled trial designed to determine whether amiodarone or the ICD will decrease overall mortality in patients with coronary artery disease or non-ischemic cardiomyopathy who are in New York Heart Association (NYHA) class II or III heart failure with a left ventricular ejection fraction ≤35%.[49] The primary end point in SCD-HeFT is total mortality.

The Defibrillator in Acute Myocardial Infarction Trial (DINAMIT) is a randomized comparison of ICD therapy versus no ICD therapy in survivors of acute myocardial infarction at risk of sudden cardiac death.[50] The study aims to enroll 675 patients shortly after their infarction (day 6 to day 40) who have reduced left ventricular function (LVEF ≤ 0·35) and impairment of cardiac autonomic function, shown by depressed heart rate variability (standard deviation of normal to normal R–R intervals 70 ms) or elevated average 24 hour heart rate (mean 24 hour R–R interval 750 ms, assessed by Holter monitoring). Patients will be followed for approximately 3 years on average, with subsequent data analysis based on the intent to treat principle. Primary outcome is all-cause mortality.

Results from SCD-Heft and DINAMIT are expected during 2003. At present the evidence of superiority of ICD in patients with low (≥30%) left ventricular ejection fraction is confined to the partially reported results of MADIT II, but counterbalanced by a neutral effect from CABG-Patch.

However, the MADIT II result is likely to be important because of the simple clear design of that study and the clear result in favor of ICD therapy. Left ventricular dysfunction is a major determinant of the degree to which patients can benefit from the ICD. In the secondary prevention trials CIDS and AVID, and in MADIT I, the benefit of the ICD is much greater in these patients with poor LV function than in those whose LV is well preserved. The results of MADIT II, which enrolled patients with severe LV dysfunction, add further evidence in support of this view. Although the occurrence of a sustained ventricular arrhythmia remains the main indication for an ICD today, it is likely that in the future reduced LV function will be the primary determinant of need.

> **Recommendation**
>
> **Grade A** The ICD is indicated for patients with coronary artery disease and LVEF ≤ 30%.

Combined ICD and antiarrhythmic drug therapy

ICDs and antiarrhythmic drugs should not be considered as exclusive alternatives.[51] In fact, many ICD patients receive concomitant antiarrhythmic therapy to help control supraventricular tachyarrhythmia, recurrent ventricular arrhythmia and frequent ICD shocks. Indeed, the ICD does not prevent VT/VF, only its fatal consequences. Conversely, the ICD is able to protect patients from the occasional proarrhythmic action of antiarrhythmic drugs. In one recent placebo controlled trial sotalol was shown to be effective in preventing shocks in ICD patients.[52]

Cost of ICD therapy

The high cost of modern ICD systems is a considerable obstacle against their wider use in many areas, making the treatment available to only a minor proportion of those at risk. The cost effectiveness of ICD implantation was analyzed for two trials.[53,54] In MADIT the ICD treatment showed increased costs compared to the drug arm, mainly owing to initial costs (US$44 600 for ICD *v* US$18 900 for non-ICD). The cost of follow up was non-significantly higher for the non-ICD arm (US$1915 *v* US$1384). ICD therapy resulted in a cost of US$27 000 for every life year saved. In CIDS, the cost per year of life saved was much higher, at about US$130 000. The main reason for the difference in cost effectiveness between MADIT and CIDS was the estimates of efficacy, the costs being similar. The more modest estimate of ICD benefit in CIDS resulted in much lower cost effectiveness. In a subsequent analysis of CIDS for patients with LVEF <35% (in whom ICD implantation was associated with a greater survival benefit), the cost of 1 year of life gained was quite reasonable (between US$60 000 and US$ 90 000). Sheldon *et al.*[55] indicated that appropriate risk stratification by simple clinical risk factors (age ≥70, LVEF ≤35% and NYHA class III) in the CIDS population reduced the cost per year of life saved to about US$40 000.

Summary

Sudden death due to ventricular arrhythmia is an important health problem against which considerable progress has been made in the past 15 years. Both drugs and devices have been shown to reduce the risk of arrhythmic death. Patients with advanced coronary or myocardial disease are at high risk of arrhythmic death and should be treated with ACE inhibitors and β blockers. Those with symptomatic heart failure should receive spironolactone. The ICD clearly further reduces the risk of arrhythmic death in those at high risk, and should be used both in patients surviving sustained VT or VF and in those with very severe left ventricular dysfunction.

Summary of recommendations

Grade A Where antiarrhythmic drugs are to be used to prevent the recurrence of ventricular tachyarrhythmia, amiodarone and sotalol are superior to class I antiarrhythmic agents.

Grade A β Blockers are indicated in all patients with prior myocardial infarction or congestive heart failure.

Grade A ACE inhibitors and spironolactone should be used in patients with congestive heart failure.

Grade A Amiodarone is the antiarrhythmic drug of choice where there is an above average risk of proarrhythmia.

Grade A Class I antiarrhythmics should be avoided in patients with coronary artery disease or left ventricular dysfunction.

Grade A ICD is the treatment of choice for patients with cardiac arrest or sustained ventricular tachycardia.

Grade A The ICD is indicated for patients with coronary artery disease with LVEF≤30%.

Grade B The ICD may be considered for patients with LVEF≤40% and with inducible sustained VT.

References

1. Huikuri HV, Castellanos A, Myerburg RJ. Sudden death due to cardiac arrhythmias. *N Engl J Med* 2001;**345**:1473–82.
2. Bayes de Luna A, Coumel P, Leclercq JF. Ambulatory sudden cardiac death: mechanisms of production of fatal arrhythmia on the basis of data from 157 cases. *Am Heart J* 1989;**117**:151–9.
3. Albert CM, Ruskin JN. Risk stratifiers for sudden cardiac death (SCD) in the community: primary prevention of SCD. *Cardiovasc Res* 2001;**50**:186–96.
4. Steinbeck G, Andresen D, Bach P *et al.* A comparison of electrophysiologically guided antiarrhythmic drug therapy with beta-blocker therapy in patients with symptomatic, sustained ventricular tachyarrhythmias. *N Engl J Med* 1992;**327**:987–92.
5. Mason JW. A comparison of seven antiarrhythmic drugs in patients with ventricular tachyarrhythmias. Electrophysiologic Study versus Electrocardiographic Monitoring Investigators. *N Engl J Med* 1993;**329**:452–8.
6. Mason JW. A comparison of electrophysiologic testing with Holter monitoring to predict antiarrhythmic-drug efficacy for ventricular tachyarrhythmias. Electrophysiologic Study versus Electrocardiographic Monitoring Investigators. *N Engl J Med* 1993;**329**:445–51.
7. Greene HL. The CASCADE Study: randomized antiarrhythmic drug therapy in survivors of cardiac arrest in Seattle. CASCADE Investigators. *Am J Cardiol* 1993;**72**:70F–4F.
8. International mexiletine and placebo antiarrhythmic coronary trial: I. Report on arrhythmia and other findings. Impact Research Group. *J Am Coll Cardiol* 1984;**4**:1148–63.
9. The Cardiac Arrhythmia Suppression Trial (CAST) Investigators. Preliminary report: effect of encainide and flecainide on mortality in a randomized trial of arrhythmia suppression after myocardial infarction. *N Engl J Med* 1989;**321**:406–12.
10. Teo KK, Yusuf S, Furberg CD. Effects of prophylactic antiarrhythmic drug therapy in acute myocardial infarction. An overview of results from randomized controlled trials. *JAMA* 1993;**270**:1589–95.
11. Cairns JA, Connolly SJ, Roberts R, Gent M. Randomised trial of outcome after myocardial infarction in patients with frequent or repetitive ventricular premature depolarisations: CAMIAT. Canadian Amiodarone Myocardial Infarction Arrhythmia Trial Investigators. *Lancet* 1997;**349**:675–82.
12. Julian DG, Camm AJ, Frangin G *et al.* Randomised trial of effect of amiodarone on mortality in patients with left-ventricular dysfunction after recent myocardial infarction: EMIAT. European Myocardial Infarct Amiodarone Trial Investigators. *Lancet* 1997;**349**:667–74.
13. Amiodarone Trials Meta-Analysis Investigators. Effect of prophylactic amiodarone on mortality after acute myocardial infarction and in congestive heart failure: meta-analysis of individual data from 6500 patients in randomised trials. *Lancet* 1997;**350**:1417–24.
14. Connolly SJ. Evidence-based analysis of amiodarone efficacy and safety. *Circulation* 1999;**100**:2025–34.
15. Boutitie F, Boissel JP, Connolly SJ *et al.* Amiodarone interaction with beta-blockers: analysis of the merged EMIAT (European Myocardial Infarct Amiodarone Trial) and CAMIAT (Canadian Amiodarone Myocardial Infarction Trial) databases. The EMIAT and CAMIAT Investigators. *Circulation* 1999;**99**:2268–75.
16. Waldo AL, Camm AJ, deRuyter H *et al.* Effect of D-sotalol on mortality in patients with left ventricular dysfunction after recent and remote myocardial infarction. The SWORD Investigators. Survival With Oral D-Sotalol. *Lancet* 1996;**348**:7–12.
17. Torp-Pedersen C, Moller M, Bloch-Thomsen PE *et al.* Dofetilide in patients with congestive heart failure and left ventricular dysfunction. Danish Investigations of Arrhythmia and Mortality on Dofetilide Study Group. *N Engl J Med* 1999;**341**:857–65.
18. Torp-Pedersen C, Moller M, Bloch-Thomsen PE *et al.* Dofetilide in patients with congestive heart failure and left ventricular dysfunction. *N Engl J Med* 1999;**341**:857–65.
19. Kober L, Bloch Thomsen PE, Moller M *et al.* Effect of dofetilide in patients with recent myocardial infarction and left-ventricular dysfunction: a randomised trial. *Lancet* 2000;**356**:2052–8.
20. Camm AJ. Azimilide Postinfarct Survival Evaluation (ALIVE): Azimilide does not affect mortality in post myocardial infarction patients. http://www. online.org/HTML_src/summarybyspec. asp? dd = Clinical styId = 3

21. Yusuf S, Peto R, Lewis J, Collins R, Sleight P. Beta blockade during and after myocardial infarction: an overview of the randomized trials. *Prog Cardiovasc Dis* 1985;**27**:335–71.

22. Carson P. Beta-blocker therapy in heart failure. *Cardiol Clin* 2001;**19**:267–78, vi.

23. The Cardiac Insufficiency Bisoprolol Study II (CIBIS-II): a randomised trial. *Lancet* 1999;**353**:9–13.

24. Effect of metoprolol CR/XL in chronic heart failure: Metoprolol CR/XL Randomised Intervention Trial in Congestive Heart Failure (MERIT-HF). *Lancet* 1999;**353**:2001–7.

25. Cohn JN, Johnson G, Ziesche S *et al.* A comparison of enalapril with hydralazine-isosorbide dinitrate in the treatment of chronic congestive heart failure. *N Engl J Med* 1991;**325**:303–10.

26. Kober L, Torp-Pedersen C, Carlsen JE *et al.* A clinical trial of the angiotensin-converting-enzyme inhibitor trandolapril in patients with left ventricular dysfunction after myocardial infarction. Trandolapril Cardiac Evaluation (TRACE) Study Group. *N Engl J Med* 1995;**333**:1670–6.

27. Cleland JG, Erhardt L, Murray G, Hall AS, Ball SG. Effect of ramipril on morbidity and mode of death among survivors of acute myocardial infarction with clinical evidence of heart failure. A report from the AIRE Study Investigators. *Eur Heart J* 1997;**18**:41–51.

28. Domanski MJ, Exner DV, Borkowf CB, Geller NL, Rosenberg Y, Pfeffer MA. Effect of angiotensin converting enzyme inhibition on sudden cardiac death in patients following acute myocardial infarction. A meta-analysis of randomized clinical trials. *J Am Coll Cardiol* 1999;**33**:598–604.

29. Yusuf S, Sleight P, Pogue J, Bosch J, Davies R, Dagenais G. Effects of an angiotensin-converting-enzyme inhibitor, ramipril, on cardiovascular events in high-risk patients. The Heart Outcomes Prevention Evaluation Study Investigators. *N Engl J Med* 2000;**342**:145–53.

30. Pitt B, Zannad F, Remme WJ *et al.* The effect of spironolactone on morbidity and mortality in patients with severe heart failure. Randomized Aldactone Evaluation Study Investigators. *N Engl J Med* 1999;**341**:709–17.

31. Gruppo Italiano per lo Studio della Sopravvivenza nell'Infarto miocardico. Dietary supplementation with *n*-3 polyunsaturated fatty acids and vitamin E after myocardial infarction: results of the GISSI-Prevenzione trial. *Lancet* 1999;**354**:447–55.

32. Strickberger SA, Hummel JD, Daoud E *et al.* Implantation by electrophysiologists of 100 consecutive cardioverter defibrillators with nonthoracotomy lead systems. *Circulation* 1994;**90**:868–72.

33. PCD Investigator Group. Clinical outcome of patients with malignant ventricular tachyarrhythmias and a multiprogrammable implantable cardioverter-defibrillator implanted with or without thoracotomy: an international multicenter study. *J Am Coll Cardiol* 1994;**23**:1521–30.

34. Shepard R, Epsten A. ICD infection avoidance: science, art, discipline. In: Kroll MW LM, ed. *Implantable cardioverter defibrillator therapy: the engineering–clinical interface*. Norwell, MA: Kluwer Academic Press, 1996.

35. Rosenqvist M. Pacing techniques to terminate ventricular tachycardia. *Pacing Clin Electrophysiol* 1995;**18**:592–8.

36. Wathen MS, Sweeney MO, DeGroot PJ *et al.* Shock reduction using antitachycardia pacing for spontaneous rapid ventricular tachycardia in patients with coronary artery disease. *Circulation* 2001;**104**:796–801.

37. Wever EFD, Hauer RNW, van Capelle FJL *et al.* Randomized study of implantable defibrillator as first-choice therapy versus conventional strategy in postinfarct sudden death survivors. *Circulation* 1995;**91**:2195–203.

38. Kuck KH, Cappato R, Siebels J, Ruppel R. Randomized comparison of antiarrhythmic drug therapy with implantable defibrillators in patients resuscitated from cardiac arrest: the Cardiac Arrest Study Hamburg (CASH). *Circulation* 2000;**102**:748–54.

39. Connolly SJ, Gent M, Roberts RS *et al.* Canadian implantable defibrillator study (CIDS): a randomized trial of the implantable cardioverter defibrillator against amiodarone. *Circulation* 2000;**101**:1297–302.

40. The Antiarrhythmics versus Implantable Defibrillators (AVID) Investigators. A comparison of antiarrhythmic-drug therapy with implantable defibrillators in patients resuscitated from near-fatal ventricular arrhythmias. *N Engl J Med* 1997;**337**:1576–83.

41. Connolly SJ, Hallstrom AP, Cappato R *et al.* Meta-analysis of the implantable cardioverter defibrillator secondary prevention trials. AVID, CASH and CIDS studies. Antiarrhythmics vs Implantable Defibrillator study. Cardiac Arrest Study Hamburg. Canadian Implantable Defibrillator Study. *Eur Heart J* 2000;**21**:2071–8.

42. Moss AJ, Hall WJ, Cannom DS *et al.* Improved survival with an implanted defibrillator in patients with coronary disease at high risk for ventricular arrhythmia. Multicenter Automatic Defibrillator Implantation Trial Investigators. *N Engl J Med* 1996;**335**:1933–40.

43. Buxton AE, Lee KL, Fisher JD, Josephson ME, Prystowsky EN, Hafley G. A randomized study of the prevention of sudden death in patients with coronary artery disease. Multicenter Unsustained Tachycardia Trial Investigators. *N Engl J Med* 1999;**341**:1882–90.

44. Buxton AE, Lee KL, DiCarlo L *et al.* Electrophysiologic testing to identify patients with coronary artery disease who are at risk for sudden death. Multicenter Unsustained Tachycardia Trial Investigators. *N Engl J Med* 2000;**342**:1937–45.

45. Bigger JT Jr. Prophylactic use of implanted cardiac defibrillators in patients at high risk for ventricular arrhythmias after coronary-artery bypass graft surgery. Coronary Artery Bypass Graft (CABG) Patch Trial Investigators. *N Engl J Med* 1997;**337**:1569–75.

46. Moss AJ, Zareba W, Hall WJ *et al.* Prophylactic implantation of a defibrillator in patients with myocardial infarction and reduced ejection fraction. *N Engl J Med* 2002;**346**:877–83.

47. Bigger JT Jr, Whang W, Rottman JN *et al.* Mechanisms of death in the CABG Patch trial: a randomized trial of implantable cardiac defibrillator prophylaxis in patients at high risk of death after coronary artery bypass graft surgery. *Circulation* 1999;**99**:1416–21.

48. Moss AJ, Cannom DS, Daubert JP *et al.* Multicenter Automatic Defibrillation Implantation Trial II (MADIT II): design and clinical protocol. *Ann Noninvas Electrocardiol* 1999;**4**:83–91.

49. Bardy GH, Lee KL, Mark DB. The Sudden Cardiac Death in Heart Failure Trial: pilot study [Abstract]. *PACE* 1997;**20**:1148.

50. Hohnloser SH, Connolly SJ, Kuck KH *et al.* The defibrillator in acute myocardial infarction trial (DINAMIT): study protocol. *Am Heart J* 2000;**140**:735–9.

51. Dorian P. Combination ICD and drug treatments – best options. *Resuscitation* 2000;**45**:S3–6.

52. Pacifico A, Hohnloser SH, Williams JH *et al.* Prevention of implantable-defibrillator shocks by treatment with sotalol. D,l-Sotalol Implantable Cardioverter-Defibrillator Study Group. *N Engl J Med* 1999;**340**:1855–62.

53. Mushlin AI, Hall WJ, Zwanziger J *et al.* The cost-effectiveness of automatic implantable cardiac defibrillators: results from MADIT. *Circulation* 1998;**97**:2129–35.

54. O'Brien BJ, Goeree R, Bernard L, Rosner A, Williamson T. Cost-effectiveness of tolterodine for patients with urge incontinence who discontinue initial therapy with oxybutynin: a Canadian perspective. *Clin Ther* 2001;**23**:2038–49.

55. Sheldon R, O'Brien BJ, Blackhouse G *et al.* Effect of clinical risk stratification on cost-effectiveness of the implantable cardioverter-defibrillator: the Canadian implantable defibrillator study. *Circulation* 2001;**104**:1622–6.

42 Impact of pacemakers: when and what kind?

William D Toff, A John Camm

Introduction

The development and implementation of the first fully implantable cardiac pacemaker in 1958 transformed the outlook for patients with symptomatic bradycardia and Stokes–Adams attacks.[1] The first pacemaker recipient survived for over 43 years after receiving his initial implant. Since then, many millions of patients have benefitted from this dramatically effective form of treatment. Technological advances and innovation have enabled the development of increasingly sophisticated pacing systems, better able to simulate the normal cardiac activation sequence, and a wide variety of different pacing modes is now available.

Initially, pacemakers were only implanted for atrioventricular (AV) block, but their use was soon extended to the management of symptomatic bradycardia associated with sinus node disease. In recent years, improved understanding of pathophysiologic mechanisms has prompted the assessment of pacemaker therapy in a number of other conditions such as neurocardiogenic syncope, hypertrophic cardiomyopathy, dilated cardiomyopathy and paroxysmal atrial fibrillation. With the emergence of new indications for pacing and the availability of a vast array of different pacing modes and techniques, an evidence-based approach to the practice of cardiac pacing has become increasingly important.

Goals of cardiac pacing

The fundamental aims of cardiac pacing are to relieve symptoms, to improve the quality of life and, in some instances, to prolong survival. The achievement of these aims is mediated by improvements in hemodynamic function and functional capacity, reduction in cardiovascular morbidity, and prevention of sudden death. Any consideration of the indications for pacing and selection of the appropriate pacing mode must have regard to all of these factors and their interrelations, which are summarized in Figure 42.1. Hemodynamic differences between alternative pacing modes do not always translate into significant differences in clinical utility and a comprehensive assessment of outcome in clinical trials is therefore essential. It is important to note that inappropriate pacing or complications from pacing may result in new or worse symptoms and increased cardiovascular morbidity. This is perhaps best exemplified by the pacemaker syndrome, which is most often seen during ventricular pacing in the presence of retrograde ventriculoatrial conduction. The syndrome has aptly been described as an iatrogenic condition.[2]

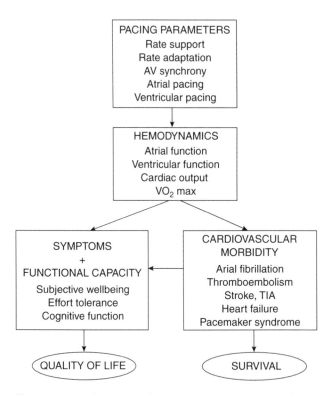

Figure 42.1 Relation of pacing parameters to clinical outcome

Current pacing practice

It is estimated that about 500 000 pacemakers per annum are implanted worldwide,[3–5] but there is considerable national and regional variation in the implant rate. In the United Kingdom, there are approximately 295 new implants per million population.[6] This is close to the median for European countries but the figure within Europe ranges from less than

100 per million (Russia) to 585 per million (Belgium).[4] The estimated new implant rate in the United States is 571 per million.[5] These variations may partly reflect differences in the age distribution and morbidity of the relevant populations but availability of resources and variations in standards of medical care and attitudes towards pacing may also be relevant. There has also been some suggestion, in the past, of inappropriate and excessive pacemaker implantation.[7]

In an effort to define appropriate pacing practice, a joint task force sub-committee of the American College of Cardiology (ACC) and the American Heart Association (AHA) published guidelines for permanent pacemaker implantation in 1984.[8] These were updated and revised in 1991[9] and again in 1998[10] (Table 42.1). The guidelines follow an evidence-based approach and include grading of the evidence supporting each recommendation. With regard to the indications for pacing, the following classification is used:

- Class I – conditions for which there is evidence and/or general agreement that pacing is beneficial, useful, and effective
- Class II – conditions for which there is conflicting evidence and/or a divergence of opinion about the usefullness/efficacy of pacing
- Class III – conditions for which there is evidence and/or general agreement that pacing is not useful/effective and in some cases may be harmful.

Class II is subdivided into Class IIa – weight of evidence/opinion is in favor of usefullness/efficacy and Class IIb – usefullness/efficacy is less well established by evidence/opinion. It is recognized that, although applicable to the "average" patient, recommendations for specific conditions may require modification to take account of patient comorbidity, limited life expectancy, and other factors that only the implanting physician can evaluate appropriately.

A working party of the British Pacing and Electrophysiology Group (BPEG) also published recommendations for pacemaker prescription in 1991.[11] These advocated general principles to guide pacemaker mode selection and made specific recommendations for optimal and alternative pacing modes in various clinical settings (Table 42.2). The recommendations regarding mode selection have, however, been criticized and attention has been drawn to their reliance on observational data from retrospective studies rather than prospective randomized clinical trials.[12] Attention has also been drawn to the financial implications of the recommendations, implementation of which might increase pacing budgets by up to 75%.[13] For whatever reason, it is clear that the BPEG recommendations have not been universally adopted in the United Kingdom[14] and there is evidence of agism, with the preferential use of optimal pacing modes only in younger patients.[15]

General principles of pacemaker mode selection
- The ventricle should be paced if there is actual or threatened atrioventricular block.
- The atrium should be paced/sensed unless contraindicated.
- Rate response is not essential if the patient is inactive or has a normal chronotropic response.
- Rate hysteresis may be valuable if the bradycardia is intermittent.

Based on recommendations of a working party of the British Pacing and Electrophysiology Group[11]

Against this background, it is pertinent to review the evidence concerning the indications for pacing and pacemaker mode selection in order fully to comprehend the basis for rational, evidence-based pacing practice. It is important to note that there have been no randomized trials to assess the efficacy of pacing in the treatment of symptomatic AV block. The absence of any satisfactory alternative therapy and the overwhelming evidence of symptom relief from observational studies over four decades render such a trial unethical and unnecessary. In the assessment of new indications for pacing and alternative pacing modes, however, observational data require critical evaluation and, where inconclusive, should be supplemented by data from carefully designed clinical trials.

Conventional indications for pacing

The principal indication for cardiac pacing is to relieve or prevent symptoms associated with bradycardia. In high grade AV block, however, there is evidence that survival may also be improved by pacing, even in the absence of symptoms, and pacing should be considered on prognostic grounds alone.

The symptoms associated with bradycardia include manifestations of limited cardiac output (tiredness, exercise intolerance, breathlessness, edema or chest discomfort), relative cerebral ischemia (transient dizziness, light-headedness, presyncope or syncope), and uncoordinated cardiac contraction (palpitation, neck or abdominal pulsation). Where significant symptoms are clearly associated with documented bradycardia, the requirement for pacing will rarely be in doubt. In other contexts, the cause of symptoms may be unclear and it is important to note that the most common symptoms are non-specific and prevalent in the elderly population, even in the absence of bradycardia.

Remediable causes of bradycardia such as acute myocardial ischemia, electrolyte imbalance, hypothyroidism or drug toxicity should always be considered before proceeding to cardiac pacing. In some instances, drugs that depress sinus node function or AV conduction may be essential and pacing may be required to enable their continued use.

Table 42.1 ACC/AHA guidelines: indications for permanent cardiac pacing[10]

Condition	Class I	Class IIa	Class IIb	Class III
Acquired AV block (adults): First degree		First degree AV block with symptoms suggestive of "pacemaker syndrome" and alleviation of symptoms with temporary AV pacing **Grade B**	Marked first degree AV block (PR > 0·3 s) in patients with LV dysfunction and symptoms of CHF in whom a more physiologic AV interval results in hemodynamic improvement **Grade C**	Asymptomatic first degree AV block **Grade B**
Second degree	Second degree AV block (any type or level) with associated symptomatic bradycardia **Grade B**	Asymptomatic type I second degree AV block at intra- or infra-His levels found incidentally at EPS **Grade B** Asymptomatic type II second degree AV block **Grade B**		Asymptomatic type I second degree block at the supra-His (AV node) level **Grade B/C**
Third degree (CHB)	CHB associated with any of: (a) Symptomatic bradycardia **Grade C** (b) Need for drugs causing symptomatic bradycardia **Grade C** (c) Documented asystole ≥3 s or escape rate <40/min in awake, symptom-free patients **Grade B/C** (d) Postablation of AV junction **Grade B/C** (e) Post operative AV block not expected to resolve **Grade C** (f) Neuromuscular disease (for example myotonic dystrophy) **Grade B**	Asymptomatic CHB at any anatomic site, with average, awake, ventricular rates ≥40/min **Grade B/C**		AV block that is expected to resolve and is unlikely to recur (for example drug toxicity, Lyme disease) **Grade B**
Chronic bifascicular or trifascicular block	Associated with intermittent CHB **Grade B** Associated with type II second degree AV block **Grade B**	Syncope not proven due to AV block when other likely causes, such as VT, have been excluded **Grade B** Incidental finding at EPS of markedly prolonged HV interval (<100 ms) in	None	Fascicular block with first degree AV block without symptoms **Grade B** Fascicular block without AV block or symptoms **Grade B**

Table 42.1 Continued

Condition	Class I	Class IIa	Class IIb	Class III
		asymptomatic patient **Grade B** Incidental finding at EPS of pacing induced infra-His block that is not physiologic **Grade B**		
AV block after the acute phase of myocardial infarction (MI)	Persistent second degree AV block in the His–Purkinje system with bilateral bundle branch block or third degree AV block within or below the His–Purkinje system after acute MI **Grade B** Transient advanced (second or third degree) infranodal AV block and associated bundle branch block. If the site of block is uncertain, an EPS may be necessary **Grade B** Persistent and symptomatic second or third degree AV block **Grade C**	None	Persistent second or third degree AV block at the AV node level **Grade B**	Transient AV block in the absence of intraventricular conduction defects **Grade B** Transient AV block in the presence of isolated left anterior fascicular block **Grade B** Acquired left anterior fascicular block in the absence of AV block **Grade B** Persistent first degree AV block in the presence of bundle branch block that is old or age indeterminate **Grade B**
Sinus node dysfunction (SND)	SND with documented symptomatic bradycardia including frequent symptomatic sinus pauses (including iatrogenic bradycardia due to essential long term drug therapy with no acceptable alternative) **Grade C**	SND, occurring spontaneously or as a result of necessary drug therapy, with heart rates <40/min when a clear association between significant symptoms consistent with bradycardia and the actual presence of bradycardia has not been documented **Grade C**	Chronic heart rates <30/min whilst awake, in minimally symptomatic patients **Grade C**	SND in asymptomatic patients, including those in whom substantial sinus bradycardia (<40/min) is due to long term drug treatment
Symptomatic chronotropic incompetence **Grade C**				SND in patients in whom symptoms suggestive of bradycardia are clearly documented not to be associated with a slow heart rate SND with symptomatic bradycardia due to non-essential drug therapy

Condition				
Hypersensitive carotid sinus syndrome and neurally mediated syncope	Recurrent syncope caused by carotid sinus stimulation; minimal carotid sinus pressure induces ventricular asystole of >3 s duration in the absence of any medication that depresses the sinus node or AV conduction **Grade C**	Recurrent syncope without clear, provocative events and with a hypersensitive cardioinhibitory response **Grade C** Syncope of unexplained origin when major abnormalities of sinus node function or AV conduction are discovered or provoked at EPS	Neurally mediated syncope with significant bradycardia reproduced by head-up tilt with or without isoproterenol or other provocative maneuvers **Grade B**	Hyperactive cardioinhibitory response to carotid sinus stimulation in the absence of symptoms Vague symptoms, such as dizziness or light-headedness, or both, with a hyperactive cardioinhibitory response to carotid sinus stimulation Recurrent syncope, light-headedness or dizziness in the absence of cardioinhibitory response Situational vasovagal syncope in which avoidance behavior is effective
Tachycardia prevention	Sustained pause-dependent VT, with or without prolonged QT, in which the efficacy of pacing is thoroughly documented **Grade C**	High risk patients with congenital long QT syndrome **Grade C**	AV re-entrant or AV node re-entrant supraventricular tachycardia not responsive to medical or ablation therapy **Grade C** Prevention of symptomatic, drug refractory atrial fibrillation **Grade C**	Frequent or complex ventricular ectopic activity without sustained VT in the absence of the long QT syndrome Long QT syndrome due to reversible causes
Hypertrophic cardiomyopathy	Class I indications for sinus node dysfunction or AV block as above **Grade C**	None	Medically refractory, symptomatic hypertrophic cardiomyopathy patients with significant resting or provoked LV outflow obstruction **Grade C**	Asymptomatic or medically controlled patients Symptomatic patients without evidence of LV outflow obstruction
Dilated cardiomyopathy	Class I indications for sinus node dysfunction or AV block as above **Grade C**	None	Symptomatic, drug refractory dilated cardiomyopathy with prolonged PR interval when acute hemodynamic studies have demonstrated hemodynamic benefit **Grade C**	Asymptomatic dilated cardiomyopathy

Table 42.1 Continued

Condition	Class I	Class IIa	Class IIb	Class III
After cardiac transplantation	Symptomatic bradyarrhythmia or chronotropic incompetence that is not expected to resolve and meets other Class I indications for permanent pacing **Grade C**	None	Symptomatic bradyarrhythmia or chronotropic incompetence that, although transient, may persist for months and require intervention	Symptomatic dilated cardiomyopathy when patients are rendered asymptomatic by drug therapy Symptomatic ischemic cardiomyopathy Asymptomatic bradyarrhythmia postcardiac transplantation
Children and adolescents	Sinus node dysfunction with correlation of symptoms during age-inappropriate bradycardia **Grade B** Advanced second or third degree AV block associated with symptomatic bradycardia, CHF or low cardiac output **Grade C** Congenital CHB with a wide QRS escape rhythm or ventricular dysfunction **Grade B** Congenital CHB in the infant with a ventricular rate <50–55/min or with congenital heart disease and a ventricular rate <70/min **Grade B/C**	Asymptomatic sinus bradycardia in a child with complex congenital heart disease where the resting heart rate is <35/min or ventricular pauses >3s occur **Grade C** Bradycardia–tachycardia syndrome needing chronic antiarrhythmic therapy other than digitalis **Grade C** Congenital CHB, beyond the first year of life, with an average heart rate <50/min, or with abrupt ventricular pauses two or three times the basic cycle length **Grade B**	Asymptomatic sinus bradycardia in an adolescent with congenital heart disease where the resting heart rate is <35/min or ventricular pauses >3s occur **Grade C** Congenital CHB in an asymptomatic neonate, child or adolescent with an acceptable rate, narrow QRS complex and normal ventricular function **Grade B**	Asymptomatic sinus bradycardia in an adolescent where the longest R–R interval is <3s and the minimum rate >40/min **Grade C** Asymptomatic type I second degree AV block **Grade C**

Postoperative advanced second or third degree AV block that is not expected to resolve, or persists at least 7 days after cardiac surgery **Grade B/C**

Sustained pause-dependent VT, with or without prolonged QT, in which the efficacy of pacing is thoroughly documented **Grade B**

Long QT syndrome with 2:1 or third degree AV block **Grade B**

Transient postoperative CHB that reverts to sinus rhythm with residual bifascicular block **Grade C**

Transient postoperative AV block with return of normal AV conduction within 7 days **Grade B**

Asymptomatic postoperative bifascicular block, with or without first degree AV block **Grade C**

Abbreviations: CHB, complete heart block; CHF, congestive heart failure; EPS, electrophysiology study; VT, ventricular tachycardia

Based on Gregoratos et al.[10]

Table 42.2   Recommended pacemaker modes

Diagnosis	Optimal	Alternative	Inappropriate
SND	AAIR	AAI	VVI/VDD
AVB	DDD	VDD	AAI/DDI
SND+AVB	DDDR/DDIR	DDD/DDI	AAI/VVI
Chronic AF+AVB	VVIR	VVI	AAI/DDD/VDD
CSS	DDI	DDD/VVI+hysteresis	AAI/VDD
MVVS	DDI	DDD	AAI/VVI/VDD

AF, atrial fibrillation; AVB, atrioventricular block; CSS, carotid sinus syndrome; MVVS, malignant vasovagal syndrome; SND, sinus node disease

Interpretation of mode acronyms:
First letter: Chamber(s) paced   A, atrium; V, ventricle; D, atrium and ventricle
Second letter: Chamber(s) sensed   A, atrium; V, ventricle; D, atrium and ventricle
Third letter: Response to sensing I, inhibition; T, triggering; D, inhibition and triggering
Fourth letter: Additional functions   R, adaptive rate

Based on recommendations of the British Pacing and Electrophysiology Group[11]

The most common causes of bradycardia requiring pacing are impaired impulse formation, as in sinus node disease, or a disturbance of cardiac conduction, as in AV block. In the United Kingdom, sinus node disease accounts for about 45% of primary implants and AV block or other conduction disturbance for about 50%.[14] The remainder includes patients paced for a variety of conditions, including carotid sinus syndrome, cardio-inhibitory forms of neurocardiogenic syncope and others. The pattern is different in the United States, where sinus node disease accounts for about 50% of primary implants and AV block for about 38%.[5] The reasons for this disparity are unclear but it may reflect different perceptions regarding the indications for pacing.

Atrioventricular block

First degree AV block

Isolated prolongation of the PR interval may be seen as a normal variant in healthy young subjects. In this context, it is most likely due to autonomic influences and has no prognostic significance.[16] In older subjects, PR prolongation is more often associated with underlying pathology, such as conducting system fibrosis or coronary artery disease but it does not usually give rise to symptoms and pacing is not generally indicated.

Occasionally, however, symptoms may arise if the PR interval is markedly prolonged. Atrial systole may then closely follow delayed ventricular systole from the previous cycle, resulting in a comparable hemodynamic disturbance to that seen in the pacemaker syndrome caused by retrograde VA conduction during ventricular pacing. The phenomenon may be accentuated during exercise as the atrial rate increases and the PR interval fails to shorten appropriately. This has been

referred to as the "pacemaker syndrome without a pacemaker"[17] or the "pseudo-pacemaker syndrome"[18] and a favorable response to dual chamber pacing has been reported.[19] In symptomatic patients with first degree AV block, the response to temporary dual chamber pacing should be assessed. If clinical and hemodynamic improvement can be demonstrated by restoration of a physiologic AV interval, permanent dual chamber pacing should be considered.[20,21] Symptomatic first degree AV block with a demonstrable improvement during temporary dual chamber pacing may reasonably be considered at least a Class II[20] and perhaps even a Class I[21] indication for pacing. **Grade B**

Second degree AV block

When second degree AV block of any type is associated with clearly attributable symptoms, pacing is indicated. In the absence of symptoms, the situation is more complex. Prognosis is thought to relate to the site of block, proximal block at the level of the AV node being more benign than distal block in the His–Purkinje system.[22] The ECG classification into Mobitz type I (Wenckebach), Mobitz type II or advanced (2:1, 3:1 or 4:1) second degree AV block is purely descriptive and the site of block cannot always be inferred although electrophysiologic studies have shown that type I block is most commonly proximal whereas type II block is almost always distal.[23] In the past, type I second degree AV block has often been regarded as benign but evidence from the Devon Heart Block and Bradycardia Survey in the United Kingdom[24] suggests that, even in asymptomatic patients, survival is significantly improved by pacing. Although this was a non-randomized, observational study, it constitutes the best available evidence and published opinion suggests that pacing should be considered in asymptomatic type I second degree AV block, particularly in older patients with structural heart disease.[25,26] In young subjects, however, asymptomatic type I second degree AV block occurring during sleep or associated with athletic training is more likely to reflect high resting vagal tone and pacing is unnecessary.[27,28] **Grade B**

Complete AV block

In symptomatic complete AV block, pacing usually, although not invariably, improves the symptoms and should always be considered. Irrespective of symptoms, however, untreated acquired complete heart block is associated with significantly impaired survival. Overall mortality may exceed 50% at one year, the outlook being worst in older patients (>80 years) and those with associated non-rheumatic structural heart disease.[29] Male sex and a history of syncope have also been associated with a worse outlook in some studies[30] but there is conflicting evidence regarding syncope.[31] Transient AV block carries a more favorable prognosis, with a 1 year mortality of 36%, compared with 70% in patients with permanent AV block,[29] but a significant proportion of patients (38–39% over median follow up of 36–54 months) progress to permanent AV block and become pacemaker-dependent when paced.[32]

Observational studies of outcome in paced patients during the early days of cardiac pacing suggested that pacing in complete AV block could improve survival to approach that of a similar age- and sex-matched group.[30] Mortality was higher in those with a history of myocardial infarction but not influenced by pre-pacing QRS duration or morphology, ventricular rate (dichotomized about 40/min) or whether AV block was intermittent or constant.[33] In a more recent study of patients aged ≥65 years, paced for symptomatic, high grade AV block, overall survival was less than expected for an age- and sex-matched cohort.[34] However, in patients aged <80 years without structural heart disease, survival was normal. Congestive heart failure, chronic obstructive pulmonary disease, age, syncope, insulin-dependent diabetes and male gender emerged as independent predictors of increased mortality. There have been no prospective randomized trials to assess the impact of pacing on survival but the high mortality of untreated complete AV block, the prevalence of symptoms, and the strength of the data from observational studies suggest that such a trial is neither ethical nor necessary. The vast majority of patients with complete AV block should be paced, whether or not they have symptoms. **Grade B**

Congenital complete AV block

The natural history and management of congenital complete AV block in infancy and childhood is beyond the scope of this review. In patients surviving to adulthood, the prognosis has previously been regarded as benign, based largely on retrospective studies of small series of patients.[35] More recent data concerning long-term follow up (7–30 years) of 102 patients with isolated congenital complete AV block, who survived without symptoms to the age of 15 years, suggest a less favorable outlook.[36] Stokes–Adams attacks occurred in 27 patients, of whom eight died (six during the first attack) and six others required cardiac resuscitation. All survivors received pacemakers. A further eight patients had repeated fainting spells requiring pacing and 27 others were paced for other reasons (fatigue, effort dyspnea, dizziness, ectopics during exercise, mitral regurgitation or slow ventricular rates). Of 40 patients followed for 30 years, only four remained asymptomatic without pacing. The only significant predictor of risk was QTc prolongation, which was seen in seven patients, all of whom had Stokes–Adams attacks and three of whom died. In contrast to previous studies, low ventricular rates, widened QRS complexes, poor chronotropic response to exercise and ectopics were not predictive of future Stokes–Adams attacks or death. These data appear to support the authors' recommendation of prophylactic pacing in adolescents and adults with congenital complete AV block, even without symptoms, notwithstanding the fact that a number of questions remain unanswered.[37] **Grade B**

Fascicular block

In asymptomatic subjects with unifascicular block (right bundle branch block, left anterior hemiblock or left posterior hemiblock), the risk of progression to high grade AV block is remote[38] and pacing is not indicated. In asymptomatic bifascicular block (left bundle branch block or right bundle branch block with left anterior or posterior hemiblock), the risk of progression to high grade AV block is in the region of 2% per annum. Prognosis is principally determined by the presence or absence of underlying structural heart disease and prophylactic pacing is not routinely indicated.[39] Progression to high grade AV block is more commonly seen in patients with a history of syncope but should not be presumed to be the cause without further assessment. If high grade AV block is documented, pacing is mandatory. When the cause of syncope remains unclear, an electrophysiology study may help to identify patients likely to benefit from pacemaker implantation. A prolonged HV interval >100 ms and His–Purkinje block during atrial pacing have high specificity for prediction of subsequent progression to high grade AV block.[40,41] Unfortunately, these are rare findings and thus of low sensitivity. Less marked HV prolongation (>70 ms) is more common but its significance is uncertain.[42] Sensitivity for disclosure of latent high grade AV block may be markedly enhanced by the use of intravenous disopyramide during the study but this is not advised in patients with impaired left ventricular function.[43] The electrophysiology study may also be of value to identify inducible ventricular tachycardia, which is a relatively common finding in patients with bundle branch block and a history of syncope.[44] This argues strongly against the empiric use of permanent pacing in this context. However, in patients with bifascicular block and a history of syncope for which no other cause is apparent despite thorough evaluation, including an electrophysiology study, empiric pacing may be the most expeditious course. This strategy is principally justified for relief of symptoms as pacing does not appear to influence mortality or the incidence of sudden death in this context.[39] **Grade B**

Atrioventricular and bundle branch block after myocardial infarction

Transient conduction disturbance is a relatively common complication of acute myocardial infarction. The acute management and indications for temporary cardiac pacing are beyond the scope of this review and will not be considered further. The long-term prognosis is principally determined by the extent of myocardial injury. When AV block complicates inferior myocardial infarction, it typically resolves within a few days and rarely persists beyond 2 or 3 weeks. In anterior infarction, however, AV block may reflect extensive septal necrosis and the prognosis is poor despite pacing.[45] Patients with high grade AV block persisting for more than 3 weeks after myocardial infarction should be considered for permanent pacing.

The occurrence of an intraventricular conduction disturbance (apart from isolated left anterior hemiblock) in patients with acute myocardial infarction identifies a group with poor short-term and long-term prognosis and an increased risk of sudden death.[46] The poor prognosis in this group, however, is mainly attributable to a high incidence of malignant ventricular arrhythmia, pump failure, and electromechanical dissociation, rather than progressive conduction disturbance. A prospective study of 50 patients randomized to pacing or control groups and followed for 5 years showed no significant difference in survival.[47] However, evidence from a retrospective multicenter study of patients with bundle branch block complicating myocardial infarction, indicates that transient high degree AV block during the acute phase is associated with a high incidence of recurrent AV block and sudden death that may be reduced by pacemaker implantation.[48,49] The risk appears to be particularly high in patients with right bundle branch block and left anterior hemiblock.[49,50] **Grade B**

Sino-atrial disease

Sino-atrial disease encompasses a wide spectrum of arrhythmia including sinus bradycardia, sinus arrest, sino-atrial block, sick sinus syndrome and the tachycardia–bradycardia syndrome in which paroxysmal atrial tachyarrhythmia alternates with bradycardia. The prognosis in sino-atrial disease is generally good unless myocardial ischemia, heart failure or systemic embolism are present.[51] Permanent pacing is indicated for the relief of symptoms that are due to bradycardia. Every effort should be made to establish a causal relationship by recording an ECG during symptoms although this may not always be possible. Occasionally, drugs needed to control tachyarrhythmia may cause or exacerbate bradycardia and pacing may be required to facilitate their continued use.

The first and only randomized trial to assess the efficacy of pacing in sick sinus syndrome has recently been reported.[52] One hundred and seven patients with symptomatic sick sinus syndrome were randomized to receive either no treatment, oral theophylline or permanent DDDR pacing. Patients were excluded in very severe cases, defined as symptomatic resting sinus rate <30/min, sinus pauses >3 s or heart failure refractory to treatment with ACE inhibitors and diuretics. During a mean follow up period of 19 months, both pacing and theophylline were associated with a lower incidence of heart failure compared with the untreated patients (3%, 3% and 17% respectively) but only pacing was associated with a significantly lower incidence of syncope (6%, 17% and 23% respectively). It is noteworthy that 14 of the 16 patients who were syncopal during follow up had a history of syncope at randomization. During follow up, 51% of patients in the control group and 42% in the theophylline group were withdrawn from the study due to syncope, overt heart failure, poorly tolerated paroxysmal tachyarrhythmia, patient wishes or drug side effects. There were no significant differences in NYHA class or symptom scores (fatigue, dizziness, and palpitation) between the groups either at baseline or after 3 months. The untreated controls showed subjective improvement, with a significant reduction of dizziness and a trend towards decreased fatigue. These findings were associated with significant increases in resting, mean and maximum heart rates, emphasizing the unpredictable natural history of the condition and the possibility of spontaneous improvement. Pacing remains the treatment of choice for patients with symptomatic sick sinus syndrome. In the absence of long-term follow up data to confirm efficacy and safety, theophylline or other pharmacologic means of chronotropic support cannot be recommended. **Grade A**

Pacing does not appear to improve survival in sino-atrial disease[53] and it is not generally indicated in asymptomatic patients. Such patients, however, should be followed closely to assess progression. Athletically trained subjects may have sinus rates as low as 30/min during sleep with pauses of almost 3 s.[54] These findings usually reflect high vagal tone and do not require pacing in the absence of symptoms. If lower rates or longer pauses are observed during sleep or if similar findings occur during the day, particularly if there is evidence of progression with time, prophylactic pacing may be justified on empiric grounds although there are no supportive data. **Grade B/C**

Mode selection in AV block and sinus node disease

AV block

The essential requirement in AV block is that the ventricle be paced. When sinus rhythm and chronotropic competence are preserved, dual chamber pacing with atrial tracking will ensure the maintenance of AV synchrony and physiologic rate adaptation. When sinus rhythm is absent or when chronotropic incompetence is present, an extrinsic sensor may be used to provide rate adaptation with either ventricular or dual chamber pacing, as appropriate.

Both dual chamber pacing[55–57] and adaptive rate single chamber pacing[58–60] have been shown to offer benefits in terms of improved hemodynamics, increased treadmill exercise tolerance and reduced symptoms when compared with single rate ventricular pacing in small randomized crossover trials. The mean patient age in most of these trials was younger than the typical paced population but similar benefits have recently been reported in patients aged 75 years or over.[61] Nonetheless, the long term clinical benefit of physiologic pacing in the elderly has been questioned.[12] Quality of life studies have yielded conflicting results although physiologic pacing does appear to offer advantages in terms of symptoms and there is considerable evidence of patient preference for physiologic modes.[62] Single chamber ventricular pacing is associated with an increased risk of pacemaker syndrome. The true incidence of this complication is unknown but estimated to be between 7 and 20%.[2] It has, however, been suggested that a subclinical form may be present in many apparently asymptomatic patients.[63] Data from a retrospective review of outcome in patients paced single or dual chamber has suggested that dual chamber pacing may confer a survival advantage in a subset of patients with congestive heart failure.[64] A more recent case–control study has confirmed this finding but showed no difference in overall survival.[65]

Sinus node disease

In isolated sino-atrial disease, rate support can be achieved by atrial, ventricular or dual chamber pacing. Small crossover studies comparing ventricular with dual chamber pacing have reported less favorable hemodynamics, worse symptomatology, and an increased risk of pacemaker syndrome.[62,66–68] Numerous retrospective studies also suggest that ventricular pacing is associated with an increased risk of atrial fibrillation, heart failure, and thromboembolism.[51,69] There is also evidence of increased mortality in ventricular paced patients.[70] Attention has been drawn to the confounding effect of selection bias on data derived almost exclusively from retrospective studies and the need for prospective randomized trials has been stressed.[71] A number of such trials have recently been completed and others are ongoing. These will be considered in the next section.

Randomized trials of pacemaker mode selection

The Danish Study

The first prospective randomized trial of pacemaker mode selection was reported from Denmark in 1994.[72] In this study, 225 patients with sick sinus syndrome were randomized to either AAI or VVI pacing and followed for a mean of 3·3 years. Neither the incidence of atrial fibrillation or stroke nor survival differed significantly between the two groups, although the incidence of a combined end point of stroke plus peripheral embolism was significantly lower in the atrial paced group. Only two of 115 patients in the VVI group required upgrade for severe pacemaker syndrome. Extended follow up of the same group of patients after a mean period of 5·5 years has subsequently been reported.[73] The previously identified benefits of atrial pacing were enhanced, with a significantly lower incidence of atrial fibrillation, thromboembolism and heart failure in the atrial paced group. All-cause mortality and mortality due to cardiovascular causes were also significantly lower in the atrial paced group. After adjustment for other pre-implant variables, there was a significant association between ventricular pacing and cardiovascular death but only a non-significant trend towards increased overall mortality. Only four of 110 patients in the atrial paced group developed second or third degree AV block, requiring pacemaker upgrade (0·6% per annum). Of these, two had right bundle branch block at the time of implant (as did four others in the atrial paced group who did not develop AV block). AV conduction, estimated as PQ interval and atrial stimulus-Q interval at atrial pacing rates of 100 and 120 min^{-1} remained stable during follow up.[74]

The Pacemaker Selection in the Elderly (PASE) Study

This trial randomized 407 patients, aged 65 or older (mean age 76 years), to ventricular or dual chamber pacing.[75] This was a *mode* randomization and all patients received DDDR pacing systems. The group included 175 patients with sinus node disease, 201 patients with AV block and 31 patients with other diagnoses. The study was powered to assess differences in health-related quality of life. As would be expected, there was marked improvement in quality of life (SF-36) after pacemaker implantation but there were no significant differences between groups in relation to pacing mode. Analysis of prespecified subgroups showed modest benefits in some quality of life domains and cardiovascular functional status (Specific Activity Scale) favoring dual chamber pacing in patients with sinus node disease. Similarly, there were trends of borderline statistical significance in clinical outcomes favoring dual chamber pacing in patients with sinus node disease but not in those with AV block (mean follow up 18 months). It is noteworthy that 26% of the patients randomized to ventricular pacing crossed over to dual chamber pacing because of symptoms attributed to pacemaker syndrome. Whilst potentially significant in itself, the high crossover rate confounds interpretation of the data, particularly in respect of clinical outcomes. The investigators reviewed the clinical, hemodynamic and electrophysiological data in the group randomized to VVIR pacing, to determine what factors might predict intolerance of VVIR pacing sufficient to prompt crossover to the DDDR mode. In a multivariate analysis, a decrease in systolic blood pressure to <110 mmHg during ventricular pacing at the time of pacemaker implantation ($P = 0.001$), use of β blockers at the time of randomization ($P = 0.01$) and non-ischemic cardiomyopathy ($P = 0.04$) were the only variables that predicted crossover.[76]

The Canadian Trial of Physiologic Pacing (CTOPP)

In the largest trial reported to date, 2568 patients aged 18 years or older (mean age 73 years), with either AV block or sinus node disease, were randomized to receive either a ventricular (VVI/R) or a physiologic pacemaker.[77] In the physiologic arm, the investigator was allowed to choose either an atrial (AAI/R) or dual chamber (DDD/R) system. Adaptive rate pacing was used in both groups if chronotropic incompetence was evident and in patients with complete AV block randomized to receive ventricular pacing. Approximately 60% of patients had AV block and 40% had sinus node disease. Over a mean follow up of 3 years there was no significant difference in the primary outcome of cardiovascular death or stroke (VVI/R 5·5% per annum v physiologic 4·9% per annum; relative risk reduction c 9·4%; 95% CI 10–25·7; $P = 0.33$). Neither was there any significant difference in all-cause mortality or inhospital admission for heart failure. There was, however, a significant, albeit modest, reduction in atrial fibrillation (defined as an episode lasting more than 15 minutes) associated with physiologic pacing (VVI/R 6·6% per annum v physiologic 5·3% per annum; relative risk reduction 18·0%; 95% CI 0·3–32·6; $P = 0.05$), the difference starting to emerge after 2 years' follow up. The difference was greater in respect of chronic atrial fibrillation, which was defined as AF still present 1 week after the index episode (VVI/R 3·84% per annum v physiologic 2·80% per annum; relative risk reduction 27·1%; 95% CI 5·5–43·6; $P = 0.016$).[78] Perioperative complications were more common with physiologic pacing (VVI/R 3·8% v physiologic 9·0%; $P < 0.001$) mainly in relation to the pacing lead(s). There was no difference in functional capacity, assessed by a 6 minute walk test at 6 month follow up, even in those patients (c 37%) who were pacemaker dependent.[79] The investigators attempted to identify baseline characteristics that might predict benefit from physiologic pacing on the risk of stroke or death due to cardiovascular causes. There was a trend

suggesting that younger patients (<74 years) might benefit from physiologic pacing.

Subgroup analysis of the CTOPP data suggests that the benefits of physiologic pacing may be influenced by pacemaker dependency.[80] This was assessed in 87% of the enrolled patients by recording the unpaced heart rate at the first follow up visit (2–8 months postimplant). In patients with unpaced heart rates $\leq 60 \text{ min}^{-1}$, the incidence of cardiovascular death or stroke was lower with physiologic pacing (VVI/R 6·4% per annum v physiologic 4·1% per annum; relative risk reduction 35·5%; 95% CI 12–53). By contrast, the treatment effect of physiologic pacing was slightly negative in patients with unpaced heart rates $>60 \text{ min}^{-1}$ (VVI/R 4·1% per annum v physiologic 4·3% per annum; relative risk reduction −1·9%; 95% CI 50–31). The difference in treatment effect between the two groups was of only borderline significance ($P = 0.058$) but the fact that the 95% confidence interval in the group with unpaced heart rates $\leq 60 \text{ min}^{-1}$ does not include zero, suggests a qualitative interaction between treatment effect and pacemaker dependency in respect of the primary outcome. Significant subgroup effects were also observed for the outcomes of cardiovascular death and total mortality but not for stroke/emboli or hospitalization for congestive heart failure. Although the reduction in relative risk of atrial fibrillation with physiologic pacing was larger in the group with unpaced heart rates $\leq 60 \text{ min}^{-1}$ than in the group with unpaced heart rates $>60 \text{ min}^{-1}$, the difference was not statistically significant ($P = 0.22$) due to a modest reduction in the latter group.

A quality of life substudy in 269 patients also showed the influence of pacemaker dependency.[81] Quality of life, assessed by a disease specific instrument, the Quality of Life Assessment Package (QLAP), and the generic SF-36, improved between implant and 6 month follow up. The improvement was similar in patients with ventricular and physiologic pacing when all subjects were considered. However, when only pacemaker-dependent subjects were considered, improvements were greater with physiologic than with ventricular pacing although the difference was only detected with the disease specific QLAP and not with the generic SF-36.

The Mode Selection Trial (MOST)

This large trial was designed to assess the benefits of rate adaptive, dual chamber pacing compared with rate adaptive, single chamber, ventricular pacing in patients with sick sinus syndrome.[82,83] Two thousand and ten patients aged ≥ 21 years were implanted with a DDDR pacing system and the pacing mode was randomized to VVIR or DDDR. The primary end point was death or non-fatal stroke. Secondary outcomes included health-related quality of life and cost effectiveness, atrial fibrillation and the development of pacemaker syndrome. During a median follow up of

33·1 months, there was no significant difference in the incidence of death (VVIR 21%; DDDR 20%) or stroke (VVIR 5%; DDDR 4%). However, the DDDR group did have a lower incidence of atrial fibrillation (VVIR 27%; DDDR 21%). Heart failure scores were also significantly improved but this did not result in a lower incidence of hospitalization for heart failure (VVIR 12%; DDDR 10%). Quality of life (assessed by the SF-36 questionnaire) was significantly better in the DDDR group. Crossover from VVIR to DDDR mode occurred in 31·4% (18·3% for pacemaker syndrome).

The Pacemaker Atrial Tachycardia (PAC-A-TACH) Trial

The Pacemaker Atrial Tachycardia (PAC-A-TACH) trial assessed the effect of pacing modality on atrial tachyarrhythmia recurrence in patients with the tachycardia–bradycardia syndrome.[84] This was a mode randomization study in 198 patients (median age 72 years), all of whom received dual chamber, rate adaptive pacemakers programmed to either VVIR or DDDR pacing. After a median of 23·7 months follow up, 44% of patients crossed over from VVIR to DDDR (due to pacemaker syndrome in 28% and atrial tachyarrhythmia in 13%) and 9% crossed over from DDDR to VVIR (due to recurrent atrial tachyarrhythmia in 7% and atrial lead problems in 2%). Intention-to-treat analysis showed no significant difference in atrial tachyarrhythmia recurrence rates at 1 year (VVIR 43%; DDDR 48%; $P=0·09$). Quality of life was assessed at randomization and at 6 month follow up using the Duke Activity Status Index and SF-36. Perhaps unsurprisingly, in view of the high crossover rate, there was no significant difference between the groups at 6 months in either intention-to-treat analysis or on-treatment analysis of those patients remaining in randomized mode.[85] Mortality, a secondary outcome, was noted to be significantly higher in the VVIR group and the trial was stopped after follow up of approximately 2 years in all patients. Cumulative mortality was 21% in the VVIR group and 5% in the DDDR group ($P<0·001$). Pacing mode (risk ratio 4·3; 95% CI 1·6–11·4; $P=0·004$) and prior history of MI (risk ratio 3·1; 95% CI 1·4–6·7; $P=0·006$) were identified as independent predictors of mortality.[86]

Ongoing trials

Three additional mode selection trials are ongoing. The United Kingdom Pacing and Cardiovascular Events (UKPACE) trial aims to compare the clinical impact and cost utility of single and dual chamber pacing in elderly patients (≥70 years) with high-grade AV block.[87] Two thousand and twenty-one patients have been randomized to receive either single (randomly assigned to VVI or VVIR) or dual chamber pacemakers. The primary end point is all-cause mortality.

Secondary outcomes include quality of life, exercise capacity, cardiovascular events and cost utility. Follow up is for a minimum of 3 years and will conclude in September 2002.

The Systematic Trial of Pacing to Prevent Atrial Fibrillation (STOP-AF) aims to assess the ability of physiologic pacing to prevent atrial fibrillation in patients aged ≥18 years with sick sinus syndrome.[88] All patients are implanted with a dual chamber pacemaker and randomized to programming in either atrial-based (AAI or DDD) or ventricular pacing modes Recruitment was closed after 227 patients had been enrolled.[89] The study, which uses sequential trial methodology to allow greater power with a limited sample size, includes an adaptive rate arm for patients with chronotropic incompetence. The primary end point is permanent atrial fibrillation resistant to DC cardioversion. Secondary outcomes include congestive heart failure, pacemaker syndrome, change of mode for lead problems, and death.

The DANPACE study aims to examine the relative merits of single lead atrial pacing (AAIR) and dual chamber pacing (DDDR) in 1900 patients aged ≥18 years with sick sinus syndrome with bradycardia (including tachycardia–bradycardia syndrome).[90] The primary outcome measure will be all-cause mortality. Secondary outcomes will include cardiovascular mortality, atrial fibrillation, thromboembolism, quality of life and economic evaluation. Recruitment is scheduled to be completed by December 2005, with follow up to December 2007.

Comment and recommendations

The results of the prospective randomized trials that have been reported to date, suggest that the clinical benefits of physiologic or dual chamber pacing may previously have been overstated. There is, however, consistent evidence of a modest but significant reduction in atrial fibrillation, particularly in its chronic form. It might be anticipated that this would translate, over time, into a lower incidence of stroke, thromboembolism and death. This was observed in the extended follow up of the Danish study but not in PASE, CTOPP or MOST. It may be relevant that significant differences in the occurrence of atrial fibrillation only occurred after 2 years in CTOPP, suggesting that the mean 3 year follow up may have been insufficient for differences in these other outcomes to emerge. For this reason, the CTOPP investigators embarked on an extended follow up for an additional 3 years, which concluded during 2001. The preliminary results show a persistent reduction of AF with physiologic pacing (20·1% relative risk reduction; $P=0·009$) but no difference in cardiovascular death, stroke or total mortality after a mean follow up of 6 years.[91]

When considering sinus node disease, it is important to note that the Danish study was the only one to use single-lead atrial pacing as the sole physiologic comparator. PASE and MOST used exclusively dual chamber devices and in CTOPP only 5·2% of the patients randomized to physiologic pacing received an atrial pacemaker. Preservation of synchronized left and right ventricular activation with atrial pacing may confer benefits that are not assured with dual chamber pacing, even when careful attention is given to optimal programming.[92] The presence of a, generally redundant, ventricular lead with dual chamber pacing might also be deleterious. The DANPACE study should ultimately provide the necessary data to clarify the relative merits of atrial and dual chamber pacing in sinus node disease.

With regard to quality of life, the advantage of physiologic pacing appears modest, as assessed by standard measures. However, interpretation of the data is complicated by the divergent estimates of mode intolerance, as judged by the investigator, between those trials in which the mode randomization was achieved by software programming (PASE, PAC-A-TACH and MOST) and those in which it was achieved by implantation of different hardware (the Danish study and CTOPP). Each design has strengths and weaknesses[93] but software randomization trials are more vulnerable to the effect of investigator bias. In the software randomization trials, crossover rates ranged from 26% to 44%, whereas in the hardware randomization trials, they did not exceed 5%. The significance of these disparities is uncertain. Further data will be forthcoming from the UKPACE trial, which includes detailed assessment of quality of life and the incidence of the pacemaker syndrome.

The completed and ongoing trials include a cumulative total of over 7000 patients. In order to determine the true value of physiologic pacing and to identify patient sub-groups that may derive particular benefit, a meta-analysis of the pooled data is being planned. The data presented to date, suggest a modest benefit in favor of dual chamber pacing, which must be weighed against a higher perioperative complication rate. Cost utility will be a further consideration that may influence mode selection and relevant economic data from CTOPP, MOST and UKPACE are awaited. **Grade A**

Pending the outcome of the ongoing trials and further analysis of those that have already reported, continued adherence to current guidelines (see Table 42.2) is recommended. Current guidelines[11] recommend the avoidance of single chamber ventricular pacing. In AV block, dual chamber pacing is the preferred mode, with rate adaptation if there is evidence of chronotropic incompetence. In sino-atrial disease, atrial-based pacing, in some form, is preferable. When AV conduction is intact, single chamber adaptive rate atrial (AAIR) pacing is regarded as the optimal mode, as it preserves both atrioventricular synchrony and a normal ventricular activation pattern. Retrospective analysis of pooled data from 28 studies has shown a low risk of subsequent AV block (0·6% per annum)[94] and this is supported by data from the Danish study.[74] Dual chamber pacing may thus be unnecessary for many patients[95] although some

physicians prefer to implant a DDDR pacing system with programming to AAIR mode, a mode conversion option or AV search hysteresis.[96] When a single chamber atrial pacing system is proposed, assessment of AV conduction at the time of implant to ensure preservation of 1:1 conduction during atrial pacing at 140/min is customary and prudent. When AV block coexists with sino-atrial disease, dual chamber pacing in DDDR mode is recommended. In patients with a history of paroxysmal atrial tachyarrhythmia, DDI pacing is preferable to avoid rapid ventricular tracking. The recent introduction of mode-switching pacemakers capable of switching from DDD/DDDR to DDI/DDIR mode on detection of atrial tachyarrhythmia has offered an attractive alternative.

New indications for pacing

Neurocardiogenic syncope

Neurocardiogenic syncope describes the clinical syndromes of syncope resulting from inappropriate autonomic responses, manifested as abnormalities in the control of peripheral vascular resistance and heart rate.[97] It is thought to account for the largest proportion of faints in clinical practice. The most common forms are carotid sinus syndrome and vasovagal syncope but other related syndromes include cough, deglutition, and micturition syncope. The pathophysiologic mechanisms are not fully understood but carotid sinus massage[98,99] and tilt-table testing[100] have emerged as useful diagnostic tools in carotid sinus syndrome and vasovagal syncope respectively, enabling abnormal reflex responses to be categorized as cardioinhibitory (asystole >3 s, bradycardia or AV block), vasodepressor (fall in systolic blood pressure >50 mmHg) or mixed. This has invited assessment of the utility of cardiac pacing which might be expected to benefit patients with predominantly cardioinhibitory or mixed responses.

Carotid sinus syndrome

Early reports of pacing in carotid sinus syndrome confirmed its efficacy in some patients but persistent symptoms were seen in those in whom there was a significant vasodepressor response or hypotension during ventricular pacing.[101] The latter was improved by AV sequential pacing and it was suggested that this was the appropriate mode in patients with mixed responses. Attention has been drawn to the variable natural history of the condition, which may remit spontaneously, and the importance of a control group when evaluating therapy has been emphasized.[102] A prospective randomized trial of pacing in patients with severe carotid sinus syndrome has subsequently been reported.[103] Sixty patients were randomized to pacing (VVI in 18 and DDD in 14 patients) or no therapy (28 patients). During a mean follow up of 36 months, syncope recurred in 16 (57%) of the non-paced group and in only three (9%) of the paced group. Nineteen patients (68%) in the non-paced group were eventually paced because of the severity of symptoms. Pacing is now the treatment of choice in all but the mildest forms of carotid sinus syndrome. Recent evidence suggests that carotid sinus syndrome is underdiagnosed and that comprehensive assessment of patients presenting with syncope, dizziness or falls may identify a significant number of otherwise unrecognized patients who may benefit from pacing.[104]

In the Syncope And Falls in the Elderly – Pacing And Carotid sinus Evaluation (SAFE PACE) trial, 24 264 patients with falls or syncope were identified from a total of 71 299 emergency room attendees aged ≥50 years during a 29 month period.[105] Patients with evident extrinsic or medical explanations for falling and those with cognitive impairment were excluded, leaving a residuum of 3384 non-accidental fallers. Of these, 1624 consented to and underwent carotid sinus massage, yielding 257 patients with cardioinhibitory or mixed carotid sinus hypersensitivity. One hundred and seventy five patients (mean age 73 years) were randomized to pacing or no pacing and followed for one year, to test the hypothesis that dual chamber pacing, with a rate-drop response algorithm, might reduce the frequency of further falls. Paced patients were significantly less likely to fall (odds ratio 0·42; 95% CI 0·23–0·75) than controls. Syncope and injurious events were also less frequent in the paced group.

SAFE-PACE 2[106] is a larger scale, multicenter, randomized controlled trial that is currently in progress, to further evaluate the preliminary observations from SAFE PACE in a wider cultural setting. Patients are eligible if they have had two or more unexplained falls (± up to one syncopal episode) and if they have a cardioinhibitory response to carotid sinus massage. Two hundred and twenty six patients will be randomized to receive either a pacemaker or an implantable loop recorder with long-term diagnostic capability, which will clarify the relationship between symptoms and arrhythmia in the non-paced patients. The primary outcome is the number of patients who fall during a 2 year follow up period. Secondary outcomes include frequency of falls, dizziness and presyncope, health and mental status (as perceived by the patient and the informant), injury rates, use of healthcare facilities, hospital admission, change in residential circumstances and cognitive function.

Comment and recommendations

Recurrent syncope caused by carotid sinus hypersensitivity is a class I indication for pacing and recurrent syncope without clear provocative events and with CICSH is a class IIa indication for pacing (see Table 42.1). Further data are required to clarify the role of pacing in patients with a history of recurrent falls (without clear evidence of syncope) and CICSH. For the time being, it should be regarded as experimental and its use should be restricted to the confines of randomized clinical trials. **Grade A/C**

Vasovagal syndrome

Pacing has also been evaluated in the so-called "malignant" form of vasovagal syndrome, characterized by recurrent syncope with only brief or absent prodromal symptoms. Evidence from several studies using temporary pacing during tilt-table testing indicates that pacing rarely prevents vasovagal syncope. The limited efficacy of pacing reflects the fact that hypotension precedes the onset of bradycardia in most patients. However, dual chamber pacing does attenuate the evolution of the final and most extreme degrees of hypotension and may thereby prolong the symptomatic presyncopal period in selected patients with a documented cardioinhibitory component.[107] A retrospective review of 37 patients receiving predominantly dual chamber pacemakers, followed for a mean of 50·2 months, reported symptomatic improvement in 89% with 62% remaining free of syncope and 27% being completely asymptomatic. The collective syncopal burden was reduced from 136 to 11 episodes per year.[108] This was an uncontrolled study but a number of multicenter prospective randomized trials have subsequently been initiated.

The North American Vasovagal Pacemaker Study[109,110] randomized patients with a history of frequent syncope (≥6 lifetime episodes) and a positive (cardioinhibitory) tilt test to receive either DDI pacing with a pacemaker incorporating a specialized rate-drop sensing algorithm, or no pacing. The rate-drop sensing algorithm is designed to detect the characteristic pattern of onset of bradycardia that is seen in vasovagal syndrome. The fall in heart rate is typically more marked than occurs with natural diurnal fluctuation yet less precipitous than that seen at the onset of complete AV block or asystole. On detection of a characteristic rate drop, pacing commences with a high initial intervention rate that gradually decreases.[111] It had been intended to enroll 284 patients, but the North American study was stopped towards the end of a 2 year pilot phase (May 1997) due to substantial benefit in the paced group. By that time, 54 patients had been enrolled and randomized, in equal numbers, to receive pacing or no pacing. Syncope recurred in 22% of patients who were paced compared with 70% of those who were not. This corresponds to a relative risk reduction of 85·4% (95% CI 59·7–94·7; $2P = 0.000022$). Mean time to syncope was 112 days in the paced patients and 54 days in the non-paced patients. There was, however, no significant effect on presyncope, which was reported by 63% of paced patients and 74% of non-paced patients. The relatively small study size, resulting from early termination, resulted in some imbalance in important baseline characteristics. For example, the median number of previous syncopal episodes (lifetime experience) was lower in the paced group than in the non-paced group (14 *v* 35) as was the median number of episodes in the previous year (3 *v* 6). However, the authors report that the relative risk reduction was essentially unchanged when the analysis was adjusted for differences in baseline variables.

The Vasovagal International Study (VASIS) Group has subsequently reported a multicentre European trial of similar design.[112] Forty-two patients with at least three syncopal episodes in the preceding 2 years and a positive cardio inhibitory response to tilt testing were randomized to DDI pacing with rate hysteresis ($n=19$) or no pacing ($n=23$). Recruitment was slower than anticipated and there appears to have been a bias towards the inclusion of more severely affected patients. Syncope recurred in only one (5%) of the paced patients but in 14 (61%) of the unpaced patients ($P=0\cdot0006$). The median time to first syncope in the unpaced group was 5 months.

The Syncope Diagnosis and Treatment (SYDIT) study assessed the relative efficacy of dual chamber pacing with a rate-drop sensing algorithm and pharmacologic therapy with atenolol.[113] Patients were eligible if they had at least three syncopal episodes in the preceding 2 years and a positive response to tilt testing (syncope with relative bradycardia). The study was terminated after 93 patients had been enrolled, as an interim analysis showed a significant effect in favor of pacing. Syncope recurred in only 4·3% of the paced group (after a median of 390 days) compared with 25·5% of the pharmacologically treated group (after a median of 135 days), giving an odds ratio of 0·133 (95% CI 0·028–0·632; $P=0\cdot004$).

Less encouraging results have recently been presented from the second Vasovagal Pacemaker Study (VPS II).[114] The inclusion criteria were similar to those of the first VPS but in contrast to both that study and VASIS, it was double blinded. All patients received a pacemaker and were randomized to DDD pacing with a rate-drop response algorithm ($n=48$) or no pacing (ODO mode) ($n=52$). During a 6 month follow up, syncope recurred in 30% of the paced group, compared with 40% of the non-paced group. This equates to a relative risk reduction of 28·7% but the difference was not statistically significant (one-sided $P=0\cdot153$). However, the event rate in the non-paced group was lower than expected and the study thus lacked sufficient power to draw a firm conclusion.

Comment and recommendations

The impressive results from the first VPS, VASIS and SYDIT studies require cautious interpretation. Enrolled patients had a substantial burden of previous syncope and a positive tilt-test with syncope (or presyncope) and relative bradycardia. There was, in addition, a suggestion of selection bias towards more severely affected and older patients. The applicability of the results to less severely affected patients and those of younger age is uncertain and these concerns are highlighted by the inconclusive results of VPS II. The accumulated data do, however, suggest that pacing should be considered in patients with severe symptoms refractory to conservative measures and drug therapy. The contrasting results of the second VPS raise the possibility of a placebo effect associated with the pacemaker implantation procedure in the earlier

trials. Further clarification of the role of pacing may come from the Vasovagal Syncope and Pacing (SYNPACE) trial, in which every patient will receive a pacemaker and then be randomized to pacing "on" or "off" until the first recurrence of syncope or the end of follow up (at least 12 months).[115] Further data are also required to clarify the relative efficacy of pharmacologic therapy, such as β blockers, disopyramide, scopolamine, alpha agonists, selective serotonin reuptake inhibitors and others, which although largely disappointing, have been of benefit to some patients.[116] **Grade A**

Hypertrophic cardiomyopathy

The ability of pacing at the right ventricular apex to reduce the left ventricular outflow tract (LVOT) gradient in patients with hypertrophic obstructive cardiomyopathy has been recognized for over 30 years.[117] The benefits are thought to be due to eccentric or abnormal activation of the septum which may increase the LVOT diameter and decrease systolic anterior movement of the mitral valve during systole. A resurgence of interest was prompted by the development of sophisticated dual chamber pacemakers able to optimize ventricular filling by preservation of AV synchrony and maximize ventricular capture by the programming of a short AV delay. In some cases, drug therapy or ablation of the AV node may be required to prolong intrinsic AV conduction for maintenance of optimal LA-LV timing, whilst permitting maximal right ventricular pre-excitation by pacing.

Initial clinical studies showed encouraging results over the short and medium term with decreased symptoms and improved exercise capacity associated with reductions of LVOT gradient in the region of 60%.[118–121] An intriguing finding was the observation, in some series, of geometrical and functional changes, suggesting that left ventricular remodeling may occur after prolonged pacing. Decreased thickness of the anterior septum and the anterolateral wall of the left ventricle have been reported, with persistence of at least partial gradient reduction on pacemaker inhibition, for a period related to the duration of pacing.[122–124]

Three prospective randomized trials have subsequently been completed. All used a similar design with blinded crossover between active (DDD) and inactive (AAI backup at 30/min) pacing modes after 3 months.

A study performed at the Mayo Clinic[125] enrolled 21 patients with severe symptoms, refractory to drug therapy. The LVOT gradient decreased to a mean of 55 mmHg during DDD pacing, compared with 76 mmHg at baseline and 83 mmHg during the AAI phase. Quality of life scores and exercise duration during DDD pacing were significantly improved from baseline but not significantly different from those during the AAI phase. Overall, 63% of patients had symptomatic improvement during DDD pacing but 42% also improved during the AAI phase. In 5%, symptoms were worse during DDD pacing. The symptomatic improvement during the AAI phase suggests that there is an important placebo effect associated with pacemaker implantation, underscoring the importance of randomized trials in assessing this form of treatment.

The European Pacing In Cardiomyopathy (PIC) study reported similar findings in a larger group of 83 similarly selected patients.[126] It was, however, a prerequisite for enrollment that patients had a reduction in peak pressure gradient of >30 mmHg during an acute trial of dual chamber pacing. LVOT gradient decreased to a mean of 30 mmHg during DDD pacing compared with 59 mmHg at baseline. Exercise duration was not significantly increased, except for a subgroup of patients with more severely limited exercise tolerance (<10 minutes of the Bruce protocol) during the inactive (AAI backup) phase. Dyspnea, angina and functional class improved during active pacing compared with the inactive phase and 95% of patients preferred pacing. A placebo effect was once again seen, with significant improvement in symptoms compared to baseline even during the inactive AAI backup phase.[126,127] Subsequent activation of pacing, however, resulted in significant improvement in symptoms and quality of life scores and, conversely, inactivation resulted in significant deterioration. Following the crossover phase, patients remained in their preferred mode for 6 months and were re-evaluated one year after the baseline assessment. Seventy-six patients opted for active pacing. The observed gradient reduction was sustained at 1 year, with further improvement in symptoms already favorably influenced and in some additional quality of life domains.[128,129]

The Multicenter Study of Pacing Therapy for Hypertrophic Cardiomyopathy (M-PATHY) randomized 44 patients (mean age 53 years) with severe refractory symptoms to 3 months each of active (DDD) and inactive (AAI backup at 30/min) pacing in a double-blind crossover study design.[130] After 6 months, all patients were offered an additional 6 months of active pacing in an uncontrolled and unblinded fashion. In the crossover phase, there were no significant differences in subjective or objective measures of symptoms or exercise capacity including NYHA functional class, quality of life, treadmill exercise time or peak oxygen consumption between active and inactive pacing. As in previous studies, however, many patients reported symptomatic improvement after pacemaker implantation suggesting a potent placebo effect. After 6 months of unblinded pacing, functional class and quality of life were improved compared with baseline ($P<0.01$) but peak oxygen consumption was unchanged. Left ventricular outflow tract gradient decreased with active pacing from a mean of 82 mmHg to 48 mmHg ($P<0.001$) but there was marked variability in response between patients. The gradient was decreased in 57% of patients but unchanged or increased in 43%. In contrast to reports from earlier studies, there was no evidence of remodeling as assessed by change in left ventricular wall thickness. Analysis of individual patient data showed that all of the six patients who completed the study and showed clinical benefit were aged 65 years or older.

Comment and recommendations

The role of dual chamber pacing in the management of patients with hypertrophic obstructive cardiomyopathy remains controversial. The accumulated data from the various studies suggest that pacing cannot be considered as primary or routine treatment. It may benefit some patients with significant symptoms refractory to drug therapy and obviate or delay the need for septal ablation or surgery but there is no evidence that it reduces the risk of sudden death or alters the long-term clinical course. A trial of pacing is certainly an option to consider in patients at high operative risk, particularly if elderly, before proceeding to surgery and in those for whom expert surgery is unavailable. Although some studies have shown a correlation of gradient reduction during temporary dual-chamber pacing with that observed during long-term follow up, the acute hemodynamic response is not a reliable predictor of symptomatic or functional improvement and temporary pacing studies are thus of little value in patient selection.[121,122,130] **Grade A**

Dilated cardiomyopathy

Conventional pacing

During the past decade, the use of dual chamber pacing in patients with heart failure but no bradyarrhythmic indication for pacing has been extensively explored. This was initially prompted by the suggestion that dual chamber pacing with a short AV delay might improve cardiac function in dilated cardiomyopathy by improving the relationship between atrial and ventricular systole, thereby decreasing presystolic, mitral and tricuspid regurgitation and increasing ventricular filling time.[131] Initial hemodynamic and clinical studies yielded encouraging results[132,133] but others failed to show any significant benefit.[134,135] It might be anticipated that patients with first-degree heart block would be most likely to benefit and this has been confirmed in hemodynamic[136] and short-term clinical studies.[137] Other criteria that may predict benefit from short AV delay pacing in this context include prolonged QRS duration, functional mitral regurgitation ≥450 ms, ventricular filling time <200 ms and early cessation of transmitral flow with concomitant diastolic mitral regurgitation on Doppler echocardiography.[138,139] During temporary pacing, responders will have an increase in systolic blood pressure and an increase in mitral regurgitation velocity (indicating a higher left ventricular systolic pressure and lower left atrial pressure), but despite these findings, the clinical outcome with pacing cannot be predicted with certainty.[139]

Alternative and multisite pacing

Recognition that pacing at the right ventricular apex is associated with an abnormal ventricular activation pattern that might offset the advantage gained from the restoration of AV synchrony, prompted the assessment of alternative pacing sites within the right ventricle. Some investigators found acute hemodynamic benefit with pacing of the right side of the interventricular septum at an optimal AV delay,[140] whereas others, pacing the septal wall of the right ventricular outflow tract, did not.[141] A 3 month crossover trial in 16 patients with atrial fibrillation or flutter and AV block (post-ablation or spontaneous), showed no symptomatic or hemodynamic benefit from right ventricular outflow tract pacing compared with apical pacing.[142] The acute hemodynamic effect of combined pacing at two right ventricular sites (apex and outflow tract) has also been assessed.[143] No significant benefit was observed despite narrowing of the QRS. It has been suggested that individualized selection of the optimal septal pacing site (to minimize the QRS duration) might prove more effective.[144] Encouraging results have recently been reported with permanent His-bundle pacing. Significant improvement in hemodynamic function and NYHA class were observed during a mean 2 year follow up in a group of patients with chronic atrial fibrillation and severe dilated cardiomyopathy.[145] This technique requires further validation in a prospective controlled study.

Cardiac resynchronization therapy (CRT)

Recent interest has focused on the use of three or four chamber pacing with synchronized biventricular activation in an atrial tracking mode with optimized AV delay, particularly in patients with abnormalities of AV or intraventricular conduction. Biatrial synchronization may also be used in the presence of interatrial conduction delay. Up to 40% of patients with severe heart failure have intraventricular conduction delay.[146] This results in asynchronous contraction of the left and right ventricles, which may adversely affect hemodynamic function. CRT aims to reverse these changes by resynchronizing left and right ventricular activation and by ensuring AV synchrony with an optimal AV delay if sinus rhythm is preserved. The potential hemodynamic benefit of biventricular pacing was first described in 1983[147] but it was not until 1994 that the clinical application of the technique was reported in a patient with severe drug-refractory congestive heart failure.[148] Early case reports documented short-term clinical and hemodynamic improvement in patients with class III and IV heart failure using three or four chamber atriobiventricular pacing.[148–150] Acute hemodynamic studies have demonstrated decreased pulmonary capillary wedge pressure and increased peak LV dP/dt, systolic blood pressure and cardiac index during biventricular pacing.[150–154] Similar or greater improvements in some parameters were also reported with LV pacing alone.[151,153,154] The early studies of biventricular pacing used an epicardial pacing lead, implanted by limited thoracotomy or thoracoscopy, to pace the left

ventricle, with a standard endocardial lead in the right ventricle. This approach has been superseded by the development of a technique for pacing the left ventricle by means of a lead introduced transvenously via the coronary sinus, with the tip located in one of the posterior or lateral cardiac veins overlying the left ventricular free wall.[155] A coronary sinus angiogram is often used to create an anatomical map to guide placement of the specialized leads that have been developed for this type of pacing.[156]

Non-randomized studies of CRT

Encouraging preliminary data regarding the clinical utility of CRT were reported from two non-randomized studies. The InSync study[157] was an uncontrolled safety and efficacy study of synchronized biventricular pacing using a purpose designed pacing system. The device used incorporated a Y-adaptor, offering pacing channels for the right atrium, the right ventricle and the left ventricle, the latter being paced transvenously via the coronary sinus and cardiac veins. The study included 81 patients (mean age 66 years) with symptomatic cardiac decompensation, NYHA class III ($n = 43$) or class IV ($n = 25$), refractory to medical therapy, QRS duration >150 ms, ejection fraction <35% and LV end-diastolic diameter (EDD) >60 mm. Implantation was technically successful in 84% of patients with a low requirement for re-intervention. There were significant improvements at 1 and 3 month follow up (compared with baseline) in NYHA functional class, quality of life (Minnesota Living with Heart Failure Score) and distance covered during a 6 minute walk. There were, however, seven deaths (including four sudden deaths) between 11 and 127 days post-implant. Follow up to 1 year has subsequently been reported and confirmed sustained clinical benefit in the survivors.[158]

The French pilot study experience (1994–1997) comprised a series of 50 patients (mean age 68 years) with refractory class III ($n = 26$) or class IV ($n = 34$) heart failure, EF<35%, LV EDD >60 mm and QRS duration >150 ms.[159] Mean follow up was 15·4 months (range 1–48 months). There were 20 deaths in this series but with only two exceptions, these patients were in NYHA class IV at entry (one third of the total cohort were in a terminal phase, requiring permanent IV inotropic support). Deaths were classified as being due to progressive pump failure ($n = 11$), sudden cardiac death ($n = 6$) or non-cardiac cause ($n = 3$). Significant improvements during follow up were reported in functional status, exercise tolerance (in the 16 patients able to exercise at baseline) and ejection fraction.

Randomized trials of CRT

A number of randomized clinical trials have been initiated in Europe and the USA to assess further the efficacy of CRT in dilated cardiomyopathy.

The Pacing Therapy in Congestive Heart Failure (PATH-CHF) Trial – The PATH-CHF trial, was a single-blind randomized, crossover controlled trial designed to evaluate the effects of pacing on acute hemodynamic function and to assess chronic clinical benefit in patients with NYHA class III or IV congestive heart failure despite optimal medical therapy.[160] Patients were required to have a QRS duration ≥120 ms and a PR interval ≥150 ms. An epicardial lead was attached to the apex or midlateral segment of the left ventricle via a limited thoracotomy and endocardial leads were sited in the right atrial appendage and right ventricle. During the acute phase of the study, right and left univentricular pacing were compared with biventricular pacing, at a variety of pre-selected AV delays, using a randomized crossover design. Overall, biventricular and LV pacing increased LV dP/dt and pulse pressure more than right ventricular pacing. LV pacing increased LV dP/dt more than biventricular pacing.[153] Pacing site had a greater influence on hemodynamics than the AV delay. During the chronic phase of the study, 42 patients were randomized to either atriobiventricular pacing or the best atriouniventricular mode (determined during the acute phase) for a 4 week period. This was followed by a 4 week wash-out phase without pacing and a further 4 weeks in the alternate mode. Compared with baseline, active pacing showed significant benefits in terms of oxygen consumption at peak exercise and at anaerobic threshold and distance covered during a 6 minute walk (the primary end points).[161] Quality of life, assessed by the Minnesota Living with Heart Failure questionnaire, and NYHA functional class were also significantly improved. There was evidence of a placebo or carry-over effect, in that improvements during the first phase of active pacing were not eliminated during the subsequent wash-out period. There was, however, a further significant improvement during the second active pacing period, implying a genuine treatment effect. On completion of the crossover phase, patients were assigned to the best chronic pacing mode and followed for 1 year. During that time, the number of days spent in hospital for heart failure was significantly lower than in the year before implantation.[162]

The Multisite Stimulation In Cardiomyopathy (MUSTIC) Trial – The MUSTIC trial used a blinded crossover between active and inactive pacing (12 weeks in each mode) to assess biventricular pacing.[163] In this study, the left ventricular lead was introduced transvenously to a lateral or posterior cardiac vein. The initial implant success rate was 92%. Patients had severe but stable heart failure due to idiopathic or ischemic LV systolic dysfunction (NYHA class III) despite optimal medical therapy, ejection fraction <35%, LV EDD >60 mm, QRS duration >150 ms and no conventional indication for pacing. Sixty-seven patients in sinus rhythm were enrolled, of whom nine were withdrawn before randomization for various reasons (failed implantation, five; unstable

heart failure, two; pre-existing indication for pacing, one; sudden death whilst the device was inactive, one). Ten patients failed to complete the two crossover periods. In the 48 patients who completed the study, the 6 minute walking distance (the primary end point) improved by 23% (P<0·001) after 3 months biventricular pacing. Quality of life scores (Minnesota Living with Heart Failure questionnaire) improved by 32% (P<0·001), peak oxygen uptake by 8% (P<0·03) and hospitalizations were decreased by two thirds (P<0·05). Active pacing was preferred by 85% of the patients (P<0·001). At the end of the crossover phase, patients were programmed to their preferred mode and reassessed at 1 year. The clinical benefits were maintained.[164] The MUSTIC study had a separate limb for patients in atrial fibrillation and preliminary results from the 41 patients (of 64 enrolled) who completed the crossover phase have been presented.[165] Trends were observed in favor of biventricular pacing but the results did not achieve statistical significance. This contrasts with the findings in a non-randomized study in which patients with atrial fibrillation showed greater benefit than those in sinus rhythm.[166] In the latter study, the AV node was systematically ablated in the patients with AF, in order to provide complete and permanent biventricular capture. Some benefit may thus have been due to improved rate control. Conversely, patients in the MUSTIC AF study may have failed fully to benefit from CRT if rate control was inadequate and resynchronization only intermittent. The Optimal Pacing SITE (OPSITE) study will address this issue by sequentially comparing right ventricular pacing, first with LV and then with biventricular pacing, using a crossover design, in patients undergoing "ablate and pace" therapy for permanent atrial fibrillation, with and without impaired LV function.[167]

The Multicenter Insync Randomized Clinical Evaluation (MIRACLE) – MIRACLE is the largest trial of biventricular pacing reported to date.[168] This was a prospective, multicentre, double-blind, randomized controlled trial in patients with NYHA class III or IV chronic heart failure, ejection fraction ≤35%, LV EDD ≥55 mm, QRS duration ≥130 ms, on optimal and stable medical therapy. Preliminary results have been presented.[169] A total of 266 patients, successfully implanted with a transvenous CRT pacing system were randomized to active CRT (n=134) or control (VDD mode at 30/min; n=132) and followed for 6 months. The initial implant success rate was 93%. In the CRT group, there were eight deaths and one patient withdrawal. In the control group there were 10 deaths, two early crossovers and one other withdrawal. Amongst those who completed the study there were significant improvements in 6 minute walk distance with CRT (mean increase 39 m; P=0·033). NYHA functional class improved by a mean of 0·8 in the CRT group, with 65% attaining class I or II, compared with 30% in the control group (P<0·001). In the quality of life assessment (Minnesota Living with Heart Failure questionnaire), there was evidence of a marked placebo effect with improvement in the control group also but the improvement in the CRT group (mean 19 points) was significantly greater ($P = 0.013$). Treadmill exercise time was also significantly increased with CRT (c 2 mins) and there was a borderline significant increase in peak VO_2.

Further evidence of the efficacy of CRT is provided by the data reported on 1000 patients enrolled in the European CONTAK registry[170] and 190 patients enrolled in the Italian InSync registry.[171] These show similar outcomes to those in the other non-randomized studies and clinical trials.

In addition to the benefits of CRT described above, there is evidence that it may reduce norepinephrine levels[172] and sympathetic activity.[173] These effects may explain the apparent antiarrhythmic effect of CRT. In one crossover study, a diminished frequency of ventricular ectopy was noted during CRT, compared with that during sinus rhythm or right ventricular pacing.[174] Similarly, in the VENTAK-CHF study, CRT decreased the frequency of appropriate antitachycardia therapy delivery in patients with an implantable cardioverter defibrillator (ICD) with biventricular pacing capability.[175] A number of recently completed and ongoing trials will provide further evidence of the short-term clinical impact of CRT in patients with severe heart failure, some or all of whom are implanted with a biventricular ICD. These include CONTAK-CD, InSync ICD, MIRACLE ICD, PATH CHF-II and PACMAN.

Comment and recommendations

There is considerable evidence that CRT can improve hemodynamics, symptoms, quality of life and functional capacity in selected patients with advanced heart failure and intraventricular conduction delay. There is also some evidence that the need for hospitalization may be diminished.
Grade A

To date, the evidence has come from relatively small and short-term studies in which all patients have received a device and outcomes have been compared pre- and post-implant or with the device alternately active and inactive. In order to define the true clinical utility of CRT, there is a pressing need for large-scale randomized trials comparing morbidity and mortality in patients receiving CRT (in addition to optimal medical therapy) and in patients receiving optimal medical therapy alone. Two such trials are ongoing. The Cardiac Resynchronization for Heart Failure (CARE-HF) trial in Europe will enrol 800 patients with stable class III or IV chronic heart failure due to LV systolic dysfunction, EF ≤ 35%, dilated LV (EDD ≥30 mm/m height) and either QRS duration ≥150 ms or QRS duration ≥120 ms with echocardiographic evidence of dysynchrony.[176] Patients will be randomized to optimal medical therapy alone

or combined with CRT and followed for a minimum of 18 months. The primary end point is all-cause mortality or cardiovascular hospitalization. Secondary end points include all-cause mortality, hospitalization for heart failure, NYHA class at 90 days and quality of life at 90 days (including a generic measure, the EuroQol EQ-5D). Echocardiographic and neurohormonal parameters will also be assessed, as will cost effectiveness. The Comparison of Medical Therapy, Pacing and Defibrillation in Chronic Heart Failure (COMPANION) trial in the USA will enroll 2200 patients with stable class III or class IV heart failure, at least one hospitalization in the preceding year, EF ≤ 35%, LV EDD ≥ 60 mm, QRS duration ≥120 ms and PR interval >150 ms.[177] This is a three-limb study, in which patients will be randomized to optimal medical therapy alone or combined with CRT or combined with CRT and ICD backup (ratio 1:2:2). Minimum follow up will be 1 year. The primary end point is all-cause mortality and hospitalization. Secondary end points include cardiac morbidity, quality of life and peak VO_2. The results from these trials should be available by 2004. In the meantime, no firm recommendations can be made regarding the place of CRT in clinical practice. Further data are also required to clarify numerous unresolved issues regarding patient selection, the optimal LV pacing site, the relative merits of LV and biventricular pacing, the role of combined CRT and ICD therapy and cost utility. Technological developments are also needed to simplify LV lead placement and shorten the procedure time.

Atrial fibrillation

The influence of pacing mode selection on the incidence of atrial fibrillation (AF) in patients paced for sick sinus syndrome or AV block has been discussed above, as has the occasional need for pacing to permit antiarrhythmic drug therapy. The limited success of drug therapy in suppressing paroxysmal AF has prompted the assessment of various pacing strategies, even in patients with no other indication for pacemaker implantation. Possible mechanisms by which pacing might suppress AF in this context include reduction of bradycardia, overdrive suppression of atrial premature beats, elimination of compensatory pauses and reduction in interatrial or intra-atrial conduction delay and dispersion of refractoriness that might otherwise favor re-entry.

Atrial rate support

In selected patients with the vagally mediated, pause-dependent, form of atrial fibrillation, permanent atrial rate support has been shown to be of benefit although concomitant drug therapy may still be required.[178] In a broader context, the use of atrial-based pacing to prevent paroxysmal atrial fibrillation in patients selected for ablation of the AV node was assessed in the Atrial Pacing Periablation for Prevention of Paroxysmal Atrial Fibrillation (PA[3]) study.[179] The first phase of the study enrolled 97 patients with at least three episodes of paroxysmal AF in the previous year (the most recent within 3 months), all of whom were refractory to or intolerant of drug therapy and being considered for total AV node ablation. Patients were implanted with a DDDR pacemaker and randomized to atrial pacing (DDIR with lower rate 70/min) or no pacing (DDI 30/min). The use of the DDI mode in both groups activated the high-rate atrial diagnostic features of the pacemaker, which were used to determine the primary outcome. Diagnostic counters were reset after a 2 week run-in period, intended to permit stabilization of drug therapy and allow for short-term effects of lead placement on arrhythmia frequency. Patients and pacemaker diagnostics were reviewed 3 months post-implant and crossover from inactive to active pacing or progression to AV node ablation was permitted in the event of intolerable recurrent symptomatic AF. Time to first recurrence of AF (≥ 5 min) was similar in the two groups and the AF burden was lower in the non-paced group. The study suggests that rate-adaptive atrial pacing does not prevent recurrence of drug-refractory paroxysmal AF, in the short-term, in patients without symptomatic bradycardia. It is noteworthy that AV node ablation was deferred in 29% of patients in each group. Whilst the significance of this observation is unclear, it lends some support to the strategy of implanting a pacemaker and reviewing the patient before proceeding to planned ablation, rather than undertaking both procedures in one session.

The second phase of the PA[3] study considered the optimal pacing mode postablation and tested the hypothesis that DDDR pacing as compared with VDD pacing reduces the time to first recurrence, the frequency and the duration of paroxysmal AF postablation.[180] Sixty-seven patients were randomized to receive DDDR pacing (lower rate 70/min) with mode switch to DDIR, or VDD pacing (lower rate 60/min to favor preservation of AV synchrony) with mode switch to VVIR. There was a crossover at 6 months and total follow up of one year. Antiarrhythmic drugs were usually discontinued after pacemaker implantation. There was a progressive increase in the prevalence of persistent AF (approximately 30–35% at 6 months) and the AF burden with time but there were no statistically significant differences between the groups in time to recurrence, frequency or total burden of AF. By one year, 43% of patients had permanent AF. The study suggests that physiologic (DDDR) pacing, compared with ventricular pacing, does not prevent the recurrence of paroxysmal AF or progression to permanent AF after AV node ablation in patients with frequent paroxysmal AF. It is possible that the findings might be different if concomitant antiarrhythmic drug therapy were used, as there is evidence from randomized trials that "ablate and pace" therapy, although better than drug therapy for relief of symptoms,

is associated with a higher incidence of permanent AF.[181,182] It is also possible that a higher pacing rate, to achieve more continuous overdrive, might have been more effective.

Atrial overdrive pacing

Overdrive pacing at higher rates in the right atrial appendage has been assessed in patients with paroxysmal AF and pacemakers implanted for conventional indications. In one study, 18 patients with DDDR mode-switching pacemakers, implanted for a variety of indications, were randomly assigned to pacing at 60, 75 and 90/min with crossover after intervals of 2 months.[183] The pacemaker Holter functions were used to assess the percentage of time spent in AF and/or the number of mode-switch episodes according to the device capability. When ranked according to the amount of AF, there was no significant difference in the amount of AF according to the pacing rate. Six patients were intolerant of pacing at 90/min and one other had increased angina. In another study, 27 patients with DDDR pacemakers, implanted for sick sinus syndrome, were randomized to two 3 month single-blinded crossover periods. In one, the pacemaker base rate was set to 60/min and in the other it was set to 10 beats/min above the mean heart rate (range 70–96/min; mean $\pm$ S.D. 75 ± 7/min). Pacemaker software recorded the number and duration of AF episodes, which were not significantly different between the two periods.[184] These findings contrast with an earlier report in which atrial overdrive was found to decrease the incidence of atrial arrhythmia in a study of 22 patients with frequent episodes and DDD pacemakers implanted for conventional indications.[185] However, even in that study, the sub-group with brady-tachy syndrome (all of whom had prior atrial tachyarrhythmia apparently not controlled by drug therapy) showed least benefit. Encouraging results have recently been reported from a randomized crossover study of medium (c 80/min) and high rate (c 90/min) right atrial overdrive pacing in 42 patients with paroxysmal AF but no conventional indication for pacing. Symptomatic (ECG verified) episodes of AF were less frequent during medium (1·42/ week; $P = 0·005$) and high rate (1·36/week; $P = 0·006$) pacing than with no pacing (2·56/week).[186]

Rate-adaptive atrial pacing

The generally disappointing results in most studies of overdrive pacing may partly reflect a failure to achieve consistent or sustained overdrive. The mean or median percentage atrial pacing was below 75% in all of the studies described above. In this regard, the impact of sensor-driven rate adaptation has been examined in a prospective randomized crossover trial comparing DDD with DDDR pacing (3 months in each mode) in 78 patients with frequent symptomatic paroxysmal AF, brady-tachy syndrome and chronotropic incompetence.[187] The percentage of atrial pacing was significantly higher in DDDR mode compared with DDD mode ($81 \cdot 1 \pm 20 \cdot 5$ and $73 \cdot 7 \pm 20 \cdot 0$ respectively; $P < 0 \cdot 01$). There was a non-significant trend towards fewer symptomatic episodes in the DDDR mode. There were also fewer mode-switching episodes ($91 \pm 109 \cdot 8$ v 120 ± 120 over 3 months; $P < 0 \cdot 05$). However, no data were available regarding the duration of the episodes, so the AF burden is unknown. Rate-adaptive pacing would only be expected to confer an advantage during periods of increased activity, as is reflected in the relatively modest increase in the overall percentage of atrial pacing. A novel implementation of sensor-driven rate-adaptive pacing in this context is the use of fixed-rate overdrive pacing but with an Automatic Rest Rate function to allow overdrive pacing to continue but at a lower rate during periods of physical or mental inactivity. Preliminary results from a randomized crossover trial, comparing DDDR pacing with and without activation of the overdrive algorithm, in 78 patients show a reduction in the number and duration of mode switching episodes.[188]

Atrial pacing algorithms

A number of specific pacemaker algorithms have been developed to try and enhance the antiarrhythmic efficacy of atrial pacing. One example uses overdrive pacing, triggered by the occurrence of atrial premature beats, to eliminate post-extrasystolic pauses and suppress further ectopy.[189] Another uses dynamic atrial overdrive (DAO) to maintain a pacing rate just above the intrinsic sinus rate. Preliminary results from a randomized crossover study (ADOPT-A), comparing DDDR pacing with the algorithm "on" or "off" in 250 patients with paroxysmal AF and a conventional indication for pacing, have been presented.[190] There was a significant reduction in AF burden as assessed from symptomatic (ECG verified) episodes. The Consistent Atrial Pacing (CAP) algorithm also aims to achieve sustained overdrive pacing, whilst avoiding excessively high rates that might compromise patient tolerance, by continuously updating the atrial escape interval. In a randomized crossover study in 15 patients receiving DDDR pacing for sick sinus syndrome, the algorithm achieved $86 \pm 28\%$ atrial pacing, was well tolerated and decreased the number of premature atrial contractions. There was, however, no significant reduction in AF as assessed by the number of mode-switching episodes.[191] In a similar study of 61 patients receiving DDDR pacing for brady-tachy syndrome, the algorithm was well tolerated, decreased the number of premature atrial contractions and achieved $96 \pm 7\%$ atrial pacing but there was no significant reduction in symptomatic AF or mode-switching episodes.[192] In a sub-group of 31 patients who had less than 90% atrial pacing during standard DDDR pacing, the algorithm increased atrial pacing from $60 \pm 26\%$ to $97 \pm 3\%$ and mode-switch episodes decreased from $1 \cdot 23 \pm 1 \cdot 27$ to $0 \cdot 75 \pm 1 \cdot 1$

($P < 0 \cdot 0001$). The CAP algorithm has subsequently been combined with two others (rate stabilization and post mode switching overdrive) in a device that also includes anti-tachycardia pacing capability. Preliminary clinical results in 31 patients with conventional pacing indications and atrial tachyarrhythmia, showed a reduction in the mean number of arrhythmia episodes but the total arrhythmia burden was unchanged.[193] Encouraging results have recently been presented from the Atrial Fibrillation Therapy (AFT) study, which assessed the efficacy of a device incorporating a combination of four preventive pacing algorithms.[194] The study included 372 patients with drug-refractory paroxysmal AF, with and without conventional indications for pacing. Conventional DDD pacing (at 40, 70 and 85/min) and DDDR pacing (at 70 and 85/min) did not significantly influence AF burden, mean duration of sinus rhythm or AF recurrence. In contrast, the AF preventive algorithm significantly improved all of these outcomes, when compared with DDD pacing at 70/min. Further studies in this area are ongoing.[195]

Biatrial pacing

It has been postulated that reduced dispersion of refractoriness might decrease the propensity to paroxysmal AF in susceptible patients and the efficacy of various multisite pacing techniques has been examined. Encouraging results were obtained with the use of biatrial synchronization in patients with advanced interatrial conduction delay and drug refractory atrial flutter and fibrillation.[196,197] Pacing leads were positioned in the right atrium and within the mid or distal coronary sinus to pace right and left atria simultaneously in triggered (AAT) mode. This strategy was subsequently evaluated in the Synchronized Biatrial Pacing (SYNBIAPACE) study.[198] This was a prospective randomized crossover study in which 42 patients (mean age 64 years) with a history (≥ 1 year) of recurrent drug-refractory AF and intra-atrial conduction delay (P wave duration ≥ 120 ms and interatrial conduction time ≥ 100 ms) spent 3 months in each of three pacing modes. Synchronous biatrial pacing at 70/min was compared with single site high right atrial DDD pacing at 70/min and the same at 40/min (the "inhibited" or control mode). Biatrial pacing was achieved using leads in the high right atrium and the mid or distal coronary sinus connected via a "Y"-bifurcated adapter to the atrial port of a bipolar DDDR pacemaker, incorporating a resynchronization algorithm to trigger atrial synchronous pacing after every sensed atrial event ("AAT" mode). There was no statistically significant difference between the three modes in either time to first arrhythmia recurrence (the primary end point) or time spent in atrial arrhythmia, although there was a trend favoring biatrial pacing. This was a relatively small study with short follow up in a highly selected group of patients and data from further studies are awaited to clarify the role of this pacing modality.

Dual site atrial pacing

An alternative approach that has been explored is the use of dual site atrial pacing, in DDDR mode, with leads in the high right atrium and at the coronary sinus os. Preliminary studies reported an increase in the arrhythmia-free interval and greater benefit than single site pacing at either site.[199] The same group subsequently reported on a series of 30 patients entered into a prospective but non-randomized, sequential, crossover comparison of single and dual site atrial pacing (3–6 month periods) with extended follow up (25–41 months) in the latter mode.[200] Arrhythmia free interval was significantly increased by dual site pacing as compared with single site pacing, either in the high right atrium or at the coronary sinus ostium, which was itself superior to a pre-implant control period. Single site pacing was of comparable efficacy at either site. Dual site pacing was achieved by connecting the high right atrial and coronary sinus ostial electrodes via a Y-connector to the atrial channel of a conventional DDDR pacemaker, the pacing rate being set to achieve overdrive with at least 80% of atrial events being paced. The technique has subsequently been evaluated in the Dual Site Atrial Pacing to Prevent AF (DAPPAF) study.[201] This was a randomized crossover comparison of dual site atrial pacing, single site high right atrial pacing and a support pacing control period (DDI 50/min or VDI), at 6 month intervals, in 120 patients with a history of paroxysmal AF and a bradyarrhythmic indication for pacing. Patient tolerance and adherence to the pacing mode was superior with dual site pacing compared with support pacing ($P < 0.001$) and high right atrial pacing ($P = 0.006$). There was a non-significant trend towards greater freedom from any symptomatic AF recurrence (the primary end point) with dual site pacing (hazard ratio 0.715, $P = 0.07$) but not with high right atrial pacing ($P = 0.19$), compared with support pacing. There was no significant difference between dual site and high right atrial pacing. Combined symptomatic and asymptomatic AF frequency, measured by device datalogs, was significantly reduced during dual site pacing, compared with high right atrial pacing ($P < 0.01$). However, in antiarrhythmic drug treated patients, dual site pacing increased symptomatic AF free survival compared to support pacing ($P = 0.011$) and high right atrial pacing (hazard ratio 0.669, $P = 0.06$).[202]

Another prospective randomized trial, the New Indication for Pacing Prevention of AF (NIPP AF) study, examined whether dual site atrial pacing with atrial overdrive near the intrinsic rate, could reduce AF recurrence in patients with paroxysmal AF, refractory to a fixed regimen of sotalol, and no bradycardic indication for pacing.[203] Twenty-two patients were randomized in crossover fashion to 12 weeks of high right atrial pacing at 30/min or dual site pacing (high right atrium and coronary sinus os) with an overdrive algorithm. The time to the first clinical AF recurrence was prolonged (15 ± 17 to 50 ± 35 days, $P = 0.006$) and total AF burden was reduced ($45 \pm 34\%$ v $22 \pm 29\%$, $P = 0.04$) by dual site pacing with overdrive. However, there was no significant difference in symptoms or quality of life.

Alternative site atrial pacing

Encouraging preliminary results have recently been reported from studies of single site pacing of the interatrial septum. In an acute study comparing right atrial appendage pacing with dual site, septal or coronary sinus os pacing, the duration of atrial activation was found to be shorter and comparable at each of the latter sites.[204] This suggests that the benefits of dual site pacing might be attained without the added complexity of a second lead. Baillin *et al* randomized 120 patients with a conventional indication for pacing and a history of recurrent paroxysmal AF to pacing either the interatrial septum in the region of Bachmann's bundle or the right atrial appendage.[205] Septal pacing was associated with a shorter P wave duration and a higher rate of survival free from chronic AF at one year, compared with right atrial appendage pacing (75% v 47%; $P < 0.05$). Padeletti *et al* randomized 46 patients with paroxysmal AF and sinus bradycardia to DDD(R) pacing with the atrial lead either on the interatrial septum at the triangle of Koch or in the right atrial appendage.[206] Within each group, a crossover comparison was made with a constant atrial pacing (CAP) algorithm "on" or "off". The number of paroxysmal AF episodes per month was lower in both groups with the CAP algorithm "on" but septal pacing was associated with a significantly lower frequency of AF episodes and AF burden with or without CAP. The same group have also reported success with the use of interatrial septal pacing to prevent early recurrence of AF after DC cardioversion in patients with a prior history of early recurrence (within 2–24 hours).[207]

Comment and recommendations

The use of pacing as a primary antiarrhythmic strategy in the management of AF is not yet justified by the available data. Interpretation of the data is confounded by heterogeneity of the pattern of the arrhythmia, the clinical characteristics of the patients and the end points and outcome measures in the various studies. In patients with conventional indications for pacing, the use of a device with preventive algorithms may be justified in selected cases. Similarly, multisite or alternative site atrial pacing may be worthy of consideration in some patients, such as those with evidence of intra- or interatrial conduction delay. These pacing modalities appear to be most effective when used as hybrid therapy with antiarrhythmic drugs. Indeed, it may be that much of the benefit in some of the studies is attributable to the facilitation of increased antiarrhythmic drug therapy by pacing. In the future, improved understanding and characterization of different patterns and modes of onset of AF may facilitate a customized approach to treatment. For the time being, the value of device therapy in AF remains unproven. **Grade A**

Long QT syndrome

Patients with the long QT syndrome are at high risk of syncope and sudden death, usually due to polymorphic ventricular tachycardia. There are compelling data from observational studies[208,209] and from the International Long QT Syndrome Registry[210,211] indicating that cardiac pacing, with concomitant β blockade, may reduce the rate of recurrent syncope and sudden death. The registry data, from 124 patients who were paced for the long QT syndrome, indicate approximately a 50% reduction in the incidence of cardiac events. Interpretation of the data is confounded by the initiation or increase of β blockers at the time of pacing in some patients. However, 30 patients were identified in whom a pacemaker was implanted after failure of β blockers but without an increase in drug dosage. In this subset, there was a significant reduction in the incidence of syncope, confirming the independent benefit of pacing. It is important to note that pacing should not be implemented without concomitant β blocker therapy and that β blockers should not be stopped. Of the 10 registry patients in whom β blockers were withdrawn after pacemaker implantation, three died suddenly during 2 years' follow up. The benefit of pacing is thought to be due to the prevention of bradycardia and pauses together with rate-related shortening of the QT interval. Unfortunately, for pacing to be effective, relatively high rates (>80/min) may be required[212] with the attendant disadvantage of reduced battery life and the potential risk of tachycardia induced cardiomyopathy.[213]

Careful attention to pacemaker programming is essential.[214] Features that allow slowing of the heart rate below the programmed lower rate limit, such as hysteresis and sleep functions, should be programmed "off". Similarly, rate hysteresis search (a feature that extends the atrial escape interval periodically to search for intrinsic sinus activity) and algorithms that extend the postventricular atrial refractory period after ventricular premature beats, should be disabled, as they may favor the occurrence of pauses. Specific rate-smoothing algorithms that are capable of preventing post-extrasystolic pauses may be useful in this context.[215] There is some indirect experimental and clinical evidence to suggest that pacing might be of particular value in patients with the LQT3 genotype,[216–218] which is particularly associated with increased dispersion of repolarization during bradycardia and with arrhythmia occurring during sleep.[219] This has not been explored in clinical studies and it should not be inferred that other genotypes will not benefit from pacing. Further data are required to clarify the extent to which therapy in the long QT syndrome can be guided by genotype. Pacing should be considered as an adjuvant to β blockade in all patients

with long QT syndrome and high grade AV block and whenever there is evidence of pause-dependent malignant arrhythmias. In selected patients, an implantable cardioverter defibrillator may also be indicated and the same device may be used for prophylactic pacing. **Grade B**

Post-cardiac transplantation

Bradycardia, usually due to transient sinus node dysfunction or AV block, may occur in almost two thirds of patients in the first few weeks following orthotopic cardiac transplantation.[220] Recovery from transient AV block usually occurs within 16 days but transient sinus node dysfunction may persist for several weeks and the optimal time for consideration of permanent pacemaker implantation is uncertain.[221] In some cases, temporary treatment with oral theophylline may avert the need for permanent pacing.[222] The proportion of transplant recipients receiving permanent pacing for persistent bradycardia ranges from 4% to 29% in different centres.[223] The variation may reflect differences in the incidence of bradycardia and the criteria for permanent pacing although differences in surgical technique may also be relevant.[224] In paced transplant recipients, bradycardia often resolves and pacemaker usage decreases during the first few months.[225] Deferring consideration of permanent pacing until 3 weeks after transplantation may mean that some patients with transient sinus node dysfunction are spared unnecessary pacemaker implantation. Deferral is also associated with a commensurate increase in pacemaker usage in those paced. However, even with this strategy, less than half of those using their pacemakers at 3 months continue to do so at 6 months and there are no clear predictive factors to guide patient selection.[226]

Following heterotopic cardiac transplantation, the donor and recipient hearts beat independently of one another, the denervated donor heart typically beating at a faster rate. Competitive contraction of the two hearts may be deleterious and left ventricular function in the recipient heart is improved when the two hearts beat out of phase. Acute studies have shown that paced linkage of the two hearts to produce consistent counterpulsation may result in significant functional improvement.[227] This technique has recently been evaluated in a chronic study using permanent dual chamber pacemakers with the atrial channel connected to the donor atrium and the "ventricular" channel connected to the recipient atrium.[228] Paced linkage was associated with significant improvements in symptoms, general health, energy, levels of activity and maximum cardiac output in the donor heart. **Grade A**

Sleep apnea

Sleep apnea with hypersomnolence is a relatively common disorder that is estimated to affect 2% to 4% of middle-aged adults, although asymptomatic forms with abnormal findings on polysomnography may be five times more frequent.[229]

The condition is associated with an increased risk of hypertension and cardiovascular disease, including bradyarrhythmia.[230] It has been noted that recognition and treatment of the condition in patients with transient but profound asymptomatic bradycardia, occurring only at night or whilst sleeping during the day, may reduce the need for pacemaker implantation, provided that advanced disease of the sinus node or AV conducting system have been excluded.[231]

Conversely, there have been anecdotal reports of improvements in sleep-disordered breathing following pacemaker implantation in patients with sinus node dysfunction and AV block.[232] Following similar observations in some patients receiving atrial overdrive pacing for the suppression of atrial tachyarrhythmia, the efficacy of atrial overdrive has been assessed in a randomized crossover trial.[233] A group of 152 patients with dual chamber pacemakers, implanted for conventional indications, was screened for symptoms of sleep-disordered breathing. Of 47 such patients that were identified, 26 underwent polysomnography and sleep apnea was confirmed in 15, all of whom had either sinus node disease or brady-tachy syndrome as their underlying diagnosis. Patients underwent polysomnographic studies on three consecutive nights. The first night provided a baseline evaluation to quantify the frequency and type of apnea or hypopnea. On the second night, the patients were randomly assigned to either backup ventricular pacing (40/min), to allow a predominantly spontaneous rhythm, or atrial overdrive pacing at a rate 15 beats/min faster than the baseline nocturnal heart rate. On the third night, the alternate mode was assessed. The mean sinus rate during spontaneous rhythm was 57 ± 5/min at baseline and the mean rate during atrial overdrive pacing was 72 ± 3/min. The hypopnea index (number of episodes divided by hours of sleep) was 9 ± 4 during spontaneous rhythm and 3 ± 3 during atrial overdrive ($P < 0.001$). For both apnea and hypopnea, the index was 28 ± 22 during spontaneous rhythm and 11 ± 14 ($P < 0.001$) during atrial overdrive.

The mechanism underlying the apparent improvement with pacing is unclear. The authors postulate that increased sympathetic activity during pacing might counteract sustained increases in vagal tone. Perhaps surprisingly, both obstructive and central forms of sleep apnea were improved, which may suggest a central mechanism affecting both respiratory rhythm and pharyngeal motor neuron activity.[234] It is noteworthy that 11 of the 15 patients had some degree of impairment of LV function but even the four patients with normal LV function showed more than a 50% reduction in the sleep apnea index. It remains unknown whether patients with sleep apnea but without conventional indications for pacing would show similar benefit and it would be premature to suggest a role for cardiac pacing in this condition. The study does, however, suggest that atrial overdrive might be of value in patients with sleep apnea who are already being paced for sinus node disease or brady-tachy syndrome.

Arrhythmia diagnosis

In recent years, the increasing sophistication and memory capacity of cardiac pacemakers has introduced the possibility of an important diagnostic role. In patients with syncope, the cause of which remains unknown after appropriate investigation, implantation of a pacemaker with diagnostic capabilities may enable the occurrence and cause of bradycardia to be identified whilst providing a therapeutic safety net.[235] Single chamber diagnostic devices capable of detecting the occurrence of bradycardia have been available for several years and dual chamber devices with diagnostic algorithms are now also available and enable the mechanism of bradycardia to be identified in many cases.[236]

In patients with known or suspected tachyarrhythmia, the Holter and telemetry functions of dual chamber pacemakers may be used to facilitate arrhythmia diagnosis. They also enable the frequency and natural history to be determined and the efficacy of antiarrhythmic therapy to be assessed.[237] In devices with the capability of switching from atrial tracking modes to non-tracking modes on detection of atrial tachyarrhythmia, mode-switch counters may serve a similar function, whilst the change in mode avoids the risk of rapid paced ventricular rates.

Conclusions

The role of cardiac pacing in symptomatic bradycardia is well established yet questions remain regarding appropriate mode selection in the conditions for which it is most often used, namely AV block and sino-atrial disease. Data from recent randomized trials have enriched the evidence base but further analysis and the results from ongoing trials must be awaited before the outstanding questions can be answered. Technological advances and innovation have greatly expanded the possibilities for sophisticated pacing with better emulation of normal physiology, yet for many of these developments, evidence of clinical utility is limited. In recent years, improved diagnostic techniques have increased understanding of the pathophysiology of other conditions, identifying many possible new roles for pacing as a therapeutic modality. The advent of large scale clinical trials to the field of cardiac pacing offers an opportunity both to test well-constructed hypotheses regarding established indications and to evaluate new ones, in order to provide a solid evidence base to guide future practice.

References

1. Elmqvist R, Senning A. An implantable pacemaker for the heart. In: Smith CN, ed. *Medical electronics* (Proceedings of the Second International Conference on Medical Electronics, Paris, 1959). London: Illiffe, 1960.

2. Travill CM, Sutton R. Pacemaker syndrome: an iatrogenic condition. *Br Heart J* 1992;**68**:163–6.

3. Mond HG. The world survey of cardiac pacing and cardioverter defibrillators: Calendar year 1997 – Asian Pacific, Middle East, South America, and Canada. *PACE* 2001;**24**:856–62.

4. Ector H, Rickards AF, Kappenberger L *et al.* The world survey of cardiac pacing and implantable cardioverter defibrillators: Calendar year 1997 – Europe. *PACE* 2001;**24**:863–8.

5. Bernstein AD, Parsonnet V. Survey of cardiac pacing and implanted defibrillator practice patterns in the United States in 1997. *PACE* 2001;**24**:842–55.

6. Cunningham AD (National Pacemaker Database, 2001). Personal communication.

7. Greenspan AM, Kay HR, Berger BC *et al.* Incidence of unwarranted implantation of permanent cardiac pacemakers in a large medical population. *N Engl J Med* 1988;**318**:158–63.

8. Frye RL, Collins JJ, DeSanctis RW *et al.* Guidelines for permanent cardiac pacemaker implantation, May 1984: A report of the Joint American College of Cardiology/American Heart Association Task Force on Assessment of Cardiovascular Procedures (Sub-committee on Pacemaker Implantation). *Circulation* 1984;**70**:331A–9A.

9. Dreifus LS, Fisch C, Griffin JC *et al.* Guidelines for implantation of cardiac pacemakers and antiarrhythmia devices. A report of the American College of Cardiology/American Heart Association Task Force on Assessment of Diagnostic and Therapeutic Cardiovascular Procedures (Committee on Pacemaker Implantation). *Circulation* 1991;**84**:455–67.

10. Gregoratos G, Cheitlin MD, Conill A *et al.* ACC/AHA Guidelines for implantation of cardiac pacemakers and antiarrhythmia devices. A report of the American College of Cardiology/American Heart Association Task Force on Practice Guidelines (Committee on Pacemaker Implantation). *J Am Coll Cardiol* 1998 (in press).

11. Clarke M, Sutton R, Ward D *et al.* Recommendations for pacemaker prescription for symptomatic bradycardia: report of a working party of the British Pacing and Electrophysiology Group. *Br Heart J* 1991;**66**:185–91.

12. Petch M. Who needs dual chamber pacing? *BMJ* 1993;**307**:215–16.

13. de Belder MA, Linker NJ, Jones S, Camm AJ, Ward DE. Cost implications of the British Pacing and Electrophysiology Group's recommendations for pacing. *BMJ* 1992;**305**:861–5.

14. National Pacemaker Database (United Kingdom and Republic of Ireland). *Annual Report* 2000. London: British Pacing and Electrophysiology Group.

15. Aggarwal RK, Ray SG, Connelly DT, Coulshed DS, Charles RG. Trends in pacemaker mode prescription 1984–1994: a single centre study of 3710 patients. *Heart* 1996;**75**:518–21.

16. Bexton RS, Camm AJ. First degree atrioventricular block. *Eur Heart J* 1984;**5**(Suppl. A):107–9.

17. Chirife R, Ortega DE, Salazar AL. "Pacemaker syndrome" without a pacemaker. Deleterious effects of first-degree AV block. *RBM* 1990;**12**:22.

18. Zornosa JP, Crossley GH, Haisty WK Jr *et al.* Pseudo-pacemaker syndrome: a complication of radiofrequency ablation of the AV junction. *PACE* 1992;**15**:590.

19. Mabo P, Varin C, Vauthier M. Deleterious hemodynamic consequences of isolated long PR intervals: correction by DDD pacing. *Eur Heart J* 1992;**13**:225.

20. Barold SS. Indications for permanent cardiac pacing in first-degree AV block: class I, II, or III? *PACE* 1996;**19**:747–51.

21. Wharton JM, Ellenbogen KA. Atrioventricular conduction system disease. In: Ellenbogen KA, Kay GN, Wilkoff BL, eds. *Clinical cardiac pacing*. Philadelphia: WB Saunders, 1995.

22. Dhingra RC, Denes P, Wu D *et al.* The significance of second degree atrioventricular block and bundle branch block. *Circulation* 1974;**49**:638–46.

23. Puech P, Grolleau R, Guimond C. Incidence of different types of AV-block and their localisation by His bundle recordings. In: Wellens HJJ, Lie KI, Janse MJ, eds. *The conduction system of the heart: structure, function and clinical implications*. Philadelphia: Lea & Febiger, 1976.

24. Shaw DB, Kekwick CA, Veale D, Gowers J, Whistance T. Survival in second degree atrioventricular block. *Br Heart J* 1985;**53**:587–93.

25. Campbell RWF. Chronic Mobitz type I second degree atrioventricular block: has its importance been underestimated? *Br Heart J* 1985;**53**:585–6.

26. Connelly DT, Steinhaus DM. Mobitz type I atrioventricular block: an indication for permanent pacing? *PACE* 1996;**19**:261–4.

27. Grossman M. Second degree heart block with Wenckebach phenomenon: its occurrence over a period of several years in a young healthy adult. *Am Heart J* 1958;**56**:607–10.

28. Meytes I, Kaplinsky E, Yahini JH, Hanne-Papara N, Neufeld HN. Wenckebach A-V block: a frequent feature following heavy physical training. *Am Heart J* 1975;**90**:426–30.

29. Johansson BW. Complete heart block. A clinical hemodynamic and pharmacological study in patients with and without an artificial pacemaker. *Acta Med Scand* 1966;**180**(Suppl. 451):1–127.

30. Edhag O, Swahn Å. Prognosis of patients with complete heart block or arrhythmic syncope who were not treated with artificial pacemakers. *Acta Med Scand* 1976;**200**:457–63.

31. Rosenqvist M, Nordlander R. Survival in patients with permanent pacemakers. *Cardiol Clin* 1992;**10**:691–703.

32. Rosenqvist M, Edhag KO. Pacemaker dependence in transient high grade atrioventricular block. *PACE* 1984;**7**:63–70.

33. Ginks W, Leatham A, Siddons H. Prognosis of patients paced for chronic atrioventricular block. *Br Heart J* 1979;**41**:633–6.

34. Shen WK, Hammill SC, Hayes DL *et al.* Long-term survival after pacemaker implantation for heart block in patients ≥65 years. *Am J Cardiol* 1984;**74**:560–4.

35. Campbell M, Emanuel R. Six cases of congenital heart block followed for 34–40 years. *Br Heart J* 1966;**59**:587–90.

36. Michaëlsson M, Jonzon A, Riesenfeld T. Isolated congenital complete atrioventricular block in adult life. *Circulation* 1995;**92**:442–9.

37. Friedman RA. Congenital AV block. Pace me now or pace me later? *Circulation* 1995;**92**:283–5.

38. Rowlands DJ. Left and right bundle branch block, left anterior and left posterior hemiblock. *Eur Heart J* 1984;**5**(Suppl. A):99–105.

39. McAnulty JH, Rahimtoola SH, Murphy E *et al*. Natural history of "high-risk" bundle branch block. Final report of a prospective study. *N Engl J Med* 1982;**307**:137–43.

40. Scheinman MM, Peters RW, Sauvé MJ *et al*. Value of the H-Q interval in patients with bundle branch block and the role of prophylactic permanent pacing. *Am J Cardiol* 1982;**50**: 1316–22.

41. Dhingra RC, Wyndham C, Bauernfeind RA *et al*. Significance of block distal to His bundle induced by atrial pacing in patients with chronic bifascicular block. *Circulation* 1979; **60**:1455–64.

42. Ward DE, Camm AJ. Atrioventricular conduction delays and block. In: Ward DE, Camm AJ, eds. *Clinical electrophysiology of the heart*. London: Edward Arnold, 1987.

43. Englund A, Bergfeldt L, Rosenqvist M. Disopyramide stress test: a sensitive and specific tool for predicting impending high degree atrioventricular block in patients with bifascicular block. *Br Heart J* 1995;**74**:650–5.

44. Click RL, Gersch BJ, Sugrue DD *et al*. Role of electrophysiologic testing in patients with symptomatic bundle branch block. *Am J Cardiol* 1987;**59**:817–23.

45. Ginks WR, Sutton R, Oh W, Leatham A. Long-term prognosis after acute anterior infarction with atrioventricular block. *Br Heart J* 1977;**39**:186–9.

46. Col JJ, Weinberg SL. The incidence and mortality of intraventricular conduction defects in acute myocardial infarction. *Am J Cardiol* 1972;**29**:344–50.

47. Watson RDS, Glover DR, Page AJF *et al*. The Birmingham trial of permanent pacing in patients with intraventricular conduction disorders after acute myocardial infarction. *Am Heart J* 1984;**108**:496–501.

48. Hindman MC, Wagner GS, JaRo M *et al*. The clinical significance of bundle branch block complicating acute myocardial infarction. 1. Clinical characteristics, hospital mortality and one-year follow up. *Circulation* 1978;**58**:679–88.

49. Hindman MC, Wagner GS, JaRo M *et al*. The clinical significance of bundle branch block complicating acute myocardial infarction. 2. Indications for temporary and permanent pacemaker insertion. *Circulation* 1978;**58**:689–99.

50. Ritter WS, Atkins J, Blomqvist CG, Mullins CB. Permanent pacing in patients with transient trifascicular block during acute myocardial infarction. *Am J Cardiol* 1976;**38**:205–8.

51. Sutton R, Kenny RA. The natural history of sick sinus syndrome. *PACE* 1986;**9**:1110–14.

52. Alboni P, Menozzi C, Brignole M *et al*. Effects of permanent pacemaker and oral theophylline in sick sinus syndrome. The THEOPACE study: a randomized controlled trial. *Circulation* 1997;**96**:260–6.

53. Shaw DB, Holman RR, Gowers JI. Survival in sino-atrial disorder (sick-sinus syndrome). *BMJ* 1980;**280**:139–41.

54. Talan DA, Bauernfeind RA, Ashley WW, Kanakis C Jr, Rosen KM. Twenty-four hour continuous ECG recordings in long-distance runners. *Chest* 1982;**82**:19–24.

55. Kruse I, Arnman K, Conradson T-B, Rydén L. A comparison of the acute and long-term hemodynamic effects of ventricular inhibited and atrial synchronous ventricular inhibited pacing. *Circulation* 1982;**65**:846–55.

56. Perrins EJ, Morley CA, Chan SL, Sutton R. Randomized controlled trial of physiological and ventricular pacing. *Br Heart J* 1983;**50**:112–17.

57. Boon NA, Frew AJ, Johnston JA, Cobbe SM. A comparison of symptoms and intra-arterial ambulatory blood pressure during long term dual chamber atrioventricular synchronous (DDD) and ventricular demand (VVI) pacing. *Br Heart J* 1987;**58**:34–9.

58. Benditt DG, Mianulli M, Fetter J *et al*. Single-chamber cardiac pacing with activity-initiated chronotropic response: evaluation by cardiopulmonary exercise testing. *Circulation* 1987;**75**: 184–91.

59. Lipkin DP, Buller N, Frenneaux M *et al*. Randomized crossover trial of rate responsive Activitrax and conventional fixed rate ventricular pacing. *Br Heart J* 1987;**58**:613–16.

60. Smedgård P, Kristensson B-E, Kruse I, Rydén L. Rate-responsive pacing by means of activity sensing versus single rate ventricular pacing: a double-blind cross-over study. *PACE* 1987;**10**:902–15.

61. Hargreaves MR, Channon KM, Cripps TR, Gardner M, Ormerod OJM. Comparison of dual chamber and ventricular rate responsive pacing in patients over 75 with complete heart block. *Br Heart J* 1995;**74**:397–402.

62. Linde C. How to evaluate quality-of-life in pacemaker patients: problems and pitfalls. *PACE* 1996;**19**:391–7.

63. Sulke N, Dritsas A, Bostock J *et al*. "Subclinical" pacemaker syndrome: a randomized study of symptom free patients with ventricular demand (VVI) pacemakers upgraded to dual chamber devices. *Br Heart J* 1992;**67**:57–64.

64. Alpert MA, Curtis JJ, Sanfelippo JF *et al*. Comparative survival after permanent ventricular and dual chamber pacing for patients with chronic high degree atrioventricular block with and without pre-existent congestive heart failure. *J Am Coll Cardiol* 1986;**7**:925–32.

65. Linde-Edelstam C, Gullberg B, Norlander R *et al*. Longevity in patients with high degree atrioventricular block paced in the atrial synchronous or the fixed rate ventricular inhibited mode. *PACE* 1992;**15**:304–13.

66. Rediker DE, Eagle KA, Homma S, Gillam LD, Harthorne JW. Clinical and hemodynamic comparison of VVI versus DDD pacing in patients with DDD pacemakers. *Am J Cardiol* 1988;**61**:323–9.

67. Mitsuoka T, Kenny RA, Au Yeung T *et al*. Benefits of dual chamber pacing in sick sinus syndrome. *Br Heart J* 1988; **60**:338–47.

68. Hummel J, Barr E, Hanich R *et al*. DDDR pacing is better tolerated than VVIR in patients with sinus node disease. *PACE* 1990;**13**:504.

69. Camm AJ, Katritsis D. Pacing for sick sinus syndrome – a risky business? *PACE* 1990;**13**:695–9.

70. Rosenqvist M, Brandt J, Schuller H. Long-term pacing in sinus node disease: effects of stimulation mode on cardiovascular morbidity and mortality. *Am Heart J* 1988;**116**:16–22.

71. Lamas GA. Pacemaker mode selection and survival: a plea to apply the principles of evidence-based medicine to cardiac pacing practice. *Heart* 1997;**78**:218–20.

72. Andersen HR, Thuesen L, Bagger JP, Vesterlund T, Thomsen PE. Prospective randomized trial of atrial versus ventricular pacing in sick-sinus syndrome. *Lancet* 1994;**344**:1523–8.

73. Andersen HR, Nielsen JC, Thomsen PEB *et al*. Long-term follow up of patients from a randomized trial of atrial versus ventricular pacing for sick sinus syndrome. *Lancet* 1997; **350**:1210–16.

74. Andersen HR, Nielsen JC, Bloch Thomsen PE *et al.* Atrioventricular conduction during long-term follow up of patients with sick sinus syndrome. *Circulation* 1998;**98**: 1315–21.

75. Lamas GA, Orav EJ, Stambler BS *et al.* Quality of life and clinical outcomes in elderly patients treated with ventricular pacing as compared with dual-chamber pacing. *N Engl J Med* 1998;**338**:1097–104.

76. Ellenbogen KA, Stambler BS, Orav EJ *et al.* Clinical characteristics of patients intolerant to VVIR pacing. *Am J Cardiol* 2000;**86**:59–63.

77. Connolly SJ, Kerr CR, Gent M *et al.* Effects of physiologic pacing versus ventricular pacing on the risk of stroke and death due to cardiovascular causes. *N Engl J Med* 2000;**342**:1385–91.

78. Skanes AC, Krahn AD, Yee R *et al.* Progression to chronic atrial fibrillation after pacing: The Canadian Trial of Physiologic Pacing. *J Am Coll Cardiol* 2001;**38**:167–72.

79. Connolly SJ, Talajic M, Roy D *et al.* The effect of pacemaker selection on functional capacity in the Canadian Trial of Physiologic Pacing (CTOPP). *Circulation* 1999;**100**(Suppl. I): I-465.

80. Tang ASL, Roberts RS, Kerr C *et al.* Relationship between pacemaker dependency and the effect of pacing mode on cardiovascular outcomes. *Circulation* 2001;**103**:3081–5.

81. Woodend K, Tang SI, Irvine J *et al.* Pacemaker dependency conditions the QoL benefits of physiological over VVI pacing: Canadian Trial of Physiologic Pacing (CTOPP). *Circulation* 1999;**100**(Suppl. I):I-20.

82. Lamas GA, Lee K, Sweeney M *et al.* The Mode Selection Trial (MOST) in sinus node dysfunction: design, rationale, and baseline characteristics of the first 1000 patients. *Am Heart J* 2000;**140**:541–51.

83. Lamas GA, Lee KL, Sweeney MO *et al.* Ventricular pacing or dual chamber pacing for sinus-node dysfunction. *N Engl J Med* 2002;**346**:1854–62.

84. Wharton JM, Sorrentino RA, Campbell P *et al.* Effect of pacing modality on atrial tachyarrhythmia recurrence in the tachycardia-bradycardia syndrome: preliminary results of the Pacemaker Atrial Tachycardia Trial. *Circulation* 1998; **98**(Suppl. I):I-494.

85. Keating E, Grill C, Hafley G, Sorrentino RA, Lee KL, Wharton JM. Effect of pacing modality on quality of life in patients with the tachycardia-bradycardia syndrome. *J Am Coll Cardiol* 1999;**33**(Suppl. A):153A.

86. Wharton JM, Sorrentino RA, Criger D *et al.* Predictors of death in VVI-R and DDD-R paced patients with the tachycardia-bradycardia syndrome. *J Am Coll Cardiol* 1999;**33**(Suppl. A): 153A.

87. Toff WD, Skehan JD, de Bono DP, Camm AJ. The United Kingdom Pacing and Cardiovascular Events (UKPACE) trial. *Heart* 1997;**78**:221–3.

88. Charles RG, McComb JM. Systematic trial of pacing to prevent atrial fibrillation (STOP-AF). *Heart* 1997;**78**:224–5.

89. Charles RG. Personal communication.

90. Andersen HR. Personal communication.

91. Kerr CR, Connolly SJ, Roberts RS *et al.* Effect of pacing mode on cardiovascular death and stroke. The Canadian Trial of Physiologic Pacing: long-term follow up. *PACE* 2002;**24**:553.

92. Andersen HR, Nielsen JC. Pacing in sick sinus syndrome – need for a prospective, randomized trial comparing atrial with dual chamber pacing. *PACE* 1998;**21**:1175–9.

93. Gribbin GM, McComb JM. Pacemaker trials: software or hardware randomization? *PACE* 1998;**21**:1503–7.

94. Rosenqvist M, Obel IWP. Atrial pacing and the risk for AV block: is there a time for change in attitude? *PACE* 1989; **12**:97–101.

95. Santini M, Ricci R. Is AAI or AAIR still a viable mode of pacing? *PACE* 2001;**24**:276–81.

96. Barold SS. Permanent single chamber atrial pacing is obsolete. *PACE* 2001;**24**:271–5.

97. Quan KJ, Carlson MD, Thames MD. Mechanisms of heart rate and arterial blood pressure control: implications for the pathophysiology of neurocardiogenic syncope. *PACE* 1997; **20**:764–74.

98. Morley CA, Sutton R. Carotid sinus syncope. *Int J Cardiol* 1984;**6**:287–93.

99. Brignole M, Menozzi C. Methods other than tilt testing for diagnosing neurocardiogenic (neurally mediated) syncope. *PACE* 1997;**20**:795–800.

100. Kenny RA, Ingram A, Bayliss J, Sutton R. Head-up tilt: a useful test for investigating unexplained syncope. *Lancet* 1986;**i**:1352–5.

101. Morley CA, Perrins EJ, Grant P *et al.* Carotid sinus syncope treated by pacing. Analysis of persistent symptoms and role of atrioventricular sequential pacing. *Br Heart J* 1982;**47**:411–18.

102. Sugrue DD, Gersh BJ, Holmes DR, Wood DL, Osborn MJ, Hammill SC. Symptomatic "isolated" carotid sinus hypersensitivity: natural history and results of treatment with anticholinergic drugs or pacemaker. *J Am Coll Cardiol* 1986;**7**: 158–62.

103. Brignole M, Menozzi C, Lolli G, Bottoni N, Gaggioli G. Long-term outcome of paced and nonpaced patients with severe carotid sinus syndrome. *Am J Cardiol* 1992;**69**:1039–43.

104. Dey AB, Bexton RS, Tynan MM, Charles RG, Kenny RA. The impact of a dedicated "syncope and falls" clinic on pacing practice in Northeastern England. *PACE* 1997;**20**:815–17.

105. Kenny RAM, Richardson DA, Steen N, Bexton RS, Shaw FE, Bond J. Carotid sinus syndrome: a modifiable risk factor for nonaccidental falls in older adults (SAFE PACE). *J Am Coll Cardiol* 2001;**38**:1491–6.

106. Kenny RA, for the SAFE PACE 2 study group. SAFE PACE 2: Syncope And Falls in the Elderly – Pacing And Carotid Sinus Evaluation. *Europace* 1999;**1**:69–72.

107. Petersen MEV, Sutton R. Cardiac pacing for vasovagal syncope: a reasonable therapeutic option? *PACE* 1997;**20**:824–6.

108. Petersen MEV, Chamberlain-Webber R, Fitzpatrick AP *et al.* Permanent pacing for cardioinhibitory malignant vasovagal syndrome. *Br Heart J* 1994;**71**:274–81.

109. Sheldon RS, Gent M, Roberts RS, Connolly SJ. North American Vasovagal Pacemaker Study: study design and organisation. *PACE* 1997;**20**:844–8.

110. Connolly SJ, Sheldon R, Roberts RS, Gent M on behalf of the Vasovagal Pacemaker Study Investigators. The North American Vasovagal Pacemaker Study (VPS). A randomized trial of permanent cardiac pacing for the prevention of vasovagal syncope. *J Am Coll Cardiol* 1999;**33**:16–20.

111. Sutton R, Petersen MEV. First steps towards a pacing algorithm for vasovagal syncope. *PACE* 1997;**20**:827–8.

112. Sutton R, Brignole M, Menozzi C *et al.* Dual-chamber pacing in the treatment of neurally mediated tilt-positive

cardioinhibitory syncope. Pacemaker versus no therapy: a multicenter randomized study. *Circulation* 2000;**102**: 294–9.

113.Ammirati F, Colivicchi F, Santini M for the Syncope Diagnosis and Treatment Study Investigators. Permanent cardiac pacing versus medical treatment for the prevention of recurrent vasovagal syncope. A multicenter, randomized, controlled trial. *Circulation* 2001;**104**:52–7.

114.Presentation by S.J. Connolly. North American Society of Pacing and Electrophysiology, 23rd Annual Scientific Sessions, San Diego, USA, 11 May 2002.

115.Raviele A, Giada F, Sutton R *et al.* The Vasovagal Syncope and Pacing (Synpace) trial: rationale and study design. *Europace* 2001;**3**:336–41.

116.Raviele A, Themistoclakis S, Gasparini G. Drug treatment of vasovagal syncope. In: Blanc JJ, Benditt D, Sutton R, eds. *Neurally mediated syncope: pathophysiology, investigations, and treatment.* Armonk, NY: Futura, 1996.

117.Bourdarias JP, Lockhart A, Ourbak P *et al.* Hemodynamique des cardiomyopathies obstructives. *Arch Mal Coeur* 1964; **57**:737–8.

118.McDonald K, McWilliams E, O'Keefe B *et al.* Functional assessment of patients treated with permanent dual-chamber pacing as a primary treatment for hypertrophic cardiomyopathy. *Eur Heart J* 1988;**9**:893–8.

119.Fananapazir L, Cannon RO, Tripodi D, Panza JA. Impact of dual-chamber permanent pacing in patients with obstructive hypertrophic cardiomyopathy with symptoms refractory to verapamil and beta-adrenergic blocker therapy. *Circulation* 1992;**85**:2149–61.

120.Jeanrenaud X, Goy JJ, Kappenberger L. Effects of dual-chamber pacing in hypertrophic obstructive cardiomyopathy. *Lancet* 1992;**339**:1318–23.

121.Slade AKB, Sadoul N, Shapiro L *et al.* DDD pacing in hypertrophic cardiomyopathy: a multicentre clinical experience. *Heart* 1996;**75**:44–9.

122.Daubert JC. Pacing and hypertrophic cardiomyopathy. *PACE* 1996;**19**:1141–2.

123.Fananapazir L, Epstein ND, Curiel RV, Panza JA, Tripodi D, McAreavey D. Long-term results of dual-chamber (DDD) pacing in obstructive hypertrophic cardiomyopathy: evidence for progressive symptomatic and hemodynamic improvement and reduction of left ventricular hypertrophy. *Circulation* 1994;**90**:2731–42.

124.Pavin D, Gras D, De Place C, Leclercq C, Mabo P, Daubert C. Long-term effect of DDD pacing in patients with hypertrophic obstructive cardiomyopathy: is there a left ventricular remodelling? *PACE* 1996;**19**:680.

125.Nishimura RA, Trusty JM, Hayes DL *et al.* Dual-chamber pacing for hypertrophic cardiomyopathy: a randomized, double-blind, crossover trial. *J Am Coll Cardiol* 1997;**29**: 435–41.

126.Kappenberger L, Linde C, Daubert C *et al.* Pacing in hypertrophic obstructive cardiomyopathy. A randomized crossover study. *Eur Heart J* 1997;**18**:1249–56.

127.Linde C, Gadler F, Kappenberger L, Ryden L, for the PIC Study Group. Placebo effect of pacemaker implantation in obstructive hypertrophic cardiomyopathy. *Am J Cardiol* 1999;**83**:903–7.

128.Kappenberger LJ, Linde C, Jeanrenaud X *et al.* Clinical progress after randomized on/off pacemaker treatment for hypertrophic obstructive cardiomyopathy. *Europace* 1999; **1**:77–84.

129.Gadler F, Linde C, Daubert C, McKenna WJ *et al.* Significant improvement of quality of life following atrioventricular synchronous pacing in patients with hypertrophic obstructive cardiomyopathy. Data from 1 year of follow up. *Eur Heart J* 1999;**20**:1044–50.

130.Maron BJ, Nishimura RA, McKenna WJ, Rakowski H, Josephson ME, Kieval RS. Assessment of permanent dual-chamber pacing as a treatment for drug-refractory symptomatic patients with obstructive hypertrophic cardiomyopathy: a randomized, double-blind, crossover study (M-PATHY). *Circulation* 1999;**99**:2927–33.

131.Brecker SJD, Xiao HB, Sparrow J, Gibson D. Effects of dual-chamber pacing with short atrioventricular delay in dilated cardiomyopathy. *Lancet* 1992;**340**:1308–12.

132.Hochleitner M, Hörtnagl H, Fridrich L, Gschnitzer F. Long-term efficacy of physiologic dual-chamber pacing in the treatment of end-stage idiopathic dilated cardiomyopathy. *Am J Cardiol* 1992;**70**:1320–5.

133.Auricchio A, Sommariva L, Salo RW, Scafuri A, Chiariello L. Improvement of cardiac function in patients with severe congestive heart failure and coronary artery disease by dual chamber pacing with shortened AV delay. *PACE* 1993; **16**:2034–43.

134.Linde C, Gadler F, Edner M *et al.* Results of atrioventricular synchronous pacing with optimized delay in patients with severe congestive heart failure. *Am J Cardiol* 1995;**75**: 919–23.

135.Gold MR, Feliciano Z, Gottlieb SS, Fisher ML. Dual-chamber pacing with a short atrioventricular delay in congestive heart failure: a randomized study. *J Am Coll Cardiol* 1995;**26**: 967–73.

136.Nishimura RA, Hayes DL, Holmes DR Jr, Tajik AJ. Mechanism of hemodynamic improvement by dual-chamber pacing for severe left ventricular dysfunction: an acute Doppler and catheterisation hemodynamic study. *J Am Coll Cardiol* 1995; **25**:281–8.

137.Paul V, Cowell R, Morris-Thurgood J *et al.* First-degree heart block in heart failure: is this a class I indication for dual-chamber pacing? *PACE* 1995;**18**:906.

138.Brecker SJD, Gibson DG. What is the role of pacing in dilated cardiomyopathy? *Eur Heart J* 1996;**17**:819–24.

139.Glikson M, Hayes DL, Nishimura RA. Newer clinical applications of pacing. *J Cardiovasc Electrophysiol* 1997;**8**: 1190–203.

140.Cowell R, Morris-Thurgood J, Ilsley C, Paul V. Septal short atrioventricular delay pacing: additional hemodynamic improvements in heart failure. *PACE* 1994;**17**:1980–3.

141.Gold M, Shorofsky SR, Metcalf MD, Feliciano Z, Fisher ML, Gottlieb S. The acute hemodynamic effects of right ventricular septal pacing in patients with congestive heart failure secondary to ischemic or idiopathic dilated cardiomyopathy. *Am J Cardiol* 1997;**79**:679–81.

142.Victor F, Leclerq C, Mabo P *et al.* Optimal right ventricular pacing site in chronically implanted patients. *J Am Coll Cardiol* 1999;**33**:311–16.

143. Buckingham TA, Candinas R, Schläpfer J *et al.* Acute hemody-namic effects of atrioventricular pacing at differing sites in the right ventricle individually and simultaneously. *PACE* 1997;**20**:909–15.

144. Schwaab B, Fröhlig G, Alexander C *et al.* Influence of right ventricular stimulation site on left ventricular function in syn-chronous ventricular pacing. *J Am Coll Cardiol* 1999; **33**:317–23.

145. Deshmukh P, Casavant DA, Romanyshyn M, Anderson K. Permanent, direct His-bundle pacing. *Circulation* 2000; **101**:869–77.

146. Wilensky RL, Yudelman P, Cohen AI *et al.* Serial electrocar-diographic changes in idiopathic dilated cardiomyopathy con-firmed at necropsy. *Am J Cardiol* 1988;**62**:276–83.

147. de Teresa E, Chamorro JL, Pulpon LA *et al.* An even more physiological pacing. Changing the sequence of activation. In: Steinbech K, Glogar D, Laszkovics A *et al*, eds. *Cardiac pacing.* (Proceedings of the VIIth World Symposium on Cardiac Pacing). Darmstadt, Germany: Steinkopff Verlag, 1983.

148. Cazeau S, Ritter P, Bakdach S *et al.* Four chamber pacing in dilated cardiomyopathy. *PACE* 1994;**17**:1974–9.

149. Bakker PF, Meijburg H, de Jonge N *et al.* Beneficial effects of biventricular pacing in congestive heart failure. *PACE* 1994;**17**:820.

150. Cazeau S, Ritter P, Lazarus A *et al.* Multi-site pacing for end-stage heart failure. *PACE* 1996;**19**:1748–57.

151. Blanc JJ, Etienne Y, Gilard M *et al.* Evaluation of different ven-tricular pacing sites in patients with severe heart failure. *Circulation* 1997;**96**:3273–7.

152. Leclercq C, Cazeau S, Le Breton H *et al.* Acute hemody-namic effects of biventricular DDD pacing in patients with end-stage heart failure. *J Am Coll Cardiol* 1998;**32**: 1825–31.

153. Auricchio A, Stellbrink C, Block M *et al.* Effect of pacing chamber and atrioventricular delay on acute systolic function of paced patients with congestive heart failure. *Circulation* 1999;**99**:2993–3001.

154. Kass DA, Chen C-H, Curry C *et al.* Improved left ventri-cular mechanics from acute VDD pacing in patients with dilated cardiomyopathy and ventricular conduction delay. *Circulation* 1999;**99**:1567–73.

155. Daubert JC, Ritter P, Le Breton H *et al.* Permanent left ven-tricular pacing with transvenous leads inserted into the coro-nary veins. *PACE* 1998;**21**:239–45.

156. Walker S, Levy T, Rex S, Brant S, Paul V. Initial United Kingdom experience with the use of permanent, biventricular pacemakers. Implantation procedure and technical considera-tions. *Europace* 2000;**2**:233–9.

157. Gras D, Mabo P, Tang T *et al.* Multisite pacing as a supple-mental treatment of congestive heart failure: preliminary results of the Medtronic Inc. InSync study. *PACE* 1998; **21**:2249–55.

158. Gras D, Ritter P, Lazarus A *et al.* Long-term outcome of advanced heart failure patients with cardiac resynchronisation therapy. *PACE* 2000;**23**:658.

159. Daubert JC, Cazeau S, Leclercq C. Do we have reasons to be enthusiastic about pacing to treat advanced heart failure? *Eur J Heart Failure* 1999;**1**:281–7.

160. Auricchio A, Stellbrink C, Sack S *et al.* The Pacing Therapies for Congestive Heart Failure (PATH-CHF) study: rationale, design, and endpoints of a prospective randomized multicen-ter study. *Am J Cardiol* 1999;**83**:130D–5D.

161. Auricchio A, Stellbrink C, Sack S *et al.* Long-term clinical effect of haemodynamically optimised cardiac resynchroniza-tion therapy in patients with heart failure and ventricular conduction delay. *J Am Coll Cardiol* 2002;**39**:2026–33.

162. Auricchio A, Stellbrink C, Sack S *et al.* PATH CHF study: reduced hospitalization days due to heart failure. *Europace* 2001;**2**:B49.

163. Cazeau S, Leclercq C, Lavergne T *et al.* Effects of multisite biventricular pacing in patients with heart failure and intraventricular conduction delay. *N Engl J Med* 2001; **344**:873–80.

164. Linde C, Leclercq C, Rex S *et al.* Long-term benefits of biven-tricular pacing in congestive heart failure: results from the MUltisite STimulation In Cardiomyopathy (MUSTIC) study. *J Am Coll Cardiol* 2002;**40**:111–18.

165. Daubert JC, Linde C, Cazeau S, Kappenberger L, Sutton R, Bailleul C. Clinical effects of biventricular pacing in patients with severe heart failure and chronic atrial fibrillation: results from the Multisite Stimulation in Cardiomyopathy – MUSTIC Study Group. *Circulation* 2000;**102**(Suppl. 2): II–693.

166. Leclercq C, Victor F, Alonso C *et al.* Comparative effects of permanent biventricular pacing for refractory heart failure in patients with stable sinus rhythm or chronic atrial fibrillation. *Am J Cardiol* 2000;**85**:1154–6.

167. Brignole M, Gammage M. An assessment of the optimal ven-tricular pacing site in patients undergoing "ablate and pace" therapy for permanent atrial fibrillation. *Europace* 2001; **3**:153–6.

168. Abraham WT. Rationale and design of a randomized clinical trial to assess the safety and efficacy of cardiac resynchroniza-tion therapy in patients with advanced heart failure: the Multicenter InSync Randomized Clinical Evaluation (MIR-ACLE). *J Cardiac Failure* 2000;**6**:369–80.

169. Abraham WT, Fisher WQ, Smith AL *et al.* Cardiac resynchro-nization in chronic heart failure. *N Engl J Med* 2002; **346**:1845–53.

170. Auricchio A, Pappone C, Schalij MJ, Neuzner J, Padeletti L, Maertens S. Sustained benefit of resynchronization therapy in large patient cohort. *Europace* 2001;**2**(Suppl. B):B48.

171. Zardini M, Tritto M, Bargiggia G *et al.* The InSync Italian Registry: analysis of clinical outcome and considerations on the selection of candidates to left ventricular resynchroniza-tion. *Eur Heart J* 2000;**2**(Suppl. J):J16–J22.

172. Saxon LA, DeMarco T, Chatterjee K, Kerwin WF, Boehmer J. Chronic biventricular pacing decreases serum norepinephrine in dilated heart failure patients with the greatest sympathetic activation at baseline. *PACE* 1999;**22**:830.

173. Hamdan MH, Zagrodzky JD, Joglar JA *et al.* Biventricular pacing decreases sympathetic activity compared with right ventricular pacing in patients with depressed ejection fraction. *Circulation* 2000;**102**:1027–32.

174. Walker S, Levy T, Rex S *et al.* Usefulness of suppression of ventricular arrhythmia by biventricular pacing in severe con-gestive cardiac failure. *Am J Cardiol* 2000;**86**:231–3.

175. Higgins SL, Yong P, Scheck D *et al.* Biventricular pacing diminishes the need for implantable defibrillator therapy. *J Am Coll Cardiol* 2000;**36**:824–7.

176. Cleland JG, Daubert JC, Erdmann E *et al.* The CARE-HF study (CArdiac REsynchronisation in Heart Failure study): rationale, design and end-points. *Eur J Heart Fail* 2001;**3**:481–9.

177. Bristow MR, Feldman AM, Saxon LA. *Heart* failure management using implantable devices for ventricular resynchronization: Comparison of Medical Therapy, Pacing, and Defibrillation in Chronic Heart Failure (COMPANION) trial. *J Cardiac Failure* 2000;**6**:276–85.

178. Coumel P, Friocourt P, Mugica J, Attuel P, Leclerq JF. Long term prevention of vagal atrial arrhythmias by atrial pacing at 90/min: experience with 6 cases. *PACE* 1983;**6**:552–60.

179. Gillis AM, Wyse DG, Connolly S *et al.* Atrial pacing periablation for prevention of paroxysmal atrial fibrillation. *Circulation* 1999;**99**:2553–8.

180. Gillis AM, Connolly SJ, Lacombe P *et al.* Randomized crossover comparison of DDDR versus VDD pacing after atrioventricular junction ablation for prevention of atrial fibrillation. *Circulation* 2000;**102**:736–41.

181. Brignole M, Gianfranchi L, Menozzi C *et al.* Assessment of atrioventricular junction ablation and DDDR mode-switching pacemaker versus pharmacological treatment in patients with severely symptomatic paroxysmal atrial fibrillation: a randomized controlled study. *Circulation* 1997;**96**:2617–24.

182. Marshall HJ, Harris ZI, Griffith MJ, Holder RL, Gammage MD. Prospective randomized study of ablation and pacing versus medical therapy for paroxysmal atrial fibrillation: effects of pacing mode and mode-switch algorithm. *Circulation* 1999;**99**:1587–92.

183. Ward KJ, Willett JE, Bucknall C, Gill JS, Kamalvand K. Atrial arrhythmia suppression by atrial overdrive pacing: pacemaker Holter assessment. *Europace* 2001;**3**:108–14.

184. Levy T, Walker S, Rex S, Paul V. Does atrial overdrive pacing prevent paroxysmal atrial fibrillation in paced patients? *Int J Cardiol* 2000;**75**:91–7.

185. Garrigue S, Barold SS, Cazeau S *et al.* Prevention of atrial arrhythmias during DDD pacing by atrial overdrive. *PACE* 1998;**21**:1751–9.

186. Wiberg S, Lonnerholm S, Jensen S *et al.* Effect of right atrial overdrive pacing on symptomatic attacks of atrial fibrillation: a multicenter randomized study. *PACE* 2001;**24**:554.

187. Bellocci F, Spampinato A, Ricci R *et al.* Antiarrhythmic benefits of dual chamber stimulation with rate-response in patients with paroxysmal atrial fibrillation and chronotropic incompetence. *Europace* 1999;**1**:220–5.

188. Funck RC, Adamec R, Lurje L *et al.* Atrial overdriving is beneficial in patients with atrial arrhythmias: first results of the PROVE study. *PACE* 2000;**23**:1891–3.

189. Murgatroyd FD, Nitzsché R, Slade AKB *et al.* A new pacing algorithm for overdrive suppression of atrial fibrillation. *PACE* 1994;**17**:1966–73.

190. Ip J, Beau S, Cameron D, for the ADOPT A Investigators. Early results of ADOPT A: Dynamic Atrial Overdrive™ pacing to treat paroxysmal atrial fibrillation. *PACE* 2001;**24**:615.

191. Lam CTF, Lau CP, Leung SK *et al.* Efficacy and tolerability of continuous overdrive atrial pacing in atrial fibrillation. *Europace* 2000;**2**:286–91.

192. Ricci R, Santini M, Puglisi A *et al.* Impact of consistent atrial pacing algorithm on premature atrial complex number and paroxysmal atrial fibrillation recurrences in brady-tachy syndrome: a randomized prospective cross over study. *J Intervent Cardiac Electrophysiol* 2001;**5**:33–44.

193. Israel CW, Lawo T, Lemke B, Grönefeld G, Hohnloser SH. Atrial pacing in the prevention of paroxysmal atrial fibrillation. *PACE* 2000;**23**:1888–90.

194. Presentation by A.J. Camm, on behalf of the AF Therapy study group. European Society of Cardiology, XXIII Congress, Stockholm, September 2001.

195. Anselme F, Saoudi N, Cribier A. Pacing in prevention of atrial fibrillation: the PIPAF studies. *J Intervent Cardiac Electrophysiol* 2000;**4**:177–84.

196. Daubert C, Mabo P, Berder V. Arrhythmia prevention by permanent atrial resynchronization in advanced interatrial block. *Eur Heart J* 1990;**11**:237.

197. Daubert C, Mabo P, Berder V *et al.* Permanent dual atrium pacing in major interatrial conduction block: a four years experience. *PACE* 1993;**16**:885.

198. Mabo P, Daubert JC, Bouhour A, on behalf of the SYNBIAPACE Study Group. Biatrial synchronous pacing for atrial arrhythmia prevention: the SYNBIAPACE study. *PACE* 1999;**22**:755.

199. Saksena S, Prakash, Hill M *et al.* Prevention of recurrent atrial fibrillation with chronic dual-site right atrial pacing. *J Am Coll Cardiol* 1996;**28**:687–94.

200. Delfaut P, Saksena S, Prakash A, Krol RB. Long-term outcome of patients with drug refractory atrial flutter and fibrillation after single- and dual-site right atrial pacing for arrhythmia prevention. *J Am Coll Cardiol* 1998;**32**:1900–8.

201. Fitts SM, Hill MR, Mehra R *et al.* Design and implementation of the Dual Site Atrial Pacing to Prevent Atrial Fibrillation (DAPPAF) clinical trial. DAPPAF Phase 1 Investigators. *J Intervent Cardiac Electrophysiol* 1998;**2**:139–44.

202. Saksena S, Filipecki A. Atrial pacing to prevent atrial fibrillation: is there any evidence of its real efficacy? In: Raviele A, ed. *Cardiac arrhythmias 2001* (Proceedings of the 7th International Workshop on Cardiac Arrhythmias, Venice, 2001). Milan: Springer, 2001.

203. Lau CP, Tse HF, Yu CM *et al.* Dual-site atrial pacing for atrial fibrillation in patients without bradycardia. *Am J Cardiol* 2001;**88**:371–5.

204. Bennett DH. Comparison of the acute effects of pacing the atrial septum, right atrial appendage, coronary sinus os, and the latter two sites simultaneously on the duration of atrial activation. *Heart* 2000;**84**:193–6.

205. Baillin SJ, Adler S, Giudici M. Prevention of chronic atrial fibrillation by pacing in the region of Bachmann's bundle: results of a multicenter randomized trial. *J Cardiovasc Electrophysiol* 2001;**12**:912–17.

206. Padeletti L, Pieragnoli P, Ciapetti C *et al.* Randomized crossover comparison of right atrial appendage pacing versus interatrial septum pacing for prevention of paroxysmal atrial fibrillation in patients with sinus bradycardia. *Am Heart J* 2001;**142**:1047–55.

207. Padeletti L, Porciani MC, Michelucci A *et al*. Prevention of short term reversible chronic atrial fibrillation by permanent pacing at the triangle of Koch. *J Intervent Cardiac Electrophysiol* 2000;**4**:575–83.

208. Moss AJ, Liu JE, Gottlieb S *et al*. Efficacy of permanent pacing in the long QT syndrome. *Circulation* 1991;**84**:1524–9.

209. Eldar M, Griffin JC, Van Hare GF *et al*. Combined use of beta-adrenergic blocking agents and long-term cardiac pacing for patients with the long QT syndrome. *J Am Coll Cardiol* 1992;**20**:830–7.

210. Schwartz PJ. *The Long QT Syndrome*. New York: Futura, 1997.

211. Zareba W, Priori SG, Moss AJ *et al*. Permanent pacing in the long QT syndrome patients. *PACE* 1997;**20**:1097.

212. Viskin S, Alla SR, Baron HV *et al*. Mode of onset of torsade de pointes in congenital long QT syndrome. *J Am Coll Cardiol* 1996;**28**:1262–8.

213. Klein H, Levi A, Kaplinsky E, DiSegni E, David D. Congenital long-QT syndrome: deleterious effect of long-term high-rate ventricular pacing and definitive treatment by cardiac transplantation. *Am Heart J* 1996;**132**:1079–81.

214. Viskin S. Cardiac pacing in the long QT syndrome: review of available data and practical recommendations. *J Cardiovasc Electrophysiol* 2000;**11**:593–600.

215. Viskin S, Fish R, Roth A, Copperman Y. Prevention of torsade de pointes in the congenital long QT syndrome: use of a pause prevention pacing algorithm. *Heart* 1998;**79**:417–19.

216. Priori SG, Napolitano C, Cantù F, Brown AM, Schwartz PJ. Differential response to Na⁺ channel blockade, α-adrenergic stimulation, and rapid pacing in a cellular model mimicking the SCN5A and HERG defects present in the long-QT syndrome. *Circ Res* 1996;**78**:1009–15.

217. Schwartz PJ, Priori SG, Locati EH *et al*. Long QT syndrome patients with mutations of the SCN5A and HERG genes have differential responses to Na⁺ channel blockade and to increases in heart rate. *Circulation* 1995;**92**:3381–6.

218. Shimizu W, Antzelevitch C. Sodium channel block with mexiletine is effective in reducing dispersion of repolarization and preventing torsade des pointes in LQT2 and LQT3 models of the long-QT syndrome. *Circulation* 1997;**96**:2038–47.

219. Schwartz PJ, Priori SG, Spazzolini C *et al*. Genotype-phenotype correlation in the long-QT syndrome: gene-specific triggers for life-threatening arrhythmias. *Circulation* 2001; **103**:89–95.

220. Jacquet L, Ziady G, Stein K *et al*. Cardiac rhythm disturbances early after orthotopic heart transplantation: prevalence and importance of the observed abnormalities. *J Am Coll Cardiol* 1990;**16**:832–7.

221. Holt ND, Tynan MM, Scott CD, Parry G, Dark JH, McComb JM. Permanent pacemaker use after cardiac transplantation: completing the audit cycle. *Heart* 1996;**76**:435–8.

222. Bertolet BD, Eagle DA, Conti JB, Mills RM, Belardinelli L. Bradycardia after heart transplantation: reversal with theophylline. *J Am Coll Cardiol* 1996;**28**:396–9.

223. Miyamoto Y, Curtiss EI, Kormos RL, Armitage JM, Hardesty RL, Griffith BP. Bradyarrhythmias after heart transplantation. *Circulation* 1990;**82**(Suppl. IV):313–17.

224. DiBiase A, Tse TM, Schnittger I, Wexler L, Stinson EB, Valantine HA. Frequency and mechanism of bradycardia in cardiac transplant recipients and need for pacemakers. *Am J Coll Cardiol* 1991;**67**:1385–9.

225. Heinz G, Kratochwill C, Schmid S *et al*. Sinus node dysfunction after orthotopic heart transplantation: the Vienna experience 1987–1993. *PACE* 1994;**17**:2057–63.

226. Scott CD, Omar I, McComb JM, Dark JH, Bexton RS. Long-term pacing in heart transplant recipients is usually unnecessary. *PACE* 1991;**14**:1792–6.

227. Morris-Thurgood J, Cowell R, Paul V *et al*. Hemodynamic and metabolic effects of paced linkage following heterotopic cardiac transplantation. *Circulation* 1994;**90**:2342–7.

228. Morris-Thurgood J, Paul VE, Dyke C *et al*. Chronic linkage after heterotopic heart transplantation. *Transplant Proc* 1997;**29**:580.

229. Young T, Palta M, Dempsey J, Skatrud J, Weber S, Badr S. The occurrence of sleep-disordered breathing among middle-aged adults. *N Engl J Med* 1993;**328**:1230–5.

230. Stegman SS, Burroughs JM, Henthorn RW. Asymptomatic bradyarrhythmias as a marker for sleep apnea: appropriate recognition and treatment may reduce the need for pacemaker therapy. *PACE* 1996;**19**:899–904.

231. Grimm W, Koehler U, Fus E *et al*. Outcome of patients with sleep apnea-associated severe bradyarrhythmias after continuous positive airway pressure therapy. *Am J Cardiol* 2000; **86**:688–92.

232. Kato I, Shiomi T, Sasanabe R *et al*. Effects of physiological cardiac pacing on sleep-disordered breathing in patients with chronic bradydysrhythmias. *Psychiatry Clin Neurosci* 2001; **55**:257–8.

233. Garrigue S, Bordier P, Jaïs P *et al*. Benefit of atrial pacing in sleep apnea syndrome. *N Engl J Med* 2002;**346**: 404–12.

234. Gottlieb DJ. Cardiac pacing – a novel therapy for sleep apnea? *N Engl J Med* 2002;**346**:444–5.

235. Murdock CJ, Klein GJ, Yee R, Leitch JW, Teo WS, Norris C. Feasibility of long-term electro-cardiographic monitoring with an implanted device for syncope diagnosis. *PACE* 1991;**13**: 1374–8.

236. Lascault G, Barnay C, Cazeau S, Frank R, Medvedowsky JL. Preliminary evaluation of a dual chamber pacemaker with bradycardia diagnostic functions. *PACE* 1995;**18**: 1636–43.

237. Cazeau S, Ritter P, Nitzsché R, Limousin M, Mugica J. Diagnosis of atrial arrhythmias using the Holter function of a new DDD pacemaker. *PACE* 1994;**17**:2106–13.

43 Syncope

David G Benditt, Cengiz Ermis, Keith G Lurie, Scott Sakaguchi

Introduction

Syncope is a symptom consisting of the sudden loss of both consciousness and postural tone, with subsequent spontaneous recovery. Syncopal episodes must be differentiated from other conditions in which real or apparent loss of consciousness may occur, such as seizures, sleep disturbances, accidents, and some psychiatric conditions. Establishing the basis for syncope is essential in order to ascertain prognosis and develop an effective treatment strategy.

Typically syncopal events are brief. Loss of consciousness rarely lasts longer than 10 or 20 seconds, and recovery is relatively prompt and usually unassociated with retrograde amnesia. Some forms of syncope are ushered in by a premonitory phase. This is especially the case with the vasovagal faint, in which lightheadedness, sweatiness, nausea and a feeling of being short of breath are not uncommon, especially in the younger fainter. Additionally, postsyncope recovery may be characterized by a prolonged period of fatigue and listlessness; this feature is once again most commonly associated with the vasovagal faint. As a result, depending upon the manner in which the medical history is elicited, the total duration of "syncope" is often reported to have been quite long. The latter is particularly the case in elderly individuals, in whom recollection of the events may be poor.

To date, with the exception of four recently completed pacing trials in patients with recurrent vasovagal faints, the evaluation and treatment of syncope has not been the subject of large-scale clinical study. Diagnostic strategies have been based largely on experience derived from multiple relatively small single-center non-randomized studies.

Certain syncope-related clinical issues have been subject to "expert task force" review and recommendation by professional and/or scientific societies. The American College of Cardiology task force report on tilt-table testing[1] and the recently published European Society Task Force on Syncope Evaluation[2] are examples of these processes. On the other hand, most current recommendations regarding evaluation and treatment of specific disorders associated with syncope (for example, sinus node dysfunction, AV block, ventricular arrhythmias) are based on compilations of uncontrolled and often retrospective experiences.

In several important clinical scenarios, such as acquired complete heart block, and syncope associated with life-threatening ventricular tachyarrhythmias, evidence of treatment efficacy (that is prevention of syncope recurrences) appears to be adequately substantiated despite the absence of randomized controlled trials. On the other hand, in conditions such as neurally mediated vasovagal syncope the efficacy of current pharmacologic treatments is less certain, and multicenter randomized studies are very much needed.

This chapter focuses on the diagnosis and treatment of the principal clinical conditions associated with syncope. The primary objectives are (1) to identify the most common causes of syncope, (2) to outline a practicable strategy for evaluation of the syncope patient, and (3) to define appropriate directions for treatment. Throughout, an attempt has been made to characterize the status of current clinical evidence related to each of these topics.

Epidemiologic considerations

Studies examining the population frequency of syncope have tended to comprise relatively small numbers of subjects in selected populations, such as the military or tertiary care medical centers or solitary medical practices. Consequently, the true incidence of syncope in the population as a whole remains uncertain. Nevertheless, a number of reports suggest that syncope accounts for approximately 1–3% of emergency room visits and from 1 to 6% of general hospital admissions in the United States,[3,4] and has a prevalence of 15–30% in selected young individuals such as military recruits.[2]

In terms of a broader population sample, the Framingham Study (in which biennial examinations were carried out over a 26 year period in 5209 free-living individuals) reported the occurrence of at least one syncopal event in approximately 3% of men and 3·5% of women.[5] The first occurred at an average age of 52 years (range 17–78 years) for men and 50 years (range 13–87 years) for women. Further, although syncope occurred at virtually all ages, its prevalence increased with advancing age, from eight per 1000 person-examinations in the 35–44 year old age group to approximately 40 per 1000 person-examinations in the ≥75 year age group. Indeed, among elderly patients confined to long-term care institutions the annual incidence may be as high as 6%. Additionally, among patients who have experienced syncope the recurrence of symptoms was reported to be very common. Several reports provide solid estimates suggesting that recurrences are to be expected in about 30% of individuals.[5–7]

Classification of the causes of syncope

Box 43.1 provides a classification of causes of syncope based on the approximate frequency with which they may be expected to occur in a general internal medicine or family practice. However, the diagnostic problem is complicated by the fact that more than one cause often contributes to the clinical picture. For example, syncope in valvular aortic stenosis is not due solely to a narrowed orifice restricting cardiac output: inappropriate reflex vasodilation and/or primary cardiac arrhythmias often play an important role. Similarly, syncope in association with certain brady- and tachyarrhythmias depends in part on neural reflex factors. For example, the ability to initiate vasoconstriction in response to an arrhythmic stress seems to be an important factor in determining whether the affected individual is able to tolerate the stress or becomes lightheaded or syncopal.[8,9]

Box 43.1 Apparent transient loss of consciousness: diagnostic classification

Syncope

Neurally mediated reflex syncope
- Vasovagal faint
- Carotid sinus syncope
- Cough syncope and related disorders
- Gastrointestinal, pelvic or urologic origin

Orthostatic syncope
- Chronic blood/plasma loss (hemorrhage, diarrhea, Addison's disease, pheochromocytoma)
- Primary autonomic failure syndromes (for example, pure autonomic failure, multiple system atrophy, Parkinson's disease with autonomic failure)
- Secondary autonomic failure syndromes (diabetic neuropathy, amyloid neuropathy)
- Drugs and alcohol

Primary cardiac arrhythmias
- Sinus node dysfunction (including bradycardia/tachycardia syndrome)
- AV conduction system disease
- Paroxysmal supraventricular and ventricular tachycardias
- Implanted device (pacemaker, ICD) malfunction

Structural cardiovascular or cardiopulmonary disease
- Cardiac valvular disease/ischemia
- Acute myocardial infarction
- Obstructive cardiomyopathy
- Subclavian steal syndrome
- Pericardial disease/tamponade
- Pulmonary embolus

- Pulmonary hypertension

Cerebrovascular
- Vascular steal syndromes
- Seizure disorders
- Panic attacks
- Hysteria

Miscellaneous conditions – not true syncope

Disorders resembling syncope
- Seizures
- Psychogenic 'syncope' (somatization disorders)

Disorders resembling syncope, but usually without complete loss of consciousness
- Hyperventilation (hypocapnia)
- Hypoglycemia
- Acute hypoxemia

In general terms, the classification of the causes of syncope leads to some reasonable conclusions regarding diagnostic testing strategies. It is apparent that attention should be focused on obtaining as detailed as possible medical history of the event(s), assessing the potential role of drugs in precipitating symptoms, and determining the presence or absence of structural heart disease. Neurologic studies (for example, EEG, MRI/CT) should be de-emphasized in the initial evaluation of the syncope patient in the absence of abnormal neurologic signs on physical examination or a clearcut history of seizure disorder.

Neurally mediated reflex syncope

In the various forms of neurally mediated reflex syncope (Box 43.2) systemic hypotension occurs primarily as a result of inappropriate neural reflex activity. In certain cases syncope is principally the result of parasympathetically induced bradycardia or asystole (so-called cardioinhibitory syncope) (Figure 43.1). In others, symptomatic hypotension is due primarily to inappropriate vasodilation (that is vasodepressor syncope). In most cases, however, both phenomena contribute;[1,2,8,10–12] in these latter cases the bradycardia is often modest but is none the less abnormal, given the severity of the hypotension (that is relative bradycardia).

Box 43.2 Neurally mediated reflex syncopal syndromes

Emotional syncope (common or "vasovagal" faint, "malignant" vasovagal faint)

Carotid sinus syncope

Cough, sneeze syncope

Exercise, postexercise variant

Gastrointestinal stimulation
   Swallow syncope, defecation syncope

Glossopharyngeal neuralgia

Postmicturition syncope

Raised intrathoracic pressure, airway stimulation
   Brass wind instrument-playing, weightlifting

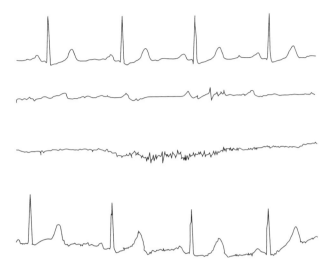

Figure 43.1 Continuous single-channel electrocardiographic recording during an episode of spontaneous vasovagal syncope. A characteristic finding is the presence of sinus bradycardia in conjunction with AV block, indicating the occurrence of concomitant cardioinhibition despite hypotension induced by bradycardia.

The vasovagal faint and carotid sinus syndrome are the most common forms of neurally mediated syncope. The vasovagal faint (also known as the "common faint") may be triggered by any of a variety of factors, including unpleasant sights, pain, extreme emotion and prolonged standing. Vasovagal syncope may often be suspected in the presence of a "typical" medical history, but often the history is not definitive. In such cases, tilt-table testing is the most important supportive diagnostic test.[1,8,10–12] Carotid sinus syndrome is probably the second most common form of the neurally mediated syncopal syndromes, but is often overlooked in clinical practice. Recent experience suggests that carotid sinus syndrome may be an important cause of non-accidental "falls" in older individuals.[13] Consequently, this often overlooked diagnosis warrants careful consideration in all older patients who faint or present with falls and/or injuries that are not readily accounted for.

Despite the apparent "mixed" bradycardia–vasodilation picture observed during diagnostic evaluation (especially during tilt-table testing), substantial recent published clinical experience suggests that bradycardia might be more important than previously believed during spontaneous syncope epsiodes, especially in vasovagal fainters. In this regard, the VPS1 study utilized a relatively complex system to identify bradycardia.[14] The VASIS trial used a more intuitive classification scheme.[15,16] In both cases, randomized controlled trials versus conventional medical treatment at the time showed pacing to be highly effective in a subset of relatively symptomatic individuals with recurrent vasovagal faints. An additional pacemaker versus β adrenergic drug treatment

trial[17] also ended in favor of pacing. Finally, in partial explanation of these observations, the recently reported ISSUE trial results indicated that tilt-table testing (for reasons as yet unknown) may overestimate the importance of the vasodilation component in vasovagal fainters.[18] Bradycardia was far more frequent than initially suspected, based on observations made using implantable loop recorders (Reveal®, Medtronic Inc., Minneapolis, MN, USA).

The occurrence of syncope (or unexplained "falls") without warning in older persons should lead to consideration of carotid sinus syndrome. The condition is probably present when symptoms are reproduced during firm linear carotid sinus massage (usually best undertaken with the patient in the upright position, carefully secured on a tilt-table) in conjunction with asystole, paroxysmal AV block, and/or a marked drop in systemic arterial pressure.[13] In the absence of symptom reproduction, a pause of 5 seconds or longer is probably sufficient to support the diagnosis (assuming other etiologies of syncope have been excluded to the extent that it is possible to do so).

Orthostatic syncope

The abrupt assumption of an upright posture often results in presyncopal symptoms (that is transient "gray-out") even in apparently healthy individuals, but frank syncope is thought to be uncommon. However, syncope may occur in some cases, especially in elderly or less physically fit individuals, or in patients who are volume depleted.

Iatrogenic factors such as excessive diuresis or the aggressive prescription of antihypertensive drugs are probably by far the most important contributors to the development of posturally related syncope. Less often, primary forms of autonomic nervous system dysfunction are the cause. Some of the more important of these include pure autonomic failure, multiple system atrophy, and Parkinson's disease with autonomic failure.[14] Although these conditions are rare, their recognition and study may provide valuable information of importance to a much larger group of patients who have disorders with less well defined defects, including neurally mediated hypotension and the postural tachycardia syndromes (POTS). Furthermore, as these often overlooked disturbances and their potentially subtle manifestations become more widely appreciated, they will be identified more often. For instance, Low *et al*[19] reviewed their experience in 155 patients referred for assessment of suspected orthostatic hypotension. Their findings revealed that among the most severely affected symptomatic patients ($n = 90$, mean age 64 years), pure autonomic failure accounted for 33%, multisystem atrophy for 26% and autonomic/diabetic neuropathy for 31%. Finally, secondary autonomic dysfunction due to neuropathies associated with chronic diseases (for example, diabetes mellitus), toxic agents (for example, alcohol) or infections (Guillain–Barré syndrome) are relatively common and may also cause syncope in association with orthostatic hypotension.

Tilt-table testing facilities may be helpful in identifying patients susceptible to syncope associated with orthostatic hypotension. However, the diagnosis of the various forms of autonomic failure using tilt-table and other autonomic testing procedures[19-22] requires a level of experience which is currently not widely available.

Primary cardiac arrhythmias

Primary cardiac arrhythmias – that is, those rhythm disturbances arising as a result of cardiac conduction system disturbances, anomalous electrical connections or myocardial disease – are important causes of syncope. In general terms, the arrhythmias most often associated with syncope or near-syncope are the bradyarrhythmias accompanying sinus node dysfunction (also termed "sick sinus syndrome"[23,24]) or AV block, and the tachyarrhythmias of ventricular origin.

Sinus node dysfunction

Sinus node dysfunction comprises various sinus node and/ or atrial arrhythmias that result in persistent or intermittent periods of inappropriately slow (sinus bradycardia, sinus pauses, sinoatrial exit block) or fast heart beating (most often atrial fibrillation or atrial flutter)[23-25] (Figure 43.2). In terms of syncope, the bradyarrhythmias appear to be the more important culprits. For example, among 56 patients with either severe bradyarrhythmias or bradycardia–tachycardia syndrome described by Rubenstein *et al*,[25] 25 (45%) presented with syncope and an additional 15 (27%) reported various presyncopal symptoms. In the vast majority of these cases (80%), bradyarrhythmias were considered to be the principal responsible rhythm disturbance.

In general terms, sinus node dysfunction may be considered as intrinsic or extrinsic in nature. Intrinsic sinus node dysfunction is, for the most part, closely associated with underderlying structural disturbances in the atria (for example, fibrosis, chamber enlargement). Atrial changes accompanying the aging process need also to be included in the intrinsic category. In the case of extrinsic sinus node

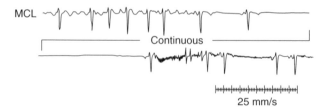

Figure 43.2 Electrocardiographic recording during a spontaneous "dizzy" spell. A prolonged pause following spontaneous termination of atrial fibrillation is a typical feature of sinus node dysfunction.

dysfunction, autonomic nervous system influences, cardioactive drugs and/or metabolic disturbances may be the principal cause (perhaps acting in conjunction with some degree of intrinsic abnormality). Of the extrinsic contributors, drug-induced disturbances due to β adrenergic receptor blockers, calcium channel blockers, membrane-active antiarrhythmics (especially amiodarone, sotalol, flecainide and propafenone) and the antiepileptic drug carbamazepine (Tegretol®) have been recognized causes of bradycardia.[23,26,27] Extrinsic factors may also play a role in initiating or aggravating atrial tachyarrhythmias (for example, so-called vagally mediated atrial fibrillation, induction of atrial fibrillation following administration of adenosine), but their importance in terms of causing syncope in this manner is probably minor.

Disturbances of atrioventricular (AV) conduction

Disturbances of AV conduction range from prolongation of AV conduction time (first degree AV block) to intermittent failure of AV impulse transmission (second degree AV block) to complete conduction failure (third degree AV block). For practical purposes, isolated first degree AV block is not usually a cause of syncopal symptoms (pseudo-pacemaker syndrome accompanying fixed long PR intervals being a possible exception). However, first degree AV block in the presence of a wide QRS complex suggests more severe conduction system disease, and raises the possibility that higher grades of AV block may be occurring from time to time. Similarly, although isolated Mobitz type I second degree AV block is an unlikely cause of syncope, its presence in the setting of a wide QRS leads to the risk that periods of higher grade AV block may be occurring from time to time. As a rule, however, it is the more severe forms of acquired AV block (that is, Mobitz type II, "high grade" and complete AV block) that are most closely associated with syncopal symptoms. In these cases the cardiac rhythm may become dependent on often unreliable subsidiary pacemaker sites. Syncope (reported in 38–61%[28,29]) occurs because of the long delay before these pacemakers begin to "fire" consistently. In addition, these subsidiary pacemaker sites often have relatively slow rates (typically 25–40 beats/min) and are easily suppressed by drugs that patients may be taking (for example, β adrenergic blockers); consequently syncope or presyncope occurs as a result of a transient period of inadequate cerebral perfusion. In contrast to acquired forms of AV block, congenital complete AV block has generally been considered to be more benign and less often the cause of syncope. Recently, however, the benign nature of this condition has been questioned. Michaelson *et al*[30] suggest that syncope is more common and mortality greater in congenital AV block patients than had previously been suspected.

Syncope in patients with various forms of bundle branch block and fascicular block depends both on the risk of developing high grade or complete AV block, as well as on the risk of occurrence of ventricular tachyarrhythmias. As a rule, in chronic infranodal conduction system disease, such as most forms of bifascicular block, progression to more severe AV block is slow. However, the risk increases the longer the duration of the HV interval (normal range 35–55 ms), and is particularly great for HV intervals >100 ms[31,32] (Figure 43.3). Nevertheless, despite clearcut evidence for severe conduction system disease, syncope in these patients may in fact be the result of ventricular tachycardia owing to the usual coexistence of conduction system disease with severe left ventricular dysfunction.[32] Invasive electrophysiologic testing is probably the most helpful way to address this latter concern in individual patients.

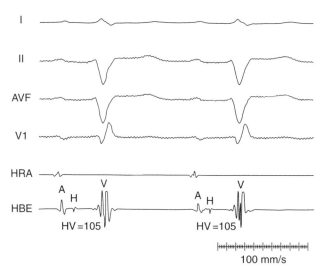

Figure 43.3 Electrocardiographic and intracardiac recordings illustrating first degree AV block and bifascicular block in conjunction with a prolonged HV interval. Syncope in this setting suggests an intermittent AV block origin. Proof requires further evaluation.

Ventricular tachyarrhythmias

Ventricular tachyarrhythmias have been reported to be responsible for syncope in up to 20% of patients referred for electrophysiologic assessment. Risk factors include underlying structural heart disease, evident conduction system disease, and congenital or drug-induced long QT syndrome (Figure 43.4). Tachycardia rate, status of left ventricular function, and the efficiency of peripheral vascular constriction

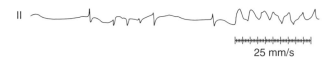

Figure 43.4 Electrocardiographic recording illustrating polymorphic VT in a patient with recurrent syncope and presyncope. The arrhythmia morphology is suggestive of *torsade de pointes*.

determine whether the arrhythmia will induce syncopal symptoms.

Non-sustained ventricular tachycardia is a common finding during ambulatory electrocardiographic monitoring, especially in patients with structural heart disease. As a result, such a finding during the assessment of a syncope patient has not in the past been considered very helpful in the absence of documented concomitant symptoms. However, this conventional view is changing, especially in patients with severely diminished left ventricular function, given the recently reported MUSTT results.[33] Consequently, in the absence of other causes of syncope, the potential role of non-sustained ventricular tachycardia warrants additional testing, particularly electrophysiologic study with concomitant hemodynamic recordings. In fact, based on the combined findings of MUSTT and MADIT 2,[34] one may argue that an implantable defibrillator may be warranted independent of electrophysiologic study when severe left ventricular dysfunction is present (as assessed by an ejection fraction <35%).

A persisting perplexing problem is the appropriate approach to be taken when syncope occurs in patients with severe underlying left ventricular dysfunction (for example, dilated cardiomyopathy) in the absence of documented ventricular tachyarrhythmia. Recent evidence suggests that there is high risk for symptom recurrence and probably sudden death.[35,36] Prophylactic placement of an implantable cardioverter defibrillator (ICD) is becoming increasingly frequently recommended, although confirmation of the reasonableness of this strategy must await completion of the SCD-HEFT study.

Long QT syndrome (LQTS) presents a special form of ventricular tachycardia risk, known for its presentation as syncope. LQTS may not be among the most common causes of syncope, but must always be borne in mind. Syncope is primarily due to *torsade de pointes*, a form of polymorphic ventricular tachycardia characterized by an undulating ECG waveform produced by a shifting QRS axis in the setting of QT interval prolongation (acquired or congenital in origin). The acquired form of LQTS is by far the more common, and is most frequently the result of drugs that prolong the QT interval. *Torsade* in this setting is most often seen during periods of bradycardia (for example, sleep) or following pauses in the cardiac rhythm (for example, post PVC) which accentuate the QT interval. Some of the best-known offending drugs/agents are listed in Box 43.3. Congenital, idiopathic or familial LQTS is caused by mutations in cardiac ion channels that contribute to the action potential repolarization process. Congenital LQTS is a very infrequent cause of syncope, but its identification can be life saving. Affected individuals have QT prolongation and a high risk of recurrent syncope and sudden cardiac death due to *torsade de pointes*. An international registry for LQTS was established in 1979;[37] among 235 probands reported in a 1991 report, the annual rate of recurrent syncope and probable LQTS-related death was 5% and 0·9%, respectively.[38] Syncope and sudden death in this setting is frequently associated with emotional or physical arousal, such as may be triggered by fear, loud noises or exertion.[37,38] Heterogeneity in clinical presentation exists, however, so that in other individuals *torsade de pointes* occurs because of bradycardia or during sleep in conjunction with rate-dependent QT interval prolongation.[39]

Box 43.3 Drugs/agents implicated in QT prolongation and *torsade de pointes*
Antiarrhythmic agents
Class IA
Quinidine
Procainamide
Disopyramide
Class III
Sotalol
Ibutilide
N-Acetylprocainamide (NAPA)
Dofetilide
Amiodarone (relatively low risk)
Antianginal agents
Bepridil (removed from market in USA)
Psychoactive agents
Phenothiazines
Thioridazine
Tricyclic antidepressants
Amitriptyline
Imipramine
Antibiotics
Erythromycin
Pentamidine
Fluconazole
Antiemetics
Droperidol
Non-sedating antihistamines
Terfenadine
Astemizole
Miscellaneous
Cisapride (removed from market in USA)
Arsenic

Supraventricular tachyarrhythmias

The supraventricular tachycardias are generally considered to be less frequent causes of syncope than are ventricular tachyarrhythmias. Supraventricular tachycardias are reported to be the cause of syncope in about 15% of patients referred for electrophysiologic evaluation.[40] The rate of the tachycardia, the volume status and posture of the patient at time of onset of the arrhythmia, the presence of associated structural cardiopulmonary disease, and the integrity of reflex peripheral vascular compensation are key factors determining whether hypotension of sufficient severity to cause syncope occurs.[9] As a rule, if symptoms of syncope or near-syncope do develop, it is at the onset of a paroxysmal tachycardia, before vascular compensation can evolve. However, syncope may also occur at the termination of tachycardia if a pause ensues prior to restoration of a stable atrial rhythm.

Structural cardiovascular or cardiopulmonary disease

Structural cardiac or cardiopulmonary disease is often present in syncope patients, particularly those in older age groups. However, in these cases it is the arrhythmias associated with structural disease that are more often the cause of the symptoms. In terms of syncope directly attributable to structural disease, probably the most common is that which occurs in conjunction with acute myocardial ischemia or infarction. Other relatively common acute medical conditions associated with syncope include pulmonary embolism and pericardial tamponade. The basis of syncope in these conditions is multifactorial, including both the hemodynamic impact of the specific lesion and neurally mediated reflex effects. The latter is especially important in the setting of acute ischemic events, exemplified by the bradycardia and hypotension often associated with inferior wall myocardial infarction.[8]

Syncope may also occur and be a presenting feature in conditions in which there is fixed or dynamic obstruction to left ventricular outflow (for example, aortic stenosis, hypertrophic obstructive cardiomyopathy).[8] In such cases symptoms are often provoked by physical exertion, but may also develop if an otherwise benign arrhythmia should occur (such as atrial fibrillation). The basis for the faint is partly inadequate blood flow owing to the mechanical obstruction. However, especially in the case of valvular aortic stenosis, ventricular mechanoreceptor mediated bradycardia and vasodilatation are thought to be important contributors.[8,41] In obstructive cardiomyopathy neural reflex mechanisms may also play a role, but the occurrence of atrial tachyarrhythmias (particularly atrial fibrillation) or ventricular tachycardia (even at relatively modest rates) is often a trigger for syncopal events.

On rare occasion subclavian "steal" syndrome or severe carotid artery disease may be the cause of syncope. Other even less common causes include left ventricular inflow obstruction in patients with mitral stenosis or atrial myxoma, right ventricular outflow obstruction, and right to left shunting secondary to pulmonic stenosis or pulmonary hypertension.

Cerebrovascular, neurologic and psychiatric disturbances

Cerebrovascular disease and neurologic disturbances (for example, seizure disorders) are rarely the cause of true syncope.[2,42] More often, these conditions result in a clinical picture that may be mistaken for syncope but which can be distinguished by careful history taking and neurologic examination. On occasion certain seizure disorders (particularly of the temporal lobe) may so closely mimic (or induce) neurally mediated reflex bradycardia and hypotension that differentiation from "true" syncope is difficult. In such cases a diagnostic EEG is necessary (recognizing that not all forms of epilepsy will be detected by EEG). More often, a number of important features help differentiate seizures from true syncope:

● Seizures tend to be positionally independent, whereas syncope is most commonly associated with upright posture.
● Seizures are often preceded by an aura, whereas syncope is not.
● Seizures are often immediately accompanied by convulsive activity and incontinence, whereas in true syncope any abnormal motor activity is less severe and incontinence is unusual.[43,44]
● Seizures are typically followed by a confusional period, whereas true syncope is typically followed by prompt restoration of mental state (although fatigue may persist, especially in the case of vasovagal syncope).

Nevertheless, despite these diagnostic features the failure of "seizures" to respond to conventional treatment must result in reconsideration of a cardiac cause (particularly a cardiac arrhythmia).[43,44]

Transient disturbances of cerebrovascular blood flow may initiate a true syncopal spell. For example, cerebrovascular spasm (possibly as part of a migraine syndrome) may present with what appears to be a syncopal episode. In the latter case, other historical features of migraine and migraine susceptibility may suggest the diagnosis. On the other hand, it has recently been proposed that cerebrovascular spasm may be a cause of apparently "normotensive" syncope without migraine.[45,46] If this proves to be relatively common, then it will be necessary to reassess the nature of the diagnosis in many patients, particularly those where the syncope is currently considered to be psychogenic in origin.

Syncope may be mimicked by anxiety attacks, hysteria or other psychiatric disturbances. Anxiety attacks are frequently associated with hyperventilation and hypocapnia. Hysteria, however, tends to be characterized by its occurring in the presence of onlookers and being unassociated with marked alterations of heart rate, systemic pressure or skin color. Currently, however, despite the apparent frequency of these conditions in patients referred for evaluation of "syncope",[47] they must be considered only after other conditions have been carefully excluded.

Miscellaneous causes

Severe hyperventilation resulting in hypocapnia and transient alkalosis may be the most frequent "syncope-like" condition in this category. In these patients anxiety may be an important coexisting feature, but its presence alone is not sufficient to establish a diagnosis. The association of emotional upset or anxiety with syncope is also common in vasovagal fainters, and is a reasonable secondary event in any patient experiencing a syncopal episode.

Metabolic and endocrine disorders rarely cause true syncope. More often such conditions may be responsible for confusional states or behavioral disturbances. Nevertheless, making a clearcut distinction between such symptoms and syncope may not be possible by history alone. As a rule, though, unlike true syncope, conditions such as diabetic coma, or severe hypoxia or hypercapnia do not resolve in the absence of active therapeutic intervention.

Strategy for the diagnostic evaluation

The goal of diagnostic testing is to establish a sufficiently strong correlation between syncopal symptoms and detected abnormalities to permit both an assessment of prognosis and initiation of an appropriate treatment plan (Figure 43.5). To this end, the first step is to obtain a detailed medical history, including interviewing knowledgeable bystanders and relatives. Next, a physical examination along with certain basic tests (electrocardiogram (ECG) and echocardiogram) should be undertaken to ascertain whether there is evidence of underlying structural heart disease. Exercise testing may be included if syncope occurs with exertion, or if ischemic heart disease is suspected. Thereafter, the need for further specialized diagnostic testing will vary depending on a variety of factors, including the certainty of the initial clinical impression; findings during physical examination; the number and frequency of syncopal events reported; the occurrence of injury or accident; family history of syncope or sudden death; and the potential risks associated with the individual's occupation (for example, commercial vehicle driver, machine operator, professional athlete, sign painter, surgeon) or avocation (for example, skier, swimmer) that might be encountered if syncope recurred.

As a rule, if structural heart disease is deemed to be absent by initial evaluation, then tilt-table testing in conjunction with related assessment of autonomic nervous system function is the most useful diagnostic test, as neurally mediated vasovagal syncope and orthostatic hypotension are by far the most frequent causes of syncope in this setting. On the other hand, if abnormal cardiac findings are identified, their functional significance should be characterized by hemodynamic and/or angiographic assessment. Furthermore, because arrhythmias are a common cause of syncope in patients with structural cardiac disease, assessing the patient's susceptibility to tachy- and bradyarrhythmias by various non-invasive (for example, ambulatory electrocardiography, signal averaged electrocardiogram, SAECG) and invasive electrophysiologic

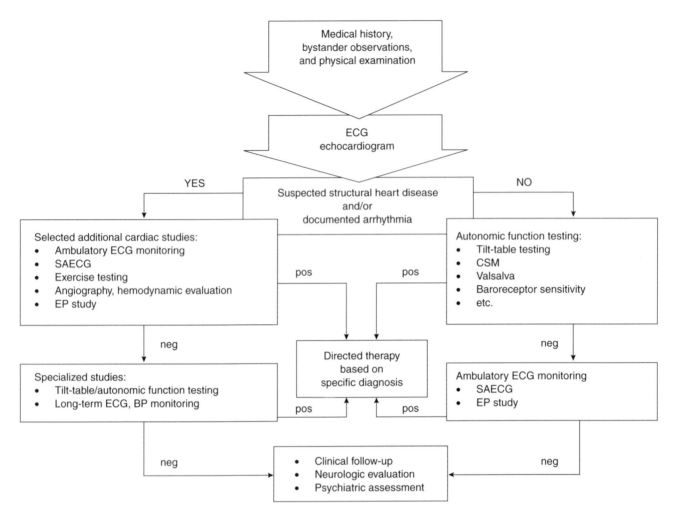

Figure 43.5 A practical strategy for the clinical evaluation of syncope

testing is warranted. Tilt-table testing would follow if the diagnosis remained in doubt.[1] Strong evidence supports the view that only infrequently should specialized neurologic studies be ordered early in the evaluation (for example, if the history were more suggestive of a seizure disorder).[1,42,43] In some cases the diagnosis can only be obtained by long-term ambulatory electrocardiographic monitoring, occasionally necessitating placement of an implantable loop recorder.[48–50]

Electrocardiographic recordings

Because cardiac arrhythmias are so frequently the cause of syncope, ECG documentation during a spontaneous syncopal event is highly desirable. In this regard, the 12-lead ECG is usually too brief to capture a specific cause. However, findings such as ventricular pre-excitation or QT interval prolongation may suggest a diagnosis. If it is feasible at all, obtaining ECG documentation during spontaneous symptoms often necessitates prolonged ambulatory monitoring

by Holter or event recorders. Exercise testing is usually of limited utility unless the syncopal events are clearly exertionally related by history. However, in rare instances exercise testing may permit the detection of rate-dependent AV block, exertionally related tachyarrhythmias, or the exercise-associated variant of neurally mediated syncope.[8,51,52] Finally, although the signal averaged electrocardiogram (SAECG) cannot provide direct evidence for the cause of syncope, such testing may be helpful in patients with ischemic heart disease if "normal": a normal SAECG tends to exclude susceptibility to ventricular tachyarrhythmias.[53]

Imaging techniques

Echocardiography rarely provides a definitive basis for syncope. None the less, the echocardiogram is invaluable, given the importance of identifying underlying structural heart disease in patients with syncope. Further, in some cases the echocardiogram may provide direct clues to the cause if, for example, hypertrophic obstructive cardiomyopathy, severe valvular aortic stenosis, intracardiac tumor (for example, myxoma) or anomalous origin of one or more coronary arteries are detected. Ultrasound techniques also are appropriately employed to assess vascular disturbances detected on physical examination. Thus, assessment of the carotid and/or subclavian system may be an appropriate step in selected individuals. Other imaging modalities, such as radionuclide imaging, are reserved for specific clinical indications.

Clinical electrophysiologic testing

Electrophysiologic testing for assessment of syncope has been the subject of many reports. Although there are no large randomized studies, there is reasonably strong evidence to indicate that electrophysiologic testing is most likely to be diagnostic in individuals with underlying structural heart disease[34,54-58]. **Grade B** For example, in a review by Camm and Lau,[40] testing was clearly more successful in patients with structural cardiac disease (71%) than in patients without (36%). However, care must be taken in interpreting the findings of electrophysiologic testing. Fujimura *et al*[59] summarized the outcomes of electrophysiologic testing in syncope patients in whom bradyarrhythmias were known to be the cause. Among 21 patients with known symptomatic AV block or sinus pauses, electrophysiologic testing only correctly identified 3 of 8 patients with documented sinus pauses (sensitivity 37·5%) and 2 of 13 patients with documented AV block (sensitivity 15·4%). On the other hand, although firm evidence is lacking, the induction of re-entry supraventricular or ventricular tachycardia in a syncope patient is highly likely to be significant. These arrhythmias are rarely inconsequential bystanders; however, demonstration of their hemodynamic significance in an individual patient may necessitate their induction with the patient in an appropriately secured upright tilt position.

Head-up tilt-table testing

So far, the head-up tilt table test is the only diagnostic tool to have been subjected to sufficient clinical scrutiny to assess its effectiveness in the evaluation of vasovagal syncope. The evidence supporting its utility in this setting is convincing, and an ACC expert task force has provided guidelines regarding indications for and the methodology of appropriate use of the tilt-table laboratory[1]. **Grade B** Such testing, especially when undertaken in the absence of drugs, appears to discriminate well between symptomatic patients and asymptomatic control subjects.[60-65] For example, de Mey and Enterling[60] reported only eight instances of hypotension bradycardia among 40 apparently normal subjects (20%). Similarly, during a 45 minute drug-free tilt at 60°, Raviele *et al*[62] noted that none of 35 control subjects developed syncope. In regard to the potential impact of provocative pharmacologic agents on the specificity of tilt testing, Natale

et al[65] found that tilt-table testing at 60, 70 and 80° exhibited specificities of 92%, 92% and 80%, respectively, when low doses of isoproterenol were used. In summary, there is very strong evidence to suggest that tilt-table testing at angles of 60–70° in the absence of pharmacologic provocation exhibits a specificity of approximately 90%. In the presence of pharmacologic provocation test specificity may be reduced, but none the less remains in a range that permits the test to be clinically useful as a diagnostic procedure.

The combination of tilt-table testing and invasive electrophysiologic testing has substantially enhanced diagnostic capabilities in syncope patients. Sra *et al*[58] reported the results of electrophysiologic testing in conjunction with head-up tilt testing in 86 consecutive patients referred for evaluation of unexplained syncope. Electrophysiologic testing was abnormal in 29 (34%) of patients, with the majority of these (21 patients) being inducible sustained monomorphic ventricular tachycardia. Among the remaining patients, head-up tilt testing proved positive in 34 cases (40%), whereas 23 patients (26%) remained undiagnosed. In general, patients exhibiting positive electrophysiologic findings were older, more frequently male, and exhibited lower ventricular ejection fractions and higher frequency of evident heart disease than was the case in patients with positive head-up tilt tests or patients in whom no diagnosis was determined.

In a further evaluation of the combined use of electrophysiologic testing and head-up tilt testing in the assessment of syncope, Fitzpatrick *et al*[66] analyzed findings in 322 patients. Conventional electrophysiologic testing provided a basis for syncope in 229 of 322 cases (71%), with 93 patients having a normal electrophysiologic study. Among the patients with abnormal electrophysiologic findings, AV conduction disease was diagnosed in 34%, sinus node dysfunction in 21%, carotid sinus syndrome in 10% and an inducible sustained tachyarrhythmia in 6%. In the 93 patients with normal electrophysiologic studies, tilt-table testing was undertaken in 71 cases and reproduced syncope, consistent with a vasovagal faint, in 53 (75%).

Neurologic studies

Conventional neurologic laboratory studies (EEG, head CT and MRI) have had a relatively low yield in unselected syncope patients. For instance, among the 433 syncope evaluations reviewed by Kapoor[42] the EEG proved helpful in only three cases. Consequently, these studies should be restricted to those situations in which other clinical observations suggest organic nervous system disease (see discussion earlier). On the other hand, given the importance of orthostatic and dysautonomic causes of syncope, tilt-table testing and other tests of autonomic function have an increasingly important role to play (see earlier discussion). In regard to the latter, a wide range of disorders associated with orthostatic intolerance (see earlier) are now being recognized by virtue of tilt-table testing and autonomic studies. These include postural orthostatic tachycardia syndrome (POTS), orthostatic hypotension (of various etiologies), inappropriate sinus tachycardia, chronic fatigue syndrome, and the neurally mediated faints. Syncope has been associated with each of these disorders, although the mechanism of the faint is often unclear. It is reasonable to assume that the sophistication of this classification and the frequency with which these conditions are recognized will increase as further experience in their diagnosis and treatment is derived.

Treatment

Prevention of syncope recurrences depends critically on establishing an accurate etiologic diagnosis. Thereafter, the treatment strategy may encompass a wide range of approaches, including reassurance and education, as well as pharmacologic and device therapies. The effectiveness of treatment varies, however, depending upon the specific diagnosis. Thus, the evidence supporting the utility of cardiac pacing in carotid sinus syncope and acquired AV block is substantial. **Grade B** On the other hand, evidence favoring the effectiveness of pharmacologic management in vasovagal syncope is much more arguable (**Grade C**, with the possible exception of β adrenergic blockade and midodrine – **Grade B**), as large-scale randomized controlled treatment trials have yet to be undertaken.

In the case of neurally mediated syncopal syndromes, treatment initially comprises education regarding the avoidance of triggering events (for example, hot crowded environments, dehydration, effects of cough etc.), recognition of premonitory symptoms, and maneuvers to abort the episode (for example, a supine posture). Additionally, if possible, strategies should address trigger factors directly (for example, suppressing the cause of cough in cough syncope).

In vasovagal syncope, most patients require primarily reassurance and education. However, when symptoms are recurrent or severe, or threaten lifestyle or occupation, a more aggressive treatment strategy is needed. In some highly motivated patients with recurrent vasovagal symptoms, the prescription of progressively prolonged periods of enforced upright posture (so-called "tilt-training") or other physical maneuvers may be useful in reducing susceptibility.[67-69] For most symptomatic patients, however, pharmacologic approaches have been favored. "Volume expanders" (for example, electrolyte-containing "sports" drinks, fludrocortisone, salt tablets) are among the safest initial approaches (excluding patients with baseline hypertension), but have not been subjected to controlled study. **Grade C** β Adrenergic blocking drugs have been the subject of more detailed study and appear to be useful in younger fainters. **Grade B** Other potentially helpful agents include midodrine (a vasoconstrictor), disopyramide, and

serotonin reuptake inhibitors. However, experience with any of these drugs is currently slight.[70-79] The few small controlled studies that have been reported (atenolol, cafedrine, disopyramide, scopolamine and etilefrine) all have methodologic problems. Midodrine may be an exception in that several single center studies, including a well designed controlled trial in which volume served as a control, tend to support its effectiveness[76-79]. **Grade B**

Cardiac pacing has proved highly successful in carotid sinus syndrome **Grade B** and is acknowledged to be the treatment of choice when bradycardia has been documented.[80] More recently, the role of pacing in vasovagal syncope has received increasing attention. In this regard, strong supportive evidence of efficacy of cardiac pacing in selected patients with vasovagal syncope has been provided in the report of the North American vasovagal pacemaker study,[14] the findings of the VASIS trial in Europe,[15] and in the study by Ammirati *et al*[17] A fourth study, VPS2, was recently reported (NASPE 2002). Although the full report is not available, pacing benefit appeared to have been less (about 30% syncope risk reduction at 6 months) than for the other studies. **Grade A**

Syncope patients qualified for inclusion in the North American study if they had both a positive head-up tilt test and either or both of (1) at least six syncopal episodes preceding the tilt test; or (2) at least one syncope recurrence within 6 months of a positive tilt test. Additionally, during the tilt test patients had to exhibit degrees of bradycardia exceeding certain pre-established thresholds. Syncope recurrence rate was substantially less in the pacemaker group than in control patients, resulting in an actuarial 1 year rate of recurrent syncope of approximately 18·5% for pacemaker patients and 59·7% for controls. However, the study was not without limitations, and a further follow up study addressing many of these limitations (particularly the potential placebo effect of a pacemaker implantation procedure) has been completed, but the results are not yet public. The results of the pacing arm of the VASIS trial[74] were similar to those of the North American Study. Finally, Ammirati *et al*[17] reported results in 93 patients (over 55 years of age) who had experienced three or more syncopal events over a 2 year period and who had positive tilt tests with evidence of bradycardia. Patients were randomized to either pacing (DDD mode with rate-drop algorithm, $n = 46$) or β adrenergic blocker therapy ($n = 47$). Paced patients had two syncope recurrences during a mean follow up of 390 days, whereas β blocker treated patients had 12 syncopal recurrences over a mean follow up of 135 days. Thus, cardiac pacing may play a useful role in severe cases with recurring periods of symptomatic cardioinhibition. **Grade A** In contrast, excluding carotid sinus syndrome, discussed above, experience with pacing in other forms of neurally mediated syncope has been too limited to permit comment.

The treatment of patients with orthostatic syncope is similar to that of the neurally mediated syncopal syndromes. However, greater emphasis must be given to modifying any potentially contributory drug treatments (for concomitant conditions). Further, physical maneuvers designed to ameliorate problems associated with upright posture seem to be helpful, although randomized controlled trials are not yet available. For instance, prescribed periods of upright posture (so-called "tilt-training"), antigravitational hose, and elevation of the bed head at night have a role to play in the treatment plan.[81] In terms of pharmacologic treatment, the mainstay has been attempted chronic expansion of central circulating volume. To this end, increased salt in the diet and/or use of salt retaining steroids (that is principally fludrocortisone) is usually the first step. **Grade C** Additional benefit has been reported with the use of agents such as erythropoietin in order to increase circulating blood volume. A further element in the strategy is reduction of the tendency for central volume to be displaced to the lower extremities with upright posture. To this end vasoconstrictors have been employed, although with limited success owing to the tendency for tachyphylaxis to develop. **Grade C** Of greatest current interest is midodrine.[76–79] Cardiac pacing at relatively rapid rates may prove valuable in certain very difficult cases, but this option has not been very wide accepted to date.

In the treatment of primary cardiac arrhythmias, especially the bradycardias and hypotensive tachyarrhythmias, strong clinical evidence supports the importance of treatment interventions for symptom prevention. The evidence unquestionably supports the importance of cardiac pacemaker therapy in patients with syncope due to bradyarrhythmias, whether due to sinus node dysfunction or to AV conduction disturbances.[82–87] **Grade B** In the case of paroxysmal supraventricular tachyarrhythmias (PSVT) there is little in the way of long-term follow up studies examining the efficacy of conventional antiarrhythmic drug treatment when the presenting feature was syncope. However, at present such patients are no longer usually treated in that fashion because of the frequency of drug-related side effects, issues of compliance, expense, and the availability of effective alternatives. Specifically, transcatheter ablation has become a very cost-effective treatment option[88] and, in PSVT associated with syncope, is probably the treatment of choice. **Grade B**

In the case of syncope due to ventricular tachycardia (VT), the almost ubiquitous presence of underlying left ventricular dysfunction increases the proarrhythmic risk associated with antiarrhythmic drug therapy (reported 5–15% incidence with Class 1 agents). Consequently, pharmacologic therapeutic strategies often involve early consideration of Class 3 agents (particularly amiodarone, given its proarrhythmia risk of 2% or less, and its generally well tolerated hemodynamic impact). However, given the difficulty of ensuring effective prophylaxis in this often high-risk patient population, the use of transcatheter ablation and implantable pacemaker cardioverter defibrillators (ICDs) is becoming increasingly important. Currently, ablation techniques are appropriate first choices in only a few forms of ventricular tachycardia, specifically symptomatic patients with right ventricular outflow tract tachycardia and bundle branch re-entry tachycardia. Although multicenter trials of this strategy have not been undertaken, the evidence is compelling for pursuing ablation in the former and reasonably strong in the latter (bundle branch re-entry, where an ICD may also be warranted in the setting of severe left ventricular dysfunction). **Grade B** In the future, ablation techniques may be used more extensively as mapping technology improves and energy delivery systems evolve. Nevertheless, it is probable that the frequent concomitant presence of poor left ventricular function may necessitate consideration of an ICD as well in these settings, despite successful ablation.

With regard to implantable devices for symptomatic ventricular tachyarrhythmias, several prospective treatment trials (MADIT, AVID, MUSTT and MADIT 2) provide evidence in favor of the efficacy of ICD compared to conventional pharmacologic approaches.[33,34,89,90] Although these studies did not directly target syncope patients, it is reasonable to extend the observations to those syncope patients in whom ventricular tachyarrhythmias and poor left ventricular function are identified. **Grade B** Furthermore, reports examining this issue retrospectively in fainters provide support for early ICD implantation. For instance, among patients with severe left ventricular dysfunction, Middlekauff et al[91,92] noted that the presence of a history of syncope was accompanied by both a significantly higher 1 year mortality (65% v 25% in comparable patients without syncope) and a greater tendency toward sudden death (45% of deaths v 12% in comparable patients).

In the subset of patients in whom structural cardiovascular or cardiopulmonary disease is the cause of syncope, treatment is best directed at amelioration of the specific structural lesion or its consequences. Thus, in syncope associated with myocardial ischemia, pharmacologic therapy and/or revascularization is clearly the appropriate strategy in most cases. Similarly, when syncope is closely associated with surgically addressable lesions (for example, valvular aortic stenosis, atrial myxoma, congenital cardiac anomaly), a direct corrective approach is often feasible. On the other hand, when syncope is caused by certain difficult to treat conditions, such as primary pulmonary hypertension or restrictive cardiomyopathy, it is often impossible to ameliorate the underlying problem adequately. Even modifying outflow gradients in hypertrophic obstructive cardiomyopathy (HOCM) is not readily achieved surgically. In the latter condition the effectiveness of standard pharmacologic therapies remains uncertain, and despite ongoing controversy recent success with cardiac pacing techniques offers considerable promise to symptomatic individuals.[93–95] **Grade C**

Cost effectiveness

Syncope occurs in all age groups. Further, syncope can masquerade as other things (for example, falls, unexplained injuries[13]), thereby causing considerable morbidity and lifestyle disturbance. Consequently, lost productivity, economic derangement and loss of vocation are important considerations and should be evaluated along with medical cost burden when assessing the manner in which syncope is to be evaluated and treated.

In 1982, Kapoor *et al*[96] identified a need for a more cost-effective approach to syncope evaluation. At that time, the average cost for evaluating syncope patients was estimated to be US$2600. However, as the actual etiology was determined in only relatively few cases, the real cost was far greater (approximately US$24 000 per specific diagnosis). Given inflation, and the more widespread proliferation of diagnostic imaging procedures, conventional electrophysiologic testing and tilt-table testing, it is reasonable to assume that the per patient expenditure has increased at least twofold in the past decade, an estimate approximately confirmed by Calkins *et al*[97] On the other hand, given the marked improvement in the frequency with which a specific diagnosis is now obtained, the cost per specific diagnosis is probably considerably lower now than was the case in 1982. Autonomic testing appears to have played an important role in improving both diagnostic capability and cost effectiveness.[98]

Summary

Syncope is a common medical problem with several potential causes and a tendency to a relatively high recurrence rate. Further, there is strong evidence for the view that prognosis is of particular concern among the subset of syncope patients with underlying organic cardiac or vascular disease. Consequently, assessment of each patient must be thorough, with particular attention being paid to the recognition and evaluation of structural cardiac and/or vascular disease. When structural disease is thought likely, hemodynamic and angiographic studies are needed. Syncope in the absence of structural heart or vascular disease is more often neurally mediated in origin, and autonomic function testing (particularly tilt-table testing) should be an early step in establishing the diagnosis. Specialized neurologic testing has proved useful in only a small minority of cases.

The treatment of syncope has been the subject of relatively few large-scale clinical trials. Nevertheless, when structural cardiovascular disturbances or primary cardiac arrhythmias are the cause of syncope, appropriately directed therapy (for example, valve replacement, pacemaker or ICD implantation) is essential and likely to be highly effective. On the other hand, documentation of pharmacologic treatment efficacy (with the possible exception of midodrine)

in vasovagal faints, orthostatic hypotension and dysautonomic states, and the various neurologic and psychiatric conditions that can mimic syncope, is less well established. Pacemaker therapy, on the other hand, has been very thoroughly studied in vasovagal syncope and appears to be very effective in selected hard to treat patients (although controversy remains[99]), but patient acceptance is, not surprisingly, a significant hurdle among younger individuals.

Key points: the evaluation of the syncope patient

- The goals
  - Establish a correlation between symptoms and abnormalities
  - Assess prognosis
  - Initiate appropriate treatment plan
- Key steps
  - Obtain detailed medical history (including bystanders/relatives)
  - Identify underlying structural heart disease
- Factors determining need for further tests
  - Evidence for structural disease
  - Certainty of the initial clinical impression
  - Number and frequency of syncopal events
  - Occurrence of injury or accident
  - Family history of syncope or sudden death
  - Occupation, avocation

Acknowledgment

The authors would like to thank Wendy Markuson and Barry LS Detloff for their assistance in the preparation of the manuscript.

References

1. Benditt DG, Ferguson DW, Grubb BP *et al.* Tilt-table testing for assessing syncope. An American College of Cardiology expert consensus document. *J Am Coll Cardiol* 1996;**28**:263–75.
2. Brignole M, Alboni P, Benditt D *et al.* Guidelines on management (diagnosis and treatment) of syncope. *Eur Heart J* 2001;**22**:1256–306.
3. Gendelman HE, Linzer M, Gabelman M *et al.* Syncope in a general hospital population. *NY State J Med* 1983;**83**:116–65.
4. Wayne HH. Syncope: physiological considerations and an analysis of the clinical characteristics in 510 patient. *Am J Med* 1961;**30**:418–38.
5. Savage DD, Corwin L, McGee DL *et al.* Epidemiologic features of isolated syncope: The Framingham Study. *Stroke* 1985;**16**:626–9.
6. Kapoor WN, Karpf M, Wieand S *et al.* A prospective evaluation and follow-up of patients with syncope. *N Engl J Med* 1983;**309**:197–204.

7. Bass EB, Elson JJ, Fogoros RN, Peterson J, Arena VC, Kapoor WN. Long-term prognosis of patients undergoing electrophysiologic studies for syncope of unknown origin. *Am J Cardiol* 1988;**62**:1186–91.

8. Benditt DG, Goldstein MA, Adler S, Sakaguchi S, Lurie KG. Neurally mediated syncopal syndromes: pathophysiology and clinical evaluation. In: Mandel WJ, ed. *Cardiac Arrhythmias*, 3rd edn. Philadelphia: JB Lippincott, 1995.

9. Leitch JW, Klein GJ, Yee R *et al.* Syncope associated with supraventricular tachycardia: an expression of tachycardia or vasomotor response. *Circulation* 1992;**85**:1064–71.

10. Kenny RA, Bayliss J, Ingram A, Sutton R. Head up tilt: a useful test for investigating unexplained syncope. *Lancet* 1986;**1**:1352–4.

11. Almquist A, Goldenberg IF, Milstein S *et al.* Provocation of bradycardia and hypotension by isoproterenol and upright posture in patients with unexplained syncope. *N Engl J Med* 1989;**320**:346–51.

12. Sutton R, Petersen M, Brignole M, Ravieli A, Menozzi C, Giani P. Proposed classification for tilt induced vasovagal syncope. *Eur J Cardiac Pacing Electrophysiol* 1992;**2**:180–3.

13. Kenny RAM, Richardson DA, Steen N *et al.* Carotid sinus syndrome: a modifiable risk factor for nonaccidental falls in older adults (SAFE PACE). *J Am Coll Cardiol* 2001;**38**:1491–6.

14. Connolly SJ, Sheldon R, Roberts RS, Gent M. Vasovagal pacemaker study investigators. The North American vasovagal pacemaker study (VPS): a randomized trial of permanent cardiac pacing for the prevention of vasovagal syncope. *J Am Coll Cardiol* 1999;**33**:16–20.

15. Sutton R, Brignole M, Menozzi C *et al.* for the VASIS investigators. Dual-chamber pacing is efficacious in treatment of neurally-mediated tilt-positive cardioinhibitory syncope. Pacemaker versus no therapy: a multicenter randomized study. *Circulation* 2000;**102**:294–9.

16. Brignole M, Menozzi C, Del Rosso A *et al.* New classification of haemodynamics of vasovagal syncope: beyond the VASIS classification. Analysis of the pre-syncopal phase of the tilt test without and with nitroglycerin challenge. Vasovagal Syncope International Study. *Europace* 2000;**2**:66–76.

17. Ammirati F, Colivicchi F, Santini M *et al.* Permanent cardiac pacing versus medical treatment for the prevention of recurrent vasovagal syncope. A multicenter, randomized, controlled trial. *Circulation* 2001;**104**:52–6.

18. Moya A, Brignole M, Menozzi C *et al.* and ISSUE Investigators. Mechanism of syncope in patients with isolated syncope and in patients with tilt-positive syncope. *Circulation* 2001;**104**:1261–7.

19. Low PA, Opfer-Gherking TL, McPhee BR *et al.* Prospective evaluation of clinical characteristics of orthostatic hypotension. *Mayo Clin Proc* 1995;**70**:617–22.

20. Bannister R. Chronic autonomic failure with postural hypotension. *Lancet* 1979;**ii**:404–6.

21. Low PA. Autonomic nervous system function. *J Clin Neurophysiol* 1993;**10**:14–27.

22. Weiling W, van Lieshout JJ. Investigation and treatment of autonomic circulatory failure. *Curr Opin Neurol Neurosurg* 1993;**6**:537–43.

23. Benditt DG, Sakaguchi S, Goldstein MA *et al.* Sinus node dysfunction: pathophysiology, clinical features, evaluation and treatment. In: Zipes DP, Jalife J, eds. *Cardiac Electrophysiology. From Cell to Bedside*, 2nd edn. Philadelphia: WB Saunders, 1995.

24. Kaplan BM, Langendorf R, Lev M, Pick A. Tachycardia–bradycardia syndrome (so-called "sick sinus syndrome"). *Am J Cardiol* 1973;**26**:497–508.

25. Rubenstein JJ, Schulman CL, Yurchak PM *et al.* Clinical spectrum of the sick sinus syndrome. *Circulation* 1972;**6**:5–13.

26. Benditt DG, Benson DW Jr, Dunnigan A *et al.* Drug therapy in sinus node dysfunction. In: Rapaport E, ed. *Cardiology Update* 1984. New York: Elsevier, 1984.

27. Linker NJ, Camm AJ. Drug effects on the sinus node. A clinical perspective. *Cardiovasc Drugs Ther* 1988;**2**:165–70.

28. Rowe JC, White PD. Complete heart block: a follow-up study. *Ann Intern Med* 1958;**49**:260–70.

29. Penton GB, Miller H, Levine SA. Some clinical features of complete heart block. *Circulation* 1956;**13**:801–24.

30. Michaelsson M, Jonzon A, Riesenfeld T. Isolated congenital complete atrioventricular block in adult life. *Circulation* 1995;**92**:442–9.

31. Scheinman MM, Peters RW, Sauve MJ *et al.* Value of H-Q interval in patients with bundle branch block and the role of prophylactic permanent pacing. *Am J Cardiol* 1982;**50**:1316–22.

32. Dhingra RC, Denes P, Wu D *et al.* Syncope in patients with chronic bifascicular block. *Ann Intern Med* 1974;**81**:302–6.

33. Buxton AE, Lee KL, Fisher JD, Josephson ME, Prystowsky EN, Hafley G, for the Multicenter Unsustained Tachycardia Trial Investigators. *N Engl J Med* 1999;**341**:1882–90.

34. Moss AJ, Zareba W, Hall WJ *et al.* Prophylactic implantation of a defibrillator in patients with myocardial infarction and reduced ejection fraction. *N Engl J Med* 2002;**346**:877–83.

35. Swerdlow CD, Winkle RA, Mason JW. Determinents of survival in patients with ventricular tachyarrhythmias. *N Engl J Med* 1983;**308**:1436–42.

36. Middelkauff HR, Stevenson WG, Stevenson LW, Saxon LA. Syncope in advanced heart failure: high risk of sudden death regardless of origin of syncope. *J Am Coll Cardiol* 1993;**21**:110–16.

37. Moss AJ, Schwartz PJ, Crampton RS *et al.* The long QT syndrome: prospective longitudinal study of 328 families. *Circulation* 1991;**84**:1136–44.

38. Schwartz PJ *et al.* Stress and sudden death: the case of the long QT syndrome. *Circulation* 1991;**83**(Suppl II):71–80.

39. Tobe TJM *et al.* Late potentials in bradycardia-dependent long QT syndrome associated with sudden death during sleep. *J Am Coll Cardiol* 1992;**19**:541–9.

40. Camm AJ, Lau CP. Syncope of undetermined origin: diagnosis and management. *Prog Cardiol* 1988;**1**:139–56.

41. Johnson AM. Aortic stenosis, sudden death, and the left ventricular baroreceptors. *Br Heart J* 1971;**33**:1–5.

42. Kapoor W. Evaluation and outcome of patients with syncope. *Medicine* 1990;**69**:160–75.

43. Grubb BP, Gerard G, Rousch K *et al.* Differentiation of convulsive syncope and epilepsy with head up tilt table testing. *Ann Intern Med* 1991;**115**:871–6.

44. Zaidi A, Crampton S, Clough P, Scheepers B, Fitzpatrick AP. Misdiagnosis of epilepsy – many seizure-like episodes have a cardiovascular cause. *PACE* 1999;**22**:814[Abstract].

45. Grubb BP, Gerard G, Roush K *et al*. Cerebral vasoconstriction during head-upright tilt induced vasovagal syncope: a paradoxic and unexpected response. *Circulation* 1991;**84**: 1157–64.

46. Njemanze PC. Cerebral circulation dysfunction and hemodynamic abnormalities in syncope during upright tilt test. *Can J Cardiol* 1993;**9**:238–42.

47. Linzer M, Varia I, Pontinen M *et al*. Medically unexplained syncope: relationship to psychiatric illness. *Am J Med* 1992; **92**:18–25.

48. Krahn AD, Klein GJ, Norris C, Yee R. The etiology of syncope in patients with a negative tilt table and electrophysiologic testing. *Circulation* 1995;**92**:1819–24.

49. Krahn A, Klein GJ, Yee R, Skanes AC. Randomized assessment of syncope trial. Conventional diagnostic testing versus a prolonged monitoring strategy. *Circulation* 2001;**104**: 46–51.

50. Krahn AD, Klein GJ, Yee R, Takle-Newhouse T, Norris C, the Reveal Investigators. Use of an exended monitoring strategy in patients with problematic syncope. *Circulation* 1999;**99**: 406–10.

51. Sakaguchi S, Shultz J, Remole C, Adler S, Lurie K, Benditt D. Syncope associated with exercise, a manifestation of neurally-mediated syncope. *Am J Cardiol* 1995;**75**:476–81.

52. Calkins H, Seifert M, Morady F. Clinical presentation and long term follow up of athletes with exercise-induced vasodepressor syncope. *Am Heart J* 1995;**129**:1159–64.

53. Kuchar DL, Thorburn CW, Sammel NL. Signal-averaged electrocardiogram for evaluation of recurrent syncope. *Am J Cardiol* 1986;**58**:949–53.

54. DiMarco JB, Garan H, Hawthorne WJ *et al*. Intracardiac electrophysiologic techniques in recurrent syncope of unknown cause. *Ann Intern Med* 1981;**95**:542–8.

55. Akhtar M, Shenasa M, Denker S, Gilbert CJ, Rizwi N. Role of cardiac electrophysiologic studies in patients with unexplained recurrent syncope. *PACE* 1983;**6**:192–201.

56. Morady F, Shen E, Schwartz A *et al*. Long-term follow-up of patients with recurrent unexplained syncope evaluated by electrophysiologic testing. *J Am Coll Cardiol* 1983; **2**:1053–9.

57. Denes P, Ezri MD. The role of electrophysiologic studies in the management of patients with unexplained syncope. *PACE* 1985;**8**:424–35.

58. Sra JS, Anderson AJ, Sheikh SH *et al*. Unexplained syncope evaluated by electrophysiologic studies and head-up tilt testing. *Ann Intern Med* 1991;**114**:1013–19.

59. Fujimura O, Yee R, Klein GJ *et al*. The diagnostic sensitivity of electrophysiologic testing in patients with syncope caused by bradycardia. *N Engl J Med* 1989;**321**:1703–7.

60. deMey C, Enterling D. Assessment of the hemodynamic responses to single passive head-up tilt by non-invasive methods in normotensive subjects. *Meth Find Exp Clin Pharmacol* 1986;**8**:449–57.

61. Fitzpatrick A, Theodorakis G, Vardas P *et al*. The incidence of malignant vasovagal syndrome in patients with recurrent syncope. *Eur Heart J* 1991;**12**:389–94.

62. Raviele A, Gasparini G, DiPede F, Delise P, Bonso A, Piccolo E. Usefulness of head-up tilt test in evaluating patients with syncope of unknown origin and negative electrophysiologic study. *Am J Cardiol* 1990;**65**:1322–7.

63. Grubb BP, Temesy-Armos P, Hahn H, Elliott L. Utility of upright tilt table testing in the evaluation and management of syncope of unknown origin. *Am J Med* 1991;**90**:6–10.

64. Grubb BP, Wolfe D, Samoil D *et al*. Recurrent unexplained syncope in the elderly: the use of head-upright tilt table testing in evaluation and management. *J Am Geriatr Soc* 1992; **40**:1123–8.

65. Natale A, Akhtar M, Jazayeri M *et al*. Provocation of hypotension during head-up tilt testing in subjects with no history of syncope or presyncope. *Circulation* 1995;**92**:54–8.

66. Fitzpatrick A, Theodorakis G, Vardas P, Sutton R. Methodology of head-up tilt testing in patients with unexplained syncope. *J Am Coll Cardiol* 1991;**17**:125–30.

67. Ector H, Reybrouck T, Heidbuchel H, Gewillig M, Van de Werf F. Tilt training: a new treatment for recurrent neurocardiogenic syncope or severe orthostatic intolerance. *PACE* 1998; **21**:193–6.

68. Di Girolamo E, Di Iorio C, Leonzio L, Sabatini P, Barsotti A. Usefulness of a tilt training program for prevention of refractory neurocardiogenic syncope in adolescents. A controlled study. *Circulation* 1999;**100**:1798–1801.

69. Wieling W, Van Lieshout JJ, Van Leeuwen AM. Physical maneuvers that reduce postural hypotension in autonomic failure. *Clin Autonom Res* 1993;**3**:57–65.

70. Fitzpatrick AP, Ahmed R, Williams S *et al*. A randomized trial of medical therapy in malignant vasovagal syndrome or neurally-mediated bradycardia/hypotension syndrome. *Eur J Cardiac Pacing Electrophysiol* 1991;**1**:991–1202.

71. Brignole M, Menozzi C, Gianfranchi L *et al*. A controlled trial of acute and long-term medical therapy in tilt-induced neurally mediated syncope. *Am J Cardiol* 1992;**70**:339–42.

72. Morillo CA, Leitch JU, Yee R *et al*. A placebo-controlled trial of intravenous and oral disopyramide for prevention of neurally mediated syncope induced by head-up tilt. *J Am Coll Cardiol* 1993;**22**:1843–8.

73. Moya A, Permanyer-Miralda G, Sagrista-Sauleda J *et al*. Limitations of head-up tilt test for evaluating the efficacy of therapeutic interventions in patients with vasovagal syncope: results of a controlled study of etilefrine versus placebo *J Am Coll Cardiol* 1995;**25**:65–9.

74. Mahanonda N, Bhuripanyo K, Kangkagate C *et al*. Randomized double-blind placebo-controlled trial of oral atenolol in patients with unexplained syncope and positive upright tilt table results. *Am Heart J* 1995;**130**:1250–3.

75. Jankovic J, Gilden JL, Hiner BC, Brown DC, Rubin M. Neurogenic orthostatic hypotension: a double-blind placebo-controlled study with midodrine. *Am J Med* 1993; **95**:38–48.

76. Sra J, Maglio C, Biehl M *et al*. Efficacy of midodrine hydrochloride in neurocardiogenic syncope refractory to standard therapy. *J Cardiovasc Electrophysiol* 1997;**8**:42–6.

77. Samniah N, Sakaguchi S, Lurie KG, Iskos D, Benditt DG. Efficacy and safety of midodrine hydrochloride in patients with refractory vasovagal syncope. *Am J Cardiol* 2001;**88**: 80–3.

78. Perez-Lugones A, Schweikert R, Pavia S *et al*. Usefulness of midodrine in patients with severely symptomatic neurocardiogenic syncope: a randomized control study. *J Cardiovasc Electrophysiol* 2001;**12**:935–8.

79. Ward CR, Gray JC, Gilroy JJ, Kenny RA. Midodrine: a role in the management of neurocardiogenic syncope. *Heart* 1998; **79**:45–9.

80. Benditt DG, Remole S, Asso A *et al.* Cardiac pacing for carotid sinus syndrome and vasovagal syncope. In: Barold SS, Mugica J, eds. *New Perspectives in Cardiac Pacing, 3*. Mount Kisco, NY: Futura, 1993.

81. Bannister R, Mathias C. Management of postural hypotension. In: Bannister R, ed. *Autonomic Failure. A Textbook of Clinical Disorders of the Autonomic Nervous System*. Oxford: Oxford University Press, 1988.

82. Benditt DG, Peterson M, Lurie K *et al.* Cardiac pacing for prevention of recurrent vasovagal syncope. *Ann Intern Med* 1995;**122**:204–9.

83. Petersen MEV, Chamberlain-Webber R, Fitzpatrick AP *et al.* Permanent pacing for cardioinhibitory malignant vasovagal syndrome. *Br Heart J* 1994;**71**:274–81.

84. Perrins EJ, Astridge PS. Clinical trials and experience. In: Ellenbogen KA, Kay GN, Wilkoff BL, eds. *Clinical Cardiac Pacing*. Philadelphia: WB Saunders, 1995.

85. Stangl K, Wirtzfeld A, Seitz K *et al.* Atrial stimulation (AAI): long-term follow-up of 110 patients. In: Belhassen B, Feldman S, Copperman Y, eds. *Cardiac Pacing and Electrophysiology. Proceedings of the VIIIth World Symposium on Cardiac Pacing and Electrophysiology*. Jerusalem: R & L Creative Communications, 1987.

86. Rosenqvist M, Brandt J, Schuller H. Long-term pacing in sick sinus node disease: effects of stimulation mode on cardiovascular morbidity and mortality. *Am Heart J* 1988;**116**:16–22.

87. Andersen HR, Thuesen L, Bagger JP *et al.* Prospective randomised trial of atrial versus ventricular pacing in sick-sinus syndrome. *Lancet* 1994;**344**:1523–8.

88. Naccarelli GV, Dougherty AH, Jalal S, Shih H-T, Wolbrette D. Paroxysmal supraventricular tachycardia: comparative role of therapeutic methods – drugs, devices, and ablation. In: Saksena S, Luderitz B, eds. *Interventional Electrophysiology. A Textbook*, 2nd edn. Armonk, NY: Futura, 1996.

89. Moss AJ, Hall WJ, Cannom DS *et al.* Improved survival with an implanted defibrillator in patients with coronary disease at high risk for ventricular arrhythmia. *N Engl J Med* 1996; **335**:1933–40.

90. The Antiarrhythmics versus Implantable Defibrillators (AVID) Investigators. A comparison of antiarrhythmic drug therapy with implantable defibrillators in patients resuscitated from near-fatal ventricular arrhythmias. *N Engl J Med* 1997; **337**:1576–83.

91. Middelkauff HR, Stevenson WG, Stevenson LW, Saxon LA. Syncope in advanced heart failure: high risk of sudden death regardless of origin of syncope. *J Am Coll Cardiol* 1993; **21**:110–16.

92. Middelkauff HR, Stevenson WG, Saxon LA. Prognosis after syncope: impact of left ventricular function. *Am Heart J* 1993;**125**:121–7.

93. Fananapazir L, Epsterin ND, Curiel RV *et al.* Long-term results of dual-chamber (DDD) pacing in obstructive cardiomyopathy. Evidence for progressive symptomatic and hemodynamic improvement and reduction of left ventricular hypertrophy. *Circulation* 1994;**90**:2731–42.

94. Kappenberger L, Linde C, Daubert C *et al.* Pacing in hypertrophic obstructive cardiomyopathy. A randomized crossover trial. *Eur Heart J* 1997;**18**:1249–56.

95. Nishimura RA, Hayes DL, Ilstrup DM *et al.* Effects of dual-chamber pacing on systolic and diastolic function in patients with hypertrophic cardiomyopathy. *J Am Coll Cardiol* 1996; **27**:421–30.

96. Kapoor W, Karpf M, Maher Y *et al.* Syncope of unknown origin: the need for a more cost-effective approach to its evaluation. *JAMA* 1982;**247**:2687–91.

97. Calkins H, Byrne M, El-Atassi R, Kalbfleisch S, Langberg JJ, Morady F. The economic burden of unrecognized vasodepressor syncope. *Am J Med* 1993;**95**:473–9.

98. Mathias CJ, Deguchi K, Schatz I. Autonomic-function investigations aid in the diagnosis of the cause of syncope and presyncope. *Lancet* 2001;**357**:348–53.

99. van Dijk N, Harms MP, Linzer M, Wieling W. Treatment of vasovagal syncope: pacemaker or crossing legs? *Clin Autonom Res* 2000;**10**:347–9.

44 Cardiopulmonary resuscitation

Nicola E Schiebel, Roger D White

Cardiopulmonary resuscitation interventions are used worldwide in attempts to restore spontaneous circulation in victims of sudden cardiac arrest. Healthcare providers frequently follow algorithmic advanced cardiac life support guidelines[1] in their approach to the four basic cardiac arrest rhythms: ventricular fibrillation (VF), pulseless ventricular tachycardia (VT), pulseless electrical activity (PEA), and asystole. Despite these guidelines, considerable clinical expertise and judgment are required in their application. This is partly because underlying causes for the arrest must always factor into clinical decisions, and may require deviations from the algorithms. The other concern is that definitive high quality evidence supporting specific interventions may be lacking and, therefore, alternatives may be acceptable. The reasons for this are many, but the key issue is that cardiac arrest outcomes are extremely difficult to study. They are relatively rare events, have many underlying causes, and issues of obtaining informed consent can make research difficult if not impossible. Some external evidence is available, though, and the practicing clinician should be aware of it. The focus of this chapter will be on the research evidence base for management of sudden cardiac death. An understanding and appraisal of this evidence will assist clinicians in deciding whether it applies to the individual patient and allow them to integrate it into resuscitation decisions most appropriately.

Monophasic *v* biphasic defibrillation

The termination of ventricular fibrillation by externally applied electricity was a major breakthrough in cardiac resuscitation. First described in 1956,[2] it has proved to be a remarkably effective treatment for an otherwise universally fatal arrhythmia. **Grade A** Multiple studies support the concept that the earlier the defibrillation is performed, the greater the probability of survival to hospital discharge.[3–5] **Grade A** As a result of this, a major focus in the past 10 years has been finding ways to improve access to early defibrillation, not only in the hospital, but in the community. The concept of public access defibrillation (defibrillation by trained non-medical personnel, including laypersons) has been strengthened by the development of automated external defibrillators (AEDs).[1] It has been recognized, however, that widespread dissemination of AED

training and equipment will require devices that are small, light, inexpensive, easy to use, and capable of being stored for long periods without recharging.[6] This goal has motivated manufacturers to develop alternative waveforms with equal or greater efficacy in an effort to reduce defibrillator energy requirements and thus confer benefits in size, weight, cost, and battery life. One such advance is the introduction of lower energy biphasic waveforms, first commercially available in 1996 for external defibrillation.

The technology of defibrillation waveforms is complex. The classic monophasic waveform delivers current that flows in one direction. Two monophasic waveforms have been marketed and vary in the speed with which they return to the zero voltage point. The damped sinusoidal waveform (MDS) returns to baseline gradually, whereas the truncated exponential (MTE) returns instantaneously. Adequate research has not been done to determine if one type is superior. The recommended energy for monophasic defibrillation in the 2000 American Heart Association (AHA) guidelines is an escalating dose of 200 J, 200–300 J, then 360 J.[1]

Biphasic waveforms first deliver current in one direction and then the current is reversed and flows in the opposite direction for the duration of the discharge. As with monophasic waveforms, biphasic waveforms have different morphologies (Figures 44.1 and 44.2). Most deliver lower energy

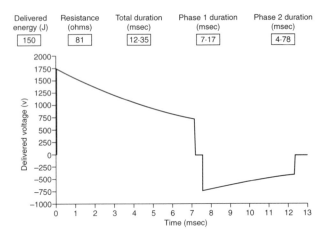

Figure 44.1 Biphasic truncated exponential waveform delivering non-escalating 150 J. Data from a patient event are included in the figure.

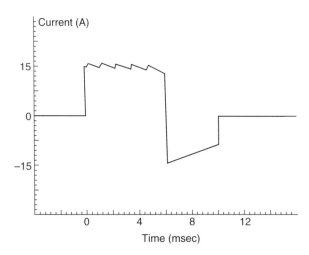

Figure 44.2 Rectilinear biphasic waveform delivering a relatively constant current during the first phase. The phasic durations are fixed at 6 and 4 msec. The figure depicts a 120 J shock delivered into a 50 ohm impedance.

defibrillation (usually 120–200 J) than their monophasic counterparts. The first device approved for clinical use employed a truncated exponential (BTE) waveform delivering non-escalating 150 J shocks, and most available data have been derived from experience with this waveform (Figure 44.1). Biphasic waveform defibrillators also incorporate an impedance compensation mechanism that alters waveform morphology based on impedance measurements during actual defibrillation. Evaluation of the evidence on biphasic waveforms is complicated further by the availability of a rectilinear biphasic waveform (120–200 J) (Figure 44.2) and traditional escalating high energy (200–360 J) BTE waveforms.

BTE waveforms have been shown to be superior to monophasic waveforms for internal defibrillation. Lower defibrillation thresholds and higher rates of defibrillation are well documented with these waveforms for internal defibrillations.[7,8] **Grade A** As a result, implantable cardioverter defibrillators (ICDs) are only available now with low energy biphasic waveforms.

Transthoracic biphasic waveforms have been developed and tested in patients undergoing electrophysiologic studies (EPS) and ICD implantation.[9–11] These multicenter, randomized, blinded, prospective studies were carried out by first inducing ventricular fibrillation, and then measuring the success rate of transthoracic "rescue" shocks. The accepted definition for defibrillation success is the termination of VF for a designated period (5–30 seconds, depending on the researchers). By this definition, a successful postshock rhythm can be any non-VF activity, including asystole. The energies tested included 115 and 130 J BTE shocks using impedance compensation and a 171 J Gurvich biphasic waveform. The BTE shocks were compared with 200 J and 360 J MDS waveforms,[10,11] and a 215 J MDS waveform

was the comparison for the Gurvich waveform.[9] Evidence from these studies confirms that low energy biphasic shocks achieve at least the same defibrillation success rates on the first shock as 200–215 J monophasic shocks in VF of short duration (20–30 seconds). **Grade A** Furthermore, in a small subgroup of these patients, investigators looked at ECG abnormalities in the immediate postshock period.[12] They found that ECG ST-segment elevation was significantly greater with 200 J MDS waveform shocks than with either the 115 J or 130 J BTE shocks. **Grade A** This suggests that the lower energy shocks may cause less myocardial injury or ischemia.

These efficacy data are encouraging, but several factors make VF episodes outside of the EPS lab different. The etiology is clearly different, with ischemia a frequent cause of arrest. The duration of VF is invariably longer in the typical cardiopulmonary arrest. The higher levels of tissue hypoxia and acidosis that result could potentially make defibrillation more difficult. Also, laboratory evidence in a dog model suggests that the longer the duration of VF the more difficult it is to defibrillate.[13] A final concern is that the outcome most widely accepted to define resuscitation success – survival to hospital discharge[14,15] – may not be affected by the defibrillation success rate on the first shock in the EPS lab.

Unfortunately, minimal data evaluating biphasic defibrillation in settings outside the EPS lab are available at this time. A randomized, multicenter, non-concealed, non-blinded trial in Europe compared 150 J BTE shocks with 200–360 J monophasic escalating shocks in out-of-hospital cardiac arrest victims. In this study 115 out-of-hospital cardiac arrest patients presented with VF and were shocked with an AED. AEDs were prospectively randomized according to defibrillation waveform on a daily basis. The primary end point was the percentage of patients with VF as the initial monitored rhythm who were defibrillated in the first series of ≤3 shocks. In the biphasic waveform group 96% of 54 patients were defibrillated, whereas 59% of the 61 patients in the monophasic waveform group were defibrillated ($P < 0.0001$; 95% CI 24–51). A higher percentage of patients (76%) achieved return of spontaneous circulation (ROSC) after biphasic defibrillation compared with monophasic defibrillation (54%, $P = 0.01$). There was no difference in survival rate to admission or hospital discharge. However, due to the small size of the study, little can be concluded regarding these last two outcomes.[16] **Grade A** Also, 80% of the patients in the monophasic group were defibrillated with a monophasic truncated exponential waveform; there is some evidence that this waveform is less effective than the monophasic damped sine waveform.[17]

The evidence supporting biphasic waveforms in VF arrests is strengthened by data from multicenter out-of-hospital case series reports. These studies demonstrated that a single 150 J impedance compensating BTE shock defibrillated the initial VF episode in 86–89% of patients.[18,19] They also reported that, of all VF episodes that received up to three shocks, 97–99% were terminated with three or fewer shocks. **Grade B** Termination of VF into an organized rhythm or asystole was the definition of success. These data compare favorably with the data from short duration VF in the EPS laboratory, where first shock defibrillation rates varied from 86% to 100% in three studies.[9–11]

In a recent evidence-based review by the AHA, it was noted that "research has not clearly established an expected success rate for out-of-hospital monophasic defibrillation".[20] A rough estimate can be derived, however, by reviewing what data are available. In 1996, Behr *et al* did a retrospective review of 86 patients treated for witnessed out-of-hospital VF who received one of two different monophasic waveforms. The first shock defibrillation rate for the 200 J MTE waveform was reported to be 43% and for the 200 J MDS waveform was 66%.[17] Although the first shock defibrillation rates were significantly different, survival to hospital discharge was not. In another prospective randomized trial by Weaver *et al*, first shock defibrillation rates for MDS waveforms at 175 J and 320 J were reported to be 61% for both energy levels.[21] Schneider *et al* reported a first shock defibrillation rate of 59% for the monophasic waveform arm in their prospective randomized study.[16]

The consistency of these rates across several studies suggests that biphasic waveforms have higher rates of defibrillation efficacy compared with monophasic waveforms. The real clinical question, however, is how do these results for initial defibrillation rates influence ultimate outcomes in terms of survival to hospital discharge. Clearly, good comparative out-of-hospital data on monophasic versus biphasic waveforms for management of VF do not exist to answer this question. However, patients who regain pulses with only defibrillation shocks have a very high survival rate when compared with patients who need advanced life support interventions (97% *v* 19%). **Grade B** These observations affirm the benefit of defibrillation as the definitive intervention in cardiac arrest caused by ventricular fibrillation.[22]

The present AHA guideline for the monophasic waveform energy sequence 200 J to 300 J to 360 J has been acknowledged by the AHA to be "largely speculative and based on common-sense extrapolation from animal data and human case series".[20] At the present time, the AHA guidelines have designated initial low energy (150 J) non-progressive impedance-adjusted biphasic waveform shocks a Class IIa recommendation (acceptable and useful; good to very good supporting evidence).[1] With the available evidence at this time, it is difficult to unequivocally state that biphasic waveforms are superior to monophasic, but they certainly appear to be at least equivalent. In fact, the question of superiority appears now to be moot, since only biphasic waveforms are being marketed for external defibrillators, following the experience with waveforms for ICDs. Both escalating

and non-escalating biphasic energy defibrillators are now marketed, but few data exist comparing their efficacy.[1]

Drugs in cardiac arrest

On close review of the literature to date, there is little evidence that the administration of any drug improves survival to hospital discharge in cardiac arrest.[23] As a result, the International Guidelines for 2000 stress that during cardiac arrest "drug administration must be secondary to other interventions".[1] Once CPR, defibrillation, and proper airway management are established, certain drugs are considered by "standard practice" to be potentially useful. Recent research has gathered new information about some of these medications as well as some new medications that might be potentially useful. These drugs include epinephrine, vasopressin, amiodarone, and lidocaine.

Epinephrine

Historically, epinephrine has been used in resuscitation of all cardiac arrest rhythms.[1] Although considerable animal data exist supporting its use, no randomized, prospective, placebo-controlled trials have been done in humans to determine its efficacy. In a non-randomized cohort study over an 11 year period, Herlitz *et al* examined the use of epinephrine (adrenaline) in out-of-hospital VF.[24] During this observation period, some of the prehospital staff were authorized to give epinephrine and some were not. A total of 1203 cases were reviewed, with epinephrine administration in 417 (35%). In patients who experienced sustained VF, those who received epinephrine were hospitalized alive more frequently ($P < 0.01$). However, survival to hospital discharge did not differ significantly. When the subgroup of patients who converted to asystole or PEA was reviewed, similar results were observed. Those who received epinephrine were more likely to be hospitalized alive ($P < 0.001$). However, survival to discharge was not significantly different. **Grade B** Given the widespread acceptance of epinephrine as a "standard of care" in refractory VF, asystole and PEA, it is doubtful that better quality evidence of its efficacy will be available in the near future.

Despite the paucity of evidence supporting the use of epinephrine in cardiac arrest, considerable research has been done comparing high-dose epinephrine (0·07–0·20 mg/kg) with standard-dose epinephrine (1 mg every 3–5 minutes). A total of eight randomized trials have been done involving more than 9000 cardiac arrest patients.[25–32] The findings are consistently the same. High-dose protocols result in higher rates of return of spontaneous circulation during initial resuscitation. However, no difference can be found when survival to hospital discharge and final neurologic outcome are compared. **Grade A** The higher doses have not clearly been shown to be harmful, but would likely confer added costs to healthcare systems by increasing hospitalization in hopeless situations.

Vasopressin

Vasopressin has been introduced in the 2000 guidelines as an acceptable alternative to epinephrine in refractory VF/pulseless VT.[1] It is a naturally occurring hormone that in high doses acts as a potent non-adrenergic vasoconstrictor. The theoretical advantage to vasopressin is that it lacks some of the potentially detrimental β adrenergic effects of epinephrine in the postresuscitation setting. In a human study, Rivers *et al* documented a dose-dependent impairment of systemic oxygen delivery and myocardial dysfunction from epinephrine.[33] Animal models have further demonstrated that these β adrenergic effects increase myocardial work and impair coronary perfusion.[34,35] In addition, Lindner *et al* have demonstrated that endogenous vasopressin levels were higher in patients who survived after CPR than in those with no ROSC.[36]

Adrenergic agents are believed to exert a beneficial effect during cardiac arrest by α receptor mediated increases in myocardial and cerebral blood flow.[37] Evidence from both animal and human studies demonstrates that a minimum coronary perfusion pressure (CPP) is required to achieve any ROSC.[38,39] In an animal cardiac arrest model, vasopressin has been shown to increase CPP during CPR.[40] From basic science research, then, it would appear to be a very promising agent for cardiac arrest.

Unfortunately, only two randomized trials exist that examined its efficacy in human cardiac arrest. Lindner *et al* prospectively randomized 40 out-of-hospital patients in VF to receive epinephrine (1 mg IV) or vasopressin (40 U IV) as the primary drug if initial defibrillation was unsuccessful. They reported four outcomes: successful resuscitation (ROSC and measurable blood pressure on admission to hospital), survival for at least 24 hours, survival to hospital discharge, and mean Glasgow Coma Score at hospital discharge. Only one of the four outcomes – survival for at least 24 hours – reached statistical significance ($P = 0.02$). However, none of the other outcomes was significantly different, and no statistical correction was done for the multiple comparisons.[41] **Grade A**

A larger trial ($n = 200$) by Stiell *et al* randomized inhospital adult cardiac arrests to receive one dose of vasopressin (40 U IV) or epinephrine (1 mg IV) as the initial vasopressor. Initial rhythms were VF, pulseless VT, PEA, or asystole. When comparing vasopressin with epinephrine, survival did not differ for hospital discharge (12% *v* 14%, respectively; 95% CI for absolute increase in survival $-11.8-7.8\%$) or 1 hour survival (39% *v* 35%, 95% CI $10.9-17$) (Table 44.1).[42] It is important to at least note some differences in baseline characteristics of the two groups that might have affected the outcomes. More of the patients in the epinephrine group were in monitored settings (emergency department or intensive care) than in the vasopressin group (49% *v* 36%). Clearly this might favor outcomes in the epinephrine group. Also, only 42/200 presented with initial VF/VT, making the ultimate outcomes for the whole group less favorable and resulting in the likelihood of demonstrating less benefit. Despite these issues, the preliminary human evidence is disappointing, and has at this point failed to detect even a modest trend favoring vasopressin over epinephrine. **Grade A** The more fundamental clinical question, however, may be whether any drug actually improves survival. Given that

Table 44.1 Survival and adverse outcomes

Outcome measure	Vasopressin ($n = 104$)	Epinephrine ($n = 96$)	P	Percentage absolute difference (95% CI)
Primary survival measures				
1 hour	40 (39%)	34 (35%)	0·66	3·1 (−10·5−17·3)
Hospital discharge	12 (12%)	13 (14%)	0·67	−2·0 (−11·6−7·8)
Other survival measures				
Any return of pulse	62 (60%)	57 (59%)	0·97	0·2 (−14·0−14·5)
Pulse > 20 min	45 (43%)	38 (40%)	0·60	3·7 (−10·6−17·9)
24 hours	27 (26%)	23 (24%)	0·74	2·0 (−10·6−14·6)
30 days	13 (13%)	13 (14%)	0·83	−1·0 (−11·0−8·9)
Adverse outcomes				
Tachyarrhythmias	10 (10%)	8 (8%)	0·75	1·3 (−7·2−9·8)
Uncontrolled hypertension	0	0	–	–
Mesenteric infarction	0	0	–	–

epinephrine has never been adequately studied, it is entirely possible that both drugs are equally ineffective (or possibly equally harmful) for improving survival in cardiac arrest.

Amiodarone and lidocaine

The use of lidocaine (lignocaine) for refractory VF/pulseless VT is largely based on historical use of the drug to prevent VF in acute MI.[43] Only one retrospective prehospital trial provides some supporting evidence for its use in VF/pulseless VT, demonstrating an improved survival to hospital admission rate.[44] Another retrospective study suggests that lidocaine has a detrimental effect on ROSC.[23] More recently, the prophylactic use of lidocaine in acute MI has been shown to be associated with increased morbidity and to cause more serious arrhythmias than it prevents.[45,46] Additionally, it has been established in experimental models that lidocaine increases energy requirements for defibrillation.[47–49] More study needs to be done to determine the role of lidocaine in cardiac arrest, and it should be recognized that current practice has no sound evidence base.

The ARREST trial is the only randomized, prospective, placebo-controlled trial that addresses the efficacy of an antiarrhythmic in cardiac arrest. Out-of-hospital cardiac arrest patients with VF (or pulseless VT) who had not responded after receiving three or more shocks and 1 mg of epinephrine, were randomly assigned to receive 300 mg of amiodarone or placebo (*n* = 540). The rate of admission to hospital with a perfusing rhythm was higher in the amiodarone group (44% *v* 34% of placebo; *P* = 0·03). Among the patients who

achieved ROSC, more in the amiodarone group experienced significant hypotension (59% *v* 48% of placebo; *P* = 0·04) or bradycardia (41% *v* 25%; *P* = 0·004). Ultimately there was no difference in survival rate to hospital discharge (13·4% of amiodarone *v* 13·2% of placebo).[50] **Grade A**

The most recent data comparing amiodarone and lidocaine in shock-resistant ventricular fibrillation were obtained in a randomized blinded trial in out-of-hospital cardiac arrest (ALIVE trial). In this study 348 patients were randomized to receive amiodarone (or placebo) or lidocaine (or placebo). The primary end point was survival to hospital admission. In the amiodarone group 22·7% of 179 patients survived to admission, whereas 11·0% of 165 patients in the lidocaine group survived (*P* < 0·0043; odds ratio 2·37; 95% CI 1·30–4·33). In patients with VF as the initial rhythm, 25·2% of amiodarone versus 13·5% of lidocaine patients survived to admission (*P* = 0·02). However, survival to discharge was not different between the two groups.[51]

The role of amiodarone in VF/pulseless VT has generated considerable controversy. It is cumbersome to dilute and administer, and in the ARREST trial required an average of 13 (and up to 21) minutes from the time of medic arrival to administration.[50] The drug cannot be provided in preloaded syringes because it adheres to plastic surfaces. Significant hypotension and bradycardia often accompany ROSC, complicating postresuscitation management. Finally, the cost of the drug is considerable, and can be prohibitive for prehospital services to stock. The consensus opinion by the most recent AHA guidelines is that the evidence for amiodarone, while better than any other antiarrhythmic, is only "fair".

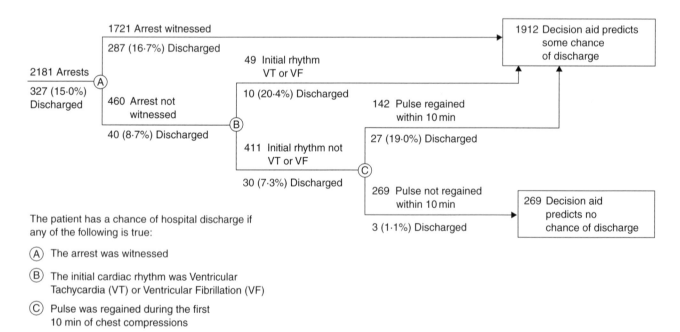

The patient has a chance of hospital discharge if any of the following is true:

(A) The arrest was witnessed

(B) The initial cardiac rhythm was Ventricular Tachycardia (VT) or Ventricular Fibrillation (VF)

(C) Pulse was regained during the first 10 min of chest compressions

Figure 44.3 Utilization of a decision aid to the validation set of attempted resuscitations. (From van Walraven C, Forster AJ, Parish DC *et al* Validation of a clinical decision aid to discontinue in-hospital cardiac arrest resuscitations. *JAMA* 2001;**285**:1602–6)

They comment that "this practice decision (to use amiodarone), must be made with a clear awareness that the evidence – powerful in design – was weak in the conclusions".

Termination of resuscitation

Physicians involved in resuscitation invariably will be called upon to make the difficult decision of when to stop resuscitative efforts. Multiple factors come into play, with the ultimate decision involving a complex interaction of patient and physician variables. The most important single factor associated with poor outcomes is prolonged time of resuscitation. As time spent increases, chance of neurologically intact survival diminishes. A simple clinical decision aid has also been derived and recently validated for inhospital arrests. It involves assessing three simple parameters: whether the arrest was witnessed *or* the initial cardiac rhythm was either VF or VT *or* patients regained a pulse during the first 10 minutes of chest compressions. If none of these three variables was present, the aid predicts no chance of discharge.[52,53]

The validation was completed on data from 2181 inhospital cardiac arrest attempts over a 10 year period in a community hospital. Overall, 327 (15%) of patients survived to hospital discharge: 324 of these patients were predicted to survive (99·1%; 95% CI 97·1–99·8). In 269 (12·3%) resuscitations, patients were predicted not to survive. Only three of these patients (1·1%) were discharged and none was able to function independently. The negative likelihood ratio was 0·064 (Figure 44.3).[53] **Grade B** Ideally, prospective testing in another inhospital setting would further ensure its validity, but it does provide clinicians with some parameters to help them make complex decisions on individual cases.

References

1. International consensus on science, American Heart Association. Guidelines 2000 for cardiopulmonary resuscitation and emergency cardiovascular care. *Circulation* 2000; **102**(Suppl. I):I60–165.
2. Zoll PM, Linenthal AJ, Gibson W, Paul MH, Normal LR. Termination of ventricular fibrillation in man by internally applied electric countershock. *N Engl J Med* 1956;**254**: 727–32.
3. Stiell IG, Wells GA, DeMaio VJ *et al.* Modifiable factors associated with improved cardiac arrest survival in a multicenter basic life support/defibrillation system: OPALS Study Phase I results. Ontario Prehospital Advanced Life Support. *Ann Emerg Med* 1999;**33**:44–50.
4. Larsen MP, Eisenberg MS, Cummins RO, Hallstrom AP. Predicting survival from out-of-hospital cardiac arrest: a graphic model. *Ann Emerg Med* 1993;**22**:1652–8.
5. Eisenberg MS, Copass MK, Hallstrom AP *et al.* Treatment of out-of-hospital cardiac arrest with rapid defibrillation by emergency medical technicians. *N Engl J Med* 1980;**302**:1379–83.
6. Weisfeldt ML, Kerber RE, McGoldrick RP *et al.* American Heart Association report on the Public Access Defibrillation Conference, December 8–10, 1994. Automatic External Defibrillation Task Force. *Circulation* 1995;**92**:2740–7.
7. Bardy GH, Ivey TD, Allen MD, Johnson G, Mehra R, Greene HL. A prospective randomized evaluation of biphasic versus monophasic waveform pulses on defibrillation efficacy in humans. *J Am Coll Cardiol* 1989;**14**:728–33.
8. Winkle RA, Mead RH, Ruder MA *et al.* Improved low energy defibrillation efficacy in man with the use of a biphasic truncated exponential waveform. *Am Heart J* 1989;**117**:122–7.
9. Greene HL, DiMarco JP, Kudenchuk PJ *et al.* Comparison of monophasic and biphasic defibrillating pulse waveforms for transthoracic cardioversion. *Am J Cardiol* 1995;**75**:1135–9.
10. Brady GH, Marchlinski FE, Sharma AD *et al.* Multicenter comparison of truncated biphasic shocks and standard damped sine wave monophasic shocks for transthoracic ventricular defibrillation. *Circulation* 1996;**94**:2507–14.
11. Bardy GH, Gliner BE, Kudenchuk PJ *et al.* Truncated biphasic pulses for transthoracic defibrillation. *Circulation* 1995;**91**: 1768–74.
12. Reddy RK, Gleva MJ, Gliner BE *et al.* Biphasic transthoracic defibrillation causes fewer ECG ST-segment changes after shock. *Ann Emerg Med* 1997;**30**:127–34.
13. Yakatis RW, Ewy GA, Otto CW, Taren DL, Moon TE. Influence of time and therapy on ventricular defibrillation in dogs. *Crit Care Med* 1980;**8**:157–63.
14. Cummins RO, Chamberlain D, Hazinski MF *et al.* Recommended guidelines for reviewing, reporting, and conducting research on in-hospital resuscitation: the in-hospital "utstein style". *Circulation* 1997;**95**:2213–39.
15. Cummins RO, Chamberlain DA, Abramson NS *et al.* Recommended guidelines for uniform reporting of data from out-of-hospital cardiac arrest: the utstein style. *Circulation* 1991;**84**:960–75.
16. Schneider T, Martens PR, Paschen H *et al.* Multi-center, randomized, controlled trial of 150-J biphasic shocks compared with 200- to 360-J monophasic shocks in the resuscitation of out-of-hospital cardiac arrest victims. *Circulation* 2000;**102**: 1780–7.
17. Behr JC, Hartley LL, York DK, Brown DD, Kerber RE. Truncated exponential versus damped sinusoidal waveform shocks for transthoracic defibrillation. *Am J Cardiol* 1996;**78**: 1242–5.
18. Poole JE, White RD, Kanz KG *et al.* Low-energy impedance-compensating biphasic waveforms terminate ventricular fibrillation at high rates in victims of out-of-hospital cardiac arrest. *J Cardiovasc Electrophysiol* 1997;**8**:1373–85.
19. Gliner BE, Jorgenson DB, Poole JE *et al.* Treatment of out-of-hospital cardiac arrest with a low-energy impedance-compensating biphasic waveform automatic external defibrillator. *Biomed Instrument Technol* 1998;**32**:631–44.
20. Cummins RO, Hazinski MF, Kerber RE *et al.* Low-energy biphasic waveform defibrillation: evidence-based review applied to emergency cardiovascular care guidelines. *Circulation* 1998; **97**:1654–67.
21. Weaver W, Cobb L, Copass M *et al.* Ventricular defibrillation: a comparative trial using 175-J and 320-J shocks. *N Engl J Med* 1982;**307**:1101–6.

22. White RD, Hankins DG, Bugliosi TF. Seven years' experience with early defibrillation by police and paramedics in an emergency medical services system. *Resuscitation* 1998;**39**:145–51.

23. van Walraven C, Stiell IG, Wells GA, Herbert PC, Vandenheen K. The OTAC Study Group. Do advanced cardiac life support drugs increase resuscitation rates from in-hospital cardiac arrest? *Ann Emerg Med* 1998;**32**:544–53.

24. Herlitz J, Ekstrom L, Wennerblom B, Axelsson A, Bang A, Holmberg S. Adrenaline in out-of-hospital ventricular fibrillation. Does it make a difference. *Resuscitation* 1995;**29**: 195–201.

25. Brown CG, Martin DR, Pepe PE *et al*. The Multicenter High-dose Epinephrine Study Group. A comparison of standard-dose and high-dose epinephrine in cardiac arrest outside the hospital. *N Engl J Med* 1992;**327**:1051–5.

26. Stiell IG, Hebert PC, Weitzman BN *et al*. High-dose epinephrine in adult cardiac arrest. *N Engl J Med* 1992;**327**: 1045–50.

27. Callaham M, Madsen CD, Barton CW, Saunders CE, Pointer J. A randomized clinical trial of high-dose epinephrine and norepinephrine vs standard-dose epinephrine in prehospital cardiac arrest. *JAMA* 1992;**268**:2667–72.

28. Lindner KH, Ahnefeld FW, Prengel AW. Comparison of standard and high-dose adrenaline in the resuscitation of asystole and electromechanical dissociation. *Acta Anaesthesiol Scand* 1991;**35**:253–6.

29. Lipman J, Wilson W, Kobilski S *et al*. High-dose adrenaline in adult in-hospital asystolic cardiopulmonary resuscitation: a double-blind randomized trial. *Anaesth Intens Care* 1993; **21**:192–6.

30. Choux C, Gueugniaud PY, Barbieux A *et al*. Standard doses versus repeated high doses of epinephrine in cardiac arrest outside the hospital. *Resuscitation* 1995;**29**:3–9.

31. Sherman BW, Munger MA, Foulke GE, Rutherford WF, Panacek EA. High-dose versus standard-dose epinephrine treatment of cardiac arrest after failure of standard therapy. *Pharmacotherapy* 1997;**17**:242–7.

32. Gueugniaud PY, Mols P, Goldstein P *et al*. A comparison of repeated high doses and repeated standard doses of epinephrine for cardiac arrest outside the hospital. *N Engl J Med* 1998;**339**:1595–601.

33. Rivers E, Wortsman J, Rady M, Blake H, McGeorge F, Buderer N. The effect of the total cumulative epinephrine dose administered during human CPR on hemodynamic, oxygen transport, and utilization variables in the postresuscitation period. *Chest* 1994;**106**:1499–507.

34. Ditchey RV, Lindenfeld J. Failure of epinephrine to improve the balance between myocardial oxygen supply and demand during closed-chest resuscitation in dogs. *Circulation* 1988; **78**: 382–9.

35. Lindner KH, Ahnefeld F, Schuerman W, Bawdler IM. Epinephrine and norepinephrine in cardiopulmonary resuscitation – effects in myocardial oxygen delivery and consumption. *Chest* 1990;**97**:1458–62.

36. Lindner KH, Haak T, Keller A, Bothner U, Lurie KG. Release of endogenous vasopressors during and after cardiopulmonary resuscitation. *Heart* 1996;**75**:145–50.

37. Michael JR, Guerci AD, Koehler RC *et al*. Mechanisms by which epinephrine augments cerebral and myocardial perfusion during cardiopulmonary resuscitation in dogs. *Circulation* 1984;**69**:822–35.

38. Paradis NA, Martin GB, Rivers EP *et al*. Coronary perfusion pressure and the return of spontaneous circulation in human cardiopulmonary resuscitation. *JAMA* 1990;**263**:1106–13.

39. Lindner KH, Ahnefeld FW, Bawdler IM. Comparison of different doses of epinephrine on myocardial perfusion and resuscitation success during cardiopulmonary resuscitation in a pig model. *Am J Emerg Med* 1991;**9**:27–31.

40. Barbar SI, Berg RA, Hilwig RW, Kern KB, Ewy GA. Vasopressin versus epinephrine during cardiopulmonary resuscitation: a randomized swine outcome study. *Resuscitation* 1999;**41**:185–92.

41. Linder KH, Dirks B, Strohmenger HU, Prengel AW, Lindner IM, Lurie KG. Randomized comparison of epinephrine and vasopressin in patients with out-of-hospital ventricular fibrillation. *Lancet* 1997;**349**:535–7.

42. Stiell IG, Hebert PC, Wells GA *et al*. Vasopressin versus epinephrine for in-hospital cardiac arrest: a randomized controlled trial. *Lancet* 2001;**358**:105–9.

43. Lie KI, Wellens HJ, van Capelle FJ, Durrer D. Lidocaine in prevention of primary ventricular fibrillation: a double-blind, randomized study of 212 consecutive patients. *N Engl J Med* 1974;**291**:1324–6.

44. Herlitz J, Ekstrom L, Wennerblom B *et al*. Lidocaine in out-of-hospital ventricular fibrillation: does it improve survival? *Resuscitation* 1997;**33**:199–205.

45. Sadowski ZP, Alexander JH, Skrabucha B *et al*. Multicenter randomized trial and a systematic overview of lidocaine in acute myocardial infarction. *Am Heart J* 1999;**137**:792–8.

46. Alexander JH, Grayer CB, Sadowski Z *et al*. The GUSTO-I and GUSTO-IIb Investigators. Prophylactic lidocaine use in acute myocardial infarction: incidence and outcomes from two international trials. *Am Heart J* 1999;**137**:799–805.

47. Dorian P, Fain ES, Davy JM, Winkle RA. Lidocaine causes a reversible, concentration-dependent increase in defibrillation energy requirements. *J Am Coll Cardiol* 1986;**8**:327–32.

48. Echt DS, Black JN, Barbey JT, Coxe DR, Cato E. Evaluation of anti-arrhythmic drugs in defibrillation energy requirements in dogs: sodium channel block and action potential prolongation. *Circulation* 1998;**79**:1106–17.

49. Babbs CF, Yim GK, Whistler SJ, Tacker WA, Geddes LA. Elevation of ventricular defibrillation threshold in dogs by antiarrhythmic drugs. *Am Heart J* 1979;**98**:345–50.

50. Kudenchuk PJ, Cobb LA, Copass MK *et al*. Amiodarone for resuscitation after out-of-hospital cardiac arrest due to ventricular fibrillation. *N Engl J Med* 1999;**341**:871–8.

51. Dorian P, Cass D, Schwartz B, Cooper R, Gelaznikas R, Barr A. Amiodarone as compared with lidocaine for shock-resistant ventricular fibrillation. *N Engl J Med* 2002;**346**:884–90.

52. van Walraven C, Forster AJ, Stiell IG. Derivation of a clinical decision rule for the discontinuation of in-hospital cardiac arrest resuscitations. *Arch Intern Med* 1998;**158**:129–34.

53. van Walraven C, Forster AJ, Parish DC *et al*. Validation of a clinical decision aid to discontinue in-hospital cardiac arrest resuscitations. *JAMA* 2001;**285**:1602–6.

Part IIIe

Specific cardiovascular disorders: Left ventricular dysfunction

Salim Yusuf, Editor

Grading of recommendations and levels of evidence used in *Evidence-based Cardiology*

GRADE A

Level 1a   Evidence from large randomized clinical trials (RCTs) or systematic reviews (including meta-analyses) of multiple randomized trials which collectively has at least as much data as one single well-defined trial.

Level 1b   Evidence from at least one "All or None" high quality cohort study; in which ALL patients died/failed with conventional therapy and some survived/succeeded with the new therapy (for example, chemotherapy for tuberculosis, meningitis, or defibrillation for ventricular fibrillation); or in which many died/failed with conventional therapy and NONE died/failed with the new therapy (for example, penicillin for pneumococcal infections).

Level 1c   Evidence from at least one moderate-sized RCT or a meta-analysis of small trials which collectively only has a moderate number of patients.

Level 1d   Evidence from at least one RCT.

GRADE B

Level 2   Evidence from at least one high quality study of non-randomized cohorts who did and did not receive the new therapy.

Level 3   Evidence from at least one high quality case–control study.

Level 4   Evidence from at least one high quality case series.

GRADE C

Level 5   Opinions from experts without reference or access to any of the foregoing (for example, argument from physiology, bench research or first principles).

A comprehensive approach would incorporate many different types of evidence (for example, RCTs, non-RCTs, epidemiologic studies, and experimental data), and examine the architecture of the information for consistency, coherence and clarity. Occasionally the evidence does not completely fit into neat compartments. For example, there may not be an RCT that demonstrates a reduction in mortality in individuals with stable angina with the use of β blockers, but there is overwhelming evidence that mortality is reduced following MI. In such cases, some may recommend use of β blockers in angina patients with the expectation that some extrapolation from post-MI trials is warranted. This could be expressed as Grade A/C. In other instances (for example, smoking cessation or a pacemaker for complete heart block), the non-randomized data are so overwhelmingly clear and biologically plausible that it would be reasonable to consider these interventions as Grade A.

Recommendation grades appear either within the text, for example, **Grade A** and **Grade A1a** or within a table in the chapter.

The grading system clearly is only applicable to preventive or therapeutic interventions. It is not applicable to many other types of data such as descriptive, genetic or pathophysiologic.

45 Prevention of congestive heart failure and treatment of asymptomatic left ventricular dysfunction

RS McKelvie, CR Benedict, Salim Yusuf

Epidemiology of heart failure

Over the past three decades, epidemiological studies have been increasingly used to identify the cause of major chronic degenerative diseases such as systemic hypertension and atherosclerosis.[1] Early studies on the prevalence and incidence of heart failure were drawn from private practice, hospital wards, and admissions to hospitals.[1] Also, data from survey studies were used to determine the prevalence rate of heart failure.[2] The prevalence of heart failure shows some disparity among the published studies, although generally the results are similar in demonstrating an increase with age.[3-7] Prevalence increases from approximately 0·7 cases/1000 persons in the younger age group (<50 years old) to approximately 27 cases/1000 in the older age group, (>65 years old) and approximately 63 cases/1000 in those over 75 years old.[8] The incidence is greater in men than in women and increases progressively with age.[5,6,9-11] The incidence in younger men (<50 years old) is approximately 1 case/1000 persons per year, increasing in the older age group (>65 years old) to 11/1000 per year, with an incidence of approximately 17/1000 persons per year in men 85 years or over.[12] In women the incidence increases in the younger age group (<50 years old) from 0·4/1000 persons per year to 5/1000 per year in older individuals (>65 years old), with an incidence of approximately 10/1000 persons per year in women 85 years or over.[12]

There are a number of reasons why some disparity has been observed among these studies examining incidence and prevalence in heart failure patients. The studies differ with regard to sampling methods (population based *v* cohort based), geography and demographics, case finding methods (medical record review versus systematic questionnaires and examinations), and diagnostic criteria.[13] Even though these differences are responsible for the disparities between studies, they also provide a more robust database and complementary information.

Once a diagnosis of heart failure has been made the prognosis has been uniformly observed to be relatively poor.[7,14-16] Croft *et al*[14] obtained Medicare hospital claims records from 1984 to 1986 and beneficiary enrollment data for 1986 to 1992 from the Health Care Financing Administration. The 1 year survival for black men (*n* = 6186) was 68%, for white men (*n* = 64 918) was 64%, for black women (*n* = 9097) was 71%, and for white women (*n* = 90 038) was 69%. Five year survival for black men was 24%, for white men 21%, for black women 30%, and for white women 29%. Mosterd *et al*[7] examined the prognosis for heart failure in the general population (*n* = 5255; 59·3% women) as part of the Rotterdam Study. In this study 1 year survival for men was 91% and for women was 87%, and survival at 5 years was 56% and 61%, respectively. Cowie *et al*[16] examined the survival of patients with a new diagnosis of heart failure. The total study population was 151 000 as of February 1996 (this was the midpoint of identification of cases, which ran from April 1995 to December 1996) and follow up for death was complete for all 220 cases to June 1997. One month survival for this group was 81%, 3 month survival was 75%, and 12 month survival was 62%.

Although there are some differences between these studies, and also clinical drug trials[17,18] in which 1 year mortality has been reported to be approximately 12%, there are several possible explanations for these discrepancies. Survival outcomes at 1 year will be related to whether the study is based on identifying patients with a new diagnosis (incidence) of heart failure or patients with a diagnosis of heart failure (prevalence) on entry into the study. Clinical drug trials usually take stable heart failure patients, and such patients would be considered "natural survivors" as they have survived the early high-risk period. This would also be true for any surveys of the general population that examined patients who on entry had a diagnosis of heart failure, such as the study by Mosterd *et al*[7] Also, clinical trials tend to recruit a select group of patients with a better prognosis than the general population of patients with heart failure. The typical age of patients in a drug trial is on average approximately 65 years, compared to the general population of heart failure patients with an average age of approximately 75 years.[19,20] Heart failure is often associated with considerable comorbidity, but patients with these types of problems are less likely to be recruited into clinical drug studies. Thus these biases, seen especially in clinical drug trials, make the prognosis of heart failure appear much better than it actually is for most patients. These findings emphasize the imperative need to identify and aggressively treat patients with left ventricular dysfunction to prevent them developing heart failure.

Epidemiology of asymptomatic left ventricular dysfunction

Studies assessing the epidemiology of heart failure have largely identified symptomatic individuals because identification of these patients is based on clinical criteria and does not require measurement of left ventricular (LV) function.[13] Asymptomatic patients with LV dysfunction have therefore not been included in these studies. Consequently, the available data on the prevalence of patients with asymptomatic LV dysfunction are limited, even though treatment of these patients may be expected to significantly improve their outcome.[21] There have been several studies that screened the general population looking for the presence of asymptomatic LV dysfunction.[8,22–26]

In 1992 McDonagh *et al* measured the ejection fraction in 1467 people aged 25–74 years during a survey of coronary risk factors.[22] The mean ejection fraction in people defined as not having cardiovascular disease was 47%, and 34% was two standard deviations below the mean. Of the 2·9% with an ejection fraction of ≤30%, half had no symptoms. The frequency of both left ventricular systolic dysfunction and symptoms was greater in older age groups, increasing sharply up to the age of 45 and less sharply thereafter (Table 45.1). Of the 7·7% of individuals with an ejection fraction of 35%, 77% were asymptomatic. Of those with definite left ventricular systolic dysfunction (Table 45.1) the proportion with symptoms increased with age. The group with left ventricular systolic dysfunction had a greater

prevalence of ischemic heart disease and hypertension than did the group with normal ventricular function (Table 45.2).

Mosterd *et al*[8] performed a population based cohort study examining the presence of symptomatic and asymptomatic left ventricular systolic dysfunction in the general population of individuals who were 55 years of age or older. A total of 2823 persons had M mode echocardiographic assessments and the echocardiograms of 556 participants were deemed inadequate to measure left ventricular dimensions reliably. The prevalence of left ventricular systolic dysfunction (fractional shortening ≤25%) in the 2267 persons with analyzable echocardiograms was 3·7% (95% CI 2·9–4·5). Overall, the prevalence in men (*n* = 1028) was 5·5% (95% CI 4·1–7·0) and in women (*n* = 1239) was 2·2% (95% CI 1·4–3·2). The age-adjusted prevalence of left ventricular dysfunction was approximately 2·5 times higher in men (OR 2·7, 95% CI 1·7–4·3). The relationship between left ventricular systolic function and symptoms/ signs of heart failure was examined in the 1698 individuals (771 men) in whom information on the presence of heart failure and echocardiographic data were available. Of the 35 individuals who had heart failure by symptoms and signs, only 10 (29%, 95% CI 15–46) had echocardiographic evidence of left ventricular systolic dysfunction. Interestingly, of the 60 individuals with left ventricular dysfunction by echocardiographic criteria only 24 (40%, 95% CI 28–53) were found to have at least one of the cardinal symptoms or signs of heart failure (shortness of breath, ankle edema or pulmonary edema): therefore 60% had asymptomatic left ventricular systolic dysfunction. Persons with left ventricular systolic dysfunction had more frequently sustained a myocardial infarction, undergone coronary artery bypass graft surgery or PTCA and were more likely to have angina pectoris.

Morgan *et al*[23] performed a cross-sectional survey to assess the prevalence and clinical characteristics of left ventricular systolic dysfunction among 817 elderly patients in a general practice setting. Echocardiography was used to

Table 45.1 Prevalence of definite left ventricular systolic dysfunction (EF ≤ 30%) by age according to the presence of symptoms (adapted with permission from McDonagh TA *et al*. Symptomatic and asymptomatic left ventricular systolic dysfunction in an urban population. *Lancet* 1997;350:829–33)

	Proportion with definite left ventricular systolic dysfunction (%) Age group (years)				
	25–34	35–44	45–54	55–64	65–74
Men	(*n* = 122)	(*n* = 135)	(*n* = 138)	(*n* = 158)	(*n* = 155)
Symptomatic	0	0	1·4	2·5	3·2
Asymptomatic	0	0·7	4·4	3·2	3·2
Women	(*n* = 126)	(*n* = 162)	(*n* = 159)	(*n* = 149)	(*n* = 164)
Symptomatic	0	0	1·2	2·0	3·6
Asymptomatic	0	0	1·2	0	1·3

Table 45.2   Risk factors for left ventricular systolic dysfunction in symptomatic and asymptomatic participants (adapted with permission from McDonagh TA *et al*). Symptomatic and asymptomatic left ventricular systolic dysfunction in an urban population. *Lancet* 1997;350:829–33)

Risk factor	Symptomatic % with RF (*n*)		OR (95% CI)	*P* value	Asymptomatic % with RF (*n*)		OR (95% CI)	*P* value
	LVSD present	LVSD absent			LVSD present	LVSD absent		
IHD								
All IHD	95% (21)	43% (197)	25 (3·6–100)	<0·001	71% (21)	17% (1138)	12·5 (4·5–33·3)	<0·001
MI	50% (22)	15% (20)	5·9 (2·3–14·3)	<0·001	14% (21)	2% (1167)	6·7 (1·8–25)	0·02
Angina	62% (21)	26% (206)	4·5 (1·8–11·1)	<0·001	43% (21)	6% (1155)	11·1 (4·5–25)	<0·001
ECG ischemia	77% (22)	25% (201)	10 (3·3–33·3)	<0·001	50% (20)	13% (1151)	6·7 (2·8–16·7)	<0·001
ECG abnormal	77% (22)	8% (201)	9·1 (3·1–25)	<0·001	60% (20)	18% (1151)	7·1 (2·8–16·7)	<0·001
Hypertension	80% (20)	53% (151)	3·1 (1·1–8·9)	0·02	67% (21)	36% (1227)	3·5 (1·4–8·5)	0·004
Valvular abnormality	25% (12)	6% (194)	5·5 (1·3–25)	<0·001	0% (14)	4% (1093)	–	0·99

Abbreviations: CI, confidence interval; IHD, ischemic heart disease; LVSD, definite left ventricular systolic dysfunction; MI, myocardial infarction; *n*, number in subgroups; OR, odds ratio; RF, risk factor

assess ventricular function in this group of patients aged 70–84 years. Left ventricular function was assessed qualitatively as normal, mild, moderate or severe dysfunction. In 667 (82%) of the patients a measurement of ejection fraction could be made. The mean ejection fraction for normal left ventricular function was 66·3% ± (SD) 13·5%, 47·7% ± 12·0% for mild dysfunction, 38·3% ± 8·1% for moderate dysfunction, and 26% ± 7·9% for severe dysfunction. The prevalence of left ventricular systolic dysfunction was higher in men (12·8%, 95% CI 9·6–16·6) than in to women (2·9%, 95% CI 1·8–5·0). The overall prevalence of all grades of left ventricular systolic dysfunction was 7·5% (95% CI 5·8–9·5). Prevalence was more than twice as great at age ≥ 80 years (men 20·5%, 95% CI 12·0–31·6; women 5·4%, 95% CI 1·8–12·2) than at ages 70–74 years (men 9·4%, 95% CI 5·5–14·7; women 2·2%, 95% CI 0·6–5·5), but the relative difference between men and women was preserved (20·5% *v* 5·4%; *P* < 0·05). At all ages the prevalence of left ventricular systolic dysfunction was much greater in men than in women (OR 5·1, 95% CI 2·6–10·1). About half (48%, 29/61 patients) of all patients with left ventricular systolic dysfunction had previous heart failure documented in their medical charts; thus 52% of the patients did not have documented heart failure and would have been considered to have asymptomatic left ventricular systolic dysfunction. Multivariate analysis demonstrated

that the probability of having any grade of echocardiographically abnormal left ventricular function was increased by a previous history of heart failure, myocardial infarction, stroke, angina, age and male gender. Gardin *et al*[26] as part of the Cardiovascular Health Study, assessed cardiac function in 5201 people between the ages of 65 and 100 years old. Left ventricular systolic function was reported in a qualitative/semi-quantitative fashion, with cardiac function being assessed as normal or abnormal. The prevalence of abnormal cardiac function was greater (*P* < 0·001) in men (6·3%) than in women (1·8%); increased with age (*P* < 0·001) from 2·3% for ages 65–69 years to 5·5% for 80 years and older; and was greater (*P* < 0·001) in those with clinical coronary heart disease (10·5%) than in either those with only hypertension (1·7%) or those with neither clinical heart disease or hypertension (0·5%). In the Strong Heart Study left ventricular systolic function was assessed in 3184 adults who were middle-aged and older[25] (range 45–74 years, with a mean of 60 years). The prevalence of mild left ventricular systolic dysfunction (left ventricular ejection fraction <40%) was 2·9%, and 72% of these individuals had no evidence of heart failure.

Clearly the prevalence of asymptomatic left ventricular dysfunction in the general population is substantial, as it is similar to that found for symptomatic left ventricular systolic dysfunction. Furthermore, when patients are screened for left ventricular systolic dysfunction, at least 50% of the cases are found in patients without a previous history of heart failure. These data are only recently being realized because most of the previous studies used signs and symptoms to identify patients with cardiac dysfunction, and there were no systematic evaluations of cardiac function performed. These studies further demonstrate that even in the elderly asymptomatic left ventricular dysfunction is high. The studies are consistent in demonstrating that those individuals with asymptomatic left ventricular dysfunction are more often men with a history of ischemic heart disease and hypertension.

Although the presence of asymptomatic LV systolic dysfunction is relatively common in the general population, a program of screening unselected individuals to identify such patients cannot currently be recommended. A more prudent approach would be to screen individuals who are at a greater risk of developing LV systolic dysfunction, such as those known to have ischemic heart disease or hypertension. Criteria that can be used to assess the risk of developing LV systolic dysfunction will be outlined below.

Left ventricular diastolic dysfunction

It is also very important to recognize that a great number of patients with symptoms and signs of heart failure do not have evidence of left ventricular systolic dysfunction. These findings highlight the possibility that many patients with typical symptoms of heart failure may have preserved left ventricular systolic function. Impaired LV diastolic function, whether by itself or in the presence of LV systolic dysfunction, is gaining more recognition as a potentially important contributor to the progression of LV systolic dysfunction and the development of symptomatic heart failure. The prevalence of normal ventricular systolic performance in patients with heart failure varies widely, from 13% to 74%, with the majority of studies reporting a value of 40–50%.[27–32] Normal ventricular systolic function with heart failure is more prevalent in patients over 65 years of age than those 65 or under, among hypertensive patients, and in women.[27–32] Studies report an annual mortality associated with diastolic heart failure of 3–9%, which is lower than that of patients with systolic heart failure.[27,29] However, other studies have demonstrated that the annual mortality for heart failure patients with associated preserved left ventricular systolic function is as great as in heart failure patients with impaired left ventricular systolic function.[28,30,33,34] In light of these studies to date, there is no doubt that left ventricular diastolic dysfunction represents a significant clinical problem, in terms of both prevalence and prognosis. A lack of consensus remains among physicians regarding what constitutes LV diastolic dysfunction measured by non-invasive techniques.[27] There is therefore a need

to develop a consensus for diagnostic criteria of diastolic heart failure which could then be used to provide a better estimate of its prevalence and prognosis. There is also a need for randomized clinical trials to determine the appropriate treatment for patients with established LV diastolic dysfunction.

Factors that lead to the development of heart failure

Even though angiotensin-converting enzyme (ACE) inhibitors have been demonstrated to decrease the morbidity and mortality associated with heart failure the event rate for symptomatic heart failure remains very high, and other measures are required. The results from the Survival and Ventricular Enlargement (SAVE) trial[35] and the Prevention trial of the Studies of Left Ventricular Dysfunction (SOLVD)[21] demonstrate that the onset of heart failure can be prevented or delayed in patients with asymptomatic or minimally symptomatic LV systolic dysfunction with the use of ACE inhibitors (Figure 45.1). Recent data from the Heart Outcomes Prevention Evaluation study (HOPE) demonstrated a reduction in the incidence of heart failure in patients with no evidence of impaired left ventricular systolic

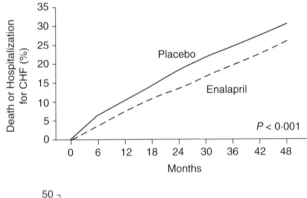

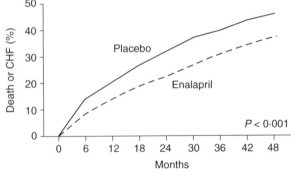

Figure 45.1 Death or hospitalization for heart failure and death or development of heart failure in the Prevention Trial from SOLVD. (From SOLVD Investigators, *N Engl J Med* 1993; **327**:685–91, with permission.)

function.[36] The combined findings from the ACE inhibitor studies suggest benefit for patients who are at high risk for heart failure, irrespective of the degree of left ventricular systolic dysfunction.[36,37] Aggressive treatment of the risk factors responsible for heart failure would also be potentially useful to prevent the development of left ventricular systolic dysfunction or the progression to symptomatic heart failure. Therefore, the most effective method to decrease mortality may be to identify patients who have asymptomatic LV dysfunction and treat them early to prevent the progression to symptomatic LV dysfunction. A number of factors have been identified which help predict whether an individual may have or develop LV dysfunction.

Hypertension

Hypertension has for many years been known to be an important risk factor for the development of heart failure.[5,9,11,38,39] In both men and women, hypertension is associated with a three- to fourfold increase in the risk of heart failure for individuals between 35 and 64 years, and approximately twofold increase for individuals over 65 years of age.[5,40] Although the relative risk is higher in the younger age group, the absolute excess risk is higher in the older age group, reflecting greater absolute risk differences.[40] Multivariate analyses have revealed that hypertension (systolic blood pressure of ≥ 140 mmHg or a diastolic of ≥ 90 mmHg, or current treatment of high blood pressure) is associated with a high population-attributable risk for coronary heart failure (CHF) accounting for 39% of cases in men and 59% in women.[39] Hypertension represents a continuous risk variable with no clear cut-off point below which CHF will not develop. Over four decades of observation there has been no significant change in the frequency of hypertension as an attributable cause of heart failure.[19] The results of more recent studies, such as the Heart Outcomes Prevention Evaluation (HOPE)[36] and the Perindopril Protection against Recurrent Stroke Study (PROGRESS)[41] studies, suggest that for high-risk patients it may be beneficial to lower blood pressure even if it is already within the "normal" range. Furthermore, a recent reanalysis of 20 years of blood-pressure data from the Framingham Heart Study suggests that the degree of benefit expected from a decrease in blood pressure may have been underestimated.[42] Therefore, hypertension remains an important risk factor for the development of heart failure.

Left ventricular hypertrophy

The presence of LV hypertrophy has been well documented as a risk factor for the development of heart failure, even after controlling for hypertension.[39] ECG evidence of LV hypertrophy criteria is associated with increased risk of CHF that is greater than the risk associated with cardiac enlargement on chest radiography. Data from Framingham demonstrate that the age-adjusted biennial rate of developing heart failure in men with ECG evidence of LV hypertrophy was 71/1000 patients aged 35–64 years and 102/1000 individuals aged 65–94 years, which was greater than that found when cardiac enlargement was present radiographically in men in the same age groups: 16/1000 individuals and 56/1000 individuals, respectively.[43] This suggests that the ECG findings reflect ischemia in addition to anatomical hypertrophy.[43] A recent report, based on a substudy from the Losartan Intervention For End (LIFE) point reduction in hypertension study, found that in hypertensive patients with clinical evidence of coronary artery disease (CAD) LV hypertrophy identifies those individuals with structural and functional cardiac abnormalities with a high risk for the development of heart failure.[44] Furthermore, in this study exceptionally high levels of myocardial oxygen demand were found in this group, and this may be additive to the ischemic effect in these patients. A recent study by Matthew *et al*[45] based on analysis of data from the HOPE study demonstrated the importance of LV hypertrophy as a predictor for the risk of developing heart failure. In this study of patients with normal or controlled blood pressure those with ECG evidence of LV hypertrophy had a much greater risk of developing heart failure (15·4% with ECG–LV hypertrophy versus 9·3% without ECG–LV hypertrophy; $P < 0.0001$). LV hypertrophy is associated with a 15-fold increase in the incidence of heart failure in men 64 years of age or under and a fivefold increase in men 65 or older.[40] In women, LV hypertrophy is associated with a 13-fold increase in heart failure for the younger age group and a fivefold increase for the older age group.[40] Although the relative risk is higher in the younger age group, the absolute excess in risk is higher in the older age group, reflecting greater absolute risk differences.

Smoking

Cigarette smoking has been found in 42% of men and 24% of women who develop heart failure.[40] In men the relationship between cigarette smoking and the development of heart failure is greater in the younger age group than in the older age group.[5,40] Multivariate analyses have demonstrated smoking to be a strongly significant independent risk factor for the development of heart failure in men, even in the older age group.[5] The relationship between cigarette smoking and the risk of developing heart failure in women is inconsistent, although there has been a trend to an increase in relative risk in older women.[40] Therefore the data would suggest that smoking is a risk factor for the development of heart failure, and in fact the hazardous effects may be underestimated, as not all studies have taken into account changes in smoking habits over time, and this could lead to an underestimation of the number of smokers in the older age groups.[5]

Hyperlipidemia

There is some evidence to suggest a relationship between elevated triglyceride levels and the development of heart failure;[5] a high ratio of total cholesterol to high density lipoprotein (HDL) cholesterol is also associated with an increased incidence of heart failure.[40] The investigators in the Simvastatin Survival Study (4S) Group Trial found that patients in the simvastatin group had a significantly lower incidence (6·2%) of heart failure than those in the placebo group (8·5%).[46] Interestingly, a higher triglyceride concentration and a lower HDL concentration predicted the development of heart failure. These results further support the importance of lipid abnormalities as a factor responsible for the development of heart failure.

Diabetes mellitus

Diabetes mellitus is a well established risk factor for the development of coronary artery disease. Over the past 25 years, diabetes mellitus has been recognized as a factor responsible for the development of heart failure,[5,9,11,38,39] working through an independent mechanism rather than the simple acceleration of coronary atherosclerosis.[1] The presence of fibrosis in the hearts of patients with diabetes mellitus has been described and it is thought to be due to diabetic microangiopathy.[47] The prevalence of diabetes mellitus in heart failure patients has been reported to be approximately 22%.[48] The Randomized Evaluation of Strategies for Left Ventricular Dysfunction (RESOLVD) study in 663 CHF patients found a 27% prevalence of documented diabetes, whereas 23% ($n = 111$ patients) of non-diabetic patients had an elevated fasting glucose $\geq 6·1$ mmol/l, and 11% ($n = 53$ patients) of these had fasting glucose concentrations in the diabetic range (fasting glucose $\geq 7·0$ mmol/l).[49] Therefore, approximately 44% of these patients had either known diabetes mellitus or abnormal fasting glucose levels. This suggests that most studies have underestimated the importance of glucose abnormalities in heart failure. Diabetes mellitus is more common in women than in men with heart failure,[40,50] and women with diabetes mellitus have a greater risk of developing heart failure than do men with diabetes mellitus.[40] Following a myocardial infarction, patients with diabetes mellitus who develop heart failure have more severe symptoms than those without diabetes mellitus who develop heart failure.[51] For any given level of infarct size, patients with diabetes mellitus had a lower ejection fraction than those without diabetes mellitus (Yusuf *et al*, unpublished data). In the SOLVD trial in patients with asymptomatic LV dysfunction, diabetes mellitus is an independent predictor of the development of heart failure and mortality.[52] Furthermore, the patients with diabetes mellitus treated with enalapril had a greater mortality than those without diabetes mellitus treated

with enalapril, indicating that although ACE inhibitors benefit this subgroup of patients, diabetes mellitus still remains a significant predictor of outcome. However, in both cases patients on enalapril had lower rates of mortality than with placebo.

Therefore, these data indicate that abnormalities of glucose metabolism in CHF patients should be aggressively searched for and perhaps treated.

Microalbuminuria

In the Heart Outcomes Prevention Evaluation (HOPE) trial, microalbuminuria was found to be a predictor of heart failure and other cardiovascular events in patients with and without diabetes mellitus.[53] In this group at high risk of a cardiovascular event, microalbuminuria increased the adjusted relative risk of hospitalization for heart failure by 3·23-fold (95% CI 2·54–4·10).

Vital capacity

A low or a decrease in vital capacity over time has been found to be associated with an increased risk of developing heart failure.[43] The abnormality probably reflects the lungs, being congested with blood as a result of LV dysfunction. However, the relationship between vital capacity and the development of heart failure has not been a consistent finding in all studies.[5]

Heart rate

In hypertensive patients, resting heart rate was a predictor of the future development of heart failure.[54] The risk of heart failure increased with the heart rate in a continuous graded fashion, from an age-adjusted biennial rate of 14·6/1000 patients at heart rates less than 64 beats per minute (bpm) to a rate of 62·2/1000 patients at heart rates greater than 85 bpm. This may indicate asymptomatic LV dysfunction and subtle activation of the neuroendocrine system.

Obesity

Obesity has been reported to be an independent risk factor for the development of heart failure.[5,55] This finding would support efforts directed at dietary modification to promote weight loss and also help correct lipid abnormalities. A study by Schirmer *et al*[56] demonstrated that body mass index (BMI) was a very important variable for categorizing subjects as having LV hypertrophy: the odds of having LV hypertrophy increased in relation to the increase in BMI. These data further suggest that obesity may contribute to the development of heart failure.

Pathophysiologic abnormalities in asymptomatic LV dysfunction that predict the development of CHF

Neuroendocrine activation

Symptomatic heart failure is characterized by the activation of several neuroendocrine systems.[57–61] The well documented finding that ACE inhibitor therapy improves survival in patients with heart failure and reduces the rates of new heart failure in patients with asymptomatic LV dysfunction[21] further suggests that neurohormones play an important role in the pathogenesis of symptomatic heart failure.[17,62] A substudy of the SOLVD trial demonstrated that the median values for plasma norepinephrine, plasma atrial natriuretic factor (ANF), plasma arginine vasopressin (AVP) and plasma renin activity (PRA) were significantly higher in patients with asymptomatic LV dysfunction than in

age and gender matched normal control individuals, with symptomatic patients having the highest neurohumoral values (Figure 45.2).[63] Plasma norepinephrine levels appear to increase early in the development of LV dysfunction, whereas the increase in PRA seems to occur only when the patients are taking diuretics. The degree of LV dysfunction is one of the mechanisms for activation of neurohormones, as patients with an ejection fraction greater than 0·45 and pulmonary congestion on chest radiography were found to have only minimal neurohormonal activation and a modest increase in AVP and PRA.[64]

In the SOLVD Prevention trial, plasma norepinephrine level was the strongest predictor of the future development of heart failure.[65] This finding was independent of LV ejection fraction, NYHA class, age, sex, cause of heart failure, treatment assignment to placebo or enalapril, or prerandomization ANF or PRA levels. Plasma norepinephrine levels above the median of 393 pg/ml were associated with

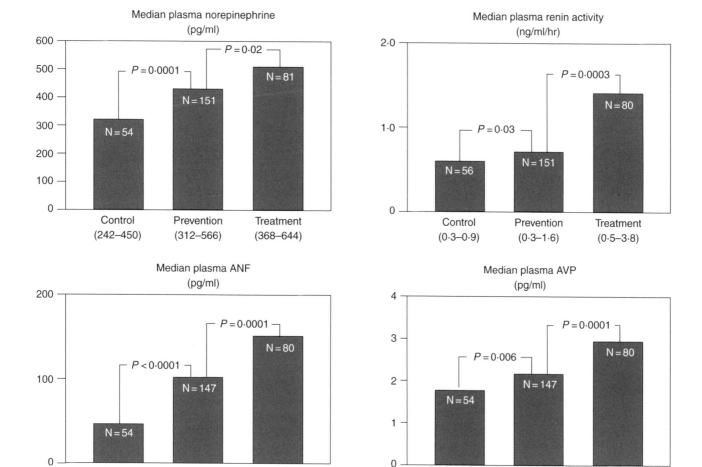

Figure 45.2 Comparison of norepinephrine, plasma renin activity, plasma atrial natriuretic factor (ANF) and plasma arginine vasopressin (AVP) in healthy control subjects, patients with asymptomatic left ventricular dysfunction and patients with symptomatic heart failure. (From Francis GS *et al*, *Circulation* 1990;**82**:1724–9, with permission.)

a relative risk of 2·59 (*P*= 0·002) for all-cause mortality, 2·55 (*P*= 0·005) for hospitalization for heart failure, 1·88 (*P*= 0·002) for the development of heart failure, 1·92 (*P*= 0·001) for ischemic events, and 2·59 (*P*= 0·005) for myocardial infarction (Figure 45.3). PRA and ANP were not as useful for predicting clinical outcome because although trends were observed for these hormones, they were not statistically significant. These data are very important because they suggest that modulating the release or effect of plasma norepinephrine early in patients with asymptomatic left ventricular dysfunction may improve prognosis and prevent heart failure and perhaps ischemic events.

A recent study examines the location of adrenergic activity in patients with early heart failure.[66] In this study a selective increase was found in cardiac adrenergic drive in patients with early heart failure. This preceded the augmented sympathetic outflow to the kidneys and skeletal muscle found in advanced heart failure. These data collectively indicate that activation of the sympathetic system in early heart failure is causally related to the syndrome and that drugs such as β blockers may be of value.

Recent data from the Australia–New Zealand Heart Failure Group has demonstrated that in patients with chronic ischemic LV dysfunction plasma N-terminal-brain natriuretic peptide (N-BNP) concentration is an independent predictor of mortality and heart failure events.[67] Other evidence suggests that natriuretic peptides may be of use to screen for and improve the ability to diagnose heart failure.[68–70]

Cardiac dilation and remodeling

The process of LV remodeling in the setting of a prior myocardial infarction leading to ventricular dilation has been well described.[71–76] Even several years after the initial cardiac insult, or remote from the precipitating cause of heart failure, this process continues progressively with continuing left ventricular dilation.[77–80] Among asymptomatic patients the rate of progression of ventricular dilation and systolic dysfunction is slower than in symptomatic patients.[77–80] It seems likely that asymptomatic and symptomatic patients represent a continuum of pathology, with the rate of progression of ventricular dilation accelerating

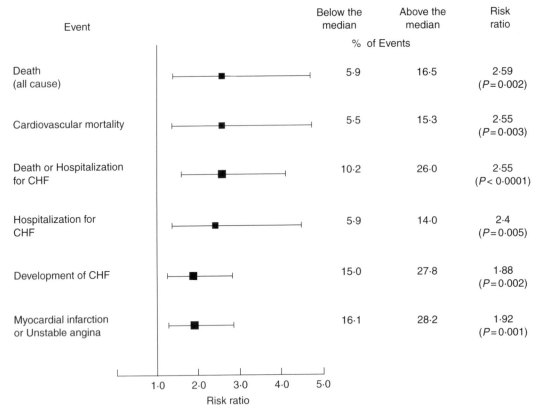

Figure 45.3 Effect of plasma norepinephrine level on all-cause mortality, cardiovascular mortality, development of heart failure, hospitalization for heart failure, and development of ischemic events. For each group, the increase in risk is shown as a percentage. Horizontal lines indicate the 95% CI. Size of each square is proportional to the number of events in that group. Vertical line corresponds to a finding of no effect. (From Bendict CR *et al*, *Circulation* 1996;**94**:690–7, with permission.)

at later stages. Although the exact stimuli affecting these changes in myocardial structure remain unknown, increased myocardial wall stress has been postulated to represent an initiating factor. Activation of the renin–angiotensin system appears to play an important role in the pathogenesis of ventricular remodeling by contributing to the increase in wall stress, and possibly by direct myocardial effects.[81–83]

The progression of LV dysfunction in asymptomatic patients can be insidious. When an initial insult causes the loss of large amounts of myocardium, the ejection fraction decreases and the end-diastolic volume increases (Figure 45.4). This increase in end-diastolic dimension is accompanied by relative thinning of the wall and an increase in wall stress.[84] As the compensatory remodeling process evolves the ventricle dilates further, but as hypertrophy develops, wall thickness increases and the ejection fraction may recover slightly. The degree of hypertrophy is never sufficient to normalize left ventricular wall stress. The results from SOLVD support this hypothesis, because in all patients studied the systolic and diastolic wall stresses were markedly augmented at baseline.[85] Neurohumoral systems are chronically activated in asymptomatic patients.[63] Because the mechanical and neurohumoral stimuli for hypertrophy continue to be activated, the remodeling process continues at a slow rate in asymptomatic patients with LV dysfunction. Furthermore, the ejection fraction may be maintained, probably because of new contractile units in

the LV walls. Ventricular function is stable for a while until the rate of ventricular dilation increases and ejection fraction further declines. This is supported by data from the SOLVD treatment trial.[78] Hypertrophy is unable to keep pace with LV dilation, wall thickness decreases and wall stress increases, rapidly resulting in a decrease in ejection fraction despite further LV dilation. Therefore, even when the asymptomatic patient with LV dysfunction appears stable, there are significant changes taking place in the heart which ultimately result in the progression of LV dysfunction to symptomatic heart failure.

Clinical factors predicting the development of symptomatic heart failure in asymptomatic LV dysfunction

The SOLVD prevention trial was the first large study to examine the clinical outcome in 4228 patients with asymptomatic LV dysfunction, of whom 2117 with EF ≤ 35% were randomized to the placebo group (2111 to ACE inhibitors) and were followed for an average of 37·4 months (range 14·6–62 months). Of these 2117 patients 70% had an EF between 26 and 35%, 26·1% had an EF between 16 and 25%, and 3·9% had an EF ≤ 15%. By NYHA functional classification 67% of the patients were in class I and 33% were in class II. None were receiving treatment for heart failure.

During the follow-up period for this population, there were 334 (15.8%) deaths, 640 (30·2%) developed congestive heart failure and 273 (12·9%) had a first hospitalization for heart failure. Using the Cox multivariate model we examined the prognostic usefulness of several clinical, echocardiographic and neurohormonal parameters in predicting the subsequent clinical outcome in these patients. In a subset of these 2117 patients the prognostic usefulness of plasma neurohormones – plasma norepinephrine (PNE), ANF, AVP and PRA – and echocardiographic parameters – end-diastolic volume (EDV) and end-systolic volume (ESV) – were also examined. Key findings are summarized below.

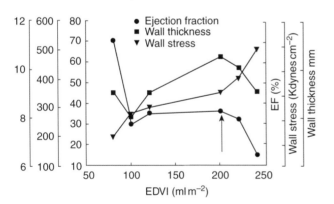

Figure 45.4 Hypothesis proposed to explain the changes in ejection fraction (EF), systolic wall stress, and wall thickness in relation to the progression of the myocardial insult. Under normal conditions, the EF is well above 50% and the wall stress is low. Immediately after the myocardial insult, EF and wall thickness decrease while wall stress increases. As the ventricle dilates, EF may recover slightly as a result of hypertrophy. The ventricle finally reaches a point that the rate and extent of dilation exceeds the capacity to hypertrophy, resulting in a rapid increase in wall stress (arrow). This would result in a decline in EF and a rapid deterioration of clinical status. (From Pouleur HG *et al*, *J Am Coll Cardiol* 1993;**22**(Suppl. A):43A–8A with permission.)

Age

Increasing age was a significant risk factor for mortality in patients with asymptomatic LV dysfunction. For every 10 year increase in age the risk ratio for mortality was 1·2 (95% CI 1·08–1·32; $P < 0·0014$), for hospitalization for CHF was 1·24 (95% CI 1·10–1·38; $P < 0·0005$) and for the development of CHF was 1·20 (95% CI 1·10–1·27; $P < 0·0001$).

Sex

Unlike age, sex was not a prognostic variable for developing clinical end points. For example, the mortality rate in males was 16·06%, whereas in females it was 13·5%, which was not significantly different. Similarly, hospitalization for CHF was 12·6% in males and 15·2% in females, and development of CHF was 28·9% in males and 30·4% in females, both of which were not significantly different. However, these results must be interpreted with caution because the SOLVD prevention trial consisted predominantly of males (~80%), which could have limited the ability to detect differences based on gender.

Ejection fraction

For a 5% lower EF, the risk ratio for mortality was 1·20 (95% CI 1·13–1·29; $P < 0.0001$), for hospitalization for CHF was 1·28 (95% CI 1·18–1·38; $P < 0.0001$), and for development of CHF was 1·20 (95% CI 1·13–1·26; $P < 0.0001$).

NYHA functional class

The NYHA functional class was not a risk factor for mortality but was a significant risk factor for risk of hospitalization for CHF (risk ratio 1·66; 95% CI 1·24–2·22; $P < 0.0007$) and the development of CHF symptoms (risk ratio 1·48; 95% CI 1·16–1·89; $P < 0.0016$).

Etiology of heart failure

Patients with an ischemic or non-ischemic etiology for asymptomatic LV dysfunction had similar outcomes with respect to mortality (15% v 13·2%), hospitalization for heart failure (11·5% v 13·9%) and development of heart failure (37% v 40·3%). Hypertension was not a significant contributor for the development of clinical events. In contrast, the presence or absence of diabetes mellitus was a major risk factor for mortality (risk ratio 1·89; 95% CI 1·27–2·24; $P = 0.0003$), hospitalization for heart failure (risk ratio 1·98; 95% CI 1·46–2·69; $P = 0.0001$) and for the development of heart failure (risk ratio 2·06; 95% CI 1·58–2·59; $P < 0.0001$). A current (but not past) history of smoking increased the risk of death (risk ratio 1·21; 95% CI 1·10–1·32; $P < 0.001$) but had only a weak and non-significant impact on the development of heart failure.

Cardiothoracic ratio

Increased cardiothoracic ratio (>0·50) was a univariate risk factor for the development of clinical end points, but in the multivariate model it failed to reach statistical significance, most probably owing to the impact of ejection fraction in this model.

Neurohormonal predictors

Previous studies in patients with symptomatic LV dysfunction have indicated that several neurohormones, including PNE,

PRA and ANF, are increased, and both PNE and ANF may be useful for predicting clinical outcomes, including mortality, in these patients. However, it is important to note that these studies have not determined whether the neurohormonal activation present is a cause or consequence of heart failure in these patients. In contrast, examination of the prognostic usefulness of neurohormones in patients with asymptomatic LV dysfunction may help us to determine whether the neurohormonal system could possibly play a role in the progression of the heart failure syndrome. In a subset of 514 patients with asymptomatic LV dysfunction from the SOLVD prevention trial, PNE, but not PRA, ANF or AVP, was found to be significantly associated with heart failure events and predicted the development of subsequent ischemic events (see Figure 45.3).[65] It is important to note that development of an interim ischemic event has previously been shown to worsen clinical outcome in this population.[60] Unlike PNE, the other neurohormones failed to predict the occurrence of subsequent clinical events in patients with asymptomatic LV dysfunction, which suggests that adrenergic activation in patients with LV dysfunction may be an early event.

Echocardiographic predictors

Over 40 years ago Linzbach[86] described structural dilation of the LV as the morphological basis for the development of congestive heart failure. More recent studies on ventricular remodeling support this concept.

Greenberg et al[79] have examined the changes in echocardiographic parameters in patients with LV dysfunction in a subset of the SOLVD trial. In the placebo treated group there was a significant increase in the end-diastolic volume from baseline after 4 months (200 ± 42 ml v 208 ± 43 ml; $P = 0.025$) and after 1 year of follow up (200 ± 42 ml v 210 ± 46 ml; $P = 0.003$). The end-systolic volume increased significantly from baseline after 4 months (148 ± 38 ml v 155 ± 43 ml, $P = 0.028$) and 1 year of follow-up (148 ± 38 ml v 156 ± 42 ml, $P = 0.014$). Vasan et al[87] reported from the Framingham study database that in asymptomatic individuals increases in LV internal dimension (both end-systolic and end-diastolic volumes) were important predictors for subsequent development of congestive heart failure.

In summary, there are a number of factors that increase the risk of developing LV dysfunction, whereas the variables of LV size, ejection fraction, increased PNE, age, and the etiology of LV dysfunction (diabetes mellitus), are important independent risk factors for the development of clinical heart failure events (Box 45.1).

Prevention of symptomatic heart failure

Although a number of clinical trials have documented that pharmacologic therapy reduces mortality in patients with

Box 45.1 Factors related to the development and prognosis of asymptomatic left ventricular dysfunction

- Ischemic heart disease
- Hypertension
- Left ventricular hypertrophy
- Smoking
- Hyperlipidemia
- Diabetes mellitus
- Microalbuminuria
- Low or decreased vital capacity over time
- Elevated resting heart rate
- Obesity
- Age
- Ejection fraction
- Plasma norepinephrine
- Cardiac dilatation

symptomatic heart failure, the prognosis of this condition remains poor.[6,17,19,35,62,88–90] These results suggest that the greatest opportunity for reducing the incidence and excess mortality of heart failure is through preventive strategies.

Treatment of hypertension

Grade A1a The development of heart failure in the setting of hypertension could be due to a number of reasons, including activation of the renin–angiotensin–aldosterone system, acute or chronic subendocardial ischemia, inappropriately high wall stress, and alterations in the peripheral circulation.[91] A number of studies have demonstrated that the treatment of hypertension substantially reduces the risk for the development of heart failure.[11,92–96] A meta-analysis by Psaty et al[97] demonstrated that CHF was effectively prevented with low-dose diuretic therapy (relative risk 0·58; 95% CI 0·44–0·76), high-dose diuretic therapy (relative risk 0·17; 95% CI 0·07–0·41), and β-blocker therapy (relative risk 0·58; 95% CI 0·40–0·84). More recently the Blood Pressure Lowering Treatment Trialists Collaboration[98] performed a prespecified overview of 15 trials comparing active treatment regimens with placebo, trials comparing more intensive versus less intensive blood pressure lowering strategies, and trials comparing treatment regimens based on different drug classes. The pooled data from these studies demonstrated that ACE inhibitors, calcium antagonists and other blood pressure lowering drugs significantly reduced cardiovascular death and major cardiovascular events. There was a trend to a reduced incidence of heart failure with ACE inhibitor therapy (RR 0·84, 95% CI 0·68–1·04), calcium antagonists (RR 0·72, 95% CI 0·48–1·07), and when more intensive blood pressure strategies were compared to less intensive strategies (RR 0·78, 95% CI 0·53–1·15). Although there was no clear evidence of a reduction in the risk of heart failure as defined, the 95% CI

did not exclude possible benefits of moderate magnitude among the assigned therapies. The small number of heart failure events would have limited the ability to detect any true benefits of these therapies. In the case of ACE inhibitors several other randomized trials have provided clear evidence that heart failure is prevented in other high-risk situations,[37] and in a large trial of high-risk patients there was a benefit of ACE inhibitors when a wider definition was used for heart failure.[36] The findings that calcium antagonists may not be as effective to prevent heart failure as other antihypertensive agents (such as diuretics, β blockers, ACE inhibitors or clonidine) despite similar blood pressure control was reported in a meta-analysis by Pahor et al[99] of nine eligible trials comprising 27 743 participants, in which those individuals assigned to calcium antagonists had a significantly higher risk of developing heart failure (RR 1·25, 95% CI 1·07–1·46, P 0·005) than those assigned to other drug therapy. Interestingly, in this overview analysis calcium antagonists were found to be potentially less effective than a diuretic or β blocker (RR 1·12, 95% CI 0·95–1·33), and ACE inhibitors were found to be potentially more effective than a calcium antagonist (RR 0·82, 95% CI 0·67–1·00) for preventing heart failure. Therefore, aggressive management of hypertension will help reduce the risk of developing heart failure. However, the data would suggest that hypertensive patients should be treated either alone or in combination with diuretic, β blocker or ACE inhibitor to most effectively reduce the risk of developing heart failure.

Lipid lowering therapy to prevent congestive heart failure

Grade A1d It has been clearly demonstrated that lipid lowering therapy significantly reduces mortality in patients with coronary artery disease.[100] A recent report from the 4S Study Group suggests that lipid lowering treatment with simvastatin ($n = 2223$) compared to placebo ($n = 2221$) prevents the onset of heart failure.[46] In this study, 189 patients (8·5%) in the placebo group were diagnosed with CHF during follow up, compared to 147 (6·2%) in the simvastatin group, resulting in a 27% ($P < 0.003$) reduction in the incidence of CHF for the simvastatin group. Further studies are required to determine whether this reduction is related to the effect of lipid lowering on coronary artery disease, or is exerted through another independent mechanism.

Prevention of myocardial ischemia

Grade A1a Treatment strategies should also be directed at preventing ischemia in patients with heart failure. In heart failure patients it has been demonstrated that the occurrence of a new myocardial infarction increases the risk of subsequent death by up to eight times, and that one third of all deaths are preceded by a major ischemic event.[101] Similar data have been reported by Rutherford *et al*[102] from the SAVE trial. These data emphasize that reductions in ischemic events should be an integral part of the management of patients with LV dysfunction. Although not formally examined in patients with asymptomatic LV dysfunction, β blockers may be very useful to reduce the development of symptomatic heart failure. β Blockers are commonly used to treat patients with findings of myocardial ischemia. Studies of β-blocker therapy in patients with symptomatic heart failure have demonstrated improvements in LV ejection fraction and decreases in cardiac dilatation.[103–105] Studies in patients following myocardial infarction have demonstrated that β blockers reduce mortality and morbidity when initiated relatively earlier following an acute myocardial infarction.[106,107] Furthermore, the relative benefit on mortality after a myocardial infarction is similar in the presence or absence of heart failure, although the absolute benefit may be greater in the former because of the higher event rate.[107] Retrospective analyses of the SAVE database in postmyocardial infarction patients[108] and the SOLVD trial involving patients mainly from the prevention trial (Exner *et al* 1999) demonstrated that the beneficial effects of β-blocker therapy were additional to those of ACE inhibitor therapy. The recently published Carvedilol Post-Infarct Survival Control in LV Dysfunction (CAPRICORN) study has further prospectively demonstrated that the β blocker carvedilol used in patients following myocardial infarction complicated by LV dysfunction reduces the frequency of all-cause and cardiovascular mortality, and recurrent non-fatal myocardial infarctions.[109] These beneficial effects were additional to those of evidenced-based treatments for acute myocardial infarction, including ACE inhibitors. In trials of patients with symptomatic heart failure β blockers have been shown to reduce mortality and reduce the incidence of repeat episodes of heart failure or hospitalizations for heart failure.[90] Based on these data it may be advisable to use β-blocker therapy in patients found to have asymptomatic LV dysfunction, with the expectation that progression to symptomatic LV dysfunction should be significantly reduced. Prospective randomized trials are required to assess whether β-blocker therapy would be beneficial to reduce the risk of developing symptomatic heart failure in patients with asymptomatic LV dysfunction or those with other markers of high cardiovascular risk.

ACE inhibitors in asymptomatic LV dysfunction or other markers of high risk

Grade A1a There have been a number of trials demonstrating the effects of ACE inhibitors to reduce mortality and morbidity in patients with heart failure.[37,110] Therapy with ACE inhibitors in patients with asymptomatic LV dysfunction[21] has been shown to significantly reduce the total

number of deaths or cases of CHF (risk reduction 29%; 95% CI 21–36), and also to reduce the total number of deaths or hospitalizations for CHF (risk reduction 20%; 95% CI 9–30). The recently published HOPE data further define which patients would benefit from ACE inhibitor therapy.[36] In patients at high risk for a cardiovascular event who did not have LV dysfunction or heart failure on admission to the study, ramipril decreased the incidence of heart failure (ramipril 417 *v* placebo 535; RR 0·77, 95% CI 0·67–0·87; *P* < 0·001). Therefore, an ACE inhibitor should be routinely administered to any patient with LV dysfunction (ejection fraction < 0·40) and to those patients meeting the HOPE study criteria who do not have a contraindication to this form of therapy.

Conclusions

The population incidence and prevalence of CHF are relatively high. CHF is associated with significant mortality, morbidity and poor quality of life for the patient. This is a progressive disorder, and at present there are relatively few therapies that slow or prevent its progression. Asymptomatic LV dysfunction occurs in 1–5% of the population, depending on the prevalence of other cardiovascular risk factors. Although routine screening of the general population cannot be justified, screening of high-risk individuals may be of value. Risk factors for the development of CHF have been identified, and these could be used to determine those who are at greatest risk for the development of LV dysfunction and ultimately symptomatic CHF.

Suggested approach to identify and treat patients with asymptomatic left ventricular dysfunction

1. Determine those at greatest risk of developing left ventricular dysfunction:
   - Hypertension
   - Left ventricular hypertrophy
   - Diabetes mellitus and/or impaired glucose tolerance
   - Hyperlipidemia (hypertriglyceridemia and low HDL)
   - Previous extensive myocardial infarction
   - Age
   - Smoking
   - Obesity
2. Assess cardiac function using radionuclide ventriculography or quantitative echocardiography.
3. If ejection fraction < 40% then start ACE inhibitors in all tolerant patients. Modify other risk factors (for example, diabetes, hypertension, dyslipidemia) and treat symptoms of myocardial ischemia.

4. If ejection fraction ≥ 40% then counsel patients, modify risk factors (for example, diabetes, hypertension etc.), treat symptoms of myocardial ischemia, and treat those meeting the HOPE study criteria with an ACE inhibitor.

These individuals should receive appropriate counseling, lifestyle advice and therapy to alter risk factors for cardiovascular disease and CHF. The fact that the prognosis from CHF remains so poor makes it clear that the greatest opportunity to reduce its incidence and the attendant high mortality is through strategies directed towards preventing its development.

References

1. Smith WM. Epidemiology of congestive heart failure. *Am J Cardiol* 1985;**55**:3A–8A.
2. Gibson TC, White KL, Klainer LM. The prevalence of congestive heart failure in two rural communities. *J Chronic Dis* 1966;**19**:141–52.
3. Parameshwar J, Shackell MM, Richardson A, Poole-Wilson PA, Sutton GC. Prevalence of heart failure in three general practices in north west London. *Br J Gen Pract* 1992; **42**:287–9.
4. Schocken DD, Arrieta MI, Leaverton PE, Ross EA. Prevalence and mortality rate of congestive heart failure in the United States. *J Am Coll Cardiol* 1992;**20**:301–6.
5. Eriksson H, Svärdsudd K, Larsson B *et al.* Risk factors for heart failure in the general population: the study of men born in 1913. *Eur Heart J* 1989;**10**:647–56.
6. Rodeheffer RJ, Jacobsen SJ, Gersh BJ *et al.* The incidence and prevalence of congestive heart failure in Rochester, Minnesota. *Mayo Clin Proc* 1993;**68**:1143–50.
7. Mosterd A, Cost B, Hoes AW *et al.* The prognosis of heart failure in the general population: The Rotterdam Study. *Eur Heart J* 2001;**22**:1318–27.
8. Mosterd A, Hoes AW, Bruijne de MC *et al.* Prevalence of heart failure and left ventricular dysfunction in the general population. The Rotterdam Study. *Eur Heart J* 1999; **20**:447–55.
9. McKee PA, Castelli WP, McNamara PM, Kannel WB. The natural history of congestive heart failure: the Framingham Study. *N Engl J Med* 1971;**285**:1441–6.
10. Remes J, Reunanen A, Aromaa A, Pyörälä K. Incidence of heart failure in eastern Finland: a population-based surveillance study. *Eur Heart J* 1992;**13**:588–93.
11. Yusuf S, Thom T, Abbott RD. Changes in hypertension treatment and in congestive heart failure mortality in the United States. *Hypertension* 1989;**13**(Suppl. I):I-74–9.
12. Cowie MR, Wood DA, Coats AJS *et al.* Incidence and aetiology of heart failure. *Eur Heart J* 1999;**20**:421–8.
13. Yamani M, Massie BM. Congestive heart failure: insights from epidemiology, implications for treatment. *Mayo Clin Proc* 1993;**68**:1214–18.
14. Croft JB, Giles WH, Pollard RA *et al.* Heart failure survival among older adults in the United States: a poor prognosis for an emerging epidemic in the medicare population. *Arch Intern Med* 1999;**159**:505–10.
15. Senni M, Tribouilloy CM, Rodeheffer RJ *et al.* Congestive heart failure in the community: trends in incidence and survival in a 10-year period. *Arch Intern Med* 1999; **159**: 29–34.
16. Cowie MR, Wood DA, Coats AJS *et al.* Survival of patients with a new diagnosis of heart failure: a population based study. *Heart* 2000;**83**:505–10.
17. The SOLVD Investigators. Effect of enalapril on survival in patients with reduced left ventricular ejection fractions and congestive heart failure. *N Engl J Med* 1991;**325**:293–302.
18. CIBIS-II Investigators and Committees. The cardiac insufficiency bisoprolol study II (CIBIS-II): a randomized trial. *Lancet* 1999;**353**:9–13.
19. Ho KKL, Anderson KM, Kannel WB, Grossman W, Levy D. Survival after the onset of congestive heart failure in Framingham Heart Study subjects. *Circulation* 1993; **88**:107–15.
20. Cowie MR, Mosterd A, Wood DA *et al.* The epidemiology of heart failure. *Eur Heart J* 1997;**18**:208–25.
21. The SOLVD Investigators. Effect of enalapril on mortality and the development of heart failure in asymptomatic patients with reduced left ventricular ejection fractions. *N Engl J Med* 1992;**327**:685–91.
22. McDonagh TA, Morrison CE, Lawrence A *et al.* Symptomatic and asymptomatic left-ventricular systolic dysfunction in an urban population. *Lancet* 1997;**350**:829–33.
23. Morgan S, Smith H, Simpson I *et al.* Prevalence and clinical characteristics of left ventricular dysfunction among elderly patients in general practice setting: cross sectional survey. *BMJ* 1999;**318**:368–72.
24. Petrie M, McMurray J. Changes in notions about heart failure. *Lancet* 2001;**358**:432–4.
25. Devereux RR, Roman MJ, Paranicas M *et al.* A population-based assessment of left ventricular systolic dysfunction in middle-aged and older adults: the Strong Heart Study. *Am Heart J* 2001;**141**:439–46.
26. Gardin JM, Siscovick D, Anton-Culver H *et al.* Sex, age, and disease affect echocardiographic left ventricular mass and systolic function in the free-living elderly. The Cardiovascular Health Study. *Circulation* 1995;**91**:1739–48.
27. Vasan RS, Benjamin EJ, Levy D. Prevalence, clinical features, and prognosis of diastolic heart failure: an epidemiologic perspective. *J Am Coll Cardiol* 1995;**26**:1565–74.
28. McAlister FA, Teo KK, Taher M *et al.* Insights into the contemporary epidemiology and outpatient management of congestive heart failure. *Am Heart J* 1999;**138**:87–94.
29. Vasan RS, Larson MG, Benjamin EJ *et al.* Congestive heart failure in subjects with normal versus reduced left ventricular ejection fraction: prevalence and mortality in a population-based cohort. *J Am Coll Cardiol* 1999;**33**:1948–55.
30. Tsutsui H, Tsuchihashi M, Takeshita A. Mortality and readmission of hospitalized patients with congestive heart failure and preserved versus depressed systolic function. *Am J Cardiol* 2001;**88**:530–3.
31. Ritzman DW, Gardin JM, Gottdiener JS *et al.* Importance of heart failure with preserved systolic function in patients ≤ 65 years of age. *Am J Cardiol* 2001;**87**:413–9.
32. Dauterman KW, Go AS, Rowell R *et al.* Congestive heart failure with preserved systolic function in a statewide sample of community hospitals. *J Cardiac Failure* 2001;**7**:221–8.

33. McDermott MM, Feinglass J, Lee PI *et al.* Systolic function, readmission rates, and survival among consecutively hospitalized patients with congestive heart failure. *Am Heart J* 1997; **134**:728–36.

34. Senni M, Tribouilloy CM, Rodeheffer RJ, Jacobsen SJ, Evans JM, Bailey KR, Redfield MM. Congestive heart failure in the community. Trends in medicine and survival in a 10 year period. *Arch Intern Med* 1999; **159**:29–34.

35. Pfeffer MA, Braunwald E, Moyé LA *et al.* Effect of captopril on mortality and morbidity in patients with left ventricular dysfunction after myocardial infarction: results of the Survival and Ventricular Enlargement trial. *N Engl J Med* 1992; **327**:669–77.

36. The Heart Outcomes Prevention Evaluation (HOPE) Study Investigators. Effects of an angiotensin-converting-enzyme inhibitor, ramipril, on cardiovascular events in high-risk patients. *N Engl J Med* 2000; **342**:145–53.

37. Flather MD, Yusuf S, Kober L *et al.* for the ACE-Inhibitor Myocardial Infarction Collaborative Group. Long-term ACE-inhibitor therapy in patients with heart failure or left-ventricular dysfunction: a systematic overview of data from individual patients. *Lancet* 2000; **355**:1575–81.

38. Kannel WB, Castelli WP, McNamara PM, McKee PA, Feinleib M. Role of blood pressure in the development of congestive heart failure: the Framingham Study. *N Engl J Med* 1972; **287**:781–7.

39. Levy D, Larson MG, Ramachandran S *et al.* The progression from hypertension to congestive heart failure. *JAMA* 1996; **275**:1557–62.

40. Ho KKL, Pinsky JL, Kannel WB, Levy D. The epidemiology of heart failure: the Framingham Study. *J Am Coll Cardiol* 1993; **22**(Suppl. A):6A–13A.

41. PROGRESS Collaborative Group. Randomized trial of a perindopril-based blood-pressure-lowering regimen among 6105 individuals with previous stroke or transient ischaemic attack. *Lancet* 2001; **358**:1033–41.

42. Clarke R, Shipley M, Lewington S *et al.* Underestimation of risk associations due to regression dilution in long-term follow-up of prospective studies. *Am J Epidemiol* 1999; **150**:341–53.

43. Kannel WB. Epidemiological aspects of heart failure. *Cardiol Clin* 1989; **7**:1–9.

44. Zabalgoitia M, Berning J, Koren MJ *et al.* for the LIFE Study Investigators. Impact of coronary artery disease on left ventricular systolic function and geometry in hypertensive patients with left ventricular hypertrophy (The LIFE Study). *Am J Cardiol* 2001; **88**:646–50.

45. Matthew J, Sleight P, Lonn E *et al.* for the Heart Outcomes Prevention Evaluation (HOPE) Investigators. Reduction of cardiovascular risk by regression of electrocardiographic markers of left ventricular hypertrophy by the angiotensin-converting enzyme inhibitor ramipril. *Circulation* 2001; **104**:1615–21.

46. Kjekshus J, Pedersen TR, Olsson AG, Faergeman O, Pyörälä K on behalf of the 4S Study Group. The effects of simvastatin on the incidence of heart failure in patients with coronary heart disease. *J Cardiac Failure* 1997; **3**:249–54.

47. van Hoeven KH, Factor SM. A comparison of the pathological spectrum of hypertensive, diabetic, and hypertensive-diabetic heart disease. *Circulation* 1990; **82**:848–55.

48. Bangdiwala SI, Weiner DH, Bourassa MG *et al.* for the SOLVD Investigators. Studies of left ventricular dysfunction (SOLVD) registry: rationale, design, methods and description of baseline characteristics. *Am J Cardiol* 1992; **70**:347–53.

49. Suskin N, McKelvie RS, Burns RJ *et al.* Glucose and insulin abnormalities relate to functional capacity in patients with congestive heart failure. *Eur Heart J* 2000; **21**:1368–75.

50. Johnstone D, Limacher M, Rousseau M *et al.* for the SOLVD Investigators. Clinical characteristics of patients in studies of left ventricular dysfunction (SOLVD). *Am J Cardiol* 1992; **70**:894–900.

51. Herlitz J, Malmberg K, Karlson BW, Rydén L, Hjalmarson Å. Mortality and morbidity during a five-year follow-up of diabetics with myocardial infarction. *Acta Med Scand* 1988; **224**:31–8.

52. Shindler DM, Kostis JB, Yusuf S *et al.* for the SOLVD Investigators. Diabetes mellitus, a predictor of morbidity and mortality in the Studies of Left Ventricular Dysfunction (SOLVD) Trials and Registry. *Am J Cardiol* 1996; **77**:1017–20.

53. Gerstein H, Mann JFE, Yi Q *et al.* for the HOPE Study Investigators. Albuminuria and risk of cardiovascular events, death, and heart failure in diabetic and non-diabetic individuals. *JAMA* 2001; **286**:421–6.

54. Kannel WB. Epidemiology of heart failure in the United States. In: Poole-Wilson PA, Colucci WS, Massie BM, Chatterjee K, Coats AJS, eds. *Heart failure. Scientific principles and clinical practice.* New York: Churchill Livingstone, 1997.

55. Sorlie P, Gordon T, Kannel WB. Body build and mortality: the Framingham Study. *JAMA* 1980; **243**:1828–31.

56. Schirmer H, Lunde P. Rasmussen K. Prevalence of left ventricular hypertrophy in a general population. The Tromsø Study. *Eur Heart J* 1999; **20**:429–38.

57. Francis GS, Goldsmith SR, Levine TB, Olivari MT, Cohn JN. The neurohumoral axis in congestive heart failure. *Ann Intern Med* 1984; **101**:370–7.

58. Cohn JN, Levine TB, Olivari MT *et al.* Plasma norepinephrine as a guide to prognosis in patients with chronic congestive heart failure. *N Engl J Med* 1984; **311**:819–23.

59. Gottlieb SS, Kukin ML, Ahern D, Packer M. Prognostic importance of atrial natriuretic peptide in patients with chronic heart failure. *J Am Coll Cardiol* 1989; **13**:1534–9.

60. Levine TB, Francis GS, Goldsmith SR, Simon A, Cohn JN. Activity of the sympathetic nervous system and renin–angiotensin system assessed by plasma hormone levels and their relationship to hemodynamic abnormalities. *Am J Cardiol* 1982; **49**:1659–66.

61. Curtiss C, Cohn JN, Vrobel T, Franciosa JA. Role of renin–angiotensin system in systemic vasoconstriction of chronic congestive heart failure. *Circulation* 1978; **58**:763–70.

62. The CONSENSUS Trial Study Group. Effect of enalapril on mortality in severe congestive heart failure. *N Engl J Med* 1987; **316**:1429–35.

63. Francis GS, Benedict C, Johnstone DE *et al.* for the SOLVD Investigators. Comparison of neuroendocrine activation in patients with left ventricular dysfunction with and without congestive heart failure. A substudy of the Studies of Left Ventricular Dysfunction (SOLVD). *Circulation* 1990; **82**:1724–9.

64. Benedict CR, Weiner DH, Johnstone DE *et al.* for the SOLVD Investigators. Comparative neurohormonal responses in patients with preserved and impaired left ventricular ejection fraction: results of the Studies of Left Ventricular Dysfunction (SOLVD) Registry. *J Am Coll Cardiol* 1993;**22**(Suppl. A): 146A–53A.

65. Benedict CR, Shelton B, Johnstone DE *et al.* for the SOLVD Investigators. Prognostic significance of plasma norepinephrine in patients with asymptomatic left ventricular dysfunction. *Circulation* 1996;**94**:690–7.

66. Rundqvist R, Elam M, Bergmann-Sverrisdottir Y, Eisenhofer G, Friberg P. Increased cardiac adrenergic drive precedes generalized sympathetic activation in human heart failure. *Circulation* 1997;**95**:169–75.

67. Richards AM, Doughty R, Nicholls MG *et al.* for the Australia–New Zealand Heart Failure Group. Plasma N-terminal pro-brain natriuretic peptide and adrenomedullin: prognostic utility and prediction of benefit from carvedilol in chronic ischemic left ventricular dysfunction. Australia–New Zealand Heart Failure Group. *J Am Coll Cardiol* 2001; **37**: 1781–7.

68. Smith JA, Bruusgaard D, Bodd E, Hall C. Relations between medical history, clinical findings and plasma N-terminal proatrial natriuretic peptide in patients in primary health care. *Eur J Heart Failure* 2001;**3**:307–13.

69. Kelly R, Struthers AD. Are natriuretic peptides clinically useful as markers of heart failure? *Ann Clin Biochem* 2001;**38**:94–102.

70. Sagnella GA. Measurement and importance of plasma brain natriuretic peptide and related peptides. *Ann Clin Biochem* 2001;**38**:83–93.

71. Eaton LW, Weiss JL, Bulkley RH, Garrison JB, Weisfeldt ML. Regional cardiac dilatation after acute myocardial infarction: recognition by two-dimensional echocardiography. *N Engl J Med* 1979;**300**:57–62.

72. Fletcher PJ, Pfeffer JM, Pfeffer MA, Braunwald E. Left ventricular diastolic pressure–volume relations in rats with healed myocardial infarctions: effects on systolic function. *Circ Res* 1981;**49**:618–26.

73. Erlebacher JA, Weiss JL, Easton LW, Kallman C, Weisfeldt ML, Bulkley BH. Late effects of acute infarct dilatation on heart size: a two dimensional echocardiographic study. *Am J Cardiol* 1982;**49**:1120–6.

74. Roberts CS, MacLean D, Maroko P, Kloner RA. Early and late remodelling of the left ventricle after acute myocardial infarction. *Am J Cardiol* 1984;**54**:407–10.

75. McKay RG, Pfeffer MA, Pasternak RC *et al.* Left ventricular remodelling after myocardial infarction. A corollary to infarction expansion. *Circulation* 1986;**74**:693–702.

76. Sharpe N, Murphy J, Smith H, Hannan S. Treatment of patients with symptomless left ventricular dysfunction after myocardial infarction. *Lancet* 1988;**i**:255–9.

77. Konstam MA, Kronenberg MW, Rousseau MF *et al.* for the SOLVD Investigators. Effects of the angiotensin converting enzyme inhibitor enalapril on the long-term progression of left ventricular dilatation in patients with asymptomatic systolic dysfunction. *Circulation* 1993;**88**:2277–83.

78. Konstam MA, Rousseau MF, Kronenberg MW *et al.* for the SOLVD Investigators. Effects of the angiotensin converting enzyme inhibitor enalapril on the long-term progression of left ventricular dysfunction in patients with heart failure. *Circulation* 1992;**86**:431–8.

79. Greenberg B, Quiñones MA, Koilpillai C *et al.* for the SOLVD Investigators. Effects of long-term enalapril therapy on cardiac structure and function in patients with left ventricular dysfunction. Results of the SOLVD echocardiography substudy. *Circulation* 1995;**91**:2573–81.

80. Koilpillai C, Quiñones MA, Greenberg B *et al.* for the SOLVD Investigators. Relation of ventricular size and function to heart failure status and ventricular dysrhythmia in patients with severe left ventricular dysfunction. *Am J Cardiol* 1996; **77**:606–11.

81. Litwin SE, Litwin CM, Raya TE, Warner AL, Goldman S. Contractility and stiffness of non-infarcted myocardium after coronary ligation in rats: effects of chronic angiotensin converting enzyme inhibition. *Circulation* 1991;**83**:1028–37.

82. Pfeffer JM, Pfeffer MA, Braunwald E. Influence of chronic captopril therapy on the infarcted left ventricle of the rat. *Circ Res* 1985;**57**:84–95.

83. Jugdutt BI, Schwarz-Michorowski BL, Khan M. Effect of long-term captopril therapy on left ventricular remodelling and function during healing of canine myocardial infarction. *J Am Coll Cardiol* 1992;**19**:713–21.

84. Pouleur HG, Konstam MA, Udelson JE, Rousseau MF for the SOLVD Investigators. Changes in ventricular volume, wall thickness and wall stress during progression of left ventricular dysfunction. *J Am Coll Cardiol* 1993;**22**(Suppl. A):43A–8A.

85. Pouleur H, Rousseau MF, van Eyll C *et al.* for the SOLVD Investigators. Cardiac mechanics during development of heart failure. *Circulation* 1993;**87**(Suppl. IV):IV-14–20.

86. Linzbach AJ. Heart failure from the point of view of quantitative anatomy. *Am J Cardiol* 1960;**5**:370–82.

87. Vasan RS, Larson MG, Benjamin EJ, Evans JC, Levy D. Left ventricular dilation and the risk of congestive heart failure in people without myocardial infarction. *N Engl J Med* 1997; **336**:1350–5.

88. Cohn JN, Archibald DG, Ziesche S *et al.* Effect of vasodilator therapy on mortality in chronic congestive heart failure: results of a Veterans Administration Cooperative Study. *N Engl J Med* 1986;**314**:1547–52.

89. Cohn JN, Johnson G, Ziesche S *et al.* A comparison of enalapril with hydralazine-isosorbide dinitrate in the treatment of chronic congestive heart failure. *N Engl J Med* 1991; **325**:303–10.

90. Brophy JM, Joseph L, Rouleau JL. β-Blockers in congestive heart failure. A Bayesian meta-analysis. *Ann Intern Med* 2001;**134**:550–60.

91. Litwin SE, Grossman W. Mechanisms leading to the development of heart failure in pressure-overload hypertrophy. *Heart Failure* 1992;April/May:48–54.

92. Veterans Administration Cooperative Study Group on Antihypertensive Agents. Effects of treatment on mortality in hypertension: results in patients with diastolic blood pressures averaging 115 through 129 mmHg. *JAMA* 1967; **202**: 1028–34.

93. Veterans Administration Cooperative Study Group on Antihypertensive Agents. Effects of treatment on morbidity in hypertension, II: results in patients with diastolic blood

pressure averaging 90 through 114 mmHg. *JAMA* 1970; **213**:1143–51.

94. Furberg CD, Yusuf S. Effect of drug therapy on survival in chronic heart failure. *Adv Cardiol* 1986;**34**:124–30.

95. The Systolic Hypertension in the Elderly Research Group. Prevention of stroke by antihypertensive drug treatment in older persons with isolated systolic hypertension: final results of the Systolic Hypertension in the Elderly Program (SHEP). *JAMA* 1991;**265**:3255–64.

96. Cutler JA, Psaty BM, MacMahon S, Furberg CD. Public health issues in hypertension control: what has been learned from clinical trials. In: Laragh JH, Brenner BH, eds. *Hypertension: Pathophysiology, diagnosis and management.* New York: Raven Press, 1995.

97. Psaty BM, Smith NL, Siscovick DS *et al.* Health outcomes associated with antihypertensive therapies used as first-line agents. A systematic review and meta-analysis. *JAMA* 1997; **277**:739–45.

98. Blood Pressure Lowering Treatment Trialists Collaboration. Effects of ACE-inhibitors, calcium antagonists, and other blood-pressure-lowering drugs: results of prospectively designed overviews of randomized trials. *Lancet* 2000;**355**:1955–64.

99. Pahor M, Psaty BM, Alderman MH *et al.* Health outcomes associated with calcium antagonists compared with other first-line antihypertensive therapies: a meta-analysis of randomized controlled trials. *Lancet* 2000;**356**:1949–54.

100. Scandinavian Simvastatin Survival Study Group. Randomized trial of cholesterol lowering in 4444 patients with coronary heart disease: the Scandinavian Simvastatin Survival Study (4S). *Lancet* 1994;**344**:1383–9.

101. Yusuf S, Pepine CJ, Garces C *et al.* Effect of enalapril on myocardial infarction and unstable angina in patients with low ejection fractions. *Lancet* 1992;**340**:1173–8.

102. Rutherford JD, Pfeffer MA, Moyé LA *et al.* Effects of captopril on ischemic events after myocardial infarction. *Circulation* 1994;**90**:1731–8.

103. The RESOLVD Investigators. Effects of metoprolol CR in patients with ischemic and dilated cardiomyopathy. The Randomized Evaluation of Strategies for Left Ventricular Dysfunction Pilot Study. *Circulation* 2000;**101**:378–84.

104. Australia–New Zealand Heart Failure Research Collaborative Group. Effects of carvedilol, a vasodilator–β blocker, in patients with congestive heart failure due to ischemic heart disease. *Circulation* 1995;**92**:212–18.

105. Kukin ML, Kalman J, Charney RH *et al.* Prospective, randomized comparison of effect on long-term treatment with metoprolol or carvedilol on symptoms, exercise, ejection fraction, and oxidative stress in heart failure. *Circulation* 1999;**99**:2645–51.

106. Held P. Effects of beta-blockers on ventricular dysfunction after myocardial infarction. Tolerability and survival effects. *Am J Cardiol* 1993;**71**:39C.

107. Houghton T, Freemantle N, Cleland JGF. Are beta-blockers effective in patients who develop heart failure soon after myocardial infarction? A meta-regression analysis of randomized trials. *Eur J Heart Failure* 2000;**2**:333–40.

108. Vantrimpont P, Rouleau JL, Wun CC *et al.* for the SAVE Investigators. Additive beneficial effects of beta-blockers to angiotensin-converting enzyme inhibitors in the survival and ventricular enlargement (SAVE) study. *J Am Coll Cardiol* 1997;**29**:229–36.

109. Exner DV, Dries DL, Waclawia MA *et al.* Beta-adrenergic blocking agent use and mortality in patients with asymptomatic and symptomatic left ventricular systolic dysfunction: a post-hoc analysis of the studies of left ventricular dysfunction. *J Am Coll Cardiol* 1999;**33**:916–23.

110. The CARPRICORN Investigators. Effect of carvedilol on outcome after myocardial infarction in patients with left ventricular dysfunction: the CAPRICORN randomised trial. *Lancet* 2001;**357**:1385–90.

111. McKelvie RS, Yusuf S. Large trials and meta-analyses. In: Poole-Wilson PA, Colucci WS, Massie BM, Chatterjee K, Coats AJS, eds. *Heart failure. Scientific principles and clinical practice.* New York: Churchill Livingstone, 1997.

46 Management of overt heart failure

Bert Andersson, Karl Swedberg

The cardiac muscle may be exposed to various ischemic, hemodynamic, metabolic, or toxic conditions that eventually lead to the clinical syndrome of congestive heart failure (CHF). Given a certain severity, any cardiac disorder will ultimately lead to heart failure. Further, many non-cardiac disorders will result in heart failure, alone or in combination with cardiovascular conditions. Last, but not least, progressive deterioration of cardiac function with age further increases the susceptibility to develop heart failure. Taken together, the aforementioned circumstances, in a continuously aging population, may explain why CHF is one of the most common, and most costly, diseases in Western society.

CHF is a potentially lethal condition. It has been evident during the past decade that whilst we are in possession of some drugs that may improve cardiac function and symptoms as well as survival, other agents are simultaneously capable of impairing long-term survival. Furthermore, as with other treatment traditions, we lack modern documentation about the oldest drugs, such as diuretics. In this chapter we intend to cover the present knowledge regarding evidence-based medical therapies in CHF.

Cardiac glycosides

Digitalis is the oldest of the drugs used in the treatment of CHF today. It has been used for at least 200 years. Although all internists, general practitioners, and cardiologists have profound experience with this drug, the mode of action is still partly unknown. The main action of the drug is thought to be exerted by action on the plasma membrane Na^+/K^+-ATPase, increasing intracellular concentrations of Na^+ and Ca^+. A variety of autonomic effects have been shown in acute experimental studies.

Acute effects in CHF

Older uncontrolled studies have suggested that digitalis produced beneficial hemodynamic effects in patients with decompensated heart failure, expressed as a decrease in pulmonary capillary wedge pressure, an increase in cardiac output, and a fall in heart rate.[1,2] It appears that the effect of digitalis on hemodynamics is dependent on the hemodynamic state of the patient. Whereas positive effects have been observed in decompensated heart failure, the effects in

normal subjects are largely negligible.[3,4] Although the slowing of heart rate would be of benefit in diastolic heart failure without systolic dysfunction, there are no data to support the use of digoxin in diastolic heart failure. On the contrary, on a theoretical basis, the increase in intracellular Ca^+ and increase in contractility may be harmful to the hypertrophic heart. Although digoxin has been found to act synergistically in combination with different vasodilators, no such effects were seen in combination with dobutamin. Ferguson showed that acute administration of digitalis restored baroreceptor function and caused a decrease in sympathetic activity.[5,6] Goldsmith *et al* were not able to reproduce these results with regard to norepinephrine kinetics or baroreceptor function.[7] Both increase and decrease in neurohormonal activity has been reported following acute digoxin administration.

Chronic digitalis therapy

The first double-blind placebo-controlled trial with chronic digoxin treatment was published in 1977.[8] In a crossover design, 46 patients were randomized; about one third were in atrial fibrillation. Sixteen patients deteriorated while on placebo, eight of whom improved after being switched over to digoxin. In a 3 month trial, Fleg *et al* could not show any superior effect of digitalis treatment over placebo, although the majority of patients on digitalis deteriorated after discontinuation of the drug.[9] Improvement of myocardial function in patients with mild heart failure was demonstrated by Taggart *et al*[10] Other studies have shown positive effects of digoxin on clinical heart failure symptoms, echocardiographic findings, and exercise capacity, in particular in patients with more advanced left ventricular dysfunction.[11–13]

The trials mentioned above were small, and the first large study was the Captopril-Digoxin Multicenter Research Group trial.[14] In this study 300 patients with relatively mild heart failure were compared using captopril, digoxin, or placebo. Digoxin and captopril were equally effective in preventing hospitalization or an increase in diuretic dosages. Although digoxin-treated patients showed a significant increase in ejection fraction, in contrast to the captopril group, digoxin did not improve exercise capacity as much as captopril. In another study with 433 patients with mild heart failure, the German and Austrian Xamoterol Study Group investigated the effect of digoxin together with xamoterol and placebo. Digoxin improved clinical indices of heart failure but not exercise capacity.[15]

Several trials have used a withdrawal design for the placebo-treated patients. Di Bianco *et al* compared digoxin with milrinone in a 3 month multicenter trial in 230 patients with moderate to severe heart failure.[16] The digoxin-treated patients showed a significant improvement in left ventricular function and exercise capacity compared with the placebo group. Furthermore, digoxin was significantly less prone to induce arrhythmias compared with milrinone.

In the PROVED trial a randomized double-blind withdrawal of digoxin was investigated in 88 patients with NYHA class II–III.[17] More placebo patients had worsening heart failure with an increase in the need for diuretics and hospitalization, and an impairment in exercise capacity and LV function. In a similar study – the RADIANCE trial – 178 patients with CHF were investigated during digoxin withdrawal compared with maintained digoxin therapy.[18] The results were also similar to those of the PROVED trial, with placebo patients showing a statistically significant deterioration in cardiac function, hospitalization, quality of life and exercise capacity.

It should be noted that the withdrawal study design is inferior compared with prospective treatment studies. Because of the selection of responders and exclusion of non-responders who have suffered from deterioration or even lethal arrhythmias during digoxin treatment, the study design will result in different answers.

The Digitalis Investigators Group (DIG) study is the largest study in CHF. It is the only survival study of digoxin. The effect of digoxin was studied in a multicenter, prospective, randomized, placebo-controlled, double-blind trial in 7788 patients with mild to moderate heart failure and sinus rhythm.[19] Among the investigated patients, 6800 had signs of systolic dysfunction expressed as ejection fraction of <45%. The remaining 998 patients might be considered to have diastolic dysfunction. There was no effect on the primary end point of all-cause mortality (odds ratio 1·0). Digoxin significantly reduced the number of hospitalizations from worsening heart failure.

Documented value of digoxin

Proven indication: always acceptable **Grade A**

- Symptomatic left ventricular systolic heart failure and sinus rhythm. Symptomatic improvement, improved exercise capacity and decreased hospitalization for heart failure
- CHF with atrial fibrillation. Heart rate control

Acceptable indication but of uncertain efficacy and may be controversial **Grade A**

- Symptomatic heart failure due to diastolic dysfunction

Not proven: potentially harmful (contraindicated) **Grade A**

- Bradycardia and atrioventricular block
- Significant ventricular arrhythmias
- Renal dysfunction
- Electrolyte disturbances, hypokalemia in particular

Taken together, present data on digoxin suggest that this drug induces small but beneficial effects on cardiac function, morbidity, and symptoms. There is a neutral effect on all-cause mortality, with a possibly lower incidence of deaths from worsening heart failure, balanced by an increase in arrhythmic and myocardial infarction deaths. However, the therapeutic window is narrow, and the potential risk for serious arrhythmias cannot be ignored.

Diuretics

Fluid retention is a consistent finding in almost every patient with CHF. The need for reduction of blood volume in patients with edema was recognized several hundred years ago. Drugs with mild diuretic effects, such as mercury salts, carbonic anhydrase inhibitors, and thiazides, have all been used. A more substantial way of inducing diuresis was achieved when the loop-diuretics were introduced, and this class of drugs has since been the cornerstone of heart failure treatment.[20] The compensatory fluid retention, as a response to lower cardiac output and reduced kidney perfusion,[21] might be of some benefit in restoring optimal preload in the earlier states of CHF. A further increase in intracavitary pressure increases wall stress in the myocardium with a parallel increase in oxygen consumption and energy expenditure. The elevation of venous pressure shifts the hydrostatic balance across the capillary wall toward a net filtration of fluid to the extracellular space, and finally to the formation of edema. The edema impairs the transportation of oxygen, nutritive substances, and waste products, which ultimately leads to organ failure. In the case of pulmonary edema, the decrease in oxygen uptake affects all organs in the body. The decrease in renal blood flow stimulates the renin system, which leads to secretion of angiotensin and aldosterone. Other neurohormones that promote retention of sodium and water include vasopressin, norepinephrine, and prostaglandins.[22] Sodium excretion is promoted by atrial natriuretic factor, dopamine, and prostacyclin.

Acute neuroendocrine and hemodynamic effects

In patients with pulmonary edema, intravenous furosemide is normally followed by a prompt response and relief of symptoms. There have not been consistent findings regarding the mode of action of loop-diuretics in the acute phase of decompensated heart failure. The reduction in filling pressures occurs even before diuresis is initiated,[23–25] and has been attributed to vasodilation. However, arterial vasoconstriction has also been found, alone or in combination with venodilation.[26–28] Regarding cardiac output, an increase, no change, or a decrease has been reported. Although furosemide is the most thoroughly tested loop-diuretic, there are others available, including bumetanide,[29] ethacrynic acid,[30] piretanide,[31] and toresemide.[32] There is little information about the acute neuroendocrine effects of diuretics. The effects on vascular tone suggest signs of neuroendocrine modulation. Venodilation may be due to the release of renal vasodilator prostaglandins.[33]

Chronic neuroendocrine and hemodynamic effects

Most long-term studies have involved a small number of patients and used a variety of drugs and doses. The first study to give information with oral diuretics was performed in a small number of patients with valvular heart disease.[24] Hydrochlorthiazide was administered and resulted in a reduction in weight, pulmonary artery pressure, arterial pressure, heart rate, and cardiac output at rest as well as during exercise. Results from other studies have yielded similar results, with different diuretics, including furosemide,[34] piretanide,[35] torasemide,[36] and amiloride.[37] Chronic neuroendocrine effects are less well studied. Oral furosemide treatment has been associated with a reduction in norepinephrine concentration and a profound increase in plasma renin activity, angiotensin, and plasma aldosterone concentration.[38,39]

Effects on survival

No study has been performed examining the effect of diuretics on long-term survival. There has been some concern raised regarding the potential neurohormonal activation by diuretics. However, any long-term neuroendocrine activation has not been demonstrated. Further, it should be kept in mind that studies showing positive survival effects in heart failure – with ACE inhibitors, β blockers or vasodilators – have all used diuretics as background treatment.

Documented value of diuretics

Proven indication: always acceptable **Grade A**
- Symptomatic improvement in case of congestion. Improvement of exercise capacity

Acceptable indication but of uncertain efficacy and may be controversial **Grade B**
- Long-term treatment in conjunction with other drugs for heart failure, such as ACE inhibitors, vasodilators and β blockers

Not proven: potentially harmful (contraindicated) **Grade C**
- Heart failure without congestion or edema
- Severe decompensated hypokalemia or hyperuricemia

Clinical management

It is clear that diuretics reduce symptoms in CHF. The effect on symptoms has been formally tested in trials with furosemide and torasemide.[40,41] Further, it has been

observed that the effects of ACE inhibitors may require the coadministration of diuretics.[42,43] Diuretics are also more effective in relieving edema and congestive symptoms than ACE inhibitors when given as single therapy.[44] Through an increase in urinary excretion of electrolytes, diuretics are prone to induce hypokalemia, hyponatremia, hypocalcemia, hypomagnesemia, and metabolic alkalosis.[45] The need for potassium supplements might be diminished by using potassium-sparing diuretics, such as amiloride or aldosterone. ACE inhibitors act synergistically with potassium-sparing diuretics, which may produce hyperkalemia. The addition of a potassium-sparing diuretic to a loop-diuretic will further increase diuresis. Additionally, the diuretic effect of a loop-diuretic is boosted by other diuretics acting at different sites in the nephron. Therefore, the combination of a loop-diuretic with a thiazide enhances the diuretic effect.

It is difficult to foresee a future situation when diuretics are no longer needed in the treatment arsenal of CHF. Further, the obvious need for relief of edema and fluid retention will prevent the launching of any long-term survival study. With reference to the multiple side effects produced by electrolyte disturbances it is advisable to keep the diuretic dosages as low as possible, and aim for combination therapies in which dosages are minimized.

Aldosterone receptor blockers

Aldosterone plays an important role in the pathophysiology of heart failure, facilitating sodium retention and potassium loss. Further, it activates the sympathetic nervous system and stimulates myocardial and vascular fibrosis, and is a component of the circulating renin–angiotensin–aldosterone system.[46–49]

Although aldosterone antagonists have diuretic effects they differ from other diuretic agents in that they are neuroendocrine antagonists, and thereby have a potential to be effective in the long-term treatment of patients with CHF. Spironolactone is an old drug that has been used for decades as a potassium-sparing agent. However, the long-term clinical effects in the treatment of CHF was not tested until recently. The concept of aldosterone antagonism was studied in the RALES study where 1663 patients in NYHA class III or IV were randomized to spironolactone or placebo.[50] Spironolactone was initiated with 25 mg/day with adjustments to 12·5 or 50 mg depending on serum potassium. Ninety five per cent of the patients were on ACE inhibitors while only 11% had a background therapy of β blockers. The trial was discontinued early after a mean follow up period of 24 months because of beneficial effect of spironolactone. There were 386 (46%) deaths in the placebo group and 284 (35%) in the spironolactine group; RR 0·70 (95% CI 0·60–0·82), $P < 0.001$. The lower risk was attributed to both a lower risk from progressive heart failure and sudden death from cardiac causes. The RALES trial demonstrates that improved antagonism of the renin–angiotensin system by spironolactone reduces the risk of both morbidity and mortality in CHF. To reduce endocrine side effects by spironolactone, a selective aldosterone receptor blocker (eplerenone) is now tested in patients with CHF.

Documented value of spironolactone

Proven indication: always acceptable **Grade A**
- Improvement of survival in severe CHF
- Reduction of morbidity in severe heart failure

Acceptable indication but of uncertain efficacy and may be controversial **Grade B**
- Reduction of morbidity in mild to moderate heart failure
- Reduction of mortality in mild to moderate heart failure

Not proven: potentially harmful (contraindicated) **Grade C**
- Hyperkalemia

Vasodilators

Vasodilation reduces left ventricular afterload and preload, and these beneficial effects were observed in 1956,[51,52] but it was not until the 1970s that the concept was widely accepted.[53,54] The first drugs used were pure vasodilators, such as nitroprusside, nitroglycerin, and phentolamine. Later, agents with combined effects were developed. Examples of combination therapies are the inotropic drugs with simultaneous vasodilation, such as dobutamine, and ACE inhibitors, which are reviewed in another section of this chapter.

Reduction of afterload and preload in CHF improves the left ventricular performance according to the Frank–Starling relation with less myocardial oxygen demand and increased cardiac output.[55,56] Further, vasodilation might reduce valvular regurgitation by means of afterload reduction. Vasodilation may improve organ dysfunction by acting directly on selected vascular beds, such as the coronary and the renal vasculature.

Acute vasodilator therapy

Nitroglycerin and nitroprusside are the drugs most commonly used for acute short-term vasodilation therapy in heart failure.

Nitroglycerin

Nitroglycerin causes smooth muscle cell relaxation and vasodilation of arterial and venous vessels through action on guanylate cyclase and the generation of cyclic guanosine monophosphate.[57] Nitrates can be used as sublingual tablet, lingual–buccal spray, or as intravenous infusion. Administration causes reduction in left ventricular filling pressures within 3–5 minutes, mainly by venodilation and lowering of preload.[58–63] Further, nitroglycerin reduces systemic vascular resistance and afterload, with ensuing improvement in cardiac output. Although the effect of nitroglycerin on coronary blood flow has not been studied in CHF, it is conceivable that nitrate therapy favorably affects myocardial perfusion and oxygen supply/demand ratio.[64,65] Acute nitrate administration appears to be especially useful in cases of elevated filling pressures and ischemic conditions, such as in ischemic cardiomyopathy and myocardial infarction.

Nitroprusside

Nitroprusside generates nitric oxide and nitrosothiols, which stimulate guanylate cyclase to increase intracellular cGMP. The smooth muscle cell relaxation is rapidly induced after administration. Sodium nitroprusside is converted to cyanide and is metabolized to thiocyanate. Thiocyanate may accumulate and lead to thiocyanate toxicity during prolonged nitroprusside therapy. As compared to nitroglycerin, nitroprusside is far more potent and causes a more pronounced arterial vasodilation.[61] The most prominent effect of nitroprusside is the arterial vasodilation with afterload reduction. There are minor effects on renal and hepatosplanchnic vasculature.[61] In contrast to nitroglycerin, nitroprusside may induce a coronary steal phenomenon.[66] Nitroprusside is best employed in cases of acute heart failure after cardiac surgery or myocardial infarction, or in patients waiting for a more definitive intervention, such as valvular surgery. Further, nitroprusside has been used to stabilize patients with chronic heart failure and to determine their optimal level of vasodilation.[67] Owing to its potent vasodilation property, nitroprusside may cause adverse hypotension, especially in cases of inadequate filling pressure. Thiocyanate and cyanide toxicity is rare during short term administration (≤ 3 micrograms/kg/min for less than 72 hours).

Hemodynamic effects of long-term vasodilator therapy

Nitrates and hydralazine

Oral nitroglycerin and hydralazine have been studied, either alone or in combination therapy. The effects on left ventricular function and hemodynamics are similar to the acute effects of vasodilators described above.[68–71]

Hydralazine was available as an antihypertensive agent when vasodilator therapy was adopted as a therapeutic strategy in CHF. Hydralazine acts as a dominant arterial vasodilator, but has probably also mild inotropic properties, which might be due to a reflex activation of sympathetic activity.[72,73] This inotropic action might be responsible for a less favorable effect on myocardial oxygen consumption counteracting the unloading effects of vasodilation.[74,75]

The addition of a nitrate to hydralazine causes a greater effect on the reduction in filling pressures than can be achieved by hydralazine alone.[76] In view of the beneficial action of nitrates on coronary dynamics, a nitrate should be added to hydralazine therapy in patients with significant coronary artery disease.[77] Although hydralazine–nitrate therapy was marginally superior to ACE inhibitor in improving exercise capacity, this combination displayed worse tolerability.[78]

Calcium-channel blockers

Besides its vasodilatory effect, the first generation calcium-channel blocker nifedipine possesses negative inotropic effects. Deleterious effects with regard to hemodynamics, neurohormonal activation, and disease progression have been demonstrated in several trials.[79] Diltiazem has been associated with deterioration, no change, or improvement in hemodynamic function. In a postinfarction study, patients with heart failure did not benefit from verapamil treatment, in contrast to patients without heart failure.[80] Furthermore, the effects of diltiazem were unfavorable in patients with CHF in conjunction with myocardial infarction in a large placebo-controlled trial in 1237 patients.[81] Second generation calcium-channel blockers have not been extensively studied in patients with heart failure, but there are indications of a risk for clinical deterioration with drugs such as nisoldipine and nicardipine.[82,83] The second generation calcium-channel blocker felodipine caused vasodilation and an increase in cardiac output during 8 weeks of treatment in a placebo-controlled trial.[84]

Other vasodilators

Other potent vasodilators, such as prazosin, minoxidil, and epoprosternol, are discussed in the next section regarding survival. These drugs are currently not used in the long-term management of CHF.

Effects on survival

Hydralazine and isosorbide dinitrate

The V-HeFT I was the first placebo-controlled clinical trial to study the effect of a vasodilator on survival in patients with chronic heart failure. The study recruited 642 patients with mild to moderate heart failure, and randomized to receive placebo, prazosin hydrochloride, or the combination of hydralazine hydrochloride and isosorbide dinitrate. Two years after randomization, the survival in the hydralazine-isosorbide treated group was significantly better than the

placebo group ($P < 0.028$). For the entire follow up, the difference was not significant ($P = 0.093$). The mortality rate in the prazosin group was not different from the placebo group.[85]

The second V-HeFT study examined the efficacy of hydralazine and isosorbide with that of enalapril. There were 804 patients, randomized to the two treatment strategies. Two years after randomization, the all-cause mortality was 18% in the enalapril group as compared with 25% in the hydralazine-isosorbide group ($P = 0.016$). For the total follow up, the difference was not significant ($P = 0.08$).

Calcium-channel blockers

Felodipine was studied in the V-HeFT III study, in which the effect on survival was neutral.[86] Amlodipine, a third generation calcium-channel blocker, was investigated in the PRAISE trial.[87] A total of 1153 patients with NYHA class III–IV were randomized, including 421 patients with non-ischemic dilated cardiomyopathy. The overall effect on mortality as well as on the combined end point mortality and hospitalization was neutral. Whereas the mortality was unchanged in the subgroup with ischemic heart failure, there were significantly fewer end points in the non-ischemic group treated with amlodipine as compared to patients on placebo (22% v 35%, $P < 0.001$). However, this was not expected prior to the conduct of the study and the hypothesis was assessed in the PRAISE-2 trial among patients with non-ischemic CHF.[88] Patients with non-ischemic etiology of CHF in NYHA class IIIb or IV ($n = 1652$) were randomized to placebo or amlodipine 10 mg/day. There was no significant difference in all-cause or cardiac mortality and cardiac event rates between the two groups. Combining the data of PRAISE-1 and PRAISE-2 suggest a complete prognostic neutrality. However, based on these trials amlodipine and felodipine may be safely used to treat angina or hypertension in patients with CHF, if other proven drugs such as ACE inhibitors and β blockers are ineffective or not tolerated.

Other vasodilators

Flosequinan is a vasodilator with a combined venous and arterial effect, with a possible positive inotropic and chronotropic effect. A large multicenter trial (PROFILE) was launched to study the effects on survival in heart failure patients. However, this study had to be stopped prematurely, because of an increase in mortality in the flosequinan-treated patients.[89] Additionally, the prostacyclin epoprostenol might improve hemodynamics, but has been shown to have an adverse effect on mortality in severe heart failure.[90]

Documented value of vasodilators

Proven indication: always acceptable **Grade A**

- Short-term reduction of afterload in cases with acute heart failure
- The combination hydralazine-isosorbide dinitrate can be used for long-term treatment in patients who do not tolerate ACE inhibitors

Acceptable indication but of uncertain efficacy and may be controversial **Grade B**

- Third generation calcium-channel blockers may be used for symptomatic treatment of conditions such as angina pectoris or hypertension

Not proven: potentially harmful (contraindicated) **Grade C**

- Vasodilators other than hydralazine-isosorbide dinitrate and third generation calcium-channel blockers may increase mortality during long-term treatment
- Treatment of patients with concomitant significant aortic or mitral stenosis

Most vasodilators can improve hemodynamics on a short-term basis. Besides the combination of hydralazine and isosorbide dinatrate, the long-term effects of different vasodilators are either neutral or detrimental. The majority of studies have shown harmful effects with calcium-channel blockers in CHF, with the exception for felodipine and amlodipine where the effects on survival have been neutral. It is therefore suggested that vasodilators other than ACE inhibitors may be used to relieve symptoms and to acutely improve the hemodynamic condition. The effects on survival are less favorable as compared with ACE inhibitors, but hydralazine-isosorbide dinitrate may be used in patients who do not tolerate ACE inhibitors.

Drugs affecting the renin–angiotensin system

Angiotensin converting enzyme (ACE) inhibitors

ACE inhibitors have been introduced for the treatment of heart failure within the past decade. Their potential value was suggested by studies showing improved symptomatology,[91] hemodynamics[92,93] and survival.[94] It was hypothesized that ACE inhibitors might attenuate left ventricular remodeling after myocardial infarction[95,96] and thus possibly prevent the progression to symptomatic heart failure. Neuroendocrine activation has been shown to be of prognostic importance[97] and ACE inhibitors have the potential of modulating this activation.[98] Several studies have reported results on the effects of ACE inhibitors on survival in patients with clinical heart failure, following acute myocardial infarction generally and following myocardial infarction with left ventricular dysfunction or heart failure.

Survival trials

CONSENSUS included 253 patients in NYHA class IV randomized to placebo or enalapril. After a follow up of 6 months (primary objective), the overall mortality was reduced by 27% ($P=0 \cdot 003$). Number of days for hospital care was reduced and NYHA classification significantly improved with enalapril.[94]

In the largest study, the Studies of Left Ventricular Treatment (SOLVD) trial, 2569 patients with symptomatic heart failure NYHA class II–III received placebo or enalapril besides conventional heart failure therapy.[99] The average follow up was 41.4 months. Mortality was significantly reduced from 40% to 35% ($P=0 \cdot 0036$). Hospitalizations for heart failure were also reduced. The largest reduction in mortality occurred among deaths attributed significantly to progressive heart failure. Symptoms and quality of life assessed by questionnaire were improved.[100]

In the Survival and Ventricular Enlargement (SAVE) trial, 2231 patients with ejection fraction of 40% or less, but without overt heart failure or symptoms of myocardial ischemia, were randomly assigned treatment with captopril or placebo.[101] Mortality from all causes was 20% in the captopril group and 25% in the placebo group (RR 19%, $P=0 \cdot 019$).

In the TRACE study 1749 patients with left ventricular dysfunction were randomly assigned treatment with placebo or the ACE inhibitor trandolapril.[102] Treatment was initiated 3–7 days from the onset of myocardial infarction. All-cause mortality in the placebo group was 42·3% and 34·7% in the trandolapril group, a 22% relative reduction of mortality ($P=0 \cdot 00065$).

In the AIRE study, 2006 patients with clinical evidence of heart failure any time after the index infarction, were randomly allocated to treatment with ramipril or placebo on day 3–10 from the onset of infarction.[103] Clinical evidence of heart failure was defined as at least one of the following: signs of left ventricular failure on chest radiograph, bilateral auscultatory crackles extending at least one third of the way up the lung fields in the absence of chronic pulmonary disease, or auscultatory evidence of a third heart sound with persistent tachycardia. The average follow up was 15 months with a minimum of 6 months. Mortality from all causes at the end of the study was 17% in the ramipril group and 23% in the placebo group (RR 27%, $P=0 \cdot 002$).

Improved blockade of the renin–angiotensin system was tested in the ATLAS trial. Patients with CHF ($n=3164$) and ejection fraction <30% were randomized to a low dose of lisinopril (2.5–5·0 mg/day) or a high dose (32.5–35 mg/day) for a median of 45·7 months.[104] There were 717 deaths in the low-dose group versus 666 in the high-dose group (hazard ratio 0·92; $P=0 \cdot 128$) for the high dose. The combined end point of all-cause mortality or hospitalization for any reason showed a hazard ratio of 0·88 (95% CI 0·82–0·96),

($P=0.002$). The side effects and tolerability were similar in the two groups.

These findings indicate that patients with heart failure should generally not be maintained on very low doses of an ACE inhibitor, and suggest that a difference in efficacy between intermediate and high doses of an ACE inhibitor is likely to be very small. Thus, patients should be titrated to dose levels observed in trials, that is lisinopril or enalapril at least 16–18 mg/day. The value of additional dose levels such as >20 mg/day lisinopril is uncertain but supported by the results of the ATLAS trial.

A recent meta-combined analysis of individual patients from five large randomized studies with ACE inhibitors was presented by Flather and coworkers. Three of these studies were postinfarction trials, enrolling 5966 patients, in a total of 12 763 cases. The risk of death was significantly lower in the ACE inhibitor-treated group (23% *v* 27%; odds ratio 0.80, 95% CI 0.74–0.87), as was the risk of re-infarctions (8.9% *v* 11%; odds ratio 0.79, 95% CI 0.70–0.89). The treatment benefits were independent of age, sex, and baseline treatment.[105]

Trials on exercise capacity

There are many trials that have focused on this objective. An extensive review of these trials has recently been published[106] and indicated that these agents improve exercise capacity, as well as symptoms in patients with chronic CHF. Changes in exercise capacity are consistent with changes in symptoms.

Trials on hemodynamics

ACE inhibitors were documented in early studies to induce beneficial hemodynamic responses. These effects included a vasodilatory effect and an increased cardiac output, increased stroke volume, and reduced pulmonary wedge pressure.[92,93]

Trials on prevention

A reduced incidence of heart failure by ACE inhibitors has been demonstrated in several trials. In the prevention arm of the SOLVD study,[99] the incidence of heart failure and the number of hospitalizations were reduced and similar findings were reported in SAVE.[101] In an overview of ACE inhibitor trials,[107] the preventive potential of ACE inhibitors is clearly demonstrated.

The potential antiatherosclerotic effect of ACE inhibitors, suggested from experimental animal studies, is supported by observations from the SOLVD[108] and SAVE[101] studies, in which the incidence of myocardial infarction and unstable angina were reduced. The HOPE trial tested the hypothesis that the ACE inhibitor ramipril might favorably influence survival in patients with different atherosclerotic conditions and in patients with high-risk diabetes mellitus ($n=9297$).[109]

These patients were considered not to have CHF at inclusion. The primary composite end point of myocardial infarction, stroke, or death from cardiovascular causes was significantly reduced in the treatment group (651 *v* 826 end points; RR 0.78; 95% CI 0.70–0.86, $P<0.001$). Ramipril also reduced the risk of heart failure (9.1% *v* 11.6%; RR 0.77, $P<0.001$). Thus, even though this was not a study on CHF patients, ramipril appeared to protect high-risk atherosclerotic and diabetic patients from future development of CHF and other cardiovascular complications.

Cost effectiveness

Enalapril therapy for patients with heart failure (SOLVD) was cost effective and justified by added benefits compared to other vasodilator therapy.[110] In asymptomatic patients with left ventricular dysfunction after an acute myocardial infarction (SAVE), captopril was cost effective in patients aged 50–80 years compared to other interventions.[111] Ramipril therapy for patients with clinical heart failure after acute myocardial infarction appears highly cost effective when assessed using data from the AIRE study.[112] ACE inhibitor treatment was considered cost effective in an evaluation of five independent studies regarding economic analysis.[113]

Documented value of ACE inhibitors

Proven indication: always acceptable **Grade A**

- Symptomatic chronic heart failure and documented systolic myocardial dysfunction. Improved survival and reduced morbidity have been demonstrated. Symptoms will be attenuated and exercise capacity improved
- Following acute myocardial infarction with clinical signs of heart failure or significant systolic dysfunction (ejection fraction <40%). Improved survival and reduced morbidity have been demonstrated
- Prevention of cardiovascular events, including heart failure, in patients with atherosclerotic disease, or in patients with diabetes mellitus and additional risk factors

Acceptable indication but of uncertain efficacy and may be controversial **Grade C**

- Heart failure from diastolic dysfunction

Not proven: potentially harmful (contraindicated) **Grade C**

- Treatment of patients with significant aortic or mitral stenosis
- Treatment of patients with hypotension (systolic blood pressure <80 mmHg)
- Treatment of patients with pronounced renal dysfunction

Clinical perspective

All patients with documented left ventricular systolic dysfunction (ejection fraction < 35–40%) should be considered for treatment with an ACE inhibitor. In symptomatic patients this should be considered first-line therapy in addition to a diuretic agent. Treatment should be continued long term. Patients with clinical CHF should be maintained on ACE inhibitor treatment in combination with a diuretic.

Contraindications to ACE inhibitors include hypotension (in general systolic blood pressure < 80 mmHg), pronounced renal dysfunction (serum creatinine > 250 micromol/1), history of angioneurotic edema, and important valve stenosis.

The dosage to be used should be titrated from a low dose and increased to the moderate high levels employed in clinical trials. If no hypotension or renal dysfunction develops, titration up to enalapril 10 mg 2×/day, captopril 50 mg 2×/day ramipril 10 mg/day, trandolapril 4 mg 4×/day, quinapril 10 mg 2×/day will be most effective.

Angiotensin II receptor (AT₁) antagonists

As ACE inhibition does not provide complete blockade from the synthesis of angiotensin II, a more effective blockade has been postulated by a specific antagonism at the receptor (AT$_1$) level. Hemodynamic effects of losartan have been similar to the effects of enalapril in comparative trials.[114] In a pilot trial, ELITE, patients with heart failure were randomized to losartan 50 mg/day or captopril 50 mg 3×/day for 48 weeks.[115] The primary end point was renal dysfunction. The effect on serum creatinine did not differ between the two groups. The secondary end point, death and/or hospitalization for heart failure, was 9·4% in the losartan group and 13·2% in the captopril group ($P = 0.075$). The difference was entirely due to a 46% decrease in total mortality among losartan-treated patients, 8·7% and 4·8% respectively ($P = 0.035$).

In an attempt to confirm the findings from the ELITE study, ELITE-II was conducted in 3152 class II–IV patients with ejection fractions (EF) of <40%, randomized to losartan 50 mg/day or captopril 50 mg 3×/day.[116] There was no significant difference in all-cause mortality or sudden death (hazard ratio 1·13; 95% CI 0·95–1·35, $P = 0.16$). Significantly fewer patients in the losartan group discontinued study treatment because of adverse effects (9·7 v 14·7%; $P < 0.001$).

In RESOLVD, there were no differences between groups receiving candesartan and enalapril in exercise tolerance, ventricular function, or symptomatic status over 43 weeks.[117] However, combined therapy with candesartan plus enalapril markedly reduced ventricular volumes and improved ejection fraction over 43 weeks compared to either candesartan or enalapril alone. There was greater inhibition of aldosterone levels with the combination at 20 weeks, but this difference narrowed at 43 weeks. The study was too small to examine the impact of clinical outcomes.

In the Val-HeFT study 5010 patients in class II–IV and EF of <40% were randomized to placebo or valsartan.[7] Dose levels were increased to 160 mg 2×/day. Background therapy with an ACE inhibitor was present in 93%. There was no effect on all-cause mortality (484 in the placebo group v 495 in the valsartan group; RR 1·02, 95% CI 0·90–1·15, $P = 0.8$). In the other primary end point, mortality or hospitalizations, there was a significant reduction from 801 (32.1%) to 723 (28·8%) (RR 0·87, 95% CI 0·79–0·96, $P = 0.009$). In a subgroup analysis patients on a background therapy with a β blocker were found to have an increased risk when given valsartan. A similar observation was observed in ELITE-II. On the other hand, patients in the RESOLVD study had an improvement in left ventricular function when metoprolol was added to enalapril or candesartan or the combination. Therefore, these apparent subgroup interactions should be viewed with considerable caution.

The newer trials with angiotensin receptor blocker (ARBs) are suggestive, but do not offer definitive proof that ARBs can be used for symptomatic treatment of patients with heart failure who do not tolerate ACE inhibitors. As yet, the documentation regarding survival benefits is not as good as for ACE inhibitors.

Documented value of AT₁-receptor antagonists
Proven indication: always acceptable **Grade A**
- Symptomatic treatment of patients with heart failure who do not tolerate ACE inhibitors
Acceptable indication but of uncertain efficacy and may be controversial **Grade C**
- Symptomatic treatment in patients who do not tolerate β blockers
Not proven and potentially harmful **Grade C**
- Treatment of patients with a background therapy of both an ACE inhibitor and a β blocker

---

Non-digitalis inotropic drugs

In CHF it is often apparent that the heart suffers from inotropic failure. It is therefore not surprising that vast efforts have been invested in order to develop drugs that might increase contractility or the state of inotropy. Although several drugs with inotropic activity are available today, it has become increasingly evident that these drugs are associated with important negative effects.

There are inotropic agents in different classes according to their mode of action.[118] Cardiac glycosides affect sarcolemmal ions through the effects on ion channels or ion pumps. These drugs are covered in another section of this chapter. Other drugs increase the intracellular level of cyclic adenosine monophosphate (cAMP), either by receptor stimulation (β adrenergic agonists), or by decreasing cAMP breakdown (phosphodiesterase inhibitors). One class of agents affects intracellular calcium mechanisms by release of sarcoplasmic reticulum calcium, or by increasing the sensitivity of contractile proteins to calcium. Further, there are inotropic drugs with multiple mechanisms of action.

β Agonist drugs

Dobutamine

Drugs with β receptor agonist properties induce an increase in intracellular cAMP activity by stimulation of cellular receptors. Already during the 1960s patients with cardiogenic shock were treated with β receptor agonists isoproterenol and norepinephrine.[119] It was realized that both drugs had potential negative effects, such as an increased risk for arrhythmias or – in the case of norepinephrine – an untoward vasoconstriction. The development of dobutamine, a drug that is a modification of the isoproterenol molecule, resulted in an agent with β_1, β_2 and α_1 adrenergic activity.[120] Dobutamine induces vasodilation in combination with an increase in contractility, leading to an increase in stroke volume and cardiac output.[121–123] An enhancement of contractility is usually associated with an increase in myocardial oxygen consumption.[124] Side effects, such as arrhythmias or an unfavorable blood pressure response, are usually modest. Dobutamine can only be administered intravenously, in doses from 2 micrograms/kg/min up to 20–25 micrograms/kg/min.[125] It has been noticed that dobutamine may decrease β receptor sensitivity,[126,127] and prolonged infusion over 96 hours has been associated with a decrease in the hemodynamic effect by as much as 50%.[128] Beneficial short-term action encouraged investigators to use the drug in patients with chronic heart failure on an outpatient basis. Intermittent therapy was found to increase quality of life and hemodynamics.[129] However, a clinical trial had to be stopped prematurely because of an increase in mortality in the dobutamine-treated group.[130]

Dopamine

Dopamine (DA) is an adrenergic agonist with predominantly β_1 receptor activity.[131,132] This drug increases contractility with minor effects on heart rate or blood pressure. At low doses (0·5–2·0 micrograms/kg/min), DA acts on DA receptors, while at doses above 5·0 micrograms/kg/min it has effects through β_1 receptors, and at higher doses also through α receptors. Infusion at low doses causes dilation of smooth muscles in renal, mesenteric, and coronary arteries, leading to an increase in diuresis.[133,134]

Ibopamine

Ibopamine is an orally active dopaminergic agonist, with the active metabolite epinine *N*-methyldopamine acting on DA_1 and DA_2 receptors. This agent had positive hemodynamic effects in terms of an increase in cardiac output, a reduction

in systemic vascular resistance, and no effect on heart rate.[135,136] In a study with digoxin and ibopamine in 161 patients with mild to moderate chronic heart failure, it was observed that ibopamine had some positive effects in patients with less ventricular dysfunction, and no effects on mortality.[137] To evaluate the long-term effects of ibopamine, a study (PRIME-II) was initiated in 1906 patients with NYHA class III–IV heart failure. However, the study was terminated prematurely because of an increase in mortality in the ibopamine group: 25% (232 of 953) in the ibopamine group died versus 20% (193 of 953) in the placebo group (RR 1·26, 95% CI 1·04–1·53, $P = 0·017$).[138]

Xamoterol

Xamoterol is a drug with β adrenergic blocking effects and high partial agonist activity, and long-term effects are similar to those of other inotropic agents. A multicenter trial had to be discontinued because of an increase in mortality in the active treatment group: 32 of 352 (9·1%) patients in the xamoterol group and 6 of 164 (3·7%) patients in the placebo group died ($P = 0·02$).[139]

Phosphodiesterase inhibitors

Through inhibition of cAMP breakdown, the phosphodiesterase inhibitors bypass the β receptor pathway. The first phosphodiesterase inhibitor was amrinone, a drug with inotropic and vasodilatory effects. During infusion, amrinone induced afterload reduction, a decrease in filling pressures, increase in cardiac index, and also an increased rate of contractility and relaxation.[140–142] The major side effect is thrombocytopenia. Similarily, the related agent milrinone has been found to enhance myocardial contractility, besides having potent vasodilatory effects,[143–145] but without thrombocytopenia.[146] The short-term effects of another agent – enoximone – have been similar to those of other phosphodiesterase inhibitors.[147–149] As phosphodiesterase inhibitors elicit intracellular effects through other pathways than β adrenergic drugs, it has been hypothesized that the combination of these two classes of drugs would enhance myocardial performance. Results from clinical trials have supported this concept.[150,151]

Whereas short-term administration may improve myocardial performance and clinical condition in CHF,[145,152] the long-term effects of phosphodiesterase inhibitors have been discouraging. Oral phosphodiesterase administration has been tested in several trials for chronic heart failure, all of which have demonstrated no beneficial effect or a substantial increase in mortality in patients receiving the investigated drug.[16,153–155] In the PROMISE trial 1088 class III–IV patients were given milrinone or placebo. There was a 28% increase in mortality in patients treated with milrinone (95% CI 1–61%, $P=0·038$).[153]

Calcium-sensitizing drugs

Pimobendan is the most thoroughly studied drug in this class of inotropics. The effect is mediated by an increase in the affinity of troponin C for intracellular calcium.[156,157] Pimobendan inhibits phosphodiesterase and thereby has effects similar to those of milrinone.[156,158] In clinical trials pimobendan has been shown to exert improvement in cardiac index, exercise performance, and quality of life.[159,160] However, treatment effects did not show congruity among different doses, and there was also a tendency toward increased mortality in a large 24 week trial.[161]

Vesnarinone is a drug with muliple actions. It is a synthetic quinolinone derivative that in part inhibits phosphodiesterase, with simultaneous effects on transmembrane ion transports. This drug seemed to have effects on contractility without increasing the heart rate,[162,163] which made it an interesting candidate for long-term therapy in heart failure. Furthermore, it was demonstrated that vesnarinone might inhibit the production of cytokines, including tumor necrosis factor (TNF-α).[164] A moderate size trial with two doses of vesnarinone was started in 1989. Whereas the 120 mg treatment arm had to be stopped prematurely because of a significant increase in mortality in the active treatment group (16 deaths *v* three deaths in the 60 mg arm and six deaths in the placebo group), the 60 mg group continued. Unexpectedly, on completion of the study it was shown that 60 mg of vesnarinone was associated with a reduction in the combined end point mortality or cardiovascular morbidity (26 of 239 *v* 50 of 238; RR 50%, 95% CI 20–69, $P = 0.003$).[165] This study was followed by a larger placebo-controlled trial (VEST), with 3800 patients. However, the study was stopped early because of a 26% increase in mortality in patients treated with 60 mg of vesnarinone.[166]

Levosimendan is a new calcium-sensitizing agent with properties similar to pimobendan. This drug has, so far, been tested in short-term studies, and no long-term survival studies have been presented. Levosimendan was compared with dobutamine in 151 patients. A 10 minute bolus was followed by a 24 hour infusion of 0.05–0.6 micrograms/kg/min. Dobutamine was given as an open-label infusion (6 micrograms/kg/min). The primary efficacy variable was the proportion of patients showing an increase in stroke volume, a decrease in pulmonary capillary wedge pressure, or an increase in cardiac output. The response rate to levosimendan ranged from 50% at the lowest dose to 88% at the highest dose (compared with placebo 14% and dobutamine 70%).[167] In another study, levosimendan was compared with placebo in 146 patients in NYHA class III–IV. The dose range was 0.1–0.4 micrograms/kg/min. Treatment caused dose-dependent decreases in right and left ventricular filling pressures and mean arterial pressure. There were minor increases in heart rate at higher doses and symptoms improved as compared with placebo.[168] Thus, short-term

infusion (up to 24 hours) of levosimendan (0.05–0.2 micrograms/kg/min) is well tolerated and leads to favorable hemodynamic effects. Further, there are unpublished data suggesting that levosimendan might have long-term favorable effects in patients with myocardial infarction and heart failure.

The clinical effects appear to be similar to those of phosphodiesterase inhibitors, although experimental data suggest that no adverse effects on myocardial metabolism occur with levosimendan. No comparable studies have been conducted between levosimendan and a phosphodiesterase inhibitor, and long-term data are still required before the clinical value can be established.

Documented value of inotropic drugs
Proven indication: always acceptable
- Short-term improvement of symptoms in patients with severe heart failure   **Grade A**
- Bridging towards more definitive surgical treatment, such as cardiac transplantation   **Grade C**

Acceptable indication but of uncertain efficacy and may be controversial   **Grade C**
- Intermittent short-term treatment in chronic heart failure

Not proven: potentially harmful (contraindicated)   **Grade A**
- Long-term treatment in chronic heart failure. These drugs increase the risk of mortality.

It should be obvious from the summary above that different inotropic drugs, with a wide variety of modes of action, may improve symptoms and cardiac function on a short-term basis. However, inotropic drugs increase the risk of mortality. Whether these detrimental long-term effects could be abolished in the development of any other compound is unclear.

Anti-adrenergic agents

β Adrenergic blockade

Clinicians have generally been cautious in using β blockers in patients with CHF, even though investigators in the early 1970s were already proposing a possible beneficial effect of β blockers in such cases.[169,170] However, data have been gathered during recent years indicating that this class of drugs may have a significant contribution to make in the heart failure treatment armamentarium of the near future.

Early case reports suggested that β blockers had a potential to elicit overt heart failure in some cases.[171,172] However, although the possibility of such an adverse reaction has been of concern, there are no placebo-controlled trials that have proven that β blockers are detrimental in congestive heart failure. On the contrary, analysis of several myocardial infarction studies has shown that patients with signs of CHF showed a similar or better response to β blockers than did patients without heart failure.[173–175]

Hemodynamic effects

The short-term effects of β adrenergic blockade differs markedly from the long-term effects, which might be one explanation for the difficulties in understanding the mode of action during long-term therapy. After IV administration, there is a rapid reduction in heart rate, contractility, and blood pressure, with ensuing fall in cardiac output.[176–179] However, intraventricular volumes, stroke volume, and ejection fraction are unaffected.[177,178] β Blockers with vasodilating properties cause an acute reduction in afterload with reduction in filling pressures.[176–179] During 1–3 months of treatment, positive diastolic effects have been observed and these effects probably precede full effects on cardiac systolic function.[178,180]

During long-term treatment (3–12 months), β blockers induce myocardial improvement, as expressed by an increase in ejection fraction, cardiac output, and exercise capacity.[181–185] Similar to ACE inhibitors, β blockers attenuate left ventricular remodeling.[186–188] In the RESOLVD trial, metoprolol CR/XL was compared with placebo over 24 weeks in 426 patients receiving either an ARB (candesartan) or an ACE inhibitor (enalapril) or the combination. There was a significant improvement in measures of LV function in the β blocker treated group with an attenuation in the increase in LV dimensions.[189]

Effects of neurohormones

Acute administration of metoprolol causes a reflex increase in peripheral catecholamines without alteration of the transmyocardial gradient.[178] With radioactive labeling of norepinephrine, the non-selective β blocker propranolol was shown to reduce myocardial norepinephrine spillover as compared to the β_1 selective blocker metoprolol.[190] There are sparse data on the long-term effects of β adrenergic blockade on neurohormonal activation, but some studies suggest a beneficial reduction in peripheral norepinephrine level.[191–195] A decrease in renin–angiotensin activity has been noted, while the levels of atrial natriuretic peptides might increase on a short-term basis.[189]

Effects on quality of life and hospitalizations

A reduction of the need for hospitalizations has been demonstrated in studies with bisoprolol,[196] metoprolol,[197] and carvedilol.[198] Quality of life was improved in the Metoprolol in Dilated Cardiomyopathy (MDC) trial.[199] Whereas both patient and physician global assessments of heart failure symptoms improved, quality of life scores were not improved in the US carvedilol studies or in the MERIT-HF study.[200–202] In the Australian–New Zealand study, there was a tendency towards worse symptoms.[187] Further, carvedilol has been shown to reduce the progression towards overt heart failure.[187]

Effects on survival

One of the first studies of β blockers in congestive heart failure showed a reduced mortality in patients treated by β blockade as compared with historical controls.[169] Not until 1993, when the MDC trial was published, did additional information on clinical outcome become available. This study showed a trend towards a 34% reduction in the combined end point deaths and need for heart transplantation ($P=0.058$) in 383 patients with idiopathic dilated cardiomyopathy, treated with placebo or metoprolol.[199] A late follow up of this study has recently demonstrated that this trend was also maintained, or possibly reinforced, regarding all-cause mortality and actual cardiac transplantations 3 years after randomization.[203] In the CIBIS study, bisoprolol was used in a placebo-controlled trial in 641 patients. Overall there was a non-significant reduction in mortality (RR 0·80, 95% CI 0·56–1·15, $P=0.22$).[204] Four studies in the USA, investigating different effects of carvedilol, were combined in a total of 1094 patients with varying degrees of heart failure, and demonstrated a lower mortality in the carvedilol group (22 of 696 [3·2%] *v* 31 of 398 [7·8%] deaths; RR 65%, 95% CI 39–80, $P<0.01$).[205] However, there was no statistically beneficial effect of carvedilol regarding survival in the Australia–New Zealand trial of 415 patients with chronic heart failure of varying etiology.[206] None of the aforementioned trials was designed to specifically study mortality, and the number of events in each trial was relatively modest.

The first study designed to test the potential survival benefits of long-term β blockade was the CIBIS-II study. The β_1 selective antagonist bisoprolol was tested versus placebo in 2647 patients in NYHA III–IV and with an ejection fraction of ≤35.[196] Study drug was initiated with 1·25 mg/day being progressively increased to 10 mg/day over 3 months. The study was stopped by the safety committee after a mean follow up of 1·3 years. All-cause mortality was significantly lower with bisoprolol than with placebo (156 [11·8%] *v* 228 [17·3%]; hazard ratio 0·66, 95% CI 0·54–0·81, $P<0.0001$. There were significantly fewer sudden deaths among patients on bisoprolol than in those on placebo (3·6% *v* 6·3%; hazard ratio 0·56, $P=0.001$).

In the MERIT-HF trial metropolol controlled release/extended release (CR/XL) was compared in 3991 patients with chronic heart failure in NYHA class II–IV and an ejection fraction of <0·40· Background therapy including an ACE inhibitor or an ARB was present in 95% of the patients. Treatment was initiated with metoprolol CR/XL 12.5–25 mg/day and titrated for 6–8 weeks up to target dose of 200 mg/day. The study was also stopped early on the recommendation of the independent safety committee. Mean follow up time was 1 year. All-cause mortality was lower in the metoprolol group than in the placebo group: 145 (7·2% per patient-year of follow up) versus 217 deaths

(11·0%) (RR 0·66, 95% CI 0·53–0·81, *P*=0·0009). There were fewer sudden deaths in the metoprolol CR/XL group than in the placebo group (79 *v* 132; RR 0·59, *P*=0·0002) and fewer deaths from worsening heart failure (30 *v* 58; RR 0·51, *P*=0·0023).[197]

In the BEST trial the effects of the non-selective β blocker bucindolol was compared with placebo in 2708 patients with CHF in NYHA class III–IV.[207] Bucindolol was initiated with 3 mg 2×/day and titrated up over 6–8 weeks to 50–100 mg 2×/day. The study was prematurely terminated by the safety committee. Mortality was reduced from 447 deaths to 409 deaths (RR 0·91, 95% CI 0·88–1·02, *P*=0·12). In a subgroup analysis there was a heterogeneous response among groups analyzed. Patients with NYHA class IV or ejection fraction below 20% did not appear to benefit. Furthermore, in a subgroup of African-Americans there was a 17% excess mortality suggesting a lack of benefit among these patients. However, these were post hoc analyses and not prespecified end points.

The recently reported COPERNICUS trial was performed in 2289 patients with symptomatic chronic heart failure with symptoms at rest or at minimal exertion.[198] Carvedilol was initiated with 3·125 mg ×2/day and titrated to 25 mg ×2/day. There was a significant reduction in all-cause mortality from 190 (18·5% per patient-year) to 130 (11·4%) with a hazard ratio of 0·65 (95% CI 0·52–0·81); *P*=0·0001. The effect was consistent among a number of prespecified subgroups.

In a post hoc subgroup analysis of patients in the MERIT-HF study with similar characteristics as the patients in the COPERNICUS trial, with an EF of <0·25 and NYHA class III–IV, there was a comparable reduction in all-cause mortality (45 [11%] *v* 72 [18%] deaths; hazard ratio 0·61, 95% CI 0·11–0·58, *P*=0·0086).[208]

All three large β blocker studies (CIBIS-II, MERIT-HF, COPERNICUS) had been stopped early because of clear evidence of benefit and therefore resulted in limited long-term experience with this treatment. Nevertheless, these trials have extended the documentation for survival benefit with β adrenergic blockers to more than 15 000 patients. Overall experience from these trials is that treatment has been possible to initiate with high tolerability during the titration phase. As the BEST trial showed somewhat different results than the other three trials and also compared with the meta-analysis by Doughty *et al*[209] there is a suggestion that these agents differ in their effect. Several smaller trials have been published comparing metoprolol and carvedilol. A recent crossover study suggested that there are differences with respect to receptor effects, while long-term clinical effects were comparable.[210] This is further explored in the COMET trial where carvedilol and metoprolol are compared in 3042 patients. The trial finishes its follow up in October 2002, and results are expected by the end of 2002. The effects of

β blockers in the elderly are currently being studied in the SENIORS trial where nebivalol is being compared with placebo in patients above 70 years of age and with chronic heart failure.

In the situation of heart failure secondary to acute myocardial infarction, there are data from several older large post myocardial infarction trials that β blockers would be beneficial also when symptoms of heart failure are present.[173–175] These findings were first tested prospectively in the CAPRICORN study, in which carvedilol or placebo was given to 1959 patients with a recent myocardial infarction and signs of left ventricular dysfunction (EF ≤40%).[211] There was no effect on the primary end point mortality or cardiovascular hospitalization (hazard ratio 0·92, 95% CI 0·80–1·07), but there was a statistically significant reduction in all-cause mortality, 166 (15%) versus 151 (12%) deaths (hazard ratio 0·77, 95% CI 0·60–0·98, *P*=0·03). The risk reduction was of similar magnitude as previous post myocardial infarction trials with β blockers.

Documented value of β blockers
Proven indication: always acceptable **Grade A**
- To improve long-term survival in patients with mild to severe heart failure
- To improve cardiac function and symptoms in patients with symptomatic chronic heart failure, already on conventional treatment with ACE inhibitors (or an ARB), diuretics or digitalis
- To improve outcome in patients with acute myocardial infarction and left ventricular dysfunction with or without symptomatic heart failure
- Symptomatic treatment of patients with heart failure who do not tolerate ACE inhibitors

Acceptable indication but of uncertain efficacy and may be controversial **Grade C**
- Symptomatic heart failure from diastolic dysfunction

Not proven: potentially harmful (contraindicated) **Grade C**
- Acute decompensated heart failure
- CHF with pronounced hypotension and/or bradycardia

Clinical perspective

Drug titration and intolerance

Due to initial negative inotropic effects, treatment with β blockers requires a slow titration procedure. Parallel to myocardial recovery, β blocker dosages can usually safely be increased. It has been noticed that patients with simultaneous marked hypotension and tachycardia, expressing severe decompensation, may not tolerate β blockers. Nevertheless, figures of intolerance have been low in randomized trials, comparable to those of ACE inhibitors. Starting doses with different β blockers have been: bisoprolol 1·25 mg/day; carvedilol 3·125–6.25 mg 2×/day; metoprolol

12.5–25 mg/day. Doses are increased every 1–2 weeks, when doses are doubled, until maintenance doses of full conventional β blockade are achieved.

Although a reduction in heart rate probably is important, it has not been possible to adequately identify responders from non-responders to β blocker therapy. In cases with significant obstructive pulmonary disease, β blockers should be used with caution, and a selective β blocker would be preferred.

Central nervous system modulators

Moxonidine

Reduction of the sympathetic nervous system activity can also be achieved by stimulating receptors within the central nervous system. Studies in this area has been performed with clonidine[212] and moxonidine. Moxonidine has been documented in several phase II and III trials. In a study over 12 weeks in 97 patients, Swedberg and coworkers demonstrated a significant attenuation of plasma norepinephrine levels.[213] With a sustained release preparation of moxonidine, a more prolonged and effective reduction of plasma norepinephrine was obtained in 265 subjects.[214] The reduction was 40–50%, achieved within 3 weeks from initiation. However, in a large phase III trial with moxonidine sustained release (MOXCON) an early increase in death rate and adverse events in the moxonidine SR group led to premature termination of the trial because of safety concerns after 1934 patients had been entered. Final analysis revealed 54 deaths (5·5%) in the moxonidine SR group and 32 deaths (3·1%) in the placebo group. Survival curves revealed a significantly ($P = 0.005$) worse outcome in the moxonidine SR group. Hospitalization for heart failure, acute myocardial infarction, and adverse events were also more frequent in the moxonidine SR group.[215] This trial terminated the efforts to explore whether CNS inhibition of adrenergic activation could be an alternative to β adrenergic blockade in heart failure.

Antiarrhythmic drugs in heart failure

Although progressive pump dysfunction is a common cause of death in heart failure, sudden death is probably the most common reason, and has been considered responsible in 25–50% of all deaths.[216–219] Besides a few cases of primary asystole, the majority of sudden deaths are due to ventricular arrhythmias.[220] The issue of antiarrhythmic therapy in heart failure patients has therefore been of major interest. Internal cardioversion defibrillators are now used for prevention of sudden death from ventricular arrhythmias, and the use of these therapeutic devices is dealt with elsewhere in this book.

Most antiarrhythmics cause a depression of left ventricular function. Although frequent and complex ventricular arrhythmias may be predictive of sudden death, left ventricular dysfunction is a more powerful predictor.[221] Furthermore, these drugs may have a proarrhythmic effect, especially in cases of left ventricular dysfunction. In the CAST study the efficacy of antiarrhythmic drugs in patients with left ventricular dysfunction after myocardial infarction and with complex ventricular arrhythmias was evaluated. Patients who responded with attenuation of arrhythmias after drug testing were randomized to encainide, flecainide, or moricizine. The results showed an increase in mortality in patients treated with these agents.[222] Amiodarone is a class III antiarrhythmic drug with no or little negative inotropic effect. Previous promising smaller trials encouraged larger trials, such as the GESICA study. In this study, 516 patients with heart failure on conventional treatment were randomized to open label amiodarone treatment ($n = 260$) or conventional treatment ($n = 256$). Both sudden deaths and deaths due to heart failure were reduced, comprising in total 87 deaths in patients on amiodorone and 106 in the placebo group ($P = 0.02$).[223] However, these results were not reproduced in another study in patients with CHF and asymptomatic ventricular arrhythmias.[224] In this study 674 patients were investigated, but amiodarone treatment was not associated with reduction of overall mortality or mortality from sudden death. Two other parallel studies have recently been finished, in which amiodarone was used in patients with a recent myocardial infarction and left ventricular dysfunction.[225,226] In addition, patients in the CAMIAT study had complex ventricular arrhythmias. Although all-cause mortality was not significantly lower in the treatment groups, both studies showed a reduction in arrhythmic deaths. A meta-analysis of 13 amiodarone trials demonstrated a significant reduction in total mortality (10·9 *v* 12.3% per year; OR 0·87 [95% CI 0·78–0·99], $P = 0.03$) and in arrhythmic deaths (4·0 *v* 5·7% per year; OR 0·71 [95% CI 0·59–0·85], $P = 0.0003$).[227,228]

Sotalol, a β blocker with class III antiarrhythmic properties, has not been found to reduce deaths from ventricular arrhythmias. On the contrary, a study with the non-β blocker isoform *d*-sotalol in postmyocardial patients had to be terminated in advance because of an increased mortality in the sotalol group.[229]

ACE inhibitors reduce the risk of progressive heart failure deaths. The possibility of ACE inhibitors to affect arrhythmias has been reviewed.[230] In some of the heart failure trials there has also been a reduction in the rate of sudden deaths.[78,231] However, these findings were not confirmed in the SOLVD trial.[232] The most impressive effects on sudden deaths have been found in the large survival studies with β blockers. Consistent effects were found with all three agents, bisoprolol, metoprolol, and carvedilol.[196–198]

Documented value of antiarrhythmic therapy in heart failure

Proven indication: always acceptable **Grade A**

- β Adrenergic blockade in patients with congestive heart failure

Acceptable indication but of uncertain efficacy and may be controversial **Grade B**

- Prevention of arrhythmic deaths in patients with ventricular arrhythmias

Not proven: potentially harmful (contraindicated) **Grade A**

- Class I antiarrhythmic drugs in patients with asymptomatic ventricular arrhythmias and heart failure
- Class III antiarrhythmic drugs, besides amiodarone

Mechanical devices and pacing

Different kinds of left ventricular mechanical assist devices (LVADs) have been studied for several years and they have been in clinical use since at least early 1990s.[233] Long-term effects have been unclear. A randomized trial has been presented in this context. In REMATCH (Randomized Evaluation of Mechanical Assistance for the Treatment of Congestive Heart failure), 129 patients with advanced heart failure in NYHA class IV were randomized to optimal medical management or LVAD (HeartMate).[234] No patient was eligible for heart transplantation. The objectives were to assess effects on survival and quality of life. The mean age was 67 years and the average ejection fraction 17%.

Kaplan–Meier survival analysis showed a reduction of 48% in the risk of death from any cause in the group that received left ventricular assist devices as compared with the medical therapy group (RR 0.52, 95% CI 0.34–0.78, $P = 0.001$). The rates of survival at 1 year were 52% in the device group and 25% in the medical therapy group ($P = 0.002$), and the rates at 2 years were 23% and 8% ($P = 0.09$), respectively. The frequency of serious adverse events in the device group was 2.35 times (95% CI 1·86–2.95) that in the medical therapy group, with a predominance of infection, bleeding, and malfunction of the device. The quality of life was significantly improved at 1 year in the device group assessed as SF-36 and Beck Depression Inventory. There was also a non-significant improvement in Minnesota Living with Heart Failure.

The study shows that LVADs can prolong life and improve quality of life in severe heart failure. The treatment effect is

---

Table 46.1   Key recommendations

Aim of treatment	Class of drug	Level of evidence
Symptomatic improvement of congestion, improvement of exercise capacity	Diuretics	Grade A
Reduction of mortality in mild to moderate heart failure	Angiotensin converting enzyme inhibitors	Grade A
	β Adrenergic blockers	Grade A
Reduction of mortality in severe heart failure	Angiotensin converting enzyme inhibitors	Grade A
	β Adrenergic blockers	Grade A
	Spironolactone	Grade A
Reduction of mortality in patients not tolerating an ACE inhibitor	Angiotensin-II receptor 1 blockers	Grade B
Reduction of morbidity and symptoms in mild–severe heart failure	Angiotensin converting enzyme inhibitors	Grade A
	β Adrenergic blockers	Grade A
	Angiotensin-II receptor 1 blockers	Grade A
	Spironolactone	Grade A
	Digitalis	Grade A
Short-term improvement of symptoms in patients with severe CHF. Bridging towards more definitive surgical treatment, such as cardiac transplantation	Non-digitalis inotropic drugs	Grade A
Prevention of arrhythmic deaths in patients with symptomatic ventricular arrhythmias	Amiodarone	Grade B
Bridging towards heart transplantation in terminal heart failure	Left ventricular assist device	Grade B

limited in time and there was no significant improvement after 2 years. The important question is to evaluate the cost effectiveness of this expensive therapy in relation to other treatments. The published information suggests that the treatment costs were considerable. **Grade B**

There are several surgical approaches to heart failure including revascularization, left ventricular reconstruction, cardiomyoplasty and mitral valvular repair. However, the clinical studies have not been controlled, and yet the partial left ventricular ventriculotomy (Batista) and cardiomyoplasty have even been classified as not recommended. **Grade C**

Besides conventional indication for antibradycardia pacing, other pacing modalities have been tried for patients with CHF. A dual chamber pacing with shortening of the atrioventricular conduction has been investigated in a small series. More recently, so called resynchronization therapy using pacing of both the right and the left ventricles has been introduced. There are promising results from smaller studies showing improved left ventricular function and symptomatology.[237–239] Larger randomized studies are now in progress testing this concept on clinical outcomes.

Concluding remarks

In the treatment of CHF there are two main classes of drugs – ACE inhibitors and β blockers – with solid and consistent documentation for reduction of morbidity and mortality. Furthermore, spironolactone has recently been accepted by the scientific community to be of value in this respect. The ARBs have not sufficient documentation to be placed on an equal status with ACE inhibitors. However, the ARBs are widely accepted as a substitute when patients are not tolerating an ACE inhibitor (Table 46.1). The concept of neurohormonal blockade is also evaluated in studies on endothelin receptor blockers and vasopeptidase inhibitors. Some of these trials are imminent. The development of devices and surgical methods are today somewhat more uncertain.

References

1. Ribner B, Plucinski DA, Hsieh AM *et al.* Acute effects of digoxin on total systemic vascular resistance in congestive heart failure due to dilated cardiomyopathy. *Am J Cardiol* 1985;**56**:896.
2. Gheorghiade M, St Clair J, St Clair C, Beller GA. Hemodynamic effects of intravenous digoxin in patients with severe heart failure initially treated with diuretics and vasodilators. *J Am Coll Cardiol* 1987;**9**:849.
3. Cohn K, Selzer A, Kersh ES *et al.* Variability of hemodynamic response to acute digitalization in chronic cardiac failure due to cardiomyopathy and coronary artery disease. *Am J Cardiol* 1975;**31**:461.
4. Braunwald E. Effects of digitalis on the normal and the failing heart. *J Am Coll Cardiol* 1985;**5**:51A.
5. Ferguson DW, Berg WJ, Sanders JS *et al.* Sympathoinhibitory responses to digitalis glycosides in heart failure patients. *Circulation* 1989;**80**:65–77.
6. Ferguson DW. Baroreflex-mediated circulatory control in human heart failure. *Heart Failure* 1990;**6**:3.
7. Goldsmith SR, Simon AB, Miller E. Effect of digitalis on norepinephrine kinetics in congestive heart failure. *J Am Coll Cardiol* 1992;**20**:858–63.
8. Dobbs SN, Kenyon WI, Dobbs RJ. Maintenance digoxin after an episode of heart failure. Placebo controlled trial in outpatients. *BMJ* 1977;**1**:749.
9. Fleg L, Gottlieb SH, Lakatta EG. Is digoxin really important in compensated heart failure? *Am J Med* 1982;**73**:244.
10. Taggart AJ, Johnston GD, McDevitt DG. Digoxin withdrawal after cardiac failure in patients with sinus rhythm. *J Cardiovasc Pharmacol* 1983;**5**:229.
11. Lee DCS, Johnston RA, Bingham JB *et al.* Heart failure in outpatients. A randomized trial of digoxin versus placebo. *N Engl J Med* 1982;**306**:699.
12. Guyatt GH, Sullivan MJJ, Fallen EL *et al.* A controlled trial of digoxin in congestive heart failure. *Am J Cardiol* 1988;**61**:371.
13. Haerer W, Bauer U, Hetzel M, Fehske J. Long-term effects of digoxin and diuretics in congestive heart failure. Results of a placebo-controlled randomized double-blind study. *Circulation* 1988;**78**:53.
14. The Captopril-Digoxin Multicenter Research Group. Comparative effects of therapy with captopril and digoxin in patients with mild moderate heart failure. *JAMA* 1988;**259**:539–44.
15. German and Austrian Xamoterol Study Group. Double-blind placebo-controlled comparison of digoxin and xamoterol in chronic heart failure. *Lancet* 1988;**i**:489.
16. DiBianco R, Shabetai R, Kostuk W *et al.* A comparison of oral milrinone, digoxin, and their combination in the treatment of patients with chronic heart failure. *N Engl J Med* 1989;**320**:677–83.
17. Uretsky BF, Young JB, Shahidi FE *et al.* Randomized study assessing the effect of digoxin withdrawal in patients with mild to moderate chronic congestive heart failure: results of the PROVED Trial. *J Am Coll Cardiol* 1993;**22**:955–62.
18. Packer M, Gheorghiade M, Young JB *et al.* Withdrawal of digoxin from patients with chronic heart failure treated with angiotensin-converting enzyme inhibitors. *N Engl J Med* 1993;**329**:1–7.
19. Perry G, Brown E, Thornton R *et al.* The effect of digoxin on mortality and morbidity in patients with heart failure. *N Engl J Med* 1997;**336**:525–33.
20. Stason WR, Cannon PJ, Heinemann HO, Laragh JH. Furosemide: a clinical evaluation of diuretic action. *Circulation* 1966;**34**:910–20.
21. Cody RJ, Ljungman S, Covit AB *et al.* Regulation of glomerular filtration rate in chronic congestive heart failure patients. *Kidney Int* 1988;**34**:361–7.
22. Francis GS, Goldsmith SR, Levine TB, Olivari MT, Cohn JN. The neurohumoral axis in congestive heart failure. *Ann Intern Med* 1984;**101**:370–7.

23. Lal S, Murtagw JG, Pollock AM, Fletcher E, Binnion PF. Acute hemodynamic effects of furosemide in patients with normal and raised left atrial pressures. *Br Heart J* 1969;**31**: 711–17.

24. Stampfer M, Epstein SE, Beiser D, Braunwald E. Haemodynamic effects of diuresis at rest and during intense uprights exercise in patients with impaired cardiac function. *Circulation* 1968;**37**:900–11.

25. Magrini F, Niarchos AP. Hemodynamic effects of massive peripheral edema. *Am Heart J* 1983;**105**:90–4.

26. Francis GS, Siegel RM, Goldsmith SR *et al.* Acute vasoconstrictor response to intravenous furosemide in patients with chronic congestive heart failure. *Ann Intern Med* 1985; **103**:1–6.

27. Dikshit K, Vyden JK, Forrester JS *et al.* Renal and extrarenal hemodynamic effects of furosemide in congestive heart failure after myocardial infarction. *N Engl J Med* 1973;**288**: 1087–90.

28. Nelson GIC, Ahuja RC, Silke B, Taylor SH. Haemodynamic effects of furosemide and its influence on repetitive rapid volume loading in acute myocardial infarction. *Eur Heart J* 1983;**4**:706–11.

29. Verma SP, Silke B, Reynolds G *et al.* Immediate effects of bumetanide on systemic haemodynamics and left ventricular volume in acute and chronic heart failure. *Br J Clin Pharmacol* 1987;**24**:21–32.

30. Ramirez A, Abelman WH. Haemodynamic effects of diuresis by ethacrynic acid. *Ann Intern Med* 1968;**121**:320–7.

31. Valette H, Hebert JL, Apoil E. Acute haemodynamic effects of a single intravenous dose of piretanide in congestive heart failure. *Eur J Clin Pharmacol* 1983;**24**:163–7.

32. Fiehring H, Achhammer I. Influence of 10 mg torasemide iv and 20 mg furosemide iv on the intracardiac pressures in patients with heart failure at rest and during exercise. *Prog Pharmacol Clin Pharmacol* 1990;**8**:87–104.

33. Mackay IG, Muir AL, Watson ML. Contribution of prostaglandins to the systemic and renal vascular response to frusemide in normal man. *Br J Clin Pharmacol* 1984;**17**: 513–19.

34. Ikram H, Chan W, Espiner EA, Nicholls ME. Haemodynamic and humoral responses to acute and chronic frusemide therapy in congestive heart failure. *Clin Sci* 1980;**59**:443–9.

35. Haerer W, Bauer U, Sultan N. Acute and chronic effects of a diuretic monotherapy with piretanide in congestive heart failure – a placebo controlled trial. *Cardiovasc Drugs Ther* 1990;**4**:515–22.

36. Podszus T, Piesche L. Effect of torasemide on pulmonary and cardiac haemodynamics after oral treatment of chronic heart failure. *Prog Pharmacol Clin Pharmacol* 1990;**8**:157–66.

37. Cheitlin MD, Byrd R, Benowitz N. Amiloride improves haemodynamics in patients with chronic congestive heart failure treated with chronic digoxin and diuretics. *Cardiovasc Drugs Ther* 1991;**5**:719–26.

38. Francis GS, Benedict C, Johnstone DE *et al.* Comparison of neuroendocrine activation in patients with left ventricular dysfunction with and without congestive heart failure. *Circulation* 1990;**82**:1724–9.

39. Bayliss J, Norell M, Canepa-Anson R, Sutton G, Poole-Wilson P. Untreated heart failure: clinical and neuroendocrine effects of introducing diuretics. *Br Heart J* 1987;**57**:17–22.

40. Achhammer I. Long-term efficacy and tolerance of torasemide in congestive heart failure. *Prog Pharmacol Clin Pharmacol* 1990;**8**:127–36.

41. Dusing R, Piesche L. Second-line therapy of congestive heart failure with torasemide. *Prog Pharmacol Clin Pharmacol* 1990;**8**:105–20.

42. Odemuyiwa O, Gilmartin J, Kenny D, Hall RJC. Captopril and the diuretic requirements in moderate and severe chronic heart failure. *Eur Heart J* 1989;**10**:586.

43. Anand IS, Kalra GS, Ferrari R *et al.* Enalapril as initial and sole treatment in severe chronic heart failure with sodium retention. *Int J Cardiol* 1990;**28**:341.

44. Richardson A, Bayliss J, Scriven AJ *et al.* Double-blind comparison of captopril alone against furosemide plus amiloride in mild heart failure. *Lancet* 1987;**ii**:709.

45. Cody RJ, Kubo SH, Pickworth KK. Diuretic treatment for the sodium retention of congestive heart failure. *Arch Intern Med* 1994;**154**:1905–14.

46. Laragh JH. Hormones in the pathogenesis of congestive heart failure: vasopressin, aldosterone, angiotensin II. *Circulation* 1962;**25**:1015–23.

47. Swedberg K, Eneroth P, Kjekshus J, Wilhelmsen L, for the CONSENSUS trial study group. Hormones regulating cardiovascular function in patients with severe congestive heart failure and their relation to mortality. *Circulation* 1990;**82**:1730–6.

48. Weber KT, Brilla CG. Pathological hypertrophy and cardiac interstitium. Fibrosis and renin-angiotensin-aldosterone system. *Circulation* 1991;**83**:1849–65.

49. Young M, Fullerton M, Dilley R, Funder J. Mineralocorticoids, hypertension, and cardiac fibrosis. *J Clin Invest* 1994;**93**: 2578–83.

50. Pitt B, Zannad F, Remme WJ, Cody R, Castaigne A, Perez A *et al.* The effect of spironolactone on morbidity and mortality in patients with severe failure. Randomized Aldactone Evaluation Study Investigators. *N Engl J Med* 1999;**341**: 709–17.

51. Eichna LW, Sobel BJ, Kessler RH. Hemodynamic and renal effects produced in congestive heart failure by the intravenous administration of a ganglionic blocking agent. *Trans Assoc Am Phys* 1956;**69**:207–13.

52. Burch GE. Evidence for increased venous tone in chronic heart failure. *Arch Intern Med* 1956;**98**:750–66.

53. Zelis R, Mason DT, Braunwald E. A comparison of the effects of vasodilator stimuli on peripheral resistance vessels in normal subjects and in patients with congestive heart failure. *J Clin Invest* 1968;**47**:960–70.

54. Majid PA, Sharma B, Taylor SH. Phentolamine for vasodilator treatment of severe heart failure. *Lancet* 1971;**ii**:719–24.

55. Franciosa JA, Guiha NH, Limas CJ, Rodriguera E, Cohn JN. Improved left ventricular function during nitroprusside infusion in acute myocardial infarction. *Lancet* 1972;**i**:650–4.

56. Cohn JN, Franciosa JA. Vasodilator therapy of cardiac failure. *N Engl J Med* 1977;**297**:27–31.

57. Tsai SC, Adamik R, Manganiello VC, Moss J. Effects of nitroprusside and nitroglycerin on cGMP content and PGI2 formation in aorta and vena cava. *Biochem Pharmacol* 1989; **38**:61–5.

58. Lavine SJ, Campbell CA, Held AC, Johnson V. Effect of nitroglycerin-induced reduction of left ventricular filling pressure

on diastolic filling in acute dilated heart failure. *J Am Coll Cardiol* 1989;**14**:233–41.

59. Mason DT, Braunwald E. The effects of nitroglycerin and amyl nitrate on arteriolar and venous tone in the human forearm. *Circulation* 1965;**32**:755–65.

60. Armstrong PW, Armstrong JA, Marks GS. Pharmacokinetic-hemodynamic studies of intravenous nitroglycerin in congestive heart failure. *Circulation* 1980;**62**:160–6.

61. Leier CV, Bambach D, Thompson MJ *et al.* Central and regional hemodynamic effects of intravenous isosorbide dinitrate, nitroglycerin, and nitroprusside in patients with congestive heart failure. *Am J Cardiol* 1981;**48**:1115–23.

62. Flaherty JT, Reid PR, Kelly DT *et al.* Intravenous nitroglycerin in acute myocardial infarction. *Circulation* 1975;**51**:132–9.

63. Ludbrook PR, Byrne JD, Kurnik PB, McKnight RC. Influence of reduction of preload and afterload by nitroglycerin on left ventricular diastolic pressure-volume relation and relaxation in man. *Circulation* 1977;**56**:937–43.

64. DeMarco T, Chatterjee K, Rouleau JL, Parmley WW. Abnormal coronary hemodynamics and myocardial energetics in patients with chronic heart failure caused by ischemic heart disease and dilated cardiomyopathy. *Am Heart J* 1988;**115**:809–15.

65. Unverferth DV, Magorien RD, Lewis RP, Leier CV. The role of subendocardial ischemia in perpetuating myocardial failure in patients with nonischemic congestive cardiomyopathy. *Am Heart J* 1983;**105**:176–9.

66. Chiariello M, Gold HK, Leinbach RC, David MA, Maroko PR. Comparison between the effects of nitroprusside and nitroglycerin on ischemic injury during acute myocardial infarction. *Circulation* 1976;**54**:766–73.

67. Stevenson LW, Dracup KA, Tillisch JH. Efficacy of medical therapy tailored for severe congestive heart failure in patients transferred for urgent cardiac transplantation. *Am J Cardiol* 1989;**63**:461–4.

68. Chatterjee K, Ports TA, Brundage BH *et al.* Oral hydralazine in chronic heart failure: sustained beneficial hemodynamic effects. *Ann Intern Med* 1980;**92**:600–4.

69. Franciosa JA, Nordstrom LA, Cohn JN. Nitrate therapy for congestive heart failure. *JAMA* 1978;**240**:443–6.

70. Miller RR, Awan NA, Maxwell KS, Mason DT. Sustained reduction of cardiac impedance and preload in congestive heart failure with the antihypertensive vasodilator prazosin. *N Engl J Med* 1977;**297**:303–7.

71. Franciosa JA, Jordan RA, Wilen MM, Leddy CL. Minoxidil in patients with chronic left heart failure: contrasting hemodynamic and clinical effects in a controlled trial. *Circulation* 1984;**70**:63–8.

72. Leier CV, Desch CE, Magorien RD *et al.* Positive inotropic effects of hydralazine in human subjects. Comparison with prazosin in the setting of congestive heart failure. *Am J Cardiol* 1980;**46**:1039–44.

73. Rouleau JL, Chatterjee K, Benge W, Parmley WW, Hiramatsu B. Alterations in left ventricular function and coronary hemodynamics with captopril, hydralazine, and prazosin in chronic ischemic heart failure, a comparative study. *Circulation* 1982;**65**:671–8.

74. Daly P, Rouleau JL, Cousineau D, Burgess JH, Chatterjee K. Effects of captopril and a combination of hydralazine and

isosorbide dinitrate on myocardial sympathetic tone in patients with severe congestive heart failure. *Br Heart J* 1986;**56**:152–7.

75. Magorien RD, Unverferth DV, Brown GP, Leier CV. Dobutamine and hydralazine. Comparative influences of positive inotropy and vasodilation on coronary blood flow and myocardial energetics in nonischemic congestive heart failure. *J Am Coll Cardiol* 1983;**1**:499–505.

76. Massie B, Chatterjee K, Werner J *et al.* Hemodynamic advantage of combined administration of hydralazine orally and nitrates nonparenterally in the vasodilator therapy of chronic heart failure. *Am J Cardiol* 1977;**40**:794–801.

77. Packer M, Meller J, Medina N, Yushak M, Gorlin R. Provocation of myocardial ischemia events during initiation of vasodilator therapy for severe chronic heart failure. Clinical and hemodynamic evaluation of 52 consecutive patients with ischemic cardiomyopathy. *Am J Cardiol* 1981;**48**:939–46.

78. Cohn JN, Johnson G, Ziesche S *et al.* A comparison of enalapril with hydralazine-isosorbide dinitrate in the treatment of chronic congestive heart failure. *N Engl J Med* 1991;**325**:303–10.

79. Elkayam U, Amin J, Mehra A *et al.* A prospective, randomized, double-blind, crossover study to compare the efficacy and safety of chronic nifedipine therapy with that of isosorbide dinitrate and their combination in the treatment of chronic congestive heart failure. *Circulation* 1990;**82**:1954–61.

80. Danish Study Group on Verapamil in Myocardial Infarction. Secondary prevention with verapamil after myocardial infarction. *Am J Cardiol* 1990;**66**:331–401.

81. Iida K, Matsuda M, Ajisaka R *et al.* Effects of nifedipine on left ventricular systolic and diastolic function in patients with ischemic heart disease. *Japan Heart J* 1987;**28**:495–506.

82. Barjon JN, Rouleau JL, Bichet D, Juneau C, De Champlain J. Chronic renal and neurohumoral effects of the calcium-entry blocker nisoldipine in patients with congestive heart failure. *J Am Coll Cardiol* 1987;**9**:622–30.

83. Gheorghiade M, Hall V, Goldberg D, Levine TB, Goldstein S. Long-term clinical and neurohormonal effects of nicardipine in patients with severe heart failure on maintenance therapy with angiotensin converting enzyme inhibitors. *J Am Coll Cardiol* 1991;**17**:274A.

84. Dunselman PHJM, Kuntze CEE, Van Bruggen A *et al.* Efficacy of felodipine in congestive heart failure. *Eur Heart J* 1989;**10**:354–64.

85. Cohn JN, Archibald DG, Ziesche S *et al.* Effect of vasodilator therapy on mortality in chronic congestive heart failure. *N Engl J Med* 1986;**314**:1547–52.

86. Cohn JN, Ziesche SM, Smith R *et al.* Effect of the calcium antagonist felodipine has supplementary vasodilator therapy in patients with chronic heart failure treated with enalapril: V-HeFT III. *Circulation* 1997;**96**:856–63.

87. Packer M, O'Connor CM, Ghali JK *et al.* Effect of amlodipine on morbidity and mortality in severe chronic heart failure. *N Engl J Med* 1996;**335**:1107–14.

88. Thackray S, Witte K, Clark AL, Cleland JG. Clinical trials update: OPTIME-CHF, PRAISE-2, ALL-HAT. *Eur J Heart Fail* 2000;**2**:209–12.

89. Packer M, Rouleau J, Swedberg K *et al.* Effect of flosequinan on survival in chronic heart failure. *Circulation* 1993;**88**:301.

90.McKenna WJ, Swedberg K, Zannad F *et al.* Experience of chronic intravenous epoprostenol infusion in end-stage cardiac failure:results of FIRST. *Eur Heart J* 1994;**15**:I-36.

91.Sharpe DN, Murphy J, Coxon R, Hannan SF. Enalapril in patients with chronic heart failure: a placebo-controlled, randomized, double-blind study. *Circulation* 1984;**70**:271–8.

92.DiCarlo L, Chatterjee K, Parmley WW *et al.* Enalapril A new angiotensin converting inhibitor in chronic heart failure:acute and chronic hemodynamic evaluations. *J Am Coll Cardiol* 1983;**2**:865–71.

93.Packer M, Medina N, Yushak M, Lee WH. Usefulness of plasma renin activity in predicting haemodynamic and clinical responses and survival during long term converting enzyme inhibition in severe chronic heart failure. Experience in 100 consecutive patients. *Br Heart J* 1985;**54**:298–304.

94.The Consensus Trial Study Group. Effects of enalapril on mortality in severe congestive heart failure. *N Engl J Med* 1987;**316**:1429–35.

95.Sharpe N, Murphy J, Heather S, Hannan S. Treatment of patients with symptomless left ventricular dysfunction after myocardial infarction. *Lancet* 1988;**i**:255–9.

96.Pfeffer JM, Pfeffer MA. Angiotensin converting enzyme inhibition and ventricular remodeling in heart failure. *Am J Med* 1988;**84**:37–44.

97.Swedberg K, Eneroth P, Kjekshus J, Wilhelmsen L for the CONSENSUS Trial Study Group. Hormones regulating cardiovascular function in patients with severe congestive heart failure and their relation to mortality. *Circulation* 1990;**82**: 1730–6.

98.Packer M. The neurohormonal hypothesis: a theory to explain the mechanism of disease progression in heart failure. *J Am Coll Cardiol* 1992;**20**:248–54.

99.The SOLVD Investigators. Effect of enalapril on mortality and the development of heart failure in asymptomatic patients with reduced left ventricular ejection fractions. *N Engl J Med* 1992;**327**:685–91.

100.Rogers WJ, Johnstone DE, Yusuf S *et al.* Quality of life among 5025 patients with left ventricular dysfunction randomized between placebo and enalapril: the studies of left ventricular dysfunction. *J Am Coll Cardiol* 1994;**23**:393–400.

101.Pfeffer MA, Braunwald E, Moyé LA *et al.* Effect of captopril on mortality and morbidity in patients with left ventricular dysfunction after myocardial infarction. *N Engl J Med* 1992;**327**:669–77.

102.Kober L, Torp-Pedersen C, Carlsen JE *et al.* A clinical trial of the angiotensin-converting-enzyme inhibitor trandolapril in patients with left ventricular dysfunction after myocardial infarction. *N Engl J Med* 1995;**333**:1670–6.

103.The Acute Infarction Ramipril Efficacy (AIRE) Study Investigators. Effect of ramipril on mortality and morbidity of survivors of acute myocardial infarction with clinical evidence of heart failure. *Lancet* 1993;**342**:821–8.

104.Packer M, Poole-Wilson PA, Armstrong PW *et al.* Comparative effects of low and high doses of the angiotensin-converting enzyme inhibitor, lisinopril, on morbidity and mortality in chronic heart failure. ATLAS Study Group. *Circulation* 1999; **100**:2312–18.

105.Flather MD, Yusuf S, Kober L *et al.* Long-term ACE-inhibitor therapy in patients with heart failure or left-ventricular dysfunction: a systematic overview of data from individual patients. ACE-Inhibitor Myocardial Infarction Collaborative Group. *Lancet* 2000;**355**:1575–81.

106.Narang R, Swedberg K, Cleland JG. What is the ideal study design for evaluation of treatment for heart failure? Insights from trials assessing the effect of ACE inhibitors on exercise capacity. *Eur Heart J* 1996;**17**:120–34.

107.Garg R, Yusuf S. Overview of randomized trials of angiotensin-converting enzyme inhibitors on mortality and morbidity in patients with heart failure. *JAMA* 1995;**273**: 1450–6.

108.Yusuf S, Pepine CJ, Garces C *et al.* Effect of enalapril on myocardial infarction and unstable angina in patients with low ejection fractions. *Lancet* 1992;**340**:1173–8.

109.Yusuf S, Sleight P, Pogue J, Bosch J, Davies R, Dagenais G. Effects of an angiotensin-converting-enzyme inhibitor, ramipril, on cardiovascular events in high-risk patients. The Heart Outcomes Prevention Evaluation Study Investigators. *N Engl J Med* 2000;**342**:145–53.

110.Paul SD, Kuntz KM, Eagle KA, Weinstein MC. Costs and effectiveness of angiotensin converting enzyme inhibition in patients with congestive heart failure. *Arch Intern Med* 1994;**154**:1143–9.

111.Tsevat J, Duke D, Goldman L *et al.* Cost effectiveness of captopril therapy after myocardial infarction. *J Am Coll Cardiol* 1995;**26**:914–19.

112.Martinez C, Ball SG. Cost effectiveness of ramipril therapy for patients with clinical evidence of heart failure after acute myocardial infarction. *Br J Clin Pract* 1995;**78**(Suppl.): 26–32.

113.McMurray J, Davie A. The pharmacoeconomics of ACE inhibitors in chronic heart failure. *Pharmacoeconomics* 1996;**9**:188–97.

114.Dickstein K, Chang P, Willenheimer *et al.* Comparison of the effects of losartan and enalapril on clinical status and exercise performance in patients with moderate or severe chronic heart failure. *J Am Coll Cardiol* 1995;**26**:438–45.

115.Pitt B, Segal R, Martinez FA *et al.* Randomised trial of losartan versus captopril in patients over 65 with heart failure (Evaluation of losartan in the elderly study, ELITE). *Lancet* 1997;**349**:747–52.

116.Pitt B, Poole-Wilson PA, Segal R *et al.* Effect of losartan compared with captopril on mortality in patients with symptomatic heart failure: randomised trial – the Losartan Heart Failure Survival Study ELITE II. *Lancet* 2000;**355**:1582–7.

117.McKelvie RS, Yusuf S, Pericak D *et al.* Comparison of candesartan, enalapril, and their combination in congestive heart failure: randomized evaluation of strategies for left ventricular dysfunction (RESOLVD) pilot study. The RESOLVD Pilot Study Investigators. *Circulation* 1999;**100**:1056–64.

118.Feldman AM. Classification of positive inotropic agents. *J Am Coll Cardiol* 1993;**22**:1233–7.

119.Smith JH, Oriol A, Morch J *et al.* Hemodynamic studies in cardiogenic shock. Treatment with isoproterenol and metaraminol. *Circulation* 1967;**35**:1084–91.

120.Tuttle RR, Mills J. Dobutamine. Development of a new catecholamine to selectively increase cardiac contractility. *Circ Res* 1975;**36**:185–96.

121.Meyer SL, Curry GC, Donsky MS *et al.* Influence of dobutamine on hemodynamics and coronary blood flow in patients with and without coronary artery disease. *Am J Cardiol* 1976;**38**:103–8.

122.Akhtar N, Midulic E, Cohn JN, Chaudry MH. Hemodynamic effect of dobutamine in patients with severe heart failure. *Am J Cardiol* 1975;**36**:202–5.

123.Leier CV, Webel J, Buch CA. The cardiovascular effects of the continuous infusion of dobutamine in patients with severe cardiac failure. *Circulation* 1977;**56**:468–72.

124.Pozen RG, DiBianco R, Katz RJ *et al.* Myocardial metabolic and hemodynamic effects of dobutamine in heart failure complicating coronary artery disease. *Circulation* 1981;**63**:1279–85.

125.Leier CV, Unverferth DV, Kates RE. The relationship between plasma dobutamine concentrations and cardiovascular responses in cardiac failure. *Am J Med* 1979;**66**:238–42.

126.Colucci WS, Denniss AR, Leatherman GF. Intracoronary infusion of dobutamine to patients with and without severe congestive heart failure. *J Clin Invest* 1988;**81**:1103–10.

127.Bristow MR, Port JD, Hershberger RE, Gilbert EM, Feldman AM. The β-adrenergic receptor-adenylate cyclase complex as a target for therapeutic intervention in heart failure. *Eur Heart J* 1989;**10**:45–54.

128.Unverferth DV, Blanford M, Kates RE, Leier VI. Tolerance to dobutamine after a 72-hour continuous infusion. *Am J Med* 1980;**69**:262–6.

129.Applefeld MM, Newman KA, Grove WR *et al.* Intermittent continuous outpatient dobutamine infusion in the management of congestive heart failure. *Am J Cardiol* 1983;**51**:455–8.

130.Dies F, Krell MJ, Whitlow P *et al.* Intermittent dobutamine in ambulatory outpatients with chronic cardiac failure. *Circulation* 1986;**74**:II-38–II-38.

131.Goldberg LI. Cardiovascular and renal actions of dopamine. Potential clinical application. *Pharmacol Rev* 1972;**241**:1–29.

132.Goldberg LI, Volkman PH, Kohli JD. A comparison of the vascular dopamine receptor with other dopamine receptors. *Annu Rev Pharmacol Toxicol* 1978;**18**:57–79.

133.Rajfer SI, Goldberg LI. Dopamine in the treatment of heart failure. *Eur Heart J* 1982;**3**:103–6.

134.Lockhandwala MF, Barrett RJ. Cardiovascular dopamine receptors. Physiological pharmaceutical and therapeutic implications. *J Auton Pharmacol* 1982;**2**:189–215.

135.Caponetto S, Terrachini V, Canale C *et al.* Long-term treatment of congestive heart failure with oral ibopamine: effects of rhythm disorders and neurohormonal alterations. *Cardiology* 1990;**77**:43–8.

136.Itoh H, Taniguchi K, Tsajibayashi R, Koike A, Sato Y. Hemodynamic effects and pharmacokinetics of long-term therapy with ibopamine in patients with chronic heart failure. *Cardiology* 1992;**80**:356–60.

137.van Veldhuisen DJ, Man in't Veld AJ, Dunselman PHJM *et al.* Double-blind placebo-controlled study of ibopamine and digoxin in patients with mild to moderate heart failure: results of the Dutch Ibopamine Multicenter Trial (DIMT). *J Am Coll Cardiol* 1993;**22**:1564–73.

138.Hampton JR, van Veldhuisen DJ, Kleber FX *et al.* Randomised study of effect of ibopamine on survival in patients with advanced severe heart failure. *Lancet* 1997;**349**:971–7.

139.The Xamoterol in Severe Heart Failure Study Group. Xamoterol in severe heart failure. *Lancet* 1990;**336**:1–6.

140.Alousi AA, Farah AE, Lesher GY, Opalka CJJ. Cardiotonic activity of amrinone-WIN 40680 [5-amino-3,4′bipyridin-6(1H)-one]. *Circ Res* 1979;**45**:666–77.

141.Millard RW, Dube G, Grupp G *et al.* Direct vasodilator and positive inotropic actions of amrinone. *J Mol Cell Cardiol* 1980;**12**:647–52.

142.Firth B, Ratner AV, Grassman ED *et al.* Assessment of the inotropic and vasodilator effects of amrinone versus isoproterenol. *Am J Cardiol* 1984;**54**:1331–6.

143.Rettig GF, Schieffer HJ. Acute effects of intravenous milrinone in heart failure. *Eur Heart J* 1989;**10**:39–43.

144.Baim DS, McDowell AV, Cherniles J *et al.* Evaluation of a new bipyridine inotropic agent – milrinone – in patients with severe congestive heart failure. *N Engl J Med* 1983;**309**:748–56.

145.Klocke RK, Mager G, Kux A *et al.* Effects of a twenty-four hour milrinone infusion in patients with severe heart failure and cardiogenic shock as a function of the hemodynamic initial condition. *Am Heart J* 1991;**121**:1965–73.

146.Kinney EL, Ballard JO, Carlin B, Zelis R. Amrinone-mediated thrombocytopenia. *Scand J Haematol* 1983;**31**:376–80.

147.Cowley AJ, Stainer K, Fullwood L, Muller AF, Hampton JR. Effects of enoximone in patients with heart failure uncontrolled by captopril and diuretics. *Int J Cardiol* 1990;**28**:S45–S53.

148.Bristow MR, Renlund DG, Gilbert EM, O'Connell JB. Enoximone in severe heart failure: clinical results and effects on β-adrenergic receptors. *Int J Cardiol* 1990;**28**:S21.

149.Herrmann HC, Ruddy TD, Dec GW *et al.* Diastolic function in patients with severe heart failure: comparison of the effects of enoximone and nitroprusside. *Circulation* 1987;**75**:1214–21.

150.Gage J, Rutman H, Lucido D, LeJemtel TH. Additive effects of dobutamine and amrinone on myocardial contractility and ventricular performance in patients with severe heart failure. *Circulation* 1986;**74**:367–73.

151.Uretsky BF, Lawless CE, Verbalis JG *et al.* Combined therapy with dobutamine and amrinone in severe heart failure. *Chest* 1987;**92**:657–62.

152.Anderson JL. Hemodynamic and clinical benefits with intravenous milrinone in severe chronic heart failure. Results of a multicenter study in the United States. *Am Heart J* 1991;**121**:1956–64.

153.Packer M, Carver JR, Rodeheffer RJ *et al.* Effect of oral milrinone on mortality in severe chronic heart failure. *N Engl J Med* 1991;**325**:1468–75.

154.Uretsky BF, Jessup M, Konstam MA *et al.* Multicenter trial of oral enoximone in patients with moderate to moderately severe congestive heart failure. *Circulation* 1990;**82**:774–80.

155.DiBianco R, Shebetai R, Silverman BD *et al.* Oral amrinone for the treatment of chronic congestive heart failure. Results of a multicenter randomized double-blind and placebo-controlled withdrawal study. *J Am Coll Cardiol* 1984;**4**:855–66.

156.Hagemeijer F. Calcium sensitization with pimobendan. Pharmacology, haemodynamic improvement, and sudden death in patients with chronic congestive heart failure. *Eur Heart J* 1993;**14**:551–66.

157. Fujino K, Sperelakis N, Solaro RJ. Sensitization of dog and guinea pig heart myofilaments to calcium activation and the inotropic effect of pimobendan. Comparison with milrinone. *Circ Res* 1988;**63**:911–22.

158. Böhm M, Morano I, Pieske B *et al.* Contribution of cAMP-phosphodiesterase inhibition and sensitization of the conctractile proteins for calcium to the inotropic effects of pimobendan in the failing human heart. *Circ Res* 1991;**68**: 689–701.

159. Katz SD, Kubo SH, Jessup M *et al.* A multicenter, randomized, double-blind, placebo-controlled trial of pimobendan, a new cardiotonic and vasodilator agent, in patients with severe congestive heart failure. *Am Heart J* 1992;**123**: 95–103.

160. Kubo SH, Gollub S, Bourge R *et al.* Beneficial effects of pimobendan on exercise tolerance and quality of life in patients with heart failure. *Circulation* 1992;**85**:942–9.

161. Just H, Hjalmarson Å, Remme WJ *et al.* pimobendan in congestive heart failure. Results of the PICO trial. *Circulation* 1995;**92**:722.

162. Schwartz A, Wallick ET, Lee SW *et al.* Studies on the mechanism of action of 3,4-dihydro-6-4-(3,4-dimethoxybenzoyl)-1-piperazinyl-2(1H)-quinolinone (OPC-8212), a new positive inotropic drug. *Arzneimittelforschung* 1984;**34**:384–9.

163. Yamashita S, Hosokawa T, Kojima M *et al. In vitro* and *in vivo* studies of 3,4-dihydro-6-[4-(3,4-dimethoxybenzoyl)-1-piperazinyl]-2(1H)-quinolinone on myocardial oxygen consumption in dogs with ischemic heart failure. *Japan Circ J* 1986;**50**:659–66.

164. Matsumori A, Shioi T, Yamada T, Matsui S, Sasayama S. Vesnarinone, a new inotropic agent, inhibits cytokine production by stimulated human blood from patients with heart failure. *Circulation* 1994;**89**:955–8.

165. Feldman AM, Bristow MR, Parmley WW *et al.* Effects of vesnarinone on morbidity and mortality in patients with heart failure. *N Engl J Med* 1993;**329**:149–55.

166. Otsuka America, PNC. Letter to VEST Investigators, 29 July 1996.

167. Nieminen MS, Akkila J, Hasenfuss G, Kleber FX, Lehtonen LA, Mitrovic V *et al.* Hemodynamic and neurohumoral effects of continuous infusion of levosimendan in patients with congestive heart failure. *J Am Coll Cardiol* 2000;**36**: 1903–12.

168. Slawsky MT, Colucci WS, Gottlieb SS *et al.* Acute hemodynamic and clinical effects of levosimendan in patients with severe heart failure. Study Investigators. *Circulation* 2000; **102**:2222–7.

169. Swedberg K, Waagstein F, Hjalmarson Å, Wallentin I. Prolongation of survival in congestive cardiomyopathy by beta-receptor blockade. *Lancet* 1979;**i**:1375–6.

170. Waagstein F, Hjalmarson Å, Varnauskas E, Wallentin I. Effect of chronic beta-adrenergic receptor blockade in congestive cardiomyopathy. *Br Heart J* 1975;**37**:1022–36.

171. Sloand EM, Thompson BT. Propranolol-induced pulmonary edema and shock in a patient with pheochromocytoma. *Arch Intern Med* 1984;**144**:173–4.

172. Greenblatt DJ, Koch-Weser J. Adverse reactions to propranolol in hospitalized patients. *Am Heart J* 1973;**86**: 478–84.

173. Herlitz J, Hjalmarson Å, Holmberg S *et al.* Development of congestive heart failure after treatment with metoprolol in acute myocardial infarction. *Br Heart J* 1984;**51**:539–44.

174. Chadda K, Goldstein S, Byington R, Curb JD. Effect of propranolol after acute myocardial infarction in patients with congestive heart failure. *Circulation* 1986;**73**:503–10.

175. Olsson G, Rehnqvist N. Effect of metoprolol in postinfarction patients with increased heart size. *Eur Heart J* 1986;**7**: 468–74.

176. Gilbert EM, Anderson JL, Deitchman D *et al.* Long-term β-blocker vasodilator therapy improves cardiac function in idiopathic dilated cardiomyopathy: a double-blind, randomized study of bucindolol versus placebo. *Am J Med* 1990;**88**: 223–9.

177. DasGupta P, Lahiri A. Can intravenous beta blockade predict long-term haemodynamic benefit in chronic congestive heart failure secondary to ischaemic heart disease? *Clin Invest* 1992;**70**:S98–S104.

178. Andersson B, Lomsky M, Waagstein F. The link between acute haemodynamic adrenergic beta-blockade and long-term effects in patients with heart failure. *Eur Heart J* 1993;**14**: 1375–85.

179. Haber HL, Simek CL, Gimple LW *et al.* Why do patients with congestive heart failure tolerate the initiation of beta-blocker therapy. *Circulation* 1993;**88**:1610–19.

180. Andersson B, Caidahl K, Di Lenarda A *et al.* Changes in early and late diastolic filling patterns induced by long-term adrenergic beta-blockade in patients with idiopathic dilated cardiomyopathy. *Circulation* 1996;**94**:673–82.

181. Woodley SL, Gilbert EM, Anderson JL *et al.* β-blockade with bucindolol in heart failure caused by ischemic versus idiopathic dilated cardiomyopathy. *Circulation* 1991;**84**:2426–41.

182. Eichhorn EJ, Bedotto JB, Malloy CR *et al.* Effect of β-adrenergic blockade on myocardial function and energetics in congestive heart failure. *Circulation* 1990;**82**:473–83.

183. Bristow MR, O'Connell JB, Gilbert EM *et al.* Dose-response of chronic β-blocker treatment in heart failure from either idiopathic dilated or ischemic cardiomyopathy. *Circulation* 1994;**89**:1632–42.

184. Eichhorn EJ, Heesch CM, Risser RC, Marcoux L, Hatfield B. Predictors of systolic and diastolic improvement in patients with dilated cardiomyopathy treated with metoprolol. *J Am Coll Cardiol* 1995;**25**:154–62.

185. Metra M, Nardi M, Giubbini R, Cas LC. Effects of short- and long-term carvedilol administration on rest and exercise hemodynamic vaiables, exercise capacity and clinical conditions in patients with idiopathic dilated cardiomyopathy. *J Am Coll Cardiol* 1995;**24**:1678–87.

186. Hall SA, Cigarroa CG, Marcoux L *et al.* Time course of improvement in left ventricular function, mass and geometry in patients with congestive heart failure treated with beta-adrenergic blockade. *J Am Coll Cardiol* 1995;**25**:1154–61.

187. Australia-New Zealand Heart Failure Research Collaborative Group. Effects of carvedilol, a vasodilator-β-blocker, in patients with congestive heart failure due to ischemic heart disease. *Circulation* 1995;**92**:212–18.

188. Groenning BA, Nilsson JC, Sondergaard L, Fritz-Hansen T, Larsson HB, Hildebrandt PR. Antiremodeling effects on the left ventricle during beta-blockade with metoprolol in the

treatment of chronic heart failure. *J Am Coll Cardiol* 2000; **36**:2072–80.

189. The RESOLVD Investigators. Effects of metoprolol CR in patients with ischemic and dilated cardiomyopathy: the randomized evaluation of strategies for left ventricular dysfunction pilot study. *Circulation* 2000;**101**:378–84.

190. Newton GE, Parker JD. Acute effects of β_1-selective and nonselective β-adrenergic receptor blockade on cardiac sympathetic activity in congestive heart failure. *Circulation* 1996;**94**:353–8.

191. Andersson B, Blomström-Lundqvist C, Hedner T, Waagstein F. Exercise hemodynamics and myocardial metabolism during long-term beta-adrenergic blockade in severe heart failure. *J Am Coll Cardiol* 1991;**18**:1059–66.

192. Nemanich JW, Veith RC, Abrass IB, Stratton JR. Effects of metoprolol on rest and exercise cardiac function and plasma catecholamines in chronic congestive heart failure secondary to ischemic or idiopathic cardiomyopathy. *Am J Cardiol* 1990;**66**:843–8.

193. Eichhorn EJ, McGhie AI, Bedotto JB et al. Effects of bucindolol on neurohormonal activation in congestive heart failure. *Am J Cardiol* 1991;**67**:67–73.

194. Andersson B, Hamm C, Persson S et al. Improved exercise hemodynamic status in dilated cardiomyopathy after beta-adrenergic blockade treatment. *J Am Coll Cardiol* 1994;**23**: 1397–404.

195. Yoshikawa T, Handa S, Anzai T et al. Early reduction of neurohumoral factors plays a key role in mediating the efficacy of beta-blocker therapy for congestive heart failure. *Am Heart J* 1996;**131**:329–36.

196. CIBIS-II Investigators and Committees. The Cardiac Insufficiency Bisoprolol Study II (CIBIS-II): a randomised trial. *Lancet* 1999;**353**:9–13.

197. The MERIT-HF Study Group. Effect of metoprolol CR/XL in chronic heart failure: Metoprolol CR/XL Randomised Intervention Trial in Congestive Heart Failure (MERIT-HF). *Lancet* 1999;**353**:2001–7.

198. Packer M, Coats AJ, Fowler MB et al. Effect of carvedilol on survival in severe chronic heart failure. *N Engl J Med* 2001; **344**:1651–8.

199. Waagstein F, Bristow MR, Swedberg K et al. Beneficial effects of metoprolol in idiopathic dilated cardiomyopathy. *Lancet* 1993;**342**:1441–6.

200. Colucci WS, Packer M, Bristow MR et al. Carvedilol inhibits clinical progression in patients with mild symptoms of heart failure. *Circulation* 1996;**94**:2800–6.

201. Packer M, Colucci WS, Sackner-Bernstein JD et al. Double-blind, placebo-controlled study of the effects of carvedilol in patients with moderate to severe heart failure. The PRECISE Trial. *Circulation* 1996;**94**:2793–9.

202. Hjalmarson A, Goldstein S, Fagerberg B et al. Effects of controlled-release metoprolol on total mortality, hospitalizations, and well-being in patients with heart failure:the Metoprolol CR/XL. Randomized Intervention Trial in congestive heart failure (MERIT-HF). MERIT-HF Study Group. *JAMA* 2000; **283**:1295–302.

203. Andersson B, for the MDC Study Group. 3-year follow-up of patients randomised in the Metoprolol in Dilated Cardiomyopathy trial. *Lancet* 1998;**351**:1180–1.

204. CIBIS Investigators and Committees. A randomized trial of β-blockade in heart failure. The Cardiac Insufficiency Bisoprolol Study (CIBIS). *Circulation* 1994;**90**:1765–73.

205. Packer M, Bristow MR, Cohn JN et al. The effect of carvedilol on morbidity and mortality in patients with chronic heart failure. *N Engl J Med* 1996;**334**:1349–55.

206. Australia/New Zealand Heart Failure Research Collaborative Group. Randomised, placebo-controlled trial of carvedilol in patients with congestive heart failure due to ischaemic heart disease. *Lancet* 1997;**349**:375–80.

207. The Beta-Blocker Evaluation of Survival Trial Investigators. A trial of the beta-blocker bucindolol in patients with advanced chronic heart failure. *N Engl J Med* 2001;**344**: 1659–67.

208. Goldstein S, Fagerberg B, Hjalmarson Å et al. Metoprolol controlled release/extended release in patients with severe heart failure: Analysis of the experience in the MERIT-HF study. *J Am Coll Cardiol* 2001;**38**:932–8.

209. Doughty RN, MacMahon S, Sharpe N. Beta-blockers in heart failure:promising or proved? *J Am Coll Cardiol* 1994;**23**: 814–21.

210. Maack C, Elter T, Nickenig G et al. Prospective crossover comparison of carvedilol and metoprolol in patients with chronic heart failure. *J Am Coll Cardiol* 2001;**38**:939–46.

211. Dargie HJ. Effect of carvedilol on outcome after myocardial infarction in patients with left-ventricular dysfunction: the CAPRICORN randomised trial. *Lancet* 2001;**357**:1385–90.

212. Manolis AJ, Olympios C, Sifaki M et al. Suppressing sympathetic activation in congestive heart failure. A new therapeutic strategy. *Hypertension* 1995;**26**: 719–24.

213. Swedberg K, Bergh CH, Dickstein K, McNay J, Steinberg M. The effects of moxonidine, a novel imidazoline, on plasma norepinephrine in patients with congestive heart failure. Moxonidine Investigators. *J Am Coll Cardiol* 2000;**35**: 398–404.

214. Swedberg K, Bristow MR, Cohn JN et al. The effects of moxonidine SR, an imidazoline agonist, on plasma norepinephrine in patients with chronic heart failure. *Circulation* 2002 (in press).

215. Jones CG, Cleland JGF. Meeting report – the LIDO, HOPE, MOXCON and WASH studies. *Eur J Heart Fail* 1999;**1**: 425–31.

216. Kannel WB, Plehn JF, Cupples LA. Cardiac failure and sudden death in the Framingham study. *Am Heart J* 1988;**115**: 869–75.

217. Kjekshus J. Arrhythmias and mortality in congestive heart failure. *Am J Cardiol* 1990;**64**:42I–48I.

218. Andersson B, Waagstein F. Spectrum and outcome of congestive heart failure in a hospitalized population. *Am Heart J* 1993;**126**:632–40.

219. Packer M. Sudden unexpected death in patients with congestive heart failure: a second frontier. *Circulation* 1985;**72**: 681–5.

220. Stevenson WG, Stevenson LW, Middlekauff HR, Saxon LA. Sudden death prevention in patients with advanced ventricular dysfunction. *Circulation* 1993;**88**:2593–61.

221. Bigger TJJ, Fleiss JL, Kleiger R et al. The relationship between ventricular arrhythmias, left ventricular dysfunction and mortality in the two years after myocardial infarction. *Circulation* 1984;**69**:250–8.

222. Cardiac Arrhythmia Suppression Trial (CAST) Investigators. Preliminary report. Effect of encainide and flecainide on mortality in a randomized trial of arrhythmia suppression after myocardial infarction. *N Engl J Med* 1989;**321**:406–10.

223. Doval HC, Nul DR, Grancelli HO *et al.* Randomised trial of low-dose amiodarone in severe congestive heart failure. *Lancet* 1994;**344**:493–8.

224. Singh SN, Fletcher RD, Fisher SG *et al.* Amiodarone in patients with congestive heart failure and asymptomatic ventricular arrhythmia. *N Engl J Med* 1995;**333**:77–82.

225. Julian DG. Randomised trial of effect of amiodarone on mortality in patients with left-ventricular dysfunction after recent myocardial infarction: EMIAT. *Lancet* 1997;**349**:667–74.

226. Cairns JA. Randomised trial of outcome after myocardial infarction in patients with frequent or repetitive ventricular premature depolarisations: CAMIAT. *Lancet* 1997;**349**:675–82.

227. Amiodarone Trials Meta-Analysis Investigators. Effect of prophylactic amiodarone on mortality after acute myocardial infarction and in congestive heart failure: meta-analysis of individual data from 6500 patients in randomised trials. Amiodarone Trials Meta-Analysis Investigators. *Lancet* 1997;**350**:1417–24.

228. Connolly SJ. Meta-analysis of antiarrhythmic drug trials. *Am J Cardiol* 1999;**84**:90R–3R.

229. Waldo AL, Camm AJ, deRuyter H *et al.* Effect of D-sotalol on mortality in patients with left ventricular dysfunction after recent and remote myocardial infarction. *Lancet* 1996;**348**: 7–12.

230. Pahor M, Gambassi G, Carbonin P. Antiarrhythmic effects of ACE inhibitors. A matter of faith or reality? *Cardiovasc Res* 1994;**28**:7–12.

231. Newman TJ, Maskin CS, Dennick LG *et al.* Effects of captopril on survival in patients with heart failure. *Am J Med* 1988;**84**:140–4.

232. The SOLVD investigators. Effect of enalapril on survival in patients with reduced left ventricular ejection fractions and congestive heart failure. *N Engl J Med* 1991;**325**:293–302.

233. McCarthy PM, Smedira NO, Vargo RL *et al.* One hundred patients with the HeartMate left ventricular assist device: evolving concepts and technology. *J Thorac Cardiovasc Surg* 1998;**115**:904–12.

234. Louis AA, Manousos IR, Coletta AP, Clark AL, Cleland JG. Clinical trials update: The Heart Protection Study, IONA, CARISA, ENRICHD, ACUTE, ALIVE, MADIT II and REMATCH. *Eur J Heart Fail* 2002;**4**:111–16.

235. Remme WJ, Swedberg K. Guidelines for the diagnosis and treatment of chronic heart failure. *Eur Heart J* 2001;**22**: 1527–60.

236. Iskandrian AS, Mintz GS. Pacemaker therapy in congestive heart failure: a new concept based on excessive utilization of the Frank-Starling mechanism. *Am Heart J* 1986;**112**: 867–70.

237. Auricchio A, Stellbrink C, Block M *et al.* Effect of pacing chamber and atrioventricular delay on acute systolic function of paced patients with congestive heart failure. The Pacing Therapies for Congestive Heart Failure Study Group. The Guidant Congestive Heart Failure Research Group. *Circulation* 1999;**99**:2993–3001.

238. Moss AJ, Hall WJ, Cannom DS *et al.* Improved survival with an implanted defibrillator in patients with coronary disease at high risk for ventricular arrhythmia. Multicenter Automatic Defibrillator Implantation Trial Investigators. *N Engl J Med* 1996;**335**:1933–40.

239. Cazeau S, Leclercq C, Lavergne T *et al.* Effects of multisite biventricular pacing in patients with heart failure and intraventricular conduction delay. *N Engl J Med* 2001;**344**: 873–80.

47 Acute myocarditis and dilated cardiomyopathy

Barbara A Pisani, John F Carlquist

Definition of myocarditis

"Myocarditis is an inflammatory disease of the myocardium which is diagnosed by established histological, immunological and immunochemical criteria." It is an inflammatory cardiomyopathy associated with cardiac dysfunction.[1] There are a variety of etiologic causes of myocarditis and the exact pathophysiologic mechanism remains to be elucidated.

Immunopathogenesis of myocarditis

A broad spectrum of infectious and non-infectious agents have been associated with myocarditis (Boxes 47.1–47.3). The application of virologic, serologic, and, most recently, molecular biologic methods has substantiated epidemiologic observations of an infectious cause in many cases. While there are limited clinical data, there has been significant animal research into the etiology and pathophysiology of myocarditis. Coxsackie A and B viruses have been the most frequently implicated infectious agents in myocarditis. However, serologic studies suggestive of recent infection with Coxsackie virus are found in only about 40% of cases.[2] Similarly, it is uncommon to recover virus in culture from myocardial tissue obtained during or after acute myocarditis despite serologic evidence suggestive of viral infection.[3,4] Molecular genetic methods have continued to provide evidence for antecedent viral infection in some cases of myocarditis. Bowles *et al*[6] using Northern hybridization identified Coxsackie B-specific RNA in nucleic acid extracts of myocardial tissue from nine of 17 patients with histologically proven myocarditis or inflammatory cardiomyopathy.

The use of the polymerase chain reaction (PCR) has produced variable results. Although some studies have found Coxsackie B or other enteroviral sequences in myocardial tissue from cases of cardiomyopathy or myocarditis by PCR,[7] others have failed to find any evidence of persistent Coxsackie B RNA in similar specimens[8] or have found a high frequency of enteroviral RNA in control specimens.[9] In a comparison of 34 children with myocarditis and 17 controls with congenital heart disease, 68% of 38 myocardial specimens had viral genome detected with PCR. There was a predominance of adenovirus when compared with adults.

Box 47.1 Common etiologies of myocarditis

Infectious
- Adenovirus
- Coxsackie virus
- Cytomegalovirus
- Epstein–Barr virus
- HIV-1
- Borrelia (Lyme's disease)
- Toxoplasmosis

Drug induced
- Amphetamines
- Anthracyclines (especially doxorubicin)
- Catecholamines
- Cocaine
- Cyclophosphamide
- Interleukin 2

Systemic diseases
- Crohn's disease
- Kawasaki disease
- Sarcoidosis
- Systemic lupus erythematosus
- Ulcerative colitis
- Cardiac rejection
- Giant cell myocarditis
- Peripartum myocarditis

Hypersensitivity
- Hydrochlorothiazide
- Methyldopa
- Penicillins
- Sulfadiazine
- Sulfamethoxazole

All control specimens and blood specimens were negative.[10] In a group of 40 postorthotopic heart transplant patients, 32% (41 samples) of 129 specimens obtained as a routine surveillance screen to rule out rejection had viral amplification with PCR. Of these, 16 were positive for CMV, 14 for adenovirus, six for enterovirus, three for parvovirus, and two for herpes simplex. In 13 of 21 patients with positive PCR, histologic scores also were consistent with moderate to severe rejection.[11] Matsumori[12] compared 36 patients with heart muscle disease and 40 consecutive patients who underwent cardiac catheterization. In six patients (16·7%)

Box 47.2   Uncommon infectious etiologies of myocarditis

Viral
- Arbovirus (dengue fever, yellow fever)
- Arenavirus (Lassa fever)
- Coronavirus
- Echovirus
- Encephalomyocarditis virus
- Hepatitis B
- Herpes virus
- Influenza virus
- Junin virus
- Mumps virus
- Poliomyelitis virus
- Rabies
- Respiratory syncytial virus
- Rubella virus
- Rubeola virus
- Vaccinia virus
- Varicella virus
- Variola virus

Bacterial
- Brucellosis
- *Campylobacter jejuni*
- *Chlamydia trachomatis*
- Clostridia
- Diphtheria
- Franciscella (Tularemia)
- Gonococcus
- Hemophilus
- Legionella
- Listeria
- Meningococcus
- *Mycobacteria* (*tuberculosis, avium-intercellulare, leprae*)
- Mycoplasma
- Pneumococcus
- Psittacosis
- Salmonella
- Staphylococcus
- Streptococcus
- *Tropheryma whippelii* (Whipple's disease)

Fungal
- Aspergillus
- Actinomycetes
- Blastomyces
- Candida
- Coccidioides
- Cryptococcus
- *Fusarium oxysporum*
- Histoplasma
- Mucormycosis
- Norcardia
- Sporothrix

Rickettsial
- *Rickettsia rickettsii* (Rocky Mountain spotted fever)
- *Coxiella burnetii* (Q fever)
- Scrub typhus
- Typhus

Spirochetal
- Leptospira
- Syphilis

Helminthic
- Cysticercus
- Echinococcus
- Schistosoma
- Toxocara (visceral larva migrans)
- Trichinella

Protozoal
- Entamoeba
- Leishmania

with dilated cardiomyopathy versus one patient (2·5%) with ischemic heart disease, hepatitis C was detected. Of these six patients, three had hepatitis C RNA identified on endomyocardial biopsy by the competitive nested PCR technique. The initial presentation in two patients was 'flu-like syndrome followed by heart failure (endomyocardial biopsy positive for myocarditis in one patient). The third patient presented with chronic heart failure. Thus, the accumulating evidence strongly implicates an antecedent or perhaps persistent or latent viral infection in the pathogenesis of myocarditis. However, the inability to convincingly establish one or a few etiologic agents in all cases suggests that other factors, such as immunologic and/or genetic, are contributory.

The difficulty in recovering infectious agents or even evidence of an ongoing infection in cases of lymphocytic myocarditis has prompted the speculation that this is at least partly autoimmune in etiology. Perhaps the best evidence for an autoimmune component in the progression of the disease comes from murine models of Coxsackie B3-induced myocarditis in susceptible animal strains. This experimental disease shows histologic resemblance to human disease[13–19] and has been useful in examining the immunologic and genetic elements of myocarditis. Original studies of this model showed a biphasic illness in which early (5–7 days postinfection) viral myocyte damage was supplanted later (9–45 days) by mononuclear interstitial infiltration and chronic inflammation.[19,20] During the early phase, infectious virus was readily recovered from the myocardium; during the postinfectious phase, infectious virus was not recoverable. It is noteworthy that genetic factors dictated the susceptibility to the development of the late phase disease[19,20] as well as the susceptibility to the initial viral infection. This animal model closely resembles the currently held model for clinical disease in humans.

The nature of the antigen(s) that initiate and perpetuate the immune response in myocarditis is not known with certainty. The hypothesis of molecular mimicry is frequently invoked to explain the occurrence of autoimmune disease following an infection. Within the framework of this hypothesis, an immune response to a dominant epitope

Box 47.3 Uncommon non-infectious causes of myocarditis

Drug-induced

Toxic myocarditis
- Amphetamines
- Arsenic
- Chloroquine
- Ephedrine[5]
- Emetine
- 5-Fluorouracil
- Interferon α
- Lithium
- Paracetamol
- Thyroid hormone

Hypersensitivity myocarditis
- Acetazolamide
- Allopurinol
- Amphotericin B
- Carbamazepine
- Cephalothin
- Chlorthalidone
- Colchicine
- Diclofenac
- Diphenhydramine
- Furosemide
- Indomethacin
- Isoniazid
- Lidocaine
- Methysergide
- Oxphenbutazone
- Para-aminosalicylic acid
- Phenindione
- Phenylbutazone
- Phenytoin
- Procainamide
- Pyribenzamine
- Ranitidine
- Reserpine
- Spironolactone
- Streptomycin
- Tetracycline
- Trimethaprim

Toxins
- Arsenic
- Carbon monoxide
- Copper
- Iron
- Lead
- Mercury
- Phosphorus
- Scorpion stings
- Snake venom
- Spider bites
- Wasp stings

Systemic diseases
- Arteritis (giant cell, Takayasu)
- β thalassemia major
- Churg–Strauss vasculitis
- Cryoglobulinemia
- Dermatomyositis
- Diabetes mellitus
- Hashimoto's thyroiditis
- Mixed connective tissue disease
- Myasthenia gravis
- Periarteritis nodosa
- Pernicious anemia
- Pheochromocytoma
- Polymyositis
- Rheumatoid arthritis
- Scleroderma
- Sjögren's syndrome
- Thymoma
- Wegener's granulomatosis

Other
- Eosinophilic myocarditis
- Genetic
- Granulomatous myocarditis
- Head trauma
- Hypothermia
- Hyperpyrexia
- Ionizing radiation
- Mononuclear myocarditis

expressed by an infectious agent could induce disease following infection. In the event that a similar or cross-reacting epitope is also present on host cells, tissue damage might result.[21] Coxsackie B3 antibodies that cross-react with myosin have been described.[22] In addition, antibodies against myosin are frequently found in experimental myocarditis.[23,24] An alternative hypothesis is that immune reactivity to self antigens results from the aberrant expression of normally sequestered epitopes or upregulation of epitopes normally expressed at a density that favors tolerance.[25] Thus, an autoimmune component of disease pathology appears to be involved in the experimental model of the disease and, in all likelihood, is etiologic in clinical disease as well. However, the same etiologic pathway may not be followed in all cases of myocarditis. This may explain the failure to identify a consistent underlying immunopathologic picture in most cases of clinical myocarditis.

It appears, therefore, that the etiology of myocarditis is heterogeneous; likewise, a variety of immune effector mechanisms have been identified in myocarditis, further underscoring the heterogeneity of the disease. The earliest potential effector mechanism to be described in myocarditis was the production of autoantibodies to normal cellular antigens. A broad variety of tissue antigens have been identified as targets for autoantibodies. Among these are the β adrenergic receptor,[26] the adenine nucleotide translocator,[27] laminin,[28] branched chain ketoacid dehydrogenase,[29] heat shock protein-60 (HSP-60),[30] and sarcolemmal epitopes.[31] Although antibodies to these antigens are frequently identified in association with myocarditis, their significance is not known. They may function in the pathogenesis of the disease or they may be epiphenomena arising in conjunction with the principal pathogenic process. Perhaps these antibodies do not initiate myocyte damage/dysfunction, but contribute to pathology at later stages of the disease.

Dilated cardiomyopathy: background and pathogenesis

Idiopathic dilated cardiomyopathy (IDC) is characterized by dilation and impaired contraction of the left ventricle or both ventricles.[1] Dilated cardiomyopathy has been postulated to occur in some cases as a result of recognized or unrecognized myocarditis. Dec and colleagues[13–19] reported that endomyocardial biopsy examination revealed myocarditis in 66% of patients with acute dilated cardiomyopathy (of <6 months duration). In the Myocarditis Treatment Trial, only 10% of those screened with heart failure of less than 2 years duration had biopsy-proven myocarditis.[32] Nonetheless, in a substantial number of cases of IDC no identifiable etiologic process can be ascribed. Viral infections have been frequently implicated in IDC, as in myocarditis. Several serologic studies have found increased prevalence or levels of antibodies to Coxsackie B in cases of IDC.[33–36] Recent investigations have used the very sensitive PCR to search for persistent enteroviral RNA in IDC cases with equivocal results. Among the various studies, a wide percentage range of IDC cases with demonstrable enteroviral RNA has been reported (0–32%); in comparison, 0–38% of biopsies from non-IDC cases also have been reported positive for enteroviral RNA.[7,37] Thus, the finding of persistent virus or viral RNA in IDC does not appear to be specific for the disease, although the overall consensus continues to favor an inciting infection in many cases.

A great deal of evidence is suggestive of autoimmune or autoimmune-like mechanisms in the pathogenesis of IDC. A spectrum of autoantibodies against similar cellular components as were identified for acute myocarditis has been found among cases of IDC. The principal cellular components reactive with antiheart antibodies associated with IDC are the adenine nucleotide translocator,[37] β adrenoceptors,[26] myosin,[38] laminin,[28] actin, tropomyosin, and heat shock protein-60 (HSP-60).[30] However, antibodies reactive with tissue antigens are often present in the circulation of asymptomatic individuals.[39] Thus, the source and significance of these antibodies relative to the pathology of IDC remain a mystery.

One of the most frequently examined aspects of IDC is the proposed linkage between disease frequency and the genes of the major histocompatibility complex (MHC). Such

evidence would strengthen the argument for an immunologic component in IDC and establish a genetic component as well. The most frequently described linkage between IDC and MHC genes in Caucasian populations has been with class II alleles. Four of five independent studies identified a positive association of IDC with HLA DR4.[40] An association between HLA DR4 and anti-β receptor antibodies also has been noted.[24] Linkage with other class II alleles has been described in other ethnic groups,[41] underscoring possible ethnic differences. These studies strongly implicate genetically controlled immunologic factors with possible immune reactivity to tissue antigens in the pathogenesis of IDC. The specific predisposing HLA-related locus/loci, however, may depend on the genetic background (ethnicity) as well as the specific vector (viral strain) involved. Conflicting findings regarding the association of HLA DR4 with familial cardiomyopathy have been reported. One study observed an association of DR4 with familial disease,[42] whereas a separate study found no such association.[43]

Despite inconclusive findings implicating HLA DR4 or any HLA allele in IDC, the genetic contribution to familial disease is incontrovertible. The possibility exists that a proportion of sporadic cases may, indeed, represent familial disease of incomplete penetrance (that is, not all gene carriers exhibit the characteristic phenotype of the disease) and that disease expression may be modified by other factors either genetic or environmental. Consistent with this hypothesis, some overlap between familial and sporadic disease has been noted. A central role for dysfunctional cytoskeletal elements in the pathogenesis of dilated cardiomyopathy is emerging. Mutations in the genes for cardiac actin,[44] dystrophin,[45] desmin,[46] and lamin A/C[47] have been found to cosegregate with disease in affected families. A mutated δ-sacroglycan gene, the product of which associates with the dystrophin complex, has been identified in both familial and sporadic cases of dilated cardiomyopathy. Additionally, exon 8 C/T polymorphism of endothelin type A gene has been implicated in sporadic cases of dilated cardiomyopathy.[48] In aggregate, these observations have led to a proposed "common pathway" for the development of cardiomyopathy (both familial and sporadic) that involves cytoskeletal elements.[49] The association of δ-sacroglycan gene mutations with both sporadic and familial cases supports the notion of a degree of etiologic overlap between these diseases involving functional alterations in cytoskeletal elements. This notion is further supported by the finding that variations in the gene encoding the actin-binding region of the nebulette protein, a Z-disc protein is significantly increased in non-familial dilated cardiomyopathy.[50]

Cytoskeletal dysfunction in the pathogenesis of cardiomyopathy is not inconsistent with either immune-mediated or infectious etiologies. As stated above, IDC is frequently associated with antibodies to cytoskeletal elements – for example, laminin,[28] myosin,[38] actin, tropomyosin,[30] and other sarcolemmal epitopes[31] – and immunization with cardiac myosin induces disease in animal models.[51,52] The cytoskeletal common pathway hypothesis also incorporates reported enteroviral associations with the disease. Enteroviral protease 2A was demonstrated to directly cleave dystrophin producing postinfectious cardiomyopathy in a mouse model.[53] Thus, the common pathway concept unifies much of the experimental, genetic and epidemiologic information surrounding myocarditis and cardiomyopathy further substantiating a relationship between these disease entities.

Epidemiology and natural history of myocarditis and IDC

The true incidence of myocarditis is unknown. In 12 747 autopsies performed in Sweden from 1975 to 1984, an incidence of 1·06% was found.[54] However, autopsies of children and young adults presenting with sudden death report an incidence as high as 17–21%.[2] In the Myocarditis Treatment Trial, 9·6% of 2333 patients with recent onset of heart failure (onset within 2 years of study enrollment) met pathologic criteria for myocarditis.[32] Of 3055 patients enrolled in the European Study of Epidemiology and Treatment of Cardiac Inflammatory Diseases (ESETCID) with suspected myocarditis, 526 (17·2%) had either histologic or immunologic evidence of acute or chronic myocarditis. However, only 74 patients met criteria for acute myocarditis.[55] There is both a seasonal variation and a male predominance. Of 136 patients with biopsy-proven myocarditis, 63% presented between December and April.[56] A 'flu-like illness within 3 months of presentation was reported by 57%.[56] Only 41% reported a similar illness within 1 month of presentation.[56] Blacks and males were noted to have a 2·5-fold increased risk.[56] Patients with acute myocarditis tend to present at a somewhat younger age (43 ± 16 years) when compared to patients with IDC (50 ± 17 years).[56]

Of the more than three million people in the United States with heart failure, 25% of cases are secondary to IDC.[57] From 1975 to 1984, Codd and colleagues[58] detected 45 cases of dilated cardiomyopathy based on echocardiography, angiography, endomyocardial biopsy, and autopsy results. The median age at the time of diagnosis was 54 years, although presentation may be in childhood, adulthood, or old age. Forty-one cases (91%) were diagnosed during life. Of these, 36 patients (88%) were symptomatic prior to diagnosis, with dyspnea being the most common symptom (75% were New York Heart Association [NYHA] functional class III–IV). Five patients (14%) had a syncopal event; 27 patients (75%) had clinical heart failure, and nine (25%) had angina. Five of the 41 patients (12%) were identified during a routine medical evaluation and

were asymptomatic. Four cases (9%) were diagnosed at autopsy although all had been symptomatic. The overall age- and sex-adjusted incidence was noted to increase from 3·9/100 000 person-years in 1975–1979 to 7·9/100 000 person-years in 1980–1984. The age- and sex-adjusted prevalence was 36·5/100 000 population. The prevalence of dilated cardiomyopathy in patients less than 55 years old was 17·9/100 000. Within this group, over one third were NYHA functional class III or IV at the time of diagnosis. The annual incidence is 5–8 cases per 100 000.[57] More recently, Felker[59] *et al* reported 51% of 1278 patients referred for symptomatic heart failure were classified as idiopathic. A histologic diagnosis was made in 16% of patients (myocarditis, $n = 117$; amyloidosis, $n = 41$; doxorubicin toxicity, $n = 16$; hemochromatosis, $n = 9$; endomyocardial fibroelastosis, $n = 1$, rheumatic carditis, $n = 1$, thrombotic thrombocytopenic purpura, $n = 1$; and interferon-induced cardiomyopathy $n = 1$). Endomyocardial biopsy in IDC yielded non-specific findings, including myocyte hypertrophy or interstitial fibrosis.

A random echocardiographic survey of 1640 patients in North Glasgow, reported a prevalence of 2·9% left ventricular dysfunction (defined as ejection fraction [EF] ≤ 30% with the Simpson's biplane rule method). Slightly less then half of the patients were asymptomatic, resulting in a population prevalence of 1·4%. There was no significant difference in mortality rate between symptomatic and asymptomatic patients.[60] The Rotterdam study reported a heart failure prevalence of 3·7% in patients 55–94 years. However, 5·5% men and 2·2% women (prevalence 2·5 times higher in men) were noted to have impaired left ventricular function fractional shortening (FS) ≤ 25%; 60% with impaired left ventricular function were asymptomatic (population prevalence 2·2%).[61] However, both studies included patients with multiple etiologies of heart failure.

Approximately 20–25% of dilated cardiomyopathy cases are classified as familial. If liberal criteria are used for the diagnosis (history of unexplained heart failure or depressed left ventricular function in a first-degree relative), up to 35% of cases may be inherited. Those with familial cardiomyopathy versus sporadic cases, are younger (51·21 ± 12·72 *v* 54·34 ± 11·98; $P < 0.03$). They more frequently have ST segment and T waves abnormalities on ECG. However, these are non-specific findings.[62] Twenty-nine per cent of asymptomatic relatives may have abnormalities on echocardiogram, including left ventricular enlargement (LVE) (≥112% predicted), depressed fractional shortening (dFS) (≤25%), or frank dilated cardiomyopathy. When compared to normal relatives, those with LVE or dFS are more likely to have an abnormal exercise stress test, with a maximal oxygen consumption (Vo_2 max) of <80%. Relatives with an abnormal Vo_2 max have a lower absolute Vo_2 max (30 ± 8 *v* 43 ± 9 cc/kg/min) than normal relatives. The occurrence of LVE with a dFS is associated with QRS duration prolongation on signal averaged ECG. At mean follow up of 39 months, 27% of those with LVE developed symptomatic dilated cardiomyopathy.[63]

An increased incidence of IDC is noted in blacks.[64,65] The cumulative survival in blacks at 12 and 24 months is 71·5% and 63·6% respectively, compared with 92% and 86·3% among whites. One year survival is adversely affected by an ejection fraction (EF) <25% or ventricular arrhythmias (<60% in both instances). Patients 60 years of age or greater had a threefold increased risk of death among both blacks and whites.[65]

Males have an increased incidence of IDC.[64,65] The male:female ratio is 3·4:1· The incidence rate for men is greater than for women within all age groups.[58] In a multi-center registry of IDC, DeMaria *et al*[66] enrolled 65 women and 238 men (male:female ratio 3·66). Patients referred for cardiac transplant were excluded. Of the various clinical char-acteristics evaluated, 10 variables were significantly different between men and women. Men more frequently had a his-tory of ethanol abuse and cigarette smoking. However, sub-group analysis revealed no influence of these variables on gender-related differences. Symptoms of heart failure were more frequently detected in women and were indicative of more advanced heart failure (NYHA class III–IV in 48%). Left bundle branch block (LBBB) was detected more frequently in women, while left anterior hemiblock (LAHB) was noted to be more common in men. There was more pronounced left ventricular dilation in women, with a slightly but not signifi-cantly higher mean myocardial thickness. Exercise tolerance was poorer in women. The median survival was 16 months for women and 19 months for men. Seven women (11%) and 17 men (7%) underwent cardiac transplantation, while 16% of women and 11% of men died from cardiac causes.

Peripartum cardiomyopathy

Peripartum cardiomyopathy (PPCM) is defined as the devel-opment of heart failure in the last month of pregnancy or within 5 months of delivery, in the absence of an identifiable cause for cardiac failure and the absence of recognizable heart disease prior to the last month of pregnancy. Additionally, left ventricular dysfunction is demonstrable by echocardiographic criteria.[67] Risk factors include age over 30, African descent, obesity, multiparity, twin gestation (7–10%), pre-eclampsia and gestational hypertension.[68,69] The incidence varies from 1 in 15000 to 1 in 100 live births.[70] PPCM is a distinct entity, rather then clinically silent cardiomyopathy, which becomes manifest owing to the hemodynamic stress of pregnancy. The incidence and natural history of the disease differs from IDC. Myocarditis has been reported in 8–76% of patients with PPCM.[68,71–73] The variability is likely due to sampling error and timing of endomyocardial biopsy, geographic variation in incidence and inclusion criteria for the diagnosis.

Other factors implicated in PPCM include abnormal immune responses to pregnancy, maladaptive responses to the stress of pregnancy, stress-activated cytokines (TNFα or interleukin-1), abnormalities of relaxin, selenium deficiency, and prolonged tocolytic therapy.[48,67] As there have been reports of familial PPCM,[74] strong consideration should be given to screening family members of patients with PPCM.

The safety of subsequent pregnancies must be carefully considered. Witlin[75] noted that of 28 patients with PPCM, five died (18% mortality), three (11%) had cardiac transplant, 18 (64%) had continued functional impairment, and two (7%) had regression of cardiomyopathy. Six women had sub-sequent pregnancies. Of these, four deteriorated clinically, one remained well compensated on therapy, and one had no recurrence. Elkayam[76] identified 44 women (23 white, 16 black, five Hispanic; aged 19–39 years) with PPCM who had subsequent pregnancies. Cardiomyopathy was diagnosed prior to delivery in seven women; in the first month post delivery in 28 women, and between 2 and 6 months post delivery in nine women. The mean time from index preg-nancy and subsequent pregnancy was 27 ± 18 months. The mean EF increased significantly from 32 ± 11% to 49 ± 12% ($P<0·001$) prior to the subsequent pregnancies. However, during the subsequent pregnancy mean EF decreased to 42 ± 13% ($P<0·001$). Twenty-eight patients had normalization of EF (>50%) prior to the subsequent pregnancy, although 21% developed heart failure during the subsequent pregnancy. Of 16 women with persistent left ventricular dysfunction, 44% developed heart failure with the subsequent pregnancy. Three women died during or after subsequent pregnancies, all with residual left ventricular dysfunction. Premature delivery (<37 weeks gestation) occurred in 13% of those who normalized the EF versus 50% in those who did not.

Women who have recovered from PPCM have a lower contractile reserve upon dobutamine challenge when compared to normal controls, despite similar baseline ven-tricular size and function.[70] This may explain recurrent symptoms with subsequent pregnancies and may be helpful in determining which patients will tolerate future pregnancy. Women whose left ventricular size and function do not return to normal, should be strongly advised against sub-sequent pregnancies.[48,67]

Mortality varies from 7% to 50%, with almost half of the deaths secondary to heart failure, arrhythmias, or thrombo-embolic events.[68,77] Almost half of the deaths occur within the first 3 months post partum. Mortality secondary to thromboembolic events is as high as 30%. Approximately 50% of patients who regain normal cardiac function do so within 6 months of initial diagnosis. Non-survivors have greater hemodynamic compromise and LV dysfunction. LV stroke work index is significantly associated with adverse events (death or transplantation; $P = 0·02$).[73]

ACE inhibitors are the mainstay of treatment post partum. They are contraindicated during pregnancy due to teratogenicity. Hydralazine and nitrates are safe alternatives during pregnancy.[67] In patients with an EF < 35%, the use of heparin during pregnancy and warfarin post partum should be considered. While the use of β blockers is not contraindicated during pregnancy, there are no data evaluating their use during pregnancy. Use of a β blocker should be considered in patients with persistent symptoms and echocardiographic evidence of left ventricular dysfunction more than 2 weeks post partum.[67] In addition, cautious use of diuretics may be necessary when sodium and fluid restriction fails. Exercise may help improve symptoms.

Midei[71] reported on the use of immunosuppressants in 18 women with PPCM. Fourteen (78%) had biopsy evidence of myocarditis. Ten patients were treated with prednisone/azathioprine and four were untreated. One patient died, despite treatment. Four patients with myocarditis improved clinically without therapy. Follow up biopsy showed near complete resolution in two. Four patients without myocarditis were not treated. Two improved and two required transplantation. After completion of treatment, biopsy, left ventricular stroke work index, and pulmonary capillary wedge pressure returned to normal in 12 (not repeated in two patients).

Bozkurt compared the use of immune globulin, 1 g/kg on 2 consecutive days in six women (NYHA II–IV; EF < 40%) with a retrospective control group of 11 patients with PPCM. Only one of 11 biopsied, had evidence of myocarditis. Four control patients had an improvement of >10% in EF, although only two were left an EF >50%; four died or had residual severe left ventricular dysfunction. Within the treatment group, all had a significantly greater improvement in EF than with conventional therapy alone($P < 0.042$); three normalized their EF.[78]

Clinical presentations

Myocarditis

The presenting symptoms and physical examination are often non-specific in both myocarditis and IDC. A history of a 'flu-like syndrome may be present in up to 90% of patients with myocarditis, although only approximately 40% report a viral syndrome within the prior month.[2] The initial presentation may be one of acute or chronic heart failure or cardiogenic shock, or may mimic an acute myocardial infarction.[79,80] Of the 3055 patients in the ESETCID study, 69% had a normal or mildly reduced EF (>45%). Dyspnea was present in 71·7%. While 31·9% had chest pain and 17·9% had arrhythmic events, 78·3% of those with an EF > 45% and 100% of those with an EF <45% had subjective clinical symptoms.[81]

The Dallas Criteria[82] (Box 47.4) were developed in order to standardize the histologic criteria for diagnosis of myocarditis (Figure 47.1), facilitating a multicenter treatment study. However, a negative biopsy does not rule out

> **Box 47.4   Dallas criteria classification of myocarditis[82]**
> **Initial biopsy**
> - *Myocarditis*: myocyte necrosis, degeneration or both in the absence of significant CAD with adjacent inflammatory infiltrate +/− fibrosis
> - *Borderline myocarditis*: inflammatory infiltrate too sparse or myocyte damage not apparent
> - *No myocarditis*
> **Subsequent biopsy**
> - Ongoing (persistent) myocarditis +/− fibrosis
> - Resolving (healing) myocarditis +/− fibrosis
> - Resolved (healed) myocarditis +/− fibrosis

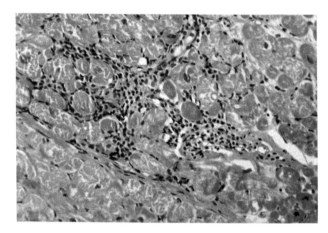

Figure 47.1   Acute myocarditis. Lymphocytic infiltrate of the myocardium with associated myocyte damage. (Hematoxylin & eosin; slide courtesy of Robert Yowell MD.)

myocarditis owing to interobserver variability, sampling error, and the temporal evolution (transient presence) of pathologic features.

Lieberman *et al*[83] proposed a clinicopathologic description of myocarditis, based on the initial manifestations, endomyocardial biopsy, and recovery (fulminant, acute, chronic active, or chronic persistent myocarditis). Patients with fulminant myocarditis had severe hemodynamic compromise, requiring vasopressors or left ventricular assist device. In addition, distinct onsets of symptoms that could be dated – fever, or viral illness within 2 weeks of hospitalization – were present (two of three criteria required). Patients were younger (aged 35 ± 16 *v* 43 ± 13; *P* = 0·05), had higher resting heart rates (100 ± 20 *v* 88 ± 21; *P* = 0·04), and higher right atrial pressures (9·9 ± 8 mmHg *v* 6·2 ± 5 mmHg; *P* = 0·02), but lower mean arterial pressures (80 ± 18 mmHg *v* 92 ± 16 mmHg; *P* = 0·005). Patients with acute myocarditis had an indistinct onset of symptoms, were hemodynamically stable or required low doses of vasopressors and were afebrile. Of 147 patients fulfilling Dallas Criteria, 15 met clinical criteria for fulminant myocarditis and 132 met criteria for acute myocarditis.

At 1 year, 93% with fulminant myocarditis survived without transplant compared to 85% with acute myocarditis. At 11 years, 93% with fulminant myocarditis survived without transplant, while 45% with acute myocarditis were alive without transplant.[84]

IDC

IDC is initially manifest by heart failure in 75–85% of patients. Ninety per cent of patients referred to a tertiary care center are NYHA functional class III–IV at presentation.[64,65] Other potential manifestations include asymptomatic cardiomegaly or left ventricular dysfunction on routine evaluation, arrhythmias or even cardiogenic shock, as in myocarditis. Patients with left bundle branch block (LBBB) have been noted to have a greater left ventricular diastolic dimension normalized for body surface area. The presence of LBBB on ECG may precede the development of cardiomyopathy in 40% of patients. LBBB may be noted on ECG for years prior to the onset of heart failure. At rest and when exercised, these patients may have a higher mean pulmonary artery pressure, although left ventricular end-diastolic volume remains normal, by comparison with normal patients.[85] Laboratory, x ray, and other diagnostic tests are helpful but may be equally non-specific, while myocyte hypertrophy, degeneration of myocytes, interstitial fibrosis, and small clusters of lymphocytes (>5 per high power field) have been noted histologically (Figure 47.2).[64,65]

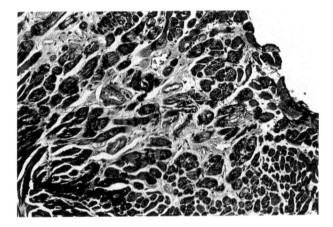

Figure 47.2 Idiopathic dilated cardiomyopathy. Myocyte hypertrophy with mild nuclear enlargement and increased interstitial collagen. (Trichrome stain; slide courtesy of Robert Yowell MD.)

Prognosis

Myocarditis

In patients with myocarditis, ECG abnormalities associated with a longer duration of illness (>1 month) include left ventricular hypertrophy (LVH), left atrial enlargement (LAE), LBBB, and atrial fibrillation (AF). The presence of an abnormal QRS complex on ECG correlates with severity of left ventricular damage and is an independent predictor of survival. LAE, AF, and LBBB also are associated with an increased mortality.[86] Higher baseline left ventricular ejection fraction (LVEF) is positively associated with survival, while intensity of conventional therapy at baseline is negatively associated with survival.[32] The presence of right ventricular (RV) dysfunction, as evidenced by abnormal RV descent on echocardiogram, was shown to be the most important predictor of death or need for cardiac transplantation in a group of 23 patients with biopsy-proven myocarditis who were followed long term.[87] In addition, a net increase in LVEF (between initial and final EF) was associated with improved survival, whereas baseline EF was not predictive of outcome. The presence and degree of left ventricular regional wall motion abnormalities did not predict the clinical course.[87]

Light microscopic findings on biopsy have not been shown to predict outcome in myocarditis. Less than 10% of biopsies repeated at 28 weeks and 52 weeks continue to show evidence of ongoing or recurrent myocarditis, regardless of therapy. However, higher baseline serum antibodies to cardiac immune globulin (Ig) G by indirect immunofluoresence were associated with a better LVEF and a smaller left ventricular end-diastolic dimension.[32] Gagliardi et al[88] followed 20 children with biopsy-proven myocarditis who were treated with cyclosporine and steroids and found that 13 of 20 had persistent myocarditis at 6 months. At 1 year, 10 patients had persistent myocarditis by endomyocardial biopsy, although ventricular size and function had improved on echocardiography. Echocardiography was unable to detect those patients with biopsy-persistent versus biopsy-resolved myocarditis. Despite histologic evidence of myocarditis, no patient died or required transplantation.

IDC

Spontaneous improvement in LVEF (over 10% points) occurs in 20–45% of patients with IDC. Improvement usually occurs within the first 6 months of presentation, but may occur up to 4 years later. Outcome is adversely affected by progressive LV enlargement, RV enlargement, and markedly reduced LVEF. Both LVEF and RV enlargement are independent predictors of survival. Mortality rates of 25–30% at 1 year are noted. Overall, the annual mortality from disease progression is 4–10% but is greater in high-risk subgroups. Twelve per cent of patients with IDC die suddenly, which accounts for 28% of all deaths.[64,65] In a retrospective study of 104 patients with dilated cardiomyopathy, Fuster et al[89] noted 77% of patients died. Two thirds of the deaths occurred within the first 2 years. Interestingly, the survival curve for the remaining patients was comparable to an age- and sex-matched control group. The 1 and 5 year mortality rates were 31% and 64%, respectively. Factors significantly associated with poorer survival were older age (97% mortality rate in patients ≥55 years), cardiothoracic ratio (86% mortality rate if the ratio was >0·55 v 40% if <0·55), cardiac index (CI) (mortality rate 89% if CI <3·0 l/min v 35% if CI >3·0 l/min) and LV end-diastolic pressure (mortality rate 87% if ≥20 mmHg). Referral bias and secular trends, new treatment modalities, and the prevalence of disease in the referral population should also be noted, as these may influence overall survival.[90]

By comparison, when one assesses the natural history of asymptomatic IDC, patients have an excellent prognosis, with a 2 year survival of 100%, a 5 year survival of 78 ± 8%, and a 7 year survival of 53 ± 10%. However, there is no improvement in survival in these patients when compared to asymptomatic patients who have previously had symptoms of heart failure. The most common reason for cardiac evaluation in this group of patients is palpitations or an abnormal chest *x* ray or ECG. When compared to patients with a prior history of congestive heart failure symptoms, these patients had a lower prevalence of cardiomegaly in chest *x* rays (31% v 57% of patients) and a smaller LV and better EF (33% v 29% EF) on echocardiography.[91]

Patients with syncope, a third heart sound, RV dysfunction, hyponatremia, elevated plasma norepinephrine, atrial natriuretic peptide or renin, a maximal systemic oxygen uptake (Vo_2) of <10–12 ml/kg/min, CI of <2·5 l/min/m^2, systemic hypotension, pulmonary hypertension, increased central venous pressure, or loss of cardiac myofilaments on high resolution microscopy show increased progression of disease and worse survival.[64,65] Patients with an elevated C-reactive protein (CRP) level (>0·5 mg/dl) and an EF <40% have a poorer 5 year survival. Of those with a CRP level >1·0 mg/dl, 62% died within five years.[92] Persistently elevated levels of troponin T (>0·02 ng/dl) are associated with more cardiac events (hospitalization, arrhythmia) and poorer survival rate.[93] Elevated levels of brain natriuretic peptide are associated with a poor prognosis and may be a useful tool to aid in the diagnosis of heart failure.[94,95]

Myocardial contractile reserve, as evaluated by change in LVEF with exercise, is an independent predictor of survival in patients with mildly symptomatic (NYHA class I or II) dilated cardiomyopathy. A change in LVEF of >4% was associated with a 75% survival versus 25% in those whose EF changed <4% with exercise.[96] Patients with greater improvements in EF with dobutamine (0·09 ± 0·06 v 0·05 ± 0·05) had a better survival at 1 year (97% v 74%; P = 0·02), 2 years (97% v 64%; P = 0·002) and 3 years (97% v 56%; P < 0·001). These patients had a shorter duration of heart failure, better functional capacity, better LV and RV EF and smaller LV size. Survivors had a greater improvement in LV and RV EF.[97] Dobutamine-induced improvements

in LVEF and LV sphericity are predictive of subsequent recovery in LV function.[98]

Coronary flow reserve is diminished in patients with dilated cardiomyopathy. Treasure *et al*[99] performed coronary angiography and Doppler flow studies of the left anterior descending (LAD) artery to estimate coronary artery flow velocities in seven normal controls and eight patients with dilated cardiomyopathy. The effect of acetylcholine and adenosine on epicardial vasoconstriction in patients with dilated cardiomyopathy was not significantly different from normal controls. However, infusion of intracoronary acetylcholine resulted in a dose-dependent increase in coronary blood flow in normal controls only, suggesting that endothelium-dependent coronary vasodilation is abnormal in dilated cardiomyopathy. There was a similar change in coronary blood flow with adenosine infusion in both groups. Impairment in both coronary microvascular response and epicardial vasodilator response to endothelial-dependant vasodilation with acetylcholine may occur early (<6 months) in the course of the disease.[100]

In infants and children the outcome of IDC is more variable. A retrospective review of 24 patients under 20 years old with IDC revealed that, in 92%, the initial manifestation was heart failure. Thirteen of the patients (54%) had onset of symptoms within 3 months of a viral syndrome although endomyocardial biopsy did not reveal active myocarditis in six. Sixty-three per cent had ECG evidence of LVH and 68% had ST-T wave abnormalities. The mean EF was 26% (5–51%). Fifteen patients died (63%). The cumulative survival was 63% at 1 year, 50% at 2 years, and 34% at 5 years of follow up. Death was most frequently due to progressive heart failure. Of the nine patients who survived, the symptoms resolved in 3–24 months. Severe mitral regurgitation was a predictor of poor outcome. Survivors more frequently had viral symptoms within the preceding 3 months.[101] Five year survival rates of 64–84% have been reported.[64,65] Sudden death is rare.[64,65] A recent review of hospital records in children from the West of Scotland identified 53 patients with IDC or myocarditis who were <12 years old. Of the 39 IDC cases, 38 were diagnosed in life. There were 15 males (M:F ratio = 1:1·6) and 64% were <1 year of age. Coxsackie viral antibodies were positive in 21%. Mitral regurgitation was present in 74% and 77% had cardiomegaly in *x* rays. Twelve patients died, all within a year; 50% within the first week of presentation. Survival was higher if fractional shortening (FS) was >15% (11/28 survived v 1/10 survivors), as was mean survival (12·2 years v 9·6 years, respectively). Of the 12 who survived, all became asymptomatic and LV size returned to normal in 10 patients. Myocarditis was diagnosed at autopsy in nine of 14 patients who presented within 10 days of illness onset; one additional patient died 4 days after diagnosis. Actuarial survival was 29% at 1 and 9 years. All survivors became asymptomatic.[102]

Comparison of IDC and myocarditis

Grogan *et al*[103] compared 27 patients with active ($n = 17$) or borderline ($n = 10$) myocarditis with 58 IDC patients. A viral illness was reported within the previous 3 months in 40% of patients with myocarditis versus 19% of the IDC patients. The EF was lower ($25 \pm 11\%$) in the group with IDC compared to the myocarditis group ($38 \pm 19\%$). Sixty-three per cent of the patients with IDC were NYHA functional class III–IV compared with only 30% of the patients with myocarditis. There was no difference in survival even when results were analyzed for the presence of active myocarditis, borderline myocarditis, or IDC (54% 5 year survival with IDC *v* 56% with myocarditis).

Summary

While multiple causal factors have been implicated in both myocarditis and IDC, the precise etiology and pathophysiology remain unknown. Spontaneous improvement in left ventricular function may be noted with both myocarditis and IDC. Survival is similar (approximately 55% at 5 years) in both.

Treatment

Treatment of myocarditis: clinical and experimental

General supportive measures for patients with myocarditis include a low sodium diet; discontinuation of ethanol, illicit drug use, and smoking; and salt restriction, especially in the presence of heart failure. Recommendations for the limitation of physical activity are based on the murine model of Coxsackie B3 myocarditis, in which forced exercise during the acute phase of illness was associated with increased inflammatory and necrotic lesions (although there was no effect on death rate).[103] The Task Force[104] on myopericardial diseases recommends a convalescent period of approximately 6 months after onset of clinical manifestations before a return to competitive sports.

Antiviral therapy

The use of the antiviral ribaviron[105] in a murine (DBA/2) model of encephalomyocarditis (ECM) myocarditis improved survival and decreased myocardial viral titers when used in higher doses (200 or 400 mg/kg/day). Therapy resulted in fewer myocardial lesions, more pronounced inhibition of viral replication, a reduced inflammatory response, and less myocardial damage. However, treatment was started immediately after viral inoculation. There are no human studies of antiviral therapy to date and the ability to detect and begin therapy immediately upon onset is limited in the clinical setting.

Angiotensin converting enzyme inhibition

Although there are multiple studies on the use of ACE inhibitors in heart failure (including patients with IDC), their utility in myocarditis has been studied only in the murine model. Studies of Coxsackie B3 myocarditis in CD1 mice reported that early treatment with captopril (starting on day 1 of infection) resulted in less inflammatory infiltrate, myocardial necrosis, and calcification. Heart weight, heart to body weight ratio, and liver congestion diminished. Even when therapy was begun later (10 days after inoculation), a beneficial effect – a reduction in left ventricular mass and liver congestion – was noted.[106]

A comparison of the ACE inhibitors captopril 7·5 g/kg/day and enalapril 1 mg/kg/day with the angiotensin II receptor blocker losartan 60 mg/kg/day in a murine model of ECM myocarditis revealed that only captopril and losartan, started 1 week after viral inoculation, resulted in decreased heart weight, body weight, heart weight to body ratio, and hypertrophy. Left ventricular cavity dimension decreased with the use of captopril and losartan 12 mg/kg/day or 60 mg/kg/day. These results are consistent with an improvement in heart failure and left ventricular hypertrophy. There was less necrosis with enalapril and captopril. However, the inflammatory score was reduced only by captopril.[77]

β Blockers

Similarly, β blockers have been studied in myocarditis only in murine models. Metoprolol was compared with saline in a murine model of acute Coxsackie B3 myocarditis, starting on the day of viral inoculation and continuing for 10 days. The result was an *increased* 30 day mortality (60% *v* 0%) in metoprolol-treated mice associated with *increased* viral replication and myocyte necrosis.[107] The β blocker carteolol has been studied in a murine model (BALB/C and DBA/2 strains) of acute, subacute, and chronic ECM myocarditis. Metoprolol was compared with carteolol in the chronically infected group. There was no difference in survival between mice whose treatment was started on the day of viral inoculation, compared to therapy begun 14 days later. In chronically infected mice, carteolol resulted in a reduction in heart weight and heart weight to body ratio (not seen with metoprolol), and improved histopathologic scores (diminished wall thickness, cavity dimension, fiber diameter, cell necrosis, fibrosis, cellular infiltration, and calcification), suggesting that carteolol may prevent the development of lesions similar to those found in dilated cardiomyopathy.[108] The results suggest that early initiation of β blockers may be harmful, whereas in the chronic stages of illness β blockers improve manifestations of heart failure. In addition, non-cardioselective β blockers may be preferable.

Calcium-channel blockers

In a murine model of ECM induced myocarditis, verapamil pretreatment was associated with a reduction in microvascular necrosis, fibrosis, and calcification. Similar changes were noted if treatment was begun 4 days after viral inoculation. The development of microvascular constriction and microaneurysm formation was prevented when compared to controls. This suggests a possible role for calcium signaling and microvascular spasm in the pathogenesis of this form of viral myocarditis. Verapamil did not reduce mortality although the severity of illness and time to death were delayed.[109] There have been no human myocarditis trials with calcium-channel blockers to date.

Non-steroidal anti-inflammatory agents

The use of ibuprofen during the acute phase of murine Coxsackie B3 myocarditis resulted in significant exacerbation of myocardial inflammation, necrosis, and viral replication, when compared to control mice.[110,111]

Vesnarinone

Vesnarinone suppressed TNF α, resulting in a reduction in myocardial necrosis, when given at a dose of 50 mg/kg, in a murine model of ECM myocarditis. At lower doses (10 mg/kg) the mortality rate was reduced in comparison to control mice, although both groups began to experience mortality on day 5 after viral inoculation.[112]

Immunosuppressants

The data supporting an immunologic basis of myocarditis have resulted in multiple treatment trials of immunosuppressants. The largest of these trials, the Myocarditis Treatment Trial,[32] screened 2333 patients with heart failure of less than 2 years' duration: 214 patients (10%) had endomyocardial biopsy evidence of myocarditis by the Dallas Criteria; 111 had a qualifying LVEF of <45%. Patients were initially divided into three treatment groups: prednisone/azathioprine, prednisone/cyclosporine, and no immunosuppressant treatment. The prednisone/azathioprine group was subsequently eliminated because of limited numbers of patients. Patients were treated for 24 weeks, during which time conventional heart failure therapy was continued. At both 28 and 52 weeks, no difference in pulmonary capillary wedge pressure or change in LVEF was observed (Figure 47.3). In addition, there was no significant change in LVEF in treated patients as compared with untreated (Figure 47.3). At 1 and 5 years, there was no difference in survival between groups or need for cardiac transplantation (Figure 47.4). On multivariate analysis, better baseline LVEF, less intensive conventional therapy, and

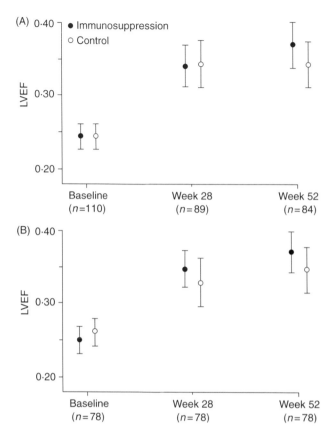

Figure 47.3 Mean (±SE) left ventricular ejection fraction (LVEF) in the immunosuppression and control groups at baseline, week 28, and week 52. (A) shows the mean values for all available studies at each time, with the numbers of patients indicated at the bottom of the panel. There was no difference between the two groups in the mean LVEF at baseline, week 28, or week 52 (P = 0.97, P = 0.95, and P = 0.45, respectively). (B) shows the mean values for the 78 patients for whom data were available at all three times. Again, there was no significant difference between the groups (P = 0.51, P = 0.60, and P = 0.50, respectively). (Adapted with permission from Mason *et al.*[32])

shorter illness duration were independent predictors of improvement in LVEF during follow up. Immunologic variables (cardiac IgG, circulating IgG, natural killer and macrophage activity, helper T cell level) were not associated with measures of cardiac function. A higher peripheral CD2$^+$ T lymphocyte count was associated with a higher risk of death. At 5 years the combined end point of death or transplantation was 56%.

Gagliardi *et al*[88] followed 20 children with biopsy-proven myocarditis who were treated with cyclosporine and prednisone. At 1 year, 10 of 20 patients still had histologic evidence of myocarditis. No patient died or required transplantation. However, there was no control group.

Certain subgroups might nonetheless benefit from immunosuppressant therapy, including those with giant

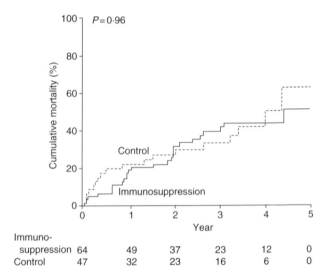

Figure 47.4 numbers at risk:

	0	1	2	3	4	5
Immuno-suppression	64	49	37	23	12	0
Control	47	32	23	16	6	0

Figure 47.4 Actuarial mortality (defined as deaths and cardiac transplantations) in the immunosuppression and control groups. The numbers of patients at risk are shown at the bottom. There was no significant difference in mortality between the two groups. (Adapted with permission from Mason *et al.*[32])

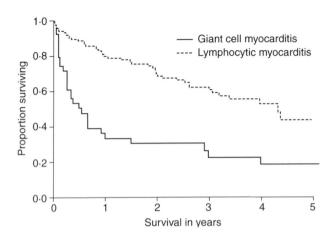

Figure 47.5 Kaplan–Meier survival curves for patients with giant cell myocarditis, showing the duration of survival among 38 patients in whom giant cell myocarditis was diagnosed by endomyocardial biopsy or by examination of a section of ventricular apex. Survival was significantly longer among patients with lymphocytic myocarditis (*P* < 0·001 by the log rank test for each comparison). (Adapted with permission from Cooper *et al.*[113])

cell myocarditis, hypersensitivity myocarditis, or cardiac sarcoidosis. With a multicenter database, Cooper[113] reviewed 63 patients with giant cell myocarditis. There was no difference in the number of men versus women, or the age of men versus women. The mean age at onset was 42·6 ± 12·7 years. Eighty-eight per cent were white and 19% had an associated autoimmune disorder. Five patients (8%) had either Crohn's disease or ulcerative colitis, which preceded the onset of myocarditis. Seventy-five per cent presented with heart failure. Approximately half had sustained refractory ventricular tachycardia during the course of the illness. The rate of death or cardiac transplantation was 89% by 3 years. Median survival was 5·5 months from symptom onset to death or transplantation. The median survival in patients treated with corticosteroids was 3·8 months versus 3·0 months in untreated patients. However, patients treated with corticosteroids and azathioprine had an average survival of 11·5 months. Cyclosporine in combination with corticosteroids, corticosteroids/azathioprine, or corticosteroids/azathioprine/OKT3 survived an average of 12·6 months. Survival was unaffected by sex, age, or time to presentation. Cardiac transplantation was performed in 34 patients. Nine (26%) died during an average 3·7 years of follow up. Five of these deaths occurred within 30 days of transplantation. Nine patients had recurrent giant cell myocarditis in the transplanted heart, after an average of 3 years post transplantation. Comparison with 111 patients in the Myocarditis Treatment Trial revealed cumulative mortality was greater in patients with giant cell myocarditis (Figure 47.5). The ongoing Giant Cell Myocarditis Treatment Trial will assess the efficacy of standard medical therapy

versus standard care, in addition to therapy with muromonab-CD3 (OKT3), cyclosporine and corticosteroids.

Other potential indications for a trial of immunosuppressant therapy include failure of myocarditis to resolve, progressive LV dysfunction despite conventional therapy, continued active myocarditis on biopsy or fulminant myocarditis that does not improve within 24–72 hours of full hemodynamic support, including mechanical assistance. Myocarditis associated with a known immune-mediated disease, such as systemic lupus erythematosus, may also benefit from immunosuppressive therapy.

These studies call into question the value of routine endomyocardial biopsy and immunosuppressant therapy in adults and children. Immunologic testing may be a more sensitive method of diagnosis and may reduce the sampling error noted with routine histology but awaits development and validation. Consideration of endomyocardial biopsy should be given whenever these specific immunosuppressant-responsive conditions are present or suspected. However, the low incidence of light microscopic evidence of histologic inflammatory disease, the fact that there is no specific therapy for most cases of myocarditis, and the fact that there are potential complications related to the procedure suggest that *routine* endomyocardial biopsy is not warranted.[114]

Smaller studies have used differing immunosuppressant regimens. Kühl *et al*[115] treated 31 patients with biopsies classified as immunohistologically positive (more than two cells per high power field and expression of adhesion molecules), negative Dallas Criteria, and LV dysfunction. Patients were treated with corticosteroids plus conventional therapy for 3 months followed by gradual tapering of methylprednisolone doses over 24 weeks (following biopsy and LVEF response). Therapy was associated with an improvement in EF in 64% and improved NYHA functional class in 77%. Four patients (12%) had no change in EF despite improvement in inflammatory infiltrates. Three patients (9%) had no change in EF or inflammatory infiltrates. However, study conclusions are limited by the absence of a control group. These findings also reinforce the suggestion that light microscopy may not be the gold standard for the diagnosis of myocarditis or evaluation of therapy. Hopefully, new advances in immunohistochemistry will increase diagnostic and prognostic sensitivity and specificity.

Drucker *et al*[116] retrospectively reviewed 46 children with congestive cardiomyopathy and Dallas Criteria of borderline or definite myocarditis: 21 patients were treated with IV IgG (2 g/kg over 24 hours) and were compared to 25 historic controls. Of the treated patients, four received a second dose of IgG and two were also treated with prednisone. Of the control patients, three received prednisone and two of these three patients also received cyclosporin. One died, one underwent heart transplantation, and one had persistent LV dysfunction. Overall survival was not improved although there was a trend toward improvement in 1 year survival in the treated group. In the IgG group, the mean LV end-diastolic dimension was not significantly different from normal after 3 months. Fractional shortening improved in both groups but returned to normal only in the IgG group. Improvement in ventricular function persisted after adjustment for age, biopsy status, and use of ACE inhibitors and inotropes.

In a comparative study of interferon-α, thymomodulin, and conventional therapy in patients with biopsy-proven myocarditis or IDC, an improvement in the treatment groups was reported for EF (at rest and during exercise), maximum exercise time, functional class, and ECG abnormalities. Three of 12 conventionally treated patients died (one suddenly and two from heart failure), compared with one of 13 treated with interferon-α (sudden death in an IDC patient) and one of 13 treated with thymomodulin (of embolic cerebrovascular accident).[117] The use of intravenous immune globulin in 10 patients (NYHA III–IV) with symptoms of <6 months duration resulted in an improvement in LVEF (Figure 47.6) and functional improvement (NYHA I–II at 1 year of follow up) in all nine patients who survived, regardless of biopsy results.[118]

Ahdoot *et al* reported on five children aged 15 months to 16·5 years, four with histologic evidence of acute myocarditis, who were treated with OKT3 (0·1 mg/kg/IV push for 10–14 days), IV IgG (2 mg/kg over 24–48 hours) and corticosteroids. Three patients also received cyclosporine (for 6 months), three received azathioprine (while maintained on cyclosporine) and one received methotrexate (for 2 months). All presented with severe heart failure, requiring

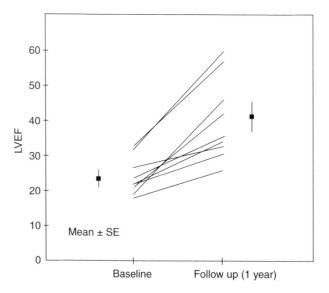

Figure 47.6 Change in LVEF (*P* = 0.003) in patients treated with IV immune globulin. All patients demonstrated functional improvement and at 1 year follow up were NYHA class I or II. No patient has been re-hospitalized for congestive failure. (Adapted with permission from McNamara *et al.*[118])

inotropic and ventilatory support. Four had life-threatening arrhythmias. Four required temporary mechanical circulatory support. One patient died from a thromboembolic event. EF normalized in the four surviving patients. After a mean follow up of 28·8 months (3–56 months), there were no heart failure recurrences or progression to dilated cardiomyopathy.[119]

Perhaps alternative immunosuppressant regimens and different diagnostic criteria may be more successful in demonstrating the usefulness of immunosuppressants. Other immunosuppressants have been studied in the murine model. The use of cyclophosphamide (CYA) in a murine model of Coxsackie B3 myocarditis revealed that therapy begun at the time of viral inoculation resulted in less severe cardiac lesions compared to controls but no improvement in mortality. When therapy was begun later (8 days after viral inoculation), survival was worse in the CYA group despite improvement in cardiac lesions. When therapy was begun even later (day 21), there was no difference in survival or in cardiac infiltrates compared with controls.[120] In a murine model of EMC viral myocarditis, the use of tumor necrosis factor (TNF) resulted in greater myocardial viral content and more extensive myocardial necrosis and cellular infiltration. Anti-TNF monoclonal antibody did not alter mortality or prevent myocardial lesions unless given *before* viral infection.[121] There are no human studies with these agents. Preliminary data on the development of an enterovirus vaccine using chimeric Coxsackie virus B3 in a murine model of myocarditis suggest an attenuation of viral replication and diminished inflammatory infiltrates.[122]

Cardiac transplantation

An analysis of outcome of 14 055 cardiac transplant recipients did not confirm the initial concern that there is a worse outcome if transplantation is performed during the acute stage of myocarditis. One year actuarial survival in all groups transplanted (IDC, myocarditis, peripartum cardiomyopathy *v* other diagnoses) was 80%.[123] Nonetheless, myocarditis may recur in the transplanted heart.[124]

Treatment of IDC: clinical and experimental

The same general supportive measures used in myocarditis are applicable in the management of IDC, except that moderate exercise is encouraged once heart failure symptoms have stabilized. Mild to moderate dynamic exercise is preferable to isometric exercise.[125]

Vasodilators, ACE inhibitors, and angiotensin receptor antagonists

The beneficial effects of vasodilators (hydralazine and isosorbide dinitrate) and ACE inhibitors on symptomatic improvement and reduction in mortality have been shown in multiple large clinical trials.[126-130] Trials have included 15–18% of enrolled patients with a diagnosis of IDC.[126-130] These trials have documented a reduction in cardiac size, improvement in functional class, and a reduction in total and cardiovascular mortality. In addition, there is a reduction in the number of hospitalizations.[126-130]

The use of enalapril in asymptomatic patients (EF < 35%) resulted in a *non-significant* decrease in mortality. However, there was a reduction in the incidence of heart failure and related hospital admissions. The time to development of heart failure was shown to be prolonged from 8·3 months to 22·3 months.[128,129] The survival benefit of enalapril was found to be superior to the combination of hydralazine plus isosorbide dinitrate in the Second Vasodilator-Heart Failure Trial (V-HeFT-2).[130]

A short trial (8 weeks) comparing the angiotensin receptor II antagonist (ARB) losartan with enalapril in 166 patients with NYHA class III–IV and an EF of <35% suggested comparable efficacy based on results of 6 minute walk test, dyspnea fatigue index, neurohumoral activation (norepinephrine and atrial natriuretic factor levels), laboratory evaluation, and adverse events.[131] In a comparison of losartan (titrated to 50 mg/day) with captopril (50 mg 3×/day) in 722 NYHA class II–IV patients over the age of 65, a 32% relative risk reduction of death and/or hospital admission was observed with the use of losartan (Evaluation of Losartan in the Elderly Study [ELITE]).[132] There was no difference in the number of hospital admissions for heart failure or improvement in functional class. This suggests that losartan may be used as an alternative to, if not

preferred to, ACE inhibitors. However, there was no significant difference in mortality, sudden death or resuscitated deaths in the follow up study (ELITE II). While the study failed to show the superiority of losartan, the drug is a safe and effective alternative in patients who cannot tolerate ACE inhibitors.[133]

The Valsartan Heart Trial Investigators[134] reported no significant difference in survival in 5010 patients with class II–IV heart failure (31% IDC) treated with valsartan plus ACE inhibitors versus placebo and ACE inhibitors. However there was a 13% lower incidence of the combined end points of mortality and cardiac arrest necessitating resuscitation, hospitalization for heart failure or need for intravenous inotropes and vasodilators. There was significant improvement in heart failure symptoms and quality of life. Of note, on post hoc analysis, valsartan had an adverse effect on mortality in patients on a combination of ACE inhibitor and β blocker (*P* < 0·009). Whether this is a true interaction requires further investigation. Thus, ARBs should be considered an alternative in patients intolerant of ACE inhibitors.[114]

Digitalis

Although the use of digitalis has long been a standard in the treatment of heart failure, only recently have large trials been conducted to assess its safety and efficacy adequately. Withdrawal trials of digitalis in patients with a depressed LVEF treated with diuretics and/or ACE inhibitors, in sinus rhythm, with mild to moderate heart failure, have shown a worsening of exercise performance and NYHA class, lower quality of life score, a need for additional drug therapy, more overall hospitalizations and hospitalizations for heart failure, and an increase in emergency room visits for heart failure compared with patients continued on digitalis. Patients who continued the use of digitalis had an increased time to treatment failure, higher LVEF, and lower heart rate and body weight. Its effect on mortality is neutral, with a balanced reduction in heart failure deaths and an increase in sudden arrhythmic deaths.[135-137] However, digoxin reduced hospitalization for heart failure.[137] Perhaps, unexpectedly, these results were similar in a group of patients with an EF of 45%.[137] The symptomatic benefit of therapy was greatest in patients with an EF of 25%, NYHA class III–IV, and in those with cardiomegaly. Idiopathic dilated cardiomyopathy was the etiology of heart failure in approximately 15–40% of patients enrolled in these trials.[135-137]

Immunosuppressants

The use of immunosuppressants is not as well studied in IDC as in myocarditis. Patients with IDC felt to be immune reactive, based on cellular infiltrate, Ig or complement deposition, elevated sedimentation rate, or a positive gallium scan, were randomized to treatment with prednisone and compared to untreated controls by Parillo *et al*[138] At 3 months, there was an improvement in EF, but this was not sustained at 9 months.[138] In another study, the use of interferon-α or thymomodulin in IDC appeared to improve EF (at rest and during exercise), maximum exercise time, functional class, and ECG abnormalities when compared with conventional therapy alone.[117]

Ten patients with recent onset of heart failure and biopsy consistent with borderline myocarditis in one patient, non-specific inflammation in one patient, and six with no cellular infiltrate received IV IgG. There was an improvement in both LVEF (Figure 47.6), and functional classification (NYHA I–II at 1 year of follow up) in all nine patients who survived.[118] Conversely, the IMAC investigators randomized 62 patients with recent onset IDC to IV IgG (2g/kg) or placebo. Sixteen per cent had biopsy evidence of cellular inflammation. The improvement noted in EF was identical in both groups. There was no significant difference in event-free survival or functional capacity between the two groups.[139]

Using immunohistological criteria as the basis to qualify for immunosuppressive therapy, Wojnicz *et al* randomized 84 heart failure patients with increased HLA expression on endomyocardial biopsy specimens to therapy with prednisone (1 mg/kg/day, which was tapered to 0·2 mg/kg/day for 90 days) and azathioprine (1 mg/kg for 100 days) versus placebo. Fifty-eight patients completed the study. There was no difference in cardiac death, transplantation or hospital re-admission rate, although the immunosuppressant group had a significant improvement in EF, left ventricular diastolic dimension, and NYHA functional class.[140]

Since the development of autoantibodies may play a role in the initiation and progression of IDC, immunoadsorption for their removal may be of benefit. Felix *et al* randomized 18 patients with severe heart failure to immunoadsorption (IA) followed by IgG (0·5g/kg) substitution versus conventional therapy. Myocarditis was excluded in all patients. There was a significant decline in β receptor antibody levels in the IA group, when compared to baseline levels ($P < 0·01$) and when compared to conventionally treated patients ($P < 0·01$). In addition, there were significant improvements in hemodynamics. Cardiac index and stroke volume index increased, while pulmonary and systemic vascular resistance decreased. These changes persisted for 3 months. The hemodynamic improvements were associated with significant improvements in EF ($P < 0·01$) and functional class ($P < 0·05$). However, this was a small study and follow up was only 3 months.[141]

Since a specific diagnosis is infrequently made in cases of dilated cardiomyopathy (approximately 17% of cases),[59] routine endomyocardial biopsy is not recommended in all heart failure patients.[114] The benefits of endomyocardial biopsy should outweigh the overall risks associated with the procedure, reported at 4·4–8%, although death from myocardial perforation is uncommon (0·02–0·4%).[59,142] As the diagnostic yield and likelihood of therapy being altered

by the histopathologic results is low, biopsy should be considered in patients with rapid clinical deterioration, new arrhythmias, history, or symptoms suggestive of secondary causes of dilated cardiomyopathy, or who fail to improve after 1 week of conventional therapy.[114,142]

Growth hormone

Preliminary data suggested growth hormone (GH) might be of therapeutic benefit in patients with IDC. In a recent pilot study, there was an improvement in quality of life, increased maximal exercise capacity, and increased LV mass and wall thickness, with resultant decreased wall stress, decreased chamber size; improved hemodynamics and systolic performance, and decreased myocardial oxygen consumption.[143] However, Isgaard[144] conducted a randomized double blind study of recombinant GH in 22 patients with heart failure of various etiologies. After 3 months of treatment, there was no improvement in systolic or diastolic function or exercise capacity. Plasma markers of neuroendocrine activation (renin activity, aldosterone, angiotensin II, adrenaline, noradrenaline) remained unchanged.

Calcium-channel blockers

The Prospective Randomized Amlodipine Survival Evaluation (PRAISE) trial[145] enrolled 1153 patients with NYHA class III–IV heart failure and an EF of <30%. Treatment with the calcium-channel blocker amlodipine was compared to placebo. On subgroup analysis, patients with dilated cardiomyopathy had a 31% reduction in fatal and non-fatal events and a 46% lower risk of death, although there was no significant reduction in overall mortality or fatal and non-fatal events. The follow up study (PRAISE II) showed no survival benefit with the use of amlodipine (presented at American College of Cardiology Scientific Sessions 15 March, 2000 in Anaheim, CA). Its use in heart failure should be limited to patients with hypertension and angina despite standard heart failure therapy.[114]

Cardiomyopathic Syrian hamsters are known to develop progressive focal myocardial necrosis, similar to lesions found in human cardiac diseases. In these hamsters, the process begins at 1 month of age, ultimately leading to heart failure. Using silicone rubber perfusion studies, Factor and colleagues[146] were able to document microvascular vasoconstriction, diffuse vessel narrowing, and lumenal irregularity associated with adjacent areas of myocytolytic necrosis. They were able to prevent the development of cellular necrosis by pretreatment of 30 day old hamsters (the period when they normally develop these lesions) with verapamil. When treatment was begun at a later time (90 or 150 days), there was no alteration in scar or necrosis. However, verapamil had a positive effect on microvascular spasm, regardless of when treatment was begun, suggesting abnormal cellular calcium metabolism may be involved in the pathogenesis. Comparable human studies have not been done. These studies lend further support to the potential role of calcium and microvascular spasm.

β Blockers

Initial trials of the use of β blockers in IDC, while uncontrolled, suggested improved cardiac function and survival when they were added to digitalis and diuretics in patients with moderate to severe heart failure.[147] In addition, the withdrawal of such therapy appeared to result in the development of worsening heart failure.[147]

The long-term effects of metoprolol were studied in an early double-blind, randomized study of limited size.[148] Patients also were frequently receiving treatment with digoxin, diuretics, and vasodilators. Patients had symptomatic heart failure with a baseline EF of 49%. In the metoprolol-treated group, a significant improvement in functional class, exercise capacity, mean EF, and LV end-diastolic dimension was observed.[148] The subsequent larger Metoprolol in Dilated Cardiomyopathy (MDC) Trial[149] in symptomatic patients with an EF of <40% showed a reduction in the composite end point of death or need for transplantation. However, all of the derived benefit was secondary to a reduction in cardiac transplantation, with no independent effect on all-cause mortality. Additional benefit was observed in several other measures; ejection fraction, pulmonary capillary wedge pressure, quality of life, exercise duration, and NYHA functional class improved significantly. The number of hospital re-admissions for all patients and re-admissions per patient were reduced with metoprolol. In a substudy of the Randomized Evaluation of Strategies of Left Ventricular Dysfunction (RESOLVD), of 450 patients with an EF of ≤0·40, there was about a 50% risk reduction in mortality ($P = 0.052$) and a significant improvement in EF with metoprolol CR compared to placebo over 20 weeks. There was no impact on cardiovascular or total hospitalizations.[150]

The Cardiac Insufficiency Bisoprolol Study (CIBIS)[151] tested bisoprolol in heart failure and found no difference in sudden death or death from documented venous thrombosis. On subgroup analysis, there was a reduction in mortality in IDC patients and those with NYHA class IV. There was also an improvement in functional status and fewer hospitalizations in patients treated with bisoprolol. The follow up study (CIBIS-II) enrolled 2647 patients with class III or IV heart failure and an EF of <35%. The study was terminated early because of a significant mortality benefit in patients treated with bisoprolol (11·8% *v* 17·3%; $P < 0.0001$). All-cause mortality was lower and there were fewer sudden deaths in the treated group (3·6% *v* 6·3%; $P = 0.0011$). In addition, fewer patients were hospitalized in the treatment group ($P = 0.0006$). The beneficial effects of therapy were independent of the etiology or severity of heart failure.[152]

The α/β blocker carvedilol has been tested in patients with an EF of ≤35% (NYHA classes II–IV), on digitalis, an ACE inhibitor, and diuretics, and was associated with a 65% reduction of all-cause mortality (not a prospective end point), a 27% reduction in hospitalization, and a 38% reduction in the combined end points of death and hospitalization (primary end point, progression of heart failure). The reduction in mortality was independent of age, sex, cause of heart failure, EF, exercise tolerance, systolic blood pressure, and heart rate.[153] Subsequent studies have confirmed the beneficial effects of carvedilol on survival and improvement in symptomatology in patients with moderate to severe heart failure on a background of ACE inhibitors, diuretics, and digitalis. Additionally, mean EF increased by 5%. There was however, no significant improvement in exercise performance.[154]

The Metoprolol CR/XL Randomized Intervention Trial in Congestive Heart Failure (MERIT-HF) enrolled 3991 patients with class III–IV heart failure and an EF of ≤40%. Patients were randomized to long-acting metoprolol or placebo after a 2 week single-blind run-in period; 90% of patients were on diuretics and ACE inhibitors. Approximately 63% were on digitalis. There was a significant reduction in all-cause hospitalization and total mortality (19% risk reduction). There was a 32% risk reduction in death or need for heart transplantation. The number of hospitalizations (451 *v* 317) and hospitalization days (5303 days *v* 3401 days) due to heart failure were significantly reduced when compared to the placebo group. There was a significant improvement in functional class and patient sense of well being, when these criteria were assessed by patients and their physicians.[155] Given the mounting evidence supporting their use, it is recommended that patients with symptomatic LV dysfunction receive treatment with β blockers. Initiation of therapy should begin in stable patients with no or minimal evidence of volume overload and without recent need of IV inotropic agents. Most recent guidelines also recommend their use in patients with asymptomatic LV dysfunction.[114]

Aldactone

The Randomized Aldactone Evaluation Study (RALES) Investigators trial randomized 1663 patients with severe heart failure (class III–IV at time of randomization; EF <35%; 46% non-ischemic etiology). All patients were on a loop diuretic, >90% on an ACE inhibitor, and >70% on digitalis. Patients randomized to aldactone had a 30% reduction in risk of death. The mortality reduction was a result of lower risk of death from heart failure and sudden death. In addition, there was a 30% reduction in the risk of hospitalization. Of those on placebo, 33% noted improvement in heart failure symptoms and 48% had worsening heart failure symptoms, as compared to 41% and 38% of patients, respectively on aldactone ($P < 0.001$).[156]

Inotropes

Multiple trials of different inotropes, both oral and IV (intermittent or continuous), with various dose ranges, have failed to result in an improvement in survival in patients with heart failure, although several agents may provide transient symptomatic improvement.[157–160] Thus, routine use of these agents cannot be recommended.[114]

Amiodarone

Over 40% of cardiac deaths occur suddenly, presumably from arrhythmias. Both the Grupo de Estudio de la Sobrevida en la Insuficiencia Cardiaca en Argentina (GESICA)[118] and the Survival Trial of Antiarrhythmic Therapy in Congestive Heart Failure (CHF-STAT)[162] assessed the efficacy of amiodarone therapy in heart failure patients with asymptomatic ventricular arrhythmias.

GESICA[161] enrolled patients with NYHA class III–IV symptoms, an LVEF <35%, who were treated with routine heart failure therapy. The presence or absence of non-sustained ventricular tachycardia on Holter was noted. Patients were prospectively randomized to amiodarone 600 mg/day for 14 days, followed by 300 mg/day for 2 years. A total of 516 (260 in the amiodarone group) patients were enrolled. Within the amiodarone group, there was a 23% risk reduction (RR) in progressive heart failure. There was a 27% RR of sudden death, although there was no difference in non-cardiac deaths. There was also a 31% RR in death or heart failure admissions. On subgroup analysis, the effect of amiodarone was similar regardless of sex, functional class (NYHA class II–IV), and the presence or absence of non-sustained ventricular tachycardia. In addition, a larger proportion of amiodarone-treated patients were in the better functional classes.

CHF-STAT[162] enrolled 674 patients (336 amiodarone treated) with heart failure, >10 PVC/hour (unaccompanied by symptoms), with an EF <40% (PVC = premature ventricular complex). Patients were treated with amiodarone 800 mg/day for 2 weeks, then 400 mg/day for 50 weeks, followed by 300 mg/day until study completion. In contrast to the GESICA trial, there was no significant reduction in heart failure deaths, sudden deaths, or non-cardiac deaths. Survival was unaffected by the suppression of PVCs or elimination of venous thrombosis. Amiodarone-treated patients had a significant improvement in LVEF at 6 months although this did not affect survival. When data were analyzed based on the etiology of heart failure, there was a trend toward improved mortality in non-ischemic patients ($P = 0.07$). The difference between these two studies may be related to the different proportion of patients with coronary artery disease in the two trials and the fact that CHF-STAT but not GESICA was double-blind placebo-controlled. The Sudden Cardiac Death in Heart Failure Trial

(SCD-HeFT) will examine the role of standard care versus standard care with amiodarone or defibrillator.

Overview of treatment measures

While general supportive measures, with a period of no exercise, are recommended in the treatment of myocarditis, no specific therapies have been approved. ACE inhibitors, β blockers, and calcium-channel blockers have only been studied in animal models. The routine use of immunosuppressants is not supported by the Myocarditis Treatment Trial, although some subgroups may benefit, and other regimens may prove beneficial (Table 47.1).

Supportive measures are also suggested in IDC and exercise is encouraged. Multiple trials support the use of vasodilators, ACE inhibitors, β blockers and digoxin, when appropriate, in IDC (Table 47.2). Angiotensin receptor blockers (ARBs) or nitrates alone, or in combination with hydralazine, may be used as alternatives in patients who cannot be given ACE inhibitors.[114] There are insufficient data to support the use of immunosuppressants for the treatment of IDC. Further studies on the use of selected calcium-channel blockers are underway (PRAISE-II). The routine use of prophylactic antiarrhythmics is also unsupported. Transplantation is a valid treatment option for patients with

Table 47.1 Grading of recommendations and levels of evidence for the treatment of myocarditis

Treatment	Level of evidence	Grade
Supportive measures	5	C
Immunosuppressants	1d,[32] 2,[88] 3,[116] 4[115,118,119]	B
Cardiac transplantation	2, 5	A

Table 47.2 Grading of recommendations and levels of evidence for treatment of dilated cardiomyopathy

Treatment	Level of evidence	Grade
Supportive measures	5	C
β Blockers	1a	A
ACE inhibitors	1a	A
Vasodilators	1a	A
Angiotensin receptor blockers	1a	B
Digitalis	1a	A
Aldactone	1a	A
Amiodarone	1a	B
Transplantation	2, 5	A

end stage IDC and/or refractory myocarditis, although myocarditis may recur. Mechanical circulatory support may be used as a bridge to transplant in patients with low cardiac output states, those dependant on intravenous inotropic support, or with intractable ventricular arrhythmias, or patients who are NHYA class IV with refractory symptoms.[163]

References

1. Richardson P, McKenna W, Bristow M *et al.* Report of the 1995 World Health Organization/International Society and Federation of Cardiology Task Force on the Definition and Classification of Cardiomyopathies. *Circulation* 1996;**93**: 841–2.

2. Taylor DO, Mason JW. Myocarditis. In: Parmley W, Chatterjee K, Cheitlin MD *et al.,* eds. *Cardiology.* Philadelphia: Lippincott-Raven, 1995.

3. Daly K, Richardson PJ, Olsen EGJ *et al.* Acute myocarditis: role of histological and virological examination in the diagnosis and assessment of immunosuppressive treatment. *Br Heart J* 1984;**51**:30–5.

4. Parillo JE, Aretz HT, Palacios I, Fallon, Block PC. The results of transvenous endomyocardial biopsy can frequently be used to diagnose myocardial diseases in patients with idiopathic heart failure: endomyocardial biopsies in 100 consecutive patients revealed a substantial incidence of myocarditis. *Circulation* 1984;**69**:93–101.

5. Theoharides TC. Sudden Death of a Healthy College Student Related to Ephedrine Toxicity From Ma Huang-Containing Drink. *J Clin Psychopharmacol* 1997;**17**:437–9.

6. Bowles NE, Richardson PJ, Olsen EGJ, Archard LC. Detection of Coxsackie-B-virus-specific RNA sequences in myocardial biopsy samples from patients with myocarditis and dilated cardiomyopathy. *Lancet* 1986;**i**:1120–3.

7. Jin O, Sole MJ, Butany JW *et al.* Detection of enterovirus RNA in myocardial biopsies from patients with myocarditis and cardiomyopathy using gene amplification by polymerase chain reaction. *Circulation* 1990;**82**:8–16.

8. Grasso M, Arbustini E, Salini E *et al.* Search of Coxsackie B3 RNA in idiopathic dilated cardiomyopathy using gene amplification by polymerase chain reaction. *Am J Cardiol* 1992;**69**: 658–64.

9. Weiss LM, Liu X-F, Chang KL, Billingham ME. Detection of enteroviral RNA in idiopathic dilated cardiomyopathy and other human cardiac tissues. *J Clin Invest* 1992;**90**:156–9.

10. Martin AB, Webber S, Fricker FJ *et al.* Acute myocarditis rapid diagnosis by PCR in children. *Circulation* 1994;**90**:330–9.

11. Schowengerdt KO, Jiyuan N, Denfield SW *et al.* Diagnosis, surveillance, and epidemiologic evaluation of viral infections in pediatric cardiac transplant recipients with the use of the polymerase chain reaction. *J Heart Lung Transplant* 1996;**15**: 111–23.

12. Matsumori A, Matoba Y, Sasayama S. Dilated cardiomyopathy associated with hepatitis C virus infection. *Circulation* 1995; **92**:2519–25.

13. Dec GW, Palacios IF, Fallon JT *et al.* Active myocarditis in the spectrum of acute dilated cardiomyopathies. Clinical features, histologic correlates, and clinical outcome. *N Engl J Med* 1985;**312**:885–90.

14. Herskowitz A, Beisel KW, Wolfgram LJ, Rose NR. Coxsackie virus B3 murine myocarditis: wide pathologic spectrum in genetically defined inbred strains. *Human Pathol* 1985;**16**: 671–3.

15. Fenoglio JJ, Ursell PC, Kellog CF, Drusin RE, Weiss MB. Diagnosis and classification of myocarditis by endomyocardial biopsy. *N Engl J Med* 1983;**310**:12–18.

16. Godman GC, Bunting H, Melnick JL. The histopathology of Coxsackie virus infection in mice. 1. Morphologic observations with four different viral types. *Am J Pathol* 1952;**28**: 223–45.

17. Woodruff JF. Viral myocarditis. *Am J Pathol* 1980;**101**: 427–79.

18. Olsen EGJ. Endomyocardial biopsy. *Br Heart J* 1978;**40**:95–8.

19. Wolfgram LJ, Beisel KW, Herskowitz A, Rose NR. Variation in the susceptibility of congenic inbred mice to Coxsackie B3 induced myocarditis among different strains of mice. *J Immunol* 1986;**136**:1846–52.

20. Herskowitz A, Wolfgram LJ, Rose NR, Beisel KW. Coxsackie B3 myocarditis: a pathologic spectrum of myocarditis in genetically defined inbred strains. *J Am Coll Cardiol* 1987;**9**: 1131–9.

21. Bhardwaj V, Kumar V, Geysen HM, Sercarz EE. Degenerate recognition of a dissimilar antigenic peptide by MBP-reactive T cells: implications for thymic education and autoimmunity. *J Immunol* 1993;**151**:5000–10.

22. Cunningham MW, Antone SM, Gulizia JM *et al.* Cytotoxic and viral neutralizing antibodies cross react with streptococcal M protein enteroviruses and human cardiac myosin. *Proc Natl Acad Sci USA* 1992;**89**:1320–4.

23. Alvarez FL, Neu N, Rose NR, Craig SW, Beisel KW. Heart-specific autoantibodies induced by Coxsackie virus B3: identification of heart autoantigens. *Clin Immunol Immunopathol* 1987;**43**:129–39.

24. Neu N, Beisel KW, Traystman MD, Rose NR, Craig SW. Autoantibodies specific for the cardiac myosin isoform are found in mice susceptible to Coxsackie B3-induced myocarditis. *J Immunol* 1987;**138**:2488–92.

25. Dahl AM, Beverley PCL, Stauss HJ. A synthetic peptide derived from the tumor-associated protein mdm2 can stimulate autoreactive, high avidity cytotoxic T lymphocytes that recognize naturally processed protein. *J Immunol* 1996;**157**: 239–46.

26. Limas CJ, Goldenberg IF, Limas C. Autoantibodies against beta-adrenoreceptors in human dilated cardiomyopathy. *Circ Res* 1989;**64**:97–103.

27. Schultheiss HP, Schulze K, Huhl U, Ulrich G, Klingenberg M. The ADP/ATP carrier as a mitochondrial autoantigen – facts and perspectives. *Ann NY Acad Sci* 1986;**488**:44–64.

28. Wolff PG, Kühl U, Schultheiss HP. Laminin distribution and autoantibodies to laminin in dilated cardiomyopathy and myocarditis. *Am Heart J* 1989;**117**:1303–9.

29. Ansari AA, Herskowitz A, Danner DJ. Identification of mitochondrial proteins that serve as targets for autoimmunity. *Circulation* 1988;**78**(Suppl.):457 (Abstract).

30. Latif N, Baker CS, Dunn MJ *et al.* Frequency and specificity of antiheart antibodies in patients with dilated cardiomyopathy

detected using SDS-PAGE and Western blotting. *J Am Coll Cardiol* 1993;**22**:1378–84.

31. Maisch B, Bauer E, Cirsi M, Kochsiek K. Cytolytic cross-reactive antibodies directed against the cardiac membrane and viral proteins in Coxsackie B3 and B4 myocarditis. *Circulation* 1993;**87**(Suppl.V):IV-49–IV-65.

32. Mason JW, O'Connell JB, Herskowitz A *et al*. A clinical trial of immunosuppressive therapy for myocarditis. *N Engl J Med* 1995;**333**:269–75.

33. Muir P, Tizley AJ, English TAH *et al*. Chronic relapsing pericarditis and dilated cardiomyopathy: serological evidence of persistent enterovirus infection. *Lancet* 1989;**1**:804–7.

34. Cambridge G, MacArthur CG, Waterson AP, Goodwin JF, Oakley CM. Antibodies to Coxsackie B viruses in congestive cardiomyopathy. *Br Heart J* 1979;**41**:692–6.

35. Kawai C. Idiopathic cardiomyopathy: a study on the infection-immune theory as a cause of the disease. *Japan Circ J* 1971; **35**:765–70.

36. Schwaiger A, Umlauft F, Weyrer K *et al*. Detection of enteroviral ribonucleic acid in myocardial biopsies from patients with idiopathic dilated cardiomyopathy by polymerase chain reaction. *Am Heart J* 1993;126:406–10.

37. Schultheiss HP, Bolte HD. Immunological analysis of auto-antibodies against the adenine nucleotide translocator in dilated cardiomyopathy. *J Mol Cell Cardiol* 1985;**17**:603–17.

38. Caforio ALP, Grazzini M, Mann JM *et al*. Identification of a- and b-cardiac myosin heavy chain isoforms as major autoantigens in dilated cardiomyopathy. *Circulation* 1992; **85**:1734–42.

39. Herskowitz A, Neumann DA, Ansari AA. Concepts of autoimmunity applied to idiopathic dilated cardiomyopathy. *J Am Coll Cardiol* 1993;**22**:1385–8.

40. Carlquist JF, Hibbs JB, Edelman LS, Watt RA, Anderson JL. Coxsackie B3 myocarditis in mice: viral clearance and post-infectious mortality are not associated with increased nitric oxide production. *Circulation* 1996;**94**(Suppl.):I-468 (Abstract).

41. Nishi H, Kimura A, Koga Y, Toshima H, Sasazuki T. DNA typing of class II genes in Japanese patients with dilated cardiomyopathy. *J Mol Cell Cardiol* 1995;**27**:2385–92.

42. McKenna CJ, Codd MB, McCann HA, Sugrue DD. Idiopathic dilated cardiomyopathy: familial prevalence and HLA distribution. *Heart* 1997;**77**:549–52.

43. Olson TM, Thibodeau SN, Lundquist PA, Schaid DJ, Michels VV. Exclusion of a primary gene defect at the HLA locus in familial idiopathic dilated cardiomyopathy. *J Med Genet* 1995;**32**:876–80.

44. Olson TM, Michels VV, Thibodeau SN, Tai YS, Keating MT. Actin mutations in dilated cardiomyopathy, a heritable form of heart failure. *Science* 1998;**280**:750–2.

45. Towbin JA, Hejtmancik JF, Brink P *et al*. X-linked dilated cardiomyopathy. Molecular genetic evidence of linkage to the Duchenne muscular dystrophy (dystrophin) gene at the Xp21 locus. *Circulation* 1993;**87**:1854–65.

46. Li D, Tapscoft T, Gonzalez O *et al*. Desmin mutation responsible for idiopathic dilated cardiomyopathy. *Circulation* 1999;**100**:461–4.

47. Fatkin D, MacRae C, Sasaki T *et al*. Missense mutations in the rod domain of the lamin A/C gene as causes of dilated car-

diomyopathy and conduction-system disease. *N Engl J Med* 1999;**341**:1715–24.

48. Charron Ph, Tesson F, Poirier O. Identification of a genetic risk factor for idiopathic dilated cardiomyopathy. Involvement of a polymorphism in the endothelin receptor type a gene. *Eur Heart J* 1999;**20**:1587–91.

49. Tsubata S, Bowles KR, Vatta M *et al*. Mutations in the human delta-sacroglycan gene in familial and sporadic dilated cardiomyopathy. *J Clin Invest* 2000;**106**:655–62.

50. Arimura T, Nakamura T, Hiroi S *et al*. Characterization of the human nebulette gene: a polymorphism in an actin-binding motif is associated with nonfamilial idiopathic dilated cardiomyopathy. *Human Genet* 2000;**107**:440–51.

51. Neu N, Pummerer C, Rieker T, Berger P. T cells in cardiac myosin-induced myocarditis. *Clin Immunol Immunopathol* 1993;**68**:107–10.

52. Smith SC, Allen PM. Expression of myosin-class II major histocompatibility complexes in the normal myocardium occurs before induction of autoimmune myocarditis. *Proc Natl Acad Sci USA* 1992;**89**:9131–5.

53. Badorff C, Lee GH, Lamphear BJ *et al*. Enteroviral protease 2A cleaves dystrophin: evidence of cytoskeletal disruption in an acquired cardiomyopathy. *Nature Med* 1999;**5**:320–6.

54. Gravanis M, Sternby N. Incidence of myocarditis: a 10-year autopsy study from Malmö, Sweden. *Arch Pathol Lab Med* 1991;**115**:390–2.

55. Hufnagel G, Pankuweit S, Richter A *et al*. The European Study of Epidemiology and Treatment of Cardiac Inflammatory Diseases (ESETCID). *Herz* 2000;**25**:279–85.

56. Herskowitz A, Campbell S, Deckers J *et al*. Demographic features and prevalence of idiopathic myocarditis in patients undergoing endomyocardial biopsy. *Am J Cardiol* 1993;**71**: 982–6.

57. Brown CA, O'Connell JB. Myocarditis and idiopathic dilated cardiomyopathy. *Am J Med* 1995;**99**:309–14.

58. Codd MB, Sugrue DD, Gersh BJ, Melton LJ. Epidemiology of idiopathic dilated and hypertrophic cardiomyopathy. *Circulation* 1989;**80**:564–72.

59. Felker GM, Hu W, Hare JM. The spectrum of dilated cardiomyopathy. The Johns Hopkins experience with 1,278 patients. *Medicine* 1999;**78**:270–83.

60. McDonagh TA. Asymptomatic left ventricular dysfunction in the community. *Curr Cardiol Rep* 2000;**2**:470–4.

61. Mosterd A, Hoes AW, de Bruyne MC *et al*. Prevalence of heart failure and left ventricular dysfunction in the general population. The Rotterdam Study. *Eur Heart J* 1999;**20**:447–55.

62. Grunig E, Tasman JA, Kucherer *et al*. Frequency and phenotypes of familial dilated cardiomyopathy. *J Am Coll Cardiol* 1998;**31**:186–94.

63. Baig MK, Goldman JH, Caforio APL. Familial dilated cardiomyopathy: cardiac abnormalities are common in asymptomatic relatives and may represent early disease. *J Am Coll Cardiol* 1998;**31**:195–201.

64. Dec GW, Fuster V. Medical progress: idiopathic dilated cardiomyopathy. *N Engl J Med* 1994;**331**:1564–75.

65. Coughlin SS, Gottdiener JS, Baughman KL *et al*. Black-white differences in mortality in idiopathic dilated cardiomyopathy: the Washington DC Dilated Cardiomyopathy Study. *J Natl Med Assoc* 1994;**86**:583–91.

66. De Maria R, Gavazzi A, Recalcati F *et al.* Comparison of clinical findings in idiopathic dilated cardiomyopathy in women versus men. *Am J Cardiol* 1993;**72**:580–5.

67. Pearson GD, Veille J, Rahimtoola S *et al.* Peripartum cardiomyopathy. National Heart, Lung, and Blood Institute and Office of Rare Diseases (National Institutes of Health) Workshop Recommendations and Review. *JAMA* 2000;**2823**:1183–8.

68. Lampert MB, Lang RM. Peripartum cardiomyopathy. *Am Heart J* 1995;**130**:860–70.

69. Grogan M, Redfield MM, Bailey KR *et al.* Long-term outcome of patients with biopsy-proved myocarditis: comparison with idiopathic dilated cardiomyopathy. *J Am Coll Cardiol* 1995;**26**:80–4.

70. Lampert MB, Weinert L, Hibbard J *et al.* Contractile reserve in patients with peripartum cardiomyopathy and recovered left ventricular function. *Am J Obstet Gynecol* 1997;**176**:189–95.

71. Midei MG, DeMent SH, Feldman AM, Hutchins GM, Baughman KL. Peripartum myocarditis and cardiomyopathy. *Circulation* 1990;**81**:922–8.

72. Rizeq MN, Rickenbacher PR, Fowler MB, Billingham ME. Incidence of myocarditis in peripartum cardiomyopathy. *Am J Cardiol* 1994;**74**:474–7.

73. Felker GM, Jaeger CJ, Klodas E *et al.* Myocarditis and long-term survival in peripartum cardiomyopathy. *Am Heart J* 2000;**140**:785–91.

74. Pearl W. Familial occurrence of peripartum cardiomyopathy. *Am Heart J* 1995;**129**:421–2.

75. Witlin AG, Mabie WC, Sibai BM. Peripartum cardiomyopathy: an ominous diagnosis. *Am J Obstet Gynecol* 1997;**176**:182–8.

76. Elkayam U, Tummala PP, Rao K *et al.* Maternal and fetal outcomes of subsequent pregnancies in women with peripartum cardiomyopathy. *N Engl J Med* 2001;**344**:1567–71.

77. Araki M, Kanda T, Imai S *et al.* Comparative effects of losartan, captopril, and enalapril on murine acute myocarditis due to encephalomyocarditis virus. *J Cardiol Pharmacol* 1995;**26**:61–5.

78. Bozkat B, Villanueva F, Holubkov R *et al.* Intravenous immune globulin in the therapy of peripartum cardiomyopathy. *J Am Coll Cardiol* 1999;**34**:177–80.

79. Dec GW, Waldman H, Southern J *et al.* Viral myocarditis mimicking acute myocardial infarction. *J Am Coll Cardiol* 1992;**20**:85–9.

80. Costanzo-Nordin MR, O'Connell JB, Subramanian R, Robinson JA, Scanlon PJ. Myocarditis confirmed by biopsy presenting as acute myocardial infarction. *Br Heart J* 1985;**53**:25–9.

81. Hufnagel G, Pankuweit S, Richter A *et al.* The European Study of Epidemiology and Treatment of Cardiac Inflammatory Diseases (ESETCID). *Herz* 2000;**25**:279–85.

82. Aretz HT. Myocarditis: the Dallas Criteria. *Human Pathol* 1987;**18**:619–24.

83. Lieberman EB, Herskowitz A, Rose NR, Baughman KL. A clinicopathologic description of myocarditis. *Clin Immunol Immunopathol* 1993;**68**:191–6.

84. McCarthy RE, Boehmer JP, Hruban RH *et al.* Long term outcome of fulminant myocarditis as compared with acute (nonfulminant) myocarditis. *N Engl J Med* 2000;**342**:690–5.

85. Kuhn H, Breithardt G, Knieriern HJ *et al.* Prognosis and possible presymptomatic manifestations of congestive cardiomyopathy (COCM). *Postgrad Med J* 1978;**54**:451–9.

86. Morgera T, Di Lenarda A, Dreas L *et al.* Electrocardiography of myocarditis revisited: clinical and prognostic significance of electrocardiographic changes. *Am Heart J* 1992;**124**:455–66.

87. Mendes LA, Dec GW, Picard MH *et al.* Right ventricular dysfunction: an independent predictor of adverse outcome in patients with myocarditis. *Am Heart J* 1994;**128**:301–7.

88. Gagliardi MG, Bevilacqua M, Squitieri C *et al.* Dilated cardiomyopathy caused by acute myocarditis in pediatric patients: evolution of myocardial damage in a group of potential heart transplant candidates. *J Heart Lung Transplant* 1993;**12**:S224–S229.

89. Fuster V, Gersh BJ, Giuliani ER *et al.* The natural history of idiopathic dilated cardiomyopathy. *Am J Cardiol* 1981;**47**:525–31.

90. Redfield MM, Gersh BJ, Bailey KR, Ballard DJ, Rodeheffer RJ. Natural history of idiopathic dilated cardiomyopathy: effect of referral bias and secular trend. *J Am Coll Cardiol* 1993;**22**:1921–6.

91. Redfield MM, Gersh BJ, Bailey KR, Rodeheffer RJ. Natural history of incidentally discovered, asymptomatic idiopathic dilated cardiomyopathy. *Am J Cardiol* 1994;**74**:737–9.

92. Kaneko K, Kanda T, Yamauchi Y *et al.* C-reactive protein in dilated cardiomyopathy. *Cardiology* 1998;**91**:215–19.

93. Sato Y, Yamada T, Taniguchi R *et al.* Persistently increased serum concentrations of cardiac troponin T in patients with idiopathic cardiomyopathy are predictive of adverse outcomes. *Circulation* 2001;**103**:369–74.

94. Tsutamota T, Wada A, Maeda K *et al.* Plasma brain natriuretic peptide level as a biochemical marker of morbidity ad mortality in patients with asymptomatic or minimally symptomatic ventricular dysfunction: Comparison with plasma angiotensin II and endothelin-1. *Eur Heart J* 1999;**20**:1799–807.

95. Dao Q, Krishnaswamy P, Kasanegra R *et al.* Usefulness of a rapid, bedside test for brain natriuretic peptide in the evaluation of patients presenting to the emergency room with possible congestive heart failure. *J Am Coll Cardiol* 2000;**35**: 171A (Abstract 1049–152).

96. Nagaoka H, Isobe N, Kubota S *et al.* Myocardial contractile reserve as prognostic determinant in patients with idiopathic dilated cardiomyopathy without overt heart failure. *Chest* 1997;**111**:344–50.

97. Ramahi TM, Longo MD, Cadariu AR *et al.* Dobutamine–induced augmentation of left ventricular ejection fraction predicts survival of heart failure patients with severe non-ischaemic cardiomyopathy. *Eur Heart J* 2001;**22**:849–56.

98. Naqvi TZ, Goel RK, Forrester JS, Siegal RJ. Myocardial contractile reserve on dobutamine echocardiography predicts late spontaneous improvement in cardiac function in patients with recent onset idiopathic dilated cardiomyopathy. *J Am Coll Cardiol* 1999;**34**:1537–44.

99. Treasure CB, Vita JA, Cox DA *et al.* Endothelium-dependent dilation of the coronary microvasculature is impaired in dilated cardiomyopathy. *Circulation* 1990;**81**:772–9.

100. Mathier MA, Rose GA, Fifeer MA *et al.* Coronary endothelial dysfunction in patients with acute-onset idiopathic dilated cardiomyopathy. *J Am Coll Cardiol* 1998;**32**:216–24.

101. Taliercio CP, Seward JB, Driscoll DJ *et al.* Idiopathic dilated cardiomyopathy in the young: clinical profile and natural history. *J Am Coll Cardiol* 1985;**6**:1126–31.

102. Venugopalan P, Houston AB, Agarwal AK. The outcome of idiopathic dilated cardiomyopathy and myocaraditis in children from the West of Scotland. *Int J Cardiol* 2001;**78**:135–41.

103. Ilbäck N-G, Fohlman J, Friman G. Exercise in Coxsackie B3 myocarditis: effects on heart lymphocyte subpopulations and the inflammatory reaction. *Am Heart J* 1989;**117**:1298–302.

104. Maron BJ, Isner JM, McKenna WJ. Task Force 3: hypertrophic cardiomyopathy, myocarditis and other myopericardial diseases and mitral valve prolapse. *J Am Coll Cardiol* 1994;**24**:845–99.

105. Matsumori A, Wang H, Abelmann WH, Crumpacker CS. Treatment of viral myocarditis with ribavirin in an animal preparation. *Circulation* 1985;**71**:834–9.

106. Rezkalla S, Kloner RA, Khatib G, Khatib R. Beneficial effects of captopril in acute Coxsackie virus B3 murine myocarditis. *Circulation* 1990;**81**:1039–46.

107. Rezkalla S, Kloner RA, Khatib G, Smith FE, Khatib R. Effect of metoprolol in Coxsackie virus B3 murine myocarditis. *J Am Coll Cardiol* 1988;**12**:412–4.

108. Tominaga M, Matsumori A, Okada I, Yamada T, Kawai C. β-Blocker treatment of dilated cardiomyopathy. Beneficial effects of carvedilol in mice. *Circulation* 1991;**83**:2021–8.

109. Dong R, Liu P, Wee L, Butany J, Sole MJ. Verapamil ameliorates the clinical and pathological course of murine myocarditis. *J Clin Invest* 1992;**90**:2022–30.

110. Costanzo-Nordin MR, Reap EA, O'Connell JB, Robinson JA, Scanlon PJ. A nonsteroid anti-inflammatory drug exacerbates Coxsackie B3 murine myocarditis. *J Am Coll Cardiol* 1985;**6**:1078–82.

111. Rezkalla S, Khatib G, Khatib R. Coxsackie B3 murine myocarditis: deleterious effects of nonsteroidal anti-inflammatory agents. *J Lab Clin Med* 1986;**107**:393–5.

112. Matsui S, Matsumori A, Matoba Y, Uchida A, Sasayama S. Treatment of virus-induced myocardial injury with a novel immunomodulating agent, vesnarinone. *J Clin Invest* 1994;**94**:1212–17.

113. Cooper LT, Berry GJ, Shabetai R, for the Multicenter Giant Cell Myocarditis Study Group Investigators. Idiopathic giant-cell myocarditis – natural history and treatment. *N Engl J Med* 1997;**336**:1860–6.

114. Hunt SA, Baker DW, Chin MH *et al.* ACC/AHA Guidelines for the evaluation and management of chronic heart failure in the adult: executive summary. *J Am Coll Cardiol* 2001;**38**:2101–13.

115. Kühl U, Schultheiss HP. Treatment of chronic myocarditis with corticosteroids. *Eur Heart J* 1995;**16**:168–72.

116. Drucker NA, Colan SD, Lewis AB *et al.* δ-Globulin treatment of acute myocarditis in the pediatric population. *Circulation* 1994;**89**:252–7.

117. Miri M, Vasiljevi J, Boji M *et al.* Long-term follow up of patients with dilated heart muscle disease treated with human leucocytic interferon alpha or thymic hormones. *Heart* 1996;**75**:596–601.

118. McNamara DM, Rosenblum WD, Janosko KM *et al.* Intravenous immune globulin in the therapy of myocarditis and acute cardiomyopathy. *Circulation* 1997;**95**:2476–8.

119. Ahdot J, Galindo A, Alejos JC *et al.* Use of OKT3 for Acute myocarditis in infants and children. *J Heart Lung Transplant* 2000;**19**:1118–21.

120. Kishimoto C, Thorp KA, Abelmann WH. Immunosuppression with high doses of cyclophosphamide reduces the severity of myocarditis but increases the mortality in murine Coxsackie virus B3 myocarditis. *Circulation* 1990;**82**:982–9.

121. Yamada T, Matsumori A, Sasayama S. Therapeutic effect of anti-tumor necrosis factor-alpha antibody on the murine model of viral myocarditis induced by encephalomyocarditis virus. *Circulation* 1994;**89**:846–51.

122. Chapman NM, Tracy S. Can recombinant DNA technology provide useful vaccines against viruses which induce heart disease? *Eur Heart J* 1995;**16**:144–6.

123. O'Connell JB, Breen TJ, Hosenpud JD. Heart transplantation in dilated heart muscle disease and myocarditis. *Eur Heart J* 1995;**16**(Suppl. O):137–9.

124. Loria K, Jessurun J, Shumway SJ, Kubo SH. Early recurrence of chronic active myocarditis after heart transplantation. *Human Pathol* 1994;**25**:323–6.

125. Williams JF, Bristow MR, Fowler MB *et al.* Guidelines for the evaluation and management of heart failure. *Circulation* 1995;**92**:2764–84.

126. Cohn JN, Archibald DG, Ziesche S *et al.* Effect of vasodilator therapy on mortality in chronic congestive heart failure: results of a Veterans Administration Cooperative Study. *N Engl J Med* 1986;**314**:1547–52.

127. CONSENSUS Trial Study Group. Effects of enalapril on mortality in severe congestive heart failure: results of the Cooperative North Scandinavian Enalapril Survival Study (CONSENSUS). *N Engl J Med* 1987;**316**:1429–35.

128. SOLVD Investigators. Effect of enalapril on survival in patients with reduced left ventricular ejection fractions and congestive heart failure. *N Engl J Med* 1991;**325**:293–302.

129. SOLVD Investigators. Effect of enalapril on mortality and the development of heart failure in asymptomatic patients with reduced left ventricular ejection fractions. *N Engl J Med* 1992;**327**:685–91.

130. Loeb HS, Johnson G, Henrick A *et al.* Effect of enalapril, hydralazine plus isosorbide dinitrate, and prazosin on hospitalization in patients with chronic congestive heart failure. The V-HeFT Cooperative Studies Group. *Circulation* 1993;**87** (Suppl. 6):VI78–87.

131. Dickstein K, Chang P, Willenheimer R *et al.* Comparison of the effects of losartan and enalapril on clinical status and exercise performance in patients with moderate or severe chronic heart failure. *J Am Coll Cardiol* 1995;**26**:438–45.

132. Pitt B, Segal R, Martinez FA *et al.* Randomized trial of losartan versus captopril in patients over 65 with heart failure (Evaluation of Losartan in the Elderly Study, ELITE). *Lancet* 1997;**349**:747–52.

133. Pitt B, Poole-Wilson PA, Segal R *et al.* Effect of losartan compared with captopril on mortality in patients with symptomatic heart failure: randomised trial – The Losartan Heart Failure Survival Study ELITE II. *Lancet* 2000;**355**:1582–7.

134. Cohn JN, Tognoni G, for the Valsartan Heart Failure Trial Investigators. A randomised trial of the angiotensin-receptor blocker valsartan in chronic heart failure. *N Engl J Med* 2001;**345**:1667–75.

135. Uretsky BF, Young JB, Shahidi FE *et al*. Randomized study assessing the effect of digoxin withdrawal in patients with mild to moderate chronic congestive heart failure: results of PROVED trial. *J Am Coll Cardiol* 1993;**22**:955–62.

136. Packer M, Gheorghiade M, Young J *et al*. Withdrawal of digoxin from patients with chronic heart failure treated with angiotensin-converting-enzyme inhibitors. *N Engl J Med* 1993;**329**:1–7.

137. Digitalis Investigation Group. The effect of digoxin on mortality and morbidity in patients with heart failure. *N Engl J Med* 1997;**336**:525–33.

138. Parillo JE, Cunnion RE, Epstein SE *et al*. A prospective, randomized, controlled trial of prednisone for dilated cardiomyopathy. *N Engl J Med* 1989;**321**:1061–8.

139. McNamara DM, Holubkov R, Starling RC *et al*. Controlled trial of intravenous immune globulin in recent-onset dilated cardiomyopathy. *Circulation* 2001;**103**:2254–9.

140. Wojnicz R, Nowalany-Kozielska E, Wojciechowska *et al*. Randomized, placebo-controlled study for immunosuppressive treatment of inflammatory dilated cardiomyopathy. Two-year follow-up results. *Circulation* 2001;**104**:39–45.

141. Felix SB, Stuudt A, Dörffel WV, *et al*. Hemodynamic effects of immunoadsorption and subsequent immunoglobulin substitution in dilated cardiomyopathy. Three-month results from a randomized study. *J Am Coll Cardiol* 2000;**35**:1590–8.

142. Wu LA, Lapeyre AC, Cooper LT. Current role of endomyocardial biopsy in the management of dilated cardiomyopathy and myocarditis. *Mayo Clin Proc* 2001;**76**:1030–8.

143. Fazio S, Sabatini D, Capaldo B *et al*. A preliminary study of growth hormone in the treatment of dilated cardiomyopathy. *N Engl J Med* 1996;**334**:809–14.

144. Isgaard J, Bergh CH, Caidahl K *et al*. A placebo-controlled study of growth hormone in patients with congestive heart failure. *Eur Heart J* 1998;**19**:1704–11.

145. Packer M, O'Connor CM, Ghali JK *et al*. Effect of amlodipine on morbidity and mortality in severe chronic heart failure (PRAISE). *N Engl J Med* 1996;**335**:1107–14.

146. Factor SM, Minase T, Cho S, Dominitz R, Sonnenblick EH. Microvascular spasm in the cardiomyopathic Syrian hamster: a preventable cause of focal myocardial necrosis. *Circulation* 1982;**66**:342–54.

147. Swedberg K, Hjalmarson A, Waagstein F, Wallentin I. Preliminary communications: prolongation of survival in congestive cardiomyopathy by beta receptor blockade. *Lancet* 1979;**1**:1374–6.

148. Engelmeier RS, O'Connell JB, Walsh R *et al*. Improvement in symptoms and exercise tolerance by metoprolol in patients with dilated cardiomyopathy: double-blind, randomized, placebo-controlled trial. *Circulation* 1985;**72**:536–46.

149. Waagstein F, Bristow MR, Swedberg K. Beneficial effects of metoprolol in idiopathic dilated cardiomyopathy. *Lancet* 1993;**342**:1441–6.

150. Tsuyuki RT, Yusuf S, Rouleau JL *et al*. for the RESOLVD Study Investigators. Combination of neurohormonal blockade with ACE inhibitors, angiotensin antagonists and beta-blockers in patients with congestive heart failure: design of the Random Evaluation of Strategies for Left Ventricular Dysfunction (RESOLVD) Pilot Study. *Can J Cardiol* 1997;**13**:1166–74.

151. CIBIS Investigators and Committees. A randomized trial of β-blockade in heart failure: the Cardiac Insufficiency Bisoprolol Study (CIBIS). *Circulation* 1994;**90**:1765–73.

152. CIBIS-II Investigators and Committees. The Cardiac Insufficiency Bisoprolol Study II (CIBIS-II): a randomized trial. *Lancet* 1999;**353**:9–13.

153. Packer M, Bristow MR, Cohn JN *et al*. The effect of carvedilol on morbidity and mortality in patients with chronic heart failure. *N Engl J Med* 1996;**334**:1349–55.

154. Packer M, Colucci WS, Sackner-Bernstein JD *et al*. Double-blind, placebo-controlled study of the effects of carvedilol in patients with moderate to severe heart failure. The PRECISE Trial. *Circulation* 1996;**94**:2793–9.

155. Hjalmarson A, Goldstein S, Fagerberg B *et al*. Effects of controlled-release metoprolol on total mortality, hospitalizations, and well-being in patients with heart failure. The Metoprolol CR/XL Randomized Intervention Trial in Congestive Heart Failure (MERIT-HF). *JAMA* 2000;**283**:1295–302.

156. Pitt B, Zannad F, Remme WJ *et al*. The effect of spironolactone on morbidity and mortality in patients with severe heart failure. *N Engl J Med* 1999;**341**:709–17.

157. Simonton CA, Chatterjee K, Cody RJ *et al*. Milrinone in congestive failure: acute and chronic hemodynamic and clinical evaluation. *J Am Coll Cardiol* 1985;**6**:453–9.

158. DiBianco R, Shabetai R, Kostuk W *et al*. for the Milrinone Multicenter Trial Group. A comparison of oral milrinone, digoxin, and their combination in the treatment of patients with chronic heart failure. *N Engl J Med* 1989;**320**:677–83.

159. Uretsky BF, Jessup M, Konstam MA *et al*. for the Enoximone Multicenter Trial Group. Multicenter trial of oral enoximone in patients with moderate to moderately severe congestive heart failure. *Circulation* 1990;**82**:774–80.

160. Feldman AM, Bristow MR, Parmley WW *et al*. for the Vesnarinone Study Group. Effects of vesnarinone on morbidity and mortality in patients with heart failure. *N Engl J Med* 1993;**329**:149–55.

161. Doval HC, Nul DR, Grancelli HO *et al*. for Grupo de Estudio de la Sobrevida en la Insuficiencia Cardiaca en Argentina (GESICA). Randomised trial of low-dose amiodarone in severe congestive heart failure. *Lancet* 1994;**344**:493–8.

162. Singh SN, Fletcher RD, Fisher SG *et al*. for the Survival Trial of Antiarrhythmic Therapy in Congestive Heart Failure. Amiodarone in patients with congestive heart failure and asymptomatic ventricular arrhythmia. *N Engl J Med* 1995;**333**:77–82.

163. Stevenson LW, Kormos RL, Bourge RC *et al*. Mechanical cardiac support 2000. Current applications and future trial designs. *J Am Coll Cardiol* 2001;**37**:340–70.

48 Hypertrophic cardiomyopathy

Perry M Elliott, Rajesh Thaman, William J McKenna

Hypertrophic cardiomyopathy (HCM) is defined by the presence of left and or right ventricular hypertrophy in the absence of a cardiac or systemic cause. It predisposes to fatal cardiac arrhythmia, and is an important cause of sudden death in individuals aged less than 35 years. The following chapter reviews current data on etiology, diagnosis, and treatment of the disease, and briefly discusses areas of uncertainty.

Genetics

In the majority of cases, HCM is an autosomal dominant inherited disease caused by mutations in genes encoding cardiac sarcomeric proteins: β-myosin heavy chain on chromosome 14q11 (35%), cardiac troponin-T on chromosome 1q3 (15%), cardiac troponin-I on chromosome 19, α-tropomyosin on chromosome 15q2 (<5%), and myosin binding protein-C on chromosome 11p11·2 (15%).[1–5] Less than 1% of patients have mutations affecting the genes encoding the essential and regulatory myosin light chains (on chromosomes 3 and 12 respectively),[6] and cardiac actin on chromosome 15.[7] A further unconfirmed mutation in the gene encoding another sarcomeric protein, Titin on chromosome 2, has also been reported.[8]

A causal association between sarcomeric protein gene abnormalities and HCM is supported by a number of observations: cosegregation of mutation and disease in adult patients, the presence of mutations in patients with familial HCM but not in unrelated unaffected individuals, and an association between *de novo* mutations and sporadic disease.[9] The manner in which specific mutations result in disease is still poorly understood, but it might be expected that point mutations occurring within critical domains of sarcomeric protein molecules would result in predictable cardiac phenotypes. Preliminary studies have suggested that patients with troponin-T gene mutations tend to have mild ventricular hypertrophy and a high prevalence of sudden death, whereas most β-myosin heavy chain mutations that are associated with sudden death have at least moderate hypertrophy. Despite this, mutations affecting identical residues can result in very different clinical outcomes,[10] suggesting that other genetic and environmental factors influence disease expression. One such disease "modifier" may be angiotensin converting enzyme (ACE) gene polymorphism, with several papers suggesting that the DD genotype is associated with more severe hypertrophy than either ID or II genotypes.[11]

Recently, investigation of the functional consequences of sarcomeric protein mutations has been facilitated by the study of mutant β-myosin within human skeletal muscle. The demonstration of selective type 1 fiber atrophy, reduced shortening velocity, and impaired isometric force contraction[12,13] suggest that the characteristic myocardial pathology of HCM is a compensatory response to impaired contractile function. A mouse model, developed by introducing a [403]Arginine to glutamine α-myosin mutation, has supported this hypothesis by demonstrating cardiac dysfunction before the development of disarray and myocyte hypertrophy.[14] This study also demonstrated that male mutant mice had more extensive disease than their female counterparts, indicating that gender may also modulate phenotype expression.

Pathology

Although any pattern of ventricular hypertrophy can be seen in HCM, it is usually asymmetrically distributed, affecting the interventricular septum more than the free or posterior walls of the left ventricle.[15] Isolated right ventricular hypertrophy is unreported, but right-sided involvement in association with left ventricular hypertrophy occurs in up to a third of patients. Microscopically, HCM is characterized by disturbance of myocyte-to-myocyte orientation, with cells forming whorls around foci of connective tissue ("disarray"). Individual cells vary in size and length, and there is disruption of the normal intracellular myofibrillar architecture. Myocyte disarray is described in congenital heart disease, hypertension, and aortic stenosis, but it is more extensive in HCM, typically affecting more than 20% of ventricular tissue blocks post mortem and more than 5% of total myocardium. Other characteristic features include myocardial fibrosis and abnormal small intramural arteries.[16] The significance of the latter remains uncertain, but the presence of extensive small vessel disease in areas of fibrosis has suggested that they may cause myocardial ischemia. However, more recent data have shown that small vessel disease may be just as widespread in patients without extensive fibrosis.[17]

Pathophysiology

Hemodynamics

Systolic function is normal or "hyperdynamic" in most patients; 25% have a subaortic pressure gradient temporally associated with contact between the anterior mitral valve leaflet and the interventricular septum in systole.[18] It is thought that the mitral valve leaflet is drawn anteriorly by Venturi forces generated as blood is rapidly ejected through a narrowed left ventricular outflow tract. More recently the importance of abnormal anterior displacement of the papillary muscles during systole and other abnormalities of the mitral valve apparatus such as leaflet elongation have been recognized as contributory factors.[19,20] Although the magnitude of the outflow tract gradient is related to the time of onset and the duration of mitral valve–septal contact, its clinical significance is still debated. Several papers have shown that up to 80% of stroke volume may be ejected before a gradient develops, leading some authorities to suggest that "true" obstruction to flow does not occur.[21] In other patients, however, the presence of rapid deceleration in aortic flow at the time of septal–mitral contact, prolongation of left ventricular ejection time, and continued ventricular shortening after the onset of the outflow gradient in the absence of forward flow, suggest that the gradient is of hemodynamic significance.[22] An analysis of published hemodynamic and echocardiographic data[18] has shown that the percentage of stroke volume ejected before mitral–septal contact is inversely related to the magnitude of the gradient. Using this model, the gradient only becomes hemodynamically "significant" when it exceeds 50 mmHg.

Diastolic function

Up to 80% of patients have a range of diastolic abnormalities that include slow and prolonged isovolumic relaxation, reduced rate of rapid filling, and increased left ventricular stiffness.[23,24] The underlying cause of diastolic abnormalities are difficult to determine in individual patients, although myocardial fibrosis, left ventricular hypertrophy, myocyte disarray, myocardial ischemia, regional asynchrony, abnormal intracellular calcium fluxes, and disordered ventricular geometry may each play a role. While diastolic abnormalities are undoubtedly the cause of symptoms in many patients, they are also observed in asymptomatic individuals. A minority of patients have features resembling restrictive cardiomyopathy with severe diastolic dysfunction, markedly elevated filling pressures, mild or no hypertrophy and bi-atrial dilatation.

Myocardial ischemia

Evidence for myocardial ischemia in HCM includes reduced coronary flow reserve and lactate production during pacing or pharmacologic stress.[25,26] The etiology of myocardial ischemia in HCM is likely to be multifactorial. Abnormal intramural vessels with small lumina, increased metabolic demands of hypertrophied myocardium, elevated left ventricular filling pressures and abnormalities in diastolic filling and relaxation may all contribute.[27] Ischemia may lead to myocardial fibrosis and scarring and, as a consequence, contribute to systolic and diastolic left ventricular dysfunction. Ischemia may also be one of the factors that contribute to the multiplicity of events leading to ventricular arrhythmia and sudden death. In routine clinical practice, however, the evaluation of chest pain remains problematic because standard non-invasive screening tests, such as exercise testing and [201]thallium perfusion scintigraphy, are difficult to interpret in the presence of ventricular hypertrophy.[27–29]

Vascular responses to exercise

The physiologic response to exercise in normal individuals consists of an increase in systolic blood pressure associated with a three- to fourfold increase in cardiac output. In one third of patients with HCM the blood pressure fails to rise appropriately or may even fall during exercise, despite an appropriate increase in cardiac output. This abnormal reflex is thought to relate to the inappropriate activation of ventricular baroreceptors, which in turn leads to a withdrawal of efferent sympathetic tone resulting in a fall in systemic vascular resistance. The mechanisms responsible for baroreceptor activation are unknown but may relate to increased wall stress and myocardial ischemia.[30–32]

Clinical aspects

Epidemiology

Six studies have examined the prevalence of HCM[32–37] and, whilst comparison between them is difficult because of the different methodologies and selection criteria used (Table 48.1), most have suggested a figure of at least 0·2%. The exception[35] was based on an analysis of patient records

Table 48.1 Prevalence of hypertrophic cardiomyopathy

Author	n	Screening method	Prevalence (%)
Savage 1983[33]	3000	M-mode echo	0·30
Hada 1987[32]	12841	ECG	0·17
Maron 1994[36]	714	2D-echo	0·50
Codd 1989[35]	3250	Echo/angio	0·02
Maron 1995[34]	4111	2D-echo	0·20

from institutions in Olmsted County, Minnesota. Although, the degree of surveillance of the resident population was admirably high, the fact that we now know that many patients with HCM have normal physical examinations and are asymptomatic makes it likely that some cases escaped detection during the initial clinical screening process. Furthermore, the reliance in the early part of the study on M-mode echocardiography means that many patients with hypertrophy in those regions of the myocardium not within the "sight" of the M-mode beam may have been overlooked, and would not have been allocated to one of the diagnostic codes used to select patients.

Natural history

It remains accepted wisdom that ventricular hypertrophy in patients with HCM usually develops during periods of rapid somatic growth, sometimes during the first year of life, but more typically during adolescence.[38–42] Until quite recently it was thought that the risk of developing hypertrophy after the age of 20 was very small. However, recent data from patients with mutations in myosin binding protein-C gene suggest that disease expression may occur throughout adult life. Patients may develop symptoms at any age, or remain asymptomatic all their lives. While most patients with HCM experience an age-dependent decline in exercise capacity and left ventricular function, only 5–10% of patients go on to develop rapid symptomatic deterioration in association with myocardial wall thinning, reduced systolic performance and increase in left ventricular end-systolic dimensions. Sudden death occurs throughout life, but the precise incidence varies in different series. Data from referral institutions suggest an overall annual mortality of 2%, with a maximum of 2–4% during childhood and adolescence,[38,39] whereas studies from several outpatient-based populations[40–42] suggest a lower figure of approximately 1% per annum. Data in infants with HCM are limited, but sudden death in the first decade is thought to be uncommon.[43]

Symptoms

In referral centers, exertional and atypical chest pains occur in approximately 30% of adult patients.[38,39] Dyspnea is also common in adults, and is probably caused by elevated pulmonary venous pressure secondary to abnormal diastolic function. Paroxysmal nocturnal dyspnea may occur in patients with apparently mild hemodynamic abnormalities. Its mechanism is uncertain, but myocardial ischemia or arrhythmia may be responsible. Approximately 15–25% of patients experience syncope and 20% presyncope. In some this is caused by paroxysmal arrhythmia, left ventricular outflow tract obstruction, conduction system disease or abnormal vascular responses during exercise, but in the majority no underlying cause is identified.

Examination

In most patients with HCM, physical examination is unremarkable. Patients may have a rapid upstroke to the arterial pulse, a forceful left ventricular impulse, and a palpable left atrial beat.[38] In approximately one third of patients, there is a prominent "a" wave in the jugular venous pressure, caused by reduced right ventricular compliance. The first and second heart sounds are usually normal, but a fourth heart sound, reflecting atrial systolic flow into a "stiff" left ventricle may be present. Up to one third of patients have a systolic murmur caused by left ventricular outflow tract turbulence. Physiologic and pharmacologic maneuvers that decrease afterload or venous return (standing, Valsalva, amyl nitrate) increase the intensity of the murmur, whereas interventions that increase afterload and venous return (squatting and phenylephrine) reduce it. The majority of patients with left ventricular outflow murmurs also have mitral regurgitation. Rarely, right ventricular outflow obstruction causes a systolic murmur best heard in the pulmonary area.

Electrocardiogram

While the literature suggests that the ECG is abnormal at least 80% of patients,[44] there are no specific changes diagnostic of HCM. Abnormal QRS morphology, repolarization abnormalities, and right and left atrial enlargement are common.[38,39,44] ST segment depression is frequent during exercise and daily life,[27,28] but is difficult to interpret in the presence of baseline ECG abnormalities. Abnormal Q waves occur in 25–50% of patients,[44–46] most commonly in the inferolateral leads. Suggested causes include abnormal septal activation and myocardial ischemia. Giant negative T waves in the mid-precordial leads may be more common in Japanese patients with apical hypertrophy,[47] but they are also seen in Western patients with more extensive hypertrophy. Some patients have a short PR interval with a slurred QRS upstroke, but only a minority (approximately 5% of all patients with HCM)[48] have accessory atrioventricular pathways.

The incidence of arrhythmias detected during 48 hour ambulatory ECG monitoring is age dependent (Figure 48.1). Runs of non-sustained ventricular tachycardia (NSVT) occur in 25% of adults,[49,50] but most episodes are relatively slow, asymptomatic, and occur during periods of increased vagal tone (such as during sleep). Sustained ventricular tachycardia is uncommon and is sometimes associated with apical aneurysms.[51] Paroxysmal supraventricular arrhythmias occur in 30–50% of patients,[52] with sustained atrial fibrillation present in 5% of patients at diagnosis. A further 10% of patients develop atrial fibrillation over the subsequent 5 years.[52]

Echocardiography

When echocardiographic diagnostic criteria for HCM were established using M-mode imaging, asymmetrical

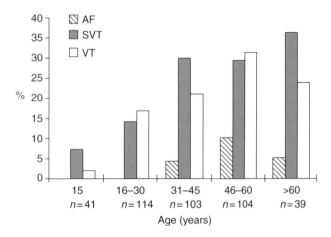

Figure 48.1 The frequency of supraventricular tachycardia (SVT), atrial fibrillation (AF), and non-sustained ventricular tachycardia (VT) at different ages in a consecutively referred population at St George's Hospital, London (unpublished data)

hypertrophy of the interventricular septum (ASH) was considered to be the *sine qua non* of the disease. However, subsequent two-dimensional echocardiographic studies have shown that any pattern of hypertrophy is compatible with the diagnosis.[53] The proportion of patients with concentric versus asymmetric hypertrophy depends on the definition employed. Thus, when a septal to posterior wall thickness ratio of 1·3:1 is used to define asymmetry, only 1–2% of patients have concentric left ventricular hypertrophy.[53] However, this proportion rises to approximately 30% when a ratio of 1·5:1 is used.[54] Criteria for abnormal wall thickness vary, but values exceeding two standard deviations from the mean corrected for age, sex, and height are generally accepted as diagnostic in the absence of any other cardiac or systemic cause. Doppler echocardiography is used to quantify the gradient across the left ventricular outflow tract using the modified Bernoulli equation:

$$\text{peak gradient} = 4V_{max}^{2}$$

where V_{max} is the maximum velocity across the left ventricular outflow tract. When it is not possible to obtain accurate Doppler measurements, the gradient can be estimated using M-mode recordings of the mitral valve and the formula:

$$\text{peak gradient} = 25(X/Y) + 25$$

where X is the duration of mitral–septal contact, and Y the period from the onset of systolic anterior motion of the mitral valve to the onset of mitral–septal contact.[18]

Cardiopulmonary responses to exercise

In most patients with HCM, peak oxygen consumption is below the predicted value corrected for age, sex, and height. This deficit is thought to relate to impaired oxygen delivery to contracting muscles and possibly abnormal peripheral oxygen utilization. Other indices of cardiopulmonary function that are often abnormal include a reduction in the anaerobic threshold and a reduced or flat oxygen pulse (Vo_2/heart rate) due to a failure to maintain an increase in stroke volume during exercise.[55] Exercise testing in HCM provides an objective assessment of exercise capacity and may also be useful in differentiating HCM from other more rare causes of ventricular hypertrophy such as mitochondrial disorders.

Cardiac catheterization

In the modern era, cardiac catheterization is performed only in patients with refractory symptoms (particularly those with severe mitral regurgitation), and in order to exclude epicardial coronary artery disease in older patients with chest pain. In addition to an outflow gradient, a variety of hemodynamic abnormalities are described including elevated left ventricular end-diastolic and pulmonary capillary wedge pressures, and a "spike and dome" appearance in the aortic waveform. Right atrial and right ventricular pressures are usually normal unless there is a substantial right ventricular outflow gradient or severe "restrictive" physiology. Resting cardiac output is typically normal or increased, except in patients with "end stage" ventricular dilatation.

In patients with hypertrophy confined to the distal left ventricle, ventriculography may show a characteristic "spade-shaped" appearance caused by the encroachment of hypertrophied papillary muscles. Coronary arteriography is usually normal, but systolic obliteration of epicardial vessels is described. Muscle bridges are also described but their relevance to an individual patient's symptoms is often difficult to assess.

Radionuclide studies

Several studies have used stress radionuclide imaging to study myocardial perfusion in patients with HCM. Fixed [201]thallium perfusion defects have been associated with increased left ventricular cavity dimensions, impaired systolic function, and reduced exercise capacity, and are thought to represent myocardial scars.[29] Reversible regional [201]thallium defects are present in over 25% of patients, but correlate poorly with symptomatic status.[27,29] It has been suggested that reversible defects are associated with a poor prognosis, but one large prospective study has failed to demonstrate any relation with medium-term outcome.[56]

Using positron emission tomography (PET) a reduction in coronary vasodilator reserve has been observed both in hypertrophied and non-hypertrophied regions of myocardium during dipyridamole-induced coronary microvascular vasodilatation.[26] The reduction in vasodilator reserve may be more pronounced in patients with a history of chest pain and ST-segment depression.[26] PET has also demonstrated subendocardial hypoperfusion after dipyridamole infusion across the septum of patients with asymmetrical septal hypertrophy. PET has been used to investigate the relationship between myocardial blood flow and metabolism using fluorine-18 labeled deoxyglucose (FDG).[57,58] Areas of blood flow/FDG mismatch thought to indicate the presence of ischemic myocardium have been described both at rest and during exercise. Other studies, however, have demonstrated selective abnormalities of glucose metabolism, independent of coronary flow[59] and, more recently, studies have suggested that heterogeneous FDG uptake may relate to regional systolic function and age.

Radionuclide angiography has been used to investigate global and regional left ventricular function in HCM, and has shown prolonged isovolumic relaxation, delayed peak filling, reduced relative volume during the rapid filling period, and increased atrial contribution to filling and regional heterogeneity in the timing, rate, and degree of left ventricular relaxation and diastolic filling.[60,61] A reduced peak filling rate has been shown to be associated with an increased disease-related mortality,[61] but its predictive value is not high and adds little to conventional risk stratification.

Differential diagnosis

In adults, unexplained left ventricular hypertrophy exceeding two standard deviations from the normal (typically, >1·5 cm) is usually sufficient to make a diagnosis of HCM. In children and adolescents the diagnosis can be more difficult as young "gene carriers" may not manifest the complete phenotype. A number of rare genetically determined disorders can present with a cardiac phenotype similar to HCM, but most are distinguished by the presence of other clinical features. Rare exceptions include patients with Friedreich's ataxia that present with cardiac disease before the onset of obvious neurological deficit,[62] Noonan syndrome patients with only very mild somatic abnormalities,[63] and patients with primary mitochondrial disease that do not have clinical evidence for neuromuscular disease (unpublished data). Recently mutations in the gene encoding the γ2 subunit of AMP-activated protein kinase (7q36) have been described in two families with left ventricular hypertrophy with Wolff–Parkinson–White syndrome. When activated, this gene functions to protect the cell from critical depletion of ATP by activating glycolysis and fatty acid uptake during hypoxic stress or extreme metabolic demand.[64] In routine clinical practice the two most commonly encountered areas of difficulty are the differentiation of HCM from "secondary" left ventricular hypertrophy as seen in hypertension and the "athlete's heart", and the more recently identified problem of incomplete penetrance in adults.

Hypertension

Left ventricular hypertrophy occurs in up to 50% of hypertensive patients. The hypertrophic response is determined by a number of factors including the degree of hypertension, sex, and race.[65] In general, patients with HCM tend to have more severe hypertrophy than hypertensives, and the presence of a maximal wall thickness of more than 2 cm in a Caucasian patient should always raise the suspicion of HCM (Table 48.2).[66,67] Concentric hypertrophy is more frequent in patients with hypertension, and asymmetric septal hypertrophy more so in HCM, but the specificity of each pattern is not high. In contrast, isolated distal ventricular hypertrophy does seem to be highly predictive of HCM. Systolic anterior motion of the mitral valve occurs in both diseases, but the combination of complete SAM with a substantial left ventricular outflow gradient and asymmetric septal hypertrophy is more indicative of HCM. A number of other echo-derived parameters such as left ventricular cross-sectional area and direction-dependent contraction have been suggested as discriminants, but these require further study.[68]

Table 48.2 Relation of the pattern of left ventricular hypertrophy to underlying etiology

	ASH[a] (%)	Distal (%)	Symmetrical (%)	Wall thickness ≥2.0 cm (%)
Sensitivity	56 (83)[b]	10	81	40 (40)
Specificity	81 (56)	100	66	93 (93)
Predictive value of positive test	83 (70)	100	58	81 (83)

[a] Defined by an interventricular septum to posterior wall thickness ratio of ≥1·5:1.
[b] Values in parentheses from Keller *et al.*
Sensitivity, specificity and predictive value of asymmetric hypertrophy (ASH and distal) in diagnosing hypertrophic cardiomyopathy and symmetrical hypertrophy in diagnosing secondary hypertrophy. The same parameters are shown for a maximal wall thickness or septal thickness of ≥2·0 cm in diagnosing HCM in patients with symmetric hypertrophy. (Taken from Shapiro *et al*[54] and Keller *et al*.[56])

Athlete's heart

While HCM is the commonest cause of unexpected sudden death in young athletes,[69,70] cardiovascular adaptation to regular training can make differentiation of the "athlete's heart" from HCM problematic. The ability to distinguish these two entities is of crucial importance, as continued competitive activity in a young person with HCM may threaten that individual's life, whereas an incorrect diagnosis of HCM in a normal athlete may unnecessarily deprive them of their livelihood. The presence of symptoms, a family history of HCM and/or premature sudden death should always raise the level of suspicion for HCM. In general, athletic training is associated with only a modest increase in myocardial mass, with <2% of elite athletes having a wall thickness >13 mm.[71] A diagnosis of HCM in an elite athlete is very likely when an individual has a left ventricular wall thickness >16 mm in men or ≥13 mm in women. Other echocardiographic features favoring a diagnosis of HCM include small left ventricular cavity dimensions (athletes tending to have increased left ventricular end-diastolic dimensions), left atrial enlargement, and the presence of a left ventricular outflow gradient.[72] Doppler evidence of diastolic impairment is also highly suggestive of HCM. The "athletic" ECG often displays voltage criteria for left ventricular hypertrophy, sinus bradycardia, and sinus arrhythmia, but Q waves, ST segment depression, and/or deep T wave inversion is highly suggestive of HCM. Incremental exercise testing may also be useful in distinguishing patients with HCM, a maximal oxygen consumption >50 ml/kg/min or 20% above the predicted maximal value being highly suggestive of athletic adaptation.[55] The type of training may also be relevant to diagnosis as hypertrophy is greatest in specific sports such as rowing and cycling. Isometric activities do not appear to cause a substantial hypertrophic response. Very occasionally a period of detraining over 3–6 months is required to distinguish HCM from the athlete's heart.

Incomplete penetrance in adults

It is increasingly recognized that some adults with sarcomeric protein mutations do not fulfill conventional echocardiographic criteria for HCM. New clinical diagnostic criteria for HCM based on the assumption that the probability of disease in a first-degree relative of a patient with HCM is 50%, have recently been proposed (Box 48.1).[75] It is important to realize that they are intended to apply only to *unexplained* ECG and echocardiographic abnormalities in first-degree adult relatives of individuals with proven HCM, and not to isolated cases of minor echocardiographic and ECG abnormalities.

HCM in the elderly

"Inappropriate" or idiopathic left ventricular hypertrophy has long been recognized in patients over the age of 65 years.[74–77] The pattern of disease in this age group is said to differ from that observed in younger patients with HCM in that symptoms occur late in life, the prognosis for most patients is relatively good, and many have mild hypertension. The echocardiographic features of HCM in the elderly are often the same as in the young, but some morphological differences are described: in comparison to their younger counterparts, patients with "elderly HCM" tend to have relatively mild hypertrophy localized to the anterior interventricular septum; the left ventricular cavity is commonly ovoid or ellipsoid rather than crescentic. Elderly patients with left ventricular outflow tract obstruction tend to have more severe narrowing of the left ventricular outflow tract, anterior displacement of the mitral valve apparatus,

---

Box 48.1 Proposed diagnostic criteria for hypertrophic cardiomyopathy in first-degree relatives of patients with definite diagnosis of hypertrophic cardiomyopathy

MAJOR	MINOR
● *Echocardiography* Left ventricular wall thickness ≥13 mm in the anterior septum or posterior wall or ≥15 mm in the posterior septum or free wall	Left ventricular wall thickness of 12 mm in the anterior septum or posterior wall, or of 14 mm in the posterior septum or free wall
Severe SAM (septal leaflet contact)	Moderate SAM (no leaflet-septal contact) Redundant MV leaflets
● *Electrocardiography* LVH + repolarization changes (Romhilt & Estes)	Complete BBB or (minor) interventricular conduction defects (in LV leads) Minor repolarization changes in LV leads
T wave inversion in leads I and aVL (≥3 mm) (with QRS-T wave axis difference ≥300), V3–V6 (≥3 mm) or II and III and aVF (≥5 mm)	
Abnormal Q waves (>40 ms or >25% R wave) in at least two leads from II, III, aVF (in the absence of left anterior hemiblock), V1–V4; or I, aVL, V5–V6	Deep S in V2 (>25 mm) Unexplained syncope, chest pain, dyspnea

It is proposed that diagnosis of hypertrophic cardiomyopathy in first-degree relatives of patients with the disease would be fulfilled in the presence of one major criterion, or two minor echocardiographic criteria, or one minor echocardiographic plus two minor ECG criteria. (From McKenna WJ *et al.*[73])

restricted anterior excursion of the anterior mitral valve leaflet in systole, and a larger area of contact between the mitral valve leaflet and the septum. Mitral valve calcification is often seen in elderly patients, but it is not associated with a greater degree of left ventricular outflow tract obstruction. The frequency of moderate to severe symptoms is similar in young and elderly patients, but the limited published evidence indicates that the elderly respond well to pharmacologic and surgical therapy and have a relatively good prognosis.[76] In spite of recent evidence demonstrating *de novo* hypertrophy in middle-aged patients with myosin binding protein-C mutations, it remains uncertain whether the majority of patients with this so-called elderly phenotype have a separate disease entity reflecting a polygenic response to hypertrophic stimuli. Hypertension is more frequent in the elderly population, but the failure to demonstrate any difference in left ventricular morphology in hypertensive and non-hypertensive HCM patients (with the possible exception of posterior wall thickness) has led some to suggest that it is not an important factor.[77] Other "hypertrophic" stimuli that may be present in older patients include increased angulation and decreased compliance of the aorta.

Risk stratification in HCM

Markers of sudden death risk in HCM

Although sudden death in HCM is a relatively uncommon event, the fact that it frequently occurs in young asymptomatic individuals gives it a particular significance to families affected by HCM and to the wider community. Clinical risk stratification in patients with HCM is based on the premise that, if sudden death can be prevented, the natural history of the disease for most patients is relatively benign. The absence of risk factors also facilitates reassurance of low risk individuals.

A number of studies have shown that individual sarcomeric protein gene mutations have different prognostic implications (Figure 48.2). For example, most families with troponin-T mutations described to date have a poor prognosis, whereas β-myosin heavy chain mutations may have a benign or malignant course. Early investigations of HCM-related α-tropomyosin disease have suggested a favorable prognosis.[79] In spite of these data, genetic testing at present has a limited role in risk stratification because the number of families studied is small, and even within families there is marked heterogeneity of disease expression.

Clinically a young age at diagnosis is associated with an increased risk of sudden death (Figure 48.3). Other recognized risk markers in this age group include a family history of multiple premature sudden deaths, and recurrent unexplained syncopal episodes.[39] More recently abnormal blood pressure responses during exercise have been shown to be

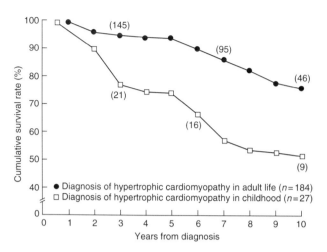

Figure 48.2 Cumulative survival from the year of diagnosis in 211 medically treated patients with hypertrophic cardiomyopathy[92]

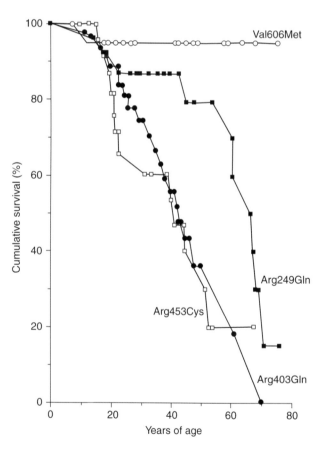

Figure 48.3 Kaplan–Meier survival curves for individuals with HCM and different gene mutations. Two β-myosin points are reported to be associated with near normal survival: Val606→Met (○) and Leu908→Val. The mutations Arg403→Gln (●), Arg453Cys (□), and Arg249Gln (■) are associated with a poorer prognosis[10]

associated with a higher mortality in patients less than 40 years of age.[30] Abnormal blood pressure responses are seen more frequently in patients with a family history of sudden death and small left ventricular cavity dimensions.[31,80]

Two recent studies have shown a correlation between severe left ventricular hypertrophy (defined as a maximal wall thickness $\geq$30 mm) and prognosis.[81,82] However, taken in isolation, left ventricular hypertrophy has a relatively low positive predictive accuracy; furthermore, the majority of patients who die suddenly have wall thickness values <30 mm. Severe left ventricular hypertrophy may be more prognostically important in the young, but further studies are required.

Two studies[49,50] have shown that NSVT in adults with HCM is associated with an increased risk of sudden death. Its clinical value is however, limited by a modest positive predictive accuracy of 22%, and a low incidence in children. Recently it has been suggested that NSVT is significant only when episodes are repetitive, prolonged and/or associated with symptoms. There are however no data to support this.

A number of other non-invasive and invasive electrophysiologic parameters have been evaluated in an attempt to further refine clinical risk stratification. QT and QTc intervals are often prolonged in patients with HCM, but no study has shown a convincing association with the risk of sudden death.[83-85] QT dispersion may be a more sensitive marker of the propensity to ventricular arrhythmia but further studies in large well-characterized populations are necessary. Abnormal signal averaged ECGs (SAECGs) are relatively common in patients with HCM and NSVT, the best predictor of NSVT being a reduced voltage ($<$150 μV) in the initial portion of the high gain QRS complex (sensitivity 95%, specificity 74%, positive predictive accuracy 64%).[86] Unfortunately, abnormal SAECGs are not associated with other clinical risk factors and do not identify patients who go on to develop sustained ventricular arrhythmia or sudden death. Similarly, while global and specific vagal components of heart rate variability (HRV) are reduced in patients with HCM and NSVT, abnormal HRV is not predictive of sudden catastrophic cardiac events.[87]

The role of programmed electrical stimulation in patients with HCM remains controversial. The largest series from a single center[48,88] reports that programmed ventricular stimulation using up to three premature stimuli in the right and/or left ventricle produces sustained ventricular arrhythmia (that is, lasting for more than 30 seconds or associated with hypotension) in 43% of patients selected on the basis of a history of previous cardiac arrest, syncope, palpitations, or non-sustained ventricular tachycardia on Holter. Inducible sustained ventricular arrhythmia was associated with a history of cardiac arrest *or* syncope and, in a subsequent study, was associated with a reduced survival. The sensitivity, specificity, and predictive accuracy for predicting subsequent cardiac events were 82%, 68%, and 17% respectively. However, almost three quarters of the patients with

sustained ventricular arrhythmias required three premature stimuli for induction. The experience in other cardiac diseases has shown that, whilst "aggressive" protocols using three or more stimuli are highly sensitive, their specificity is low. In addition 76% of patients had polymorphic ventricular tachycardia or fibrillation rather than sustained monomorphic ventricular tachycardia, which is generally thought to be a more sensitive and specific marker of sudden death risk. The interpretation of these published data in HCM and their translation into clinical practice is further complicated by the selection criteria used to select patients as "low-risk" patients were under-represented in the analysis. The general view at present is that programmed stimulation is of limited use in the assessment of risk in HCM.

Recently, the putative arrhythmogenic substrate in HCM has been investigated by analyzing changes in individual paced ECG transitions ("fractionation") recorded at three sites in the right ventricle.[89] Compared with controls, patients with a history of ventricular fibrillation have prolongation of the paced ECG at relatively long extrastimulus coupling intervals. Patients with a family history of premature sudden death or NSVT exhibit responses that span the range from "high risk" (ventricular fibrillation) to "low risk" (no adverse prognostic features).

Identification of high-risk patients

The identification of individuals at high risk of sudden death has been hampered by the inherent difficulties of studying a disease with a low prevalence and event rate. This is further compounded by the low positive predictive accuracy of most suggested risk markers for sudden death. Recent data have suggested that risk may be assessed using a small number of easily determined risk markers, specifically, non-sustained ventricular tachycardia, left ventricular wall thickness ($\geq$30 mm), abnormal blood pressure response in those under 80 years of age, family history of multiple sudden deaths, and recurrent unexplained syncope. *Patients with none of the above risk factors have <1% estimated annual risk of sudden death compared with patients with two or more risk factors who have a 4–6% annual risk of sudden death.*[90] **Grade B** Risk stratification remains problematic in those patients with a single risk factor, some of whom are clearly at increased risk of sudden death. Further work to identify which of these individuals would benefit from prophylactic therapy is required.

Management of the "high-risk" patient

There is now general agreement that low-risk adult patients – that is, those without symptoms or risk factors – can be readily identified, and in most populations represent the majority of individuals with the disease. For patients who are considered to be at high risk of sudden death,

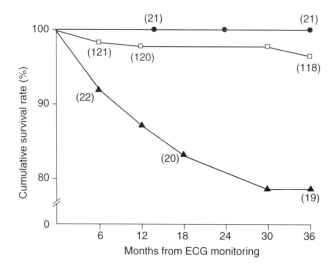

Figure 48.4 Cumulative survival curves for patients with non-sustained ventricular tachycardia treated with either conventional antiarrhythmic drugs (▲) or amiodarone (●), and for patients without non-sustained ventricular tachycardia (□).[91]

implantable cardioverter defibrillators (ICDs) are increasingly seen as the preferred therapy. The ICD has been accepted as a superior treatment to antiarrhythmic medication for the prevention of life-threatening ventricular arrhythmias and sudden death in high-risk patients with other cardiovascular diseases. Although randomized data comparing amiodarone to ICD in high-risk patients with hypertrophic cardiomyopathy are not currently available, ICDs have been shown to be effective in terminating life-threatening tachyarrhythmias. In addition the pacing capabilities of the most recent defibrillators offer protection from cardiac arrest from bradyarrhythmias. Studies have shown that low-dose amiodarone can reduce the incidence of sudden death in adults with NSVT (Figure 48.4),[91] and in children considered to be at risk,[92] although the finding of appropriate discharges in patients with ICDs already taking amiodarone suggests that the ICD may be superior in preventing sudden death. **Grade B** Approximately 30% of patients with HCM and a history of cardiac arrest have a further event within 6 years of their first episode. There is general agreement that, in patients with a history of ventricular fibrillation, arrest ICD is the preferred therapy.[93–97] In patients with multiple risk factors ICDs are increasingly seen as the preferred therapy. In patients with a single risk factor, management needs to be individualized; amiodarone or ICD may be appropriate in selected individuals.

Symptomatic therapy

Obstructive hypertrophic cardiomyopathy

Most physicians still use β blockade as the first-line drug therapy in patients with left ventricular outflow obstruction.

Grade B While some studies have suggested that up to 70% of patients improve with β blockers, high doses are frequently required and side effects may be limiting. The beneficial effects of β blockers on symptoms (principally dyspnea and chest pain) and exercise tolerance appear to result largely from a decrease in the heart rate with a consequent prolongation of diastole and increased passive ventricular filling and myocardial blood flow. By reducing the inotropic response, β blockers may also lessen myocardial oxygen demand and decrease the outflow tract gradient during exercise, when sympathetic tone is increased.

Verapamil has favorable effects on symptoms secondary to improved ventricular filling and probable reduction in myocardial ischemia. In patients with a substantial outflow tract gradient or markedly elevated pulmonary pressure (or both), verapamil should be used with caution, however, as the drug's vasodilatory effect may lead to serious hemodynamic complications. There is no evidence that the administration of β blockers and verapamil together is more advantageous than the use of either drug alone, and there is no evidence that either protects patients from sudden death.

Disopyramide reduces left ventricular outflow tract gradients and relieves symptoms by virtue of its negative inotropic properties and has been extensively used in some centers for symptomatic therapy in patients with significant outflow obstruction.[99,100] Reduction in SAM (systolic anterior motion), left ventricular ejection time and improved exercise capacity and functional status are all described but, in common with other therapies, the initial hemodynamic and clinical benefits may decrease with time. Because disopyramide may shorten the atrioventricular nodal conduction time and thus increase the ventricular rate during paroxysmal atrial fibrillation, supplementary therapy with β blockers or verapamil in low doses is advisable. The anticholinergic effects of disopyramide (dry mouth, urinary retention, glaucoma) may limit the drug's use, particularly in elderly patients.

When drug therapy fails or is only partially effective, surgery remains the "gold standard" treatment.[101–107] The most frequently performed operation is septal myotomy–myectomy in which a wedge of myocardium is excised from the upper interventricular septum via a transaortic approach. Operative mortality in experienced centers is now 1–2%, but may be higher in less experienced units. Most studies indicate that operative mortality is higher when myectomy is combined with other cardiac operations. The incidence of non-fatal complications such as conduction system disease and ventricular septal defect has declined with modification of surgical practice and the use of intraoperative transesophageal echocardiography. Some data suggest that surgery reduces or abolishes resting gradients in 95% of cases, and that 70% of patients show useful symptomatic and functional improvement. However, at least 10% continue to experience significant symptoms. Mitral valve replacement has been proposed as an alternative to myectomy, its attraction being that it avoids potential complications of ventricular septal defect and complete heart block. In a series of 58 patients, mitral valve replacement resulted in a substantial reduction in left ventricular outflow gradient, improved symptomatic class, and an actuarial survival at 3 years of 86%.[108] However, early operative mortality was 9%, and only 68% of patients were free from thromboembolism, anticoagulant-related problems, congestive cardiac failure, and reoperation. Thus mitral valve replacement, whilst successfully treating outflow tract obstruction, is usually advocated only in selected patients. These include patients with severe mitral regurgitation from intrinsic abnormalities of the valve apparatus; patients with mid-cavity obstruction from anomalous insertion of papillary muscle into the anterior mitral leaflet; and patients with only mild septal hypertrophy, which suggests that muscular resection would be associated with a high risk of septal perforation or an inadequate hemodynamic result. **Grade B** Mitral valvuloplasty has also been combined with myotomy–myectomy in some patients with particularly elongated mitral leaflets.

Dual chamber pacing has been proposed as a less invasive alternative to surgery. Several studies have described significant gradient reduction in patients treated with atrioventricular synchronous pacemakers programmed with a short atrioventricular delay to ensure constant capture of the right ventricle.[109–113] It was initially thought that pacing reduced the outflow gradient by causing paradoxical movement of the interventricular septum, but it is now realized that many aspects of ventricular activation are altered by right ventricular pacing, and it is likely that reduced or delayed septal thickening, reduced contractility, and altered papillary muscle movement contribute to gradient reduction. In general, outflow gradients can be reduced by approximately 50%, but the translation of this benefit into useful clinical improvement is very variable and unpredictable. Some workers suggest that suboptimal responses to pacing may be caused by short native PR intervals that make it impossible to achieve maximum pre-excitation simultaneously and maintain normal atrial filling of the left ventricle. This can be overcome in some patients by pharmacologically increasing the PR interval with β blockers and/or calcium antagonists, but some groups controversially advocate radiofrequency ablation of the atrioventricular node in order to achieve "optimal" AV pacing. Other unresolved issues include the significance of the appreciable placebo effect of pacing demonstrated in at least two randomized studies, the effect of long-term pacing on left ventricular wall thickness, and the role of pacing in the young. Despite the drawbacks, pacing may be an option in a minority of drug refractory patients in whom surgery poses an unacceptable operative risk.

Several centers are now examining a novel approach to gradient reduction that uses injection of alcohol into the first septal perforator branch of the left anterior descending artery to produce a "chemical myectomy".[114–116] Published data suggest that procedure-related mortality is less than 1% in experienced centers, but deaths from conduction system damage and inadvertent injection of alcohol into other myocardial segments are recognized. This later problem can be minimized by the use of intracoronary myocardial contrast echocardiography. Preliminary data indicate that significant gradient reduction and improvement in symptoms can be achieved. However, as with dual chamber pacing, the actual mechanism of gradient reduction and symptomatic improvement is likely to be more complex than the creation of a "localized" scar in the interventricular septum. The most frequent complication reported to date is complete heart block, although the incidence varies between the small numbers of centers currently performing the procedure. There has been some concern regarding the short- and long-term consequences of deliberately producing a myocardial infarct such as a possible predisposition to ventricular dysarrhythmias and progressive left ventricular wall thinning. *Long-term follow up data is not yet available in patients who have undergone pacing or alcohol septal ablation.*

Non-obstructive HCM

The treatment options in symptomatic patients without an outflow tract gradient are limited. β Blockers and calcium-channel antagonists can be used alone or in combination, and, in patients with symptoms suggestive of pulmonary venous congestion, diuretics may also be helpful. In a small number of patients with severe refractory chest pain, a variety of techniques, such as transcutaneous nerve stimulation and cardiac denervation, have been used with variable success.

For the minority of patients with HCM, who arrive at an end stage characterized by wall thinning, cavity enlargement, and systolic impairment treatment, should include standard therapeutic agents for heart failure associated with systolic dysfunction, including diuretics, ACE inhibitors, and digitalis. Ultimately these patients may become candidates for heart transplantation. **Grade C**

Management of supraventricular arrhythmia

Paroxysmal episodes of supraventricular tachycardias, such as atrial fibrillation or flutter, can lead to rapid clinical deterioration by reducing diastolic filling and cardiac output, usually as a consequence of the high ventricular rate. Conversely chronic supraventricular arrhythmias are often well tolerated if the heart rate is adequately controlled.[47] Established atrial fibrillation/flutter should be cardioverted, but when restoration of sinus rhythm is not possible, β blockers and verapamil are usually efficacious in controlling the heart rate. **Grade B** Occasionally radiofrequency ablation of the atrioventricular node and implantation of a pacemaker may be necessary in selected patients to achieve adequate rate control. In patients with recurrent supraventricular arrhythmias, treatment is indicated only if they are sustained (>30 seconds) or associated with symptoms. Specific medical therapy with low dose amiodarone (1000–1400 mg/week), or β blockers with class III action (for example, sotalol) is effective in maintaining sinus rhythm, and in controlling the ventricular rate during breakthrough episodes. The role of other drugs such as class 1 agents is uncertain. Atrial fibrillation/flutter in HCM is associated with a significant risk of thromboembolism, and anticoagulation should be considered in all patients when atrial fibrillation/flutter is sustained or recurs frequently.

Conclusion

HCM is a disorder of diverse etiology, pathology, and clinical presentation. While recent advances in molecular genetics and clinical characterization have led to greater understanding of the disease and its management, several clinical issues remain unresolved. Nevertheless, the pace of current research suggests that many of these controversies will be resolved over the next decade.

Summary 1

- The majority of cases of hypertrophic cardiomyopathy (HCM) are caused by mutations in genes encoding cardiac sarcomeric proteins.
- Although symptoms of chest pain, dyspnea, palpitation, and syncope are common, many patients are asymptomatic and may present for the first time with sudden death.
- Recurrent syncope, a family history of premature sudden death, non-sustained ventricular tachycardia during ambulatory ECG, left ventricular wall thickness ≥30 mm, and abnormal exercise blood pressure responses are associated with an increased risk of sudden death.

Summary 2

- Symptomatic patients with left ventricular outflow gradients should be initially treated with β blockers or disopyramide. If drug therapy is ineffective, patients should be considered for surgery. **Grade B**
- Pacing and alcohol septal myectomy are a viable option for patients with symptomatic left ventricular outflow gradient who are unsuitable or not keen on surgery. **Grade B**
- All patients should undergo non-invasive risk stratification using ambulatory electrocardiography and exercise testing. **Grade B**
- Low-risk adults can generally be reassured that their prognosis is good. High-risk patients require further assessment and should be considered for amiodarone or ICD therapy. **Grade B**

References

1. Kimura A, Harada H, Park J-E *et al.* Mutations in the cardiac troponin I gene associated with hypertrophic cardiomyopathy. *Nature Genet* 1997;**16**:379–82.
2. Jarcho JA, McKenna WJ, Pare JA *et al.* Mapping a gene for familial hypertrophic cardiomyopathy to chromosome 14q1. *N Engl J Med* 1989;**321**:1372–8.
3. Thierfelder L, MacRae C, Watkins H *et al.* A familial hypertrophic cardiomyopathy locus maps to chromosome 15q2. *Proc Nat Acad Sci USA* 1993;**90**:6270–4.
4. Watkins H, MacRae C, Thierfelder L *et al.* A disease locus for familial hypertrophic cardiomyopathy maps to chromosome 1q3. *Nature Genet* 1993;**3**:333–7.
5. Bonne G, Carrier L, Bercovici J *et al.* Cardiac myosin binding protein C gene splice acceptor site mutation is associated with familial hypertrophic cardiomyopathy. *Nature Genet* 1995;**11**:438–40.
6. Poetter K, Jiang H, Hassanzadeh S *et al.* Mutations in either the essential or regulatory light chains of myosin are associated with a rare myopathy in human heart and skeletal muscle. *Nature Genet* 1996;**13**:63–9.
7. Oslon TM, Doan TP, Kishimoto NY, Whitby FG, Ackerman MJ, Fananapazir L. Inherited and *de novo* mutations in the cardiac actin gene cause hypertrophic cardiomyopathy. *J Mol Cell Cardiol* 2000;**32**:1687–94.
8. Satoh M, Takahashi M, Sakamoto T, Hiroe M, Marumo F, Kimura A. Structural analysis of the titin gene in hypertrophic cardiomyopathy: identification of a novel disease gene. *Biochem Biophys Res Commun* 1999;**262**:411–17.
9. Watkins H, Thierfelder L, Hwang D, McKenna WJ, Seidman JG, Seidman CE. Sporadic hypertrophic cardiomyopathy due to *de novo* myosin mutations. *J Clin Invest* 1992;**90**:1666–71.
10. Watkins H, Rozenzweig A, Hwang DS *et al.* Characteristics and prognostic implications of myosin missense mutations in familial hypertrophic cardiomyopathy. *N Engl J Med* 1992;**326**:1108–14.
11. Lechin M, Quinones MA, Omran A *et al.* Angiotensin converting enzyme genotypes and left ventricular hypertrophy in patients with hypertrophic cardiomyopathy. *Circulation* 1995;**92**:1808–12.
12. Rayment I, Holden HM, Sellers JR *et al.* Structural interpretation of the mutations in the beta-cardiac myosin that have been implicated in familial hypertrophic cardiomyopathy. *Proc Nat Acad Sci USA* 1995;**92**:3864–8.
13. Lankford EB, Epstein ND, Fananapazir L, Sweeney HL. Abnormal contractile properties of muscle fibres expressing beta-myosin heavy chain gene mutations in patients with hypertrophic cardiomyopathy. *J Clin Invest* 1995;**95**:1409–14.
14. Geisterfer-Lowrance AA, Christe M, Conner DA, Ingwall JS, Schoen FJ, Seidman CE, Seidman JG. A mouse model of familial hypertrophic cardiomyopathy. *Science* 1996;**272**:731–4.
15. Davies MJ, McKenna WJ. Hypertrophic cardiomyopathy: pathology and pathogenesis. *Histopathology* 1995;**26**:493–500.
16. Maron BJ, Wolfson JK, Epstein SE, Roberts WC. Intramural ("small vessel") coronary artery disease in hypertrophic cardiomyopathy. *J Am Coll Cardiol* 1986;**8**:545–57.

17. Varnava AM, Elliott PM, Sharma S, McKenna WJ, Davies MJ. Hypertrophic cardiomyopathy: the interrelation of disarray, fibrosis, and small vessel disease. *Heart* 2000;**84**: 476–82.

18. Wigle ED, Sasson Z, Henderson MA *et al*. Hypertrophic cardiomyopathy: the importance of the site and extent of hypertrophy: a review. *Prog Cardiovasc Dis* 1985;**28**:1–83.

19. Levine RA, Vlahakes GJ, Lefebvre XP *et al*. Papillary muscle displacement causes systolic anterior motion of the mitral valve. Experimental validation and insights into the mechanism of subaortic obstruction. *Circulation* 1995;**91**:1189–95.

20. Klues HG, Maron BJ, Dollar AL, Roberts WC. Diversity of structural mitral valve alterations in hypertrophic cardiomyopathy. *Circulation* 1992;**85**:1651–60.

21. Sugrue DD, McKenna WJ, Dickie S *et al*. Relation between left ventricular gradient and relative stroke volume ejected in early and late systole in hypertrophic cardiomyopathy. Assessment with radionuclide cineangiography. *Br Heart J* 1984;**52**:602–9.

22. Maron BJ, Epstein SE. Clinical significance and therapeutic implications of the left ventricular outflow tract pressure gradient in hypertrophic cardiomyopathy. *Am J Cardiol* 1986; **58**:1093–6.

23. Hanrath P, Mathey DG, Siegert R, Biefield W. Left ventricular and filling patterns in different forms of left ventricular relaxation and filling patterns in different forms of left ventricular hypertrophy. An echocardiographic study. *Am J Cardiol* 1980; **45**:15–23.

24. Maron BJ, Spirito P, Green KJ, Wesley YE, Bonow RO, Arce J. Noninvasive assessment of left ventricular diastolic function by pulsed Doppler echocardiography in patients with hypertrophic cardiomyopathy. *J Am Coll Cardiol* 1987;**10**: 733–42.

25. Cannon RO, Rosing DR, Maron BJ *et al*. Myocardial ischemia in patients with hypertrophic cardiomyopathy: contribution of inadequate vasodilator reserve and elevated left ventricular filling pressures. *Circulation* 1985;**71**:234–43.

26. Camici P, Chiriatti G, Lorenzoni R *et al*. Coronary vasodilatation is impaired in both hypertrophied and non hypertrophied myocardium of patients with hypertrophic cardiomyopathy: A study with Nitrogen-13 ammonia and positron emission tomography. *J Am Coll Cardiol* 1991;**17**:879–86.

27. Cannon RO, Dilsizian V, O'Gara P *et al*. Myocardial metabolic, hemodynamic, and electrocardiographic significance of reversible thallium-201 abnormalities in hypertrophic cardiomyopathy. *Circulation* 1991;**83**:1660.

28. Elliott PM, Kaski JC, Prasad K *et al*. Chest pain during daily life in patients with hypertrophic cardiomyopathy: an ambulatory electrocardiographic study. *Eur Heart J* 1996;**17**: 1056–64.

29. O'Gara PT, Bonow RO, Maron BJ *et al*. Myocardial perfusion abnormalities in patients with hypertrophic cardiomyopathy: assessment with thallium-201 emission computed tomography. *Circulation* 1987;**76**:1214–23.

30. Sadoul N, Prasad K, Slade AKB, Elliott PM, McKenna WJ. Abnormal blood pressure response during exercise is an independent marker of sudden death in young patients with hypertrophic cardiomyopathy. *Circulation* 1997;**96**:2987–91.

31. Frenneaux MP, Counihan PJ, Caforio A, Chikamori T, McKenna WJ. Abnormal blood pressure response during exercise in hypertrophic cardiomyopathy. *Circulation* 1990; **82**:1995–2002.

32. Hada Y, Sakamoto T, Amano K *et al*. Prevalence of hypertrophy cardiomyopathy in a population of adult Japanese workers as detected by echocardiographic screening. *Am J Cardiol* 1987;**59**:183–4.

33. Savage DD, Castelli WP, Abbott RD *et al*. Hypertrophic cardiomyopathy and its markers in the general population: the great masquerader revisited: the Framingham Study. *J Cardiovasc Ultrason* 1983;**2**:41–7.

34. Maron BJ, Gardin JM, Flack JM, Gidding SS, Kurosaki TT, Bild DE. Prevalence of hypertrophic cardiomyopathy in a population of young adults. Echocardiographic analysis of 4111 subjects in the CARDIA study. Coronary Artery Risk Development in (Young) Adults. *Circulation* 1995;**92**:785–9.

35. Codd MB, Sugrue DD, Gersh BJ, Melton LJ. Epidemiology of idiopathic dilated and hypertrophic cardiomyopathy: a population based study in Olmsted County, Minnesota, 1975–1984. *Circulation* 1989;**80**:564–72.

36. Maron BJ, Peterson EE, Maron MS, Peterson JE. Prevalence of hypertrophic cardiomyopathy in an outpatient population referred for echocardiographic study. *Am J Cardiol* 1994;**73**: 577–80.

37. Maron BJ, Mathenge R, Casey SA, Poliac LC, Longe TF. Clinical profile of hypertrophic cardiomyopathy identified *de novo* in rural communities. *J Am Coll Cardiol* 1999 May; **33**(6):1590–5.

38. Frank S, Braunwald E. Idiopathic hypertrophic subaortic stenosis: clinical analysis of 126 patients with emphasis on the natural history. *Circulation* 1968;**37**:759–88.

39. McKenna WJ, Deanfield J, Faruqui A, England D, Oakley C, Goodwin J. Prognosis in hypertrophic cardiomyopathy. Role of age and clinical, electrocardiographic and haemodynamic features. *Am J Cardiol* 1981;**47**:532–8.

40. Spirito P, Chiarella F, Carratino L, Zoni-Berisso M, Bellotti P, Vecchio C. Clinical course and prognosis of hypertrophic cardiomyopathy in an outpatient population. *N Engl J Med* 1989;**320**:749–55.

41. Cecchi F, Olivotto I, Montereggi A, Santoro G, Dolara A, Maron BJ. Hypertrophic cardiomyopathy in Tuscany: clinical course and outcome in an unselected regional population. *J Am Coll Cardiol* 1995;**26**:1529–36.

42. Cannan CR, Reeder GS, Bailey KR, Melton LJ III, Gersh BJ. Natural history of hypertrophic cardiomyopathy. A population based study, 1976 through 1990. *Circulation* 1995;**92**: 2488–95.

43. Maron BJ, Tajik AJ, Ruttenberg HD *et al*. Hypertrophic cardiomyopathy in infants: clinical features and natural history. *Circulation* 1982;**65**:7–17.

44. Savage DD, Seides SF, Clark CE *et al*. Electrocardiographic findings in patients with obstructive and non-obstructive hypertrophic cardiomyopathy. *Circulation* 1978;**58**:402–9.

45. Lemery R, Kleinebenne A, Nihoyannopoulos P, Alfonso F, McKenna WJ. Q-waves in hypertrophic cardiomyopathy in relation to the distribution and severity of right and left ventricular hypertrophy. *J Am Coll Cardiol* 1990;**16**:368–74.

46. Cosio FG, Moro C, Alonso M, Saenz de la Calzada C, Llovet A. The Q-waves of hypertrophic cardiomyopathy. *N Engl J Med* 1980;**302**:96–9.

47. Yamaguchi H, Ishimura T, Nishiyama S *et al.* Hypertrophic nonobstructive cardiomyopathy with giant negative T-waves (apical hypertrophy): ventriculographic and echocardiographic features in 30 patients. *Am J Cardiol* 1979;**44**: 401–12.

48. Fananapazir L, Tracey CM, Leon MB *et al.* Electrophysiological abnormalities in patients with hypertrophic cardiomyopathy: a consecutive analysis in 155 patients. *Circulation* 1989;**80**:1259.

49. McKenna WJ, England D, Doi Y, Deanfield JE, Oakley CM, Goodwin JF. Arrhythmia in hypertrophic cardiomyopathy. 1. Influence on prognosis. *Br Heart J* 1981;**46**:168–72.

50. Maron BJ, Savage DD, Wolfson JK, Epstein SE. Prognostic significance of 24 hour ambulatory electrocardiographic monitoring in patients with hypertrophic cardiomyopathy: a prospective study. *Am J Cardiol* 1981;**48**:252–7.

51. Alfonso F, Frenneaux MP, McKenna WJ. Clinical sustained uniform ventricular tachycardia in hypertrophic cardiomyopathy: association with left ventricular apical aneurysm. *Br Heart J* 1989;**61**:178–81.

52. Robinson K, Frenneaux MP, Stockins B, Karatasakis G, Poloniecki J, McKenna WJ. Atrial fibrillation in hypertrophic cardiomyopathy: a longitudinal study. *J Am Coll Cardiol* 1990;**15**:1279–85.

53. Maron BJ, Gottdiener JS, Epstein SE. Patterns and significance of the distribution of left ventricular hypertrophy in hypertrophic cardiomyopathy: a wide angle, two-dimensional echocardiographic study of 125 patients. *Am J Cardiol* 1981;**48**:418–28.

54. Shapiro LM, McKenna WJ. Distribution of left ventricular hypertrophy in hypertrophic cardiomyopathy: a two-dimensional echocardiographic study. *J Am Coll Cardiol* 1983;**2**:437–44.

55. Sharma S, Elliott PM, Whyte G *et al.* Utility of metabolic exercise testing in distinguishing hypertrophic cardiomyopathy from physiologic left ventricular hypertrophy in athletes. *J Am Coll Cardiol* 2000;**36**:864–70.

56. Dilsizian V, Bonow RO, Epstein SE, Fananapazir L. Myocardial ischemia detected by thallium scintigraphy is frequently related to cardiac arrest and syncope in young patients with hypertrophic cardiomyopathy. *J Am Coll Cardiol* 1993;**22**:796–804.

57. Nienaber CA, Gambhir SS, Moddy FV *et al.* Regional myocardial blood flow and glucose utilization in symptomatic patients with hypertrophic cardiomyopathy. *Circulation* 1993;**87**:1580–90.

58. Grover-McKay M, Schwaiger M, Krivokapich J, Perloff JK, Phelps ME, Schelbert HR. Regional myocardial blood flow and metabolism at rest in mildly symptomatic patients with hypertrophic cardiomyopathy. *J Am Coll Cardiol* 1989;**13**: 317–24.

59. Gould KL. Myocardial metabolism by positron emission tomography in hypertrophic cardiomyopathy. *J Am Coll Cardiol* 1989;**13**:325–6.

60. Betocchi S, Bonow RO, Bacharach SL, Rosing DR, Maron BJ, Green MV. Isovolumic relaxation period in hypertrophic cardiomyopathy: assessment by radionuclide angiography. *J Am Coll Cardiol* 1986;**7**:74–81.

61. Chikamori T, Dickie S, Poloniecki JD, Myers MJ, Lavender JP, McKenna WJ. Prognostic significance of radionuclide-assessed diastolic dysfunction in hypertrophic cardiomyopathy. *Am J Cardiol* 1990;**65**:478–82.

62. Child JS, Perloff JK, Bach PM, Wolfe AD, Perlman S, Kark RA. Cardiac involvement in Friedreich's ataxia. A clinical study of 75 patients. *J Am Coll Cardiol* 1986;**7**:1370.

63. Burch M, Sharland M, Shinebourne E, Smith G, Patton M, McKenna WJ. Cardiologic abnormalities in Noonan syndrome: phenotypic diagnosis and echocardiographic assessment of 118 patients. *J Am Coll Cardiol* 1993;**22**:1189–92.

64. Blaire E, Redwood C, Ashrafian H, Oliveira M, Broxholme J, Kerr B, Salmon A, Ostram-Smith I, Watkins H. Mutations in the gamma (2) subunit of AMP-activated protein kinase cause familial HCM: evidence for the central role of energy compromise in disease pathogenesis. *Hum Mol Genet* 2001;**10**:1215–20.

65. Devereux RB. Cardiac involvement in essential hypertension. Prevalence, pathophysiology and prognostic implications. *Med Clin N Am* 1987;**71**:813–26.

66. Shapiro LM, Kleinebenne A, McKenna WJ. The distribution of left ventricular hypertrophy in hypertrophic cardiomyopathy: comparison to athletes and hypertensives. *Eur Heart J* 1985;**6**:967–74.

67. Keller H, Wanger K, Goepfrich M, Stegaru B, Buss J, Heene DL. Morphological quantification and differentiation of left ventricular hypertrophy in hypertrophic cardiomyopathy and hypertensive heart disease. *Eur Heart J* 1990;**11**:65–74.

68. Hattori M, Aoki T, Sekioka K. Differences in direction-dependent shortening of the left ventricular wall in hypertrophic cardiomyopathy and in systemic hypertension. *Am J Cardiol* 1992;**70**:1326–32.

69. Maron BJ, Roberts WC, McAllister HA, Rosing DR, Epstein SE. Sudden death in young athletes. *Circulation* 1980;**62**: 218–29.

70. Burke AP, Farb A, Virmani R, Goodin J, Smialek JE. Sports-related and non-sports related sudden cardiac death in young adults. *Am Heart J* 1991;**121**:568–75.

71. Pelliccia A, Maron BJ, Spataro A, Proschan MA, Spirito P. The upper limit of physiologic cardiac hypertrophy in highly trained elite athletes. *N Engl J Med* 1991;**324**:295.

72. Maron BJ, Pellicia A, Spirito P. Cardiac disease in young trained athletes. Insights into methods for distinguishing athlete's heart from structural heart disease, with particular emphasis on hypertrophic cardiomyopathy. *Circulation* 1995;**91**:1569.

73. McKenna WJ, Spirito P, Desnos M, Dubourg O, Komajda M. Experience from clinical genetics in hypertrophic cardiomyopathy: proposal for new diagnostic criteria in adult members of affected families. *Heart* 1997;**77**:130–2.

74. Lewis JF, Maron BJ. Clinical and morphology expression of hypertrophic cardiomyopathy in patients 65 years of age. *Am J Cardiol* 1994;**73**:1105–11.

75. Topol EJ, Traill TA, Fortuin NJ. Hypertensive hypertrophic cardiomyopathy of the elderly. *N Engl J Med* 1985:**312**: 277–83.

76. Faye WP, Taliercio CP, Ilstrup DM, Tajik AJ, Gersh BJ. Natural history of hypertrophic cardiomyopathy in the elderly. *J Am Coll Cardiol* 1990;**16**:821–6.

77. Karam R, Lever HM, Healy BP. Hypertensive hypertrophic cardiomyopathy or hypertrophic cardiomyopathy with hypertension? A study of 78 patients. *J Am Coll Cardiol* 1989;**13**: 580–4.

78. Varnava AM, Elliott PM, Baboonian C, Davison F, Davies MJ, McKenna WJ. Hypertrophic cardiomyopathy: histopathological features of sudden death in cardiac troponin T disease. *Circulation* 2001;**104**:1380–4.

79. Coviello DA, Maron BJ, Spirito P *et al.* Clinical features of hypertrophic cardiomyopathy caused by mutation of a "hotspot" in the alpha-tropomyosin gene. *J Am Coll Cardiol* 1997;**29**:635–40.

80. Elliott PM, Gimeno Blanes JR, Mahon NG, Poloniecki JD, McKenna WJ. Relation between severity of LVH and prognosis in patients with hypertrophic cardiomyopathy. *Lancet* 2001;**357**:407–8.

81. Spirito P, Bellone P, Harris KM, Bernabo P, Bruzzi P, Maron BJ. Magnitude of left ventricular hypertrophy and risk of sudden death in hypertrophic cardiomyopathy. *N Engl J Med* 2000;**342**:1778–85.

82. Counihan PJ, Frenneaux MP, Webb DJ, McKenna WJ. Abnormal vascular responses to supine exercise in hypertrophic cardiomyopathy. *Circulation* 1991;**84**:686–96.

83. Dritsas A, Sabarouni E, Gilligan D, Nihoyannopoulos P, Oakley CM. QT-Interval abnormalities in hypertrophic cardiomyopathy. *Clin Cardiol* 1992;**15**:739–42.

84. Fei L, Slade AK, Grace AA, Malik M, Camm AJ, McKenna WJ. Ambulatory assessment of the QT interval in patients with hypertrophic cardiomyopathy: risk stratification and effect of low dose amiodarone. *Pacing Clin Electrophys* 1994;**17**:2222–7.

85. Buja G, Miorelli M, Turrini P, Melacini P, Nava A. Comparison of QT dispersion in hypertrophic cardiomyopathy between patients with and without ventricular arrhythmias and sudden death. *Am J Cardiol* 1993;**72**:973–6.

86. Kulakowski P, Counihan PJ, Camm AJ, McKenna WJ. The value of time and frequency domain, and spectral temporal mapping analysis of the signal-averaged electrocardiogram in identification of patients with hypertrophic cardiomyopathy at increased risk of sudden death. *Eur Heart J* 1993;**14**:941–50.

87. Counihan PJ, Fei L, Bashir Y, Farrell TG, Haywood GA, McKenna WJ. Assessment of heart rate variability in hypertrophic cardiomyopathy. Association with clinical and prognostic features. *Circulation* 1993;**88**:1682–90.

88. Fananapazir L, Chang AC, Epstein SE, McAreavey D. Prognostic determinants in hypertrophic cardiomyopathy: prognostic evaluation of a therapeutic strategy based on clinical, Holter, hemodynamic and electrophysiological findings. *Circulation* 1992;**86**:730–40.

89. Saumarez RC, Slade AKB, Grace AA, Sadoul N, Camm AJ, McKenna WJ. The significance of paced electrocardiogram fractionation in hypertrophic cardiomyopathy. A prospective study. *Circulation* 1995;**91**:2762–8.

90. Elliott PM, Poloniecki J, Dickie S *et al.* Sudden death in hypertrophic cardiomyopathy: identification of high-risk patients. *J Am Coll Cardiol* 2000;**36**:2212–18.

91. McKenna WJ, Oakley CM, Krikler DM *et al.* Improved survival with amiodarone in patients with hypertrophic cardiomyopathy and ventricular tachycardia. *Br Heart J* 1985;**53**:412–16.

92. McKenna WJ, Deanfield JE. Hypertrophic cardiomyopathy: an important cause of sudden death. *Arch Dis Childhood* 1984;**59**:971–5.

93. Elliott PM, Sharma S, Varnava A, Poloniecki J, Rowland E, McKenna WJ. Survival after cardiac arrest or sustained ventricular tachycardia in patients with hypertrophic cardiomyopathy. *J Am Coll Cardiol* 1999;**33**:1596–601.

94. Maron BJ, Shen WK, Link MS *et al.* Efficacy of implantable cardioverter-defibrillators for the prevention of sudden death in patients with hypertrophic cardiomyopathy. *N Engl J Med* 2000;**342**:365–73.

95. Primo J, Geelen P, Brugada J *et al.* Hypertrophic cardiomyopathy: role of the implantable cardioverter defibrillator. *J Am Coll Cardiol* 1998;**31**:1081–5.

96. Silka MJ, Kron J, Dunnigan A, Dick M. Sudden cardiac death and the use of implantable cardioverter-defibrillator in paediatric patients. *Circulation* 1993;**87**:800–7.

97. Kron J, Oliver RP, Norsted S, Silka MJ. The automatic implantable cardioverter defibrillator in young patients. *J Am Coll Cardiol* 1990;**16**:896–902.

98. Elliott PM, Sharma S, Poloniecki J, Prasad K, Murd'Ah, McKenna WJ. Amiodarone and sudden death in hypertrophic cardiomyopathy. (Abstract) *Circulation* 1997;**96**:I-464.

99. Pollick C. Muscular subaortic stenosis: hemodynamic and clinical improvement after disopyramide. *N Engl J Med* 1982;**307**:997–9.

100. Pollick C. Disopyramide in hypertrophic cardiomyopathy. Hemodynamic assessment after intravenous administration. *Am J Cardiol* 1988;**62**:1248–51.

101. Morrow AG, Reitz BA, Epstein SE, Henry WL, Conkle DM, Itscoitz SB, Redwood DR. Operative treatment in hypertrophic subaortic stenosis: techniques, and the results of pre and postoperative assessments in 83 patients. *Circulation* 1975;**52**:88–102.

102. Maron BJ, Merrill WH, Freier PA, Kent KM, Epstein SE, Morrow AG. Long-term clinical course and symptomatic status of patients after operation for hypertrophic subaortic stenosis. *Circulation* 1978;**57**:1205–13.

103. Williams WG, Wigle ED, Rakowski H, Smallhorn J, LeBlanc J, Trusler GA. Results of surgery for hypertrophic obstructive cardiomyopathy. *Circulation* 1987;**76**(Suppl. V):V104–8.

104. Heric B, Lytle BW, Miller DP, Rosenkranz ER, Lever HM, Cosgrove DM. Surgical management of hypertrophic obstructive cardiomyopathy. Early and late results. *J Thorac Cardiovas Surg* 1995;**110**:195–208.

105. Robbins RC, Stinson Eb. Long-term results of left ventricular myotomy and myectomy for obstructive hypertrophic cardiomyopathy. *J Thorac Cardiovasc Surg* 1996;**111**:586–94.

106. Schulte HD, Bircks WH, Loesse B, Godehardt EAJ, Schwartzkopff B. Prognosis of patients with hypertrophic obstructive cardiomyopathy after transaortic myectomy. Late results up to 25 years. *J Thorac Cardiovasc Surg* 1993;**106**:709–17.

107. McCully RB, Nishimura RA, Tajik J, Schaff HV, Danielson GK. Extent of clinical improvement after surgical treatment of hypertrophic obstructive cardiomyopathy. *Circulation* 1996;**94**:467–71.

108. McIntosh CL, Greenberg GJ, Maron BJ, Leon MB, Cannon RO, Clark RE. Clinical and hemodynamic results after mitral valve replacement in patients with hypertrophic cardiomyopathy. *Ann Thorac Surg* 1989;**47**:236–46.

109. Slade AKB, Sadoul N, Shapiro L *et al.* DDD pacing in hypertrophic cardiomyopathy: a multicenter clinical experience. *Heart* 1996;**75**:44–9.

110. Jeanrenaud X, Goy JJ, Kappenberger L. Effects of dual-chamber pacing in hypertrophic obstructive cardiomyopathy. *Lancet* 1992;**339**:1318–23.

111. Fananapazir L, Epstein ND, Curiel RV, Panza JA, Tripodi D, McAreavey D. Long-term results of dual chamber (DDD) pacing in obstructive hypertrophic cardiomyopathy. Evidence for progressive symptomatic and hemodynamic improvement and reduction of left ventricular hypertrophy. *Circulation* 1994;**90**:2731–42.

112. Nishimura RA, Trusty JM, Hayes DL *et al.* Dual chamber pacing for hypertrophic cardiomyopathy: a randomised double-blind crossover trial. *J Am Coll Cardiol* 1997;**29**: 435–41.

113. Kappenberger L, Linde C, Daubert C *et al.* (PIC study Group). Pacing in hypertrophic obstructive cardiomyopathy. A randomised crossover study. *Eur Heart J* 1997;**18**:1249–56.

114. Sigwart U. Non-surgical myocardial reduction for hypertrophic obstructive cardiomyopathy. *Lancet* 1995;**346**:211–14.

115. Gleichman U, Seggewiss H, Faber L, Fassbender D, Schmidt HK, Strick S. [Catheter treatment of hypertrophic cardiomyopathy]. [German]. *Deut Medizin Woch* 1996;**121**:679–85.

116. Knight C, Kurbaan AS, Seggewiss H *et al.* Non-surgical reduction for hypertrophic obstructive cardiomyopathy: outcome in the first series of patients. *Circulation* 1997;**95**: 2075–81.

49 Other cardiomyopathies

José A Marin-Neto, Marcus Vinícius Simões, Benedito Carlos Maciel

Introduction

From the vast array of clinical entities that comprise the cardiomyopathies, two conditions were selected for this chapter: Chagas' heart disease and endomyocardiofibrosis.

In neither disease have large randomized controlled trials been conducted to support recommendations for therapeutic options. Knowledge of natural history and pathophysiology is based almost entirely on observational studies, mostly of the case series kind. Most are flawed by heterogeneous criteria for patient selection and investigation. Thus, particularly in Chagas' heart disease, a large volume of incomplete and biased information has been obtained, so that meta-analysis of available data has been limited to the etiologic treatment in a subgroup of patients.

Despite the paucity of evidence-based knowledge, the diseases epitomize quite different unique pathophysiological conditions. In essence, Chagas' heart disease is a myocarditis of parasitic origin, although the role of the etiologic agent in the chronic phase of the disease is still somewhat controversial. Endomyocardiofibrosis has no defined etiology or pathogenesis and reasonably good animal models exist only for the study of Chagas' disease.

There are many reasons for the lack of solid evidence-based data in both diseases. However, while the apparently low prevalence of endomyocardiofibrosis is an obvious obstacle, the high prevalence of Chagas' heart disease in many countries has not helped to produce large randomized trials on therapeutic management.

Chagas' heart disease

Epidemiology

Chagas' disease is caused by *Trypanosoma cruzi* infection. Its transmission is mainly vectoral, through the feces of infected bloodsucking insects of the family *Reduviidae* (subfamily *Triatominae*). Many case series reports have also documented that the infection can occur by transplacental and oral transmission, blood transfusion, laboratory contamination, and organ transplantation. Although virtually every organic system may be involved and megaesophagus and megacolon can produce florid clinical conditions, it is the cardiac involvement – the object of this chapter – that constitutes the most serious form of the disease.

The current prevalence of Chagas' heart disease is unknown because no recent large scale screening has been carried out even in endemic countries. Besides, the epidemiological information available from the different countries is strikingly varied. This reflects the diversity of public health programs, including the control of vectoral and transfusional transmission. Thus, a survey carried out from 1988 to 1990 in 850 municipalities of Brazil revealed that serological screening for Chagas' disease was performed in only two thirds of all blood donors.[1] Also, a review of serological surveys for Chagas' infection among blood donors conducted over the 1980s in several countries in the American continent disclosed a highly variable rate of prevalence, from 0% to 63%.[2]

Neither is case reporting reliable, even in high endemicity areas. Rough estimates by the World Health Organization, based upon limited serological surveys, suggest that 15–18 million people are infected in extensive areas of the South American subcontinent.[3] Moreover, some 65 million are at risk.

Cross-sectional epidemiological studies have been carried out in scattered areas of Brazil and Venezuela to assess the prevalence of clinical manifestations and mortality due to Chagas' heart disease. However, probably because of marked variations in the genetic background, parasite strain, climate, socioeconomic and related hygienic alimentary conditions, and healthcare measures, the prevalence of both morbidity and mortality is extremely variable even within each country.[1]

Nevertheless, Chagas' heart disease is by far the most common form of cardiomyopathy in Latin American countries. Further, because of modern migratory trends, it is likely to become ubiquitous. This tendency is shown in the United States, where based on a prevalence of 4·5% of *T. cruzi* infection detected serologically in 205 Latin American immigrants and on rough estimates of the number of such legal and illegal immigrants, 400 000–500 000 infected people are believed to be living there now.[4] Also, rural–urban migration from endemic areas in Brazil is believed to have brought half a million infected people to cities such as São Paulo and Rio de Janeiro in the past three decades.

Chagas' heart disease has a very high social impact. It has been estimated that over 750 000 years of productive life are lost annually due to premature deaths in Latin American countries, at a cost of about US$1200 million/year.[5] These figures substantiate the need for the elimination of transmission – a goal achieved in some regions[7] and proved to be a highly cost effective public health policy.

Natural history and prognostic factors

There is sound experimental, pathological, and clinical evidence that Chagas' heart disease presents two phases, acute (immediately following infection) and chronic. The long period – 10–30 years – between the acute condition and the clinically manifest chronic Chagas' heart disease is known as the indeterminate form of the disease and constitutes one of its most intriguing features. Its classical definition – now the subject of controversy[6] – requires that the patients be asymptomatic, have no physical signs of Chagas' disease, and normal ECG and radiological exploration of the chest, esophagus and colon.

Megaesophagus and megacolon are also frequently diagnosed in chagasic patients in Brazil, Argentina, and Chile, but not in Mexico, Colombia or Venezuela. The hypothesis that different *T. cruzi* strains or environmental factors may cause this difference in morbidity[8] has not been evaluated by appropriately designed studies.

The natural history of Chagas' heart disease is relatively well known from observational studies conducted mainly in endemic areas in Brazil, Argentina, and Venezuela since the early 1940s. There is also a wealth of case series reports dealing with acute Chagas' disease acquired through non-vector transmission. Most of these investigations consist of cross-sectional observations of infected people in rural areas. Very few studies have been conducted using case–control populations of chagasic and non-chagasic people.

There have also been some observational investigations focusing on the description and follow up of hospital based cohorts of chagasic patients.

Both the rural and the hospital based studies have limitations. There is usually no adequate identification of cardiac involvement provided in the rural based studies. Furthermore, because of the protracted course of heart involvement, from the acute phase to end stage heart failure, no prospective studies encompassing the whole span of the disease are available. Conversely, in hospital based studies the heart disease is often well characterized, but results could not be extended to the whole chagasic population.

Prognosis in the acute phase

Case series using serological tests in endemic areas have shown that in no more than 10% of the acute cases were clinical manifestations sufficient to make a correct diagnosis.[9] This is a major deterrent for understanding the transition from the acute to the chronic stages of Chagas' disease. However, the scarce clinical data are in general agreement with findings from experimental models of Chagas' disease.

For the minority of patients in whom the clinical diagnosis was possible, cardiac involvement occurred in around 90% of 313 successive cases; in 70–80%, cardiac enlargement was seen on x rays, contrasting with only 50% of cases showing ECG abnormalities. The severity of myocarditis was inversely proportional to age; signs of heart failure were twice as intense in children aged up to 2 years than in those aged between 3 and 5 years.[9] Mortality in the acute phase, as seen in the 313 cases, was 8·3%. This was higher than the 3–5% reported in similar studies in other endemic areas in Brazil, Argentina, and Uruguay. The ECG was normal in 63·3% of the non-fatal cases and in only 14·3% of those who died in the acute phase. Seventy-five per cent of all deaths were seen in children aged under 3 years. Heart failure was the constant finding in all fatal cases, with or without concomitant encephalitis.[9]

Survival is characterized by disappearance of symptoms and signs of heart failure within 1–3 months and normalization of the ECG in over 90% of the cases after 1 year of the infection. However, there is no evidence of spontaneous cure of the infection, as demonstrated by serial xenodiagnosis and serological tests in studies of several hundreds of chagasic patients.

Of 172 patients who were followed in Bambuí (central Brazil) for up to 40 years after the acute infection, the development of cardiac involvement (based on clinical signs, ECG, and chest x ray changes) occurred in 33·8%, 39·3%, and 58·1% for follow up periods of 10–20 years, 21–30 years, and 31–40 years respectively.[9] In another review from the same area, for 268 patients whose acute phase of the disease had been diagnosed an average of 27 years before, the general mortality for the period was 13·8%.[9]

Prognosis in the indeterminate phase

Factors that affect the varying rates of disease progression are currently unknown. A 1–3% per year rate of appearance of heart involvement has been observed in several studies. Of 400 young adults followed for 10 years, 91 (23%) showed clinical, ECG or chest x ray markers of cardiac disease. Of note, eight deaths were recorded in that period, of which only one could be ascribed to reagudization (that is, a full-blown infective illness with parasitemia) of Chagas' heart disease.[10]

Another longitudinal study in Bambui, central Brazil, contrasted the evolution of 885 young chagasic patients in the indeterminate phase for 10 years with that of 911 chagasic patients with initially abnormal ECGs in the same period. Survival after 10 years was 97·4% and 61·3% respectively for the indeterminate group and the group with cardiac involvement.[11]

A third longitudinal study in a rural Venezuelan community, with 47% prevalence of positive serology for Chagas' disease, followed 364 patients for a mean period of 4 years.

It revealed the appearance of heart disease at a rate of 1·1% per year in seropositive individuals. Mortality was 3% in the 4 years of follow up and Chagas' heart disease was the cause of death in 69% of all fatal cases.[12]

In 1973 a longitudinal study was initiated in a rural community in northeast Brazil. In the initial cross-sectional study, of 644 individuals aged >10 years, 53·7% were seropositive. The population initially described in 1973–1974 was re-examined in 1977, 1980, and 1983. The overall rate of development of abnormal ECG was 2·57% in seropositive (248) as compared to 1·25% per year in seronegative (332) individuals, a relative risk of 2 for the same geographical area. The age adjusted mortality rate was higher in seropositive (8·9/1000/year of 488 patients) than in seronegative individuals (7·8/1000/year of 509 individuals). Mortality in this study was strongly associated with ventricular conduction defects and arrhythmias.[13]

These results were obtained in chagasic populations with more than 50% of the patients younger than 20 years. It is relevant that fewer indeterminate cases are found in the older age groups because of the evolutive nature of the disease (that is, more aging patients presenting clinical signs of cardiac or digestive involvement).

Key points

- As long as the patients remain in the indeterminate phase, their prognosis is good. **Grade B2**
- After 10 years almost 80% of patients remain in the indeterminate phase of the disease and probably 50% of the entire population will have no signs of heart disease throughout their lives. **Grade B2**
- There are no clues as to why some chagasic patients remain in the indeterminate phase, while others sooner or later go through the chronic phase of heart involvement.

Prognosis of chronic Chagas' heart disease

The evidence provided by the studies mentioned above shows that the mere appearance of ECG changes entails a bad prognosis. Also, a retrospective analysis of seropositive individuals followed over 18 years revealed that right bundle branch block was three times more common in fatal cases than in survivors.[14]

Another important negative prognostic factor once heart disease is manifest is male gender. This is borne out by several studies carried out with long-term follow up of different cohorts of chagasic patients.[15]

Only two case–control follow up studies have been reported in Brazilian endemic areas. In central Brazil[16] two cross-sectional clinical assessments (1974 and 1984) included 12-lead ECG and radiological evaluation of heart size. Seropositive patients and controls were matched by age and gender. In the first cross-sectional study 264 pairs of

subjects were evaluated, of which 110 were re-examined after the 10 year follow up period with the same clinical, ECG, and chest *x* ray assessment. The incidence of heart disease in previously healthy but serologically positive individuals was 38·3% in the 10 year period. In those patients with previous heart involvement, a rate of 34·5% of deterioration was observed in the same period. In the chagasic population the overall 10 year mortality was 23%, compared to 10·3% in the controls. Moreover, cardiac mortality, including sudden death and death in heart failure, was 17% among chagasic patients and only 2·3% in the control population. Again, the overall mortality was much higher in chagasic males and largely predominated in the group aged 30–59 years.[13] The same group of investigators, applying similar methods in northeastern Brazil, showed that mortality rates were 1·6% and 0% for 125 matched pairs of respectively chagasic and non-chagasic patients followed for 4·5 years.[17] Progression of disease as assessed by ECG changes occurred in 10·4% of patients, as compared to 4·8% of controls. The hypothesis that the different morbidity and mortality rates in the two regions were due to differences in the pathogenicity characteristics of *T. cruzi* strains was not substantiated by direct evidence.

There is persuasive evidence to support the concept that the mortality associated with Chagas' disease strongly correlates with severity of the myocardial dysfunction. For example, survival 2 years after the first episode of heart failure was only 33·4% in 160 cases.[18] Of note, 10% of deaths were sudden. In addition, 98% of the deceased people were autopsied, revealing <20% prevalence of amastigote forms of *T. cruzi* in the cardiac tissue, but with a clear predominance of this finding in male patients.[18]

In a study of 107 chagasic patients followed for 10 years, a significant reduction in life expectancy, as compared to that of 22 non-chagasic patients, was detected only in those with ECG or clinical changes. A mortality rate of 82% over the 10 year follow up period was seen in the group of 34 patients with signs of heart failure at the beginning of the study. In contrast, a 65% 10 year survival was associated with ECG abnormalities but in the absence of signs of heart failure.[19]

Another study of 104 male chagasic patients admitted to hospital with heart failure revealed a mortality rate of 52% after 5 years. The strongest predictors of survival were reduced LV ejection fraction and maximal oxygen uptake during exercise.[20]

In a series of 42 patients with Chagas' heart disease in the United States 11 deaths occurred during a mean follow up of nearly 5 years, always in association with global or regional LV dysfunction. Established or developing heart failure was a strong predictor of mortality but aborted sudden death or the presence of sustained ventricular tachycardia were not predictors for mortality in this series.[21] These results conflict with the evidence from 44 chagasic patients followed for a mean period of 2 years that ventricular tachycardia detected during exercise testing is a marker of increased risk of sudden death.[22] This discrepancy probably reflects the limitations of small numbers and relatively short follow up in both studies.

Key points

- There is substantial evidence that the most important prognostic factor in established Chagas' heart disease is the degree of myocardial dysfunction. However, ECG changes also herald increased risk. **Grade B2**
- Once overt cardiac failure ensues the prognosis is poor and approaches 50% in 4 years. **Grade B2**
- It is possible – but not proven by good evidence – that ventricular dysrhythmia and sudden death play a more prominent role in mortality due to Chagas' disease than in heart failure due to other etiologies. **Grade B4**

Clinical features of Chagas' heart disease

Cardiac abnormalities are present in all stages of Chagas' disease, but their clinical expression is highly variable. The paucity of clinical indicators of the typical myocarditis of acute Chagas' disease has already been pointed out. There is also solid evidence – from necropsy studies as well as from *in vivo* investigations – that virtually all patients, even in the indeterminate phase of the disease, have some subtle degree of cardiac structural or functional involvement.[23–29]

Patients with Chagas' heart disease are classified following the criteria shown in Table 49.1. The anatomical and functional disturbances detected during life are consistent with the autopsy findings reported on several series of chagasic patients who died in the various stages of the disease.[23,24,30]

It is not uncommon for patients with ECG and marked LV regional abnormalities to be asymptomatic hard workers and capable of performing as such under laboratory conditions.[26] When symptoms occur, they are usually in the form of fatigue and exertional dyspnea, palpitations, dizziness and syncope or chest pain. These are the expression of a reduction of the cardiac reserve (including minor early signs of diastolic dysfunction), the presence of ventricular dysrhythmias, and atrioventricular block. The chest pain is usually atypical for myocardial ischemia but in sporadic cases may mimic an acute coronary syndrome.

Systemic and pulmonary embolism, arising from mural thrombi in the cardiac chambers, is a conspicuous complication of Chagas' heart disease, but post-mortem findings show they are often overlooked. In 1345 necropsies on patients with Chagas' heart disease, 595 cases (44%) had cardiac thrombi and/or visceral thromboembolism. The presence of cardiac thrombi was related to severity of ventricular enlargement. Embolism most frequently involved

lungs (36%), kidneys (36%), spleen (14%), and brain (10%).[31]

Congestive heart failure is more commonly expressed by prominent signs of systemic congestion, with less intense pulmonary congestion.[32] This peculiar feature of Chagas' heart disease is linked to early severe damage of the RV, a chamber frequently neglected in investigations of cardiac function.[33,34]

Sudden unexpected death occurs with undefined but not negligible frequency even in patients previously asymptomatic. It is usually precipitated by physical exercise and associated with ventricular tachycardia and fibrillation or, more rarely, with complete AV block. Limited evidence from autopsy studies in these patients indicates variable degrees of inflammatory and neuronal cardiac alterations.[24]

Patients with chronic Chagas' heart disease invariably have one or more positive serological tests. There is also recent and limited experience with polymerase chain reaction-based methods for detecting *T. cruzi* DNA sequences in the blood of chagasic patients. This method is likely to replace the cumbersome and unreliable method of direct demonstration of parasite infection by xenodiagnosis.[35]

ECG abnormalities are present in most patients with chronic Chagas' heart disease, mainly in the form of conduction disturbances and ventricular arrhythmias. In more advanced stages pathological Q waves are found, compatible with extensive areas of myocardial fibrosis. The combination of right bundle branch block and left anterior hemiblock is very typical in chronic Chagas' heart disease. Nevertheless, no ECG changes can be considered specific to the disease.

Many case series reports have documented the typical feature of striking segmental-wall motion abnormalities in several hundreds of chronic chagasic patients. The most characteristic lesion is the apical aneurysm, but it is the posterior basal dysynergy that best correlates with the occurrence of malignant ventricular arrhythmia. A few small retrospective studies have evaluated the correlation between ventricular arrhythmia and symptoms in Chagas' heart disease. It is apparent that complex ventricular dysrhythmia may occur in asymptomatic patients, but it is usually a conspicuous manifestation associated with poor LV function. The aneurysms are also sources of emboli.

In spite of chest pain being a common complaint in many chagasic patients, coronary angiography is usually normal. However, functional abnormalities in the myocardial blood flow regulation have been described and all types of myocardial perfusion defects have been detected in several small groups of selected patients, possibly implying microvascular coronary disturbances.[28]

Cardiac autonomic dysfunction, mainly parasympathetic, has been shown in various groups of several hundreds of chagasic patients (including those with isolated digestive disease) whose response to various autonomic tests was

Table 49.1   A clinical classification of Chagas' heart disease

	Clinical phase				
	Acute	Indeterminate		Overt heart disease	Heart failure
		IA	IB		
Symptoms	Fairly common	Absent	Absent	Minimal	Present
Physical	Usually Abnormal	Normal	Normal	May be abnormal	Abnormal
ECG changes	Common	Absent	Absent	RBBB, LAHB, AVB, PVCs	+ Q waves VT
Heart size (x rays)	Usually abnormal	Normal	Normal	Normal	Enlarged
RV function	Usually abnormal	Normal	May be depressed	Usually abnormal	Abnormal
LV diastolic function	?	?	Mild impairment	Abnormal	Abnormal
LV systolic function	Abnormal	Normal	Mild segmental dysynergy	Segmental dysynergy	Global depression
Perfusion defects	?	Mild abnormalities	Mild abnormalities	Common	Common
Autonomic function	?	May be abnormal	May be abnormal	May be abnormal	Usually abnormal
RV biopsy	Abnormal	May be abnormal	Usually abnormal	Abnormal	Abnormal
Exercise stress test	?	Normal	May be abnormal – Arrhythmia – Chronotropic deficit	May be abnormal – Arrhythmia – Chronotropic deficit	Abnormal Reduced exercise capacity
Arrhythmia/Sudden death	?	Absent	Very uncommon	May be detected	Common

Abbreviations: AVB, atrioventricular block; ECG, electrocardiogram; LAHB, left anterior hemiblock;   LV, left ventricle; PVCs, premature ventricular complexes; RBBB, right bundle branch block; RV, right ventricle; VT, ventricular tachycardia; ?, unknown

compared to that of control subjects.[28,34,36,37] However, in Chagas' disease patients, the autonomic abnormalities do not correlate with any symptoms or cause postural hypotension. Recent scintigraphic studies demonstrated early sympathetic denervation, topographically related to the segmental-wall motion and perfusional abnormalities often detected in patients with more advanced stages of disease.[38]

Pathophysiology and pathogenetic mechanisms

The clinical manifestations arising during the acute phase are closely related to parasite presence in target organs such as the gastrointestinal tract, central nervous system and heart, coexisting with high grade parasitemia. Lymphadenopathy, liver and spleen enlargement are markers of widespread immunologic reaction.

As the parasitemia abates and the systemic inflammatory reaction subsides, it is believed that a silent, relentless, focal myocarditis ensues during the indeterminate phase. In predisposed hosts, encompassing approximately 30–50% of the infected population, this chronic myocarditis may evolve to cumulative destruction of cardiac fibers and marked reparative fibrosis. During this phase ventricular arrhythmias and sudden death may rarely occur as manifestations of the underlying focal inflammatory process, and possibly, of the early autonomic denervation. The incessant myocarditis is eventually responsible for myocardial mass loss attaining critical degrees, thereby leading to regional and global ventricular remodeling, chamber dilation and setting the anatomic substrate for malignant dysrhythmia.

This hypothesis is based on experimental models for Chagas' heart disease. Additional evidence has been provided by studies correlating clinical and pathological findings in autopsied humans dying in all phases of the disease. Most studies included case series of dozens of patients for the acute and indeterminate phases and ranging from hundreds to thousands of cases for the chronic phase.

The most intriguing challenge for understanding the pathophysiology of Chagas' heart disease lies in the complex host-parasite relationship.[39,40] It is not clear why in many patients (who remain in the indeterminate phase) the myocardial aggression is controlled at low levels, whereas in others the development of full blown chronic Chagas' cardiomyopathy is triggered. In brief, *auto-immune mediated myocardial injury* is probably sustained and exacerbated by continuous antigen presentation related to *low grade persistent T. cruzi tissue parasitism.*

Evidence gathered from pathophysiological studies in animal models and in humans is consistent with the hypothesis that four main pathogenetic mechanisms participate in the genesis of chronic Chagas' heart disease:

- neurogenic mechanisms
- parasite-dependent inflammatory aggression
- microvascular disturbances
- immune mediated cardiac damage.

Neurogenic mechanisms – As discussed above, abnormal autonomic cardiac regulation, preceding the development of myocardial damage, has been conclusively shown in many functional investigations.[28,34,36,37,38,41–46] Accordingly, intense neuronal depopulation has been clearly demonstrated in several pathologic studies.[30,47]

Antibodies against autonomic receptors may be detected in experimental and human chronic Chagas' disease. Functional abnormalities in the cardiac electrogenesis can be caused by auto-antibodies against beta1-adrenergic and muscarinic M2-receptors.[42–46] It is still speculative whether receptor stimulation or inhibition thus triggered could mediate myocardial damage.

However, various kinds of evidence militate against neurogenic derangements being a main pathogenetic mechanism. Even in endemic areas cardiac denervation shows marked individual variability in intensity and frequency.[37,48] Also, no correlation has been shown between cardiac parasympathetic denervation and the extent of myocardial dysfunction or the presence of dysrhythmia. Moreover, the typical chagasic cardiomyopathy is found in geographical regions where the disease is apparently caused by parasite strains devoid of neurotropism. Interestingly, in such regions, the typical chagasic digestive syndromes – considered to be causally related to parasympathetic denervation of the esophagus and colon – are rarely described.[37] Furthermore, no follow up studies correlating autonomic regulation, myocardial function, and cardiac rhythm assessment have been reported.

In conclusion, the role of dysautonomia remains to be determined. Furthermore, the attractive hypothesis implicating autonomic impairment in triggering sudden death has never been appropriately tested.

Parasite-dependent inflammatory aggression – A direct cause-effect relationship between parasitism and inflammatory findings in the chronic phase of Chagas' heart disease was initially discarded.[47] Very low-grade parasitemia was detected by xenodiagnosis. Also, the scanty tissular nests of amastigotic *T. cruzi* bear no topographic relation with the diffuse focal inflammation, as seen by classical histopathological staining techniques.

However, more sensitive molecular biology methods have shown that parasitemia may be persistent in the chronic phase of Chagas' disease.[49,50] In myocardial biopsy specimens from chronic chagasic patients techniques using amplification of DNA sequences of *T. cruzi*[51] and immunofluorescent monoclonal antibodies[52,53] showed parasite antigens in the inflammatory infiltrates.

Microvascular disturbances – Several independent studies in animal models[54,55] and in humans with Chagas' disease,[56–59] focusing on histopathological changes, platelet activation and endothelial function disturbances support the hypothesis of microvascular abnormalities. These derangements may cause ischemic-like symptoms and transient ECG changes often detected in chagasic patients. They might also constitute the mechanism responsible for the myocardial perfusion abnormalities described in chagasic patients with angiographically normal coronary arteries.[4,28]

On the basis of the evidence from these investigations, it has been postulated that microvascular derangements could be a relevant mechanism for the amplification and perpetuation of myocardial damage triggered by the inflammatory process;[55] however, there is no information on their prognostic implications.

Immune mediated cardiac damage – Studies in humans and in animal experiments provide evidence for the role played by immunological mechanisms in chronic Chagas' heart disease. It is widely accepted that mononuclear inflammatory infiltrates seen in chronic chagasic myocarditis are the expression of cell mediated aggression. Ultrastructural microscopic studies in animal models show that immune effector cells cause lysis of non-parasitized myocardial cells.[60] Depletion of the TDC^{4+} lymphocyte subpopulation prevents myocardial injury in the murine model of Chagas' heart disease.[61] Conversely, myocardial damage is induced in non-chagasic animals, by passive transfer of TDC^{4+} lymphocytes from infected mice.[61,62] Furthermore, the identification of antigenic epitopes related to cross-reactivity between *T. cruzi* and myocardial protein has been reported.[63,64]

These findings support the notion of an organ-specific autoimmune aggression against self-antigens modified since the acute phase. Also plausible is an incessant aggression maintained by persistent presentation of cross-reacting parasite antigens to the macrophage system, as a consequence of lifelong tissue parasitism.

Key points

- The evidence gathered from pathophysiological studies in animal models and in humans is consistent with the hypothesis of immune mediated injury being a key pathogenetic mechanism in chronic Chagas' heart disease.
- The immune responses are probably related to the persisting low-grade *T. cruzi* tissue parasitism but the mechanisms triggering exacerbated responses in some cases and deterring significant immune damage in others are still unknown.
- The presence of the parasite (or its remnants) in direct topographic relation to the inflammatory foci has potential therapeutic implication.
- Microvascular disturbances probably constitute important amplification mechanisms for the inflammatory myocardial injury.
- Cardiac dysautonomia is a well characterized feature that may precede other manifestations of myocardial damage but its pathogenetic role is still debated.

Management of Chagas' heart disease

Etiologic treatment

Although recent developments in basic biochemistry of the parasite allowed the identification of potential targets for chemotherapy, such as protein prenylation, sterol, proteases and phospholipid metabolism,[65] few antitrypanosomal agents are currently available for clinical use. Nifurtimox and benznidazole have been shown to be comparable in efficacy and high incidence of side effects including dermatitis, polyneuritis, leukopenia, gastrointestinal intolerance. This often warrants discontinuation of treatment, and nifurtimox was abandoned in most centers.

Acute phase – There is consensus that in the acute phase etiologic treatment is mandatory to control symptoms and life threatening myocarditis and encephalitis. Guidelines have been developed to recommend etiologic treatment also for laboratory or surgical accidents and in organ transplant recipient and donors.[66,67] After adequate treatment a negative xenodiagnosis is found in over 90% of cases and serological tests are negative in 80%. A more recent study suggested that molecular methods can be more effective to show parasite persistence; the etiologic treatment in the acute phase led to PCR negative results in 73% of the cases, while xenodiagnosis was negative in 86% after 3 years.[68]

Despite these current recommendations, in the absence of long-term follow up trials, there is no evidence for the prevention of chronic organ damage even for patients treated in the acute phase. The impact on prognosis has not been established, again due to lack of appropriately designed follow up studies.

Chronic phase – From experimental studies there is scarce evidence for benefit of trypanocide treatment against the development of chronic tissue damage.[69] Also, evidence for potential benefits of etiologic chemotherapy in chronic human Chagas' disease is extremely limited, due mainly to misleading criteria being employed in small trials.

Besides several case-series studies, a prospective, nonrandomized, controlled trial involving 131 patients treated with benznidazole (5 mg/kg/day for 30 days) and 70 untreated patients with a mean follow up period of 8 years has been reported.[70] Progression of disease was assessed by ECG changes. Treated patients presented fewer ECG changes than the control group (4·2% *v* 30%) and less deterioration in the clinical condition (2·1% *v* 17%). These results suggest that etiologic treatment may impact favorably in the chronic phase.

However the parasitological criterion of persistent negativity of the xenodiagnosis is unreliable as this test is commonly negative in the chronic phase of Chagas' disease – 60–80% – despite the presence of overt and progressive cardiac involvement. Moreover, large fluctuations of parasitemia occur over time. There may also be bias in the trials caused by selection of patients with persistent parasitemia in the pretreatment period. Furthermore, results of experimental studies have shown that in the chronic phase the parasitemia is low or not detectable at all, while there is a predominant tissular parasitism by amastigotic forms of *T. cruzi*.

Conversely, because persistently positive serological tests may merely reflect mechanisms of immunological memory or be associated with crossreactivity to altered host antigens, results of any of the serological criteria used to assess etiological treatment are clearly inadequate. In fact, the observed rate of negativation of serological tests following treatment in the chronic phase is consistently low (4–8%) in trials suffering the same methodological limitations discussed above.

Thus, until an adequate laboratory method is available for assessment of cure, the only acceptable criteria for etiologic treatment must be based on the prevention of the appearance of the clinical manifestation or the arrest of damage already detected. For this, a long follow up period of large cohorts of patients would be required.

Using better diagnostic tests and research designs, more recent clinical trials have reported high rates of parasitologic cure in children with early chronic *T. cruzi* infection and claimed trypanocidal therapy for the indeterminate phase.[71]

A recent systematic review of studies testing the efficacy of trypanocide therapy in the chronic asymptomatic *T. cruzi* infection has been carried out.[72] Only five studies met the inclusion criteria requiring that published trials randomly allocated participants with chronic *T. cruzi* infection without symptomatic Chagas' heart disease to one or more of the trypanocidal drugs (benznidazole, nifurtimox, allopurinol) given for at least 30 days at any dose, and to control treatment with or without placebo.[71-76] Studies had to report on at least one of the following outcomes: all-cause mortality, sudden death, incidence of heart failure, side effects of treatment, ECG changes (collectively named here as "clinical outcomes") or reduction in parasite load, reduction in antibody titres to *T. cruzi* or negative seroconversion (collectively named as "parasite-related outcomes"). General characteristics of the five studies included are shown in Table 49.2. Data synthesis for pooled outcomes including all information available are shown in Figure 49.1.

The most important finding in this review was that trypanocide therapy improved parasite-related outcomes. The strongest effect was found for benznidazole that significantly reduced the proportion of positive xenodiagnosis in both children and adults and increased the rate of negative seroconversion in children, when serology was tested using the ELISA with Antigen-total stimulation (AT ELISA) technique. Allopurinol and itraconazole failed to demonstrate a significant effect on these outcomes and had severe side effects. Although these results are in favor of the use of trypanocide therapy in children and asymptomatic adults for reducing antibodies or the parasite load respectively, whether this effect will result in clinical benefit remains to be proven. None of these trials was designed primarily to assess clinical outcomes and failed to report key methodological issues. In addition, because of the variability in their designs and the small size of each trial, the meta-analysis performed for the pooled outcomes could never include all randomized participants. Thus, all observations on the effects of these agents for chronic asymptomatic *T. cruzi* infection should be interpreted in the light of the small number of participants in studies not intended to evaluate clinical outcomes. Hence, at present, no experimental evidence is available to support any recommendation on the clinical use of trypanocide therapy for improving clinical outcomes in chronic asymptomatic *T. cruzi* infection. Large randomized controlled studies encompassing

---

Table 49.2   General characteristics of included studies

Author country (year)	Participants (% IP)	Interventions (*n* randomized) dose	Outcomes[a] (Primary and secondary)
Andrade Brazil (1996)	School children (90%)	Benznidazole (64) 7·5 mg/kg/day – 8 weeks *v* placebo (65)	Seroconversion Antibodies changes
Apt Chile (1998)	Adults (70%)	Allopurinol (187) 8·5 mg/kg/day – 8 weeks *v* itraconazol (217) 6 mg/kg/day – 16 weeks *v* placebo[b] (165)	Seroconversion *n* positive xenodiagnosis ECG changes Side effects
Coura Brazil (1997)	Adults (NA)	Benznidazole (26) 5 mg/kg/day – 4 weeks *v* nifurtimox (27) 5 mg/kg/day – 4 weeks *v* placebo (24)	*n* positive xenodiagnosis
Gianella Bolivia (1997)	Adults (NA)	Allopurinol (20) 300 mg tid – 8 weeks *v* placebo (20)	*n* positive xenodiagnosis
Sosa-Estani Argentina (1998)	School children (95%)	Benznidazole (55) 5 mg/kg/day – 8 weeks *v* placebo (51)	Seroconversion Antibodies changes

[a]As stated by the authors in the report.
[b]Participants initially in placebo arm were re-allocated to one of the active arms after two months of treatment.
Abbreviations: NA, information not available; IP, indeterminate phase. Reproduced with permission[72]

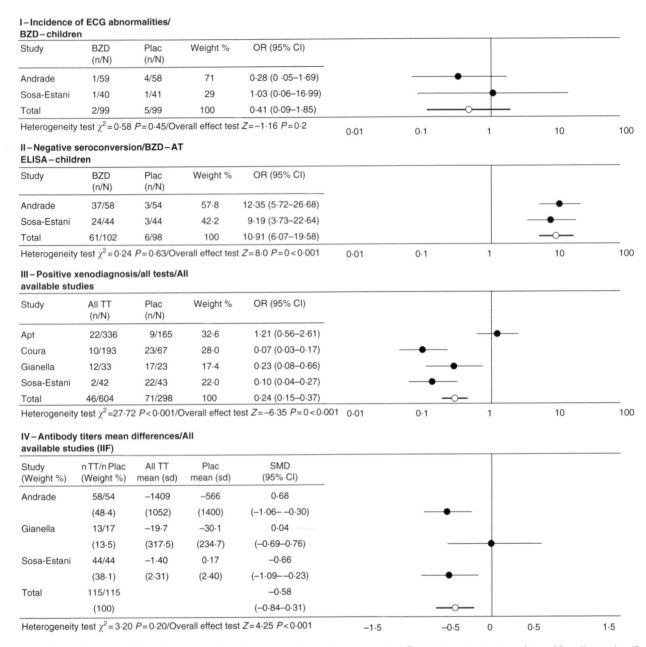

I – Incidence of ECG abnormalities/ BZD – children

Study	BZD (n/N)	Plac (n/N)	Weight %	OR (95% CI)
Andrade	1/59	4/58	71	0·28 (0·05–1·69)
Sosa-Estani	1/40	1/41	29	1·03 (0·06–16·99)
Total	2/99	5/99	100	0·41 (0·09–1·85)

Heterogeneity test $\chi^2 = 0.58$ $P = 0.45$/Overall effect test $Z = -1.16$ $P = 0.2$

II – Negative seroconversion/BZD – AT ELISA – children

Study	BZD (n/N)	Plac (n/N)	Weight %	OR (95% CI)
Andrade	37/58	3/54	57·8	12·35 (5·72–26·68)
Sosa-Estani	24/44	3/44	42·2	9·19 (3·73–22·64)
Total	61/102	6/98	100	10·91 (6·07–19·58)

Heterogeneity test $\chi^2 = 0.24$ $P = 0.63$/Overall effect test $Z = 8.0$ $P = 0 < 0.001$

III – Positive xenodiagnosis/all tests/All available studies

Study	All TT (n/N)	Plac (n/N)	Weight %	OR (95% CI)
Apt	22/336	9/165	32·6	1·21 (0·56–2·61)
Coura	10/193	23/67	28·0	0·07 (0·03–0·17)
Gianella	12/33	17/23	17·4	0·23 (0·08–0·66)
Sosa-Estani	2/42	22/43	22·0	0·10 (0·04–0·27)
Total	46/604	71/298	100	0·24 (0·15–0·37)

Heterogeneity test $\chi^2 = 27.72$ $P < 0.001$/Overall effect test $Z = -6.35$ $P = 0 < 0.001$

IV – Antibody titers mean differences/All available studies (IIF)

Study (Weight %)	n TT/n Plac (Weight %)	All TT mean (sd)	Plac mean (sd)	SMD (95% CI)
Andrade	58/54	−1409	−566	0·68
	(48·4)	(1052)	(1400)	(−1·06– −0·30)
Gianella	13/17	−19·7	−30·1	0·04
	(13·5)	(317·5)	(234·7)	(−0·69–0·76)
Sosa-Estani	44/44	−1·40	0·17	−0·66
	(38·1)	(2·31)	(2·40)	(−1·09– −0·23)
Total	115/115			−0·58
	(100)			(−0·84–0·31)

Heterogeneity test $\chi^2 = 3.20$ $P = 0.20$/Overall effect test $Z = 4.25$ $P < 0.001$

Figure 49.1 Overview of the effect, estimates for data on four outcomes pooled. Estimates are expressed as odds ratios, using the method proposed by Yusuf and Peto (Peto OR), or standardized mean differences (SMD) and its 95% confidence intervals using the fixed models statistical approach (95% CI Fixed). Antibodies mean changes are given in the units originally reported by authors. A negative sign means reduction of levels after being treated. Reproduced from Villar *et al*[72] with permission.

patients in different stages of disease have to be performed to overcome the current dilemma.

Prevention of reagudization

Trypanosomicide therapy has been shown in several cases to prevent the parasitological reactivation of Chagas' disease following corticosteroid therapy.[77] It is debatable whether primary chemoprophylaxis would be justifiable in all patients undergoing treatment with immunosuppressant drugs for associated diseases.[78]

Treatment of congestive heart failure

Hemodynamic derangements in chronic chagasic patients with heart failure are comparable to those reported in dilated cardiomyopathies of other etiologies. Similarly, the classic therapeutic interventions – sodium restriction, diuretics, digitalis, and vasodilation with nitrates and hydralazine – have been successful in relieving congestive symptoms. Small studies have documented short-term hemodynamic beneficial effects of these agents and, to a lesser extent, improvement in exercise tolerance in chronic chagasic patients. However, no studies reported improvement in survival or even in long-term outcome.

Small prospective studies on ACE inhibitors have shown promising results in heart failure complicating Chagas' disease. A multicenter, prospective, non-controlled trial assessed the impact of adding an ACE inhibitor to conventional therapy in 115 patients with heart failure (of whom 20 were chagasics). At the end of 12 weeks, irrespective of etiology, the NYHA functional class was significantly improved in most patients (85·2%).[79] A single-blind, crossover trial of ACE inhibitor and placebo for 6 weeks each, with a washout period of 2 weeks, was reported on 18 NYHA class IV chagasic patients.[80] Treatment with the ACE inhibitor was associated with significant reduction in neuro-humoral activation and ventricular arrhythmias. These results indicate a potentially beneficial role for this class of drugs in reducing active mechanisms related to sudden death. However, no long-term controlled study has assessed the impact on survival of chagasic patients treated with ACE inhibitors.

Other neuro-humoral blocking drugs such as beta adrenergics and spironolactone have not been objectively tested in any clinical trial including a large enough number of chagasic patients to permit efficacy assessment comparative to other etiologies of congestive heart failure.

Surgical treatment

Heart transplantation – Heart transplantation has been performed in small numbers of patients with refractory heart failure due to Chagas' disease. However, transplantation is limited by socioeconomic factors in the areas where the disease is endemic and by problems related to the obligatory immunosuppression.

Acute myocarditis with marked transitory LV systolic depression has previously been reported in small case series as a frequent complication in patients receiving the usual dose cyclosporin therapy.[81] Although the reactivation of acute infection was usually responsive to antiparasite therapy, the possibility of definitive damage to the allograft could not be ruled out and early concern was raised that this could constitute a severe limitation or even contraindication for heart transplantation in Chagas' disease. Nevertheless, recent data have shown more encouraging results to circumvent this limitation, through the use of reduced immunosuppression regimen. The long-term impact of heart transplantation in chagasic patients has recently been

described in a subgroup of a large cohort of 792 patients submitted to orthotopic heart transplantation in 16 centers in Brazil, The mean overall follow up period was 2·87±3·05 years, and 117 patients with chronic Chagas' heart disease constituted the subgroup. The entire cohort population also included 407 patients with idiopathic dilated cardiomyopathy and 196 with ischemic heart disease.[82] Among chagasic patients the reported criteria and contraindications for transplantation were similar to those used for non-chagasic patients, except for the detection of megacolon or megaesophagus, also considered a contraindication for transplantation. The survival rate of Chagas' disease patients at 1 and 12 years was respectively 76%, and 46%. These survival rates were statistically better in comparison with the rest of the cohort group in which the respective survival rates were 72% and 27%. It is worthy of note that reactivation of *T. cruzi* infection with myocarditis and meningoencephalitis was rarely reported, and was the cause of death, in only 0·3% of the entire chagasic cohort. Even allowing for the poor control of other relevant characteristics of chagasic and non-chagasic patients in this retrospective analysis of a cohort study, the results suggest that heart transplantation is a valid therapeutic option in end stage Chagas' heart disease with expected survival rate at least comparable to other patients submitted to this procedure.

Dynamic cardiomyoplasty – Reported experience with this procedure in chagasic patients is limited. While initial results in very few patients showed encouraging symptom and LV function improvement,[83] a survey of surgical centers in South America (112 patients of whom 96 had heart failure due to dilated cardiomyopathy and 13 due to Chagas' heart disease) was less optimistic.[84] Comparative analysis showed survival rates of 86·1% and 49·8% for patients with dilated cardiomyopathy and 40% and 9·5% for chagasic patients at 1 and 5 years follow up respectively. These results were corroborated by another recent observational study, again including a quite reduced number of chagasic patients.[85] There are no clues from these data to elucidate why the prognosis for chagasic patients was worse.

Clearly large controlled randomized trials are needed to define any value of dynamic cardiomyoplasty as a temporary approach, before refractory heart failure due to Chagas' heart disease can be treated by more radical interventions such as cardiac transplantation.[86]

Partial left ventriculectomy and synchronization therapy – The so-called Batista operation has been performed in small numbers of chagasic patients in many scattered surgical centers in Brazil, without any systematic approach specific for this disease. Because no systematic outcome information is available, and also due to the lack of consistent results with the procedure in other etiologies, currently, partial left ventriculotomy can not be recommended for the treatment of chagasic heart failure. Also, recent small case-series studies reported acute symptomatic and hemodynamic improvement after dual-chamber or multisite pacemaker implantation, but on an entirely empirical basis.

Prevention of thromboembolic events

There is very limited clinical information on the risk of embolism in patients with mural thrombus or apical aneurysm. In 65 selected patients with apical aneurysm, a follow up study ranging from 19 to 176 months documented 17 episodes of thromboembolism in 14 patients (24·5%)[87] – seven to the brain, nine to the lung and one to the iliac artery. These patients also had congestive heart failure and 11 died in the observation period. In eight of those patients, the cause of death was related to heart failure and in three it was a consequence of cerebral embolism.

Another small study in an endemic region of South America addressed the contribution of Chagas' heart disease in 69 patients having embolic strokes.[88] Of 13 patients with non-ischemic dilated cardiomyopathy, Chagas' heart disease was detected in nine (13·0%). It was the third most frequently identified cause of embolism after atrial fibrillation (29%) and rheumatic valvular heart disease (20·3%).

However, the real risk of thromboembolism in patients with Chagas' heart disease is unknown, as no specific studies have addressed this problem.

Furthermore, despite the preliminary evidence that thromboembolic events are relevant factors in the natural history of Chagas' disease, no clinical studies have been conducted to date on adequate treatment and prevention. Current recommendations for anticoagulant therapy are based on information derived from other dilated cardiomyopathies. Thus, chagasic patients presenting global LV dysfunction, atrial fibrillation, previous embolic episodes, and dyskinetic areas with detected mural thrombus are candidates for treatment with intravenous and/or oral anticoagulants. Social and economic factors limit the implementation of this treatment, however, even in chagasic patients with otherwise apparently clear indications for prevention of thromboembolism.

Management of rhythm disturbances

A wide spectrum of rhythm disturbances is one of the main hallmarks of Chagas' heart disease. Sinus node dysfunction and other atrial dysrhythmias are common findings and usually present at the early appearance of symptoms. Management of rhythm disturbances does not differ from that recommended for other cardiomyopathies, although there is no sound evidence to support any specific treatment.

Complex ventricular dysrhythmia is the most important disturbance because of its implication for sudden death. It is believed that this is more common in chagasic patients than in other dilated cardiomyopathies, but no adequate comparative study has been reported to support this hypothesis. As may be expected, there is reasonable evidence that the more complex and frequent the ventricular dysrhythmia, the worse the ventricular function. However, there is convincing evidence that complex ventricular dysrhythmia may also occur in chagasic patients with preserved global LV function. This is more remarkable when dyskinesia in the posterior basal LV region seems to provide the electrophysiologic substrate for refractory ventricular tachycardia. Although no prospective controlled trial has been conducted, the scarce experience reported suggests that this subgroup may benefit from surgical excision of fibrotic tissue following careful electrophysiologic mapping of LV dyskinetic regions. Equally limited is the reported experience with implantable cardioverter defibrillators in chagasic patients surviving episodes of sudden death.[4,89]

Except for several small case series reports, very scanty information has been published on the efficacy of pharmacological antiarrhythmic therapy in Chagas' heart disease. A prospective, double-blind, placebo-controlled, randomized crossover study in a reduced number of patients reported similar effects of disopyramide and amiodarone for controlling ventricular dysrhythmia.[90] Another prospective open, parallel, randomized study in 81 chagasic patients with ventricular dysrhythmia compared the efficacy of flecainide and amiodarone.[91] The final evaluation by Holter monitoring after 60 days showed a significant and comparable reduction in the frequency of ventricular tachycardia achieved with both flecainide (96·5%) and amiodarone (92·6%). However, the follow up was insufficient for conclusions to be drawn on the long-term efficacy or the impact of arrhythmia control on the incidence of sudden death.

Two moderately large randomized trials included chagasics among patients treated with amiodarone. The GESICA (Grupo de Estudio de la Sobrevida en la Insuficiencia Cardiaca en Argentina) study concluded after 2 years of follow up that low-dose amiodarone was effective in reducing mortality and hospital admission in patients with severe heart failure, independent of the presence of complex ventricular dysrhythmia.[92] Unfortunately, the subgroup of chagasic patients was very modest (48 of 516 patients) and subgroup analysis was not provided. Neither would it have been likely to be useful.

An ongoing prospective, multicenter, randomized, controlled study designed to evaluate the impact of amiodarone on survival of treatment of asymptomatic ventricular arrhythmia also included chagasic patients.[93] In its pilot phase, this trial enrolled 127 patients (24 with Chagas' heart disease) with LVEF <35%, presenting frequent ventricular premature complexes and/or repetitive forms of asymptomatic ventricular arrhythmia. The preliminary results after 12 months of follow up showed a significant reduction in the incidence of sudden death in the amio-darone group (7·0% *v* 20·4%). However, owing to a high dropout rate (16%), follow up data were obtained in only 106 patients. Nevertheless, it is to be hoped that the final results, recruiting a larger number of chagasic patients, will provide some helpful evidence on treating ventricular dys-rhythmia with amiodarone in Chagas' disease.

Complete atrioventricular block may also contribute to low cardiac output and cause syncope and sudden death in chagasic patients. In this situation pacemakers are used, as in other cardiac conditions. The evidence on the effects of pacemaker implantation comes from limited case series reports with historic control series of patients in whom this treatment was not possible.[89]

The common association of atrioventricular disturbances and ventricular complex dysrhythmia in the same patient also requires pacemaker implantation associated with phar-macological antiarrhythmic therapy. This management is regarded as prophylactic, although it is not based on unquestionable evidence.

Key points

- Etiologic treatment is clearly warranted for treatment of acute phase or chronic infection reactivation associated with immune-suppressive states. **Grade A/B4** Despite recent evidence supporting the participation of persist-ent tissue parasitism in the chronic phase of disease, and preliminary persuasive evidence that treatment of chronic asymptomatic patients results in benefit from the parasite outcomes point-of-view, there is no evidence that clinical outcomes are influenced. **Grade A/C, 1c and 5**
- Digitalis, diuretics and neurohumoral blocking drugs are empirically used for treating chagasic patients with heart failure. **Grade B2**
- Heart transplantation can be considered a promising treatment for refractory heart failure in Chagas' patients, even though this position is based in only one prospec-tive multicenter cohort including small number of patients. **Grade B2**
- Pharmacological, surgical, and device-based strategies for the treatment of ventricular dysrhythmia in chagasic patients are empirical and not supported by any large randomized, controlled trials. **Grade B4**

Endomyocardial fibrosis (EMF)

EMF is a restrictive cardiomyopathy with still unknown eti-ology occurring most frequently in tropical and subtropical countries. Major endocardial fibrotic involvement of the inflow portion of one or both ventricles, including the subvalvular region, leads to cavity obliteration, restriction of diastolic filling, and clinical manifestations of congestive heart failure and valvular regurgitation. A remarkably

similar cardiac involvement occurring in non-tropical coun-trieshas been described as endomyocardial disease. This is commonly named Löffler endocarditis or hypereosinophilic syndrome.

Although a still disputed issue, it has been postulated that the two conditions represent different stages of the same dis-ease.[94] Another controversial hypothesis is that eosinophil-derived factors have a toxic role in the pathogenesis of endomyocardial damage. A recent report combines circum-stantial evidence for the association of vector-borne etiology and helminth hypereosinophilia as an etiologic hypothesis for endemic EMF in tropical rain forest zones.[95]

Epidemiology and natural history

The low prevalence of EMF inhibits the study of the epi-demiology and natural history. Even the larger published series have included only around 100 patients.

Symptoms and signs

Biventricular involvement has been documented in approxi-mately half of the patients with EMF, while isolated right or left ventricular disease is variably described in 10–40% of cases in different published series. Depending upon predom-inant involvement of either chamber, symptoms and signs related to pulmonary congestion (left-sided) and systemic congestion (right-sided disease), and to mitral or tricuspid reflux, will tend to be more conspicuous.

Constrictive pericarditis is an important differential diag-nosis in EMF, especially when the right ventricle is markedly involved.[96] Demonstration of ventricular oblitera-tion by imaging techniques is essential for the diagnosis, but endomyocardial biopsy can be decisive in selected patients.

The magnitude of symptoms, the grade of ventricular obliteration (especially of the right ventricle), and the occur-rence of valvar regurgitation are important prognostic deter-minants of mortality in this disease. These clinical markers are useful in selecting patients for surgery since a good long-term prognosis has been reported for patients who have mild ventricular dysfunction and no valvular regurgitation.[97]

Surgical management

Extensive surgical excision of the fibrotic tissue, preserving or replacing the atrioventricular valves, can ameliorate symp-toms and improve hemodynamics and has been suggested to improve the long-term prognosis.[98] An operative mortality ranging from 4·6% to 25·0% has been reported in small case series studies. Ten year 70% and 17 year 55% survival rates have been respectively reported in European and Latin American series.[99,100]

It must be emphasized that no reports based on random-ized controlled trials of treatment strategies are available.

Key points

- The etiology and pathogenesis of EMF are still to be determined.
- The epidemiology, natural history, and pathophysiology are very incompletely understood, with available data based solely on retrospective evidence from small observational investigations. **Grade B4**
- Promising preliminary results obtained with surgical approaches await validation in large randomized, controlled studies before any general recommendation for improving quality of life and survival rates can be made. **Grade B4**

References

1. Wanderley DMV, Corrêa FMA. Epidemiology of Chagas' heart disease. *São Paulo Med J* 1995; **113**: 742–9.

2. Schmunis GA. *Trypanosoma cruzi*, the etiologic agent of Chagas' disease: status in the blood supply in endemic and nonendemic countries. *Transfusion* 1991;**31**:547–57.

3. WHO. *Control of Chagas' disease*. WHO Technical Report Series 811. Geneva: World Health Organization, 1991.

4. Hagar JM, Rahimtoola SH. Chagas' heart disease. *Curr Prob Cardiol* 1995;**10**:825–928.

5. Schofield CJ, Dias JCP. A cost benefit analysis of Chagas' disease control. *Mem Inst Oswaldo Cruz* 1991;**86**:285–95.

6. Acquatella H, Catalioti F, Gomez-Mancebo JR, Davalos V, Villalobos L. Long-term control of Chagas' disease in Venezuela: effects on serologic findings, electrocardiographic abnormalities, and clinical outcome. *Circulation* 1987;**76**: 556–62.

7. Prata A. Clinical and epidemiological aspects of Chagas disease. *Lancet Infect Dis* 2001;**1**:92–100.

8. Miles MA, Póvoa MM, Prata A, Cedillos RA, De Souza AA, Macedo V. Do radically dissimilar trypanosoma cruzi strains (Zymodemes) cause Venezuelan and Brazilian forms of Chagas' Disease? *Lancet* 1981;**20**:1338–40.

9. Dias JCP. Cardiopatia chagásica: história natural. In: Cançado JR, Chuster M. eds. *Cardiopatia chagásica*. Belo Horizonte Fundação: Carlos Chagas de Pesquisa Médica, 1985.

10. Dias JCP. The indeterminate form of human chronic Chagas' disease. A clinical epidemiological review. *Rev Soc Bras Med Trop* 1989;**22**:147–56.

11. Forichon E. *Contribution aux estimations de morbidité et de mortalité dans la maladie de Chagas*. Toulouse: Universite Paul-Sabatier, 1974.

12. Puigbó JJ, Rhode JRN, Barrios HG, Yépez CG. A 4-year follow up study of a rural community with endemic Chagas' disease. *Bull World Health Organ* 1968;**39**:341–8.

13. Mota EA, Guimarães AC, Santana OO *et al.* A nine year prospective study of Chagas' disease in a defined rural population in northeast Brazil. *Am J Trop Med* 1990;**42**:429–40.

14. Dias JCP, Kloetzel K. The prognostic value of the electrocardiographic features of chronic Chagas' disease. *Rev Inst Med Trop São Paulo* 1968;**10**:158–62.

15. Lima e Costa MFF, Barreto SM, Guerra HL, Firmo JOA, Uchoa E, Vidigal PG. Ageing with *Trypanosoma cruzi* infection in a community where the transmission has been interrupted: the Bambuí Health and Ageing Study (BHAS). *Int J Epidemiol* 2001;**30**:887–93.

16. Coura JR, Abreu LL, Pereira JB, Willcox HP. Morbidade da doença de chagas. IV. Estudo longitudinal de dez anos em Pains e Iguatama, Minas Gerais. *Mem Inst Oswaldo Cruz* 1985; **80**:73–80.

17. Pereira JB, Cunha RV, Willcox HP, Coura JR. Development of chronic human Chagas' cardiopathy in the hinterland of Paraìba, Brazil, in a 4·5 year period. *Rev Soc Bras Med Trop* 1990;**23**:141–7.

18. Pugliese C, Lessa I, Santos Filho A. Estudo da sobrevida na miocardite crônica de chagas descompensada. *Rev Inst Med Trop São Paulo* 1976;**18**:191–201.

19. Espinosa R, Carrasco HA, Belandria F *et al.* Life expectancy analysis in patients with Chagas' disease: prognosis after one decade (1973–1983). *Int J Cardiol* 1985;**8**:45–56.

20. Mady C, Cardoso RHA, Barreto ACP *et al.* Survival and predictors of survival in congestive heart failure due to Chagas' cardiomyopathy. *Circulation* 1994;**90**:3098–102.

21. Hagar JM, Rahimtoola SH. Chagas' heart disease in the United States. *N Engl J Med* 1991;**325**:763–8.

22. de Paola AA, Gomes JA, Terzian AB *et al.* Ventricular tachycardia on exercise testing is significantly associated with sudden cardiac death in patients with chronic chagasic cardiomyopathy and ventricular arrhythmias. *Br Heart J* 1995;**74**:293–5.

23. Laranja FS, Dias E, Nobrega G, Miranda A. Chagas' disease: a clinical, epidemiologic, and pathologic study. *Circulation* 1956;**14**:1035–59.

24. Lopes ER, Chapadeiro E, Almeida HO, Rocha A, Rocha A. Contribuição ao estudo da anatomia patológica dos corações de Chagásicos falecidos subitamente. *Rev Soc Bras Med Trop* 1975;**9**:269–82.

25. Marin-Neto JA, Simoes MV, Sarabanda AVL. Chagas' heart disease. *Arq Bras Cardiol* 1999;**72**:264–80.

26. Gallo Jr L, Maciel BC, Marin-Neto JA *et al.* Control of heart rate during exercise in health and disease. *Brazilian J Med Biol Res* 1995;**28**:1179–84.

27. Barreto ACP, Arteaga-Fernandez E. RV endomyocardial biopsy in chronic Chagas' disease. *Am Heart J* 1986;**111**:307–12.

28. Marin-Neto JA, Marzullo P, Marcassa C. Myocardial perfusion defects in chronic Chagas' disease. Assessment with thallium-201 scintigraphy. *Am J Cardiol* 1992;**69**:780–4.

29. Barreto ACP, Ianni BM. The undetermined form of Chagas' heart disease: concept and forensic implications. *São Paulo Med J* 1995;**113**:797–801.

30. Oliveira JSM. A natural human model of intrinsic heart nervous system denervation: Chagas' cardiopathy. *Am Heart J* 1985;**110**:1092–8.

31. Oliveira JSM, Araújo RRC, Mucillo G. Cardiac thrombosis and thromboembolism in chronic Chagas' heart disease. *Am J Cardiol* 1983;**52**:147–51.

32. Prata A, Andrade Z, Guimarães AC. Chagas' heart disease. In: Shaper AG, Hutt MSR, Fejfar Z, eds. *Cardiovascular disease in the tropics*. London: British Medical Association, 1974.

33. Marin-Neto JA, Marzullo P, Sousa ACS *et al.* Radionuclide angiographic evidence for early predominant right ventricular

involvement in patients with Chagas' disease. *Can J Cardiol* 1988;**4**:231–6.

34. Marin-Neto JA, Bromberg-Marin G, Pazin-Filho A, Simões MV, Maciel BC. Cardiac autonomic impairment and early myocardial damage involving the right ventricle are independent phenomena in Chagas' disease. *Int J Cardiol* 1998;**65**:261–9.

35. Britto C, Cardoso A, Silveira C, Macedo V, Fernandes O. Polymerase chain reaction (PCR) as a laboratory tool for the evaluation of the parasitological cure in Chagas' disease after specific treatment. *Medicina (B Aires)* 1999;**59**:176–8.

36. Marin-Neto JA, Gallo L Jr, Manço JC, Rassi A, Amorin DS. Mechanisms of tachycardia on standing: studies in normal individuals and in chronic Chagas' heart patients. *Cardiovasc Res* 1980;**14**:541–50.

37. Amorim DS, Marin-Neto JA. Functional alterations of the autonomic nervous system in Chagas' heart disease. *São Paulo Med J* 1995;**113**:772–83.

38. Simões MV, Pintya AO, Marin GB *et al*. Relation of regional sympathetic denervation and myocardial perfusion disturbances to wall motion impairment in Chagas' cardiomyopathy. *Am J Cardiol* 2000;**86**:975–81.

39. Rassi Jr A, Rassi A, Little WC. Chagas' heart disease. *Clin Cardiol* 2000;**23**:883–9.

40. Higuchi ML. Chronic chagasic cardiopathy: the product of a turbulent host-parasite relationship. *Rev Inst Med Trop Sao Paulo* 1997;**39**:53–60.

41. Ribeiro ALP, Moraes RS, Ribeiro JP *et al*. Parasympathetic dysautonomia precedes left ventricular systolic dysfunction in Chagas' disease. *Am Heart J* 2001;**141**:260–5.

42. Sterin-Borda L, Gorelik G, Postan M, Gonzalez CS, Borda E. Alterations in cardiac beta-adrenergic receptors in chagasic mice and their association with circulating beta-adrenoceptor-related antibodies. *Cardiovasc Res* 1999;**41**:116–25.

43. Wallukat G, Nissen E, Morwinski R, Muller J. Autoantibodies against the beta- and muscarinic receptors in cardiomyopathy. *Herz* 2000;**25**:261–6.

44. Chiale PA, Ferrari I, Mahler E *et al*. Differential profile and biochemical effects of antiautonomic membrane receptor antibodies in ventricular arrhythmias and sinus node dysfunction. *Circulation* 2001;**103**:1765–71.

45. Mahler E, Sepulveda P, Jeannequin O *et al*. A monoclonal antibody against the immunodominant epitope of the ribosomal P2beta protein of *Trypanosoma cruzi* interacts with the human beta 1-adrenergic receptor. *Eur J Immunol* 2001;**31**:2210–16.

46. Costa PCS, Fortes FSA, Machado AB *et al*. Sera from chronic chagasic patients depress cardiac electrogenesis and conduction. *Braz J Med Biol Res* 2000;**33**:439–46.

47. Köberle F. Chagas' heart disease and Chagas' syndromes: the pathology of American trypanosomiasis. *Adv Parasitol* 1968;**6**:63–116.

48. Amorim DS, Manço JC, Gallo L Jr, Marin-Neto JA. Chagas' heart disease as an experimental model for studies of cardiac autonomic function in man. *Mayo Clin Proc* 1982;**57**:48–60.

49. Avila HA, Sigman DS, Cohen LM, Millikan RC, Simpson L. Polymerase chain reaction amplification of *Trypanosoma cruzi* kinetoplast minicircle DNA isolated from whole blood lysates: diagnosis of chronic Chagas' disease. *Mol Biochem Parasitol* 1991;**48**:211–21.

50. Monteon-Padilha V, Hernandez-Becerril N, Ballinas-Verdugo MA, Aranda-Faustro A, Reyes PA. Persistence of *Trypanosoma cruzi* in chronic chagasic cardiopathy patients. *Arch Med Res* 2001;**32**:39–43.

51. Jones EM, Colley DG, Tostes S *et al*. A *Trypanosoma cruzi* DNA sequence amplified from inflammatory lesions in human chagasic cardiomyopathy. *Trans Assoc Am Phys* 1992;**105**:182–9.

52. Bellotti G, Bocchi EA, Moraes AV *et al*. *In vivo* detection of *Trypanosoma cruzi* antigens in hearts of patients with chronic Chagas' disease. *Am Heart J* 1996;**131**:301–7.

53. Anez N, Carrasco H, Parada H *et al*. Myocardial parasite persistence in chronic chagasic patients. *Am J Trop Med Hyg* 1999;**60**:726–32.

54. Morris SA, Tanowitz HB, Wittner M, Bilezikian JP. Pathophysiological insights into the cardiomyopathy of Chagas' disease. *Circulation* 1990;**83**:1900–9.

55. Rossi MA. Microvascular changes as a cause of chronic cardiomyopathy in Chagas' disease. *Am Heart J* 1990;**120**:233–6.

56. Reis DD, Jones EM, Tostes S. Expression of major histocompatibility complex antigens and adhesion molecules in hearts of patients with chronic Chagas' disease. *Am J Trop Med Hyg* 1993;**49**:192–200.

57. Torres FW, Acquatella H, Condado J, Dinsmore R, Palacios I. Coronary vascular reactivity is abnormal in patients with Chagas' heart disease. *Am Heart J* 1995;**129**:995–1001.

58. Simões MV, Ayres-Neto EM, Attab-Santos JL, Maciel BC, Marin-Neto JA. Chagas' heart patients without cardiac enlargement have impaired epicardial coronary vasodilation but no vasotonic angina. *J Am Coll Cardiol* 1996;**27**:394–5A.

59. Higuchi ML. Human chronic chagasic cardiopathy: participation of parasite antigens, subsets of lymphocytes, cytokines and microvascular abnormalities. *Mem Inst Oswaldo Cruz* 1999;**94**:263–7.

60. Andrade ZA, Andrade SG, Correa R, Sadigursky M, Ferrans VJ. Myocardial changes in acute *Trypanosoma cruzi* infection. *Am J Pathol* 1994;**144**:1403–11.

61. Santos RR, Rossi MA, Laus JL *et al*. Anti-CD4 abrogates rejection and re-establishes long-term tolerance to syngeneic newborn hearts grafted in mice chronically infected with *Trypanosoma cruzi*. *J Exp Med* 1992;**175**:29–39.

62. Ribeiro-dos-Santos R, Mengel JO, Postol E *et al*. A heart-specific CD4+ T-cell line obtained from chronic chagasic mouse induces carditis in heart-immunized mice and rejection of normal heart transplants in the absence of *Trypanosoma cruzi*. *Parasite Immunol* 2001;**23**:93–101.

63. Cunha-Neto E, Duranti M, Gruber A *et al*. Autoimmunity in Chagas' disease cardiopathy: biological relevance of a cardiac myosin-specific epitope crossreactive to an immunodominant *Trypanosoma cruzi* antigen. *Proc Natl Acad Sci* USA 1995;**92**: 3541–5.

64. Giordanengo L, Maldonado C, Rivarola HW *et al*. Induction of antibodies reactive to cardiac myosin and development of cardiac alteration in cruzipain-immunized mice and their offspring. *Eur J Immunol* 2000;**30**:3181–9.

65. Docampo R. Recent developments in the chemotherapy of Chagas' disease. *Curr Pharm Des* 2001;**7**:1157–64.

66. Cançado JR. Etiological treatment of chronic Chagas' disease. *Rev Inst Med Trop Sao Paulo* 2001;**43**:173–81.

67. Sosa-Estani S, Segura EL. Treatment of *Trypanosoma cruzi* infection in the undetermined phase. Experience and current guidelines of treatment in Argentina. *Mem Inst Oswaldo Cruz* 1999;**94**:363–5.

68. Solari A, Ortiz S, Soto A *et al.* Treatment of *Trypanosoma cruzi*-infected children with nifurtimox: a 3 year follow up by PCR. *J Antimicrob Chemother* 2001;**48**:515–19.

69. Andrade SG, Stocker-Guerret S, Pimentel AS, Grimaud JA. Reversibility of cardiac fibrosis in mice chronically infected with *Trypanosoma cruzi*, under specific chemotherapy. *Mem Inst Oswaldo Cruz* 1991;**86**:187–200.

70. Viotti R, Vigliano C, Armenti H, Segura E. Treatment of chronic Chagas' disease with benznidazole: clinical and serologic evolution of patients with long-term follow up. *Am Heart J* 1994;**127**:151–62.

71. Andrade AL, Zicker F, deOliveira RM *et al.* Randomized trial of efficacy of benznidazole in treatment of early *Trypanosoma cruzi* infection. *Lancet* 1996;**348**:1407–13.

72. Villar JC, Marin-Neto JA, Ebrahim S, Yusuf S. Trypanocidal drugs for chronic asymptomatic *Trypanosoma cruzi* infection (Cochrane Review). In: The Cochrane Library 2002; (Issue 2). Oxford: Update Software CD003463.

73. Coura JR, de Abreu LL, Faraco Willcox HP, Petana W. Estudo comparativo controlado com emprego de Benznidazole, Nifurtimox e placebo, na forma crônica da doença de Chagas, em uma área de campo com transmissão interrompida. Avaliação preliminar. *Rev Soc Bras Med Trop* 1997;**30**:139–44.

74. Gianella A, Holzman A, Lihoshi N, Barja Z, and Peredo Z. Eficacia del Alopurinol en la enfermedad de Chagas crónica. Resultados del estudio realizado en Santa Cruz, Bolivia. *Bol Cientif CENETROP* 1997;**16**:25–30.

75. Sosa-Estani S, Segura EL, Velazquez E, Ruiz AM, Porcel BM, Yampotis C. Efficacy of chemotherapy with benznidazole in children in the indeterminate phase of Chagas' disease. *Am J Trop Med Hyg* 1998;**59**:526–9.

76. Apt W, Aguilera X, Arribada A *et al.* Treatment of chronic Chagas' disease with itraconazole and allopurinol. *Am J Trop Med Hyg* 1998;**59**:133–8.

77. Rassi A, Amato Neto V *et al.* [Protective effect of benznidazole against parasite reactivation in patients chronically infected with *Trypanosoma cruzi* and treated with corticoids for associated diseases]. *Rev Soc Bras Med Trop* 1999;**32**:475–82.

78. Nishioka Sde A. [Benznidazole in the primary chemoprophylaxis of the reactivation of Chagas' disease in chronic chagasic patients using corticosteroids at immunosuppressive doses: is there sufficient evidence for recommending its use?]. *Rev Soc Bras Med Trop* 2000;**33**:83–5.

79. Batlouni M, Barretto AC, Armaganijan D *et al.* Treatment of mild and moderate cardiac failure with captopril. A multicenter trial. *Arq Bras Cardiol* 1992;**58**:417–21.

80. Roberti RR, Martinez EE, Andrade JL *et al.* Chagas' cardiomyopathy and captopril. *Eur Heart J* 1992;**13**:966–70.

81. Bocchi EA, Bellotti G, Mocelin AO *et al.* Heart transplantation for chronic Chagas' heart disease. *Ann Thorac Surg* 1996;**61**:1727–33.

82. Bochi EA, Fiorelli A. On behalf of the First Guidelines Group for Heart Transplantation of the Brazilian Society of Cardiology. The Paradox of Survival Results after Heart Transplantation for Cardiomyopathy caused by *T. cruzi. Ann Thor Surg* 2001;**71**:1833–8.

83. Jatene AD, Moreira LF, Stolf NA *et al.* Left ventricular function changes after cardiomyoplasty in patients with dilated cardiomyopathy. *J Thorac Cardiovasc Surg* 1991;**102**:132–8.

84. Moreira LF, Stolf NA, Braile DM, Jatene AD. Dynamic cardiomyoplasty in South America. *Ann Thorac Surg* 1996;**61**:408–12.

85. Braile DM, Godoy MF, Thevenard GH *et al.* Dynamic cardiomyoplasty: long-term clinical results in patients with dilated cardiomyopathy. *Ann Thorac Surg* 2000;**69**:1445–7.

86. Bocchi EA. Cardiomyoplasty for treatment of heart failure. *Eur J Heart Fail* 2001;**3**:403–6.

87. Albanesi-Filho FM, Gomes JB. O tromboembolismo em pacientes com lesão apical da cardiopatia chagásica crônica. *Rev Port Cardiol* 1991;**10**:35–42.

88. Rey RC, Lepera SM, Kohler G, Monteverde DA, Sica RE. Cerebral embolism of cardiac origin. *Medicina (Buenos Aires)* 1992;**52**:206–16.

89. Rassi Jr A, Rassi SG, Rassi A. Sudden death in Chagas' disease. *Arq Bras Cardiol* 2001;**76**:75–96.

90. Carrasco HA, Vicuna AV, Molina C *et al.* Effect of low oral doses of disopyramide and amiodarone on ventricular and atrial arrhythmias of chagasic patients with advanced myocardial damage. *Int J Cardiol* 1985;**9**:425–38.

91. Rosembaum M, Posse R, Sgammini H *et al.* Comparative multicenter clinical study of flecainide and amiodarone in the treatment of ventricular arrhythmias associated to chronic Chagas cardiopathy. *Arch Inst Cardiol Mex* 1987;**57**:325–30.

92. Doval HC, Nul DR, Grancelli HD *et al.* Randomized trial of low-dose amiodarone in severe congestive heart failure. *Lancet* 1994;**344**:493–8.

93. Garguichevich JJ, Ramos JL, Gambarte A *et al.* Effect of amiodarone therapy on mortality in patients with left ventricular dysfunction and asymptomatic complex ventricular arrhythmias: Argentine pilot study of sudden death and amiodarone (EPAMSA). *Am Heart J* 1995;**130**:494–500.

94. Olsen EGJ, Spry CJF. Relationship between eosinophilia and endomyocardial disease. *Prog Cardiovasc Dis* 1985;**27**:241–54.

95. Ogunowo PO, Akpan NA, Odigwe CO, Ekanem IA, Esin RA. Helminth associated hypereosoniphilia and tropical endomyocardiofibrosis (EMF) in Nigeria. *Acta Trop* 1998;**69**:127–40.

96. Somers K, Brenton DP, Sood NK. Clinical features of endomyocardial fibrosis of the right ventricle. *Br Heart J* 1968;**30**:309–21.

97. Barreto ACP, Luz PL, Mady C, Bellotti G, Pilleggi F. Determinants of survival in patients with endomyocardial fibrosis. *Circulation* 1988;**78**:526–30.

98. Oliveira SA, Barreto ACP, Mady C, Bellotti G, Pilleggi F. Surgical treatment of endomyocardial fibrosis: a new surgical approach. *J Am Coll Cardiol* 1990;**5416**:1246–51.

99. Schneider U, Jenni R, Turina J, Turina M, Hess OM. Long-term follow up of patients with endomyocardial fibrosis: effects of surgery. *Heart* 1998;**79**:362–7.

100. Moraes F, Lapa C, Hazin S, Tenorio E, Gomes C, Moraes CR. Surgery for endomyocardiofibrosis revisited. *Eur J Cardiothorac Surg* 1999;**15**:309–12.

Part IIIf

Specific cardiovascular disorders: Pericardial disease

Bernard J Gersh, Editor

Grading of recommendations and levels of evidence used in *Evidence-based Cardiology*

GRADE A

Level 1a   Evidence from large randomized clinical trials (RCTs) or systematic reviews (including meta-analyses) of multiple randomized trials which collectively has at least as much data as one single well-defined trial.

Level 1b   Evidence from at least one "All or None" high quality cohort study; in which ALL patients died/failed with conventional therapy and some survived/succeeded with the new therapy (for example, chemotherapy for tuberculosis, meningitis, or defibrillation for ventricular fibrillation); or in which many died/failed with conventional therapy and NONE died/failed with the new therapy (for example, penicillin for pneumococcal infections).

Level 1c   Evidence from at least one moderate-sized RCT or a meta-analysis of small trials which collectively only has a moderate number of patients.

Level 1d   Evidence from at least one RCT.

GRADE B

Level 2   Evidence from at least one high quality study of non-randomized cohorts who did and did not receive the new therapy.

Level 3   Evidence from at least one high quality case–control study.

Level 4   Evidence from at least one high quality case series.

GRADE C

Level 5   Opinions from experts without reference or access to any of the foregoing (for example, argument from physiology, bench research or first principles).

A comprehensive approach would incorporate many different types of evidence (for example, RCTs, non-RCTs, epidemiologic studies, and experimental data), and examine the architecture of the information for consistency, coherence and clarity. Occasionally the evidence does not completely fit into neat compartments. For example, there may not be an RCT that demonstrates a reduction in mortality in individuals with stable angina with the use of β blockers, but there is overwhelming evidence that mortality is reduced following MI. In such cases, some may recommend use of β blockers in angina patients with the expectation that some extrapolation from post-MI trials is warranted. This could be expressed as Grade A/C. In other instances (for example, smoking cessation or a pacemaker for complete heart block), the non-randomized data are so overwhelmingly clear and biologically plausible that it would be reasonable to consider these interventions as Grade A.

Recommendation grades appear either within the text, for example, **Grade A** and **Grade A1a** or within a table in the chapter.

The grading system clearly is only applicable to preventive or therapeutic interventions. It is not applicable to many other types of data such as descriptive, genetic or pathophysiologic.

50 Pericardial disease: an evidence-based approach to diagnosis and treatment

Bongani M Mayosi, James A Volmink, Patrick J Commerford

Pericardial disease is a potentially curable cause of heart disease that accounts for about 7% of all patients who are hospitalized for cardiac failure in Africa.[1] Although there are no good epidemiologic data on the incidence or prevalence of pericarditis in different populations,[2] hospital-based series indicate that the spectrum of pericardial disease is determined by the epidemiologic setting of the patient. In Western countries, most cases of primary pericarditis are of unknown cause, whereas tuberculosis accounts for the majority of patients in the developing world.[3,4] Thus, evidence-based guidelines should be adapted according to the prevalence of certain diseases in particular geographic areas and patient populations.

A discussion of the large number of diseases that may affect the pericardium[5] (Box 50.1) cannot be covered in this short chapter. Consequently, this overview will focus on the diagnosis and treatment of idiopathic and tuberculous pericarditides. It will, in particular, aim to examine the extent to which existing treatments are supported by evidence from well-designed prospective studies. The findings reported here are based on a comprehensive search of electronic databases and bibliographies of articles on pericarditis.

Primary acute pericardial disease

Acute pericarditis may be caused by a variety of disorders (Box 50.1). Among the secondary forms of pericarditis, the underlying disorder is usually evident before pericardial involvement. The most challenging dilemma for the physician is the patient with acute pericardial disease without apparent cause at the initial evaluation (primary acute pericardial disease). In Western series a specific etiology has been found in only 14–22% of these patients when they are subjected to a prospective diagnostic protocol (Table 50.1).[3,6]

Diagnosis

Acute pericarditis is the occurrence of two or more of the following: characteristic chest pain, pericardial friction rub (pathognomonic of acute pericarditis), and an electrocardiogram (ECG) showing characteristic ST segment elevation or typical serial changes.[7] The chest radiograph, echocardiogram, and radionuclide scans are of little diagnostic value in uncomplicated acute pericarditis.

The first step in the etiologic diagnosis of acute pericarditis consists of a search for an underlying disease that may require specific therapy. In most cases of suspected viral pericarditis, special studies for etiologic agents are not necessary because of the low diagnostic yield of viral studies and lack of specific therapy for viral disease.[7] However, a treatable condition such as *Mycoplasma*-associated pericarditis must be considered and treated with antibiotics if the serologic test is consistent with the diagnosis.[8] The Permanyer-Miralda *et al* protocol[3] for the evaluation of acute pericardial disease is discussed under "Pericardial effusion" below.

Treatment

Although there are no controlled trials, it is generally accepted that bed rest and oral non-steroidal anti-inflammatory drugs

---

Box 50.1 Causes of acute pericarditis[5]
- Malignant tumor
- Idiopathic pericarditis
- Uremia
- Bacterial infection
- Anticoagulant therapy
- Dissecting aortic aneurysm
- Diagnostic procedures
- Connective tissue disease
- Postpericardiotomy syndrome
- Trauma
- Tuberculosis
- Other
  - radiation
  - drugs inducing lupus-like syndrome
  - myxedema
  - postmyocardial infarction syndrome
  - fungal infections
  - AIDS-related pericarditis

Table 50.1   Etiology of primary acute pericarditis in the West

	Permanyer-Miralda *et al* 1985[3] (n = 231)	Zayas *et al* 1995[5] (n = 100)
Acute idiopathic pericarditis	199 (86%)	78 (78%)
Neoplastic pericarditis	13 (6%)	7 (7%)
Tuberculous pericarditis	9 (4%)	4 (4%)
Other infections	6 (3%)	3 (3%)
Collagen vascular disease	2 (0.5%)	3 (3%)
Other	2 (0.5%)	5 (5%)

(NSAIDs) are effective in most patients with acute pericarditis.[7] The use of corticosteroids for acute idiopathic pericarditis when the disease does not subside rapidly is also untested in randomized trials, but it may be unnecessary and even dangerous in acute non-relapsing pericarditis in view of the availability of other agents, such as the parenteral NSAID ketorolac tromethamine.[9] Ketorolac is an extremely potent analgesic agent that appears to cause rapid resolution of symptomatic acute pericarditis. However, the limitation of this study of 20 patients with acute pericarditis was that there was no control group for comparison.[9]

Idiopathic relapsing pericarditis is the most troublesome complication of acute pericarditis, affecting about 20% of cases. There are no established therapeutic guidelines for patients who do not respond to NSAIDs.[7] Corticosteroids provide symptomatic relief in most of these patients, but symptoms recur in many when the prednisone dosage is reduced and severe complications are associated with prolonged steroid use.[10] Claims of effectiveness have been made in small uncontrolled studies for pericardiectomy, azathioprine, high-dose oral and intravenous corticosteroids,

and colchicine (Table 50.2).[10] The results of these studies are inconsistent and the effectiveness of these potentially harmful therapeutic modalities remains to be established in well-designed randomized studies. Nevertheless, colchicine, used on the basis of its efficacy in the recurrent polyserositis seen in familial Mediterranean fever,[16] has aroused much interest following the dramatic effects which were initially reported with its use in recurrent pericarditis.[15] The accumulating experience with colchicine indicates that, whilst its long-term use is well tolerated, it is associated with a variable remission rate of 33–100% (Table 50.2), and there is a tendency for a small proportion of patients to relapse after cessation of therapy.[16] In a multicenter cohort study involving 51 patients with recurrent pericarditis who did not respond to conventional treatments, colchicine induced remission in 86%, and 60% remained recurrence-free after discontinuation of the drug.[20] These data support the use of colchicine to prevent recurrent attacks of pericarditis as an adjunct to conventional treatment, although the effectiveness of the agent remains to be evaluated in randomized controlled trials. **Grade B**

Table 50.2   Therapeutic strategies previously evaluated in recurrent pericarditis (after failure of non-steroidal anti-inflammatory drugs)

Study	Patients (n)	Therapeutic strategy evaluated	Remission rate
Fowler[10]	9	Pericardiectomy	2/9 (22%)
Hatcher[11]	24	Pericardiectomy	20/24 (83%)
Asplen[12]	2	Azathioprine	2/2 (100%)
Melchior[13]	2	IV Methylprednisolone as pulse therapy	2/2 (100%)
Marcolongo[14]	12	High-dose prednisone with aspirin	11/12 (92%) Major side effects in 3
Guindo[15] and de la Serna[16]	9	Colchicine	9/9 (100%)
Spodick[17]	8	Colchicine	3/9 (33%)
Adler[18]	8	Colchicine	4/8 (50%)
Millaire[19]	19	Colchicine	14/19 (74%)
Guindo[20]	51	Colchicine	44/51 (86%)

Pericardial effusion

The spectrum of causes of pericardial effusion is similar to acute pericarditis (Box 50.1). However, prospective studies indicate that large pericardial effusions are more likely to be a result of serious underlying illnesses such as tuberculosis and cancer, where rapid diagnosis may lead to earlier therapy and improved survival.[3] The clinical features vary depending on the rate of accumulation of the fluid, the amount of fluid that accumulates, and the stage at which the patient is first seen.

Diagnosis

The radiographic signs of pericardial effusion include an enlarged cardiac silhouette, a pericardial fat stripe, a predominant left-sided pleural effusion, and an increase in transverse cardiac diameter compared with previous chest radiographs. However, these signs cannot reliably confirm or exclude the presence of pericardial effusion, thus making radiography poorly diagnostic of pericardial effusion.[21] Similarly, ECG is useful only in that it may suggest a cardiac abnormality. The QRS complexes are usually small, with generalized T wave inversion. Electrical alternans, which suggests the presence of massive pericardial effusion, is uncommon. Even more uncommon is total electrical alternans (P-QRS-T alternation), which is pathognomonic of tamponade.[22]

Echocardiography, computed tomography (CT), and magnetic resonance imaging (MRI) can accurately detect and quantify pericardial effusion. Echocardiography, which is relatively inexpensive, sensitive (capable of detecting as little as 17 ml pericardial fluid), harmless, and widely available, is the diagnostic method of choice for pericardial effusion.[5] Furthermore, it may also provide prognostic information. A large effusion with a circumferential echo-free space of >1 cm in width at any point is reported to be a powerful predictor of tamponade[23] and intrapericardial echo images are associated with an increased likelihood of subsequent constriction.[24]

Permanyer-Miralda *et al*[3] have evolved a systematic approach for the evaluation of acute primary pericardial disease in developed countries with a low prevalence of tuberculosis (Table 50.3). It is based on a prospective study of 231 consecutive patients who were evaluated to determine the safest and most sensitive approach to the etiologic diagnosis of acute pericardial disease. The findings were confirmed in a subsequent prospective study of a similar diagnostic protocol involving 100 patients with primary pericardial disease.[5] First, these prospective studies indicate that a specific etiology is found in only 14–22% of patients with acute primary pericardial disease (Table 50.1). Secondly, while therapeutic pericardiocentesis is absolutely indicated for cardiac tamponade, it is not warranted as a routine investigation because of low diagnostic yield. The

Table 50.3 Protocol for evaluation of primary acute pericardial disease[3]

Stage	Evaluation
Stage I General studies and echocardiogram	Electrocardiogram Chest radiograph Tuberculin skin test Serologic tests
Stage II Pericardiocentesis	Therapeutic pericardiocentesis: absolutely indicated for cardiac tamponade Diagnostic pericardiocentesis: clinical suspicion of purulent or tuberculous pericarditis Illness lasting for more than 1 week
Stage III Surgical biopsy of the pericardium	"Therapeutic" biopsy: as part of surgical drainage in patients with severe tamponade relapsing after pericardiocentesis Diagnostic biopsy: in patients with more than 3 weeks illness and without an etiologic diagnosis having been reached by previous procedures
Stage IV Empirical antituberculous treatment	Fever and pericardial effusion of unknown origin persisting for more than 5–6 weeks

indications for diagnostic pericardiocentesis are the clinical suspicion of purulent or tuberculous pericarditis and those with an illness lasting longer than 1 week. Thirdly, the diagnostic yield of pericardiocentesis and pericardial biopsy is similar. Whereas biopsy is more invasive and may entail the need for general anesthesia, it is a safe procedure and direct histologic examination of the pericardium may allow immediate diagnosis in the case of tuberculosis. Furthermore, pericardial biopsy may allow a more direct visualization of the pericardium. However, even when detailed investigations are performed, including pericardioscopy and surgery, the etiology of pericardial effusion remains obscure in a significant number of patients.[25]

Cardiac tamponade

A pericardial effusion may result in the life-threatening complication of cardiac tamponade, a condition caused by compression of the heart and impaired diastolic filling of the ventricles. It is an indication for pericardiocentesis.

Cardiac tamponade is a clinical diagnosis, which is confirmed by echocardiography. The clinical examination shows elevated systemic venous pressure, tachycardia, dyspnea, and pulsus paradoxus.[26] Pulsus paradoxus may be absent in some instances such as left ventricular dysfunction, atrial septal defect, regional tamponade, and positive pressure breathing. Systemic blood pressure may be normal, decreased, or even elevated. The diagnosis is usually confirmed by the echocardiographic demonstration of a large circumferential pericardial effusion and some of the features listed in Table 50.4. However, as a diagnostic test for tamponade, echocardiography may lack both sensitivity and specificity in certain clinical situations. For example, echocardiographic features of right heart collapse may be absent in the presence of loculated effusions causing regional left ventricular compression or in patients with pulmonary hypertension. This is particularly important after cardiac surgery when the absence of a circumferential effusion and right atrial collapse and right ventricular diastolic collapse may not exclude the presence of life-threatening tamponade.[27,28] Furthermore, a dilated non-collapsing inferior vena cava and an abnormal respiratory pattern of diastolic flow are not specific signs of tamponade (Table 50.4).

Constrictive pericarditis

The etiology of constrictive pericarditis has changed over the past four decades.[29] Tuberculous constrictive pericarditis, which was a common cause of constriction worldwide before the 1960s, has since declined in incidence and is now rare in Western countries. In these countries the diminished importance of tuberculous pericarditis has been associated with a large contribution made by idiopathic cases. Postradiotherapy constriction, which was first recognized as an important disease in the 1960s, continues to feature prominently among the causes of constrictive pericarditis, while postsurgical constriction has emerged as an important cause.

Constrictive pericarditis is characterized anatomically by an abnormally thickened and non-compliant pericardium that limits ventricular filling in mid to late diastole. Consequently, nearly all ventricular filling occurs very rapidly in early diastole. This results in elevated cardiac filling pressures and the characteristic hemodynamic waveforms during which the diastolic pressures of the cardiac chambers equalize. The clinical manifestations of constrictive pericarditis, which are secondary to systemic venous congestion, mimic a variety of cardiopulmonary disorders, making the diagnosis of this condition difficult in some cases.

Diagnosis

The chest radiograph and ECG are usually abnormal, drawing attention to the heart, but the abnormalities are largely non-specific. Chest radiography may reveal a small, normal, or enlarged cardiac silhouette, pleural effusions in 60%, and pericardial calcification in 5–50% of cases.[29–31] Calcification is not specific for constrictive pericarditis, as a calcified pericardium does not necessarily imply constriction. Non-specific but generalized T wave changes are seen in most cases, while low voltage complexes occur in about 30%.

The ideal imaging technique for the accurate preoperative diagnosis of pericardial constriction would simultaneously provide both anatomic data describing the thickness of the pericardium and physiologic/hemodynamic data describing

---

Table 50.4 Echocardiographic features of cardiac tamponade[26]

Echocardiographic/Doppler criteria	Comments
1. Right heart collapse: right atrial compression, right ventricular diastolic collapse	Changes in blood volume may affect the sensitivity and specificity of right heart collapse as a sign of tamponade. False positives and false negatives may occur
2. Abnormal respiratory changes in ventricular dimensions	Inconstant finding
3. Abnormal respiratory changes in tricuspid and mitral flow velocities	May also be seen in obstructive airways disease, pulmonary embolism, and right ventricular infarction
4. Dilated inferior vena cava with lack of inspiratory collapse	Often seen with congestive heart failure and constrictive pericarditis
5. Left ventricular diastolic collapse	Frequent sign of regional cardiac tamponade and useful marker of tamponade in postoperative patients in a retrospective investigation[27]
6. Swinging heart	Not sensitive, specificity unknown

the characteristic differential diastolic filling to the left ventricle and the right ventricle with respiration. In these regards, echocardiographic findings of abnormal ventricular septal motion (septal bounce or shudder), dilated inferior vena cava, and hepatic veins in patients with right heart failure are suggestive of constrictive pericarditis. Respiratory variation in mitral inflow velocities and hepatic veins is quite characteristic for constrictive pericarditis, although the lack of respiratory variation does not exclude constrictive pericarditis. Specificity of these Doppler findings of constrictive pericarditis is enhanced by demonstrating no significant respiratory variation in the superior vena cava velocity. In patients with increased respiratory effort such as chronic obstructive pulmonary disease, which simulates the interventricular dependence resulting in similar two-dimensional and Doppler echocardiographic findings, superior vena caval velocities are markedly increased with inspiration.[32] New tissue Doppler recording of mitral annulus velocity adds more confidence in distinguishing constrictive pericarditis from restrictive process because of myocardial disease (Table 50.5).[33]

CT and MRI can demonstrate the extent and distribution of pericardial thickening. While this does not make the diagnosis of constriction, it is often very useful to know that the pericardium is abnormal in a patient in whom this diagnosis is suspected. In addition, CT or MRI features of myocardial atrophy or fibrosis predict a poor outcome following pericardiectomy.[34] A promising new imaging technique is cine-CT, which simultaneously provides both anatomic and physiologic data that may allow accurate preoperative diagnosis of pericardial constriction.[35] Unless the diagnosis is very obvious, cardiac catheterization is usually performed. The characteristic finding is equal end-diastolic pressures in the two ventricles, persisting with respiration and fluid challenge. However, the diagnosis of constrictive pericarditis remains a challenge because it is often mimicked by restrictive cardiomyopathy. A number of studies, using different techniques, have attempted to distinguish the two conditions, including studies of left ventricular filling rate, mitral and tricuspid diastolic flow patterns, pulmonary venous flow velocity, hepatic flow velocity patterns, hemodynamic

Table 50.5   The differentiation of constrictive pericarditis from restrictive cardiomyopathy

Type of evaluation	Constrictive pericarditis	Restrictive cardiomyopathy
Physical examination	Regurgitant murmurs uncommon	Regurgitant murmurs may be present
Chest radiography	Pericardial calcification may be present	Pericardial calcification absent
Echocardiography	Normal wall thickness	Increased wall thickness, thickened cardiac valves and granular sparkling texture (amyloid). Enlarged atria
	Pericardium may be thickened[a]	Pericardium usually normal
	Prominent early diastolic filling with abrupt displacement of interventricular septum due to increased ventricular interaction	
Doppler studies	Early mitral flow is reduced with onset of inspiration and reciprocal effect on tricuspid flow	No respiratory variation in diastolic flow with short deceleration time
	Expiratory increase of hepatic vein diastolic flow reversal	Inspiratory increase of hepatic vein diastolic flow reversal
		Mitral and tricuspid regurgitation may be present
	Mitral annulus velocity ≥7 cm/s	Mitral annulus velocity <7 cm/s
Cardiac catheterization	RVEDP and LVEDP usually equal	LVEDP often >5 mmHg greater than RVEDP, but may be identical
	RV systolic pressure <50 mmHg	RV systolic pressure ≥50 mmHg
	RVEDP >one third of RV systolic pressure	
Endomyocardial biopsy	May be normal or show non-specific myocyte hypertrophy or myocardial fibrosis	May reveal specific cause of restrictive cardiomyopathy
CT/MRI	Pericardium may be thickened ≥3 mm[a]	Pericardium usually normal

Abbreviations: CT, computed tomography; LV, left ventricular; LVEDP, left ventricular end-diastolic pressure; MRI, magnetic resonance imaging; RV, right ventricular; RVEDP, right ventricular end-diastolic pressure
[a] Normal thickness of the pericardium does not rule out pericardial constriction.

investigations, endomyocardial biopsy, and CT and MRI studies.[36] Table 50.5 summarizes the important differences between the two conditions. No technique is totally reliable and in some patients, the only way of making the diagnosis is to perform a pericardiectomy.[37]

Treatment

The treatment for chronic constrictive pericarditis is complete resection of the pericardium. The average hospital mortality following pericardiectomy in several series ranges from about 5% to 16%.[29,38–40] Poor outcome is related mainly to preoperative disability, the degree of constriction, and myocardial involvement. The majority of early deaths are associated with low cardiac output, which has been attributed to myocardial atrophy. Thus, early pericardiectomy is recommended in patients with non-tuberculous constrictive pericarditis before severe constriction and myocardial atrophy occur.

Among patients who survive the operation, symptomatic improvement can be expected in about 90% and complete relief of symptoms in about 50%. The 5 year survival rate ranges from 74% to 87%. Long-term survival and symptomatic relief do not appear to be influenced by age, choice of median sternotomy or left thoracotomy, or transient low output syndrome postoperatively. However, long-term survival is unfavorably influenced by the presence of severe preoperative functional disability (NYHA class III or IV, diuretic use), renal insufficiency in the preoperative state, the presence of extensive non-resectable calcifications, incomplete pericardial resection, and the presence of radiation pericarditis, which is commonly complicated by myocardial fibrosis and restrictive myocardial disease.

Tuberculous pericarditis

The prevalence of tuberculous pericarditis follows the same pattern as that of tuberculosis in general. It is the most common cause of pericarditis in developing countries where tuberculosis remains a major public health problem, but accounts for only about 5% of cases in the West.[3,4] In Africa the incidence of tuberculous pericarditis is rising as a direct result of the human immunodeficiency virus epidemic[41] and this trend is likely to occur in other parts of the world where the spread of AIDS is leading to the resurgence of tuberculosis. Tuberculosis caused by drug resistant *Mycobacterium tuberculosis* has emerged in the past few years as a serious threat to global public health, but its impact on pericardial tuberculosis has not been studied.

Tuberculous pericarditis appears to be more common in blacks than whites and males than females,[42,43] although the sex difference was reversed in the large prospective studies of Strang *et al*[30,44] The disease can occur at any age.

Tuberculous pericardial effusion

Tuberculous pericarditis is usually detected clinically either in the effusive stage or after the development of constriction. Tuberculous pericarditis has a variable clinical presentation and it should be considered in the evaluation of all instances of pericarditis without a rapidly self-limited course.[43] While tuberculous pericarditis may cause effusions that do not produce cardiac compression, more commonly there is at least some degree of cardiac compression, which may be severe, causing tamponade.

Tuberculous pericardial effusion usually develops insidiously, presenting with non-specific systemic symptoms such as fever, night sweats, fatigue, and loss of weight.[4,42,45] Chest pain, cough, and breathlessness are common.[45–47] Severe pericardial pain of acute onset characteristic of idiopathic pericarditis is unusual in tuberculous pericarditis.[42,45,48] Right upper abdominal aching due to liver congestion is also common in these patients.[4,42,45] In South African patients with tuberculous pericardial effusion, evidence of chronic cardiac compression that mimics heart failure is by far the most common presentation (Table 50.6).[4,47,49] While there is marked overlap between the physical signs of pericardial effusion and constrictive pericarditis, the presence of increased cardiac dullness extending to the right of the sternum favors a clinical diagnosis of pericardial effusion.

Diagnosis

A definite diagnosis of tuberculous pericarditis is based on the demonstration of tubercle bacilli in pericardial fluid or on histologic section of the pericardium and a probable diagnosis is made when there is proof of tuberculosis elsewhere in a patient with unexplained pericarditis. A definite or probable diagnosis is made in up to 73% of patients treated for tuberculous pericarditis.[44,50] The chest radiograph shows features of active pulmonary tuberculosis in only 30% and pleural effusion is present in 40–60% of cases.[43] The ECG is usually abnormal, drawing attention to the heart.[44,51] The ST segment elevations characteristic of acute pericarditis are usually absent. ECG findings are not specific for a tuberculous etiology.[50]

Pericardiocentesis is recommended in all patients in whom tuberculosis is suspected. The pericardial fluid is bloodstained in 80% of cases[4] and, since malignant disease and the late effects of penetrating trauma cause bloody pericardial effusion, confirmation of tuberculosis as the cause is important. The difficulty in finding tubercle bacilli in the direct smear examination of pericardial fluid is well known. Culture of tubercle bacilli from pericardial effusions can be improved considerably by inoculation of the fluid into double strength liquid Kirchner culture medium at the bedside. A prospective study of the value of the double strength liquid Kirchner culture medium in patients considered to have

Table 50.6 Physical signs documented by a single observer in 88 patients with pericardial effusion and 67 patients with constrictive pericarditis in South Africa[4]

Signs	Pericardial effusion (n = 88)	Constrictive pericarditis (n = 67)
Hepatomegaly	84 (95%)	67 (100%)
Increased cardiac dullness	83 (94%)	17 (25%)
Raised jugular venous pulse	74 (84%)	67 (100%)
Soft heart sounds	69 (78%)	51 (76%)
Sinus tachycardia	68 (77%) (Transient AF in 3)	47 (70%) (Persistent AF in 2)
Ascites	64 (73%)	60 (89%)
Apex palpable	53 (60%)	39 (58%)
Significant pulsus paradoxus	32 (36%)	32 (48%)
Edema	22 (25%)	63 (94%)
Pericardial friction rub	16 (18%)	–
Pericardial knock	–	14 (21%)
Third heart sound	–	30 (45%)
Sudden inspiratory splitting of the second heart sound	–	24 (36%)

Abbreviation: AF, atrial fibrillation

tuberculosis reported a 75% yield compared to a 53% yield with conventional culture.[52] For *Mycobacterium tuberculosis*, the radiometric method (BACTEC) permits an average recovery and drug sensitivity testing time of 18 days, compared to 38·5 days for conventional methods, but the low yield of 54% is the major disadvantage of the former method.[52] Sputum with acid-fast bacilli will be found in only about 10% of patients.[4] Gastric washings from such patients may be studied and urine culture and lymph node biopsy may also demonstrate tubercle bacilli.

In developing countries tuberculin skin testing is of little value owing to the high prevalence of primary tuberculosis, mass BCG immunizations and the likelihood of cross-sensitization from mycobacteria present in the environment.[53] Furthermore, the limited utility of the tuberculin skin test has also been documented in a prospective study performed in a non-endemic area.[43]

There is considerable urgency to establish the correct diagnosis of tuberculosis since early initiation of therapy is associated with a favorable outcome.[45] Since tubercle bacilli are often not found on stained smears of pericardial fluid[46,54] and their growth on culture requires 3–6 weeks, there is a need for other means of making an early diagnosis. Unfortunately, a rapid, simple, inexpensive, sensitive, and specific diagnostic test for pericardial tuberculosis is not available.[53] Pericardial biopsy is an important option, but a normal result does not exclude the diagnosis.

Recently, the usefulness of measuring adenosine deaminase activity for the rapid diagnosis of pericardial

tuberculosis has been reported in different study populations with consistent results showing a pericardial fluid activity of $\geq 40\,U/l$ to have a sensitivity and specificity of more than 90%.[55–57] An analysis of the largest prospective study of the usefullness of the adenosine deaminase test for the diagnosis of pericardial tuberculosis,[58] which included a wide spectrum of patients with pericardial effusion, yielded a likelihood ratio of 3·8 and 0·05 for positive and negative tests respectively (Table 50.7). Fagan's nomogram (Figure 50.1) for interpreting diagnostic test results can be used to determine the usefulness of a positive (adenosine deaminase ≥ 40) or negative (adenosine deaminase <40) test result.[59,60] Although the likelihood ratio for a positive test is 3·8, a high pretest probability of 80% is associated with a post-test probability of 95% if the adenosine deaminase result is positive. The likelihood ratio of a negative adenosine deaminase test is 0·05, which should confer conclusive changes on pretest to post-test probabilities.

In addition to the adenosine deaminase test, the measurement of interferon γ levels in pericardial fluid may offer another means of early diagnosis. A study involving 12 patients, with definite tuberculous pericardial effusion, and 19 controls indicated that elevated interferon γ measured by radioimmunoassay in pericardial aspirate is a sensitive (92%) and highly specific (100%) marker of a tuberculous etiology in patients with a pericardial effusion.[61] This promising report needs confirmation in larger studies.

The polymerase chain reaction is useful in detecting *Mycobacterium tuberculosis* DNA in pericardial fluid,[62–64]

Table 50.7 Test properties of the adenosine deaminase (ADA) assay derived from Latouf *et al*[58]

ADA level	Definite diagnosis of pericardial tuberculosis				Likelihood ratio
	Present		Absent		
	n	Proportion	*n*	Proportion	
ADA ≥40 U/l	77	77/80 = 0·963	26	26/103 = 0·253	3·80
ADA <40 U/l	3	3/80 = 0·038	77	77/103 = 0·748	0·05
Total	80		103		

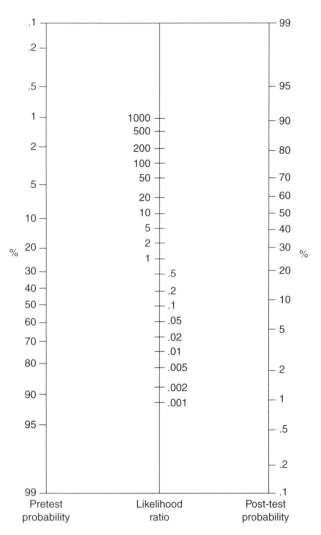

Figure 50.1 Nomogram for interpreting diagnostic test results. (Adapted from Fagan[59,60])

but the technique is less sensitive than established methods and is prone to contamination and false positive results and thus not yet suitable for routine clinical use.[53,64] At present, serum antibody tests against specific tuberculoprotein epitopes have not offered a significant diagnostic advance over other methods.[53]

Treatment

In areas and communities with a high prevalence of tuberculosis, a pericardial effusion is often considered to be tuberculous, unless an alternative cause is obvious, and treatment often has to be commenced before a bacteriologic diagnosis is established.[52] A definite diagnosis is not made in about a third of patients treated for tuberculous pericarditis and an adequate response to antituberculous chemotherapy serves as confirmation. When systematic investigation fails to yield a diagnosis in patients living in non-endemic areas, good prospective data indicate that there is no justification for starting antituberculous treatment empirically.[7] **Grade A**

Antituberculous chemotherapy dramatically increases survival in tuberculous pericarditis. In the preantibiotic era, mortality was 80–90% and currently it ranges from 8% to 17%.[47,65,66] A regimen consisting of rifampicin, isoniazid, and pyrazinamide in the initial phase of at least 2 months, followed by isoniazid and rifampicin for a total of 6 months of therapy has been shown to be highly effective in treating patients with extrapulmonary tuberculosis.[67,68] Treatment for 9 months or longer gives no better results and has the added disadvantages of increased costs and poor compliance.[68] Short-course chemotherapy is also highly effective in curing tuberculosis in HIV-infected patients,[69] although it has not been evaluated specifically in tuberculous pericarditis.

In 1988 Strang *et al*[44] reported a prospective double-blind evaluation of patients with tuberculous pericardial effusion treated with antituberculous drugs who were randomly allocated to prednisolone or placebo during the first 11 weeks of therapy (Figure 50.2): 240 patients entered the study and 198 were evaluated at 24 months; 42 patients (18%) were excluded from analysis mainly owing to loss to follow up and non-compliance with medication. In this trial, five of 97 patients given prednisolone compared with 11 of 101 given placebo died of pericarditis; seven and 17 needed repeat pericardiocentesis; three and seven open surgical drainage, and 91 and 88 had a favorable functional status at 24 months, respectively. Table 50.8 shows the outcomes for patients in the prednisolone and control groups together with the associated odds ratios (95% CI) and *P* values for the 198 patients who were analyzed in the trial. Patients treated with prednisolone were significantly less likely to

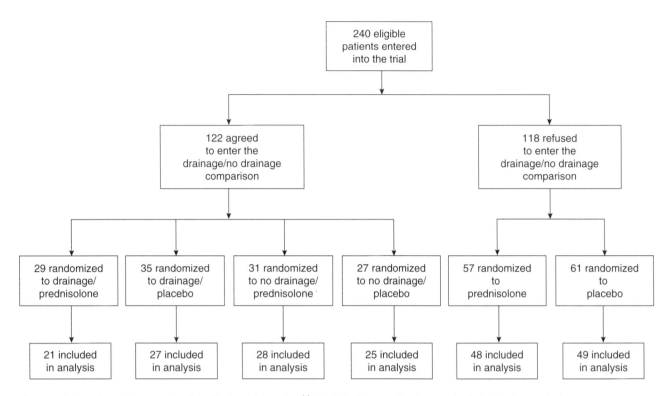

Figure 50.2 Tuberculous pericardial effusion trial profile.[44] A total of 198 patients were included in the analysis.

Table 50.8   Pericardial effusion: prednisolone versus placebo[44]

Outcome	Group prednisolone (n = 97)	Group placebo (n = 101)	Peto's odds ratio (95% CI)	P value
1. Favorable status at 24 months[a]	91/97	88/101	2·15 (0·84–5·53)	0·11
2. Repeat pericardiocentesis	7/97	17/101	0·41 (0·17–0·95)	0·04
3. Subsequent open drainage	3/97	7/101	0·45 (0·13–1·60)	0·22
4. Pericardiectomy	7/97	10/101	0·71 (0·26–1·92)	0·50
5. Total with one or more adverse events[b]	21/97	35/101	0·53 (0·29–0·98)	0·04
6. Death from pericarditis	5/97	11/101	0·46 (0·17–1·29)	0·14

[a] Patients were classified as having a favorable status if the following criteria were fulfilled or if only one was still abnormal: pulse rate ≤100, jugular venous pulse ≤5 cm, arterial pulsus paradoxus ≤10 mmHg, ascites and edema absent/just detectable, physical activity unrestricted, cardiothoracic ratio ≤55%, and electrocardiogram voltage ≥6 mm in V6 or ≥4 mm along the frontal axis.
[b] Includes outcomes numbered 2, 3, 4, and 6.

require repeat pericardiocentesis and had fewer combined adverse events than the placebo group. Although there is a suggestion that prednisolone may have a beneficial effect with regard to death from pericarditis, the 95% confidence intervals are consistent with a null effect.

It appears from these data that the adjuvant use of prednisolone in tuberculous pericarditis is associated with a reduced risk of reaccumulation of pericardial fluid and less morbidity during the treatment period, which may be clinically significant. It should, however, be noted that the

exclusion of a high proportion of randomized patients from the analysis may be a source of substantial bias in the findings reported in this study. In support of the possibility of bias, a re-analysis of this trial that includes all the participants in the groups to which they were randomized showed that the tendency for prednisolone to reduce the incidence of cardiac tamponade requiring pericardiocentesis was not statistically significant (RR = 0·43, 95% CI 0·19–1·01).[70] Similarly, the effect of prednisolone on all-cause mortality showed a promising but non-significant effect (RR = 0·53,

95% CI 0·23–1·18). Therefore, on the basis of the currently available data, prednisolone cannot be recommended for routine use in patients with tuberculous pericardial effusion. We concur with the recommendation that corticosteroids should be reserved for critically ill patients with recurrent large effusions who do not respond to pericardial drainage and antituberculous drugs alone.[31]

Grade A In the study by Strang *et al*,[44] which compared prednisolone and placebo, those who were willing were also randomized to open complete drainage by substernal pericardiotomy and biopsy under general anesthesia followed by suction drainage on admission or percutaneous pericardiocentesis as required to control symptoms and signs (Figure 50.2); 101 patients participated in this comparison. Complete open drainage abolished the need for pericardiocentesis (odds ratio 0·12, 95% CI 0·04–0·39) but did not influence the need for pericardiectomy for subsequent constriction (odds ratio 0·45, 95% CI 0·10–2·06) or the risk of death from pericarditis (odds ratio 1·51, 95% CI 0·33–6·96).

The impact of antituberculous treatment on the development of constrictive pericarditis in patients with chronic pericardial effusion of unknown cause has been investigated in a randomized trial in India:[71] Twenty-five adults were randomized in a prospective 2:1 fashion to receive either three-drug antituberculous treatment (group A) or placebo (group B) for 6 months; 21 patients (14 in group A and seven in group B) completed the study protocol, and were included in the analysis. The primary end points were the development of pericardial thickening diagnosed by CT scan and constrictive pericarditis diagnosed by cardiac catheterization. There was no significant difference between the groups in the development of the combined end point of pericardial thickening and constrictive pericarditis (group A: $n = 3$, 21·4% v group B: $n = 2$, 29·6%; P = NS); and pericardial fluid had disappeared in 10 patients (six in group A and four in group B). Thus, antituberculous treatment did not prevent the development of constrictive pericarditis and did not alter the clinical course in patients with large chronic pericardial effusions of undetermined etiology in an endemic area. However, the results of this trial should be considered with caution because of the small sample size involved. Nevertheless, the study makes a very important observation that requires further evaluation. In endemic areas antituberculous chemotherapy, which is not without hazard, is often administered to patients with large pericardial effusions in the absence of proof of tuberculosis.[4]

Recently, Hakim *et al*[72] reported the first double-blind randomized placebo controlled trial of adjunctive steroids in the treatment of effusive tuberculous pericarditis in HIV seropositive patients. This Zimbabwean study randomized 58 HIV positive patients aged 18–55 years with suspected tuberculous pericarditis to receive prednisolone ($n = 29$) or placebo ($n = 29$) for 6 weeks, in addition to standard short-course antituberculous chemotherapy. The primary end points were resolution of pericardial fluid and death over an 18-month period of observation. There was no difference in the rate of radiologic and echocardiographic resolution in pericardial effusion. By contrast, there were fewer deaths in the intervention group (5/29) compared with the placebo group (10/29), but the numbers were small and the result could have occurred by chance (RR = 0·50, 95% CI 0·19–1·28). Thus the trials of steroids for the treatment of tuberculous pericarditis suggest that prednisolone has a potentially large beneficial effect on survival in immunocompetent and HIV seropositive patients, but the individual trials were too small to be sure that this is a true effect.[70] We believe that well-designed and adequately powered trials of steroids in tuberculous pericarditis are warranted.

Tuberculous pericardial constriction

Constrictive pericarditis is one of the most serious sequelae of tuberculous pericarditis and it occurs in 30–60% of patients despite prompt antituberculous treatment and the use of corticosteroids.[42,43] Tuberculosis is the most frequent cause of constrictive pericarditis in developing countries.[3,4] The presentation is highly variable, ranging from asymptomatic to severe constriction. The diagnosis is often missed on cursory clinical examination (Table 50.6). The diastolic lift (pericardial knock) with a high-pitched early diastolic sound and sudden inspiratory splitting of the second heart sound are subtle but specific physical signs, and found in 21–45% of patients with constrictive pericarditis. These signs are often missed by the inexperienced observer unless specifically sought. Furthermore, if the investigation is not clinically guided, echocardiography has the potential to miss the signs that are suggestive of this diagnosis.

Diagnosis

Most patients with constrictive pericarditis in South Africa have the subacute variety, in which a thick fibrinous exudate fills the pericardial sac, compressing the heart and causing a circulatory disturbance. As a result, calcification of the pericardium will be absent in the majority.[30] The chest radiograph findings are non-specific. In a study reported by Strang *et al*, 70% of 143 patients had a cardiothoracic ratio greater than 55% and only 6% had a ratio greater than 75%.[30] It is uncommon to find concomitant pulmonary tuberculosis. Nonspecific but generalized T wave changes are seen in most cases, while low voltage complexes occur in about 30% of cases. Atrial fibrillation occurs in less than 5% of cases, is persistent, and usually occurs with a calcified pericardium. As with tuberculous pericardial effusion, the ECG is useful only in drawing attention to the presence of a cardiac abnormality.

Echocardiography is particularly valuable in confirming the diagnosis of subacute constrictive pericarditis. Typically, a thick fibrinous exudate is seen in the pericardial sac and is associated with diminished movements of the surface of the heart, normal sized chambers, absence of valvular heart disease, and absence of myocardial hypertrophy.[30] In time, the pericardial exudate condenses into a thick skin surrounding the heart, which usually, but not always, can be distinguished from myocardium.

Treatment

The treatment of tuberculous pericardial constriction involves the use of antituberculous drugs and pericardiectomy for persistent constriction in the face of drug therapy. In a double-blind, randomized, controlled trial in South Africa, 143 patients with tuberculous pericarditis and clinical signs of a constrictive physiology were allocated to receive prednisolone or placebo in addition to antituberculous drugs

during the first 11 weeks of treatment. (Figure 50.3)[30]: 114 patients were available for evaluation at 24 months; 20% of patients were excluded from analysis mainly due to loss to follow up and non-compliance with medication. Although clinical improvement occurred more rapidly in the prednisolone group and there was a lower mortality from pericarditis at 24 months (4% *v* 11%) and a lower requirement for pericardiectomy (21% *v* 30%), these findings were not statistically significant (Table 50.9). The remarkable finding of this study is that constriction resolved on antituberculous chemotherapy within 6 months in most patients, and only 29 (25%) of the 114 patients with constrictive pericarditis required pericardiectomy for persistent or worsening constriction.

No controlled studies have compared early pericardiectomy with late pericardiectomy in this condition. We recommend pericardiectomy if the patient's condition is static

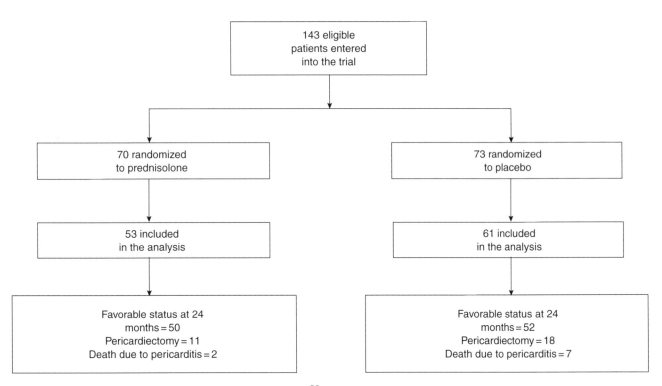

Figure 50.3 Tuberculous constrictive pericarditis trial profile[30]

Table 50.9 Constrictive pericarditis: prednisolone versus placebo[30]

Outcome	Group prednisolone (*n* = 53)	Group placebo (*n* = 61)	Peto's odds ratio (95% CI)	*P* value
1. Favorable status at 24 months[a]	50/53	52/61	2·60 (0·79–8·59)	0·116
2. Pericardiectomy	11/53	18/61	0·63 (0·27–1·47)	0·29
3. Death from pericarditis	2/53	7/61	0·35 (0·09–1·36)	0·13

[a] See note [a] in Table 50.8.

hemodynamically or deteriorating after 4–6 weeks of anti-tuberculous therapy. However, if the disease is associated with pericardial calcification, which is a marker of chronic disease, surgery should be undertaken earlier under the antituberculous drug cover. The reported risks of death with pericardiectomy in patients with tuberculous constrictive pericarditis are variable, ranging from 3% to 16%.[40,73] **Grade C**

Effusive constrictive tuberculous pericarditis

This mixed form is a common presentation in Southern Africa. There is increased pericardial pressure owing to effusion in the presence of visceral constriction and the venous pressure remains elevated after pericardial aspiration. In addition to physical signs of pericardial effusion, a diastolic knock may be detected on palpation and an early third heart sound on auscultation.

In patients with the effusive constrictive syndrome echocardiography may show a pericardial effusion between thickened pericardial membranes, with fibrinous pericardial bands apparently causing loculation of the effusion.

The treatment of effusive constrictive pericarditis is a problem because pericardiocentesis does not relieve the impaired filling of the heart and surgical removal of the fibrinous exudate coating the visceral pericardium is not possible. Antituberculous drugs should be given in the standard fashion and serial echocardiography performed to detect the development of a pericardial skin, which is amenable to surgical stripping. The place of corticosteroids in such patients is unknown.

Acknowledgments

The authors wish to acknowledge valuable comments made by Dr JK Oh on the earlier version of this chapter.

References

1. Maharaj B. Causes of congestive heart failure in black patients at King Edward VIII Hospital, Durban. *Cardiovasc J S Afr* 1991;**2**:31–2.
2. Maisch B. Pericardial diseases, with a focus on etiology, pathogenesis, pathophysiology, new diagnostic imaging methods and treatment. *Curr Opin Cardiol* 1994;**9**:379–88.
3. Permanyer-Miralda G, Sagrista-Sauleda J, Soler-Soler J. Primary acute pericardial disease: a prospective series of 231 consecutive patients. *Am J Cardiol* 1985;**56**:623–9.
4. Strang JIG. Tuberculous pericarditis. *Clin Cardiol* 1984;**7**:667–70.
5. Fowler NO. Pericardial disease. *Heart Dis Stroke* 1992;**1**:85–94.
6. Zayas R, Anguita M, Torres F *et al.* Incidence of specific etiology and role of methods for specific etiologic diagnosis of primary acute pericarditis. *Am J Cardiol* 1995;**75**:378–82.
7. Permanyer-Miralda G, Sagrista-Sauleda J, Shebatai R *et al.* Acute pericardial disease: an approach to etiologic diagnosis and treatment. In: Soler-Soler J *et al.*, eds. *Pericardial disease: new insights and old dilemmas.* Dordrecht: Kluwer Academic Publishers, 1990.
8. Farraj RS, McCully RB, Oh JK, Smith TF. *Mycoplasma*-associated pericarditis. *Mayo Clin Proc* 1997;**72**:33–6.
9. Arunsalam S, Siegel RJ. Rapid resolution of symptomatic acute pericarditis with ketorolac tromethamine: a parenteral nonsteroidal antiinflammatory agent. *Am Heart J* 1993;**125**:1455–8.
10. Fowler NO, Harbin AD. Recurrent pericarditis: follow-up of 31 patients. *J Am Coll Cardiol* 1986;**7**:300–5.
11. Hatcher CR, Logue RB, Logan WD *et al.* Pericardiectomy for recurrent pericarditis. *J Thorac Cardiovasc Surg* 1971;**62**:371–8.
12. Asplen CH, Levine HD. Azathioprine therapy of steroid responsive pericarditis. *Am Heart J* 1970;**80**:109–11.
13. Melchior TM, Ringsdal V, Hildebrandt P, Torp-Pedersen C. Recurrent acute idiopathic pericarditis treated with intravenous methylprednisolone given as pulse therapy. *Am Heart J* 1992;**123**:1086–8.
14. Marcolongo R, Russo R, Lavender F, Noventa F, Agostini C. Immunosuppressive therapy prevents recurrent pericarditis. *J Am Coll Cardiol* 1995;**26**:1276–9.
15. Guindo J, Rodriguez de la Serna A, Ramio J *et al.* Recurrent pericarditis. Relief with colchicine. *Circulation* 1990;**82**:1117–20.
16. Rodriguez de la Serna A, Guindo Soldevila J, Marti Claramunt V, Bayes de Luna A. Colchicine for recurrent pericarditis. *Lancet* 1987;**ii**:1517.
17. Spodick DH. Colchicine therapy for recurrent pericarditis. *Circulation* 1991;**83**:1830.
18. Adler Y, Zandman-Goddard G, Ravid M *et al.* Usefulness of colchicine in preventing recurrences of pericarditis. *Am J Cardiol* 1994;**73**:916–17.
19. Millaire A, deGroote P, Decoulx E *et al.* Treatment of recurrent pericarditis with colchicine. *Eur Heart J* 1994;**15**:120–4.
20. Guindo J, Adler Y, Spodick H *et al.* Colchicine for recurrent pericarditis: 51 patients followed up for 10 years. *Circulation* 1997;**96**(Suppl. I):I-29 (Abstract).
21. Eisenberg MJ, Dunn MM, Kanth N, Gamsu G, Schiller NB. Diagnostic value of chest radiography for pericardial effusion. *J Am Coll Cardiol* 1993;**22**:588–92.
22. Spodick DH. Electrical alternation of the heart. Its relation to the kinetics and physiology of the heart during cardiac tamponade. *Am J Cardiol* 1962;**10**:155–65.
23. Eisenberg MJ, Oken K, Guerrero S, Saniei MA, Schiller NB. Prognostic value of echocardiography in hospitalized patients with pericardial effusion. *Am J Cardiol* 1992;**70**:934–9.
24. Sinha PR, Singh BP, Jaipuria N *et al.* Intrapericardial echogenic images and development of constrictive pericarditis in patients with pericardial effusion. *Am Heart J* 1996;**132**:1268–72.
25. Nugue O, Millaire A, Porte H *et al.* Pericardioscopy in the etiologic diagnosis of pericardial effusion in 141 consecutive patients. *Circulation* 1996;**94**:1635–41.
26. Fowler NO. Cardiac tamponade: a clinical or an echocardiographic diagnosis? *Circulation* 1993;**87**:1738–41.

27. Chuttani K, Pandian NG, Mohanty PK *et al.* Left ventricular diastolic collapse: an echocardiographic sign of regional cardiac tamponade. *Circulation* 1991;**83**:1999–2006.

28. Chuttani K, Tischler MD, Pandian MG, Lee RT, Mohanty PK. Diagnosis of cardiac tamponade after cardiac surgery: relative value of clinical, echocardiographic and hemodynamic signs. *Am Heart J* 1994;**127**:913–18.

29. Ling LH, Oh JK, Schaff HV *et al.* Constrictive pericarditis in the modern era: evolving clinical spectrum and impact on outcome after pericardiectomy. *Circulation* 1999;**100**: 1380–6.

30. Strang JIG, Kakaza HHS, Gibson DG *et al.* Controlled trial of prednisolone as adjuvant in treatment of tuberculous constrictive pericarditis in Transkei. *Lancet* 1987;**ii**:1418–22.

31. Lorell BH. Pericardial diseases. In: Braunwald E, ed. *Heart disease: a textbook of cardiovascular medicine*. Philadelphia: WB Saunders, 1997.

32. Boonyaratavej S, Oh JK, Tajik AJ, Appleton CP, Seward JB. Comparison of mitral inflow and superior vena cava Doppler velocities in chronic obstructive pulmonary disease and constrictive pericarditis. *J Am Coll Cardiol* 1998;**32**:2043–8.

33. Ha J-W, Oh JK, Ling LH, Nishimura RA, Seward JB. Annulus paradoxus: transmitral flow velocity to mitral annular velocity ratio is inversely proportional to pulmonary capillary wedge pressure in patients with constrictive pericarditis. *Circulation* 2001;**104**:976–8.

34. Reinmuller R, Gurgan M, Erdmann E *et al.* CT and MR evaluation of pericardial constriction: a new diagnostic and therapeutic concept. *J Thorac Imaging* 1993;**8**:108–21.

35. Oren RM, Grover-McKay M, Stanford W, Weiss RM. Accurate preoperative diagnosis of pericardial constriction using cine computed tomography. *J Am Coll Cardiol* 1993; **22**:832–8.

36. Fowler NO. Constrictive pericarditis: its history and current status. *Clin Cardiol* 1995;**18**: 341–50.

37. Kushwaha SS, Fallon JT, Fuster V. Restrictive cardiomyopathy. *N Engl J Med* 1997;**336**:267–76.

38. Tirilomis T, Unverdorben S, von der Emde J. Pericardiectomy for chronic constrictive pericarditis: risks and outcome. *Eur J Cardiothor Surg* 1994;**8**:487–92.

39. McCaughan BC, Schaff HV, Piehler JM *et al.* Early and late results of pericardiectomy for constrictive pericarditis. *J Thorac Cardiovasc Surg* 1985;**89**:340–50.

40. Bashi VV, John S, Ravikumar E *et al.* Early and late results of pericardiectomy in 118 cases of constrictive pericarditis. *Thorax* 1988;**43**:637–41.

41. Cegielski JP, Ramaiya K, Lallinger GJ, Mtulia IA, Mbaga IM. Pericardial disease and human immunodeficiency virus in Dar es Salaam, Tanzania. *Lancet* 1990;**335**:209–12.

42. Schrire V. Experience with pericarditis of Groote Schuur Hospital, Cape Town: an analysis of one hundred and sixty cases over a six-year period. *S Afr Med J* 1959;**33**:810–17.

43. Sagrista-Sauleda J, Permanyer-Miralda G, Soler-Soler J. Tuberculous pericarditis: ten-year experience with a prospective protocol for diagnosis and treatment. *J Am Coll Cardiol* 1988;**11**:724–8.

44. Strang JIG, Kakaza HHS, Gibson DG *et al.* Controlled clinical trial of complete open surgical drainage and of prednisolone in treatment of tuberculous pericardial effusion in Transkei. *Lancet* 1988;**ii**:759–64.

45. Hageman JH, d'Esopo ND, Glenn WWL. Tuberculosis of the pericardium: a long-term analysis of forty-four proved cases. *N Engl J Med* 1964;**270**:327–32.

46. Fowler NO, Manitsas GT. Infectious pericarditis. *Prog Cardiovasc Dis* 1973;**16**:323–36.

47. Desai HN. Tuberculous pericarditis: a review of 100 cases. *S Afr Med J* 1979;**55**:877–80.

48. Quale JM, Lipschik GY, Heurich AE. Management of tuberculous pericarditis. *Ann Thorac Surg* 1987;**43**:653–5.

49. Heimann HL, Binder S. Tuberculous pericarditis. *Br Heart J* 1940;**2**:165–76.

50. Fowler NO. Tuberculous pericarditis. *JAMA* 1991;**266**: 99–103.

51. Schrire V. Pericarditis (with particular reference to tuberculous pericarditis). *Aust Ann Med* 1967;**16**:41–51.

52. Strang G, Latouf S, Commerford P *et al.* Bedside culture to confirm tuberculous pericarditis. *Lancet* 1991;**338**:1600–1.

53. Ng TTC, Strang JIG, Wilkins EGL. Serodiagnosis of pericardial tuberculosis. *Quart J Med* 1995;**88**:317–20.

54. Schepers GWH. Tuberculous pericarditis. *Am J Cardiol* 1962; **9**:248–76.

55. Koh KK, Kim EJ, Cho CH *et al.* Adenosine deaminase and carcinoembryonic antigen in pericardial effusion diagnosis, especially in suspected tuberculous pericarditis. *Circulation* 1994; **89**:2728–35.

56. Martinez-Vasquez JM, Ribera E, Ocana I *et al.* Adenosine deaminase activity in tuberculous pericarditis. *Thorax* 1986; **41**:888–9.

57. Komsouglu B, Goldeli O, Kulan K, Komsouglu SS. The diagnostic and prognostic value of adenosine deaminase in tuberculous pericarditis. *Eur Heart J* 1995;**16**:1126–30.

58. Latouf SE, Levetan BN, Commerford PJ. Tuberculous pericardial effusion: analysis of commonly used diagnostic methods. *S Afr Med J* 1996;**86**(Suppl.):15 (Abstract).

59. Fagan TJ. Nomogram for Bayes' theorem (C). *N Engl J Med* 1975;**293**:257.

60. Jaeschke R, Guyatt GH, Sackett DL III. How to use an article about a diagnostic test: B. What are the results and will they help me in caring for my patients? *JAMA* 1994;**271**:703–7.

61. Latouf SE, Ress SR, Lukey PT, Commerford PJ. Interferon-gamma in pericardial aspirates: a new, sensitive and specific test for the diagnosis of tuberculous pericarditis. *Circulation* 1991;**84**(Suppl.):II-149.

62. Brisson-Noel A, Gicquel B, Lecossier D *et al.* Rapid diagnosis of tuberculosis by amplification of mycobacterial DNA in clinical samples. *Lancet* 1989;**ii**:1069–71.

63. Godfrey-Faussett P, Wilkins EGL, Khoo S, Stoker N. Tuberculous pericarditis confirmed by DNA amplification. *Lancet* 1991;**337**:176–7.

64. Cegielski JP, Blythe BH, Morris AJ *et al.* Comparison of PCR, culture, and histopathology for diagnosis of tuberculous pericarditis. *J Clin Microbiol* 1997;**35**:3254–7.

65. Harvey AM, Whitehill MR. Tuberculous pericarditis. *Medicine* 1937;**16**:45–94.

66. Bhan GL. Tuberculous pericarditis. *J Infect* 1980;**2**:360–4.

67. Cohn DL, Catlin BJ, Peterson KL, Judson FN, Sbarbaro JA. A 62-dose, 6-month therapy for pulmonary and extrapulmonary tuberculosis. A twice-weekly directly-observed, cost-effective regimen. *Ann Intern Med* 1990;**112**:407–15.

68.Combs DL, O'Brien RJ, Geiter LJ. USPHS Tuberculosis Short-Course Chemotherapy Trial 21: effectiveness, toxicity and acceptability. The report of final results. *Ann Intern Med* 1990;**112**:397–406.

69.Perriens JH, St Louis M, Mukadi YB *et al.* Pulmonary tuberculosis in HIV-infected patients in Zaire: a controlled trial of treatment for either 6 months or 12 months. *N Engl J Med* 1995;**332**:779–84.

70.Mayosi BM, Volmink JA, Commerford PJ. Interventions for treating tuberculous pericarditis (Cochrane Review). In: Cochrane Collaboration. *Cochrane Library*, Issue 2. Oxford: Update Software, 2001.

71.Dwivendi SK, Rastogi P, Saran RK, Rarain VS, Puri VK, Hasan M. Antituberculous treatment does not prevent constriction in chronic pericardial effusion of undetermined aetiology. *Indian Heart J* 1997;**49**:411–14.

72.Hakim JG, Ternouth I, Mushangi E, Siziya S, Robertson V, Malin A. Double blind randomised placebo controlled trial of adjunctive prednisolone in the treatment of effusive tuberculous pericarditis in HIV seropositive patients. *Heart* 2000;**84**:183–8.

73.Pitt Fennell WM. Surgical treatment of constrictive tuberculous pericarditis. *S Afr Med J* 1982;**62**:353–5.

Part IIIg

Specific cardiovascular disorders: Valvular heart disease

Bernard J Gersh, Editor

Grading of recommendations and levels of evidence used in *Evidence-based Cardiology*

GRADE A

Level 1a   Evidence from large randomized clinical trials (RCTs) or systematic reviews (including meta-analyses) of multiple randomized trials which collectively has at least as much data as one single well-defined trial.

Level 1b   Evidence from at least one "All or None" high quality cohort study; in which ALL patients died/failed with conventional therapy and some survived/succeeded with the new therapy (for example, chemotherapy for tuberculosis, meningitis, or defibrillation for ventricular fibrillation); or in which many died/failed with conventional therapy and NONE died/failed with the new therapy (for example, penicillin for pneumococcal infections).

Level 1c   Evidence from at least one moderate-sized RCT or a meta-analysis of small trials which collectively only has a moderate number of patients.

Level 1d   Evidence from at least one RCT.

GRADE B

Level 2   Evidence from at least one high quality study of non-randomized cohorts who did and did not receive the new therapy.

Level 3   Evidence from at least one high quality case–control study.

Level 4   Evidence from at least one high quality case series.

GRADE C

Level 5   Opinions from experts without reference or access to any of the foregoing (for example, argument from physiology, bench research or first principles).

A comprehensive approach would incorporate many different types of evidence (for example, RCTs, non-RCTs, epidemiologic studies, and experimental data), and examine the architecture of the information for consistency, coherence and clarity. Occasionally the evidence does not completely fit into neat compartments. For example, there may not be an RCT that demonstrates a reduction in mortality in individuals with stable angina with the use of β blockers, but there is overwhelming evidence that mortality is reduced following MI. In such cases, some may recommend use of β blockers in angina patients with the expectation that some extrapolation from post-MI trials is warranted. This could be expressed as Grade A/C. In other instances (for example, smoking cessation or a pacemaker for complete heart block), the non-randomized data are so overwhelmingly clear and biologically plausible that it would be reasonable to consider these interventions as Grade A.

Recommendation grades appear either within the text, for example, **Grade A** and **Grade A1a** or within a table in the chapter.

The grading system clearly is only applicable to preventive or therapeutic interventions. It is not applicable to many other types of data such as descriptive, genetic or pathophysiologic.

51 Rheumatic heart disease: prevention and acute treatment

Edmund AW Brice, Patrick J Commerford

Rheumatic fever is the most important cause of acquired heart disease in children and young adults worldwide. Initiated by an oropharyngeal infection with group A β hemolytic streptococci (GAS) and following a latent period of approximately 3 weeks, the illness is characterized by an inflammatory process primarily involving the heart, joints, and central nervous system. Pathologically, the inflammatory process causes damage to collagen fibrils and connective tissue ground substance (fibrinoid degeneration) and thus rheumatic fever is classified as a connective tissue or collagen vascular disease. It is the destructive effect on the heart valves that leads to the important effects of the disease, with serious hemodynamic disturbances causing cardiac failure or embolic phenomena resulting in significant morbidity and mortality at a young age.

There have been many publications concerning the primary and secondary prevention of rheumatic fever and the treatment of the acute attack. The evidence from randomized controlled clinical trials is strongest in the field of primary prevention or the treatment of pharyngitis caused by GAS. There are few randomized trials concerning secondary prevention. In the treatment of the acute attack, most publications have been observational studies with only a small minority of randomized trials.

Epidemiology

In the developed countries of the world, the incidence of rheumatic fever fell markedly during the 20th century. For example, in the USA the incidence per 100 000 was 100 at the start of this century, 45–65 between 1935 and 1960, and is currently estimated to be approximately 2 per 100 000. This decrease in rheumatic fever incidence preceded the introduction of antibiotics and is a reflection of improved socio-economic standards, less overcrowded housing, and improved access to medical care. The current prevalence of rheumatic fever in the USA and Japan, 0·6–0·7 per 1000 population, contrasts sharply with that in the developing countries of Africa, Asia, and South America, where rates as high as 15–21 per 1000 have been reported. For example, in a study of 12 050 schoolchildren in Soweto, South Africa, a peak prevalence of rheumatic heart disease of 19·2/1000 children was reported.[1]

As GAS pharyngitis and rheumatic fever are causally related, both diseases share similar epidemiologic features. The age of first infection is commonly between 6 and 15 years. Also, the risk for developing rheumatic fever is highest in situations where GAS is more common, for example where people live in crowded conditions.

Pathogenesis

Clinical, epidemiologic, and immunologic observations tend to support strongly the causative role of untreated GAS pharyngitis in rheumatic fever. Beyond this, however, the pathogenesis of acute rheumatic fever and clinical heart disease remains unclear and several important and unexplained observations render the management of this important disease extremely difficult. These are:

- individual variability of susceptibility to GAS pharyngitis;
- individual variability of development of symptomatic GAS pharyngitis;
- individual variability of development of acute rheumatic fever after an episode of GAS pharyngitis;
- individual variation in the development of carditis and chronic rheumatic heart disease after an attack of acute rheumatic fever;
- the development of chronic rheumatic heart disease in patients who have no definite history of acute rheumatic fever.

Streptococcal skin infection (impetigo) has not been shown to cause rheumatic fever. While effective antibiotic treatment virtually abolishes the risk of rheumatic fever, in situations of untreated epidemic GAS pharyngitis up to 3% of patients develop it.[2] Worryingly, as many as a third of patients who develop rheumatic fever do so after virtually asymptomatic GAS and in more recent outbreaks, 58% denied preceding symptoms.[3] This does not augur well for the primary prevention of rheumatic fever where prompt diagnosis of GAS pharyngitis and treatment are essential.

The virulence of the streptococcal infection is dependent on the organisms' M protein serotype, which determines the antigenic epitopes shared with human heart tissue, especially sarcolemmal membrane proteins and cardiac myosin.[4] It is these variations in virulence, as a result of M protein variation, that are thought to explain the occasional outbreaks of rheumatic fever in areas of previously low incidence.[5] Other factors influencing the risk for rheumatic fever are the magnitude of the immune response and the persistence of the organism during the convalescent phase of the illness.[2]

Evidence suggests that host factors play a role in the risk for rheumatic fever. In patients who have suffered an attack of rheumatic fever, the incidence of a repeat attack is approximately 50%. A specific B cell alloantigen has been found to be present in 99% of patients with rheumatic fever versus 14% of controls.[6] Certain HLA antigens appear to be associated with increased risk for rheumatic fever. Approximately 60–70% of patients worldwide are positive for HLA-DR3, DR4, DR7, DRW53, or DQW2.[7] Such genetic markers for rheumatic fever risk may be useful to identify those in need of GAS prophylaxis. However, in view of the frequency with which these markers occur, they are unlikely to be of practical benefit in the short term.

Clinical features

While there is no specific clinical, laboratory or other test to confirm conclusively a diagnosis of rheumatic fever, the diagnosis is usually made using the clinical criteria first formulated in 1944 by T Duckett Jones[8] and subsequently modified by the Committee on Rheumatic Fever, Endocarditis, and Kawasaki Disease of the Council on Cardiovascular Disease in the Young (American Heart Association).[9] The revised criteria emphasize the importance of diagnosing *initial* attacks of rheumatic fever. The criteria are often incorrectly applied to the diagnosis of recurrent attacks, for which they were not originally intended. The diagnosis is suggested if, in the presence of preceding GAS infection, two major criteria (carditis, chorea, polyarthritis, erythema marginatum, and subcutaneous nodules) or one major and two minor criteria (fever, arthralgia, elevated erythrocyte sedimentation rate, elevated C-reactive protein, or a prolonged PR interval on ECG) are present. Evidence of preceding GAS infection, essential for the diagnosis, may be obtained from throat swab culture (only positive in approximately 11% of patients at the time of diagnosis of acute rheumatic fever)[3] or by demonstrating a rising titer of antistreptococcal antibodies, either antistreptolysin O (ASO) or anti-deoxyribonuclease B (anti-DNase B).

Prevention

The most recent recommendations on the prevention of rheumatic fever have been published by the Committee on Rheumatic Fever, Endocarditis, and Kawasaki Disease of the Council on Cardiovascular Disease in the Young (American Heart Association).[10]

Prevention of rheumatic fever may be considered to be either prevention of the initial attack (primary prevention) or prevention of recurrent attacks (secondary prevention). *True primary prevention* of rheumatic fever depends more on socioeconomic than medical factors. Upgrading housing and other aspects of urban renewal will do more toward eradicating the disease than antibiotic prophylaxis.

Primary prevention

Prevention of the initial attack of rheumatic fever depends on the prompt recognition of GAS pharyngitis and its effective treatment. Whilst it has been demonstrated that therapy initiated as long as 9 days after the onset of GAS pharyngitis can prevent an attack of rheumatic fever,[11] early treatment reduces both the morbidity and the period of infectivity.

The first report of the use of penicillin for the treatment of GAS pharyngitis and prevention of most attacks of rheumatic fever was published in 1950.[11] Over the following 40 years, attention focused on accurate diagnosis and treatment of GAS pharyngitis. A single dose of intramuscular benzathine penicillin G became the most common mode of treatment and avoided problems of non-compliance. Subsequently, as a result of the pain and possibility of allergic reaction associated with benzathine penicillin G, oral penicillin became the treatment of choice[12] and remains so today.[13] In situations where compliance with a 10 day course of oral penicillin would be unreliable, a single dose of IM benzathine penicillin G would be preferred (dosage 1·2 million U if >27 kg, otherwise 600 000 U).

Early studies established a 10 day course of oral penicillin as optimal[14,15] and this has been supported in more recent studies.[16,17] Shorter treatment periods are associated with significant decreases in bacteriological cure while longer courses of treatment do not increase cure rate.

Current recommendations[10] for penicillin therapy in children cite a dose of 250 mg ×2–3/day. These recommendations are based on trials (Table 51.1) of 250 mg given ×2–4/day resulting in equivalent cure rates.[18–21] A dose of 750 mg/day penicillin yielded significantly worse results than 250 mg ×3/day when compared in a randomized study.[22] There is no evidence available for optimal doses of penicillin in adults but 500 mg ×2–3/day is currently recommended.[10] **Grade A**

Over the past decade, many trials have been published comparing penicillin VK to a variety of other antimicrobial agents, most commonly cephalosporins and macrolides. This has been prompted by the reported increase in treatment failures with penicillin. It has been suggested that treatment failure rates of up to 38% are possible. This contention, however, has been thoroughly investigated in a study by Markowitz *et al*[23] in which treatment failure rates of penicillin were compared between two time periods,

Table 51.1 Cure rates for various penicillin dosage schedules used in treatment of streptococcal pharyngitis

Reference	Agent/dose	Bacteriologic cure rate (%)
Gerber et al. (1985)[21]	Pen V 250 mg 2×/day ×10 days	82·0
	Pen V 250 mg 3×/day ×10 days	71·5
Gerber et al. (1989)[22]	Pen V 750 mg 1×/day ×10 days	78·0
	Pen V 250 mg 3×/day ×10 days	92·0
Vann and Harris (1972)[19]	Potassium Pen G 80 000 U 2×/day ×10 days	88·0
Spitzer and Harris (1977)[20]	Pen V 500 mg 2×/day ×10 days	83·0
	Pen V 250 mg 3×/day ×10 days	84·0

Abbreviation: Pen, penicillin

1953–1979 and 1980–1993. Of the almost 2800 patients with GAS serotyping, treatment failures ranged between 10·5% and 17%, with no significant difference between each time period. It was thus concluded that the over-reporting of treatment failures was due to problems with the design of the individual studies.

An increased bateriologic cure rate for streptococcal pharyngitis by cephalosporins was demonstrated in a meta-analysis[24] of 19 randomized comparisons of a variety of cephalosporins with 10 days of oral penicillin therapy. Throat swab cultures were used to determine the presence of GAS and clearance after treatment. The results showed a statistically significant advantage of cephalosporins for which a bacteriologic cure rate of 92% was reported versus 84% for penicillin. The corresponding clinical cure rates were 95% and 89% respectively. It is suggested that the resistance of cephalosporins to penicillinase-producing anaerobes and staphylococci present in the pharyngeal flora may explain these findings. This difference in efficacy would mean that 12–13 patients would require cephalosporin treatment to potentially prevent one penicillin bacteriological treatment failure.

More recently, a multicenter comparison of 10 day therapy with cefibuten oral suspension (9 mg/kg/day in one dose) and penicillin V (25 mg/kg/day in three divided doses)[25] revealed a bacteriological cure rate of 91% versus 80% respectively (corresponding clinical cure rates were 97% v 89%). **Grade A** Shorter courses of selected cephalosporins[26] (4 or 5 days) have been shown to be effective, but current recommendations[10] suggest that further study of these regimens is required before their adoption. The cephalosporins offer statistically significant advantages over penicillin in controlled clinical trials. It remains to be demonstrated, however, whether this statistical benefit can be translated into clinical or epidemiological benefit in regions where the disease is endemic. Given the financial constraints on healthcare resources of developing nations and the considerable cost difference, it would seem that this is unlikely in the foreseeable future. Greater benefit is likely to be achieved by concerted efforts to identify, treat, and ensure compliance in large numbers of patients with the established, albeit inferior, penicillin schedules.

In patients allergic to penicillin, erythromycin has been shown to have an equivalent cure rate.[27] The recommended dosage for erythromycin estolate is 20–40 mg/kg/day in 2–4 divided doses, and for erythromycin ethylsuccinate, it is 40 mg/kg/day in 2–4 divided doses, both for 10 days.[28] **Grade A** The efficacy of erythromycin estolate is superior to that of erythromycin ethylsuccinate and is associated with fewer gastrointestinal tract side effects.[29] GAS strains resistant to erythromycin have been reported in some parts of the world.[30]

Thus, penicillin V remains the treatment of choice in non-penicillin allergic patients as it has a long record of efficacy and is probably the most cost effective option.

Appropriate antibiotic therapy in children with streptococcal pharyngitis should result in a clinical response within 24 hours – most children will become culture negative within the first or second day of treatment.[31] After completion of therapy, only patients who have persistent or recurring symptoms, or those at an increased risk for recurrence, require repeat throat swab culture. If symptomatic patients are still harboring GAS in the oropharynx, a second course of antibiotics, preferably with another agent (amoxicillin clavulanate, cephalosporins, clindamycin or penicillin and rifampicin), is recommended.[10] Failure to eradicate GAS occurs more frequently following the administration of oral penicillin than IM benzathine penicillin G.[32] Further treatment of asymptomatic patients, who are frequently chronic GAS carriers, is only indicated for those with previous rheumatic fever or their family members.

Secondary prevention

Following an initial attack of rheumatic fever, there is a high risk of recurrent attacks, which increase the likelihood of cardiac damage, and continuous antibiotic therapy is required. This is especially important as GAS infections need not be symptomatic to trigger a recurrence of rheumatic fever, nor does optimal GAS treatment preclude a recurrence. It is recommended that patients who have suffered either proven attacks of rheumatic fever or Sydenham's chorea be given long-term prophylaxis following the initial treatment to eradicate the pharyngeal GAS organisms. Recommendations regarding the duration of such prophylaxis are largely empiric and based on observational studies.

The duration of prophylaxis should be individualized and take into account the socioeconomic conditions and risk of exposure to GAS for that patient. Individuals who have suffered carditis, with or without valvular involvement, are at higher risk for recurrent attacks[33,34] and should receive prophylaxis well into adulthood and perhaps for life. If valvular heart disease persists then prophylaxis is indicated for at least 10 years after the last attack of rheumatic fever and at least until 40 years of age. Those patients who have not suffered rheumatic carditis can receive prophylaxis until 21 years of age or 5 years after the last attack.[35]

The choice of prophylactic agent has to be made with due regard for the likelihood of compliance with a regimen over a period of many years. **Grade A** Therefore, despite associated pain *(which can be ameliorated by using lidocaine as a diluent[36])*, intramuscular injection of benzathine penicillin G is the method of choice in most situations. The recommended dose is 1·2 million U every 3–4 weeks. A comparison of 3 weekly (*n* = 90) versus 4 weekly (*n* = 63) benzathine penicillin prophylaxis[37] demonstrated the superiority of the 3 weekly dosage. The only prophylaxis failure in the 3 weekly dosage group was due to partial compliance versus five true failures in the 4 weekly dosage group. A long-term follow up study[38] for a mean period of 6·4 years (range 1–12 years) in 249 consecutively randomized patients to 3 or 4 weekly regimens further supported the former schedule (0·25% *v* 1·29% prophylaxis failures respectively). Assays for penicillin levels in blood have also shown that 4 weekly dosage did not provide adequate drug levels throughout the intervening period between doses.[39] Therefore, only those considered at low risk should receive a 4 weekly dose.

Oral prophylaxis has been shown to be less effective than intramuscular penicillin G prophylaxis, even when compliance is optimal.[32] Penicillin V 250 mg ×2/day for adults and children is the recommended dose. No published data exist on other penicillins, macrolides, or cephalosporins for secondary prophylaxis of rheumatic fever. However erythromycin, at a dose of 250 mg ×2/day is usually recommended for those allergic to penicillin.

Patients who have either had prosthetic valves inserted and/or who are in atrial fibrillation require warfarin anticoagulation. This is a situation that may necessitate the use of an oral prophylaxis regimen. In such patients intramuscular injections of penicillin may carry the risk of hematoma formation, especially in patients rendered asthenic as a consequence of their underlying illness. This important circumstance is, as far as we are aware, not addressed in the literature.

Acute management

The aim of the acute treatment of a proven attack of rheumatic fever is to suppress the inflammatory response and so minimize the effects on the heart and joints, to eradicate the GAS from the pharynx, and provide symptomatic relief.

The longstanding recommendation of bed rest would appear to be appropriate, mainly in order to lessen joint pain. **Grade C** The duration of bed rest should be individually determined but ambulation can usually be started once the fever has subsided and acute phase reactants are returning towards normal. Strenuous exertion should be avoided, especially for those with carditis.

Even though throat swabs taken during the acute attack of rheumatic fever are rarely positive for GAS, it is advisable for patients to receive a 10 day course of penicillin V (or erythromycin if penicillin allergic). Although conventional, this strategy is untested. Thereafter, secondary prophylaxis should commence as described in the previous section.

The choice of anti-inflammatory agent is between salicylates and corticosteroids. **Grade A** Recently, a meta-analysis of trials comparing these two agents has been published.[40] In this review, a total of 130 publications from 1949 were assessed. While 11 studies had been randomized, only five (Table 51.2)[41–45] fulfilled the meta-analysis criteria of:

- adequate case definition by the Jones criteria;
- proper randomization to either salicylates or some form of corticosteroid;
- non-overlap of subjects between studies; and
- follow up for at least 1 year for assessment of the presence of an apical systolic murmur suggesting structural cardiac damage as a result of carditis.

The trials varied in the use of steroid agent used, either cortisone, ACTH, or prednisone.

The largest study of the five selected for the meta-analysis was that of the Rheumatic Fever Working Party where ACTH, cortisone, and aspirin were compared in a trial involving 505 children in the USA and UK.[44] This study found no long-term advantage to be associated with either therapy. While apical systolic murmurs disappeared more rapidly in the steroid-treated groups, the prevalence of a cardiac murmur at 1 year follow up was the same as for the salicylate-treated group. The erythrocyte sedimentation rate was found to normalize and nodules resolved faster in the steroid group.

When the five studies were examined in the meta-analysis, it was found that the advantage of corticosteroids over salicylates, in preventing the development of a pathologic apical

Table 51.2 Randomized trials of acute rheumatic fever treatment

Reference	Number of patients analyzed	Agent/dose	Apical murmur present at 1 year (%)
Combined Rheumatic Fever Study Group (1960)[41]	57	Prednisone 60 mg/day ×21 days then taper v ASA 50 mg/lb/day ×9 weeks, then taper	Steroids 57·1% v ASA 37%
Combined Rheumatic Fever Study Group (1965)[42]	73	Prednisone 3 mg/lb/day ×7 days then taper v ASA 50 mg/lb/day × 6 weeks	Steroids 25·3% v ASA 32·1%
Dorfman et al (1961)[43]	129	Hydrocortisone 250 mg then taper and/or ASA to 20–30 mg%	Steroids 12·5% v ASA 34·4%
Rheumatic Fever Working Party (1955)[44]	497	ACTH 80–120 U and taper v cortisone 300 mg and taper v ASA 60 mg/lb/day and taper	Steroids 48·6% v ASA 44%
Stolzer et al (1965)[45]	128	ASA 30–60 mg/lb/day ×6 weeks v cortisone 50–300 mg/day v ACTH 20–120 v mg/day	Steroids 26·3% v ASA 34·6%

systolic murmur after 1 year of treatment, was not statistically significant (estimated odds ratio 0·88, 95% CI 0·53–1·46).

All these trials may be criticized on two important points. Firstly, the method used to assess cardiac involvement was clinical with the development or persistence of an apical systolic murmur the usual criterion. It could be argued that observer error and interobserver variability of clinical methodology could invalidate the results and that the question should be re-examined using modern non-invasive techniques. It has, however, been shown that, at least during the acute phase of the illness, transthoracic two-dimensional echocardiography with color flow imaging does not add significantly to the clinical evaluation of the degree of cardiac involvement.[46] The second point relates to the duration of follow up. Lack of clinical evidence of cardiac involvement at 1 or 2 years following the initial attack of acute rheumatic fever is no guarantee that the important sequelae of valvular incompetence or stenosis will not develop in the ensuing decades.

Appropriate dosages of anti-inflammatory agents are aspirin 100 mg/kg/day in four or five divided doses or prednisone 1–2 mg/kg/day. Patients with severe cardiac involvement appear to respond more promptly to corticosteroids.[47]

The duration of therapy must be gauged from the severity of the attack, the presence of carditis, and the rate of response to treatment. Milder attacks with little or no carditis may be treated with salicylates for approximately a month or until inflammation has subsided, as assessed by clinical and laboratory evidence. More severe cases may require 2–3 months of steroid therapy before this can be gradually weaned. Up to 5% of patients may still have rheumatic activity despite treatment at 6 months. Occasionally a "rebound"

of inflammatory activity can occur when anti-inflammatory therapy is reduced, and may require salicylate treatment.

Alternative non-steroidal anti-inflammatory agents have not been adequately assessed in trials and would be of benefit only in individuals allergic to or intolerant of aspirin.

A recent prospective randomized controlled trial demonstrated no benefit for intravenous immunoglobulin over placebo when administered during the first episode of rheumatic fever.[48]

In patients whose initial attack of rheumatic fever is inadequately treated, there is a high risk that the rheumatic activity will continue and result in valvular incompetence, most commonly of the mitral valve. The end result of an ongoing rheumatic process with deteriorating valvular function is heart failure. Experience has shown that in such cases prompt surgical management[49] is the sole option and can result in the survival of up to 90% of patients.[50] It has been suggested that the reduction in cardiac workload following valve surgery results in a settling of the rheumatic process – akin to the beneficial effect observed for bed rest.

Conclusion

While questions regarding the pathogenesis of rheumatic fever remain, sufficient evidence is available to offer guidance on the appropriate prevention and acute treatment of this common illness (Table 51.3). It must be remembered that as most sufferers of this disease are in poor socioeconomic environments and in countries where resources are scarce, the regimens used must be cost effective and chosen with a view to maximizing patient compliance.

Table 51.3   Recommendations for prophylaxis and therapy

Agent	Dose	Route	Duration
Primary prevention			
Benzathine penicillin G	600 000 U if ≤27 kg, 1 200 000 U if >27 kg	Intramuscular injection	Once
Penicillin V	Children 250 mg, ×2–3/day	Oral	10 days
	Adults 500 mg ×2–3/day		
Erythromycin estolate	20–40 mg/kg/day ×2–4/day (max 1g/day)	Oral	10 days
Secondary prevention (prevention of recurrent attacks)[a]			
Benzathine penicillin G	1 200 000 U every 3 weeks (low risk, every 4 weeks)	Intramuscular injection	
Penicillin V	250 mg ×2/day	Oral	
Erythromycin	250 mg ×2/day	Oral	

Treatment of the acute attack of rheumatic fever:
- Bed rest
- Salicylates 100 mg/kg/day in 4–5 doses (in severe attacks with cardiac involvement, prednisone 1–2 mg/kg/day)
- Valve repair/replacement surgery for severe valve dysfunction.

[a] Duration of secondary prophylaxis depends on history of carditis and if valvular involvement persists. For details see text.

A recent study of the effect of a 10 year education program on the reduction of rheumatic fever incidence[51] demonstrated what can be achieved by a structured approach to patient identification, community education, and effective diagnosis and treatment. This intervention resulted in a 78% reduction in the incidence of rheumatic fever within 10 years. Much could be achieved through the establishment of similar programs where rheumatic fever is rife.

References

1. McLaren MJ, Hawkins DM, Koornhof HJ *et al.* Epidemiology of rheumatic heart disease in black schoolchildren of Soweto, Johannesburg. *BMJ* 1975;**3**:474–8.

2. Siegel AC, Johnson EE, Stollerman GH. Controlled studies of streptococcal pharyngitis in a pediatric population. 1. Factors related to the attack rate of rheumatic fever. *N Engl J Med* 1961;**265**:559–65.

3. Dajani AS. Current status of nonsuppurative complications of group A streptococci. *Pediatr Infect Dis J* 1991;**10**:S25–7.

4. Dale JB, Beachey EH. Sequence of myosin cross-reactive epitopes of streptococcal M protein. *J Exp Med* 1986;**164**:1785–90.

5. Schwartz B, Facklam RR, Breiman RF. Changing epidemiology of group A streptococcal infection in the U.S.A. *Lancet* 1990;**336**:1167–71.

6. Khanna AK, Buskirk DR, Williams RC *et al.* Presence of non-HLA B cell antigen in rheumatic fever patients and their families as defined by a monoclonal antibody. *J Clin Invest* 1989;**83**:1710–16.

7. Haffejee I. Rheumatic fever and rheumatic heart disease: the current state of its immunology, diagnostic criteria and prophylaxis. *Quart J Med* 1992;**84**:641–58.

8. Jones TD. Diagnosis of rheumatic fever. *JAMA* 1944;**126**:481–4.

9. Dajani AS, Ayoub EM, Bierman FZ *et al.* Guidelines for the diagnosis of rheumatic fever: Jones criteria, updated 1992. *JAMA* 1992;**268**:2069–73.

10. Dajani A, Taubert K, Ferrieri P *et al.* Treatment of acute streptococcal pharyngitis and prevention of rheumatic fever: a statement for health professionals. *Paediatrics* 1995;**96**:758–64.

11. Denny FW, Wannamaker LW, Brink WR, Rammelkamp CH Jr, Custer EA. Prevention of rheumatic fever: treatment of the preceding streptococci infection. *JAMA* 1950;**143**:151–3.

12. Gerber MA, Markowitz M. Management of streptococcal pharyngitis reconsidered. *Pediatr Infect Dis* 1984;**4**:518–26.

13. Nelson JD, McCracken GH Jr, Streptococcal infections (editorial). *Pediatr Infect Dis J Newsletter* 1993;**12**:12.

14. Wannamaker LW, Rammelkemp CR Jr, Denny FW *et al.* Prophylaxis of acute rheumatic fever by the treatment of the preceding streptococcal infection with varying amounts of depot penicillin. *Am J Med* 1951;**10**:673–95.

15. Breese BB. Treatment of beta haemolytic streptococcal infections in the home: relative value of available methods. *JAMA* 1953;**152**:10–14.

16. Schwartz RH, Wientzen RL, Pedreira F *et al.* Penicillin V for group A streptococcal pharyngotonsillitis: a randomised trial of seven vs. ten day therapy. *JAMA* 1981;**246**:1790–5.

17. Gerber MA, Randolf MF, Chanatry J *et al.* Five vs. ten days of penicillin V therapy for streptococcal pharyngitis. *Am J Dis Child* 1987;**141**:224–7.

18. Breese BB, Disney FA, Talpey WB. Penicillin in streptococcal infections: total dose and frequency of administration. *Am J Dis Child* 1965;**110**:125–30.

19. Vann RL, Harris BA. Twice a day penicillin therapy for streptococcal upper respiratory infections. *South Med J* 1972;**65**: 203–5.

20. Spitzer TG, Harris BA. Penicillin V therapy for streptococcal pharyngitis: comparison of dosage schedules. *South Med J* 1977;**70**:41–2.

21. Gerber MA, Spadaccini LJ, Wright LL, Deutsch L, Kaplan EL. Twice daily penicillin in the treatment of streptococcal pharyngitis. *Am J Dis Child* 1985;**139**:1145–8.

22. Gerber MA, Randolf MF, DeMeo K, Feder HM, Kaplan EL. Failure of once-daily penicillin therapy for streptococcal pharyngitis. *Am J Dis Child* 1989;**143**:153–5.

23. Markowitz M, Gerber MA, Kaplan EL. Treatment of streptococcal pharyngotonsillitis: reports of penicillin's demise are premature. *J Pediatr* 1993;**123**:679–85.

24. Pichichero ME, Margolis PA. A comparison of cephalosporins and penicillins in the treatment of group A beta-haemolytic streptococcal pharyngitis: a meta analysis supporting the concept of microbial copathogenicity. *Pediatr Infect Dis J* 1991;**10**:275–81.

25. Pichichero ME, McLinn SE, Gooch WM IIIrd *et al*. Cefibuten vs. penicillin V in group A beta-haemolytic streptococcal pharyngitis. Members of the Cefibuten Pharyngitis International Study Group. *Pediatr Infect Dis J* 1995; **14**: S102–7.

26. Aujard Y, Boucot I, Brahimi N, Chiche D, Bingen E. Comparative efficacy and safety of four-day cefuroxime axetil and ten day penicillin treatment of group A beta-haemolytic streptococcal pharyngitis in children. *Pediatr Infect Dis J* 1995;**14**:295–300.

27. Shapera RM, Hable KA, Matsen JM. Erythromycin therapy twice daily for streptococcal pharyngitis: a controlled comparison with erythromycin or penicillin phenoxymethyl four times daily or penicillin G benzathine. *JAMA* 1973;**226**: 531–5.

28. Derrick CW, Dillon HC. Erythromycin therapy for streptococcal pharyngitis. *Am J Dis Child* 1976;**130**:175–8.

29. Ginsberg CM, McCracken GH Jr, Crow SD *et al*. Erythromycin therapy for group A streptococcal pharyngitis. Results of a comparative study of the estolate and ethylsuccinate formulations. *Am J Dis Child* 1984;**138**:536–9.

30. Seppala H, Missinen A, Jarvinen H *et al*. Resistance to erythromycin in group A streptococci. *N Engl J Med* 1992;**326**: 292–7.

31. Krober MS, Bass JW, Michels GN. Streptococcal pharyngitis placebo controlled double-blind evaluation of clinical response to penicillin therapy. *JAMA* 1985;**253**:1271–4.

32. Feinstein AR, Wood HF, Epstein JA *et al*. A controlled study of three methods of prophylaxis against streptococcal infection in a population of rheumatic children. *N Engl J Med* 1959;**260**:697–702.

33. Majeed HA, Yousof AM, Khuffash FA *et al*. The natural history of acute rheumatic fever in Kuwait: a prospective six year follow up report. *J Chronic Dis* 1986;**39**:361–9.

34. Kuttner AG, Mayer FE. Carditis during second attacks of rheumatic fever – its incidence in patients without clinical evidence of cardiac involvement in their initial rheumatic episode. *N Engl J Med* 1963;**268**:1259–61.

35. Berrios X, delCampo E, Guzman B, Bisno AL. Discontinuing rheumatic fever prophylaxis in selected adolescents and young adults. *Ann Intern Med* 1993;**118**:401–6.

36. Amir J, Ginat S, Cohen YH *et al*. Lidocaine as a diluent for administration of benzathine penicillin G. *Pediatr Infect Dis J* 1998;**17**:890–3.

37. Lue HC, Wu MH, Hseih KH *et al*. Rheumatic fever recurrences: controlled study of 3-week versus 4-week benzathine penicillin prevention programs. *J Pediatr* 1986;**108**: 299–304.

38. Lue HC, Wu MH, Wang JK *et al*. Long-term outcome of patients with rheumatic fever receiving benzathine penicillin G prophylaxis every three weeks versus every four weeks. *J Pediatr* 1994;**125**:812–6.

39. Kaplan EL, Berrios X, Speth J *et al*. Pharmacokinetics of benzathine penicillin G: serum levels during the 28 days after intramuscular injection of 1 200 000 units. *J Pediatr* 1989; **115**:146–50.

40. Albert DA, Harel L, Karrison T. The treatment of rheumatic carditis: a review and meta-analysis. *Medicine (Baltimore)* 1995;**74**:1–12.

41. Combined Rheumatic Fever Study Group (RFSG). A comparison of the effect of prednisone and acetylsalicylic acid on the incidence of residual rheumatic carditis. *N Engl J Med* 1960;**262**:895–902.

42. Combined Rheumatic Fever Study Group (RFSG). A comparison of short-term intensive prednisone and acetyl salicylic acid therapy in the treatment of acute rheumatic fever. *N Engl J Med* 1965;**272**:63–70.

43. Dorfman A, Gross JI, Lorincz AE. The treatment of acute rheumatic fever. *Pediatrics* 1961;**27**:692–706.

44. Rheumatic Fever Working Party (RFWP) of the MRC, Great Britain, and the Subcommittee of Principal Investigators of the American Council on Rheumatic Fever and Congenital Heart Disease, American Heart Association. The treatment of acute rheumatic fever in children: a cooperative clinical trial of ACTH, cortisone and aspirin. *Circulation* 1955;**11**: 343–71.

45. Stolzer BL, Houser HB, Clark EJ. Therapeutic agents in rheumatic carditis. *Arch Intern Med* 1955;**95**:677–88.

46. Vasan RS, Shrivastava S, Vijayakumar M *et al*. Echocardiographic evaluation of patients with acute rheumatic fever and rheumatic carditis. *Circulation* 1996;**94**:73–82.

47. Czoniczer G, Amezcua F, Pelargonio S, Massel BF. Therapy of severe rheumatic carditis: comparison of adrenocortical steroids and aspirin. *Circulation* 1964;**29**:813–19.

48. Voss LM, Wilson NJ, Neutze JM *et al*. Intravenous immunoglobulin in acute rheumatic fever: a randomized controlled trial. *Circulation* 2001;**103**:401–6.

49. Lewis BS, Geft IL, Milo S, Gotsman MS. Echocardiography and valve replacement in the critically ill patient with acute rheumatic carditis. *Ann Thorac Surg* 1979;**27**:529–35.

50. Barlow JB, Kinsley RH, Pocock WA. Rheumatic fever and rheumatic heart disease. In: Barlow JB, ed. *Perspectives on the mitral valve*. Philadelphia: FA Davis, 1987.

51. Bach JF, Chalons S, Forier E *et al*. 10-year educational programme aimed at rheumatic fever in two French Caribbean islands. *Lancet* 1996;**347**:644–8.

52 Mitral valve disease: indications for surgery

Blasé A Carabello

Introduction

In mitral valve disease symptomatic status, ventricular functional status and the kind of operation that will ultimately be performed all affect the indication for valve surgery. This chapter will integrate these aspects into a strategy for surgical correction. It should be noted that in surgery for valve disease there are few large controlled trials of therapy. Most knowledge of the response of valve disease to surgery accrues from reports of surgical outcome in both selected and unselected patients.

Mitral regurgitation

Surgical objectives

Like all valvular lesions, mitral regurgitation imposes a hemodynamic overload on the heart. Ultimately, this overload can only be corrected by surgically restoring valve competence. For valve surgery in general, the timing of surgery has two opposing tenets. First, as surgery has an operative risk and, if a prosthesis is inserted, imposes the risks inherent in valve prosthesis, surgery should be delayed for as long as possible. Second, surgery which is delayed until the hemodynamic overload has caused irreversible left ventricular dysfunction will result in a suboptimal outcome. In some patients, far advanced left ventricular dysfunction may militate against operating at all.

The timing of valve surgery is made even more complex in mitral regurgitation, as frequently valve repair rather than valve replacement can be effected. Because valve repair does not involve the use of a valvular prosthesis, and because it also helps to preserve left ventricular function, it is applicable at the two ends of the spectrum of mitral regurgitation. Repair might be considered in asymptomatic patients with normal left ventricular function because the disease could be cured then without the need for intense follow up and without the use of a valve prosthesis.[1] At the other end of the spectrum, patients with severe impairment of left ventricular function who might not be candidates for mitral valve replacement with chordal disruption might have a good result from valve repair.[2] However, for most patients mitral valve surgery is performed for the relief of symptoms or to prevent worsening of asymptomatic left ventricular dysfunction.

Etiology

The mitral valve apparatus consists of the mitral valve annulus, the valve leaflets, the chordae tendineae and the papillary muscles. Abnormalities of any of these structures may cause mitral regurgitation. The common causes of mitral regurgitation include infective endocarditis, the mitral valve prolapse syndrome with myxomatous degeneration of the valve, spontaneous chordal rupture, rheumatic heart disease, collagen disease such as Marfan's syndrome, and coronary artery disease leading to papillary muscle ischemia or necrosis. These etiologies are especially important with regard to surgical correction. For instance, the spontaneous rupture of a posterior chorda tendinea leads to mitral valve repair in almost 100% of cases. On the other hand, severe rheumatic deformity of the valve which has led to mitral regurgitation may be irreparable, necessitating replacement.

Pathophysiology

Hemodynamic phases of mitral regurgitation

Figure 52.1 depicts the pathophysiologic phases of mitral regurgitation.[3] In the acute phase, such as might occur with spontaneous chordal rupture, there is sudden volume overload on both the left ventricle and the left atrium. The regurgitant volume, together with the venous return from the pulmonary veins, distends both chambers. Distention of the left ventricle increases use of the Frank–Starling mechanism, by which increased sarcomere stretch increases end-diastolic volume modestly and also increases left ventricular stroke work. The new orifice for left ventricular ejection (the regurgitant pathway) facilitates left ventricular emptying and end-systolic volume decreases. Acting in concert, these two effects increase ejection fraction and total stroke volume. However, as shown in Figure 52.1, panel A, if only 50% of the total stroke volume is ejected into the aorta there is a net loss of 30% of the initial forward stroke volume. At the same time, volume overload on the left atrium increases

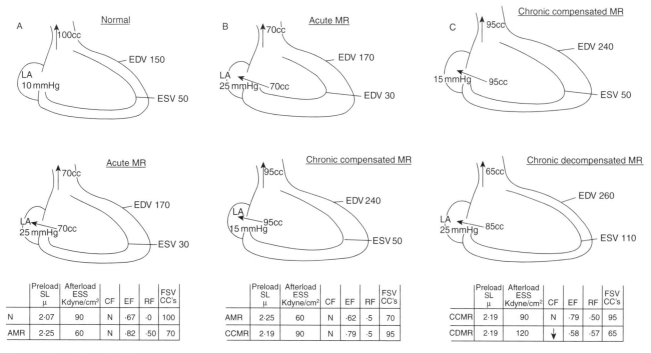

Figure 52.1 (Panel A) Normal hemodynamic state compared to acute mitral regurgitation (AMR). In AMR, total stroke volume and ejection performance increase as preload is increased and afterload is reduced. However, forward stroke volume is reduced and left atrial pressure increased. (Panel B) AMR compared to chronic compensated mitral regurgitation (CCMR). In CCMR, increased end-diastolic volume permitted by eccentric hypertrophy increases both total and forward stroke volume. Enlargement of atrium and ventricle allows increased volume to be accommodated at lower filling pressure. Increase in afterload toward normal in this state of compensation reduces ejection performance slightly. (Panel C) Chronic decompensated mitral regurgitation (CDMR) compared with CCMR: contractile function is reduced and afterload is increased in CDMR. Both reduce ejection performance and forward cardiac output. There is further cardiac dilation in CDMR, leading to worsening mitral regurgitation, further compromising pump function by reducing forward stroke volume and increasing filling pressure. CF, contractile function; EDV, end-diastolic volume; EF, ejection fraction; ESS, end-systolic stress; ESV, end-systolic volume; FSV, forward stroke volume; LA, left atrial pressure; N, normal hemodynamic state; RF, regurgitant fraction; SL, sarcomere length. (Reproduced with permission from Carabello.[3])

left atrial pressure. At this point in time the patient suffers from low output and pulmonary congestion and appears to be in left ventricular failure, although left ventricular muscle function is either normal or even augmented by sympathetic reflexes. Acute severe mitral regurgitation may lead to shock and pulmonary edema, requiring intra-aortic balloon counterpulsation and urgent mitral valve repair or replacement. However, if the patient can be maintained in a relatively stable condition, he or she may then enter the chronic compensated phase (Figure 52.1, panel B) within 3–6 months.

In the chronic compensated phase of mitral regurgitation, eccentric cardiac hypertrophy, in which sarcomeres are laid down in series, allows enlargement of the left ventricle, enhancing its total volume pumping capacity. Total stroke volume is increased, allowing normalization of forward stroke volume. Enlargement of the left atrium accommodates the volume overload at a lower pressure, eliminating pulmonary congestion. In this phase the patient may be remarkably asymptomatic, able to perform normal daily activities, and can even engage in sporting events of modest physical demands.[4]

The patient may remain in the compensated phase for months or years. However, eventually the persistent volume overload leads to a decline in left ventricular function (Figure 52.1, panel C). A loss of myofibrils or an insensitivity to cyclic AMP may be responsible, at least in part, for loss of left ventricular contractility.[5,6] In this phase, left ventricular end-systolic volume increases because the reduced force of contraction results in poor left ventricular emptying, forward stroke volume falls, and left ventricular dilation may worsen the mitral regurgitation. At this time there is re-elevation of the left atrial pressure, resulting again in pulmonary congestion. Notably, the still favorable loading conditions of mitral regurgitation (increased preload and normal afterload) permit a "normal" ejection fraction even though left ventricular dysfunction has developed.

Importance of the mitral valve apparatus

Although the contribution of the mitral valve apparatus to left ventricular function was noted by Rushmer and Lillehei decades ago,[7,8] its physiologic significance and impact on patient care have only recently received widespread appreciation. It is quite clear that the mitral valve apparatus has a wider role than simply to prevent mitral regurgitation. Rather, the apparatus is an integral part of the left ventricular internal skeleton. In early systole, tugging on the apparatus by the chordae tendineae may shorten the major axis while lengthening the minor axis, in turn augmenting preload there during the pre-ejection phase of systole. In addition, the apparatus helps to maintain the normal and efficient ellipsoid shape of the left ventricle.

Transection of the chordae causes an immediate fall in left ventricular function.[9] Until the importance of chordal preservation during mitral valve surgery was recognized, ejection fraction almost always fell following surgery. This was attributed to increased afterload from surgical closure of the low-impedance pathway which, preoperatively, had facilitated ejection into the left atrium. However, it is now clear that closure of the same low-impedance pathway in which chordal integrity is maintained results in no fall in ejection fraction, or only a modest decline, suggesting that the increased postoperative load theory is not the sole mechanism for ejection fraction falls.[2,11–13] In fact, chordal preservation can actually effect a lowering of systolic wall stress (afterload) instead of an increase as left ventricular radius decreases following surgery [stress = pressure $\times$ radius$/2 \times$ thickness].[10] Thus, chordal integrity should be maintained whenever possible. A recent randomized study demonstrated that maintenance of just the posterior apparatus lowers mortality and leads to superior postoperative function compared to posterior and anterior chordal transection.[14]

Apart from the benefits on left ventricular function, if mitral valve repair can be performed instead of replacement, operative mortality is lower, postoperative survival is better and the need for anticoagulation is removed while thromboembolism remains low.[14–17] Even if the mitral valve is so badly damaged that a prosthesis must be inserted, chordal preservation, especially of the posterior chords, can usually be performed, resulting in better ventricular function than if all the chords were removed.[10] Unfortunately, despite recognition of the importance of the mitral valve apparatus, repair is only performed in about 30% of all operations for mitral regurgitation, varying from zero in some institutions to 90% in others.

Indications for surgery

Severity of mitral regurgitation Grade B

Under most circumstances only severe mitral regurgitation is corrected surgically. Mild to moderate regurgitation (regurgitant fraction $< 40\%$) under most circumstances neither causes symptoms nor leads to left ventricular dysfunction, even over a protracted period of time. Severity is

difficult to ascertain by physical examination alone, especially in acute mitral regurgitation. As noted above, in acute mitral regurgitation there has been no time for cardiac dilation to occur. Thus, palpation of the precordium does not reveal a hyperdynamic left ventricular impulse. Although the murmur of mitral regurgitation is present, severity cannot be gauged from its intensity. In most cases of severe mitral regurgitation an S3 should be present. This finding does not necessarily indicate heart failure, but may simply be the result of a large regurgitant volume filling the left ventricle under a higher than usual left atrial pressure. In chronic mitral regurgitation there should be evidence on physical examination of an enlarged hyperdynamic left ventricle, unless the patient's size or habitus makes physical examination difficult. Failure to find evidence of an enlarged heart suggests that the mitral regurgitation is not either severe enough or chronic enough to cause left ventricular enlargement.

In chronic severe mitral regurgitation the chest radiograph should also show cardiac enlargement, and the electrocardiogram is likely to demonstrate left atrial abnormality and left ventricular hypertrophy.

In most cases, quantification of regurgitant severity is estimated during echocardiography, with Doppler interrogation of the mitral valve. In acute mitral regurgitation, transthoracic echocardiography may underestimate regurgitant severity.[18] In such cases, transesophageal echocardiography is helpful. It should be noted that Doppler flow studies visually demonstrate blood flow velocity across the mitral valve, and not true flow. Because of this, both under- and overestimation of regurgitant severity is possible. Flow mapping, which expresses the regurgitant jet in terms relative to left atrial size, has been used extensively. However, the limitations of this method are well known and the technique is semiquantitative at best.[19,20] Other methods, such as the proximal isovelocity surface area, have been employed experimentally and in clinical investigations.[21–23] In using proximal isovelocity surface area to estimate regurgitation flow, the area of convergence of the regurgitant jet on the ventricular side of the mitral valve is measured at the point of aliasing. By multiplying proximal isovelocity surface area by the known aliasing velocity, actual flow is obtained, which should be a better indication of regurgitant severity. Unfortunately, the convergence pattern is often difficult to pinpoint clinically and is not applicable in many cases. As with mitral valve repair, practice varies from center to center, with some centers routinely accurately quantifying the severity of disease[24] whereas others rely on a visual estimation.

When regurgitation severity is in doubt because of discordance between left ventricular size and the regurgitant signal, that is a small left ventricle and left atrium suggesting mild disease and a Doppler signal suggesting severe disease, the issue should be resolved at cardiac catheterization. During cardiac catheterization, hemodynamics and a left ventriculogram give additional (although also imperfect) information about the degree of mitral regurgitation. The left ventriculogram, unlike the Doppler study, visualizes the actual flow of contrast medium from the left ventricle into the left atrium. Care must be taken to inject enough contrast agent (at least 60 ml) to opacify both the enlarged left ventricle and the left atrium in mitral regurgitation. Coronary arteriography is also performed at cardiac catheterization if there is any suspicion of an ischemic etiology for mitral regurgitation, or when risk factors for coronary disease coexist.

Acute mitral regurgitation Grade C

In almost all cases of severe acute mitral regurgitation the patient is symptomatic. The acute hemodynamic changes noted above cause decreased forward output and sudden left atrial hypertension, resulting in pulmonary congestion, reduced forward flow, and the symptoms of dyspnea, orthopnea, exercise intolerance and fatigue. Vasodilator therapy may be successful in alleviating symptoms by preferentially increasing forward flow while simultaneously decreasing left ventricular size, thereby partially restoring mitral valve competence.[25] If vasodilators fail, or if the patient is so severely decompensated that hypotension contraindicates their use, intra-aortic balloon counterpulsation is necessary. In such cases surgery should follow soon after. This is especially true for the patient with ischemic mitral regurgitation. Such patients may have a volatile course, with initially mild heart failure which progresses unpredictably in severity. These patients require close follow up.[26,27] In milder cases where symptoms can be relieved by medical therapy, patients should be given a trial of medical therapy, during which they may enter the compensated chronic phase. In such cases patients may then become asymptomatic for months or years. However, one study[28] suggests that such patients are at risk of sudden death. If confirmed, this would indicate that relief of symptoms with medical therapy might be masking hemodynamic or electrical instability, and thus be dangerous.

Chronic mitral regurgitation

Symptomatic disease Grade B – The onset of symptoms of congestive heart failure, or a more subtle decrease in exercise tolerance, is usually indicative of a change in physiologic status which usually has important clinical significance. The onset of new atrial fibrillation is also probably indicative of a significant change in disease status. Further, atrial fibrillation by itself leads to increased morbidity and decreased cardiac output. In most cases, the onset of symptoms or persistent atrial fibrillation is an indication for mitral valve surgery even when objective indicators of left ventricular function do not show advancement to dysfunction. Early surgery in the mildly

symptomatic patient is especially indicated when there is a high probability that mitral valve repair can be effected. In this circumstance there is no need to delay longer, waiting for more severe symptoms or the onset of more apparent left ventricular dysfunction. A valve repair will allow improvement in lifestyle while at the same time avoiding the risks of a prosthesis. Early surgery may be especially important when mitral regurgitation is due to a flail leaflet, because this condition may be associated with a modest increase in the risk of sudden death.[29] If preoperative evaluation indicates that repair is unlikely, close follow up of the patient is indicated. If symptoms continue to worsen, or if left ventricular dysfunction develops, mitral competence should be restored.

In the patient with mild symptoms and normal left ventricular function, transesophageal echocardiography to determine valve anatomy is crucial. This procedure is the best preoperative test to define whether or not repair can be performed or if replacement will be necessary.

Assessment of left ventricular function – A major goal in the management of the patient with mitral regurgitation is to correct the lesion prior to the development of irreversible left ventricular contractile dysfunction. Unfortunately, contractility is difficult to measure clinically. Standard ejection phase indices, such as ejection fraction, which are used to gauge left ventricular function in most cardiac diseases, are confounded by the abnormal loading conditions present in mitral regurgitation, necessitating alterations in the way these indices are used.[30] Because ejection fraction is augmented by increased preload in mitral regurgitation[31] the value for ejection fraction should be supernormal in the face of normal contractility. A "normal" ejection fraction for the patient with mitral regurgitation is probably 0·65–0·75. Indeed, Enriquez-Sarano and colleagues[32] have demonstrated that once the ejection fraction falls to less than 0·60 in patients with mitral regurgitation, long-term mortality is increased, suggesting that left ventricular dysfunction has already developed at that threshold for ejection fraction.

End-systolic dimension, which is less dependent upon preload, has also been developed as an important indicator of left ventricular dysfunction in this disease. As demonstrated in Figure 52.2, when the end-systolic dimension exceeds 45 mm, the postoperative outcome is worsened.[33] This figure, or its angiographic equivalent, has been found to be predictive in other studies.[34,35] Careful evaluation of the patient with mitral regurgitation with history and physical examination, augmented by serial echocardiograms, should avoid the situation in which unrecognized left ventricular dysfunction develops. Yearly follow up is probably adequate as long as the ejection fraction exceeds 0·65 and the end-systolic dimension is less than 40 mm. If the ejection fraction is lower or the end-systolic dimension is higher, more frequent follow up is indicated. When the ejection fraction approaches 0·60 or when the end-systolic dimension approaches 45 mm, surgery should be contemplated.

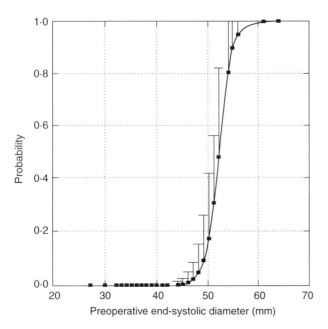

Figure 52.2 Plot of an S-shaped curve-related computed probability of postoperative death or severe heart failure to measured preoperative end-systolic diameter. Individual data coordinates are indicated by solid squares and bars represent upper 95% confidence intervals that were computed from the standard error (some points are overlapping; total *n* = 61). (Reproduced with permission from Wisenbaugh *et al.*[31])

Indications for surgery in the asymptomatic patient with mitral regurgitation

Patients with normal left ventricular function **Grade B** – At first glance the asymptomatic patient with mitral regurgitation who has normal left ventricular function would not seem to require surgery. In this patient, surgery will neither improve lifestyle nor prevent reversible left ventricular dysfunction from developing imminently. However, patients with flail leaflet may become symptomatic within the next year[29] and may be at some increased risk for sudden death.

In other cases where it is apparent that the severity of mitral regurgitation will eventually necessitate surgery, it could be argued that if mitral valve repair can be performed, little is to be gained by waiting. This circumstance is much like atrial septal defect, where at low operative mortality (less than 1%) the defect can be repaired without the use of a prosthesis before unwanted sequelae develop (in the case of atrial septal defect, persistent atrial arrhythmias and pulmonary hypertension; in the case of mitral regurgitation, left ventricular dysfunction). If this approach is taken it must be clear that repair rather than replacement can be effected. If the asymptomatic patient with normal left ventricular function is ultimately treated with a prosthesis when a repair had been anticipated, it should be considered a complication of surgery, as the unwanted risks of a prosthesis could have been at least temporarily avoided.

Asymptomatic patients with left ventricular dysfunction **Grade B** – It is the asymptomatic patient with left ventricular dysfunction at whom serial follow up is aimed. If left ventricular dysfunction has developed (ejection fraction < 0·6, endsystolic dimension > 45 mm), surgery should be performed to prevent further irreversible left ventricular dysfunction even if it entails a prosthetic valve. As left ventricular dysfunction has already been indicated by non-invasive testing in such patients, every effort should be made to spare at least part of the mitral valve apparatus to prevent a further decline in left ventricular function postoperatively.

Asymptomatic elderly patients **Grade C** – Patients over the age of 75 with mitral regurgitation are at increased risk for operative death and a poor outcome. This is especially true if replacement instead of repair is performed, or if concomitant coronary disease – a consequence of aging – is present.[12,36] Thus, elderly asymptomatic patients with mild left ventricular dysfunction should probably be managed medically. Only patients with severe symptoms in whom medical therapy is ineffective should undergo this relatively high-risk procedure. A summary of indications for surgery is given in Table 52.1.

Table 52.1   Indications for mitral surgery in asymptomatic patients with severe non-ischemic mitral regurgitation

Repair likely	Repair unlikely
Patient aged <75 with flail leaflet	—
Patient aged <75 with persistent atrial fibrillation	—
Patient aged <75 with EF <0·60 or ESD >45 mm	Patient aged < 75 with EF < 0·60 or ESD > 45 mm

Abbreviations: EF, ejection fraction; ESD, end-systolic minor axis dimension

Establishment of symptom status – Because of the insidious nature of mitral valve disease, patients may subtly alter their lifestyle to maintain their asymptomatic status. Thus, history alone may fail to identify this gradual decline in exercise tolerance. Therefore, in patients with mitral valve disease, formal exercise testing is useful to objectively quantify changes in exercise tolerance over the time of follow up and to separate truly asymptomatic patients from those who avoid situations that produce symptoms.

Far advanced disease Grade B

Occasionally patients reach the first attention of the physician when in severe congestive heart failure, with far advanced left ventricular dysfunction. Many patients in this category may benefit from surgery because correction of mitral regurgitation will lower left atrial pressure and perhaps increase forward output. However, in such cases postoperative left ventricular function will remain depressed and lifespan is likely to be shortened. It is often difficult to decide whether left ventricular dysfunction is so far advanced that surgery should not be performed. The answer to this question is predicated upon the kind of operation that is contemplated. If repair with sparing of most chordal structures can be performed, patients with an ejection fraction as low as 30% can survive surgery with postoperative ejection performance maintained at this relatively low level.[2] However, for patients with an ejection fraction <40% in whom only mitral valve replacement can be performed, operative mortality might be prohibitive. Wisenbaugh[33] has further suggested that if the end-systolic dimension exceeds 50 mm in patients with rheumatic mitral regurgitation, postoperative risk is extremely high whether repair can be effected or not.

Ischemic mitral regurgitation Grade C

The prognosis for ischemic mitral regurgitation remains substantially worse than for non-ischemic disease.[37,38] A worsened prognosis probably accrues from the automatic presence of a second potentially fatal and independently progressive cardiac disease, and from the presence of ischemic myocardial dysfunction. Guidelines for surgery are not well developed. Common sense indicates that surgery should be performed when ischemic mitral regurgitation has caused shock or intractable pulmonary congestion.

Medical therapy Grade C

Apart from the use of prophylactic antibiotics against infective endocarditis, there is no proven medical therapy for chronic mitral regurgitation. Although vasodilators are effective in treating the acute disease, no large long-term trials have been performed to examine their effect in chronic disease.

The trials that have been performed differ regarding benefit from this therapy.[39,40] Further, because afterload is not typically elevated in chronic mitral regurgitation, the physiologic underpinnings for vasodilators used for afterload reduction are less clear. In fact, vasodilators in this case might lead to cardiac atrophy, potentially putting the patient at a disadvantage when mitral valve replacement is finally performed.

Summary

Patients with acute mitral regurgitation and severe hemodynamic instability require surgical correction. In less severe situations medical therapy may allow the patient to enter the chronic compensated phase, in which surgery can be delayed.

When symptoms develop in chronic mitral regurgitation, they are usually an indication for valve surgery. This is especially true if left ventricular dysfunction is developing, or if it is certain that a mitral valve repair can be performed. In asymptomatic patients with normal ventricular function surgery should only be contemplated when there is a certainty of repair. On the other hand, if left ventricular dysfunction is developing surgery should be performed to prevent further deterioration, whether or not a repair can be effected.

Mitral stenosis

Etiology and pathophysiology

Most mitral stenosis in adults is acquired through rheumatic heart disease. In developed countries it typically appears in women in their fourth or fifth decade. In developing nations, where the rheumatic process appears to be more aggressive, stenosis may develop in adolescence or early adulthood.

As mitral stenosis worsens, a gradient develops between the left atrium and left ventricle during diastole. At the same time the stenotic valve impairs left ventricular filling, limiting cardiac output. The combination of pulmonary congestion caused by left atrial hypertension and diminished forward cardiac output caused by inflow obstruction mimics the hemodynamics of left ventricular failure, even though the left ventricle itself is usually spared from the rheumatic process, especially in developed countries.[41] However, in approximately one third of patients left ventricular ejection performance is reduced despite no impairment in contractility.[42] Reduced ejection fraction is caused by reduced preload from the impairment of left ventricular filling and from increased left ventricular afterload secondary to reflex systemic vasoconstriction in the face of decreased cardiac output. Ejection performance may return to normal shortly after mitral stenosis is relieved.[43]

Although the left ventricle is usually spared from direct involvement in this disease, the right ventricle experiences pressure overload because it supplies the hemodynamic force propelling blood across the stenotic mitral valve. Thus, as left atrial pressure rises, pulmonary pressure and right ventricular pressure also must increase, placing a pressure overload on the right ventricle. For reasons that are unclear, as the disease progresses reversible pulmonary vasoconstriction develops, leading to a worsening of pulmonary hypertension and eventually to right ventricular failure.

Indications for surgery Grade B

In most cases mitral stenosis can be relieved by balloon valvotomy, which offers results comparable to those of open commissurotomy, as shown in a randomized trial.[44] Surgery is reserved for those cases in which valve anatomy is unfavorable for balloon valvotomy, or in which balloon valvotomy has been attempted and failed. Although in some instances open surgical commissurotomy can be successful even though balloon valvotomy was predicted to be unsuccessful, the unfavorable anatomy for balloon valvotomy will also be unfavorable for commissurotomy, necessitating valve replacement. Thus when surgery is anticipated, the risks and complications of a prosthesis should also be anticipated.

The timing of surgery for mitral stenosis can largely be predicated on symptomatic status, as shown in Figure 52.3.[45]

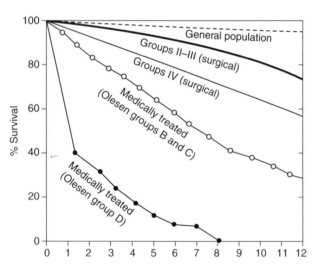

Figure 52.3 Comparison between surgical and medical treatment in patients with mitral stenosis. Groups II, III and IV, equivalent to NYHA classifications II, III and IV, are approximately similar to the groups represented by letters B, C and D, respectively. Class IV patients had better improved survival when treated surgically than did class D patients who were treated medically. Class II and III patients also had better survival when treated surgically than did the patients in groups B and C, although the difference is not as dramatic. (Reproduced with permission from Roy and Gopinath.[45])

Once more than New York Heart Association (NYHA) class II symptoms develop, mortality increases abruptly and surgery should be performed before class III symptoms appear. In addition, some studies indicate that the presence of pulmonary hypertension substantially increases operative risk,[35,46] and so surgery should be contemplated in patients who develop asymptomatic pulmonary hypertension (pulmonary artery systolic pressure >50 mmHg). When surgery precedes severe pulmonary hypertension, operative mortality, even with the insertion of a prosthesis, is 1–3%.

The most difficult situation for timing surgery arises in the young woman who wishes to bear children. In such patients in whom balloon valvotomy has already been ruled out because of unfavorable valve anatomy, the choice of prosthetic valve becomes quite difficult. If a mechanical valve is placed it will require anticoagulation, which is problematic during pregnancy. Administration of warfarin causes a particularly high incidence of fetal malformation, especially when used during the first trimester. It can be substituted by daily injections of heparin, but serious thrombotic complications have occurred in such circumstances, suggesting that this therapy is inadequate in at least some cases.[47] On the other hand, if a bioprosthesis is placed in a young woman it is likely to degenerate within a decade or sooner, forcing the patient to have a reoperation with its attendant increased surgical risk. There is no correct solution to this dilemma, and the prosthesis that is eventually inserted is chosen after lengthy consultation between patient and surgeon.

Summary Grade B

In most cases mitral stenosis can be treated successfully with balloon valvotomy. However, if this procedure is unfeasible, open commissurotomy or valve replacement is indicated for those with NYHA symptoms greater than class II, or for the development of pulmonary hypertension.

References

1. Carabello BA. Timing surgery for mitral regurgitation in asymptomatic patients. *Choices Cardiol* 1991;**5**:137–8.
2. Goldman ME, Mora F, Guarino T, Fuster V, Mindich BP. Mitral valvuloplasty is superior to valve replacement for preservation of left ventricular function. An intraoperative two-dimensional echocardiographic study. *J Am Coll Cardiol* 1987;**10**:568–75.
3. Carabello BA. Mitral regurgitation, Part 1: basic pathophysiologic principles. *Mod Concepts Cardiovasc Dis* 1988;**57**:53–8.
4. Cheitlin MD, Douglas PS, Parmley WW. 26th Bethesda Conference: recommendations for determining eligibility for competition in athletes with cardiovascular abnormalities. Task Force 2: acquired valvular heart disease. *J Am Coll Cardiol* 1994;**24**:874–80.
5. Urabe Y, Mann DL, Kent RL *et al.* Cellular and ventricular contractile dysfunction in experimental canine mitral regurgitation. *Circ Res* 1992;**70**:131–47.

6. Mulieri LA, Leavitt BJ, Martin BJ, Haeberle JR, Alpert NR. Myocardial force–frequency defect in mitral regurgitation heart failure is reversed by forskolin. *Circulation* 1993;**88**:2700–4.

7. Rushmer RF. Initial phase of ventricular systole: asynchronous contraction. *Am J Physiol* 1956;**184**:188–94.

8. Lillehei CW, Levy MJ, Bonnabeau RC. Mitral valve replacement with preservation of papillary muscles and chordae tendineae. *J Thorac Cardiovasc Surg* 1964;**47**:532–43.

9. Hansen DE, Cahill PD, DeCampli WM *et al.* Valvular-ventricular interaction: importance of the mitral apparatus in canine left ventricular systolic performance. *Circulation* 1986; **73**:1310–20.

10. Rozich JD, Carabello BA, Usher BW *et al.* Mitral valve replacement with and without chordal preservation in patients with chronic mitral regurgitation. Mechanisms for differences in postoperative ejection performance. *Circulation* 1992; **86**:1718–26.

11. David TE, Burns RJ, Bacchus CM, Druck MN. Mitral valve replacement for mitral regurgitation with and without preservation of chordae tendineae. *J Thorac Cardiovasc Surg* 1984;**88**:718–25.

12. Enriquez-Sarano M, Schaff HV, Orszulak TA *et al.* Valve repair improves the outcome of surgery for mitral regurgitation. A multivariate analysis. *Circulation* 1995;**91**:1022–8.

13. Duran CG, Pomar JL, Revuelta JM *et al.* Conservative operation for mitral insufficiency: critical analysis supported by postoperative hemodynamic studies in 72 patients. *J Thorac Cardiovasc Surg* 1980;**79**:326–37.

14. Horskotte D, Schulte HD, Bircks W, Strauer BE. The effect of chordal preservation on late outcome after mitral valve replacement: a randomized study. *J Heart Valve Dis* 1993;**2**:150–8.

15. Cohn LH, Couper GS, Aranki SF *et al.* Long-term results of mitral valve reconstruction for regurgitation of the myxomatous mitral valve. *Cardiovasc Surg* 1994;**107**:143–51.

16. Cosgrove DM, Chavez AM, Lytle BW *et al.* Results of mitral valve reconstruction. *Circulation* 1986;**74**(Suppl. I):I-82–I-87.

17. Wells FC. Conservation and surgical repair of the mitral valve. In: Wells FC, Shapiro LM, eds. *Mitral valve disease*, 2nd edn. Oxford: Butterworth–Heinemann, 1996.

18. Castello R, Fagan L Jr, Lenzen P, Pearson AC, Labovitz AJ. Comparison of transthoracic and transesophageal echocardiography for assessment of left-sided valve regurgitation. *Am J Cardiol* 1991;**68**:1677–80.

19. Smith MD, Kwan OL, Spain MG, DeMaria AN. Temporal variability of color Doppler jet areas in patients with aortic and mitral regurgitation. *Am Heart J* 1992;**123**:953–60.

20. Slater J, Gindea AJ, Freedberg RS *et al.* Comparison of cardiac catheterization and Doppler echocardiography in the decision to operate in aortic and mitral valve disease. *J Am Coll Cardiol* 1991;**17**:1026–36.

21. Recusani F, Bargiggia GS, Yoganathan AP *et al.* A new method for quantification of regurgitant flow rate using color Doppler flow imaging of the flow convergence region proximal to a discrete orifice: an in vitro study. *Circulation* 1991;**83**: 594–604.

22. Utsunomiya T, Ogawa T, Doshi R *et al.* Doppler color flow "proximal isovelocity surface area" method for estimating volume flow rate: effects of orifice shape and machine factors. *J Am Coll Cardiol* 1991;**17**:1103–11.

23. Vandervoort PM, Rivera JM, Mele D *et al.* Application of color Doppler flow mapping to calculate effective regurgitant orifice area: an in vitro study and initial clinical observations. *Circulation* 1993;**88**:1150–6.

24. Enriquez-Sarano M, Miller FA Jr, Hayes SN *et al.* Effective mitral regurgitant orifice area: clinical use and pitfalls of the proximal isovelocity surface area method. *J Am Coll Cardiol* 1995;**25**:703–9.

25. Yoran C, Yellin EL, Becker RM *et al.* Mechanisms of reduction of mitral regurgitation with vasodilator therapy. *Am J Cardiol* 1979;**43**:773–7.

26. Nishimura RA, Schaff HV, Shub C *et al.* Papillary muscle rupture complicating acute myocardial infarction: analysis of 17 patients. *Am J Cardiol* 1983;**51**:373–7.

27. Nishimura RA, Schaff HV, Gersh BJ, Holmes DR Jr, Tajik AJ. Early repair of mechanical complications after acute myocardial infarction. *JAMA* 1986;**256**:47–50.

28. Grigioni F, Enriquez-Sarano M, Ling LH *et al.* Sudden death in mitral regurgitation due to flail leaflet. *J Am Coll Cardiol* 1999;**34**:2078–85.

29. Ling LH, Enriquez-Sarano M, Seward JB *et al.* Clinical outcome of mitral regurgitation due to flail leaflet. *N Engl J Med* 1996;**335**:1417–23.

30. Eckberg DL, Gault JH, Bouchard RL, Karliner JS, Ross J Jr. Mechanics of left ventricular contraction in chronic severe mitral regurgitation. *Circulation* 1973;**47**:1252–9.

31. Wisenbaugh T, Spann JF, Carabello BA. Differences in myocardial performance and load between patients with similar amounts of chronic aortic versus chronic mitral regurgitation. *J Am Coll Cardiol* 1984;**3**:916–23.

32. Enriquez-Sarano M, Tajik AJ, Schaff HV *et al.* Echocardiographic prediction of survival after surgical correction of organic mitral regurgitation. *Circulation* 1994;**90**:830–7.

33. Wisenbaugh T, Skudicky D, Sareli P. Prediction of outcome after valve replacement for rheumatic mitral regurgitation in the era of chordal preservation. *Circulation* 1994;**89**:191–7.

34. Zile MR, Gaasch WH, Carroll JD, Levine HF. Chronic mitral regurgitation: predictive value of preoperative echocardiographic indexes of left ventricular function and wall stress. *J Am Coll Cardiol* 1984;**3**:235–42.

35. Crawford MH, Souchek J, Oprian CA *et al.* Determinants of survival and left ventricular performance after mitral valve replacement. Department of Veterans Affairs Cooperative Study on Valvular Heart Disease. *Circulation* 1990;**81**:1173–81.

36. Nair CK, Biddle WP, Kaneshige A *et al.* Ten-year experience with mitral valve replacement in the elderly. *Am Heart J* 1992;**124**:154–9.

37. Connolly MW, Gelbfish JS, Jacobowitz IJ *et al.* Surgical results for mitral regurgitation from coronary artery disease. *J Thorac Cardiovasc Surg* 1986;**91**:379–88.

38. Akins CW, Hilgenberg AD, Buckley MJ *et al.* Mitral valve reconstruction versus replacement for degenerative or ischemic mitral regurgitation. *Ann Thorac Surg* 1994;**58**: 668–75.

39. Schon HR, Schroter G, Barthel P, Schomig A. Quinapril therapy in patients with chronic mitral regurgitation. *J Heart Valve Dis* 1994;**3**:303–12.

40. Wisenbaugh T, Sinovich V, Dullabh A, Sareli P. Six month pilot study of captopril for mildly symptomatic, severe isolated mitral

and isolated aortic regurgitation. *J Heart Valve Dis* 1994;**3**:197–204.

41. Hildner FJ, Javier RP, Cohen LS *et al.* Myocardial dysfunction associated with valvular heart disease. *Am J Cardiol* 1972;**30**: 319–26.

42. Gash AK, Carabello BA, Cepin D, Spann JF. Left ventricular ejection performance and systolic muscle function in patients with mitral stenosis. *Circulation* 1983;**67**:148–54.

43. Liu C-P, Ting C-T, Yang T-M *et al.* Reduced left ventricular compliance in human mitral stenosis. Role of reversible internal constraint. *Circulation* 1992;**85**:1447–56.

44. Reyes VP, Raju BS, Wynne J *et al.* Percutaneous balloon valvuloplasty compared with open surgical commissurotomy for mitral stenosis. *N Engl J Med* 1994;**331**:961–7.

45. Roy SB, Gopinath N. Mitral stenosis. *Circulation* 1968; **38**(Suppl. V):V68–76.

46. Ward C, Hancock BW. Extreme pulmonary hypertension caused by mitral valve disease. Natural history and results of surgery. *Br Heart J* 1975;**37**:74–8.

47. Sbarouni E, Oakley CM. Outcome of pregnancy in women with valve prostheses. *Br Heart J* 1994;**71**:196–201.

53 Indications for surgery in aortic valve disease

Heidi M Connolly, Shahbudin H Rahimtoola

Evidence-based management of patients with aortic valve disease is limited by the absence of prospective randomized trials of surgery versus medical therapy. There is one prospective randomized trial evaluating patient outcome with use of a pharmacologic agent in patients with aortic valve regurgitation. However, evidence can also be obtained from retrospective studies. This evidence is extremely useful and important in the management of patients.

Sir Thomas Lewis pointed out 80 years ago the inadequacy of knowledge of prognosis in patients with heart disease. He proposed a system for prospective follow up of patients, which we now call "databases" or "registries". The latter are, of course, the major evidence used in this chapter to delineate the indications for surgery. The American College of Cardiology and American Heart Association published *Guidelines for the management of patients with valvular heart disease*.[1] This document has provided an important framework upon which clinical decisions can be based.

Aortic valve stenosis

Etiology

A wide variety of disorders may produce aortic valve obstruction;[2] however, those that result in severe stenosis in adults are:

- congenital
- acquired
  - calcific (degenerative)
  - autoimmune
- rheumatic.

The most common cause of aortic stenosis in younger adults is a congenital bicuspid valve, which is found in 1–2% of the general population. Rheumatic heart disease is still common in developing countries. In most patients aged ≥40 years, the severely stenotic valve is calcified. In patients aged ≥65 years, 90% of severely stenotic valves are tricuspid. Non-rheumatic calcified valves are thought to be "degenerative" but recent data suggest that it may be the result of an autoimmune reaction to antigens present in the valve;[3] and that the initial process may be an atherosclerotic lesion.[4,5]

Grading the degree of stenosis

The natural history of aortic stenosis is variable depending on the degree of stenosis and the rate at which it progresses. Cardiac catheterization and echocardiographic–Doppler ultrasound studies indicate the systolic pressure gradient increases on an average by 10–15 mmHg per year. The 10–15 mmHg increase is a linearized value whereas the increase is not linear but a stepwise function with periods of steady state interspersed by an increase in gradient. The range of progression is also wide. Recent data suggest that the progression of aortic stenosis may be related to cardiovascular risk factors.[6] The systolic gradient across the stenotic aortic valve is dependent on the following:

- the stroke volume (not the cardiac output because the gradient and valve area are a per beat, and not a per minute, function)
- the systolic ejection period
- systolic pressure in the ascending aorta.

The stenotic valve area is inversely related to the square root of the mean systolic gradient. Thus, measurement of valve area is an important part of the assessment of the severity of aortic valve stenosis. The valve area may decrease by as much as $0{\cdot}12 \pm 0{\cdot}19\,cm^2$ per year.[7]

Valve area is related to the body surface area and increases in larger individuals, probably because of the need for a larger stroke volume and cardiac output. The normal aortic valve area ranges from 3 to $4\,cm^2$. It is reduced to half its size before a systolic gradient occurs.[8] The orifice area has to be reduced to one third of its size before significant hemodynamic changes are seen;[9] gradients increase precipitously after that. The obvious clinical problem is that in an individual patient with aortic stenosis one usually does not know the valve area prior to the onset of disease. Echocardiography is usually the initial procedure used to confirm the presence and determine the severity of aortic valve stenosis.[10] In an experienced center the severity of aortic stenosis determined by Doppler echocardiography correlates reasonably well with the severity determined by cardiac catheterization.[11] A comprehensive echocardiographic examination in aortic valve stenosis should include assessment of the aortic valve peak and mean gradient as well as aortic valve area.[12] When the clinical picture does not correlate with the hemodynamic data obtained by Doppler echocardiography, re-evaluation by cardiac catheterization is indicated.

The outcome of patients with severe aortic valve stenosis was described by Ross and Braunwald[13] after review of seven autopsy studies published before 1955, and Horstkotte and Loogen[14] reported on 35 patients (10 of whom were asymptomatic) with aortic valve area of <0·8 cm² by cardiac catheterization who refused surgery. The findings are shown in Table 53.1.

The mortality of symptomatic patients with "severe" aortic stenosis from eight studies[15] is given in Table 53.2.

Mild aortic stenosis

The classification of the severity of aortic valve stenosis was defined in the guidelines provided by the Committee on

Valvular Heart Disease.[1] In this document aortic valve stenosis is defined as mild when the aortic valve area was >1·5 cm². In two studies, patients with aortic valve area >1·5 cm² by catheterization had no mortality on follow up. At the end of 10 years, in one study 8% had severe stenosis, and in the other 15% had a cardiac event. At the end of 20 years, aortic stenosis had become severe in only 20% and continued to be mild in 63%.[14,15]

Moderate aortic stenosis

Moderate aortic valve stenosis is defined as a valve area of >1·0–1·5 cm². In one study in which patients were followed after cardiac catheterization, the 1 year and 10 year mortality was 3% and 15%, respectively; and at 10 years 65% of patients had had a cardiac event.[15]

Severe aortic stenosis

Several criteria have been used to define severe aortic stenosis. The guidelines provided by the Committee on Valvular Heart Disease[1] describes severe aortic valve stenosis as an aortic valve area ≤1·0 cm² and a mean aortic pressure gradient, in the setting of normal cardiac output, of >50 mmHg. This definition was supported by data from a large multicenter database (492 patients) which suggested that the 1 year mortality of those with aortic valve areas after catheter balloon valvuloplasty for calcific aortic stenosis of ≤0·7 cm² versus that of those with valve areas >0·7 cm² was 37% versus 42%, respectively.[16] Kennedy and coworkers[17] reported on 66 patients with aortic valve areas of 0·7–1·2 cm² (0·92±0·15 cm²), normal left ventricular volumes and ejection fraction, whose average age was 67 years. In an average follow up of 35 months, 21% died and 32% had valve replacement; at 4 years, the actuarial incidence of death or valve replacement was 41%.[17] Thus, these studies show that patients with aortic valve areas of 0·7–1·0 cm² have an outcome without valve replacement that is not benign, and is not consonant with moderate

Table 53.1 Survival, according to symptoms, of patients with "severe" aortic stenosis

Symptoms	Average survival	
	Autopsy data[a] (years)	Post cardiac catheterization[b] (months)
Overall	3	23
Angina[c]	5	45
Syncope	3	27
Heart failure	<2	11

[a] Data of Ross and Braunwald.[13]
[b] Data of Horstkotte and Loogen.[14]
[c] Angina in patients with aortic stenosis occurs even in those without associated obstructive CAD.

Table 53.2 Mortality of symptomatic patients with "severe" aortic stenosis[15]

Authors	Year of publication	Patients (n)	Mortality follow up time (years)					
			1	2	3	5	10	11
Frank et al[23]	1973	15			36%	52%	90%	
Rapaport[84]	1975					62%	80%	
Chizner et al[85]	1980	23	26%	48%		64%		94%
Schwarz et al[30]	1982	19			79%			
O'Keefe et al[86]	1987	50	43%	63%	75%			
Turina et al[87]	1987	50	40%					
Kelly et al[88]	1988	39	38%					
Horstkotte et al[14]	1988	35			82%			

stenosis; these patients should be considered as having severe stenosis. Since gradients are frequently measured initially by Doppler ultrasound, a suggested conservative guideline for relating Doppler ultrasound gradient to severity of aortic stenosis (AS) in adults with normal cardiac output and normal average heart rate is shown in Table 53.3.

A suggested grading of the degree of aortic stenosis is given in Table 53.4.

Table 53.3 Doppler ultrasound gradient as an indicator of severe aortic stenosis (AS)

Peak gradient	Mean gradient	AS severe
≥80 mmHg	≥70 mmHg	High likely
60–79 mmHg	50–69 mmHg	Probable
<60 mmHg	<50 mmHg	Uncertain

From Rahimtoola,[15] with permission

Table 53.4 Grading of stenosis by aortic valve area (AVA)

Aortic stenosis	AVA (cm^2)	AVA index (cm^2/m^2)
Mild	>1·5	>0·9
Moderate	1·1–1·5	>0·6–0·9
Severe[a]	≤1·0	≤0·6

[a] Patients with AVAs that are at borderline values between the moderate and severe grades (0·9–1·1 cm^2; 0·55–0·65 cm^2/m^2) should be individually considered.
From Rahimtoola[15] with permission

Natural history

The duration of the asymptomatic period after the development of severe aortic stenosis is uncertain. In a study of asymptomatic patients with varying degrees of severity of aortic stenosis, 21% of 143 patients[18] with a mean age of 72 years required valve replacement within 3 months of evaluation at a referral center. At 2 years the mortality was 10% and the event rate (death/valve replacement) in the remaining patients was 26%. Moreover, it is important to recognize that most patients in this study had only *moderate* aortic stenosis. In another study of 123 asymptomatic adults,[7] also with varying grades of severity of aortic stenosis aged 63±16 years, only the actuarial probability of death or aortic valve surgery is provided. It was 7±5% at 1 year, 38±8% at 3 years and 74±10% at 5 years. The event rate at 2 years for aortic jet velocity by Doppler ultrasound of >4·0 m/s (peak gradient by Doppler ultrasound >64 mmHg) was 79±18%, for a velocity of 3·0–4·0 m/s (peak gradient 36–64 mmHg) was 66±13%, and for a velocity of <3·0 m/s

(peak gradient of <36 mmHg) was 16±16%.[7] Aortic jet velocity is influenced by the same parameters as aortic valve gradient (see above). Thus, the duration of the asymptomatic period, particularly in those aged ≥60 years, is probably very short.[19,20]

Paul Dudley White in 1951[21] credited the first recorded occurrence of sudden death to T Bonet in 1679.[22] In the past 70 years the reported incidence of sudden death in eight series has ranged from 1 to 21%. Ross and Braunwald,[13] after reviewing seven autopsy series published before 1955, concluded the incidence was 3–5%. The incidence in asymptomatic adult patients has been 33% (one in three)[23] and 30% (three of ten).[14] This information is difficult to use in clinical decision making because important data are not available – that is, the incidence by actuarial analysis of sudden death in a significant number of asymptomatic patients with severe stenosis. It is reasonable to conclude that the true incidence of sudden death in adults with severe aortic valve stenosis is unknown and that sudden death usually occurs after the onset of symptoms, however minor or minimal the symptoms may be. The incidence of sudden death is believed to be higher in children.

The development of symptoms of angina, syncope, or heart failure, changes the prognosis of the patient with aortic valve stenosis. Average survival after the onset of symptoms is <2–3 years. Nearly 80% of asymptomatic patients with peak aortic valve velocity measured by Doppler echocardiography ≥4 m/s develop symptoms within 3 years, and therefore careful clinical monitoring for the development of symptoms and progressive disease is indicated.

Management

Patients with valvular heart disease need antibiotic prophylaxis against infective endocarditis; those with rheumatic valves need additional antibiotic prophylaxis against recurrences of rheumatic fever.[24] **Grade A**

Surgery is recommended in those with severe valve stenosis and is the only specific and direct therapy for most adults with severe aortic stenosis. Rarely, in young patients, the aortic valve is suitable for balloon or surgical valvotomy. In most adults, surgery for aortic stenosis means valve replacement.[24,25] **Grade B**

The operative mortality of valve replacement is ≤5%.[25–27] In those without associated coronary artery disease, heart failure or other comorbid conditions, it is ≤2% in experienced and skilled centers.[28] Aortic valve replacement in conjunction with coronary artery bypass carries a surgical mortality of about 7%.[27] The operative mortality in those ≥70 years and in octogenarians is much higher, averaging 8% for valve replacement and 13% for those undergoing valve replacement and associated coronary bypass surgery;[25] however, operative mortality in these patients is also dependent on the associated factors listed above.[29]

Patients with associated coronary artery disease (CAD) should have coronary bypass surgery at the same time as valve replacement, because it results in a lower operative mortality (4·0% v 9·4%) and better 10 year survival (49% v 36%).[28] This was in spite of the fact that those who underwent coronary bypass surgery had more CAD (34% had three vessel disease, 11% had left main artery disease, and 38% had single vessel disease) than those who did not undergo coronary bypass surgery (13% had three vessel disease, 1% had left main disease, and 65% had single vessel disease).[28] Although this approach to CAD is generally approved, there are no randomized trials to support these recommendations. The presence of CAD, its site and severity can be estimated only by selective coronary angiography, which should be performed in all patients 35 years of age or older who are being considered for aortic valve surgery, and in those aged

<35 years if they have left ventricular dysfunction, symptoms or signs suggesting CAD, or they have two or more risk factors for premature CAD (excluding gender).[25] The incidence of associated CAD will vary considerably depending on the prevalence of CAD in the population;[15,24] in general, in persons 50 years of age or older it is about 50%.[25]

In severe aortic stenosis, valve replacement results in an improvement of survival (Figure 53.1) even if they have normal left ventricular function preoperatively.[14,30]

Normal preoperative left ventricular function remains normal postoperatively if perioperative myocardial damage has not occurred.[31] Left ventricular hypertrophy regresses toward normal;[31,32] after 2 years, the regression continues at a slower rate up to 10 years after valve replacement.[32]

In patients with excessive preoperative left ventricular hypertrophy,[33] the hypertrophy may regress slowly or not

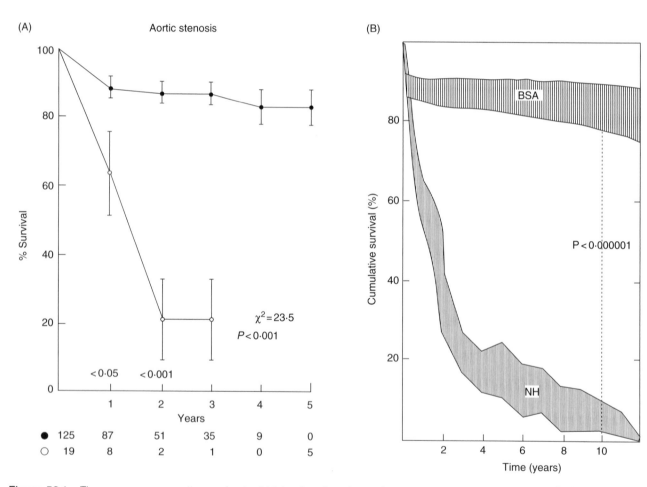

Figure 53.1 There are no prospective randomized trials of aortic valve replacement in severe aortic stenosis (AS), and there are unlikely to be any in the near future. Two studies have compared the results of aortic valve replacement with medical treatment in their own center during the same time period in symptomatic patients with normal left ventricular systolic pump function. (A) Patients who had valve replacement (closed circles) had a much better survival than those treated medically (open circles). (From Schwarz *et al*[30] with permission.) (B) Patients who were treated with valve replacement (BSA) had a better survival than those treated medically (NH). (From Horstkotte and Loogen[14] with permission.) These differences in survival between those treated medically and surgically are so large that there is a great deal of confidence that aortic valve replacement significantly improves the survival of those with severe aortic stenosis. **Grade A**

at all. Preoperatively, these patients have a small left ventricular cavity, severe increase in wall thickness, and "supernormal" ejection fraction; this occurs in 42% of women and 14% of men in those aged ≥60 years.[33] After valve replacement their clinical picture often resembles that of hypertrophic cardiomyopathy without outflow obstruction, which is a difficult clinical condition to treat, both in the early postoperative period and after hospital discharge;[33] therefore, surgery should be performed prior to development of excessive hypertrophy. Surviving patients are functionally improved.[25]

After valve replacement, the 10 year survival is ≥60% and 15 year survival is about 45%.[25,34] One half or more of the late deaths are not related to the prosthesis but to associated cardiac abnormalities and other comorbid conditions.[34] Thus, the late survival will vary in different subgroups of patients. The older patients (≥60 years) have a 12 year actuarial survival of ≥60%.[35] Relative survival refers to survival of patients compared to age- and gender-matched people in the population. The relative 10 year survival after surgery is significantly better in those aged ≥65 than in those aged ≤65 years (94% *v* 81% respectively, Figure 53.2);[36] the 94% relative survival is not significantly different from the 100% relative survival. Thus, surgery should not be denied to those ≥60–65 years old and should be performed early.[25,35–37]

Patients who present with heart failure related to aortic valve stenosis should undergo surgery as soon as possible. Medical treatment in hospital prior to surgery is reasonable but ACE inhibitors should be used with great caution in such patients, and in such a dosage that hypotension and significant fall of blood pressure is avoided. They should not be used if the patient is hypotensive. If heart failure does not respond satisfactorily and rapidly to medical therapy, surgery becomes a matter of considerable urgency.[25] Catheter balloon valvuloplasty has a very limited role in adults with calcific aortic stenosis and carries a risk of >10%. In addition, restenosis and clinical deterioration occur within 6 to 12 months. In adults with aortic stenosis, balloon valvuloplasty is not a substitute for valve replacement but can be a bridge procedure in selected patients.[38] It usually improves patients' hemodynamics and may make them better candidates for valve replacement.

The operative mortality for patients with heart failure has declined: 25 years ago the operative mortality was <20%,[39] but in the current era it is ≤10%.[40] Although this is higher than in patients without heart failure, the risk is justified, because late survival in those who survive the operation is excellent and is far superior to that which can be expected with medical therapy. The 7 year survival of patients who survive operation is 84%.[41] The 5 year survival in those without associated CAD is greater than in those with CAD (69% *v* 39%, *P* = 0·02).[40] Left ventricular function improves in most patients provided there has been no perioperative myocardial damage and becomes normal in two thirds of the patients, unless there was irreversible preoperative

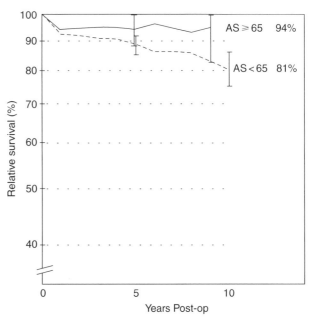

Figure 53.2 Data from the Karolinska Institute in Sweden has provided an interesting perspective on the long-term survival after valve replacement in patients with aortic stenosis (AS) aged ≥65 years. They have examined the relative survival – compared the survival of the patient who has undergone aortic valve replacement with another age and sex matched person in the same population. Actuarial survival ±95% confidence interval is shown. Patients under the age of 65 had a relative survival of 81% which is significantly lower than 100%, and is also lower than that of those aged ≥65 years. On the other hand, patients who underwent valve replacement at age ≥65 had a relative survival of 94% at the end of 10 years and this was not significantly different from 100%. These data indicate that survival following valve replacement for aortic stenosis in patients aged ≥65 is not significantly different from age- and sex-matched individuals in the population without aortic stenosis; and the late relative survival of patients aged ≥65 years is much better than that of patients aged <65. (From Lindblom *et al*[36] with permission.)

myocardial damage (Figure 53.3).[39,40] In addition, the operative survivors are functionally much improved.[39,40] Left ventricular hypertrophy and left ventricular dilation, if present preoperatively, regress toward normal.[39] Despite the excellent results of valve replacement in patients with severe aortic stenosis who are in heart failure, these results are not as good as for those who are not in heart failure; therefore, it is important to recognize that surgery should not be delayed until heart failure develops. **Grade B**

Six per cent of older patients with aortic stenosis present in cardiogenic shock.[38] The hospital mortality in such patients is near 50%. The subsequent mortality is also very high if the patients have not had their aortic stenosis relieved.[38] Thus, these patients need to be managed aggressively by emergency surgery with or without catheter balloon valvuloplasty as a "bridge" procedure.[38]

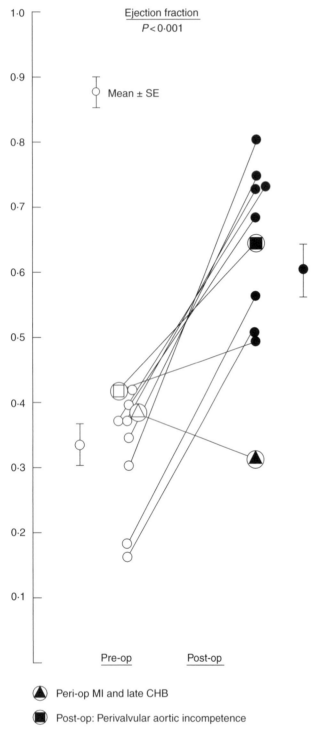

Figure 53.3 Examination of changes in LVEF in each individual patient among those who had left ventricular systolic dysfunction and clinical heart failure. After valve replacement the LVEF improved from 0·34 to 0·63. All but one patient showed an improvement in LVEF; the only patient who showed deterioration in ejection fraction suffered a perioperative myocardial infarction and had a complete heart block; and the only patient who showed only a small increase in ejection fraction had had a myocardial infarct prior to valve replacement. Note that

Boxes 53.1 and 53.2 summarize the results of valve replacement in those with severe aortic stenosis and the factors predictive of a worse postoperative survival, less recovery of left ventricular function, and less improvement of symptoms in those with severe aortic stenosis and preoperative left ventricular systolic dysfunction.[15,25,29–32,34–36,39–41]

Box 53.1   Results of valve replacement in patients with severe aortic valve stenosis
- Improved symptoms and survival in symptomatic patients, especially in those with left ventricular systolic dysfunction, clinical heart failure, and in those aged ≤65 years
- Improvement in left ventricular systolic dysfunction, which normalizes in two thirds of patients
- Regression of left ventricular hypertrophy
- Improvement in functional class, more marked in those with severe symptoms preoperatively

---

Box 53.2   Factors predictive of a less favorable outcome
- Extent and severity of associated comorbid conditions
- Presence and severity of clinical heart failure preoperatively
- Severe associated coronary artery disease
- Severity of depression of preoperative left ventricular ejection fraction
- Duration of preoperative left ventricular systolic dysfunction
- Extent of preoperative irreversible myocardial damage
- Skill and experience of operating and other associated professional teams
- Extent of perioperative myocardial damage
- Complications of a prosthetic heart valve

Patients with severe left ventricular dysfunction, low aortic valve gradient, and small calculated aortic valve area represent a difficult patient population. There is controversy regarding the best management of these patients, in part related to the difficulty differentiating patients with true severe aortic valve stenosis from patients with moderate aortic valve stenosis and severe left ventricular dysfunction. Differentiating these two patient groups may have an important impact on the management decision and the operative outcome. Thus, patients with low gradient aortic valve stenosis should not be denied aortic valve replacement. A recent series confirms that

ejection fraction normalized in two thirds of the patients and, in the two patients with the lowest ejection fraction (0·18 and 0·19), ejection fraction normalized in both. These data indicate that there is probably no lower limit of ejection fraction at which time these patients become inoperable. This also indicates that the lower the ejection fraction, the more urgent the need for valve replacement. (From Smith *et al*[39] with permission.)

the surgical mortality is high and late survival lower than expected. Importantly however, most survivors experienced improvement in functional class and ejection fraction.[42]

A small gradient across the valve may be associated with a small calculated aortic valve area that would be in a range indicating severe aortic stenosis. There are at least two possible causes for this clinical circumstance. First, there is a small or reduced stroke volume and a normal or near normal systolic ejection time; thus, the gradient is small and the calculated aortic valve area correctly indicates severe aortic stenosis. The second consideration is that the stroke volume is reduced, and thus the valve needs to open only to a small extent to allow the left ventricle to eject the small stroke volume. The calculated aortic valve area accurately reflects the extent to which the valve has opened but overestimates the severity of aortic stenosis. Use of a provocative test using an inotropic agent, such as dobutamine,[43,44,45] may allow one to make the correct differentiation between the two. Dobutamine increases systolic flow per second owing to increases in stroke volume or shortening of ejection time or both. In the first circumstance described above, dobutamine will result in an increase in gradient but the calculated valve area remains more or less unchanged. On the other hand, in the second circumstance described above, the gradient may or may not increase with dobutamine but the calculated valve area increases significantly, indicating that the stenosis is not severe. When the dobutamine test is used, it is important to measure cardiac output and simultaneous left ventricular and aortic pressures both before and during dobutamine infusion. Alternatively, the gradient and valve area may be assessed by echocardiography/Doppler during dobutamine infusion; however, one needs to be certain that cardiac output has increased significantly with dobutamine. **Grade B**

Surgery should be advised for the symptomatic patient who has severe aortic stenosis. In young patients, if the valve is pliable and mobile, simple balloon valvuloplasty or surgical commissurotomy may be feasible. Older patients and even young patients with calcified, rigid valves will require valve replacement.

In view of the dismal natural history of symptomatic patients with severe aortic stenosis, the excellent outcome after surgery, and the uncertain natural history of the asymptomatic patient, it is reasonable to recommend aortic valve replacement in select asymptomatic patients in centers with the appropriate skill and experience. The combined risk of surgery and late complications of a valve prosthesis must be weighed against the risk of sudden death. There is no consensus about valve replacement in the truly asymptomatic patient. Clearly, if the patient has left ventricular dysfunction, obstructive CAD or other valve disease that needs surgery, and has severe aortic stenosis, then aortic valve replacement should be performed. Some would recommend valve replacement in all asymptomatic patients with severe aortic stenosis, while others would recommend it in all those with

aortic valve area of $\leq 0.70\,cm^2$ and in selected patients only with aortic valve area of $0.71–1.0\,cm^2$.

Exercise testing should be avoided in symptomatic patients with aortic stenosis but has been used by some cardiologists to help determine which patients with asymptomatic aortic stenosis should be referred for aortic valve replacement.[19] In a small series, Amato and colleagues reported no serious exercise-related complications. During follow up, 6% of the asymptomatic patients (4/66) experienced sudden death; all had a positive exercise test and an aortic valve area of $\leq 0.6\,cm^2$. The exercise test was considered positive if there was a horizontal or down sloping ST segment depression of $\geq 1\,mm$ in men or $\geq 2\,mm$ in women, or an up sloping ST segment depression of $\geq 3\,mm$ in men, measured 0.08 seconds after the J point. The exercise test was also considered positive if precordial chest pain or near syncope occurred, if the ECG showed a complex ventricular arrhythmia, or if systolic blood pressure failed to rise by $\geq 20\,mmHg$ during exercise compared with baseline. **Grade B** It must be emphasized that this is a controversial issue. Some cardiologists advise against exercise testing in any patient with severe aortic valve stenosis, especially when the extent of coronary artery disease is not known.

Recommendations: aortic valve replacement/repair in severe aortic stenosis[1]

Indication	Class
• Symptomatic patients	I
• Asymptomatic patients with:	
• associated significantly obstructed CAD needing surgery	I
• other valve or aortic disease needing surgery	I
• left ventricular systolic dysfunction	IIa
• aged $\geq 60–65$ years	IIa
• abnormal response to exercise	IIa
• severe left ventricular hypertrophy ($\geq 15\,mm$)	IIb
• significant arrhythmias	IIb
• left ventricular dysfunction on exercise	IIb
• Prevention of sudden death in asymptomatic patients	III

CAD, coronary artery disease

Class I: Conditions for which there is evidence and/or general agreement that a given procedure or treatment is useful and effective.

Class II: Conditions for which there is conflicting evidence and/or a divergence of opinion about the usefullness/efficacy of a procedure or treatment.

IIa: Weight of evidence or opinion is in favor of usefullness/efficacy.

IIb: Usefullness/efficacy is less well established by evidence/opinion.

Class III: Conditions for which there is evidence and/or general agreement that the procedure/treatment is not useful, and in some cases, may be harmful.

Chronic aortic valve regurgitation

Etiology

The causes of chronic aortic regurgitation are:[46]

- aortic root/annular dilation
- congenital bicuspid valve
- previous infective endocarditis
- rheumatic
- in association with other diseases.

In developed countries, aortic root/annular dilation and congenital bicuspid valve are the commonest causes of severe chronic aortic regurgitation.

Natural history

During the first world war, Sir Thomas Lewis and his colleagues[47] at Hampstead and Colchester Military Hospitals reported to the Medical Research Council highlighting the inadequacy of the knowledge of heart disease, especially from the standpoint of prognosis. Sir Thomas Lewis proposed a system,[48] subsequently called "after histories",[48] which was a prospective follow up of patients. All patients in RT Grant's "after histories"[48] had valvular heart disease – most had aortic regurgitation – in which the patient characteristics were defined and described in detail, particularly by the degree of cardiac enlargement and the grade of cardiac failure. This probably was the start of databases or registries in cardiovascular medicine.

Chronic aortic valve regurgitation is a condition of combined volume and pressure overload. With progression of the disease, compensatory hypertrophy and recruitment of preload reserve permit the left ventricle to maintain a normal ejection performance despite the elevated afterload. The majority of patients remain asymptomatic throughout the compensated phase, which may last decades. The natural history of chronic aortic valve regurgitation can be considered by three different eras: the era of syphilis, the era of rheumatic fever/carditis, and the current era of noninvasive quantification of left ventricular function.

Era of syphilis

The data are from the 1930s and 1940s, and thus largely prior to availability of antibiotics.[49] The duration from syphilis infection to death was 20 years. The duration of the asymptomatic period after aortic regurgitation was 5 years in 60% of patients; and the 5 year survival was 95%. Once symptoms had developed, the 10 year survival ranged from 40 to 60%. Heart failure was associated with a 1 year survival of 30–50%, and 10 year survival of 6%. In a study of 161 patients reported in 1935, the 10 year survival after heart failure had developed was 34% but was 66% in those treated with arsenic.[49] Syphilis still occurs, but current therapy of syphilis is cheap and efficacious if diagnosed early. Syphilitic aortic regurgitation is

not common, and the outcome in syphilitic aortic regurgitation may be more benign in the current era.

Era of rheumatic fever/carditis

Although the incidence of rheumatic valve disease is low in developed countries, rheumatic heart disease remains the most common form of valve disease in many parts of the world. Moreover, some people now domiciled in the developed world have had their initial attack(s) of acute rheumatic fever whilst living in less developed countries.

The detection of a murmur after the episode of acute rheumatic fever averages 10 years.[49] The average interval from detection of murmur to development of symptoms is 10 years and the percentage of patients remaining symptom-free 10 years after detection of the murmur is 50%.[49]

In 1971, Spagnuolo and coworkers[50] reported the 15 year actuarial follow up of 174 young people who had a median follow up of 10 years. Patients were considered to be in a cumulative high-risk group if they had systolic blood pressure <140 mmHg and/or diastolic blood pressure >40 mmHg, moderate or marked left ventricular enlargement on chest radiography, and two of three ECG abnormalities (S in V2 + R in V5 ≥ 51 mm, ST segment depression or T wave inversion in left ventricular leads). The group's findings are summarized in Table 53.5.

Table 53.5 Reported outcome in 174 young people followed for a mean of 10 years after an episode of rheumatic fever

Symptoms/outcome	Outcome (years)	%
● Cumulative high-risk group		
● mortality	6	30
● angina	7	60
● heart failure	6	60
● mortality or angina or heart failure	6	87
● Cumulative low-risk group		
● Mortality	6	0
	15	5[a]
● Angina	5	2
● Heart failure	6	2
	15	5
● Mortality or angina or heart failure	15	8

[a] The one patient (of the 72 patients) in this subgroup who died had developed two of the three risk factors.

In 1973, Goldschlager and coworkers[51] reported on the duration of the asymptomatic period in 126 patients with varied etiology (Table 53.6).

Table 53.6 Asymptomatic period observed in 126 patients following an episode of rheumatic fever

Age group (years)	Patients symptomatic at 10 years[a] (%)
11–20	0
21–30	24
31–40	35
41–50	71
51–60	77
61–70	89

[a] Symptoms were those of dyspnea, fatigue and, less frequently, chest pain and palpitations. Patients deteriorated from NYHA functional Class I to Classes II, III, or IV. From Goldschlager *et al.*[50]

Table 53.7 Outcomes of patients with severe aortic regurgitation

Outcome	Incidence
Asymptomatic patients with normal left ventricular systolic function[52–59]	
progression to symptoms and/or left ventricular systolic dysfunction	2·4–5·7% per year (average 3·8% per year)
progression to asymptomatic left ventricular dysfunction:	
follow up at 12 month intervals[a][54]	0·9% per year
follow up at 6 month intervals[a][58]	3·4% per year
Sudden death	0·1% per year
Asymptomatic patients with left ventricular systolic dysfunction[60–61]	
progression to cardiac symptoms	>25% per year
Symptomatic patients[50,62–64]	
mortality rate	average >10% per year
angina	>10% per year
heart failure	>20% per year

[a] See text for details.

Current era

In the current era, patients have been followed after noninvasive tests (echocardiography/Doppler ultrasound, radionuclide LVEF) or after invasive studies (cardiac catheterization or angiography). Reported outcomes are shown in Table 53.7.

As outlined in Table 53.7,[52–58,64] the natural history of patients with chronic aortic valve regurgitation depends on the presence or absence of symptoms and on the status of the left ventricle. In asymptomatic patients with normal left ventricular function, data would suggest the progression to symptoms and or left ventricular systolic dysfunction in approximately 4% per year. Sudden death occurs very rarely, 0·1% per year, and asymptomatic left ventricular dysfunction occurs at a rate of 1–3% per year, depending on the frequency of follow up.

There are limited data on asymptomatic patients with reduced left ventricular systolic function. However, available data would suggest that most of these patients will develop symptoms warranting surgery within two to three years, at an average rate of >25% per year.

Limited data are available on the natural history of symptomatic patients with severe aortic valve regurgitation. These patients have a poor prognosis despite medical therapy, with reported mortality rates of 10 and 20% per year in patients with angina and heart failure, respectively.

Important limitations of some of the studies in the literature must be kept in mind. For example, the "natural history" group in one study was composed of several subsets of patients[53] and 36% of this group were on medications for symptoms. Another concern is the true rate of the development of asymptomatic left ventricular dysfunction.[54] At least 25% of patients who develop left ventricular systolic dysfunction do so before they have symptoms, thus emphasizing

the need for quantitative assessment of left ventricular systolic function at follow up in asymptomatic patients with severe aortic regurgitation and normal left ventricular systolic function. More recent studies indicate a poor outcome of symptomatic patients with medical therapy, even among those with preserved systolic function (Table 53.8).[57,65]

Sir William Broadbent[66] stated 100 years ago that "The *age* of the patient at the time when the lesion is acquired is

Table 53.8 Likelihood of symptoms or left ventricular dysfunction or death

● Left ventricular end-diastolic dimension	
≥70 mm	10% per year
<70 mm	2% per year
● Left ventricular end-systolic dimension	
≥50 mm	19% per year
End-systolic dimension >25 mm/m²	8% per year
40–49 mm	6% per year
<40 mm	0% per year

the most important consideration in prognosis ...". In asymptomatic patients with normal left ventricular systolic function, the independent predictors of symptoms, left ventricular systolic dysfunction, and death by multivariate analysis were: older age, decreasing resting LVEF, and left ventricular dimension on M-mode echocardiography.[54] However, in many of these patients, M-mode images were not obtained from two dimensionally directed echocardiograms. Very importantly, most of these dimensions were obtained in the United States, and US women have smaller left ventricular dimensions than men, even when they become symptomatic.[67] Thus, it is unlikely that the above criteria apply to women and almost certainly will not be applicable to populations of smaller body size, for example, Asians, Latin Americans, sub-Saharan Africans, and Orientals. The left ventricular dimension should be corrected to body surface area.[68] Patients also develop symptoms and/or left ventricular systolic dysfunction at a faster rate if their initial left ventricular end-diastolic volume is $\geq 150 \, ml/m^2$ when compared to those with volumes $< 150 \, ml/m^2$.[53] Older age also appears to increase the annual mortality.[68]

Patients with severe ventricular dilation when exercised have shown mean pulmonary artery wedge pressure $\geq 20 \, mmHg$ and/or exercise ejection fraction $< 0{\cdot}50$, and such patients have demonstrated reduced exercise capacity, with reduced maximum Vo_2.[69,70]

Patients who present with ventricular tachycardia, ventricular fibrillation or syncope and have inducible ventricular tachycardia on electrophysiologic studies have an 80% probability of a serious arrhythmic event up to 4 years of follow up, versus 47% in those in whom ventricular tachycardia could not be induced ($P < 0{\cdot}005$).[71]

Acute severe aortic valve regurgitation usually causes sudden severe symptoms of heart failure or cardiogenic shock. The sudden large regurgitant volume load is imposed on a normal size left ventricle causing marked elevation in left ventricular end-diastolic pressure and left atrial pressure. Echocardiography is invaluable in determining the severity and etiology of aortic valve regurgitation.[10] The etiology of acute aortic valve regurgitation may have an important impact on the treatment, which is usually emergency surgery.

Management options

Angina is a result of a relative reduction of myocardial blood flow because of an increased need or associated obstructive CAD or both.[25] It does not respond to nitrates as well as in aortic stenosis. The options are to reduce the amount of aortic regurgitation and/or to revascularize the myocardium by coronary bypass surgery or by percutaneous catheter techniques. Clinical heart failure is treated with the traditional first-line triple therapy, that is, digitalis, diuretics, and ACE inhibitors. Parenteral inotropic and vasodilator therapy may be needed for those in severe heart failure.[72] The only

direct method(s) to reduce the amount of regurgitation is by arterial dilators[73] and valve surgery – that is, valve replacement or valve repair.

Arterial dilators

In chronic aortic valve regurgitation, therapy with vasodilating agents is designed to improve forward stroke volume and reduce regurgitant volume. These effects should translate into reductions in left ventricular end-diastolic volume, wall stress, and afterload, resulting in preservation of left ventricular systolic function and reduction in left ventricular mass. These effects have been observed in small numbers of patients receiving hydralazine.[73] In a trial of 80 patients over 2 years[74] in which 36% of patients were symptomatic (NYHA class II) and were being treated with digitalis and diuretics, hydralazine produced very minor improvements of left ventricular size and function.[74] Side effects associated with long-term use of hydralazine seriously impaired compliance and only 46% of the patients completed the trial. Hydralazine is rarely used currently. Occasionally it is used for a short period of time, to tide the patient over an acute reversible complication or in preparation for elective surgery in selected patients with left ventricular dysfunction. Less consistent results have been reported with ACE inhibitors, depending on the degree of reduction in arterial pressure and end-diastolic volume. In an acute study in the catheterization laboratory, 20 patients were randomized to either oral nifedipine or oral captopril.[75] Nifedipine produced a reduction of regurgitant fraction but captopril did not. Nifedipine produced a greater increase of forward stroke volume and cardiac output and a greater fall of systemic vascular resistance. This study showed that, acutely, nifedipine was superior to an ACE inhibitor. A short-term 6 month randomized trial of a small number of patients showed that the results with captopril were similar to placebo – that is, there were no significant changes in M-mode echocardiographic left ventricular dimensions.[76]

A randomized trial of 72 patients for 12 months of long-acting nifedipine showed statistically significant reductions of left ventricular end-diastolic volume index and left ventricular mass, and increase of LVEF.[58] The role of long-acting nifedipine on *patient outcome* has been evaluated in a prospective, randomized trial of 143 asymptomatic patients with chronic, severe aortic valve regurgitation, and normal left ventricular systolic function; 69 patients were randomized to long-acting nifedipine and 74 patients to digoxin. The patients were evaluated at 6 month intervals for medication complication and had a history, physical examination, ECG, chest radiograph, and echocardiographic/ Doppler study. Two independent blinded observers read each echocardiographic/Doppler study. Criteria for valve replacement were established prior to the start of the study. If left ventricular dysfunction developed, this had to be confirmed by a repeat echocardiographic/Doppler study at 1 month and by preoperative left ventricular angiographic study. At 6 years, the need for valve replacement was 34±6% in the digoxin-treated group and 15±3% in the nifedipine-group, $P < 0.001$ (Figure 53.4).[58] Thus, for every 100 patients treated with nifedipine, 19 fewer valve replacements were needed at the end of 6 years; note that even after 6 years, the curves are not parallel and do not converge (see Figure 53.4). Compared to the digoxin group, the nifedipine-treated group demonstrated a reduction in left ventricular volume and mass. Ejection fraction increased in the digoxin arm of the trial, and left ventricular volumes and mass increased. After aortic valve replacement, 12 of 16 patients (75%) in the digoxin group and all six patients in the nifedipine group who had an abnormal LVEF before surgery had a normal ejection fraction. Eighty-five per cent of patients in the digoxin arm of the trial, who underwent valve replacement, developed an abnormal ejection fraction and only three patients had valve replacement for symptoms. Moreover, patients in the digoxin arm of the trial had an outcome similar to that reported in the natural history studies.

Long-acting nifedipine is the drug of choice for asymptomatic patients with severe chronic aortic valve regurgitation and normal left ventricular systolic function unless there is a contraindication to its use.[25] The goal of vasodilator therapy is to reduce systolic blood pressure. The dose should be increased until there is a measurable decrease in blood pressure or side effects. Vasodilator therapy is not indicated in patients with normal left ventricular dimension and/or normal blood pressure. ACE inhibitors are not of proven benefit in asymptomatic patients with severe chronic aortic valve regurgitation and normal left ventricular systolic function. **Grade A**

Valve surgery (replacement/repair)

Surgery for aortic valve regurgitation should only be considered when the degree of regurgitation is severe. However, the presence of severe aortic valve regurgitation does not mandate surgery. The critical issue is to choose the best time for surgical intervention. Aortic valve repair or replacement should be performed in most symptomatic patients irrespective of the degree of left ventricular dysfunction. Postoperative survival is better after valve replacement in symptomatic patients with normal or mildly impaired left ventricular systolic function (ejection fraction [EF] ≥ 0·45) than in those with greater impairment of left ventricular systolic function (EF < 0·45).[77] In one study, patients with preoperative left ventricular EF of ≥0·60 had a better survival than those with left ventricular EF of <0·60.[78] Extreme left ventricular dilation (end-diastolic dimension >80) associated with aortic valve regurgitation occurs primarily in men and is often associated with left ventricular dysfunction. Extreme left ventricular dilation, however, is not a marker of irreversible left ventricular dysfunction. Operative risk and late postoperative survival are acceptable in these patients.[79] In the setting of severe left ventricular dysfunction (EF <0·25), the risk of aortic valve surgery increases and potential benefits decline, since left ventricular dysfunction may be on the basis of irreversible myocardial damage. However, even in the highest risk patients, the risk of surgery and postoperative medical therapy for heart failure are usually less than the risk of long-term medical management alone. **Grade B**

Aortic valve surgery for asymptomatic patients is more controversial but is indicated in the setting of left ventricular dysfunction with an EF ≤0·50 and in the setting of severe left ventricular dilation (end-diastolic dimension >75 mm or end systolic dimension >55 mm), even if the ejection fraction is normal. The threshold values of end-diastolic and end-systolic dimension recommended for aortic valve replacement in asymptomatic patients may need to be adjusted to body surface area. In one series, it was noted that a left ventricular end-systolic dimension corrected for body surface area (LVS/BSA) of ≥25 mm/m² was associated with increased mortality when followed conservatively.[1,68,79]

After valve replacement, patients with normal preoperative left ventricular systolic function have reductions of left ventricular volumes and hypertrophy.[80] In the majority of patients with normal preoperative left ventricular function, there is an increase in EF after valve replacement, presumably because of a reduction of myocardial stress.[31,81] Left

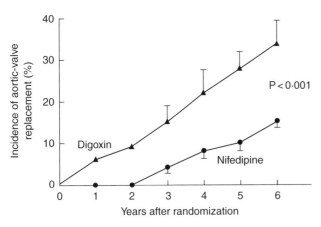

Figure 53.4 The role of long term, long acting nifedipine therapy in asymptomatic patients with severe aortic regurgitation and normal left ventricular systolic pump function was evaluated in 143 asymptomatic patients in a prospective randomized trial. By actuarial analysis, at 6 years, 34 ± 6% of patients in the digoxin group underwent valve replacement versus 15 ± 3% of those in the nifedipine group ($P < 0.001$). This randomized trial demonstrates that long term arteriolar dilator therapy with long acting nifedipine reduces and/or delays the need for aortic valve replacement in asymptomatic patients with severe aortic regurgitation and normal left ventricular systolic pump function. (From Scognamiglio *et al*[52] with permission.)

ventricular hypertrophy continues to decline for up to 5–8 years in those with normal preoperative left ventricular systolic function, but at a slower rate after 18–24 months.[31,81] Most patients are symptomatically improved and are in NYHA class I.[25]

After valve replacement in those with abnormal preoperative left ventricular systolic function (EF 0·25–0·49), there is a reduction of heart size and left ventricular end-diastolic pressure, end-diastolic and end-systolic volumes and hypertrophy.[77] Left ventricular EF improves or normalizes only if the EF was abnormal for ≤12 months prior to surgery.[81] Very early after valve replacement, there may be a reduction in EF. The left ventricular end-diastolic volume has not yet decreased but the regurgitant volume has been eliminated; this causes a decline in EF. An early decrease in left ventricular end-diastolic dimension is a good indicator of functional success of aortic valve replacement as the magnitude of reduction in end-diastolic dimension after operation correlates with the magnitude of late increase in EF.[1] Moreover, unless there is a perioperative complication, most patients are symptomatically improved and are in NYHA class I or II.[25]

Box 53.3 Results of valve replacement in patients with severe chronic aortic valve regurgitation

- Improved survival in those with mild to moderate impairment of left ventricular systolic function and in those with severe left ventricular enlargement irrespective of their symptomatic status
- Improvement in left ventricular systolic dysfunction; function normalizes if the dysfunction is of ≤12 months' duration preoperatively
- Regression of left ventricular hypertrophy
- Improvement in functional class, particularly in those with preoperative mild to moderate impairment and in those with preoperative left ventricular dysfunction

---

Box 53.4 Factors predictive of a less favorable outcome

- Extent and severity of associated comorbid conditions
- Severe obstructive coronary artery disease
- Presence and severity of clinical heart failure preoperatively
- Severity of depression of preoperative LVEF
- Duration of preoperative left ventricular systolic dysfunction
- Extent of preoperative irreversible myocardial damage
- Severity of increase in left ventricular end-diastolic and end-systolic size (left ventricular end-diastolic and end-systolic volumes of ≥210 and ≥110 ml/m², respectively, or end-diastolic and end-systolic dimensions of ≥80 mm and ≥60 mm, respectively)
- Skill and experience of operating and associated professional teams, for example, anesthetists
- Extent of perioperative myocardial damage
- Complications of a prosthetic heart valve

In those with severe symptoms and severe reduction of EF or severe left ventricular dilation preoperatively, survival as well as the beneficial effects on left ventricular function and functional class are less marked.[80,82]

Boxes 54.3 and 54.4 summarize the results of valve replacement in those with severe chronic aortic valve regurgitation and the factors predictive of a worse postoperative survival, less recovery of left ventricular function, and less improvement in symptomatic state in those with severe regurgitation and preoperative left ventricular systolic dysfunction.

There are two controversial questions regarding patients with severe aortic valve regurgitation. First, when does the symptomatic patient become inoperable? Second, when should one operate on asymptomatic patients with severe aortic valve regurgitation (assuming that associated comorbid conditions do not make the patient inoperable or at high risk for surgery)?

Severe left ventricular systolic dysfunction is the major factor that makes the patient with severe aortic valve regurgitation inoperable. In the published study of left ventricular dysfunction in which the patient and left ventricular function improved after valve replacement, the patients had an EF of 0·25–0·49.[77,80] Personal experience indicates that with skilled and experienced surgery, patients with an EF of 0·18–0·24 are improved with operation. There are limited data on the results of valve replacement in patients with severe aortic valve regurgitation and severe left ventricular systolic dysfunction with a left ventricular EF of <0·18, these patients are very high risk for conventional valve surgery and many would consider such patients inoperable.

The asymptomatic patient with severe aortic valve regurgitation poses a challenging clinical dilemma. If patients have developed left ventricular systolic dysfunction, then their outcome is poor without surgery, and left ventricular dysfunction, if present for 12 months or longer, does not normalize after surgery;[81] therefore, surgery is advisable. Patients who need surgery for associated conditions, for example, obstructive CAD, thoracic aortic disease, such as an aortic aneurysm, or another valve lesion, should have surgery for the severe aortic regurgitation. Patients who have developed severe left ventricular dilation are on the edge of developing symptoms at a high rate. One could wait for symptoms to develop and follow these patients very carefully at frequent intervals. Asymptomatic patients who do not have severe left ventricular dilation and those who do not have left ventricular dysfunction at rest or exercise should not have surgery for chronic aortic valve regurgitation. The current status of aortic valve repair prevents recommending this as an early prophylactic procedure. It is difficult to determine which aortic valves will be amenable to repair. In addition, the current rate of reoperation is at a level that prevents regular use of this procedure in asymptomatic patients with minimal left ventricular enlargement.[83]

Recommendations: aortic valve replacement/repair in severe chronic aortic regurgitation	
● **Indication**	**Class**
● Symptomatic patients with:	
● NYHA class III or IV symptoms and normal LV systolic function (LVEF ≥ 0·5)	I
● NYHA class II symptoms, preserved systolic function (LVEF ≥ 0·5) but with progressive LV dilation or declining EF at rest, or declining exercise capacity on exercise testing	I
● Canadian Heart Association class II or greater angina with or without CAD	I
● NYHA class II symptoms with preserved LV systolic function (LVEF ≥ 0·5) with stable LV size and systolic function on serial studies and stable exercise tolerance	IIa
● LV systolic dysfunction	
−LVEF 0·25–0·49	I
−LVEF 0·18–0·24	IIb
● Asymptomatic patients with:	
● LV systolic dysfunction	
−LVEF 0·25–0·49	I
−LVEF 0·18–0·24	IIb
● normal LV function and:	
● associated severe obstructive CAD needing surgery	I
● other valve or thoracic aortic disease needing surgery	I
● severe LV dilation with EDD ≥70 mm *or* ESD ≥55 mm and normal LV systolic function (LVEF ≥0·50)	IIb
● normal systolic function at rest (LVEF ≥0·5) but decline in EF (<0·50) on exercise radionuclide angiography	IIb
● normal systolic function at rest (LVEF ≥0·5) but decline in EF (<0·50) on stress echocardiography	III
● LV dilation is not severe (EDD <70 mm, ESD <50 mm)	III

Abbreviations: NYHA, New York Heart Association; EDD, end-diastolic dimension; ESD, end-systolic dimension; LVEF, left ventricular ejection fraction; EF, ejection fraction; LV, left ventricular

For definition of classes, see p. 773

References

1. Bonow R, Carabello B, de Leon A *et al.* Guidelines for the management of patients with valvular heart disease: executive summary. A report of the American College of Cardiology/American Heart Association Task Force on Practice Guidelines (Committee on Management of Patients with Valvular Heart Disease). *Circulation* 1998;**98**:1949–84.

2. Rahimtoola S. *Aortic valve stenosis*. St. Louis: CV Mosby; 1997.

3. Olsson N, Dalsgaaro C, Haegerstrand A, Rosenqvist M, Ryden L, Nilson J. Accumulation of T lymphocytes and expression of interluken-2 receptors in nonrheumatic stenotic aortic valves. *J Am Coll Cardiol* 1994;**23**:1162–70.

4. Otto C, Kuusisto J, Reichenbach D, Gown A, O'Brien K. Characterization of the early lesion of "degenerative" valvular aortic stenosis. Histological and immunohistochemical studies. *Circulation* 1994;**90**:844–53.

5. Otto C. Aortic stenosis – listen to the patient, look at the valve. *N Engl J Med* 2000;**343**:652–4.

6. Pohle K, Maffert R, Ropers D *et al.* Progression of aortic valve calcification: association with coronary atherosclerosis and cardiovascular risk factors. *Circulation* 2001;**104**:1927–32.

7. Otto C, Burwask I, Legget M *et al.* Prospective study of asymptomatic valvular aortic stenosis: clinical, echocardiographic, and exercise predictors of outcome. *Circulation* 1997;**95**:2262–70.

8. Rahimtoola S. The problem of valve prosthesis–patient mismatch. *Circulation* 1978;**58**:20–4.

9. Tobin J Jr, Rahimtoola S, Blundell P, Swan H. Percentage of left ventricular stroke workloss: a simple hemodynamic concept for estimation of severity in valvular aortic stenosis. *Circulation* 1967;**35**:868–79.

10. Cheitlin M, Alpert J, Armstrong W *et al.* ACC/AHA Guidelines for the Clinical Application of Echocardiography. A report of the American College of Cardiology/American Heart Association Task Force on Practice Guidelines (Committee on Clinical Application of Echocardiography). Developed in collaboration with the American Society of Echocardiography. *Circulation* 1997;**95**:1686–744.

11. Currie P, Seward J, Reeder G *et al.* Continuous-wave Doppler echocardiographic assessment of severity of calcific aortic stenosis: a simultaneous Doppler-catheter correlative study in 100 adult patients. *Circulation* 1985;**71**:1162–9.

12. Rahimtoola S. "Prophylactic" valve replacement for mild aortic valve disease at time of surgery for other cardiovascular disease? No. *J Am Coll Cardiol* 1999;**33**:2009–15.

13. Ross JJr, Braunwald E. Aortic stenosis. *Circulation* 1968;**36** (Suppl. IV):61–7.

14. Horstkotte D, Loogen F. The natural history of aortic valve stenosis. *Eur Heart J* 1988;(Suppl. E):57–64.

15. Rahimtoola S. *Perspective on valvular heart disease: Update II*. New York: Elsevier, 1991.

16. O'Neill W. Predictors of long-term survival after percutaneous aortic valvuloplasty: report of the Mansfield Scientific Balloon Aortic Valvuloplasty registry. *J Am Coll Cardiol* 1991;**17**:193–8.

17. Kennedy K, Nishimura R, Holmes DJ, Bailey K. Natural history of moderate aortic stenosis. *J Am Coll Cardiol* 1991;**17**:313–19.

18. Pellikka P, Nishimura R, Bailey K, Tajik A. The natural history of adults with asymptomatic, hemodynamically significant aortic stenosis. *J Am Coll Cardiol* 1990;**15**:1012–27.

19. Amato M, Moffa P, Werner K, Ramires J. Treatment decision in asymptomatic aortic valve stenosis: role of exercise testing. *Heart* 2001;**86**:361–2.

20. Rosenhek R, Binder T, Porenta G *et al.* Predictors of outcome in severe, asymptomatic aortic stenosis. *N Engl J Med* 2000;**343**:611–17.

21. White P. *Heart Disease, 4th ed.* New York: Macmillan, 1951.
22. Bonet T. *Sepulchretum, sire Anatomia Practica, 4th ed.* Geneva: Leonard Chouet; New York: Macmillan, 1951.
23. Frank S, Johnson A, Ross JJ. Natural history of valvular aortic stenosis. *B Heart J* 1973;**35**:41–6.
24. Rahimtoola S. *Aortic valve stenosis, 10th ed.* New York: McGraw-Hill, 2001.
25. Rahimtoola S. *Aortic valve regurgitation, 9th ed.* New York: McGraw-Hill, 1998.
26. Sethi GK, Miller DC, Souchek J *et al.* Clinical, hemodynamic and angiographic predictors of operative mortality in patients undergoing single valve replacement. *J Thorac Cardiovasc Surg* 1987;**93**:884–7.
27. Edwards F, Peterson E, Coombs L *et al.* Predication of operative mortality after valve replacement surgery. *J Am Coll Cardiol* 2001;**37**:885–92.
28. Mullany C, Elveback E, Frye R *et al.* Coronary artery disease and its management: influence on survival in patients undergoing aortic valve replacement. *J Am Coll Cardiol* 1987;**10**:66–72.
29. Rahimtoola S. Lessons learned about the determinants of the results of valve surgery. *Circulation* 1988;**78**:1503–7.
30. Schwarz F, Banmann P, Manthey J *et al.* The effect of aortic valve replacement on survival. *Circulation* 1982;**66**:1105–10.
31. Pantely G, Morton M, Rahimtoola S. Effects of successful uncomplicated valve replacement on ventricular hypertrophy, volume, and performance in aortic stenosis and aortic incompetence. *J Thorac Cardiovasc Surg* 1978;**75**:383–91.
32. Monrad E, Hess O, Murakami T, Nonogi H, Corin W, Krayenbuehl H. Time course of regression of left ventricular hypertrophy after aortic valve replacement. *Circulation* 1988;**77**:1345–55.
33. Carroll J, Carroll EP, Feldman T *et al.* Sex-associated differences in left ventricular function in aortic stenosis of the elderly. *Circulation* 1992;**86**:1099–107.
34. Hammermeister K, Sethi G, Henderson W, Oprian C, Kim T, Rahimtoola S. A comparison of outcomes in men 11 years after heart-valve replacement with a mechanical valve or bioprosthesis. *N Engl J Med* 1993;**328**:1289–96.
35. Murphy E, Lawson R, Starr A, Rahimtoola S. Severe aortic stenosis in patients 60 years of age and older: left ventricular function and ten-year survival after valve replacement. *Circulation* 1981;**64**(Suppl. II):184–8.
36. Lindblom D, Lindblom U, Qvist J LundströmH Long-term relative survival rates after heart valve replacement. *J Am Coll Cardiol* 1990;**15**:566–73.
37. Sprigings D, Forfar J. How should we manage symptomatic aortic stenosis in the patient who is 80 or older? *Br Heart J* 1995;**74**:481–4.
38. Rahimtoola S. Catheter balloon valvuloplasty for severe calcific aortic stenosis: a limited role. *J Am Coll Cardiol* 1994;**23**:1076–8.
39. Smith N, McAnulty J, Rahimtoola S. Severe aortic stenosis with impaired left ventricular function and clinical heart failure: results of valve replacement. *Circulation* 1978;**58**:255–64.
40. Connolly H, Oh J, Orszulak T *et al.* Aortic valve replacement for aortic stenosis with severe left ventricular dysfunction. Prognostic indicators. *Circulation* 1997;**95**:2395–2400.
41. Rahimtoola S, Starr A. *Valvular surgery.* New York: Grune and Stratton, 1982.
42. Connolly H, Oh J, Schaff H *et al.* Severe aortic stenosis with low transvalvular gradient and severe left ventricular dysfunction: result of aortic valve replacement in 52 patients. *Circulation* 2000;**101**:1940–6.
43. deFilippi C, Willett D, Brickner M *et al.* Usefulness of dobutamine echocardiography in distinguishing severe from non-severe valvular aortic stenosis in patients with depressed left ventricular function and low transvalvular gradients. *Am J Cardiol* 1995;**75**:191–4.
44. Monin J, Monchi M, Gest V, Duval-Moulin A, Dubois-Rande J, Gueret P. Aortic stenosis with severe left ventricular dysfunction and low transvalvular pressure gradients: risk stratification by low-dose dobutamine echocardiography. *J Am Coll Cardiol* 2001;**37**:2101–7.
45. Nishimura RA, Grantham JA, Connolly HM, Schaff HV, Higano ST, Holmes DR Jr. Low-output, low-gradient aortic stenosis in patients with depressed left ventricular systolic function: the clinical utility of the dobutamine challenge in the catheterization laboratory. *Circulation* 2002;**106**(Suppl. 7):809–13.
46. Rahimtoola S. *Aortic valve regurgitation.* St. Louis: CV Mosby, 1997.
47. Lewis TS. *Special Report Series of the National Health Insurance Joint Committee, Medical Research Committee, Report No. 8.* London: MRC, 1917.
48. Grant R. After histories for 10 years of a thousand men suffering from heart disease. *Heart* 1933;**16**:275–334.
49. McKay C, Rahimtoola S. *Natural history of aortic regurgitation.* New York: Kluwer, 1980.
50. Spagnuolo M, Kloth H, Taranta A, Doyle E, Pasternack B. Natural history of rheumatic aortic regurgitation. Criteria predictive of death, congestive heart failure, and angina in young patients. *Circulation* 1971;**34**:368–80.
51. Goldschlager N, Pfeifer J, Cohn K, Popper R, Selze R. Natural history of aortic regurgitation: a clinical and hemodynamic study. *Am J Med* 1973;**54**:577–88.
52. Scognamiglio R, Fasoli G, Dalla Volta S Progression of myocardial dysfunction in asymptomatic patients with severe aortic insufficiency. *Clin Cardiol* 1986;**9**:151–6.
53. Siemienczuk D, Greenberg B, Morris C *et al.* Chronic aortic insufficiency: factors associated with progression to aortic valve replacement. *Ann Intern Med* 1989;**110**:587–92.
54. Bonow R, Lakatos E, Maron B, Epstein S. Serial long-term assessment of the natural history of asymptomatic patients with chronic aortic regurgitation and normal left ventricular systolic function. *Circulation* 1991;**84**:1625–35.
55. Scognamiglio R, Fasoli G, Ponchia A, Dalla Volta S Long-term nifedipine unloading therapy in asymptomatic patients with chronic severe aortic regurgitation. *J Am Coll Cardiol* 1990;**16**:424–9.
56. Tornos M, Olona M, Permanyer-Miralda G *et al.* Clinical outcome of severe asymptomatic chronic aortic regurgitation. A long-term prospective follow-up study. *Am Heart J* 1995;**130**:333–9.
57. Ishii K, Hirota Y, Suwa M, Kita Y, Onaka H, Kawamura K. Natural history and left ventricular response in chronic regurgitation. *Am J Cardiol* 1996;**78**:357–61.
58. Scognamiglio R, Rahimtoola S, Fasoli G, Nistri S, Dalla Volta S. Nifedipine in asymptomatic patients with severe aortic regurgitation and normal left ventricular function. *N Engl J Med* 1994;**331**:689–95.

59. Henry W, Bonow R, Rosing D, Epstein S. Observations on the optimum time for operative intervention for aortic regurgitation. II. Serial echocardiographic evaluation of asymptomatic patients. *Circulation* 1980;**61**:484–92.

60. McDonald I, Jelinek V. Serial M-mode echocardiography in severe chronic aortic regurgitation. *Circulation* 1980;**62**: 1291–6.

61. Bonow R. Radionuclide angiography in the management of asymptomatic aortic regurgitation. *Circulation* 1991;**84**: I.296–I.302.

62. Hegglin R, Scheu H, Rothlin M. Aortic insufficiency. *Circulation* 1968;**38**(Suppl. 15):V77–V92.

63. Rapaport E. Natural history of aortic and mitral valve disease. *Am J Cardiol* 1975;**35**:221–7.

64. Rahimoola S. Aortic *Valve regurgitation, 10th ed.* New York: McGraw-Hill, 2001.

65. Aronow W, Ahn C, Kronzon I, Nanna M. Prognosis of patients with heart failure and unoperated severe aortic valvular regurgitation and relation to ejection fraction. *Am J Cardiol* 1994;**74**:286–8.

66. Broadbent W. Aortic incompetence. In: *Heart disease: with special reference to prognosis and treatment.* London: Baillière, Tindall & Cox, 1897.

67. Klodas E, Enriquez-Sarano M, Tajik A, Mullany C, Bailey K, Seward J. Surgery for aortic regurgitation in women: contrasting indications and outcomes compared with men. *Circulation* 1996;**94**:2472–8.

68. Dujardin K, Enriquez-Sarano M, Schaff H, Bailey K, Seward J, Tajik A. Mortality and morbidity of aortic regurgitation in clinical practice. A long-term follow-up study. *Circulation* 1999; **99**:1851–7.

69. Boucher C, Wilson R, Kanarek D *et al.* Exercise testing in asymptomatic or minimally symptomatic aortic regurgitation: relationship of left ventricular ejection fraction to left ventricular filling pressure during exercise. *Circulation* 1983;**67**: 1091–1100.

70. Kawanishi D, McKay C, Chandraratna P *et al.* Cardiovascular response to dynamic exercise in patients with chronic symptomatic mild-moderate and severe aortic regurgitation. *Circulation* 1986;**73**:62–72.

71. Martinez-Rubio A, Schwammenthal Y, Schwammenthal E *et al.* Patients with valvular heart disease presenting with sustained ventricular tachyarrhythmias or syncope: results of programmed ventricular stimulation and long-term follow-up. *Circulation* 1997;**96**:500–8.

72. Rahimtoola S. Management of heart failure in valve regurgitation. *Clin Cardiol* 1992;**15**(Suppl. I):22–7.

73. Rahimtoola S. Vasodilator therapy in chronic, severe aortic regurgitation. *J Am Coll Cardiol* 1990;**16**:430–2.

74. Greenberg B, Massie B, Bristow J *et al.* Long-term vasodilator therapy of chronic aortic insufficiency: a randomized double-blind, placebo-controlled clinical trial. *Circulation* 1988;**78**: 92–103.

75. RöthlisbergerC, Sareli P, Wisenbaugh T. Comparison of single-dose nifedipine and captopril for chronic severe aortic regurgitation. *Am J Cardiol* 1993;**72**:799–804.

76. Wisenbaugh T, Sinovich V, Dullabh A, Sareli P. Six month pilot study of captopril for mildly symptomatic, severe isolated mitral and isolated aortic regurgitation. *J Heart Valve Dis* 1994;**3**:197.

77. Greves J, Rahimtoola S, Clinic M *et al.* Preoperative criteria predictive of late survival following valve replacement for severe aortic regurgitation. *Am Heart J* 1981;**101**:300–8.

78. Cunha C, Giuliani E, Fuster V, Seward J, Brandenburg R, McGoon D. Preoperative M-mode echocardiography as a predictor of surgical results in chronic aortic insufficiency. *J Thorac Cardiovasc Surg* 1980;**79**:256–65.

79. Klodas E, Enriquez-Sarano M, Tajik A, Mullany C, Bailey K, Seward J. Optimizing timing of surgical correction in patients with severe aortic regurgitation: role of symptoms. *J Am Coll Cardiol* 1997;**30**:746–52.

80. Clark D, McAnulty J, Rahimtoola S. Valve replacement in aortic insufficiency with left ventricular dysfunction. *Circulation* 1980;**61**:411–21.

81. Bonow R, Dodd J, Maron B *et al.* Long-term serial changes in left ventricular function and reversal of ventricular dilatation after valve replacement for chronic aortic regurgitation. *Circulation* 1988;**78**:1108–20.

82. Klodas E, Enriquez-Sarano M, Tajik A, Mullany C, Bailey K, Seward J. Aortic regurgitation complicated by extreme left ventricular dilation: long-term outcome after surgical correction. *J Am Coll Cardiol* 1996;**27**:670–7.

83. Izumoto H, Kawazoe K, Ishibashi K *et al.* Aortic valve repair in dominant aortic regurgitation. *Japan J Thorac Cardiovasc Surg* 2001;**49**:355–9.

84. Rapaport E. Natural history of aortic and mitral valve disease *Am J Cardiol* 1975;**35**(Suppl. 2):221–7.

85. Chizner MA, Pearle DL, deLeon AC Jr. The natural history of aortic stenosis in adults. *Am Heart J* 1980;**99**(Suppl. 4):419–24.

86. O'Keefe JH Jr, Vlietstra RE, Bailey KR, Holmes DR Jr. Natural history of candidates for balloon aortic valvuloplasty. *Mayo Clin Proc* 1987;**62**(Suppl. 11):986–91.

87. Turina J, Hess O, Sepulcri F, Krayenbuehl HP. Spontaneous course of aortic valve disease. *Eur Heart J* 1987;**8**(Suppl. 5): 471–83.

88. Kelly TA, Rothbart RM, Cooper CM, Kaiser DL, Smucker ML, Gibson RS. Comparison of outcome of asymptomatic to symptomatic patients older than 20 years of age with valvular aortic stenosis. *Am J Cardiol* 1988:**61**(Suppl. 1):123–30.

54 Balloon valvuloplasty: aortic valve

Daniel J Diver, Jeffrey A Breall

Aortic stenosis: natural history and prognosis

Grade A There are three major etiologies for valvular aortic stenosis in the adult patient: rheumatic aortic stenosis; congenital bicuspid aortic stenosis with secondary calcification; and senile calcific or degenerative aortic stenosis. In rheumatic aortic stenosis the major pathologic feature is commissural fusion, with associated thickening and fibrosis of the valve leaflets. Symptoms may not occur until the age of 50 or 60 and are often accompanied by evidence of other valvular disease, usually mitral. Patients with congenital bicuspid aortic stenosis develop progressive narrowing and calcification of the aortic valve over time, with symptoms often present by age 40–50. Degenerative calcific (senile) aortic stenosis appears to result from years of normal mechanical stress on the aortic valve, with progressive immobilization of cusps secondary to calcium accumulation in the pockets of the aortic cusps, and eventual fibrosis. Degenerative calcific aortic stenosis is now the most common cause of aortic stenosis in patients presenting for aortic valve replacement.[1]

Most data regarding the natural history of aortic stenosis are derived from clinical experience during the presurgical era. The natural history of aortic stenosis is characterized by a long latent period marked by slowly increasing obstruction and adaptive myocardial hypertrophy. The majority of patients are free of cardiovascular symptoms until relatively late in the course of the disease. However, once patients with aortic stenosis develop symptoms of angina, syncope or heart failure, survival with medical therapy is dismal, with death occurring within 2–5 years in most patients following the development of symptoms (Figure 54.1). Average survival in patients with aortic stenosis and angina or syncope is 2–3 years, and may be as short as 1·5 years in patients with aortic stenosis who develop heart failure.[2] Concomitant atrial fibrillation decreases survival in all symptom groups.

Asymptomatic patients with aortic stenosis have an excellent prognosis and rarely die without premonitory symptoms. A study by Pellikka *et al*[4] showed that mortality was slightly higher in asymptomatic patients treated with "prophylactic" valve replacement than in patients not operated on until symptoms develop. A recent study by Otto and colleagues reported follow up of 123 patients with asymptomatic aortic stenosis. During the 2·5 year, follow up period

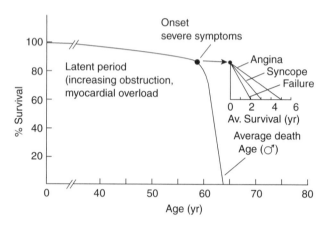

Figure 54.1 Natural history of aortic stenosis without operative treatment. (Reproduced with permission from Ross and Braunwald.[3])

there were no sudden cardiac deaths. This study suggested that the rate of hemodynamic progression and clinical outcome in adults with asymptomatic aortic stenosis may be predicted by echocardiographic aortic jet velocity. Of those patients who entered the study with a peak aortic jet velocity >4 m/s only 21% were alive and free of valve replacement 2 years later.[5]

The timing of aortic valve replacement in patients with aortic stenosis is predicated on the development of symptoms or deterioration in left ventricular performance, rather than severity of valve gradient or reduction in valve orifice area. Carabello[6] has proposed a definition of "critical" aortic stenosis as that valve area small enough to cause the symptoms of aortic stenosis that often presage sudden death: a "critical" situation indicating the need for aortic valve replacement. The aortic valve area associated with such symptom development varies significantly from patient to patient.

Aortic stenosis: natural history and prognosis

- Long latent period without symptoms
- Poor prognosis following symptom development with death in 2–5 years
- Prognosis significantly improved by valve replacement surgery.

Surgery for aortic stenosis

Grade B The initial surgical approach to treatment of aortic stenosis involved surgical valvuloplasty. In contrast to the situation with pulmonary and mitral stenosis, the stenotic aortic valve did not respond favorably to surgical valvuloplasty techniques. Closed aortic commissurotomy was associated with a high incidence of acute aortic regurgitation and operative mortality, and was abandoned after the development of open aortic valve surgical techniques. Surgical valvuloplasty under direct vision for aortic stenosis was first described in 1956, but was limited by a high rate of restenosis leading to subsequent aortic valve replacement, as well as a significant incidence of complications, including aortic regurgitation, infective endocarditis and systemic embolization.[7] Although ultrasonic decalcification and careful surgical sculpting procedures carried out under direct vision are initially effective in some patients, restenosis remains a serious problem.[8] However, open surgical valvulotomy remains an important treatment for infants and children with critical aortic stenosis, a situation where initial prosthetic valve replacement is undesirable.

The development and refinement of surgical aortic valve replacement significantly improved morbidity and mortality in patients with symptomatic aortic stenosis. Although there is no prospective randomized controlled study comparing aortic valve replacement with medical therapy in such patients, long-term follow up in high-quality case series has convincingly demonstrated the long-term benefits of aortic valve replacement, including hemodynamic improvement, regression of left ventricular hypertrophy, improvement of left ventricular function and improved survival.[9–11] Operative mortality for aortic valve replacement ranges from 2 to 8%, but may be as low as 1% in patients less than 70 years of age without significant comorbidity.

Aortic valve replacement, however, is associated with increased morbidity and mortality in certain subgroups.[10,12–15] Aortic valve replacement in the presence of left ventricular failure may be associated with perioperative mortality as high as 10–25%, and the need for emergency aortic valve replacement with operative mortality as high as 40%. Surgical risk is increased in the elderly patient, and may be increased severalfold with the need for concomitant bypass or multiple valve surgery. Although advanced age remains a strong predictor of operative death for aortic valve replacement even in recent studies, age alone is not a contraindication to aortic valve replacement in patients with aortic stenosis.[16] The Society of Thoracic Surgeons National Cardiac Surgery Database identified risk factors in nearly 50 000 patients who had valve surgery between 1994 and 1997: for patients with isolated aortic valve replacement, age was not a strong predictor of risk.[17] Fremes and colleagues[18] at the University of Toronto described the result of valve surgery in 469 consecutive patients over 70 years of age, and found that the predicted probability of operative mortality ranged from 0·9 to 76%, depending on the presence of other risk factors, including urgent operation, double valve surgery, coronary artery disease, female gender and left ventricular dysfunction. The authors suggested that elderly patients in good risk categories should be offered surgical intervention for the correction of valvular lesions, whereas alternative therapy might be indicated in patients with multiple risk factors in whom surgical mortality was prohibitively high. Levinson and colleagues at the Massachusetts General Hospital reported on aortic valve replacement for aortic stenosis in octogenarians.[19] In their cohort of 64 patients, serious comorbid non-cardiac conditions were infrequent. In-hospital mortality was 9·4%. An additional 10% of patients had permanent severe neurologic deficits and an additional 38% had a "complicated" course, marked by temporary encephalopathy, discharge to a rehabilitation facility or some combination thereof, albeit with ultimately good results. Although most survivors were ultimately free of cardiac symptoms, there was a high price to pay in terms of perioperative mortality and morbidity to achieve these results. However, recent series suggest that surgical results may be improving in very elderly patients. Rosengart and colleagues[20] compared results in 100 consecutive patients age 85 years or older who underwent open heart surgery between 1994 and 1997 with results obtained in the prior decade, and noted improvement in 30 day mortality and risk of major complications.

Therefore, while surgical aortic valve replacement has clearly improved the outcome in most patients with critical aortic stenosis, the higher risk in some patient subgroups, including the elderly, often leads to physician or patient deferral of aortic valve replacement. In an attempt to define the natural history of such patients, O'Keefe and colleagues[21] at the Mayo Clinic performed a case comparison study of 50 patients with severe, symptomatic aortic stenosis in whom surgery was declined by the patient ($n = 28$) or the physician ($n = 22$). The actuarial survival at 1, 2 and 3 years was 57, 37 and 25%, respectively. The survival of age- and sex-matched control subjects was 93, 85 and 77%, respectively ($P < 0·0001$ at each 1 year interval) (Figure 54.2). This study suggested that the natural history of untreated aortic stenosis remains dismal and has not improved in the modern era, and confirmed the necessity of evaluating alternative non-surgical therapy, such as balloon aortic valvuloplasty, in patients likely to decline aortic valve replacement, or for whom surgery is not an option.

Development of balloon aortic valvuloplasty

Grade C Children and adolescents with congenital aortic stenosis generally have non-calcified valves with commissural fusion. Because aortic valve replacement is not desirable in

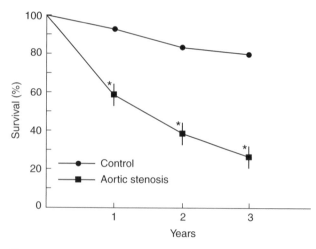

Figure 54.2 Survival among 50 patients with severe aortic stenosis who did not undergo surgical treatment, in comparison with an age- and sex-matched control group from the US population. Asterisks denote significant differences ($P < 0.0001$) between the two groups. Standard errors are shown as vertical lines. (Reproduced with permission from O'Keefe et al.[21])

this age group, commissural incision under direct vision is the preferred surgical procedure, and has been shown to confer significant hemodynamic improvement at low risk.[22] The contribution of commissural fusion to the etiology of valvular stenosis and mechanism of surgical improvement in this patient group led to the consideration of balloon aortic valvuloplasty as an alternative, non-surgical therapy.

In 1984 Lababidi and colleagues[23] reported the first series of 23 children and young adults with congenital aortic stenosis treated with percutaneous balloon aortic valvuloplasty. The patients ranged in age from 2 to 17 years. Balloon valvuloplasty was performed by the retrograde approach from the femoral artery, utilizing balloons of 10–20 mm in diameter. Percutaneous balloon dilation resulted in a decrease in the peak aortic valve gradient from 113 to 32 mmHg, with no change in cardiac output. The excellent initial results of percutaneous balloon valvuloplasty for aortic valve stenosis were confirmed by Rosenfeld and colleagues in young adults with congenital aortic stenosis. Long-term follow-up appeared to be excellent, with a 58% event-free rate at mean follow-up of 38 months,[24] although a recent multicenter study from Japan reported that progressive aortic insufficiency and recurrence of pressure gradient was not uncommon by 4 years after balloon valvuloplasty.[25]

The excellent results of balloon valvuloplasty in pediatric patients with congenital aortic stenosis led to consideration of this technique in adult patients with acquired calcific aortic stenosis. Two reports in 1986 described the first successful balloon valvuloplasty procedures in adult patients. Cribier and colleagues in France performed percutaneous balloon dilation in three elderly patients with calcific aortic

stenosis.[26] The peak aortic gradient decreased from 75 to 33 mmHg, with an increase in calculated aortic valve area from 0·5 to 0·8 cm². All patients had symptomatic improvement. McKay and colleagues[27] at the Beth Israel Hospital in Boston described two elderly patients (aged 93 and 85 years) with calcific aortic stenosis treated with balloon valvuloplasty with 12–18 mm balloons. This report likewise described a substantial reduction in the transaortic pressure gradient and a significant increase in aortic valve area, with symptomatic improvement in both patients and significant improvement in left ventricular function in one. Despite initial concern regarding the possibility of valve disruption or embolization in the calcific valves present in adult patients, no patient in either report developed emboli or a significant increase in aortic regurgitation.

Mechanism of balloon aortic valvuloplasty

Grade B To assess the safety, efficacy and mechanism of balloon aortic valvuloplasty, Safian and colleagues[28] performed balloon dilation of stenotic aortic valves in 33 postmortem specimens and in six patients undergoing aortic valve replacement, prior to removal of the stenotic valve. The cause of aortic stenosis was degenerative nodular calcification in 28 cases, calcific bicuspid aortic stenosis in eight cases, and rheumatic heart disease in three. The distribution of the etiology of aortic stenosis in this report is in concordance with the observation that degenerative calcific aortic stenosis is now the most common cause of aortic stenosis in adults presenting for aortic valve replacement.[1]

Safian and colleagues performed balloon dilation with 15–25 mm balloons in the postmortem specimens, and with 18–20 mm balloons in the surgical patients. Balloon dilation resulted in increased leaflet mobility and increased valve orifice dimensions in all patients. The mechanism of successful dilation included fracture of calcified nodules within the leaflets in 16 valves, separation of fused commissures in five valves, both in six valves, and "grossly inapparent microfractures" (or stretching) in 12 valves. Liberation of calcific debris, valve ring disruption and midleaflet tears did not occur in any valve, although valve leaflet avulsion was produced in one postmortem specimen after inflation with a clearly oversized balloon. The authors concluded that there were several mechanisms for successful balloon aortic valvuloplasty, with the predominant mechanism in a given patient depending on the etiology of the stenosis. Furthermore, it appeared that embolic phenomena and acute regurgitation were not likely to be frequent complications following valvuloplasty.

The study by Safian and colleagues suggested that the most common etiology of aortic stenosis in the balloon valvuloplasty population is degenerative nodular calcification, and that the predominant mechanism of valve dilation is fracture of calcified nodules within leaflets and leaflet stretching. Considered in conjunction with the disappointing surgical experience when stenotic aortic valves were dilated or cracked, the results of this mechanistic study predicted that there might be only mild improvement in aortic valve orifice area in patients treated with balloon aortic valvuloplasty, and that any such improvement might be short-lived. As will be seen, these implications were subsequently borne out in clinical trials.

Technical aspects

In the original reports by Cribier[26] and McKay,[27] balloon valvuloplasty was performed via the retrograde femoral approach. The most common balloon size used with the single-balloon retrograde approach is 20 mm, although smaller balloons can be used initially in small or frail patients. If no waist is produced in the inflated balloon, or if the aortic valve gradient is not sufficiently decreased by a given balloon size, a larger balloon may produce a better result.

Several modifications of the percutaneous retrograde femoral approach have been described. Block and Palacios[29] described an antegrade transseptal technique which they advocated for patients with severe iliac occlusive disease, tortuous iliac vessels or abdominal aortic aneurysm. This approach has recently been reported using the Inoue balloon, which may provide a greater increase in aortic valve area than conventional balloons[30] and which allows combined mitral and aortic valvuloplasty using a single catheter and access site.[31] A retrograde brachial approach may also be useful in such situations, although care must be taken to avoid injury to the brachial artery by the large valvuloplasty balloon. Dorros and colleagues[32] described a double-balloon technique, using both femoral arteries or a combined brachial and femoral approach. The combined diameter of the balloons used in this approach usually exceeds the diameter of the largest balloon used with single-balloon techniques. While initial results with double-balloon aortic valvuloplasty showed a greater enlargement of aortic valve area, follow-up studies showed no reduction in subsequent restenosis compared to single-balloon valvuloplasty.[33] An important recent technical advance is management of the femoral access site with preloaded suture closure devices,

which may significantly reduce the incidence of vascular complications following balloon valvuloplasty.[34,35]

Initial results of balloon aortic valvuloplasty

Single center studies

Grade B Within several years of the initial reports of balloon valvuloplasty in adult patients with aortic stenosis, several centers reported large single-center experiences.[36–39] Cribier *et al*[36] reported their initial experience with 92 adult patients with symptomatic aortic stenosis and a mean age of 75 years. The aortic valve gradient was reduced from 75 to 30 mmHg, with an increase in calculated aortic valve area from 0·5 to 0·9 cm^2. The left ventricular ejection fraction rose from 48% at baseline to 51% immediately following the procedure. The majority of patients had marked symptomatic improvement. There were three in-hospital deaths and eight late deaths.

Safian *et al*[37] reported their initial experience with balloon aortic valvuloplasty in 170 consecutive patients treated at the Beth Israel Hospital in Boston. The procedure was completed successfully in 168 patients and resulted in significant increases in mean aortic valve area (0·6–0·9 cm^2) and cardiac output (4·6–4·8 l/min) and a significant decrease in aortic valve pressure gradient (71–36 mmHg) ($P < 0·01$ for all comparisons). There were six in-hospital deaths and five patients required early aortic valve replacement. The majority of patients had marked symptomatic improvement following the procedure. The most common complication was vascular, involving the femoral access site: 40 patients required transfusion and 17 required surgical repair. Transient dysrhythmias, most commonly left bundle branch block, occurred in 28 patients. Left ventricular perforation and tamponade occurred in three patients, a marked increase in aortic regurgitation in two patients, and a non-Q wave myocardial infarction in one patient. No patient suffered a stroke.

The hemodynamic results and complications of balloon aortic valvuloplasty in several large single-center studies are summarized in Tables 54.1 and 54.2, respectively. The results are remarkable for their similarity across study sites.

Table 54.1 Acute hemodynamic results of balloon aortic valvuloplasty

Author	Patients (*n*)	Aortic valve gradient (mmHg)		Aortic valve area (cm^2)	
		Pre	Post	Pre	Post
Cribier[26]	92	75	30	0.5	0.9
Safian[28]	170	71	36	0.6	0.9
Block[29]	162	61	27	0.5	0.9
Lewin[39]	125	87	32	0.6	1.0

Table 54.2   Complications of balloon aortic valvuloplasty

Author	Patients (n)	Complications (%)					
		Death	CVA	Perforation	MI	AI	Vascular
Safian[28]	170	3·5	0	1·8	0·6	1·2	10·0
Block[29]	162	7·0	2·0	0	0	0	7·0
Lewin[39]	125	10·4	3·2	0	1·6	1·6	9·6
Total	457	6·6	1·5	0.7	0·7	0·9	8·8

Abbreviations: AI, aortic insufficiency; CVA, cerebrovascular accident; MI, myocardial infarction

In general, balloon aortic valvuloplasty resulted in a 50–70% decrease in aortic valve gradient and a 50–70% increase in aortic valve area, resulting in early symptomatic improvement in most patients. The most common complication was vascular at the access site; there was a low incidence of life-threatening procedural complications. Death during the periprocedural period occurred in about 6% of patients.

Multicenter studies

Grade B Two large multicenter studies reported the initial results of balloon valvuloplasty in adult patients with symptomatic aortic stenosis.[40,41] The Mansfield Balloon Aortic Valvuloplasty Registry[40] evaluated data from 27 clinical centers in the United States and included 492 patients treated with balloon aortic valvuloplasty between December 1986 and October 1987. The mean age of patients was 79 years. All had severe symptoms, with 92% reporting congestive heart failure. Balloon aortic valvuloplasty was performed via the femoral approach in 92% of patients, by the brachial approach in 6%, and by the transseptal approach in 2%. A single-balloon technique was used in 72% of patients. The largest balloon size was 20 mm in over half of patients.

In the Mansfield Registry, balloon aortic valvuloplasty resulted in a decrease in mean aortic valve gradient from 60 to 30 mmHg, an increase in cardiac output from 3·9 to 4·0 l/min and an increase in aortic valve area from 0·5 to 0·8 cm^2. Most patients had significant symptomatic improvement. Death occurred during the procedure in 4·9% of patients, and within 7 days of the procedure in an additional 2·6%. The most common complication (11%) was local vascular injury, requiring surgical repair in 5·7% of patients. Embolic complications, ventricular perforation resulting in tamponade, and significant increase in aortic insufficiency each occurred in 1–2% of patients, and significant arrhythmia or myocardial infarction in less than 1%. Emergency aortic valve replacement was required in 1% of patients following balloon valvuloplasty.

The National Heart Lung and Blood Institute (NHLBI) Balloon Valvuloplasty Registry enrolled 674 elderly (average

age 78 years) patients at 24 centers between November 1987 and November 1989.[41] Heart failure was the most common presenting symptom, occurring in 92% of patients; 45% of patients had angina and 35% had syncope. A single-balloon retrograde valvuloplasty technique was used in 94% of patients; the largest balloon used was 20 mm in over half. The mean gradient decreased from 55 to 29 mmHg and the aortic valve area increased from 0·5 to 0·8 cm^2, associated with symptomatic improvement in most patients. Procedural mortality was 3%; other major complications associated with the valvuloplasty procedure included cardiac arrest (5%), emergency aortic valve replacement (1%), left ventricular tamponade (2%), cerebral vascular accident (1%), systemic embolus (1%), emergency temporary pacing (5%), and ventricular arrhythmia requiring countershock (3%).

In summary, the initial results of the multicenter studies were similar to each other, and to the results of the previously described single-center studies, and suggested that balloon aortic valvuloplasty resulted in modest hemodynamic improvement and significant symptomatic improvement in many patients considered to be at high risk for aortic valve surgery.

Left ventricular function

Grade B Aortic valve replacement has been shown to improve left ventricular function in many patients with aortic stenosis and left ventricular dysfunction.[9–11] Safian and colleagues[42] at Beth Israel Hospital examined the effect of balloon aortic valvuloplasty on left ventricular performance in 28 patients with a low left ventricular ejection fraction (mean 37%), severe aortic stenosis and a mean age of 79 years. Balloon valvuloplasty resulted in significant increases in aortic valve area (0·5–0·9 cm^2), systolic pressure (120–135 mmHg), and cardiac output (4·2–4·8 l/min) ($P < 0.01$ for all comparisons), and significant decreases in transaortic pressure gradient (69–35 mmHg) and pulmonary capillary wedge pressure (24–20 mmHg) ($P < 0.01$ for both comparisons). All patients were symptomatically improved at the time of discharge.

Serial radionuclide ventriculography showed an increase in left ventricular ejection fraction from 37% prior to valvuloplasty to 44% 48 hours post procedure and 49% at 3 month follow up. However, there was substantial heterogeneity of response, with 13 patients showing progressive increases in left ventricular ejection fraction (34% to 49% to 58%, $P<0\cdot001$), whereas 15 patients showed no significant change in ejection fraction (41% to 40% to 41%, $P=$ NS) over 3 months. There was no difference between the groups with respect to age, extent of coronary disease, history of myocardial infarction, or baseline or postprocedure aortic valve area. However, peak systolic wall stress and left ventricular dimensions were higher in those patients who showed no improvement in ejection fraction. It may be that the failure to increase ejection fraction in this group is due to irreversible impairment in myocardial contractile function, secondary to previous infarction or longstanding aortic stenosis. Davidson and colleagues at Duke University also found that fewer than half of patients with a baseline left ventricular ejection fraction less than 45% showed sustained improvement following percutaneous balloon aortic valvuloplasty, even at short-term follow up.[43]

Follow up

Grade B Despite the moderate hemodynamic improvement and significant symptomatic improvement initially achieved in most patients with aortic stenosis following percutaneous balloon valvuloplasty, this technique is severely limited by the high incidence of restenosis. The Beth Israel group reported follow-up results in 170 patients (mean age 77 years) with symptomatic aortic stenosis who underwent balloon aortic valvuloplasty between October 1985 and April 1988.[37] The procedure was completed successfully in 168 patients, with significant improvement in aortic valve area and gradient. There were six in-hospital deaths and five patients required early aortic valve replacement. Follow up averaging 9·1 months was available for all 157 patients discharged from the hospital after successful valvuloplasty. In 44 patients (28%), recurrent symptoms developed a mean of 7·5 months after the procedure: 16 were treated by repeat valvuloplasty, 17 by aortic valve replacement and 11 with medical therapy. Two patients had a second restenosis, treated by aortic valve replacement in one case and by a third valvuloplasty procedure in the other. At latest follow up 103 patients (66%) were symptomatically improved, including 15 with restenosis who successfully underwent redilation. Twenty-five patients died after discharge, a mean of 6 months after balloon valvuloplasty. The most common cause of death was progressive congestive heart failure.

Repeat cardiac catheterization was performed in 35 patients in the Beth Israel follow-up cohort, including 21 with recurrent symptoms, a mean of 6 months after valvuloplasty. Significant aortic valve restenosis was found in all 21 patients with recurrent symptoms, and in eight of the 14 patients

without symptoms. If restenosis was assumed to have occurred in all 25 patients who died, and in all 44 patients with recurrent symptoms, then the "clinical" rate of restenosis following valvuloplasty was 44% at only 9 months. The probability of survival at 1 year was 74% for the entire study population. However, if both recurrent symptoms and death were considered as events, the probability of event-free survival at 1 year was only 50%.

Similarly poor long-term results with high rates of early restenosis were reported by both of the multicenter studies of balloon aortic valvuloplasty. Among the 492 patients treated with balloon valvuloplasty in the Mansfield Registry the 1 year survival rate was 64%, with an event-free survival rate of only 43%.[44] Among the 674 patients reported in the National Heart, Lung and Blood Institute Balloon Valvuloplasty Registry, survival at 1, 2 and 3 years was 55, 35 and 23%, respectively.[45] Lieberman and colleagues[46] reported long-term follow up in 165 patients undergoing balloon aortic valvuloplasty. The median duration of follow up was 3·9 years, with follow up achieved in 99% of patients. Ninety-three per cent of patients died or underwent aortic valve replacement, and 60% died of cardiac-related causes. The probability of event-free survival, defined as freedom from death, aortic valve replacement or repeat balloon aortic valvuloplasty at 1, 2 and 3 years after balloon aortic valvuloplasty, was 40%, 19% and 6%, respectively. By contrast, the probability of survival 3 years after balloon aortic valvuloplasty in a subset of 42 patients who underwent subsequent aortic valve replacement was 84%.

Mechanism of restenosis

Because the mechanism by which balloon aortic valvuloplasty increases aortic valve area appears to consist chiefly of fracture of calcified nodules within leaflets and leaflet stretching, and only rarely involves separation of commissural fusion,[28] it is not surprising that the initial improvement in aortic valve area is modest at best, and that significant and early restenosis occurs in most patients. Any element of improvement in the aortic valve area due to leaflet stretching is likely to be rapidly compromised by elastic recoil, and in fact postprocedure echocardiographic follow up suggests early loss of initial valve area in many patients.[47] Histologic examination in patients who underwent balloon aortic valvuloplasty and had subsequent valve tissue examined at the time of aortic valve replacement or necropsy, showed evidence of closing of fractures in calcified nodules by granulation tissue that may lead to valvular scarring.[48,49] The more rapid time course of this type of inflammatory response, compared to the slowly developing valvular calcification that initially led to the aortic stenosis, may explain the relatively rapid progression to symptomatic restenosis following initially successful balloon valvuloplasty.

Results of balloon aortic valvuloplasty

- Initial hemodynamic and symptomatic improvement
- Early restenosis, with recurrent symptoms
- No improvement in long-term survival or event-free survival.

Predictors of outcome following balloon aortic valvuloplasty

Grade B Following recognition of the high incidence of restenosis after balloon aortic valvuloplasty, attempts were made to identify patient subsets more likely to derive long-term benefit. Kuntz and colleagues[50] analyzed event-free survival in 205 patients who underwent balloon valvuloplasty for symptomatic critical aortic stenosis. They evaluated 40 demographic and hemodynamic variables as univariate predictors of event-free survival by Cox regression analysis, and attempted to identify independent predictors of event-free survival by stepwise multivariate analysis. The rate of event-free survival, defined as survival without recurrent symptoms, repeat balloon valvuloplasty or subsequent aortic valve replacement, was 18% over a mean follow-up period of 24 months (Figure 54.3). Direct predictors of long-term event-free survival in the univariate analysis included female gender, left ventricular ejection fraction, and left ventricular and aortic systolic pressure. Inverse

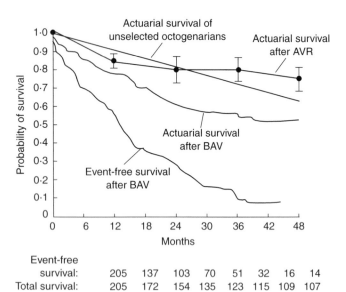

Figure 54.3 Actuarial total and event-free survival among 205 patients treated by balloon aortic valvuloplasty (BAV). Shown for comparison are the actuarial survival rates among unselected octogenarians in the United States and among octogenarians who undergo aortic-valve replacement (AVR). The numbers below the figure show how many patients were alive or alive without an event at each follow-up. (Reproduced with permission from Kuntz *et al.*[50])

predictors of event-free survival included pulmonary capillary wedge and pulmonary artery pressures. Although the pre- and postvalvuloplasty aortic valve area and aortic valve gradient were not associated with event-free survival, the per cent reduction in the peak aortic valve gradient was a strong predictor of long-term event-free survival. For patients with a left ventricular ejection fraction of less than 40% at baseline, improvement in the ejection fraction was also directly associated with event-free survival. Notably, when patients aged 80 or older were analyzed as a subgroup, univariate analysis indicated that the predictors of long-term event-free survival were the same in elderly patients as in the entire patient cohort.

In the stepwise multivariate analysis the only independent predictors of event-free survival following balloon aortic valvuloplasty were the baseline aortic systolic pressure, the baseline pulmonary capillary wedge pressure (inversely related), and the per cent reduction in the peak aortic valve gradient. A baseline aortic systolic pressure less than 110 mmHg was associated with a relative risk of late events of 2·03, and a baseline pulmonary capillary wedge pressure greater than 25 mmHg was associated with a relative risk of 1·73, compared to the risk in patients with a baseline aortic systolic pressure greater than or equal to 140 mmHg and a pulmonary capillary wedge pressure less than 18 mmHg, respectively. Furthermore, a reduction of less than 40% in the peak aortic valve gradient was associated with a relative risk of late events of 1·75, compared to the risk in patients in whom valvuloplasty produced a reduction of 55% or more in the peak aortic valve gradient.

To facilitate prediction of outcome following aortic valvuloplasty, using only information available *prior* to the procedure, Kuntz and colleagues utilized the two independent baseline hemodynamic predictors in the Cox model, and estimated the probability of event-free survival at 6, 12, 18 and 24 months for all patients (Table 54.3). According to this two-variable predictive model, patients with baseline pulmonary capillary wedge pressure less than 18 mmHg and aortic systolic pressure greater than or equal to 140 mmHg (the most favorable patient subgroup) had event-free survival rates of 65% at 1 year and 41% at 2 years. On the other hand, patients with baseline pulmonary capillary wedge pressure greater than 25 mmHg and aortic systolic pressure less than 110 mmHg had event-free survival rates of only 23% at 1 year and 4% at 2 years.

In summary, Kuntz and colleagues found that the most important predictors of event-free survival following balloon aortic valvuloplasty were factors related to baseline left ventricular performance, a finding confirmed by analysis of long-term outcome in both large multicenter balloon aortic valvuloplasty registries.[44,45] The best long-term results following valvuloplasty were observed in patients who would also have been expected to have excellent long-term results after aortic valve replacement. In fact, comparison with the

Table 54.3 Estimated event-free survival according to baseline hemodynamic variables

Pre PCWP (mmHg)	Pre AOSP (mmHg)	Event-free survival (%)			
		6 mth	12 mth	18 mth	24 mth
<18	≥140	79	65	51	41
<18	110–139	73	58	42	31
<18	<110	64	46	30	19
18–25	≥140	74	59	43	32
18–25	110–139	68	50	34	23
18–25	<110	58	38	22	13
>25	≥140	63	44	28	18
>25	110–139	55	35	19	10
>25	<110	43	23	10	4

Abbreviations: AOSP, aortic systolic pressure; PCWP, pulmonary capillary wedge pressure
Reproduced with permission from Kuntz *et al.*[50]

surgical data on aortic valve replacement in octogenarians suggests that patients with good hemodynamic performance have better survival after aortic valve replacement than after balloon aortic valvuloplasty.[19] Among patients with poor left ventricular performance or advanced heart failure, event-free survival following balloon aortic valvuloplasty was dismal and did not appear to improve the natural history of untreated aortic stenosis.[21] Therefore, even in elderly patients with advanced heart failure and higher perioperative risk,[13] aortic valve replacement may increase the likelihood of long-term survival compared to balloon aortic valvuloplasty. In such high-risk patients, however, balloon aortic valvuloplasty may have a role in providing transient hemodynamic improvement, perhaps decreasing the risk of subsequent aortic valve replacement.

Repeat balloon aortic valvuloplasty

Grade B/C In patients who are not candidates for surgery the development of restenosis following balloon aortic valvuloplasty can be managed with a repeat procedure. Studies of repeat valvuloplasty have shown that the absolute aortic valve area tends to be slightly smaller both before and after the repeat valvuloplasty, even when larger balloons or balloon combinations are used.[51] The incidence of repeat restenosis remains high: follow up of the 47 patients in the Mansfield Registry who underwent repeat valvuloplasty showed that 66% of patients had died, undergone subsequent valve replacement or required a third valvuloplasty at a mean follow up of 5 months.[52] Histologic study of valves treated with balloon valvuloplasty, and excised prior to subsequent surgery or examined at autopsy, has shown active cellular proliferation within the splits in calcified nodules, as well as foci of ossification.[48] These findings suggest

an active scarring process in response to balloon valvuloplasty, which may explain the failure to achieve better results with the use of larger balloons, and raises the possibility that balloon-induced injury to the aortic valve may accelerate the natural history of aortic stenosis.

Aortic valve surgery after balloon aortic valvuloplasty

Grade B Most surviving patients who have undergone balloon aortic valvuloplasty develop clinically significant restenosis within 1–2 years of the procedure. Many of these patients are subsequently treated with aortic valve replacement. Johnson and colleagues at the Beth Israel Hospital reported 45 patients (25% of the initial balloon valvuloplasty cohort) subsequently treated with aortic valve replacement.[53] Three patients required emergency operation immediately after unsuccessful valvuloplasty, and the remaining 42 had an elective operation at a mean of 8 months following valvuloplasty, primarily for the development of symptomatic restenosis. Despite the fact that the majority of these patients had initially undergone balloon valvuloplasty because they were considered to be at high risk for surgery, there were only four hospital deaths among the 45 patients. Three additional patients died a mean of 11 months following surgery. All surviving patients had persistent symptomatic improvement following surgery.

Lieberman and colleagues at Duke reported 40 patients (24% of the initial balloon valvuloplasty treatment group) who subsequently underwent aortic valve replacement.[54] Only one patient (2·5%) suffered a perioperative death. The probability of survival 3 years from the date of the last mechanical intervention was 75% for patients treated with balloon valvuloplasty and subsequent aortic valve replacement, compared to only 20% for patients whose restenosis was treated with repeat balloon valvuloplasty, and 13% for patients who had no further mechanical intervention after developing restenosis. The majority of surgically treated patients remained asymptomatic at last follow up. It is important to note that this study is not a randomized comparison of treatment strategies for restenosis, and the results must be interpreted in light of the probable selection bias with regard to choice of management strategy for aortic valve restenosis. Nevertheless, it appears that in this group of patients initially felt to be at high risk for aortic valve replacement, surgery could be performed with an acceptable operative risk. Furthermore, as opposed to balloon valvuloplasty, aortic valve replacement appears to offer a reasonable chance of long-term freedom from symptoms. Although these reports do not specifically address potential reduction in the risk of subsequent surgery by prior performance of balloon valvuloplasty, a beneficial effect cannot be excluded.

Balloon aortic valvuloplasty *v* aortic valve surgery

Grade B There are no randomized trials comparing balloon aortic valvuloplasty with aortic valve replacement in adult patients with critical aortic stenosis. However, Bernard and colleagues in France compared two non-randomized matched series of patients with aortic stenosis treated with either balloon aortic valvuloplasty or aortic valve replacement at the same institution between January 1986 and March 1989.[55] Forty-six patients were treated with balloon aortic valvuloplasty and 23 with aortic valve replacement with a bioprosthesis. Baseline clinical and hemodynamic parameters were similar in both groups; all patients were at least 75 years old. Follow-up was 22 months for the aortic valvuloplasty patients and 28 months for those having surgery. Among patients treated with balloon aortic valvuloplasty, three patients (6·5%) died within 5 days of the procedure, and an additional 24 (42%) died during subsequent follow up, with 16 deaths being due to recurrent heart failure. Sixteen patients (35%) underwent subsequent aortic valve replacement at a mean of 16 months following balloon valvuloplasty. At last follow up, only three valvuloplasty patients (6·5%) remained alive without subsequent aortic valve replacement. Of the patients treated with initial aortic valve replacement, two (8·7%) died in the perioperative period and an additional three (13%) died during the follow up period. All remaining patients (78%) were alive and in New York Heart Association functional class I or II at last follow up. The overall survival rate following balloon valvuloplasty was 75% at 1 year, 47% at 2 years and 33% at 5 years. By contrast, survival following surgery was 83% at 1 and 2 years and 75% at 3 and 4 years. Although selection

bias cannot be excluded in this non-randomized case comparison study, nevertheless the results strongly suggest that percutaneous balloon aortic valvuloplasty does not compare favorably with aortic valve surgery in elderly patients with aortic stenosis.

Specific indications for balloon valvuloplasty

Aortic valvuloplasty prior to non-cardiac surgery

Grade B/C Patients with severe aortic stenosis are at increased risk for significant cardiac complications during non-cardiac surgery.[56] Three studies described the role of balloon aortic valvuloplasty in the management of patients with critical aortic stenosis requiring major non-cardiac surgery.[57–59] In these studies, 29 patients with critical aortic stenosis underwent balloon aortic valvuloplasty which was complicated by procedural death due to ventricular perforation and tamponade in one patient. Valvuloplasty resulted in a significant improvement in aortic valve gradient and aortic valve area. Twenty-eight of the 29 patients underwent the planned surgical procedure under general or epidural anesthesia. All but one patient had uncomplicated non-cardiac surgery, with no significant congestive heart failure, hypotension, myocardial infarction, arrhythmia or conduction abnormality either during or immediately after surgery. One patient developed marked hypotension requiring transient intravenous pressor support during surgery for bowel carcinoma, resulting in interruption of surgery. This patient subsequently underwent aortic valve replacement and coronary artery bypass graft surgery, followed by repeat bowel resection. Procedures performed successfully following palliative balloon aortic valvuloplasty included aortic aneurysm repair, repair of hip fracture, exploratory laparotomy and thoracotomy. However, the cited reports are not randomized or case–control comparisons of preoperative balloon aortic valvuloplasty versus aortic valve replacement or medical therapy, and do not test the hypothesis that routine balloon valvuloplasty reduces the risk of non-cardiac surgery in patients with critical aortic stenosis. O'Keefe and colleagues[60] at the Mayo Clinic described 48 patients with severe aortic stenosis who underwent non-cardiac surgery (including vascular, orthopedic and abdominal procedures) without preoperative balloon valvuloplasty. There were no major perioperative complications in this group, who were managed with careful monitoring of systemic and pulmonary artery pressure during anesthesia. Therefore, the available evidence suggests that balloon valvuloplasty prior to urgent non-cardiac surgery may have greatest benefit in those patients with critical aortic stenosis and poor ventricular function, heart failure or hypotension, in whom transient hemodynamic improvement may decrease the risk of perioperative complications.

Aortic valvuloplasty as a bridge to aortic valve replacement

Grade B/C As noted earlier, many patients treated with balloon aortic valvuloplasty subsequently undergo aortic valve replacement. Early series of such patients demonstrated an acceptable operative risk and excellent surgical outcome, with long-term freedom from symptoms in most survivors.[53,54] In contrast, recent reports of cardiac surgery in octogenarians identified previous percutaneous aortic valvuloplasty as an independent predictor of hospital death following valve replacement.[61,62] However, in most patients undergoing surgery in these studies, valve replacement was performed because of failure of the initial balloon aortic valvuloplasty, which was not specifically used to stabilize the patient for subsequent surgery.

Smedira and colleagues[63] studied critically ill patients with aortic stenosis in whom balloon aortic valvuloplasty was specifically used as a bridge to aortic valve replacement. They reported five patients with severe aortic stenosis, multiple organ failure and severe hemodynamic compromise who were judged to be at excessive risk for aortic valve surgery. Balloon aortic valvuloplasty was used in these patients to provide transient hemodynamic improvement, to improve organ function, and to decrease the risk of subsequent definitive surgical correction. Following successful balloon aortic valvuloplasty and clinical stabilization, subsequent elective valve replacement was performed in all patients without complications. This report suggests that balloon aortic valvuloplasty may have a role as a bridge to subsequent aortic valve replacement for patients in whom heart failure or hypotension is so severe that the risk of primary aortic valve surgery is unacceptable.

Aortic valvuloplasty in cardiogenic shock

Grade C Of the 674 patients in the multicenter NHLBI Balloon Valvuloplasty Registry, 39 (6%) had cardiogenic shock. The largest reported series specifically describing the role of balloon aortic valvuloplasty in cardiogenic shock is that of Moreno and colleagues from the Massachusetts General Hospital.

Moreno[64] studied 21 patients with critical aortic stenosis and cardiogenic shock treated with balloon aortic valvuloplasty. All patients had major associated comorbid conditions precluding the use of emergency aortic valve replacement. The hemodynamic results were excellent, with an increase in systolic aortic pressure from 77 to 116 mmHg and an increase in aortic valve area from 0·5 to 0·8 cm^2 ($P = 0·0001$ for both comparisons). Cardiac index increased from 1·84 to 2·24 l/min/m^2 ($P = 0·06$). Nine treated patients died in hospital, two during the procedure and seven following successful valvuloplasty. Procedural complications were frequent, with five patients suffering vascular complications and one patient each developing stroke,

cholesterol embolus and aortic regurgitation requiring aortic valve replacement. Twelve patients (57%) survived and were discharged from the hospital. During follow up of 15 months, five additional patients died. Actuarial survival was 38% at 27 months. The only predictor of improved survival was the postprocedure cardiac index.

In summary, the limited published data suggest that emergency percutaneous balloon aortic valvuloplasty can be successfully performed in patients with critical aortic stenosis and cardiogenic shock. Morbidity and mortality remain high even after hemodynamically successful procedures. Given the poor long-term outcome in patients treated with balloon aortic valvuloplasty, its use in patients with cardiogenic shock should be considered a bridge to subsequent aortic valve replacement in those patients who improve sufficiently to undergo surgery at reasonable risk.

Aortic valvuloplasty in patients with low output, low gradient

Grade B Patients with left ventricular dysfunction and aortic stenosis in the presence of low cardiac output and low aortic valve gradient present a complex diagnostic and therapeutic challenge. Aortic valve surgery is associated with increased morbidity and mortality in such patients, a subset of whom have irreversible myocardial dysfunction.[10–12] Balloon aortic valvuloplasty has been proposed as a diagnostic tool in patients with aortic stenosis and low-output low-gradient hemodynamics, to distinguish those with reversible myocardial dysfunction due to abnormal loading conditions from those with irreversible myocardial dysfunction. It has been suggested that patients with low-output low-gradient hemodynamics who have a significant improvement in either ventricular function or symptoms following successful balloon aortic valvuloplasty are more likely to improve following aortic valve replacement than those patients in whom the former produces no significant benefit.

Safian and colleagues studied 28 patients with a low left ventricular ejection fraction (mean 37%) and severe aortic stenosis who underwent balloon aortic valvuloplasty.[42] On the basis of response to balloon valvuloplasty they were able to separate patients into a subset with progressive improvement in left ventricular ejection fraction, and a subset which showed no significant change in left ventricular function. Nishimura and colleagues, utilizing data from the multicenter Mansfield Aortic Valvuloplasty Registry, compared 67 patients with low-output low-gradient hemodynamics against 200 patients with a low cardiac index but not a low aortic valve gradient.[65] Patients with low-output low-gradient hemodynamics had less of a decrease in aortic valve gradient after valvuloplasty, but a similar improvement in estimated aortic valve area. However, actuarial survival at 12 months was 46% for these patients, as against 64% in the comparison cohort ($P < 0·05$). Furthermore, patients with low-gradient hemodynamics were less likely to show sustained symptomatic improvement. Therefore, as long-term outcome after balloon valvuloplasty is poor in these patients aortic valve replacement may be indicated in those in whom balloon aortic valvuloplasty produces an initial favorable response. Although these reports suggest that it may be possible to identify a subset of patients with aortic stenosis and low-output low-gradient hemodynamics likely to benefit from subsequent aortic valve replacement, the hypothesis that response to aortic valvuloplasty predicts subsequent outcome following surgery has not been tested.

Other indications

Grade C Case reports have described the use of balloon aortic valvuloplasty for the management of critical aortic stenosis in pregnancy, documenting its safe performance during pregnancy with subsequent normal births.[66] Given their age range, pregnant patients are more likely to have congenital or rheumatic aortic stenosis and therefore to have valve stenosis due to commissural fusion, which responds more favorably to balloon dilation than does the more frequently encountered degenerative calcific valvular disease. Use of balloon aortic valvuloplasty as a bridge to subsequent cardiac transplant in a patient with aortic stenosis and end-stage heart failure has also been described.[67]

Indications for balloon aortic valvuloplasty

- Symptomatic critical aortic stenosis in patients who are not candidates for aortic valve replacement
- Bridge to aortic valve replacement in patients with severe hemodynamic compromise
- Prior to urgent non-cardiac surgery
- Aortic stenosis with low-output low-gradient hemodynamics.

Conclusions

The development and analysis of balloon aortic valvuloplasty as a treatment strategy for adult patients with critical aortic stenosis offers a paradigm for the investigation of new therapeutic techniques. The initial enthusiasm for new treatment modalities, often based on arguments of physiology, first principles or small case series, is often replaced by a sobering realization of limitations and complications, revealed by careful prospective multicenter clinical trials, ultimately resulting in the development of appropriate clinical indications for the new treatment strategy. The development and investigation of balloon aortic valvuloplasty for aortic stenosis followed just such a course and illustrates the impact of careful, early prospective clinical trial data on the evolution and rapid development of appropriate indications for new therapeutic techniques.

Although valve replacement clearly improves morbidity and mortality in patients with symptomatic aortic stenosis, concern regarding the higher morbidity in high-risk subgroups led to the investigation of balloon aortic valvuloplasty as an alternative. Early evidence from both single- and multicenter series showing hemodynamic and symptomatic improvement in most patients treated with balloon valvuloplasty, led to initial widespread enthusiasm for this new technique. However, this enthusiasm was quickly tempered as subsequent follow up in these high-quality case series demonstrated a high rate of hemodynamic and clinical restenosis, and failure of balloon valvuloplasty to improve long-term or event-free survival.

Critical evaluation of the data from these large case series provided further understanding of the appropriate role of balloon valvuloplasty in the management of patients with aortic stenosis. When patients were stratified by the independent predictors of event-free survival, it became clear that those who did best with balloon aortic valvuloplasty were acceptable candidates for valve surgery and had an even better event-free survival following surgery. On the other hand, patients with baseline profiles that indicated a high risk for surgery also did extremely poorly with balloon valvuloplasty, with event-free survival that did not appear to differ from the natural history of untreated aortic stenosis. The rapid accumulation and careful analysis of clinical trial data on patients treated with balloon valvuloplasty quickly established that the treatment of choice for adult patients with symptomatic aortic stenosis is valve replacement, with balloon valvuloplasty being reserved for those in whom surgery is not possible or practical. Further refinement of the appropriate therapeutic niche for balloon aortic valvuloplasty has been aided by small case series targeted at specific indications for non-surgical therapy of aortic stenosis.

The following guidelines on appropriate utilization of balloon aortic valvuloplasty in adult patients with symptomatic critical aortic stenosis are based on case series and case–control studies, and therefore should be considered as Grade B recommendations.

Based on the available evidence, balloon aortic valvuloplasty should be considered:

1. For patients with symptomatic aortic stenosis who are not operable, or who are poor candidates for aortic valve replacement owing to severe comorbid illness or advanced age in the presence of other significant predictors of surgical risk. It should be emphasized that advanced age alone in a patient without other significant surgical risk factors is not a contraindication to aortic valve replacement. It must be further stressed that the goal of balloon aortic valvuloplasty in this patient group is transient symptomatic relief, as there is no evidence that valvuloplasty improves survival or provides long-term freedom from symptoms. **Grade B**

2. As a bridge to subsequent aortic valve replacement in patients with advanced heart failure, hypotension or cardiogenic shock, when clinical presentation suggests excessive risk for an initial surgical strategy. The goal of balloon aortic valvuloplasty in this cohort is transient hemodynamic improvement, leading to stabilization of the patient for subsequent aortic valve replacement, the only treatment shown to ultimately improve long-term survival. **Grade B**

3. For patients with critical aortic stenosis and poor ventricular function, heart failure or hypotension who require urgent or emergency non-cardiac surgery. The goal of balloon aortic valvuloplasty in this patient subset is successful completion of the required non-cardiac surgical procedure, with subsequent aortic valve replacement for the underlying aortic stenosis. **Grade B**

4. For patients with aortic stenosis, diminished left ventricular function and low-output low-gradient hemodynamics, in whom the response to initial "diagnostic" balloon valvuloplasty may help identify those likely to benefit from subsequent aortic valve replacement. **Grade B**

Given the disparity in outcome between aortic valve replacement and balloon aortic valvuloplasty in large high-quality case series and non-randomized case–control studies, it is unreasonable to pursue randomized clinical trials comparing these treatment strategies. However, the high-quality case series rapidly performed and reported in patients treated with balloon aortic valvuloplasty not only established the appropriate role for balloon valvuloplasty in the treatment of aortic stenosis, but also confirmed the value of prompt clinical investigation in the rapid development of appropriate indications for new therapeutic techniques. When the *goal* of therapy is long-term or symptom-free survival, the available clinical trial data clearly support valve replacement as the treatment of choice for aortic stenosis. However, in patients who are not candidates for or who refuse surgery, the trial data have demonstrated a role for balloon aortic valvuloplasty, albeit with the more limited goal of transient, palliative symptomatic relief, without improvement in survival or long-term symptomatic benefit.

References

1. Passik CS, Ackermann DM, Pluth JR, Edwards WD. Temporal changes in the causes of aortic stenosis: a surgical pathologic study of 646 cases. *Mayo Clin Proc* 1987;**62**:119–23.
2. Frank S, Johnson A, Ross J. Natural history of valvular aortic stenosis. *Br Heart J* 1973;**35**:41–6.
3. Ross J, Braunwald E. Aortic stenosis. *Circulation* 1968;**38** (Suppl. V):61–7.
4. Pellikka PA, Nishimura RA, Bailey KR, Tajik AJ. The natural history of adults with asymptomatic, hemodynamically significant aortic stenosis. *J Am Coll Cardiol* 1990;**15**:1012–17.
5. Otto CM, Burwash IG, Legget ME *et al.* Prospective study of asymptomatic valvular aortic stenosis. Clinical, echocardiographic, and exercise predictors of outcome. *Circulation* 1997;**95**:2262–70.
6. Carabello BA. Timing of valve replacement in aortic stenosis. Moving closer to perfection. *Circulation* 1997;**95**:2241–3.
7. Hsieh K, Keane JF, Nadas AS, Bernhard WF, Castaneda AR. Long-term follow-up of valvotomy before 1968 for congenital aortic stenosis. *Am J Cardiol* 1986;**58**:338–41.
8. McBride LR, Nannheim KS, Fiore AC *et al.* Aortic valve decalcification. *J Thorac Cardiovasc Surg* 1990;**100**:36–42.
9. Kennedy JW, Doces J, Stewart DK. Left ventricular function before and following aortic valve replacement. *Circulation* 1977;**56**:944–50.
10. Smith N, McAnulty JH, Rahimtoola SH. Severe aortic stenosis with impaired left ventricular function and clinical heart failure: results of valve replacement. *Circulation* 1978;**58**:255–64.
11. Lund O. Preoperative risk evaluation and stratification of long-term survival after valve replacement for aortic stenosis. *Circulation* 1990;**82**:124–39.
12. Magovern JA, Pennock JL, Campbell DB *et al.* Aortic valve replacement and combined aortic valve replacement and coronary artery bypass grafting: predicting high risk groups. *J Am Coll Cardiol* 1987;**9**:38–43.
13. Edmunds LH, Stephenson LW, Edie RN, Ratcliffe MB. Open-heart surgery in octogenarians. *N Engl J Med* 1988;**319**:131–6.
14. Verheul HA, Van Den Brink RBA, Bouma BJ *et al.* Analysis of risk factors for excess mortality after aortic valve replacement. *J Am Coll Cardiol* 1995;**26**:1280–6.
15. Gehlot A, Mullany CJ, Ilstrup D *et al.* Aortic valve replacement in patients aged eighty years and older: early and long-term results. *J Thorac Cardiovasc Surg* 1996;**111**:1026–36.
16. Asimakopoulos G, Edwards M, Taylor K. Aortic valve replacement in patients 80 years of age and older. Survival and cause of death based on 1100 cases: collective results from the UK Heart Valve Registry. *Circulation* 1997;**96**:3403–8.
17. Edwards FH, Peterson ED, Coombs LP *et al.* Prediction of operative mortality after valve replacement surgery. *J Am Coll Cardiol* 2001;**37**:885–92.
18. Fremes SE, Goldman BS, Ivanou J, Weisel RD, David TE, Salerno T. Valvular surgery in the elderly. *Circulation* 1989;**80**(Suppl. I):177–90.
19. Levinson JR, Akins CW, Buckley MJ *et al.* Octogenarians with aortic stenosis. Outcome after aortic valve replacement. *Circulation* 1989;**80**(Suppl. I):149–56.
20. Rosengart TK, Finnin EB, Kim DY *et al.* Open heart surgery in the elderly: results from a consecutive series of 100 patients aged 85 years or older. *Am J Med* 2002;**112**:143–77.
21. O'Keefe JH, Vlietstra RE, Bailey KR, Holmes DR. Natural history of candidates for balloon aortic valvuloplasty. *Mayo Clin Proc* 1987;**62**:986–91.
22. Kirklin JW, Barratt-Boyes BG. Congenital aortic stenosis. In: *Cardiac Surgery*, 2nd edn. New York: Churchill Livingstone, 1993.

23. Lababidi Z, Wu JR, Walls JT. Percutaneous balloon aortic valvuloplasty: results in 23 patients. *Am J Cardiol* 1984; **53**:194–7.

24. Rosenfeld HM, Landzberg MJ, Perry SB, Colan SD, Keane JF, Lock JE. Balloon aortic valvuloplasty in young adults with congenital aortic stenosis. *Am J Cardiol* 1994;**73**:1112–17.

25. Tomita H, Echigo S, Kimura K *et al.* Balloon aortic valvuloplasty in children: a multicenter study in Japan. *Jpn Circ J* 2001;**65**:599–602.

26. Cribier A, Savin T, Saondi N, Rocha P, Berland J, Letac B. Percutaneous transluminal valvuloplasty of acquired aortic stenosis in elderly patients: an alternative to valve replacement? *Lancet* 1986;**i**:63–7.

27. McKay RG, Safian RD, Lock JE *et al.* Balloon dilatation of calcific aortic stenosis in elderly patients: postmortem, intraoperative, and percutaneous valvuloplasty studies. *Circulation* 1986;**74**:119–25.

28. Safian RD, Mandell VS, Thurer RE *et al.* Postmortem and intraoperative balloon valvuloplasty of calcific aortic stenosis in elderly patients: mechanisms of successful dilation. *J Am Coll Cardiol* 1987;**9**:655–60.

29. Block PC, Palacios IF. Comparison of hemodynamic results of anterograde versus retrograde percutaneous balloon aortic valvuloplasty. *Am J Cardiol* 1987;**60**:659–62.

30. Eisenhauer AC, Hadjipetrou P, Piemonte TC. Balloon aortic valvuloplasty revisited: the role of the Inoue balloon and transseptal antegrade approach. *Cathet Cardiovasc Interv* 2000;**50**:484–91.

31. Bahl VK, Chandra S, Goswami KC. Combined mitral and aortic valvuloplasty by the antegrade transseptal approach using the Inoue balloon catheter. *Int J Cardiol* 1998;**63**:313–15.

32. Dorros G, Lewin RF, King JF, Janke LM. Percutaneous transluminal valvuloplasty in calcific aortic stenosis: the double balloon technique. *Cathet Cardiovasc Diagn* 1987;**13**:151–6.

33. Fields CD, Lucas A, Desnoyers M *et al.* Dual balloon aortic valvuloplasty, despite augmenting acute hemodynamic improvement, fails to prevent post-valvuloplasty restenosis. *J Am Coll Cardiol* 1989;**13**:148A.

34. Solomon LW, Fusman B, Jolly N, Kim A, Feldman T. Percutaneous suture closure for management of large French size arterial puncture in aortic valvuloplasty. *J Invas Cardiol* 2001;**13**:592–6.

35. Michaels AD, Ports TA. Use of a percutaneous arterial suture device (Perclose) in patients undergoing percutaneous balloon aortic valvuloplasty. *Cathet Cardiovasc Interv* 2001;**53**:445–7.

36. Cribier A, Savin T, Berland J *et al.* Percutaneous transluminal balloon valvuloplasty of adult aortic stenosis: report of 92 cases. *J Am Coll Cardiol* 1987;**9**:381–6.

37. Safian RD, Berman AD, Diver DJ *et al.* Balloon aortic valvuloplasty in 170 consecutive patients. *N Engl J Med* 1988;**319**:125–30.

38. Block PC, Palacios IF. Clinical and hemodynamic follow-up after percutaneous aortic valvuloplasty in the elderly. *Am J Cardiol* 1988;**62**:760–3.

39. Lewin RF, Dorros G, King JF, Mathiak L. Percutaneous transluminal aortic valvuloplasty: acute outcome and follow-up of 125 patients. *J Am Coll Cardiol* 1989;**14**:1210–17.

40. McKay RG, for the Mansfield Scientific Aortic Valvuloplasty Registry. Balloon aortic valvuloplasty in 285 patients: initial results and complications. *Circulation* 1988;**78**(Suppl. II):II–594.

41. McKay RG, for the NHLBI Aortic Valvuloplasty Registry. Clinical outcome following balloon aortic valvuloplasty for severe aortic stenosis. *J Am Coll Cardiol* 1989;**13**:1218.

42. Safian RD, Warren SE, Berman AD *et al.* Improvement in symptoms and left ventricular performance after balloon aortic valvuloplasty in patients with aortic stenosis and depressed left ventricular ejection fraction. *Circulation* 1988;**78**:1181–91.

43. Davidson CJ, Harrison JK, Leithe ME, Kisslo KB, Bashore TM. Failure of balloon aortic valvuloplasty to result in sustained clinical improvement in patients with depressed left ventricular function. *Am J Cardiol* 1990;**65**:72–7.

44. O'Neill WW, for the Mansfield Scientific Aortic Valvuloplasty Registry Investigators. Predictors of long-term survival after percutaneous aortic valvuloplasty: report of the Mansfield Scientific Aortic Valvuloplasty Registry. *J Am Coll Cardiol* 1991;**17**:193–8.

45. Otto CM, Mickel MC, Kenedy JW *et al.* Three year outcome after balloon aortic valvuloplasty. Insights into prognosis of valvular aortic stenosis. *Circulation* 1994;**89**:642–50.

46. Lieberman EB, Bashore TM, Hermiller JB *et al.* Balloon aortic valvuloplasty in adults: failure of procedure to improve long-term survival. *J Am Coll Cardiol* 1995;**26**:1522–8.

47. Nishimura RA, Holmes DR, Reeder GS *et al.* Doppler evaluation of results of percutaneous aortic balloon valvuloplasty in calcific aortic stenosis. *Circulation* 1988;**78**:791–9.

48. Feldman T, Glagov S, Carroll JD. Restenosis following successful balloon valvuloplasty: bone formation in aortic valve leaflets. *Cathet Cardiovasc Diagn* 1993;**29**:1–7.

49. Isner JM. Aortic valvuloplasty: are balloon-dilated valves all they are "cracked" up to be? *Mayo Clin Proc* 1988;**63**:830–4.

50. Kuntz RE, Tosteson AN, Berman AD *et al.* Predictors of event-free survival after balloon aortic valvuloplasty. *N Engl J Med* 1991;**325**:17–23.

51. Kuntz RE, Tosteson AN, Maitland LA *et al.* Immediate results and long-term follow-up after repeat balloon aortic valvuloplasty. *Cathet Cardiovasc Diagn* 1992;**25**:4–9.

52. Ferguson JJ, Garza RA, and the Mansfield Scientific Aortic Valvuloplasty Registry Investigators. Efficacy of multiple balloon aortic valvuloplasty procedures. *J Am Coll Cardiol* 1991;**17**:1430–5.

53. Johnson RG, Dhillon JS, Thurer RL, Safian RD, Wientraub RM. Aortic valve operation after percutaneous aortic balloon valvuloplasty. *Ann Thorac Surg* 1990;**49**:740–5.

54. Lieberman EB, Wilson JS, Harrison JK *et al.* Aortic valve replacement in adults after balloon aortic valvuloplasty. *Circulation* 1994;**90**(Suppl. II):II205–8.

55. Bernard Y, Etievent J, Mourand JL *et al.* Long-term results of percutaneous aortic valvuloplasty compared with aortic valve replacement in patients more than 75 years old. *J Am Coll Cardiol* 1992;**20**:796–801.

56. Goldman L, Caldera DL, Nussbaum SR. Multifactorial index of cardiac risk in noncardiac surgical procedures. *N Engl J Med* 1977;**297**:845–56.

57. Levine MJ, Berman AD, Safian RD, Diver DJ, McKay RG. Palliation of valvular aortic stenosis by balloon valvuloplasty as preoperative preparation for noncardiac surgery. *J Am Coll Cardiol* 1988;**62**:1309–10.

58. Roth RB, Palacios IF, Block PC. Percutaneous aortic balloon valvuloplasty: its role in the management of patients with aortic stenosis requiring major noncardiac surgery. *J Am Coll Cardiol* 1989;**13**:1039–41.

59. Hayes SN, Holmes DR, Nishimura RA, Reeder GS. Palliative percutaneous aortic balloon valvuloplasty before noncardiac operations and invasive diagnostic procedures. *Mayo Clin Proc* 1989;**64**:753–7.

60. O'Keefe JH, Shub C, Pettke SR. Risk of noncardiac surgical procedures in patients with aortic stenosis. *Mayo Clin Proc* 1989;**64**:400–5.

61. Kohl P, Lahaye L, Gerard P, Limet R. Aortic valve replacement in octogenarians: perioperative outcome and clinical follow-up. *Eur J Cardiovasc Surg* 1999;**16**:68–73.

62. Kolh P, Kerzmann A, Lahaye L, Gerard P, Limet R. Cardiac surgery in octogenarians: peri-operative outcome and long-term results. *Eur Heart J* 2001;**22**:1235–43.

63. Smedira NG, Ports TA, Merrick SH, Rankin JS. Balloon aortic valvuloplasty as a bridge to aortic valve replacement in critically ill patients. *Ann Thorac Surg* 1993;**55**: 914–16.

64. Moreno PR, Ik-Kyung J, Block PC, Palacios IF. The role of percutaneous aortic balloon valvuloplasty in patients with cardiogenic shock and critical aortic stenosis. *J Am Coll Cardiol* 1994;**23**:1071–5.

65. Nishimura RA, Holmes DR, Michela ME *et al*. Follow-up of patients with low output, low gradient hemodynamics after percutaneous balloon aortic valvuloplasty: the Mansfield Scientific Aortic Valvuloplasty Registry. *J Am Coll Cardiol* 1991;**17**:828–33.

66. Banning AP, Pearson JF, Hall RJ. Role of balloon dilatation of the aortic valve in pregnant patients with severe aortic stenosis. *Br Heart J* 1993;**70**:544–5.

67. Vaitkus PT, Mancini D, Herrman HC. Percutaneous balloon aortic valvuloplasty as a bridge to heart transplantation. *J Heart Lung Transplant* 1993;**12**:1062–4.

55 Balloon valvuloplasty: mitral valve

Zoltan G Turi

Introduction

Percutaneous balloon mitral valvuloplasty is the latest technique in an evolution that began with Elliot Cutler advancing a knife retrograde through the apex of the left ventricle of a beating heart in 1923.[1] Neither he nor Henry Suttar, who performed a similar procedure in England two years later received the expected accolades,[2] and there has been continuing dispute about the relative role of mitral obstruction in defining the spectrum of mitral stenosis. Sir Thomas Lewis' statement that valvotomy was based on an erroneous idea, namely that the valve is the chief source of the trouble[3] has few proponents in the modern era and relieving mitral obstruction is the *de facto* standard of care.

After a 20 year hiatus, the battlefield experience with closed heart procedures in the second world war led to the application of these techniques outside the trauma arena. Although early results were confounded by significant morbidity and mortality, closed mitral valvotomy became a routine procedure for severe mitral stenosis, and is still the treatment of choice in many parts of the world where the disease is endemic and medical facilities limited. Large series[4,5] have claimed good long-term results, but lack of systematic follow up or comprehensive objective data obscure the actual restenosis rate and survival. In a Mayo Clinic retrospective analysis[6] there was 79% 10 year and 55% 20 year survival rate with reoperation in 34% by 10 years; however nearly a quarter of patients were lost to follow up and severity of disease at baseline could only be estimated. Open commissurotomy with the potential advantages of direct vision has supplanted closed procedures in industrialized nations. Controversy remains as to its superiority[7–9] with the advantages of direct vision favoring cases where thrombus is present.

The percutaneous approach

A pediatric cardiac surgeon, Kanji Inoue, developed a double lumen atrial septostomy balloon catheter made of latex, with a mesh weave used to constrain the balloon during inflation into the classic wishbone shape depicted in Figure 55.1.[10] He then adapted the device for percutaneous balloon mitral valvuloplasty, demonstrated under direct vision in the operating room its ability to split fused mitral commissures[11] and performed the first procedure in 1982.[12]

Mechanisms of valvuloplasty

The mechanisms responsible for the benefits of balloon mitral valvuloplasty[13] arise from the substantial radial force exerted by the enlarging balloon.[14] This stretches the mitral annulus, has the capacity to split fused commissures, and occasionally results in the cracking of calcifications. The stretching mechanism has been observed intraoperatively,[15] whereas the splitting of commissures[16] and cracking of

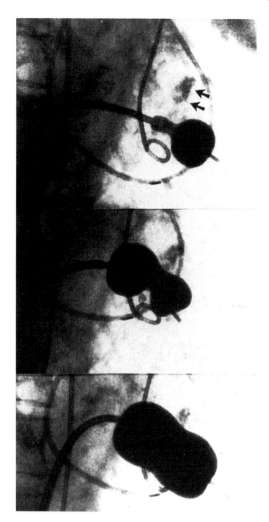

Figure 55.1 The Inoue balloon during staged deployment. From top to bottom: distal inflation with pullback against the valve; proximal inflation; full deployment. (Reprinted with permission of the American Heart Association, Inc.[38])

calcifications have been demonstrated by direct observation in excised valves.[17] The largely successful nature of balloon mitral valvuloplasty is derived from commissural splitting; balloon dilatation procedures where the other two mechanisms predominate, such as balloon valvuloplasty for calcific aortic stenosis, have less impressive short- and long-term results.

Preprocedure evaluation

The most common reason for exclusion of patients is unsuitable valve anatomy. Specific relevant physical examination findings are diminution of the first heart sound (often indicative of extensive subvalvular disease) and a hyperdynamic ventricle, suggestive of volume loading secondary to mitral or aortic regurgitation, both of which are relative contraindications to the procedure.

Non-invasive methods

The echocardiographic findings of greatest predictive value have been debated at length. The standard,[18] the Wilkins-Weyman score, incorporates a scoring system for mitral valve leaflet thickening, mobility and calcification, and severity of subvalvular disease (Table 55.1), with a score of <8 described as an "ideal" patient population, and echo scores over 12 potentially predicting poorer results. The correlation between this echo score and initial as well as long-term results is only fair, perhaps because it is a semiquantitative system based on partly subjective assessments

and because other factors not included in the system have predictive value. Thus studies have alternately confirmed[19-21] or refuted the predictive value of the Wilkins-Weyman score.[22-25] One element of the score, leaflet mobility, correlates more strongly with outcome (r value $= 0.67$) than the complete score,[26] while another element, severe calcification of the valve,[27] alone predicts a fourfold increase in cardiac complications and a 26% increase in 6 year mortality. In addition important anatomic features that predict outcome, such as eccentricity of commissural fusion and a funnel shaped subvalvular apparatus[28] (both negative predictors) are not included. Neither are presence of moderate or severe mitral regurgitation or left atrial thrombus, both relative contraindications. In univariate analysis, the scoring system does predict long-term results,[20] but so do age, presence of atrial fibrillation,[27] and severity of stenosis before and after the procedure.[29] Further, multivariate analyses that included the echo score *but not its individual components*, failed to demonstrate a single preprocedure predictor of event free survival.[30] Multivariate analysis that *includes* commissural calcification did reveal this to be a strong predictor of death, restenosis, and mitral valve replacement.[31] Perhaps the most compelling reason for routinely deriving the echo score is to allow for comparison with known data; most mitral valvuloplasty trials incorporate this or similar scoring systems. However, no absolute predictors of short- and long-term outcome have been developed.

Routine, preprocedure, transesophageal echocardiography has been recommended because of its superiority for detection of left atrial thrombus,[32] as well as other structural

Table 55.1   Grading of mitral valve characteristics from the echocardiographic examination

Grade	Mobility	Subvalvar thickening	Thickening	Calcification
1	Highly mobile valve with only leaflet tips restricted	Minimal thickening just below the mitral leaflets	Leaflets near normal in thickness (4–5 mm)	A single area of increased echo brightness
2	Leaflet mid and base portions have normal mobility	Thickening of chordal structures extending up to one third of the chordal length	Midleaflets normal, considerable thickening of margins (5–8 mm)	Scattered areas of brightness confined to leaflet margins
3	Valve continues to move forward in diastole, mainly from the base	Thickening extending to the distal third of the chords	Thickening extending through the entire leaflet (5–8 mm)	Brightness extending into the midportion of the leaflets
4	No or minimal forward movement of the leaflets in diastole	Extensive thickening and shortening of all chordal structures extending down to the papillary muscles	Considerable thickening of all leaflet tissue (>8–10 mm)	Extensive brightness throughout much of the leaflet tissue

Note. The total echocardiographic score was derived from an analysis of mitral leaflet mobility, valvar and subvalvar thickening, and calcification which were graded from 0 to 4 according to the above criteria. The total possible score ranges from 0 to 16.

Reprinted with permission from Wilkins GT, Weyman AE, Abascal VM *et al.* Percutaneous balloon dilation of the mitral valve: an analysis of echocardiographic variables related to outcome and the mechanism of dilation. *Br Heart J* **60**:299–309. © 1988 by the BMJ Publishing Group.[18]

abnormalities including vegetations or ruptured chordae. The case is most compelling in patients predisposed to clot formation such as those with spontaneous echo contrast ("smoke") on surface echocardiography and those with atrial fibrillation. The former was an independent predictor of left atrial thrombus in a prospective study of 100 patients.[33]

Cardiac catheterization

Cardiac catheterization prior to balloon commissurotomy is rarely necessary in young patients, but can be beneficial to exclude coronary artery disease in older subjects. The gradient alone is a poor proxy for assessment of severity of disease pre-valvuloplasty since it can lead to overestimation of disease with poor heart rate control or underestimation in patients who have not had fluids for many hours prior to catheterization.

Contraindications

While the usually cited contraindications are left atrial thrombus, greater than mild mitral regurgitation and severe calcification or subvalvular disease, these were largely empirically derived and can be challenged.

Thrombus

Hung[34] and others have described at least three series exceeding 90 patients total with apparent organized left atrial appendage clot who underwent uncomplicated balloon commissurotomy. However, valvuloplasty is not attempted when there is left atrial thrombus along the septum, free in the cavity, or on the surface of the valve. Using the conservative approach preferred by most interventionalists, Kang reports successful resolution of left atrial thrombi with warfarin therapy followed by balloon commissurotomy.[35]

Mitral regurgitation

The general presumption that valvuloplasty in patients with moderate or greater mitral regurgitation carried a high risk has not been prospectively tested; however, there have been two retrospective evaluations. A comparison of 25 patients with moderate mitral regurgitation and 25 age and gender matched patients with mild or no regurgitation did indeed demonstrate an increase in severe insufficiency post procedure; however, these patients had much higher echo scores and twice as frequently had severe calcification.[36] Further, while 20% of those with initially moderate mitral regurgitation developed severe regurgitation, hemodynamic improvement overall was similar, as was the incidence of post procedure mitral valve replacement. Similarly, patients with mild mitral regurgitation also had less favorable anatomy at baseline and had lower event

free survival but a similar success rate.[37] Thus, the evidence suggests that balloon commissurotomy can still be considered for these patients if they are poor risks for heart surgery. Nevertheless, a theoretical disadvantage is additional volume loading of the left ventricle when antegrade flow is improved after balloon commissurotomy, a concern in the presence of aortic regurgitation as well.

Severe calcification

Patients with symmetrical severe calcification may not respond at all to balloon commissurotomy;[22,38] those with asymmetric calcification are prone to leaflet tearing or rupture.[28] While high echo score alone does not predict the occurrence of severe mitral regurgitation,[39] one component, severe calcification, does.[40] Nevertheless, when the risk of surgery is prohibitive, growing experience with predominantly elderly patients with high echo scores and poor overall morphology has shown moderate improvement in hemodynamics and palliation of symptoms at the cost of high morbidity and mortality.[41]

Procedure

Antegrade v retrograde approaches

The predominant approach to percutaneous balloon mitral valvuloplasty is the antegrade transseptal approach. The techniques include single cylindrical balloon, Inoue, double and trefoil balloons, as well as monorail and metal valvulotomes. Inoue and the double cylindrical balloon methods account for virtually all mitral valvuloplasties performed. The procedure has also been performed retrograde.[42–44] The advantages include avoidance of transseptal puncture; however large devices are introduced into the femoral artery and balloons are passed across the submitral apparatus without balloon flotation (increasing the risk of catheter entrapment). There are no direct comparison studies between antegrade and retrograde techniques.

Inoue technique

The Inoue balloon's principal features are: a modifiable distal tip with reduced profile for transseptal passage, a nylon mesh covering that allows the balloon to straddle the mitral valve, and a compliance curve that allows the balloon to dilate over at least a 4 mm range of sizes (Figure 55.1). A stepwise approach involves evaluating the patient, typically by echocardiography, between each balloon inflation to assess for improvement and detect presence of increasing mitral regurgitation. If improvement is suboptimal and regurgitation has not occurred/increased, the size is typically increased by 1 mm increments. In reviewing 19 series reporting results of Inoue valvuloplasty, we noted a reported early success rate of 93% in a total of 7091 patients.[45,46] Success was variably defined and in some reports overlapped with severe mitral regurgitation, atrial septal defect or embolic events, but included a doubling of the valve area in most studies.

Cylindrical balloon techniques

The cylindrical balloon technique, introduced in 1985,[47] did not uniformly result in adequate gradient reduction and gave way to a double balloon method.[48] A stepwise dilation technique is also used with progressively larger balloons placed side by side until adequate gradient reduction is obtained or an increase in mitral regurgitation is noted. The results of 12 studies incorporating 1864 patients reported a 90% overall success rate.

Long-term follow up

In an extraordinary series of 4832 patients across 120 centers in China, Chen and colleagues have claimed that 98·8% of patients were in NYHA functional class I or II at a mean 32 months follow up, 99·3% success rate, and virtually no complications.[49] Restenosis was reported as 5·2% over a mean 32 months follow up. While there were likely problems with data gathering, the evidence from multiple studies of high success and low complication rates in patients with favorable anatomy is consistent.[20,50] Less favorable long-term results were reported by Cohen et al[51] for 145 patients followed for a mean of 3 years. Their 5 year event free survival was only 51% (freedom from mitral valve replacement, redilation, or death); however, a high percentage of their patients had unfavorable anatomic features. In general, these descriptive series have suffered from incomplete follow up, non-overlapping end points, and lack of serial hemodynamic measurements for assessing hemodynamics and restenosis.

Single v double cylindrical balloons

The disadvantages of single balloons are related to the conundrum of a round balloon in an elliptical orifice – resulting in lower gradient reduction. Although no randomized comparisons were made, and much of the data are from sequential individual operator series, or sequential inflations with single followed by double balloons, the latter appears to be superior in retrospective comparisons (Figure 55.2)[52–54] as well as in an *in vitro* study.[55] The increased lateral force exerted by two balloons is one presumed mechanism for the superior splitting of the laterally directed commissures. However, a comparison of effective balloon dilating area to body surface area showed that a large single balloon could have similar hemodynamic benefits as two smaller balloons. Thus, geometry is not the sole determinant.

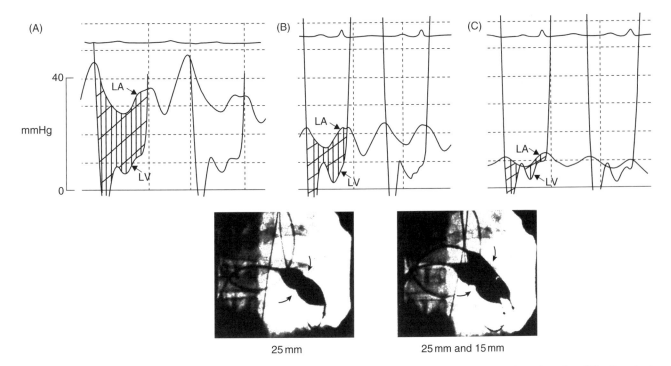

25 mm   25 mm and 15 mm

Figure 55.2 Single *v* double balloon mitral valvotomy. Note the initial modest reduction of gradient from baseline (A) after single balloon commissurotomy (B), with near complete resolution of gradient after double balloon inflation (C). (Reprinted with permission of the American Heart Association, Inc.[115])

Inoue *v* double balloon (Table 55.2)

The Inoue technique's principal advantages are simplicity and short procedure times. The Inoue balloon differs from cylindrical single balloons because of the unique balloon design. The slenderizing feature that facilitates septal passage and the dumb-bell shape of the inflated balloon have been reported by some to result in a lower incidence of atrial septal defect ($\leq 2.5\%$ *v* up to 10% for the double balloon technique)[56] and a much lower likelihood of catastrophic apical perforation.

In a prospective randomized comparison between Inoue and double balloon valvotomy, no significant differences were noted in immediate results, including complications.[57] A trend toward fewer atrial septal defects with the Inoue balloon was not significant. Because of a lack of other prospective randomized comparisons by physicians equally experienced at both techniques, questions remain unanswered. It is likely that an easier procedure with lower complication rates (the Inoue technique) is a trade off for slightly greater mitral regurgitation,[25,58] possibly because the distal portion of the balloon is oversized and may traumatize the subvalvular apparatus. There are also suggestive data that the double balloon technique, by virtue of the lateralization of forces, is advantageous in less favorable anatomy. One example is the result of dilation of asymmetrically fused commissures – where the Inoue technique has been used this led to significant risk of severe mitral regurgitation,[59] whereas with double balloon technique use this appeared to be less of a problem.[60] The disadvantages of the two balloon technique include longer procedure times, and higher risk of left ventricular apical perforation[61–64] although the higher complication rates reported[61,65] may also reflect operator experience with this more complex procedure. **Grade B**

Other techniques

Percutaneous metal mitral commissurotomy is a promising new technique being adopted primarily in a number of developing countries; a series of 153 patients was described by its inventor, Alain Cribier.[66] The device, essentially a Tubbs dilator mounted on a cable, is introduced via the right femoral venous approach and can be opened to a maximum of 40 mm. Initial results are encouraging; in particular, what appear to be relatively high postprocedure valve areas ($2.2 \pm 0.4\,\text{cm}^2$) and low rates of mitral regurgitation (severe mitral regurgitation in 1%). Randomized trials comparing this technique to balloon dilatation have not yet been published although several smaller studies have been completed. The metallic head of the device, the most expensive component, is theoretically resterilizable by autoclaving: a potential advantage in parts of the world where mitral stenosis is endemic and the cost of disposables prohibitive. **Grade B**

Additional data on the retrograde non-transseptal technique previously described by Stefanadis and colleagues have been reported[67] for the first time from multiple investigational sites. Long-term (up to 9 years) results are relatively comparable to antegrade techniques. However, significant rates of severe mitral regurgitation (3·4%) and of femoral artery injury (1·1%), as well as a relatively modest success rate (88%) in the setting of favorable echocardiography scores (7.7 ± 2.0), suggest that this procedure might best be reserved for patients where transseptal puncture has

Table 55.2 Comparative results of valvuloplasty techniques

	Inoue		Double balloon		Single balloon	
	MVA (mean ± SD)	*n*	MVA (mean ± SD)	*n*	MVA (mean ± SD)	*n*
Abdullah[117]	1·9 ± 0·4	60	2·1 ± 0·5	60		
Arora[57]	2·1 ± 0·4	310	2·2 ± 0·4	290		
Bassand[64]	2·0 ± 0·5	71	2·0 ± 0·5	161		
Kasper[118]	1·7 ± 0·7	23	2·2 ± 0·8	22		
Ortiz[119]	1·8 ± 0·4	100	2·0 ± 0·5	36		
Park[56a]	1·9 ± 0·5	59	2·0 ± 0·5	61		
Rothlisberger[120]	1·6 ± 0·6	145	1·8 ± 0·7	90		
Ruiz[121]	1·9 ± 0·3	85	2·0 ± 0·6	322		
Sharma[25]	2·2 ± 0·4	120	2·1 ± 0·5	230		
Trevino[60]	2·0 ± 0·4	157	2·1 ± 0·5	56		
Zhang[61]	1·8 ± 0·3	43	1·8 ± 0·4	43		
NHLBI[122]			2·0 ± 0·8	591	1·7 ± 0·7	114

[a]Study by Park *et al* was randomized.
Abbreviation: MVA, mitral valve area in cm^2

unique contraindications. Because of the learning curve associated with this procedure, and the fact that most patients are amenable to the antegrade approach, the long-term role of this technique is uncertain. Similarly, a series of antegrade Inoue balloon valvuloplasties via a jugular venous route had a significant associated complication rate, but represents another alternative approach.[68] Finally, Bonhoeffer and colleagues have described a monorail double balloon technique that has potential cost advantages and simplifies the standard double balloon technique; no formal comparison to other techniques has been performed.[69]

Intraprocedural transesophageal echocardiography

Use of transesophageal echocardiography during balloon mitral valvuloplasty has been recommended for early detection of major complications (severe mitral regurgitation, tamponade, and large atrial septal defect).[70] In addition, transesophageal echo can confirm needle location during transseptal puncture.[71] Finally, decreased procedure time, mitral regurgitation, and residual atrial septal defects have been described in a randomized study of fluoroscopy plus transesophageal echo versus fluoroscopy without echo during balloon commissurotomy.[72] The evidence provided by these three studies is not compelling. The latter included a 60% rate of major complications in the non-echo group, suggesting limited experience. Surface two-dimensional echocardiography is sensitive enough to detect increasing mitral regurgitation in most patients, and is an excellent tool for early appreciation of tamponade. Atrial septal defects are becoming substantially less common and are largely limited to 5 mm or smaller and resolve post procedure. Finally, transseptal puncture in experienced hands has limited risk; arguably the procedure should not be performed by those who need transesophageal echo guidance. Intracardiac echo using a transducer placed via the femoral vein may be an alternative but has not yet been tested systematically in this setting.

Complications

The learning curve is steep, which has had a major effect both on success and complication rates,[73] as well as skewing data in the literature.[56] The National Heart Lung Blood Institute (NHLBI) registry reported substantially lower rates of all major complications except acute mitral regurgitation at centers performing more than 25 cases and in the second year that sites enrolled patients; a willingness to attempt balloon commissurotomy in higher-risk subsets in the second year may explain the mitral regurgitation. A recent report compares the first 100 cases of Inoue balloon dilatation versus a subsequent 133 cases, all by the same high volume operator with extensive prior double balloon experience. The postprocedure valve area, overall success rate and complication rates were significantly improved beyond 100 cases.[74] It is likely that the best interests of patients undergoing the procedure would be served by having relatively few centers perform higher volumes.

Overall mortality has been approximately 1%, most commonly related to tamponade not only from transseptal catheterization[75] but also from fenestration of the left ventricular apex, in particular by the cylindrical balloon technique. The incidence of tamponade has ranged from 2% to 4%, severe mitral regurgitation from 1% to 6%, and cerebral vascular accident and/or thromboembolism in up to 4%. Disturbingly, magnetic resonance imaging detected new hyperintensitivity foci suggestive of cerebral infarcts in 11 of 27 patients.[76] All had been evaluated before their procedure by transesophageal echocardiography without detection of clot. Thus, embolization may be common even if not clinically apparent. The probable sources are intracavitary clot, catheter induced thrombus formation and showers of calcium.

Atrial septal defects were a significant source of early complications,[76] arising from transseptal tearing secondary to inadvertent proximal deployment of cylindrical balloons, withdrawal of winged balloons retrograde, or trauma to the septum from 5 or 8 mm balloons used to dilate the septum. Theoretically these problems should be avoidable by use of a dilator and a shorter balloon system, both features of the Inoue technique, and indeed this has been the finding.[77] It should be noted that decompression of the left atrium by a significant sized post procedure atrial septal defect may have influenced the results of some balloon valvuloplasty series and may lead operators to overestimate the mitral valve area post procedure.[78]

Predictors of outcome

Predictors of outcome were addressed in a number of non-randomized prospective and retrospective analyses. Factors predicting poorer functional class, hemodynamics, overall and event free survival were found to include age, presence of atrial fibrillation, valvular calcification, and postprocedure results, with event free survival at 6–7 years ranging from 15% (unfavorable baseline anatomy) to 83%.[79–81] Although these studies were not randomized, they incorporate a broader spectrum of patients with mitral stenosis than the randomized trials, and may represent a more "real world" assessment of results to be expected in the overall population.

Additional attention was focused on predictors of adverse outcome, in particular mitral regurgitation. Age and severity of mitral stenosis,[82] and degree of anterior leaflet retraction[83] correlated with postprocedure insufficiency. The nature of pre- and postprocedure mitral regurgitation was carefully studied in 50 patients.[84] As previously noted,

Evidence-based Cardiology

severe mitral regurgitation is typically due to leaflet tearing, while most new mitral regurgitation is typically pericommissural in origin. In addition to anatomic predictors, the steep compliance curve of the Inoue balloon was reported as a likely culprit for severe mitral regurgitation.[85] Use of balloon sizes in the upper portion of the pressure-volume curve was associated with increased mitral regurgitation; whether this finding, based on retrospective observation, is truly causal is unproven, but has been the subject of numerous anecdotal reports and several abstracts. Previous observations that patients with prior surgical commissurotomy have satisfactory but inferior results were again confirmed.[86,87]

Perhaps the most comprehensive analysis of outcome was a recently published follow up of up to 15 years in 879 patients. Severe postprocedure mitral regurgitation, echo score >8, age, prior surgical commissurotomy, NYHA functional class IV, moderate preprocedure mitral regurgitation, and elevated pulmonary artery pressures postprocedure were identified as independent predictors of adverse events at long-term follow up.[88]

Valvuloplasty for mild mitral stenosis

Several studies have looked retrospectively at the results of balloon valvuloplasty for patients with valve areas of 1·3–1·5 cm^2.[89,90] While historical comparisons suggest greater valve area increase than in patients with severe mitral stenosis, there is no evidence that the risk of occasional mortality, need for mitral valve replacement or other major morbidity warrants this approach. The possibility that early commissurotomy may adversely affect the course of the disease, including progression to pulmonary hypertension, atrial fibrillation and stroke remains a hypothesis in need of prospective investigation.[91] **Grade C**

Pregnancy

There have been multiple reports of successful balloon commissurotomy during pregnancy.[92–94] The procedure has been performed with echo guidance and without fluoroscopy[95] to avoid radiation exposure to the fetus. **Grade B**

Dilation for restenosis

Reoperation for mitral valve stenosis has long been associated with increased morbidity and mortality.[96] Several large balloon commissurotomy series have reported inferior overall results compared to de novo dilatation. Davidson reported less symptomatic improvement[97] while Jang described a 20% lower success rate (only 51% having valve area >1·5 cm^2) and nearly 20% requiring mitral valve replacement by 4 years.[98] Cohen described twice the frequency[99] and Medina

described a 10-fold increase in restenosis rates at 5 years for patients with prior commissurotomy[100] (both to approximately 20%). Most significant is the finding by Jang and colleagues that stratification by echo score resulted in nearly superimposable results for de novo and repeat commissurotomy procedures, suggesting that results are defined by valve morphology rather than history of prior commissurotomy.[98] **Grade B**

Bioprosthesis

Several case reports have described successful balloon dilatation of bioprosthetic mitral valves, although both the hemodynamic and longer term benefits were obscure in all but one.[101–103] However, bioprosthetic valves are typically similar histologically to those seen in calcific aortic stenosis: severe leaflet thickening, immobility and calcification, without commissural fusion.[104,105] **Grade B** Thus, a formal intraoperative study, examining the morphology of severely stenosed bioprosthetic valves before and after balloon dilation, revealed "completely ineffectual" dilation[106] with substantial leaflet tearing and cuspal perforation. Although the need for a percutaneous approach to the problem is great, the data do not support bioprosthetic mitral valve dilation.

Balloon v surgical commissurotomy

Randomized trials comparing balloon and surgical commissurotomy were begun early in the development phase of the percutaneous technique. Because both use blind dilation of the valve with blunt instruments, and because closed commissurotomy was the predominant procedure in countries where mitral stenosis was prevalent, the early randomized trials compared balloon and closed commissurotomy. In these studies, surgeons were typically more experienced than the operators performing balloon valvuloplasty. In 1988 we randomized 40 patients with relatively ideal anatomy and severe mitral stenosis;[107] these patients have been followed with serial catheterization and echocardiography over a 7 year period; there were similar hemodynamic improvements in both groups, sustained through 7 years (Figure 55.3), with one late death in each group and need for repeat commissurotomy in 20%.[108] The actual restenosis rate (26% in the balloon group and 35% in the surgical group) as defined by a 50% loss of the gain and a valve area <1·5 cm^2 is significantly higher than the repeat commissurotomy rate because restenosis and functional class do not correlate strongly. Thus it is likely that restenosis rates in trials that have not done formal follow up hemodynamics underestimated the true severity of disease during follow up. Two other studies have compared balloon and closed commissurotomy with shorter, non-invasive follow

476

up only; these have demonstrated balloon results superior to[73] or similar to closed commissurotomy.[109] However closed commissurotomy in the former study resulted in only a 1·3 cm² mean valve area, suggesting relatively unaggressive dilation. Finally, a randomized comparison by Ben Farhat and colleagues described superior acute results (2·2 ± 0·4 cm² *v* 1·6 ± 0·4 cm²) for balloon valvuloplasty and 4 year restenosis rate of 7% *v* 37%.[110] Thus balloon commissurotomy is at least equal and probably superior to closed surgical commissurotomy. **Grade A**

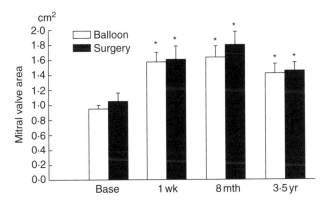

Figure 55.3 Mitral valves areas at baseline and each follow up interval over $3\frac{1}{3}$ years in patients randomized to percutaneous balloon or surgical closed mitral commissurotomy.[108] Asterisk denotes *P* < 0·001 compared with baseline.

Open commissurotomy *v* balloon

The hypothesis that open commissurotomy would be superior to balloon valvuloplasty was based on the potential benefits of direct vision, including surgical splitting and remodeling of the subvalvular apparatus, neither of which are features of closed or balloon commissurotomy. A prospective series of 100 open commissurotomy patients gathered data specifically for historical comparison to the then reported results of balloon valvuloplasty and concluded that open commissurotomy was distinctly superior.[111] The results of surgery, mean valve area 2·9 cm², exceeds expectations and may be related to technique of measurement[112] or patient selection, while mitral regurgitation was absent in all but eight cases (where it was reported to be mild), results also testimony to great operator skill but in excess of prior reports.[8] **Grade A** On the contrary, the more compelling evidence from prospective randomized studies is for similar or superior results with balloon commissurotomy. In 1989 we randomized 60 patients to a prospective comparison of balloon versus open commissurotomy.[113] Patients had near identical baseline hemodynamics but those undergoing balloon commissurotomy had superior mitral valve areas at 3 years (Figure 55.4). A possible explanation for superior results in balloon commissurotomy patients is the direct and

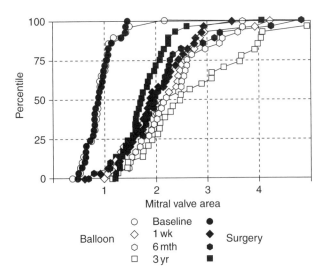

Figure 55.4 Mitral valve areas at baseline and at each follow up interval in patients randomized to balloon or open surgical commissurotomy. The values represent the percentile of patients whose valve areas are ≤ the valve areas on the abscissa. The baseline values overlap, but a shift to the right (representing higher valve areas) is seen for the balloon group at each time point. (Reprinted by permission of the *New England Journal of Medicine.* Copyright © 1994, Massachusetts Medical Society.[113])

continuous feedback to the operator of hemodynamics during catheterization laboratory procedures, which even with the advent of transesophageal monitoring in the operating room is not available to the same degree to the surgeon.

In the trial referred to earlier, Ben Farhat and colleagues report a three-way randomized comparison of balloon, closed and open surgical commissurotomy in 90 patients.[110] Most of the objective information is through 6 month follow up, although clinical status/events and valve areas are described through 7 years. Their results, which include an absence of mortality, NYHA class I function in 90% of the balloon and open mitral commissurotomy (OMC) patients, and residual valve area of 1·8 cm² in these two groups at 7 years with only 7% restenosis, are exceptionally optimistic. The results of closed commissurotomy were distinctly inferior. Because functional class correlates poorly with hemodynamics in mitral stenosis and because planimetry, the technique used here for mitral valve area assessment beyond 6 months, is subjective when the commissures are open (and was not performed by blinded investigators), the findings of this study need to be confirmed. Less optimistic data, utilizing hemodynamics and blinded interpretation, suggest that restenosis rates may be 25% by 7 years even in patients with relatively ideal valve anatomy preprocedure.[114] Nevertheless, this paper confirms that balloon valvuloplasty is at least as effective as open commissurotomy for patients with severe mitral stenosis and ideal valve anatomy.

The study's optimistic findings may perhaps in part be due to a distinguishing feature of all of the randomized comparisons of balloon versus surgical commissurotomy: single site studies that depend to a significant degree on individual physician practices and small patient populations. **Grade A**

Cost

Although formal cost comparison studies have not been reported, charges and costs at hospitals in India and in the United States have been estimated. Lau and Ruiz described cost to a United States hospital of $3000 for balloon valvuloplasty and $6000 for closed commissurotomy (assuming a hospital could be found that still performs this procedure). We published 1991 charges for balloon and closed commissurotomy in the United States and India (Figure 55.5) and demonstrated a sixfold greater expense for balloon valvuloplasty in India. However, our calculations did not include the extensive reuse of disposables in developing countries, where balloons can account for a much higher portion of the charges than physicians' fees or operating room billings. Percutaneous metallic commissurotomy, as referred to earlier, may also have a significant impact on cost considerations.

The results of the randomized trials offer compelling evidence that balloon valvuloplasty is an effective alternative to surgery for patients with good valve anatomy. Even with a number of anatomic features predicting less favorable

outcome, balloon commissurotomy, at the cost of higher risk in patients with unfavorable anatomy, still has the potential for palliation. The safety and efficacy of Inoue and double balloon valvuloplasty are not compellingly different in experienced hands and the selection of techniques should be based on operator preference, experience, and equipment availability. Low cost, avoidance of thoracotomy scar and discomfort, shorter hospitalization and excellent follow up results to date mandate consideration of balloon valvuloplasty in most patients with rheumatic mitral valve stenosis without significant contraindications. Since balloon as well as surgical commissurotomy are largely palliative procedures, percutaneous balloon valvuloplasty has the added benefit of delaying the time until eventual thoracotomy. **Grade A**

In summary, percutaneous balloon mitral valvuloplasty is a superior alternative to surgical commissurotomy for a significant subset of patients with rheumatic mitral stenosis. Careful case selection and performance of the procedure by experienced teams will have a significant impact on outcome. Both clinical and financial considerations suggest that balloon valvuloplasty is the procedure of choice for rheumatic mitral stenosis in patients with suitable anatomy. **Grade A**

Key points

- Ideal patients have severe mitral stenosis without:
  >mild mitral regurgitation, severe subvalvular disease, or severe calcification
  eccentric commissural fusion, clot in left atrium, volume loaded left ventricle
- Procedure may be of benefit in:
  <critical mitral stenosis, but evidence for favorable long-term risk–benefit ratio is lacking
  patients with unfavorable anatomy, including moderate mitral regurgitation, but with less favorable results and higher morbidity/mortality
  patients with mitral restenosis, dependent on anatomic features
  pregnant patients
- Balloon valvuloplasty is superior to closed commissurotomy and is equivalent or superior to open commissurotomy in ideal patients

---

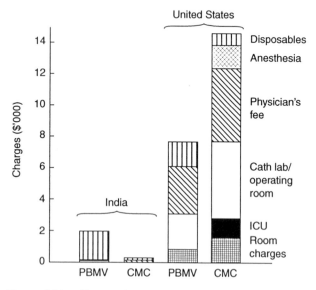

Figure 55.5 Charges for percutaneous balloon mitral valvuloplasty (PBMV) and closed surgical commissurotomy (CMC) at the Nizam's Institute of Medical Sciences in Hyderabad, India and at Harper Hospital in Detroit, MI in 1991. With the extensive reuse of disposables in developing countries, the cost of balloon valvuloplasty more closely approximates that for closed commissurotomy. (© 1993, F.A. Davis Co. Reprinted with permission.[116])

References

1. Cutler EC, Levine SA. Cardiotomy and valvulotomy for mitral stenosis. Experimental observations and clinical notes concerning an operated case with recovery. *Boston Med Surg J* 1923;**188**:1023–7.
2. Suttar HS. The surgical treatment of mitral stenosis. *BMJ* 1925;**2**:603–6.
3. Lewis T. *Diseases of the heart. 3rd edn*. London: Macmillan, 1943.
4. John S, Bashi VV, Jairaj PS *et al.* Closed mitral valvotomy: early results and long-term follow-up of 3724 consecutive patients. *Circulation* 1983;**68**:891–6.

5. Toumbouras M, Panagopoulos F, Papakonstantinou C *et al.* Long-term surgical outcome of closed mitral commissurotomy. *J Heart Valve Dis* 1995;**4**:247–50.

6. Rihal CS, Schaff HV, Frye RL, Bailey KR, Hammes LN, Holmes DR Jr. Long-term follow-up of patients undergoing closed transventricular mitral commissurotomy: a useful surrogate for percutaneous balloon mitral valvuloplasty? *J Am Coll Cardiol* 1992;**20**:781–6.

7. Scalia D, Rizzoli G, Campanile F *et al.* Long-term results of mitral commissurotomy. *J Thorac Cardiovasc Surg* 1993;**105**:633–42.

8. Villanova C, Melacini P, Scognamiglio R *et al.* Long-term echocardiographic evaluation of closed and open mitral valvulotomy. *Int J Cardiol* 1993;**38**:315–21.

9. Hickey MS, Blackstone EH, Kirklin JW, Dean LS. Outcome probabilities and life history after surgical mitral commissurotomy: implications for balloon commissurotomy. *J Am Coll Cardiol* 1991;**17**:29–42.

10. Inoue K, Kitamura F, Chikusa H, Miyamoto N. Atrial septostomy by a new balloon catheter. *Jpn Circ J* 1981;**45**:730–8.

11. Inoue K, Nakamura T, Kitamura F. Nonoperative mitral commissurotomy by a new balloon catheter. [Abstract] *Jpn Circ J* 1982;**46**:877.

12. Inoue K, Owaki T, Nakamura T, Kitamura F, Miyamoto N. Clinical application of transvenous mitral commissurotomy by a new balloon catheter. *J Thorac Cardiovasc Surg* 1984;**87**:394–402.

13. Block PC, Palacios IF, Jacobs ML, Fallon JT. Mechanism of percutaneous mitral valvotomy. *Am J Cardiol* 1987;**59**: 178–9.

14. Matsuura Y, Fukunaga S, Ishihara H *et al.* Mechanics of percutaneous balloon valvotomy for mitral valvular stenosis. *Heart Vessels* 1988;**4**:179–83.

15. Nabel E, Bergin PJ, Kirsh MM. Morphological analysis of balloon mitral valvuloplasty; intra-operative results. [Abstract] *J Am Coll Cardiol* 1990;**15**:97A.

16. Kaplan JD, Isner JM, Karas RH *et al. In vitro* analysis of mechanisms of balloon valvuloplasty of stenotic mitral valves. *Am J Cardiol* 1987;**59**:318–23.

17. McKay RG, Lock JE, Safian RD *et al.* Balloon dilation of mitral stenosis in adult patients: postmortem and percutaneous mitral valvuloplasty studies. *J Am Coll Cardiol* 1987;**9**: 723–31.

18. Wilkins GT, Weyman AE, Abascal VM, Block PC, Palacios IF. Percutaneous balloon dilatation of the mitral valve: an analysis of echocardiographic variables related to outcome and the mechanism of dilatation. *Br Heart J* 1988;**60**:299–308.

19. Desideri A, Vanderperren O, Serra A *et al.* Long-term (9 to 33 months) echocardiographic follow-up after successful percutaneous mitral commissurotomy. *Am J Cardiol* 1992;**69**:1602–6.

20. Palacios IF, Tuzcu ME, Weyman AE, Newell JB, Block PC. Clinical follow-up of patients undergoing percutaneous mitral balloon valvotomy. *Circulation* 1995;**91**:671–6.

21. Abascal VM, Wilkins GT, O'Shea JP *et al.* Prediction of successful outcome in 130 patients undergoing percutaneous balloon mitral valvotomy. *Circulation* 1990;**82**:448–56.

22. Fatkin D, Roy P, Morgan JJ, Feneley MP. Percutaneous balloon mitral valvotomy with the Inoue single-balloon catheter: commissural morphology as a determinant of outcome. *J Am Coll Cardiol* 1993;**21**:390–7.

23. Levin TN, Feldman T, Bednarz J, Carroll JD, Lang RM. Transesophageal echocardiographic evaluation of mitral valve morphology to predict outcome after balloon mitral valvotomy. *Am J Cardiol* 1994;**73**:707–10.

24. Herrmann HC, Ramaswamy K, Isner JM *et al.* Factors influencing immediate results, complications, and short-term follow-up status after Inoue balloon mitral valvotomy: a North American multicenter study. *Am Heart J* 1992;**124**:160–6.

25. Sharma S, Loya YS, Desai DM, Pinto RJ. Percutaneous mitral valvotomy using Inoue and double balloon technique: comparison of clinical and hemodynamic short term results in 350 cases. *Cathet Cardiovasc Diagn* 1993;**29**:18–23.

26. Reid CL, Chandraratna PA, Kawanishi DT, Kotlewski A, Rahimtoola SH. Influence of mitral valve morphology on double-balloon catheter balloon valvuloplasty in patients with mitral stenosis. Analysis of factors predicting immediate and 3-month results. *Circulation* 1989;**80**:515–24.

27. Zhang HP, Allen JW, Lau FY, Ruiz CE. Immediate and late outcome of percutaneous balloon mitral valvotomy in patients with significantly calcified valves. *Am Heart J* 1995;**129**: 501–6.

28. Miche E, Fassbender D, Minami K *et al.* Pathomorphological characteristics of resected mitral valves after unsuccessful valvuloplasty. *J Cardiovasc Surg* 1996;**37**:475–81.

29. Ruiz CE, Zhang HP, Gamra H, Allen JW, Lau FY. Late clinical and echocardiographic follow up after percutaneous balloon dilatation of the mitral valve. *Br Heart J* 1994;**71**:454–8.

30. Orrange SE, Kawanishi DT, Lopez BM, Curry SM, Rahimtoola SH. Actuarial outcome after catheter balloon commissurotomy in patients with mitral stenosis. *Circulation* 1997;**95**:382–9.

31. Cannan CR, Nishimura RA, Reeder GS *et al.* Echocardiographic assessment of commissural calcium: a simple predictor of outcome after percutaneous mitral balloon valvotomy. *J Am Coll Cardiol* 1997;**29**:175–80.

32. Kronzon I, Tunick PA, Glassman E, Slater J, Schwinger M, Freedberg RS. Transesophageal echocardiography to detect atrial clots in candidates for percutaneous transseptal mitral balloon valvuloplasty. *J Am Coll Cardiol* 1990;**16**:1320–2.

33. Rittoo D, Sutherland GR, Currie P, Starkey IR, Shaw TR. A prospective study of left atrial spontaneous echo contrast and thrombus in 100 consecutive patients referred for balloon dilation of the mitral valve. *J Am Soc Echocardiogr* 1994;**7**:516–27.

34. Hung JS. Cheng TO, eds. *Percutaneous balloon valvuloplasty.* Mitral stenosis with left atrial thrombi: Inoue balloon catheter technique. New York: Igaku-Shoin, 1992.

35. Kang DH, Song JK, Chae K *et al.* Comparison of outcomes of percutaneous mitral valvuloplasty versus mitral valve replacement after resolution of left atrial appendage thrombi. *Am J Cardiol* 1998;**81**:97–100.

36. Zhang HP, Gamra H, Allen JW, Lau FY, Ruiz CE. Balloon valvotomy for mitral stenosis associated with moderate mitral regurgitation. *Am J Cardiol* 1995;**75**:960–3.

37. Alfonso F, Macaya C *et al.* Early and late results of percutaneous mitral valvuloplasty for mitral stenosis associated with mild mitral regurgitation. *Am J Cardiol* 1993;**71**:1304–10.

38. Tuzcu EM, Block PC, Griffin B, Dinsmore R, Newell JB, Palacios IF. Percutaneous mitral balloon valvotomy in patients with calcific mitral stenosis: immediate and long-term outcome. *J Am Coll Cardiol* 1994;**23**:1604–9.

39. Feldman T, Carroll JD, Isner JM *et al.* Effect of valve deformity on results and mitral regurgitation after Inoue balloon commissurotomy. *Circulation* 1992;**85**:180–7.

40. Herrmann HC, Lima JA, Feldman T *et al.* Mechanisms and outcome of severe mitral regurgitation after Inoue balloon valvuloplasty. North American Inoue Balloon Investigators. *J Am Coll Cardiol* 1993;**22**:783–9.

41. Tuzcu EM, Block PC, Griffin BP, Newell JB, Palacios IF. Immediate and long-term outcome of percutaneous mitral valvotomy in patients 65 years and older. *Circulation* 1992;**85**:963–71.

42. Bahl VK, Juneja R, Thatai D, Kaul U, Sharma S, Wasir HS. Retrograde nontransseptal balloon mitral valvuloplasty for rheumatic mitral stenosis. *Cathet Cardiovasc Diagn* 1994;**33**:331–4.

43. Stefanadis C, Stratos C, Kallikazaros I *et al.* Retrograde nontransseptal balloon mitral valvuloplasty using a modified Inoue balloon catheter. *Cathet Cardiovasc Diagn* 1994;**33**:224–33.

44. Stefanadis C, Stratos C, Pitsavos C *et al.* Retrograde nontransseptal balloon mitral valvuloplasty. Immediate results and long-term follow-up. *Circulation* 1992;**85**:1760–7.

45. Lau KW, Hung JS, Ding ZP, Johan A. Controversies in balloon mitral valvuloplasty: the when (timing for intervention), what (choice of valve), and how (selection of technique). *Cathet Cardiovasc Diagn* 1995;**35**:91–100.

46. Glazier JJ, Turi ZG. Percutaneous balloon mitral valvuloplasty. *Prog Cardiovasc Dis* 1997;**40**:5–26.

47. Lock JE, Khalilullah M, Shrivastava S, Bahl V, Keane JF. Percutaneous catheter commissurotomy in rheumatic mitral stenosis. *N Engl J Med* 1985;**313**:1515–18.

48. al Zaibag M, Ribeiro PA, Al Kasab S, al Fagih MR. Percutaneous double-balloon mitral valvotomy for rheumatic mitral-valve stenosis. *Lancet* 1986;**1**:757–61.

49. Chen CR, Cheng TO. Percutaneous balloon mitral valvuloplasty by the Inoue technique: a multicenter study of 4832 patients in China. *Am Heart J* 1995;**129**:1197–203.

50. Iung B, Cormier B, Ducimetiere P *et al.* Functional results 5 years after successful percutaneous mitral commissurotomy in a series of 528 patients and analysis of predictive factors. *J Am Coll Cardiol* 1996;**27**:407–14.

51. Cohen DJ, Kuntz RE, Gordon SP *et al.* Predictors of long-term outcome after percutaneous balloon mitral valvuloplasty. *N Engl J Med* 1992;**327**:1329–33.

52. Shrivastava S, Mathur A, Dev V, Saxena A, Venugopal P, SampathKumar A. Comparison of immediate hemodynamic response to closed mitral commissurotomy, single-balloon, and double-balloon mitral valvuloplasty in rheumatic mitral stenosis. *J Thorac Cardiovasc Surg* 1992;**104**:1264–7.

53. Al Kasab S, Ribeiro PA, Sawyer W. Comparison of results of percutaneous balloon mitral valvotomy using consecutive single (25 mm) and double (25 mm and 12 mm) balloon techniques. *Am J Cardiol* 1989;**64**:1385–7.

54. Chen CG, Wang YP, Qing D, Lin YS, Lan YF. Percutaneous mitral balloon dilatation by a new sequential single- and double-balloon technique. *Am Heart J* 1988;**116**:1161–7.

55. Ribeiro PA, al Zaibag M, Rajendran V *et al.* Mechanism of mitral valve area increase by *in vitro* single and double balloon mitral valvotomy. *Am J Cardiol* 1988;**62**:264–9.

56. Complications and mortality of percutaneous balloon mitral commissurotomy. A report from the National Heart, Lung, and Blood Institute Balloon Valvuloplasty Registry. *Circulation* 1992;**85**:2014–24.

57. Park SJ, Kim JJ, Park SW, Song JK, Doo YC, Lee SJ. Immediate and one-year results of percutaneous mitral balloon valvuloplasty using Inoue and double-balloon techniques. *Am J Cardiol* 1993;**71**:938–43.

58. Arora R, Kalra GS, Murty GS *et al.* Percutaneous transatrial mitral commissurotomy: immediate and intermediate results. *J Am Coll Cardiol* 1994;**23**:1327–32.

59. Miche E, Bogunovic N, Fassbender D *et al.* Predictors of unsuccessful outcome after percutaneous mitral valvulotomy including a new echocardiographic scoring system. *J Heart Valve Dis* 1996;**5**:430–5.

60. Rodriguez L, Monterroso VH, Abascal VM *et al.* Does asymmetrical mitral valve disease predict an adverse outcome after percutaneous balloon mitral valvotomy? An echocardiographic study. *Am Heart J* 1992;**123**:1678–82.

61. Trevino AJ, Ibarra M, Garcia A *et al.* Immediate and long-term results of balloon mitral commissurotomy for rheumatic mitral stenosis: comparison between Inoue and double-balloon techniques. *Am Heart J* 1996;**131**:530–6.

62. Zhang HP, Gamra H, Allen JW, Lau FY, Ruiz CE. Comparison of late outcome between Inoue balloon and double-balloon techniques for percutaneous mitral valvotomy in a matched study. *Am Heart J* 1995;**130**:340–4.

63. Fu XY, Zhang DD, Schiele F, Anguenot T, Bernard Y, Bassand JP. Complications of percutaneous mitral valvuloplasty; comparison of the double balloon and the Inoue techniques. *Arch Mal Coeur Vaiss* 1994;**87**:1403–11.

64. Rihal CS, Nishimura RA, Reeder GS, Holmes DR Jr. Percutaneous balloon mitral valvuloplasty: comparison of double and single (Inoue) balloon techniques. *Cathet Cardiovasc Diagn* 1993;**29**:183–90.

65. Bassand JP, Schiele F, Bernard Y *et al.* The double-balloon and Inoue techniques in percutaneous mitral valvuloplasty: comparative results in a series of 232 cases. *J Am Coll Cardiol* 1991;**18**:982–9.

66. Cribier A, Eltchaninoff H, Koning R *et al.* Percutaneous mechanical mitral commissurotomy with a newly designed metallic valvulotome. *Circulation* 1999;**99**:793–9.

67. Stefanadis CI, Stratos CG, Lambrou SG *et al.* Retrograde nontransseptal balloon mitral valvuloplasty: immediate results and intermediate long-term outcome in 441 cases – a multicenter experience. *J Am Coll Cardiol* 1998;**32**:1009–16.

68. Joseph G, Baruah DK, Kuruttukulam SV, Chandy ST, Krishnaswami S. Transjugular approach to transseptal balloon mitral valvuloplasty. *Cathet Cardiovasc Diagn* 1997;**42**:219–26.

69. Bonhoeffer P, Esteves C, Casal U *et al.* Percutaneous mitral valve dilatation with the Multi-Track System. *Catheter Cardiovasc Interv* 1999;**48**:178–83.

70. Goldstein SA, Campbell A, Mintz GS, Pichard A, Leon M, Lindsay J, Jr. Feasibility of on-line transesophageal echocardiography during balloon mitral valvulotomy: experience with 93 patients. *J Heart Valve Dis* 1994;**3**:136–48.

71. Ballal RS, Mahan EF, Nanda NC, Dean LS. Utility of transesophageal echocardiography in interatrial septal puncture

during percutaneous mitral balloon commissurotomy. *Am J Cardiol* 1990;**66**:230–2.

72. Ramondo A, Chirillo F, Dan M *et al.* Value and limitations of transesophageal echocardiographic monitoring during percutaneous balloon mitral valvotomy. *Int J Cardiol* 1991; **31**:223–33.

73. Rihal CS, Nishimura RA, Holmes DR, Jr. Percutaneous balloon mitral valvuloplasty: the learning curve. *Am Heart J* 1991;**122**:1750–6.

74. Sanchez PL, Harrell LC, Salas RE, Palacios IF. Learning curve of the Inoue technique of percutaneous mitral balloon valvuloplasty. *Am J Cardiol* 2001;**88**:662–7.

75. Schoonmaker FW, Vijay NK, Jantz RD. Left atrial and ventricular transseptal catheterization review: losing skills. *Cathet Cardiovasc Diagn* 1987;**13**:233–8.

76. Rocha P, Mulot R, Lacombe P, Pilliere R, Belarbi A, Raffestin B. Brain magnetic resonance imaging before and after percutaneous mitral balloon commissurotomy. *Am J Cardiol* 1994; **74**:955–7.

77. Yoshida K, Yoshikawa J, Akasaka T *et al.* Assessment of left-to-right atrial shunting after percutaneous mitral valvuloplasty by transesophageal color Doppler flow-mapping. *Circulation* 1989;**80**:1521–6.

78. Thomas MR, Monaghan MJ, Metcalfe JM, Jewitt DE. Residual atrial septal defects following balloon mitral valvuloplasty using different techniques. A transthoracic and transoesophageal echocardiography study demonstrating an advantage of the Inoue balloon. *Eur Heart J* 1992;**13**: 496–502.

79. Petrossian GA, Tuzcu EM, Ziskind AA, Block PC, Palacios I. Atrial septal occlusion improves the accuracy of mitral valve area determination following percutaneous mitral balloon valvotomy. *Cathet Cardiovasc Diagn* 1991;**22**:21–4.

80. Lau KW, Ding ZP, Quek S, Kwok V, Hung JS. Long-term (36–63 month) clinical and echocardiographic follow-up after Inoue balloon mitral commissurotomy. *Cathet Cardiovasc Diagn* 1998;**43**:33–8.

81. Meneveau N, Schiele F, Seronde MF *et al.* Predictors of event-free survival after percutaneous mitral commissurotomy. *Heart* 1998;**80**:359–64.

82. Zhang HP, Yen GS, Allen JW, Lau FY, Ruiz CE. Comparison of late results of balloon valvotomy in mitral stenosis with versus without mitral regurgitation. *Am J Cardiol* 1998;**81**:51–5.

83. Matsubara T, Yamazoe M, Tamura Y *et al.* Progression to moderate or severe mitral regurgitation after percutaneous transvenous mitral commissurotomy using stepwise inflation technique. *J Cardiol* 1998;**31**:289–95.

84. Mueller UK, Sareli P, Essop MR. Anterior mitral leaflet retraction – a new echocardiographic predictor of severe mitral regurgitation following balloon valvuloplasty by the Inoue technique. *Am J Cardiol* 1998;**81**:656–9.

85. Rittoo D, Sutherland GR, Shaw TR. A prospective echocardiographic study of the effects of balloon mitral commissurotomy on pre-existing mitral regurgitation in patients with mitral stenosis. *Cardiology* 1998;**89**:202–9.

86. Goel PK, Garg N, Sinha N. Pressure zone used and the occurrence of mitral regurgitation in Inoue balloon mitral commissurotomy. *Cathet Cardiovasc Diagn* 1998;**43**:141–6.

87. Ito T, Suwa M, Hirota Y *et al.* Comparison of immediate and long-term outcome of percutaneous transvenous mitral

commissurotomy in patients who have and have not undergone previous surgical commissurotomy. *Jpn Circ J* 1997;**61**: 218–22.

88. Palacios IF, Sanchez PL, Harrell LC, Weyman AE, Block PC. Which patients benefit from percutaneous mitral balloon valvuloplasty? Prevalvuloplasty and postvalvuloplasty variables that predict long-term outcome. *Circulation* 2002;**105**: 1465–71.

89. Pan M, Medina A, Suarez De Lezo J *et al.* Balloon valvuloplasty for mild mitral stenosis. *Cathet Cardiovasc Diagn* 1991; **24**:1–5.

90. Herrmann HC, Feldman T, Isner JM *et al.* Comparison of results of percutaneous balloon valvuloplasty in patients with mild and moderate mitral stenosis to those with severe mitral stenosis. The North American Inoue Balloon Investigators. *Am J Cardiol* 1993;**71**:1300–3.

91. Turi ZG. Mitral balloon valvuloplasty [letter; comment]. *Cathet Cardiovasc Diagn* 1992;**25**:343–4.

92. Glantz JC, Pomerantz RM, Cunningham MJ, Woods JR Jr. Percutaneous balloon valvuloplasty for severe mitral stenosis during pregnancy: a review of therapeutic options. *Obstet Gynecol Surg* 1993;**48**:503–8.

93. Patel JJ, Mitha AS, Hassen F *et al.* Percutaneous balloon mitral valvotomy in pregnant patients with tight pliable mitral stenosis. *Am Heart J* 1993;**125**:1106–9.

94. Ribeiro PA, Fawzy ME, Awad M, Dunn B, Duran CG. Balloon valvotomy for pregnant patients with severe pliable mitral stenosis using the Inoue technique with total abdominal and pelvic shielding. *Am Heart J* 1992;**124**: 1558–62.

95. Kultursay H, Turkoglu C, Akin M, Payzin S, Soydas C, Akilli A. Mitral balloon valvuloplasty with transesophageal echocardiography without using fluoroscopy. *Cathet Cardiovasc Diagn* 1992;**27**:317–21.

96. Harken DE, Black H, Taylor WJ, Thrower WB, Ellis LB. Reoperation for mitral stenosis. A discussion of postoperative deterioration and methods of improving initial and secondary operation. *Circulation* 1961;**23**:7–12.

97. Davidson CJ, Bashore TM, Mickel M, Davis K. Balloon mitral commissurotomy after previous surgical commissurotomy. The National Heart, Lung, and Blood Institute Balloon Valvuloplasty Registry participants. *Circulation* 1992;**86**: 91–9.

98. Jang IK, Block PC, Newell JB, Tuzcu EM, Palacios IF. Percutaneous mitral balloon valvotomy for recurrent mitral stenosis after surgical commissurotomy. *Am J Cardiol* 1995; **75**:601–5.

99. Cohen JM, Glower DD, Harrison JK *et al.* Comparison of balloon valvuloplasty with operative treatment for mitral stenosis. *Ann Thorac Surg* 1993;**56**:1254–62.

100. Medina A, de Lezo JS, Hernandez E *et al.* eds. *Percutaneous balloon valvuloplasty.* Mitral restenosis: the Cordoba-Las Palmas experience. New York: Igaku-Shoin, 1992.

101. Calvo OL, Sobrino N, Gamallo C, Oliver J, Dominguez F, Iglesias A. Balloon percutaneous valvuloplasty for stenotic bioprosthetic valves in the mitral position. *Am J Cardiol* 1987;**60**:736–7.

102. Cox DA, Friedman PL, Selwyn AP, Lee RT, Bittl JA. Improved quality of life after successful balloon valvuloplasty of a stenosed mitral bioprosthesis. *Am Heart J* 1989;**118**:839–41.

103. Babic UU, Grujicic S, Vucinic M. Balloon valvoplasty of mitral bioprosthesis. *Int J Cardiol* 1991;**30**:230–2.

104. Waller BF, McKay C, VanTassel J, Allen M. Catheter balloon valvuloplasty of stenotic porcine bioprosthetic valves: Part II: Mechanisms, complications, and recommendations for clinical use. *Clin Cardiol* 1991;**14**:764–72.

105. Waller BF, McKay C, Van Tassel J, Allen M. Catheter balloon valvuloplasty of stenotic porcine bioprosthetic valves: Part I: Anatomic considerations. *Clin Cardiol* 1991;**14**:686–91.

106. Lin PJ, Chang JP, Chu JJ, Chang CH, Hung JS. Balloon valvuloplasty is contraindicated in stenotic mitral bioprostheses. *Am Heart J* 1994;**127**:724–6.

107. Turi ZG, Reyes VP, Raju BS et al. Percutaneous balloon versus surgical closed commissurotomy for mitral stenosis. A prospective, randomized trial. *Circulation* 1991;**83**:1179–85.

108. Raju BS, Turi ZG, Raju R et al. Three and one-half year follow-up of a randomized trial comparing percutaneous balloon and surgical closed mitral commissurotomy. [Abstract] *J Am Coll Cardiol* 1993;**21**:429A.

109. Arora R, Nair M, Kalra GS, Nigam M, Khalilullah M. Immediate and long-term results of balloon and surgical closed mitral valvotomy: a randomized comparative study. *Am Heart J* 1993;**125**:1091–4.

110. Ben Farhat M, Ayari M, Maatouk F et al. Percutaneous balloon versus surgical closed and open mitral commissurotomy: seven-year follow-up results of a randomized trial. *Circulation* 1998;**97**:245–50.

111. Antunes MJ, Nascimento J, Andrade CM, Fernandes LE. Open mitral commissurotomy: a better procedure? *J Heart Valve Dis* 1994;**3**:88–92.

112. Acar J. Open mitral commissurotomy or percutaneous mitral commissurotomy? [editorial]. *J Heart Valve Dis* 1994;**3**:133–5.

113. Reyes VP, Raju BS, Wynne J et al. Percutaneous balloon valvuloplasty compared with open surgical commissurotomy for mitral stenosis. *N Engl J Med* 1994;**331**:961–7.

114. Turi ZG. Percutaneous balloon valvuloplasty versus surgery: randomized comparisons. *J Interv Cardiol* 2000;**13**:395–401.

115. Palacios I, Block PC, Brandi S et al. Percutaneous balloon valvotomy for patients with severe mitral stenosis. *Circulation* 1987;**75**:778–84.

116. Turi ZG. Frankel W, Brest A, eds. *Valvular heart disease: comprehensive evaluation and treatment. 2nd edn.* Valvuloplasty. Philadelphia: F.A. Davis, 1993.

117. Abdullah M, Halim M, Rajendran V, Sawyer W, al Zaibag M. Comparison between single (Inoue) and double balloon mitral valvuloplasty: immediate and short-term results. *Am Heart J* 1992;**123**:1581–8.

118. Kasper W, Wollschlager H, Geibel A, Meinertz T, Just H. Percutaneous mitral balloon valvuloplasty – a comparative evaluation of two transatrial techniques. *Am Heart J* 1992;**124**:1562–6.

119. Ortiz FA, Macaya C, Alfonso F. Mono- versus double-balloon technique for commissural splitting after percutaneous mitral valvotomy. *Am J Cardiol* 1992;**69**:1100–1.

120. Rothlisberger C, Essop MR, Skudicky D, Skoularigis J, Wisenbaugh T, Sareli P. Results of percutaneous balloon mitral valvotomy in young adults. *Am J Cardiol* 1993;**72**:73–7.

121. Ruiz CE, Zhang HP, Macaya C, Aleman EH, Allen JW, Lau FYK. Comparison of Inoue single-balloon versus double-balloon technique for percutaneous mitral valvotomy. *Am Heart J* 1992;**123**:942–7.

122. Multicenter experience with balloon mitral commissurotomy. NHLBI Balloon Valvuloplasty Registry Report on immediate and 30-day follow-up results. The National Heart, Lung, and Blood Institute Balloon Valvuloplasty Registry Participants. *Circulation* 1992;**85**:448–61.

56 Valve repair and choice of valves

Paul J Pearson, Hartzell V Schaff

Introduction

Changes in treatment of mitral regurgitation provide a classic example of how advances in surgical technique influence the overall strategy of medical management of valvular heart disease, including both the indications for and timing of operation. In North America, degenerative diseases such as floppy valves and ruptured chordae tendineae are the most common causes of non-ischemic mitral valve regurgitation.[1–3]

Previously, clinicians observed patients with mitral regurgitation until symptoms developed or until there was evidence of left ventricular failure. Usually, operation resulted in replacement of the valve with a prosthesis. This left the patient with ventricular dysfunction, irreversible in some cases, and also the attendant prosthesis-related risks such as thromboembolism, hemorrhage caused by systemic anticoagulation, infection, and risks of mechanical failure. The advent of mitral valve repair, with its predictability and safety, lead to new criteria for intervention. Indeed, early operation for valve repair should be considered for all patients with severe mitral regurgitation.[4,5]

Timing of operation for mitral valve regurgitation

Grade B Mitral valve regurgitation often progresses slowly and because of favorable loading conditions, left ventricular dysfunction can develop even though systolic indices of left ventricular performance are maintained. Indeed, with severe mitral valve regurgitation, normal ventricular function should result in a hyperdynamic left ventricle with a supranormal ejection fraction. When the ejection fraction falls below 60% in the presence of severe mitral regurgitation, the prognosis of patients after surgical correction worsens (Figure 56.1).[4] However, the relative insensitivity of ejection fraction in gauging ventricular performance in patients with mitral regurgitation has led to the development of indices of

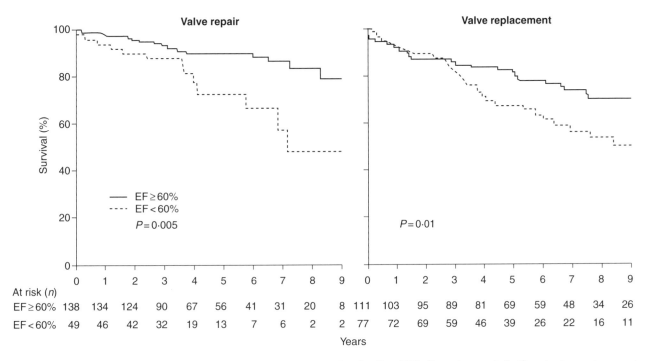

Figure 56.1 Graphs of late survival according to preoperative ejection fraction (EF) after valve repair (left) and valve replacement (right). (From Enriques-Sarano *et al*.[4])

left ventricular function that are less dependent on preload, such as end systolic dimension. Again, prognosis after valve repair or replacement is poor when preoperative left ventricular end systolic dimension exceeds 45 mm.[4] Thus, even in an asymptomatic patient with an ejection fraction greater than 60%, if left ventricular end systolic diameter approaches 45 mm, valve repair should be seriously considered.[4]

Valve repair *v* replacement

Grade A There are no prospective, randomized studies comparing outcomes after mitral valve repair with replacement for mitral regurgitation. In addition, it is often difficult to compare these two modes of surgical treatment by review of the literature because of heterogeneous patient populations.[6] Patients with anatomy favorable for valve repair may have less advanced disease when compared to those patients in whom valve replacement is necessary.[7]

However, even with these confounding factors, some generalizations can be made. First, analysis based upon adjustment for baseline differences in patient populations indicates that patients undergoing mitral valve repair have improved survival and better postoperative left ventricular function than patients undergoing mitral valve replacement (Figure 56.2).[7] In addition, patients undergoing valve repair have a lower operative mortality than their counterparts having prosthetic replacement (Table 56.1).[6] These good

Table 56.1 Operative mortality for mitral valve replacement *v* repair

	Replacement	Repair	*P*
Overall	*n* = 214 (10·3%)	*n* = 195 (2·6%)	0·002
Age ≤75 years	*n* = 39 (30·8%)	*n* = 44 (6·8%)	0·0005
Age ≥75 years	*n* = 175 (5·7%)	*n* = 151 (1·3%)	0·036

From Enriquez-Sarano *et al*[7]

results following valvuloplasty are, at least in part, due to maintenance of normal left ventricular geometry and function through preservation of the valve-chordal-papillary muscle complex.[8–11]

Importantly, valve repair and replacement have similar low rates of reoperation. A study from our clinic comparing the outcomes of 195 patients undergoing valve repair with 214 who underwent valve replacement for organic mitral regurgitation demonstrated that freedom from reoperation was 90% and 93% (repair and replacement) at 5 years and 75% and 80% at 10 years respectively (*P* = 0·47)[7] (Figure 56.3).

Valve repair can even be undertaken in some patients with calcification of the leaflets and annulus. Although this

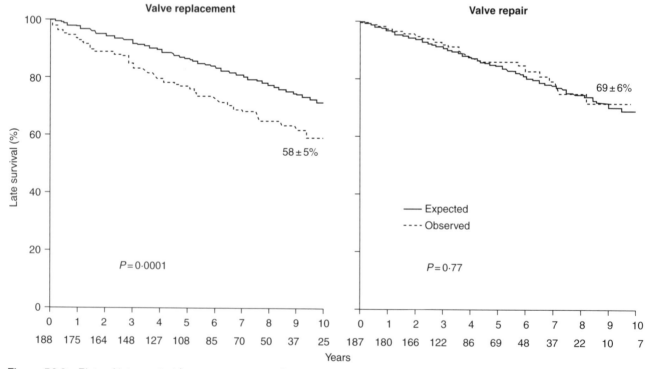

Figure 56.2 Plots of late survival (in operative survivors) of patients with valve replacement (left) and valve repair (right) compared with their expected survival. Note that in patients with valve repair, there is no difference in the expected survival, whereas in patients with valve replacement, the survival is significantly lower than expected. (From Enriquez-Sarano *et al*[7])

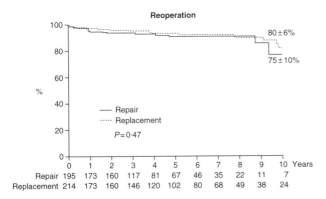

Figure 56.3 Plot of freedom from reoperation in valve repair and replacement groups. No significant difference is observed. (From Enriquez-Sarano *et al.*[7])

presents a challenge to the surgeon, repair utilizing standard techniques after tissue decalcification and debridement does not adversely affect surgical outcome.[12,13] Mitral valve repair rather than replacement is also possible in the setting of native valve endocarditis, as this results in lower hospital mortality and improved long-term outcome when compared to valve replacement.[14] Thus, valve repair for mitral regurgitation, whatever the etiology, should be the first choice of surgical correction.

Freedom from reoperation for structural valve-related degeneration has been reported as high as 90% at 10 years and 85% at 15 years following valve repair.[15] In patients who exhibit valve failure following repair, successful re-repair can be undertaken in 16–21% of patients.[16,17] Thus, the ultimate likelihood of requiring a mitral prosthesis following surgical repair of mitral regurgitation is very low.

Basic concepts of repair

Prolapse of a segment of the posterior leaflet is treated by triangular or quadrangular resection of the unsupported portion or by plication of the redundant leaflet tissue.[18,19] In patients with anterior leaflet prolapse, with or without chordal rupture, we favor chordal replacement with Gore-Tex suture.[20]

Dilation of the valve annulus almost always accompanies mitral regurgitation.[21] Progressive annular enlargement worsens regurgitation by further decreasing the area of leaflet coaptation. The dilation tends to be asymmetrical, in that it affects the mural leaflet up to the commissures.[22] Dilation changes annular shape so that the anteroposterior diameter of the valve becomes greater than the transverse diameter. Because of this, an annuloplasty procedure is an integral part of mitral valve repair. The goals of an annuloplasty are fourfold:

1. decrease annulus diameter, thereby decreasing the area that the leaflets must seal;
2. prevent further dilation of the annulus;
3. allow coaptation of the leaflets along several millimeters from their free margins, thus decreasing the probability of tears in areas where segments of leaflets or chordae were repaired;
4. restoration of normal annulus shape.

Annuloplasty is typically performed with a prosthetic ring;[23,24] we favor a partial posterior ring[25] to reorient the anterior or posterior leaflets for adequate coaptation (Figure 56.4). Postoperative valve function as assessed by degree of regurgitation, transvalvular gradient, and valve area is comparable, irrespective of which technique is utilized.[25] It should be noted that the normal mitral annulus changes size and shape during the cardiac cycle.[26–29] This "sphincter-like" function results in a reduction in valve area by 26% during systole, which is associated with a change in shape from circular to elliptical.[30] If a flexible annuloplasty is utilized for repair rather than a rigid ring, superior left ventricular systolic function can be demonstrated early and late following valve repair.[31,32]

Valve replacement

Grade B Choice of a valve prosthesis requires consideration of the qualities of the valve weighed against the patient's needs. Durability of the prosthesis is often the primary concern of the patient. Indeed, when discussing valve replacement with a patient, the most commonly asked question is "How long will it [the prosthesis] last?" For currently available mechanical valves in the United States, the answer is a qualified "forever", qualified in the sense that intrinsic material failure of mechanical valves is now extremely rare.[33] However, this does not mean that a valve might not need to be replaced because of extrinsic mechanical failure (for example, pannus ingrowth inhibiting proper function of the closure mechanism), and the patient should understand these differences. Durability of biologic valves is not so well

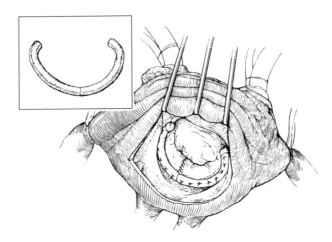

Figure 56.4 An annuloplasty ring

defined for the individual patient. Indeed, as outlined below, by their very nature, tissue valves have a limited lifespan and their use must be matched to a patient's needs.

Anticoagulation and thrombogenicity are the other major issues with prosthetic valves. Mechanical valves offer excellent durability that clearly surpasses that of currently available tissue valves, but thrombus formation and thromboembolism are recognized hazards. Anticoagulation to prevent thromboembolism introduces an incremental risk to a patient. Indeed, taken together, anticoagulant-related hemorrhage and thrombosis account for up to 75% of complications following mechanical valve replacement.[34]

Finally, when evaluating different types of cardiac valve prostheses, one must understand the concepts of valvular hemodynamics. These are directly related to valve design and determine the work the heart must expend to pump blood through the prosthesis. All currently approved prosthetic valves have a sewing ring which, with the housing of the valve, takes up a certain cross-sectional area in the path of blood flow. This "sewing ring area" is larger for the tissue valves than for the mechanical valves. The effective orifice area (EOA) of a valve is the actual area of the valve available for blood flow. If one divides the EOA by the sewing ring area, one can calculate the performance index of a given valve. The performance index of currently available porcine valves ranges from 0·35 to 0·4, pericardial valves 0·65, and tilting disc valves from 0·67 to 0·70, so that all stent mounted prosthetic valves are, by definition, stenotic compared to normal native valves. The potential for residual outflow obstruction when a small prosthetic valve is used in a large patient gives rise to the condition termed valve-prosthesis patient mismatch.[35,36] For most patients, the transvalvular gradient is small and of little clinical significance. It should be noted, however, that as the valve size decreases and the EOA concomitantly decreases, there can be a precipitous rise in the transvalvular gradient, which could cancel out the clinical improvement anticipated from valve replacement.

Two other aspects of valve function are often overlooked: dynamic and static prosthetic valve regurgitation. Dynamic regurgitant fraction is the amount of regurgitation that occurs through a valve before the occluder has a chance to close fully. This is lowest for the tilting disc valves, followed by the bileaflet prostheses; the greatest dynamic regurgitation is associated with the ball and cage prostheses.[37] Static regurgitation occurs through a valve after the valve has closed. Some static regurgitation is engineered into most valves to wash the valve components and eliminate microemboli. Bileaflet valves and Medtronic-Hall tilting disc valves have greater static regurgitation than ball and cage valves.[37] Although regurgitant volume through a normally functioning prosthesis is not important in a patient with adequate ventricular function, in the face of decreased ejection fraction, large regurgitant volumes may attenuate the hemodynamic improvement produced by valve replacement.

Mechanical valves

Grade B Currently in the United States, there are five categories of mechanical valves approved for implication by the Food and Drug Administration. These include the St Jude (St Jude Medical, Minneapolis, MN) bileaflet prosthesis, the Medtronic-Hall (Medtronic Inc, Minneapolis, MN) tilting disc valve, the CarboMedics (CarboMedics, Austin, TX) bileaflet prosthesis, the Starr-Edwards ball valve (Baxter Healthcare, Santa Ana, CA), and the Omnicarbon tilting disc valve, which evolved from the Omniscience valve. There are few prospective, randomized studies comparing outcomes between these categories of valves in the same patient populations.

Non-randomized studies and informal comparisons of published series show little difference in late patient outcome, either in morbidity or mortality, following implantation of currently approved mechanical prostheses (for review, see reference[37]). Several prospective, randomized studies comparing specific valves bear out this assertion. Schulte and associates randomized 150 consecutive patients to receive a tilting disc prosthesis or Starr-Edwards valve or mitral valve replacement; there was no significant difference in late patient survival (mean follow up 14·8 years) between the two tilting disc valves (Bjork-Shiley, Lillehei-Kaster) and a ball and cage prosthesis (Starr-Edwards).[38]

In another randomized study of 102 patients, Fiore and colleagues found no significant difference in linearized rates of valve-related events and 3 year actuarial survival between a tilting disc (Medtronic-Hall) and bileaflet (St Jude) prosthesis (Figure 56.5).[39] Even when comparing an early model tilting disc prosthesis (Bjork-Shiley) with a bileaflet prosthesis (St Jude), no significant difference in early and late survival or major bleeding complications could be demonstrated in 178 patients in a prospectively randomized, European study (mean follow up of 52 months or 778 patient-years).[40] Thus, with regard to clinical performance and hemodynamic data, there are no large randomized studies that definitively demonstrate the superiority and thus preferential selection of one mechanical prosthesis over another.

Bioprosthetic valves

Grade B The three most commonly used bioprostheses are the Hancock porcine valve (Medtronic Inc) and the Carpentier-Edwards porcine and bovine pericardial valves (Baxter Healthcare). The main drawback of the bioprosthetic valves is structural deterioration which is not a simple linear function of time as the rate of structural dysfunction steadily accelerates after 5–6 years of implantation.[41–43] Regurgitation through cusp tears associated with calcific nodules is the most frequent form of bioprosthesis failure; pure stenosis due to calcified leaflets occurs infrequently. Structural dysfunction of bioprostheses is markedly accelerated in children, adolescents, and young adults, but is attenuated in very elderly

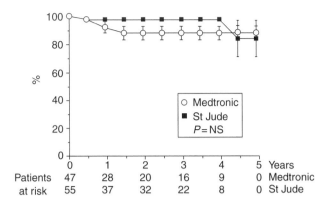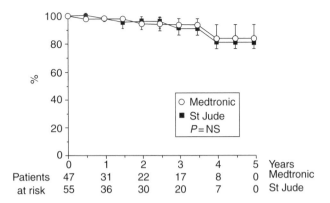

Figure 56.5 Actuarial freedom from thromboembolism (left) and hemorrhage (right) after mitral valve replacement with the St Jude and Medtronic-Hall valves (NS=not significant). (From Fiore *et al.*[39])

patients. For aortic bioprostheses, patients younger than 39–44 years of age have structurally related, event free estimates ranging from 58% to 70% at 10 years;[43–45] this drops to 33% at 15 years.[46] This is in contrast to patients over 70 years of age, who have event free estimates of 95% and 93% at 10 and 15 years following implantation.[46] Event free estimates for patients between 60 and 69 years of age, 10 years following implantation, range from 92% to 95%.[45–47]

Many investigators have compared the performance of the Hancock and the Carpentier-Edwards porcine bioprostheses. In general, no significant differences in the short- and long-term performance of these valves have been demonstrated.[48–51] Indeed, at 10 year follow up of 174 patients undergoing mitral or aortic valve replacement who were prospectively randomized to receive either a Hancock or Carpentier-Edwards porcine bioprosthesis, there were no significant differences in patient survival, durability of the prosthesis or valve-related complications.[48] These findings were confirmed in another study of 147 patients randomized to receive either the Carpentier-Edwards or Hancock porcine bioprosthesis in the mitral position. At 10 years, no significant differences in survival or valve-related complications were apparent.[52]

Previously, all commercially available bioprostheses were mounted on a stent or frame to give the relatively flaccid tissue valve a fixed base to facilitate implantation. The stent and sewing ring, however, significantly decrease the EOA and make tissue valves relatively obstructive when compared with mechanical prostheses. There has been considerable interest recently in stentless bioprosthetic valves that are inserted in much the same fashion as homografts. Hemodynamic performance of stentless bioprostheses is good and like other tissue valves, no anticoagulation is required.[53–56] In one report, 254 patients with the Toronto SPV stentless valve (St Jude Medical) were followed for 3 years and the initially favorable EOAs and transvalvular gradients were said to improve with time.[53] In addition, left ventricular mass decreased by 14·3% in the study period.

The primary mode of failure of stentless valves, like all bioprostheses, is valvular regurgitation. Indeed, 27% of 200 patients were found to have aortic insufficiency 1 year following implantation of a stentless aortic valve (PRIMA Edwards; Baxter Healthcare); however, only one patient exhibited grade 3 insufficiency.[55] In addition, in a non-randomized study of 150 patients receiving either a stentless bioprosthesis (PRIMA Edwards), a traditional bioprosthesis or a homograft, no difference in morbidity or mortality was noted between the groups after 1 year.[57] While the initial data on stentless bioprostheses in the aortic position are encouraging, further long-term studies will be needed to establish their ultimate role in the management of aortic valve disease.

Development of stentless valves for the mitral position has been difficult. Because the mitral valve annulus changes shape during the cardiac cycle, a stentless prosthesis in this location requires additional external support to maintain competence. This engineering challenge has been met by using artificial chordae to anchor the stentless valve to native papillary muscle.[58] Short-term success has been reported, but a stentless prosthesis for the mitral position should be considered as experimental.

An additional category of tissue valves currently available for implantation are homografts. These are human tissue valves (either aortic or pulmonic) that have been harvested from cadavers, sterilized antibiotically, and cryopreserved.[59,60] Homografts have many attractive features including minimal gradients, low thrombogenicity without need for anticoagulation, and low risk of infection, even when used in patients with active endocarditis.[61,62] Implantation of a homograft is considered more difficult than implantation of a stent mounted bioprosthesis and both experience of the surgeon and surgical technique appear to influence late results.[63] Freedom from reoperation due to structural deterioration of homografts has been reported to range from 83% at 8 years[64] to 86% at 14 years.[60] When valve failure occurs, it is due to the gradual development of insufficiency.

The other homograft available for aortic valve replacement is the pulmonary valve autograft (termed the Ross procedure). The Ross procedure involves excision of a patient's normal pulmonic valve (autograft) and utilizing it to replace the diseased aortic valve.[65,66] A cryopreserved human pulmonary artery homograft (allograft) is then implanted to replace the native pulmonic valve. There are many positive aspects of the operation. First, as both of the valves are tissue valves, no anticoagulation is required. Second, since the pulmonic valve autograft is not exposed to the antibiotic sterilization or cryopreservation process, it is viable and has potential for growth and long-term durability.[67,68] In one series of 195 patients, the freedom from reoperation (autograft or allograft) was reported to be 89% at 5 years.[69] Compared to allograft replacement of the aortic valve, patients receiving the pulmonary autograft have comparable hemodynamics and early-to medium-term postoperative recovery.[70]

However, there are three potential drawbacks to the pulmonary autograft. First, the operation converts single valve disease to a double valve replacement. And even if the pulmonary autograft functions perfectly, there is potential for tissue degeneration and obstruction of the pulmonary allograft; in fact, the need for right-sided valve re-replacement may be underestimated. In the best of hands and in carefully selected patients, cumulative risk of reoperation for pulmonary valve substitute approaches 20% at 20 years postoperatively.[65,71] In addition, there is a 10–20% incidence of autograft aortic insufficiency, grade 2+, following operation.[72] Long-term follow up from multiple institutions is necessary to define the safety and durability of the pulmonary autograft for aortic valve replacement.

Comparative studies of mechanical v bioprosthetic valves

Grade A In a prospective, randomized study in which 262 patients received either a mechanical (Bjork-Shiley) or porcine bioprosthesis (initially Hancock and subsequently Carpentier-Edwards) in the mitral position, actuarial survival and incidence of thromboembolism was comparable at 7 years follow up.[73] Another prospective, randomized study also demonstrated comparable survival following valve replacement with either a mechanical valve or bioprosthesis.[74] Five hundred and seventy-five men, scheduled to undergo either aortic or mitral valve replacement, were randomized either to receive a mechanical valve (Bjork-Shiley) or porcine bioprosthesis (Hancock). After 11 years, survival rates and freedom from all valve-related complications were similar for both patient groups. However, the profile of valve-related complications was different in that structural failure was only observed with the bioprosthetic valves, whereas bleeding complications were more frequent in patients with mechanical valves. Thus, while the types of complications might differ between patients with either a

bioprosthesis or mechanical valve, the actual incidence of the complications is comparable and survival is similar. As such, the choice between a bioprosthesis and a mechanical valve should be based on other factors.

Matching the patient to the prosthesis: factors in selecting a valve for implantation

Grade B Because patient survival following valve replacement is independent of the type of prosthesis used and dependent on other factors, one needs to focus on patient variables when selecting a valve. First, one must assess a patient's life expectancy after valve replacement. For patients aged 65–69 years undergoing aortic and/or mitral valve replacement, survival is approximately 53% at 10 years and 25% at 15 years; for patients 70 years of age or older, survival is 30–38% at 10 years and 25% at 15 years.[47] Coronary artery disease requiring bypass grafting at the time of valve replacement further decreases long-term survival.[75]

All other factors being equal, it has been our practice to suggest a mechanical valve to patients 70 years or younger and a bioprosthesis to those 75 years and older. In the "gray area" between 70 and 75 years, recommendations are made based upon a patient's general health and personal preference.

The other major issue related to the choice of a valve prosthesis is anticoagulation. Obviously, a mechanical valve, with its obligatory need for lifelong oral anticoagulation, would be contraindicated in a patient who:

- has bleeding tendencies
- because of geography or psychosocial issues, would be unable to monitor the level of anticoagulation
- has an occupation with a high risk of trauma
- is a female of childbearing age who desires a future pregnancy.

In these situations, one of the tissue valves would be indicated. However, if a patient is likely to require anticoagulation for some other condition such as atrial fibrillation, a large left atrium, chronic deep venous thrombosis or a mechanical prosthesis in another location, then a mechanical valve is chosen for its durability. In addition, if for some reason a patient would be at great risk for reoperation and valve re-replacement, a mechanical valve is favored.

References

1. Dare AJ, Harrity PJ, Tazelaar HD, Edwards WD, Mullany CJ. Evaluation of surgically excised mitral valves: revised recommendations based on changing operative procedures in the 1990s. *Hum Pathol* 1993;**24**:1286–93.
2. Olson LJ, Subramanian R, Ackermann DM, Orszulak TA, Edwards WD. Surgical pathology of the mitral valve: a study of 712 cases spanning 21 years. *Mayo Clin Proc* 1987;**62**:22–34.

3. Waller BF, Morrow AG, Maron BJ *et al.* Etiology of clinically isolated, severe, chronic, pure mitral regurgitation: an analysis of 97 patients over 30 years of age having mitral valve replacement. *Am Heart J* 1982;**104**:276–88.

4. Enriquez-Sarano M, Tajik AJ, Schaff HV *et al.* Echocardiographic prediction of survival after surgical correction of organic mitral regurgitation. *Circulation* 1994;**90**:830–7.

5. Ling LH, Enriquez-Sarano M, Sewrad JB *et al.* Clinical outcome of mitral regurgitation due to flail leaflet. *N Engl J Med* 1996;**355**:1417–23.

6. Perier P, Deloche A, Chauvaud S *et al.* Comparative evaluation of mitral valve repair and replacement with Starr, Bjork, and porcine valve prostheses. *Circulation* 1984;**70**:187–92.

7. Enriquez-Sarano M, Schaff HV, Orszulak TA *et al.* Valve repair improves the outcome of surgery for mitral regurgitation: a multivariate analysis. *Circulation* 1995;**91**:1022–8.

8. Goldman ME, Mora F, Guarino T, Fuster V, Mindich BP. Mitral valvuloplasty is superior to mitral valve replacement for preservation of left ventricular function: an intraoperative two-dimensional echocardiographic study. *J Am Coll Cardiol* 1987;**10**:568–75.

9. Rozich JD, Carabello BA, Usher BW *et al.* Mitral valve replacement with and without chordal preservation in patients with chronic mitral regurgitation. Mechanisms for differences in postoperative ejection performance. *Circulation* 1992;**86**:1718–26.

10. David TE, Uden DE, Strauss HD. The importance of the mitral apparatus in left ventricular function after correction of mitral regurgitation. *Circulation* 1983;**68**:1176–83.

11. David TE, Burns RJ, Bacchus CM, Druck MN. Mitral regurgitation with and without preservation of chordae tendineae. *J Thorac Cardiovasc Surg* 1984;**88**:718–25.

12. Grossi EA, Galloway AC, Steinberg BM *et al.* Severe calcification does not affect long-term outcome of mitral valve repair. *Ann Thorac Surg* 1994;**58**:685–8.

13. Carpentier AF, Pellerin M, Fuzellier JF, Relland JYM. Extensive calcification of the mitral valve annulus: pathology and surgical management. *J Thorac Cardiovasc Surg* 1996;**111**:718–30.

14. Muehrcke DD, Cosgrove DM, Lytle BW *et al.* Is there an advantage to repairing infected mitral valves? *Ann Thorac Surg* 1997;**63**:1718–24.

15. Alvarez JM, Deal CW, Loveridge K *et al.* Repairing the degenerative mitral valve: ten to fifteen year follow-up. *J Thorac Cardiovasc Surg* 1996;**112**:238–47.

16. Cerfolio RJ, Orszulak TA, Pluth JR, Harmsen WS, Schaff HV. Reoperation after valve repair for mitral regurgitation: early and immediate results. *J Thorac Cardiovasc Surg* 1996;**111**:1177–84.

17. Gillinov AM, Cosgrove DM, Lytle BW *et al.* Reoperation for mitral valve repair. *J Thorac Cardiovasc Surg* 1997;**113**:467–75.

18. Carpentier A. Cardiac valve surgery: the French connection. *J Thorac Cardiovasc Surg* 1983;**86**:323–37.

19. McGoon DC. Repair of mitral insufficiency due to ruptured chordae tendinae. *J Thorac Cardiovasc Surg* 1960;**39**:357–62.

20. David TE, Armstrong S, Sun Z. Replacement of chordae tendineae with Gore-Tex sutures: a ten-year experience. *J Heart Valve Dis* 1996;**5**:352–5.

21. Ormiston JA, Shah PM, Tei C, Wong M. Size and motion of the mitral valve annulus in man. II. Abnormalities in mitral valve prolapse. *Circulation* 1982;**65**:713–19.

22. Carpentier A. Plastic and reconstructive mitral valve surgery. In Kalmanson D, ed. *The mitral valve, a pluridisciplinary approach.* London: Publishing Science Group, 1976.

23. Carpentier A, Deloche A, Dauptain J *et al.* A new reconstructive operation for correction of mitral and tricuspid insufficiency. *J Thorac Cardiovasc Surg* 1971;**61**:1–13.

24. Duran CMG, Umbago JL. Clinical and hemodynamic performance of a totally flexible prosthetic ring for atrioventricular valve reconstruction. *Ann Thorac Surg* 1976;**22**:458–63.

25. Odell JA, Schaff HV, Orszulak TA. Early results of a simplified method of mitral valve anuloplasty. *Circulation* 1995;**92** (Suppl. II):II-150–4.

26. David TE, Strauss HD, Mesher E *et al.* Is it important to preserve the chordae tendineae and papillary muscles during mitral valve replacement? *Can J Surg* 1981;**24**:236–9.

27. Hansen DE, Cahill PD, DeCampli WM *et al.* Valvular ventricular interactions: importance of the mitral apparatus in canine left ventricular systolic performance. *Circulation* 1986;**73**:1310–20.

28. Hansen DE, Cahill PD, Derby GC, Miller DC. Relative contributions of the anterior and posterior mitral chordae tendineae to canine global left ventricular systolic performance. *J Thorac Cardiovasc Surg* 1987;**93**:45–55.

29. Sarris GE, Cahill PD, Hansen DE *et al.* Restoration of left ventricular systolic performance after reattachment of the mitral chordae tendineae. The importance of the valvular-ventricular interaction. *J Thorac Cardiovasc Surg* 1988;**95**:969–79.

30. Ormiston JA, Shah PM, Tei C, Wong M. Size and motion of the mitral annulus in man: a two-dimensional echocardiographic method and findings in normal subjects. *Circulation* 1981;**64**:113–20.

31. David TE, Komeda M, Pollick C, Burns RJ. Mitral valve annuloplasty: the effect of the type on left ventricular function. *Ann Thorac Surg* 1989;**47**:524–8.

32. Duran CG, Revuelta JM, Gaite L, Alonso C, Fleitas MG. Stability of mitral reconstructive surgery at 10–12 years for predominantly rheumatic valvular disease. *Circulation* 1988;**78**:191–6.

33. Grunkemeier GL, Rahimtoola SH. Artificial heart valves. *Annu Rev Med* 1990;**41**:251–63.

34. Edmonds LH. Thrombotic and bleeding complications of prosthetic heart valves. *Ann Thorac Surg* 1987;**44**:430–45.

35. Rahimtoola SH. The problem of valve prosthesis-patient mismatch. *Circulation* 1978;**58**:20–4.

36. Rahimtoola SH, Murphy E. Valve prosthesis-patient mismatch. A long-term sequela. *Br Heart J* 1981;**45**:331–5.

37. Akins CW. Results with mechanical cardiac valvular prostheses. *Ann Thorac Surg* 1995;**60**:1836–44.

38. Schulte HD, Horstkotte D, Bircks W, Strauer BE. Results of a randomized mitral valve replacement with mechanical prostheses after 15 years. *Int J Artif Organs* 1992;**15**:611–16.

39. Fiore AC, Naunheim KS, d'Orazio S *et al.* Mitral valve replacement: randomized trial of St. Jude and Medtronic-Hall prostheses. *Ann Thorac Surg* 1992;**54**:68–73.

40. Vogt S, Hoffmann A, Roth J *et al.* Heart valve replacement with the Bjork-Shiley and St. Jude Medical

prostheses: a randomized comparison in 178 patients. *Eur Heart J* 1990; **11**:583–91.

41. Jamieson WRE, Murno AI, Miyagishima RT *et al.* Carpentier-Edwards standard porcine bioprosthesis: clinical performance to seventeen years. *Ann Thorac Surg* 1995;**60**:999–1007.

42. Glower DD, White WD, Hatton AC *et al.* Determinants of reoperation after 960 valve replacements with Carpentier-Edwards prostheses. *J Thorac Cardiovasc Surg* 1994;**107**: 381–93.

43. Pelletier LC, Carrier M, Leclerc Y *et al.* Influence of age on late results of valve replacement with porcine bioprostheses. *J Cardiovasc Surg* 1992;**33**:526–33.

44. Cohn LH, Collins JJ Jr, DiSesa V *et al.* Fifteen-year experience with 1,678 Hancock porcine bioprosthetic heart valve replacements. *Ann Surg* 1989;**210**:435–43.

45. Jones EL, Weintraub WS, Craver JM *et al.* Ten-year experience with the porcine bioprosthetic valves; interrelationship of valve survival and patient survival in 1,050 valve replacements. *Ann Thorac Surg* 1990;**49**:370–84.

46. Burdon TA, Miller DC, Oyer PE *et al.* Durability of porcine valves at fifteen years in a representative North American population. *J Thorac Cardiovasc Surg* 1992;**103**:238–52.

47. Burr LH, Jamieson WRE, Munro AI *et al.* Porcine bioprostheses in the elderly: clinical performance by age groups and valve positions. *Ann Thorac Surg* 1995;**60**:S264–9.

48. Sarris GE, Robbins RC, Miller DC *et al.* Randomized, prospective assessment of bioprosthetic valve durability: Hancock verses Carpentier-Edwards valves. *Circulation* 1993;**88** (pt 2):55–64.

49. Bolooki H, Kaiser GA, Mallon SM, Palatianos GM. Comparison of long-term results of Carpentier-Edwards and Hancock bioprosthetic valves. *Ann Thorac Surg* 1986;**42**:494–9.

50. Hartz RS, Fisher EB, Finkelmeier B *et al.* An eight-year experience with porcine bioprosthetic cardiac valves. *J Thorac Cardiovasc Surg* 1986;**91**:910–17.

51. McDonald ML, Daley RC, Schaff HV *et al.* Hemodynamic performance of a small aortic valve bioprostheses: is there a difference? *Ann Thorac Surg* 1997;**63**:362–6.

52. Perier P, Deloche A, Chauvaud S *et al.* A ten-year comparison of mitral valve replacement with Carpentier-Edwards and Hancock porcine bioprostheses. *Ann Thorac Surg* 1989; **48**:54–9.

53. Del Rizzo DF, Goldman BS, Christakis GT, David TE. Hemodynamic benefits of the Toronto Stentless Valve. *J Thorac Cardiovasc Surg* 1996;**112**:1431–45.

54. Sintek CF, Fletcher AD, Khonsari S. Small aortic root in the elderly: use of a stentless bioprosthesis. *J Heart Valve Dis* 1996;**5**(Suppl. 3):S308–13.

55. Dossche K, Vanermen H, Daenen W, Pillai R, Konertz W. Hemodynamic performance of the PRIMA Edwards stentless aortic xenograft: early results of a multicenter clinical trial. *Thorac Cardiovasc Surg* 1996;**44**:11–14.

56. Wong K, Shad S, Waterworth PD *et al.* Early experience with the Toronto stentless porcine valve. *Ann Thorac Surg* 1995;**60**(Suppl. 2):S402–5.

57. Dossche K, Vanermen H, Wellens F *et al.* Free-hand sewn allografts, stentless (Prima Edwards) and stented (CESA) porcine

bioprostheses. A comparative hemodynamic study. *Eur J Cardiothorac Surg* 1995;**9**:562–6.

58. Deac RF, Simionescu D, Deac D. New evolution in mitral physiology and surgery: mitral stentless pericardial valve. *Ann Thorac Surg* 1995;**60**(Suppl. 2):S433–8.

59. McGriffin DC, O"Brien MF, Stafford EG *et al.* Long-term results of the viable cryopreserved allograft valve: continuing evidence for superior valve durability. *J Cardiac Surg* 1988; **3**(Suppl.):289.

60. O'Brien MF, McGriffin DC, Stafford EG *et al.* Allograft aortic valve replacement: long-term comparative clinical analysis of the viable cryopreserved and antibiotic 4 C stored valves. *J Cardiac Surg* 1991;**6**(Suppl. 4):534.

61. Tuna IC, Orszulak TA, Schaff HV, Danielson GK. Results of homograft aortic valve replacement for active endocarditis. *Ann Thorac Surg* 1990;**49**:619–24.

62. Dearani JA, Orszulak TA, Schaff HV *et al.* Results of allograft aortic valve replacement for complex endocarditis. *J Thorac Cardiovasc Surg* 1997;**113**:285–91.

63. Dearani JA, Orszulak TA, Daly RC *et al.* Comparison of techniques for implantation of aortic valve allografts. *Ann Thorac Surg* 1996;**62**:1069–75.

64. Kirklin JK, Naftel DC, Novick W *et al.* Long-term function of cryopreserved aortic valve homografts: a ten year study. *J Thorac Cardiovasc Surg* 1993;**106**:154–66.

65. Ross D, Jackson M, Davies J. Pulmonary autograft aortic valve replacement: long-term results. *J Cardiac Surg* 1991;**6**: 529–53.

66. Elkins RC, Santangelo K, Stelzer P, Randolph JD, Knott-Craig CJ. Pulmonary autograft replacement of the aortic valve: an evolution of technique. *J Cardiac Surg* 1992;**7**:108–16.

67. Gerosa G, McKay R, Ross DN. Replacement of the aortic valve or root with an autograft in children. *Ann Thorac Surg* 1991;**51**:424.

68. Walls JT, McDaniel WC, Pope ER *et al.* Documented growth of autogenous pulmonary valve translocated to the aortic valve position (letter). *J Thorac Cardiovasc Surg* 1994;**107**:1530.

69. Elkins RC, Lane MM, McCue C. Pulmonary autograft reoperation: incidence and management. *Ann Thorac Surg* 1996; **62**:450–5.

70. Santini F, Dyke C, Edwards S *et al.* Pulmonary autograft versus homograft replacement of the aortic valve: a prospective randomized trial. *J Thorac Cardiovasc Surg* 1997;**113**:894–900.

71. Ross D. Replacement of the aortic valve with a pulmonary autograft: the "switch" operation. *Ann Thorac Surg* 1991;**52**:1346.

72. Elkins RC. Editorial: pulmonary autograft – the optimal substitute for the aortic valve? *N Engl J Med* 1994;**330**:59.

73. Bloomfield P, Kitchin AH, Wheatley DJ *et al.* A prospective evaluation of the Bjork-Shiley, Hancock, and Carpentier-Edwards heart valve prostheses. *Circulation* 1993;**88**:1155–64.

74. Hammermeister KE, Sethi GK, Henderson WG *et al.* A comparison of outcomes in men 11 years after heart-valve replacement with a mechanical valve or bioprosthesis. *N Engl J Med* 1993;**328**:1289.

75. Jones EL, Weintraub WS, Craver JM *et al.* Interaction of age and coronary disease after valve replacement: implications for valve selection. *Ann Thorac Surg* 1994;**58**:378–85.

57 Diagnosis and management of infective endocarditis

David T Durack, Michael L Towns

The diagnosis and management of infective endocarditis (IE) raises many questions and clinical decisions which invite application of the principles of evidence-based medicine. Most of these have not been formally asked or answered by means of controlled clinical studies. Current practice is based upon an extensive accumulation of uncontrolled clinical experience, rather than upon validated clinical trials.

Here we will discuss common issues that arise during diagnosis and management of IE. Recommendations will be offered, along with an evidence-based grading (on an A, B, C scale) of the basis for each recommendation.

Background

Pathophysiology

Endocarditis refers to inflammation of the endocardial lining of the heart. The heart valves are most often involved, or less commonly the lining of the heart chambers (mural endocarditis). When the lesions of endocarditis (vegetations) contain micro-organisms, the associated disease is termed infective endocarditis. This general term covers the various clinical subcategories of the disease (for example, acute, subacute, prosthetic valve infection) and also the various etiologic agents (bacteria, yeasts or fungi).

The pathophysiology of this disease often begins with the formation of non-bacterial thrombotic endocarditis (NBTE). This lesion, which is sometimes called a "fibrin-platelet plug", is a receptive precursor site which may become infected by circulating organisms during the course of a bacteremia or fungemia.[1–3] NBTE is not normally found in healthy hearts, but it may develop on an endocardial lining which has been damaged by one of several mechanisms. One of the most common pathogenic mechanisms is that of a cardiac valvular lesion, such as scarring or stenosis, leading to high velocity turbulent flow across the valve, with resultant damage to the endothelial lining.[4,5] The damaged area may become a locus for deposition of fibrin and platelets, resulting in NBTE. The type of underlying cardiac valvular lesion determines where a vegetation is most likely to form on the endocardial surface. A bacteremia caused by organisms that have the capacity to adhere to this lesion, mediated by surface factors such as adhesins, may seed the NBTE and lead to development of an infected vegetation.[1–3,6]

Vegetations are the pathologic hallmark of IE.[1,2,6] They are composed of masses of organisms enmeshed with fibrin, platelets, and a variable (often scanty) inflammatory infiltrate. The vegetations may be of various sizes, and may or may not progress to cause further valvular, perivalvular, or extracardiac complications. Valvular complications may include valvular dysfunction, destruction, or obstruction. Perivalvular complications include extension of infection into adjacent structures, which may result in formation of a perivalvular abscess. Extracardiac complications most commonly result from embolic phenomena such as embolization into the coronary arteries or the systemic arterial tree, resulting in ischemia, infarcts, and sometimes secondary bleeding. Less commonly, abscesses or mycotic aneurysms may develop in various organs. Other extracardiac complications may include immune complex mediated disease such as glomerulonephritis.

Epidemiology

IE has been variously categorized in the past as acute, subacute, chronic, native valve, prosthetic valve, culture-negative, and intravenous drug abuse associated endocarditis. These terms have some value, but they may overlap. It is useful to specify the infecting organism because this allows prediction of the likely natural history, treatment requirements, and prognosis for an individual patient. Here we will briefly discuss the epidemiology of IE in the context of three main categories: native valve, prosthetic valve, and culture-negative endocarditis.[7–9]

Table 57.1 shows the etiologic agents that are most commonly isolated in native valve IE. Cases caused by virulent pathogens such as *Streptococcus pneumoniae* or *Staphylococcus aureus* may develop on previously normal valves. More often, native valve endocarditis develops in association with predisposing congenital or acquired valvular lesions, especially when caused by less virulent organisms such as the viridans streptococci.

Prosthetic valve endocarditis can be subcategorized into early (onset up to 60 days after valve replacement),

Table 57.1   Frequency of various organisms isolated in native value infective endocarditis

Organism	NVE (%)	IV drug abusers (%)	Early PVE (%)	Late PVE (%)
Streptococci	65	15	5	35
Viridans, alpha-hemolytic	35	5	<5	25
Strep. bovis (group D)	15	<5	<5	<5
Strep. faecalis (group D)	10	8	<5	<5
Other streptococci	<5	<5	<5	<5
Staphylococci	25	50	50	30
Coagulase-positive	23	50	20	10
Coagulase-negative	<5	<5	30	20
Gram-negative aerobic bacilli	<5	5	15	10
Fungi	<5	5	10	5
Miscellaneous bacteria	<5	5	5	5
Diphtheroids, propionibacteria	<1	<5	5	<5
Other anaerobes	<1	<1	<1	<1
Rickettsia	<1	<1	<1	<1
Chlamydia	<1	<1	<1	<1
Polymicrobial infection	<1	5	5	5
Culture-negative endocarditis	5–10	<5	<5	<5

These are representative figures collated from the literature; wide local variations in frequency are to be expected.
Abbreviations: NVE, native valve endocarditis; PVE, prosthetic valve endocarditis
Reproduced with permission, from Durack[7]

intermediate (onset from 2 to 12 months) or late cases (onset after one year). The observed spectrum of etiologic agents is different for the two categories, with the organisms causing late onset prosthetic valve endocarditis more closely resembling native valve subacute endocarditis, except that coagulase-negative staphylococci remain important (Table 57.1).

Culture-negative IE remains fairly common (3–30% of cases in recent series), despite improvements in blood culture techniques and culture media. Organisms that previously were difficult to recover, such as nutritionally variant streptococci and the fastidious Gram-negatives (HACEK group: *Haemophilus* spp, *Actinobacillus actinomycetemcomitans*, *Cardiobacterium hominis*, *Eikenella* spp, and *Kingella kingae*) are now routinely isolated from modern, optimized blood culture media, usually within 3–5 days. An exception to this is *Bartonella* spp which have recently been found in association with endocarditis among homeless individuals, and as a rare opportunistic infection in patients with AIDS.[10,11]

Diagnosis

Clinical manifestations

Patients with acute IE typically present with an accelerated course typified by high fever, chills, and prostration, whereas those with subacute endocarditis present more insidiously.

These patients often have a "flu-like illness" consisting of fever, chills, myalgias/arthralgias, and weakness, but there is great variability in the clinical presentation.[7]

Cardiac manifestations may dominate the clinical presentation in either acute or subacute disease, with the presence of new or worsened murmurs, or development of cardiac failure due to valvular damage. The patient may present with chest pain due to pleuritis, pericarditis or myocardial infarction resulting from coronary arterial embolism.

Extracardiac clinical manifestations consist of embolic as well as vascular phenomena. The patient may present with a headache without any definable neurologic abnormalities, or may have focal abnormalities such as areas of cerebritis, infarcts, hemorrhages or mycotic aneurysms. A cellular reaction in the cerebrospinal fluid (with or without meningismus) may also be present, although only a minority of patients have positive cerebrospinal fluid cultures. The patient may present with focal pain such as flank or left-sided upper quadrant abdominal pain due to embolic infarcts, which may at times be complicated by the formation of abscesses, especially in the spleen. There are many other potential sites for embolization with associated clinical findings, although autopsy findings show that many emboli go undetected during life.

Various other vascular phenomena may occur, including petechiae, splinter hemorrhages, Osler's nodes, Janeway lesions, or clubbing of the fingernails.

Laboratory tests

Anemia is commonly present, usually of mild to moderate severity with a normochromic, normocytic film typical of the anemia of chronic disease. Although many patients with acute or subacute endocarditis have some degree of leukocytosis, this is not a reliable laboratory finding. In approximately 90% of patients with infective endocarditis the erythrocyte sedimentation rate (ESR) is elevated; the median value is about 65 mm/h, but the range is wide and about 10% are within the normal range. Urinalysis may show microscopic hematuria and/or mild proteinuria in approximately 50% of cases, with occasional red blood cell casts and heavy proteinuria in those patients who develop immune-complex glomerulonephritis. Non-specific serologic abnormalities are common, especially positive rheumatoid factor which is seen in 30–40% of cases of the subacute form of the disease. A polyclonal increase in gammaglobulins is characteristic of active endocarditis.

Microbiology

Blood cultures remain the definitive microbiologic procedure for diagnosis of infective endocarditis.[12–15] The microorganisms isolated from blood cultures may provide the clinician with clues to the diagnosis, given the clinical setting. For example, patients who present from the community with a fever of unknown origin who have multiple positive blood cultures for viridans group streptococci, enterococci, or the HACEK organisms, should be considered to have IE until proven otherwise.[12,16,17] In addition, the temporal pattern of positive cultures may assist in the diagnosis. If three or more blood culture sets drawn at least one hour apart all are positive for the same micro-organism, this is termed "persistent bacteremia", which indicates that an endovascular infection may be present. Table 57.1 shows the leading organisms isolated from patients with acute, subacute, and prosthetic valve infective endocarditis.

What are the optimal blood culture techniques required to diagnose infective endocarditis?

Background

A positive blood culture is one of the two major diagnostic criteria for IE.[13] Therefore, blood cultures should be obtained from every patient in whom this diagnosis is suspected. Optimal techniques are required in order to minimize the number of patients with infective endocarditis that fall into the "culture-negative" category, without resorting to an excessive number of costly blood cultures.[14,15]

Evidence

Typically, the bacteremia associated with endocarditis is continuous, with 10–200 colony-forming units per milliliter

of blood.[18] If this were true in every case, it would only be necessary to draw one single sample of about one milliliter of venous blood in order to make the diagnosis. In practice, however, some patients with IE have intermittent or fluctuating bacteremia, and some have less than one organism per milliliter of blood. Therefore, the number of positive culture results is directly correlated with the number of blood samples drawn and the volume of blood in each individual sample.

Single samples should not be drawn because the most common contaminants of blood cultures, coagulase-negative staphylococci from the skin, can cause IE.[12,19–21] Therefore, a single sample drawn from a patient who might have IE, which is positive for a coagulase-negative staphylococcus, is uninterpretable.

Overall, about two thirds of all samples drawn from patients with IE are positive. This figure represents the combined results from two patient populations. The first group includes the "classical" untreated IE patient with continuous bacteremia in whom all or nearly all cultures will be positive.[22] In such patients, more than 90% will be diagnosed by the first sample drawn, rising to more than 95% from three cultures.[19–22] The second population is a mixed group in whom the proportion of positive cultures is much lower. Many of these patients have received some antibiotic treatment, such as empirical oral ampicillin or cephalosporin, which has temporarily or permanently suppressed the bacteremia and turned the blood cultures negative without curing the underlying endocarditis. Others may have difficult-to-culture organisms, fungal infections or culture-negative IE.[14]

In order to decrease the number of "culture-negative" endocarditis episodes, investigators have tried to improve the yield by drawing blood during fever spikes, or by culturing arterial instead of venous blood.[23] These practices are of marginal or no value.

The majority of clinical microbiology laboratories routinely hold their blood culture bottles for 5–7 days before issuing a negative report. Because some of the etiologic agents, for example, HACEK group organisms,[24,25] have been traditionally regarded as slow-growers, some laboratories have adopted the policy of prolonging incubation times for blood cultures to 14–21 days in cases of suspected infective endocarditis. Recent data, however, suggest that with modern, improved blood culture media this practice may be unnecessary for all but a very few organisms, such as *Bartonella* spp.[10,12,26,27]

Should transesophageal echocardiography be performed in all patients with suspected infective endocarditis?

Background

Transthoracic M-mode echocardiography (TTE) was first used for the detection of vegetations associated with endocarditis

Conclusions	Grading	Comments/references
Draw at least two sets (two separate venepunctures, with each sample divided equally between two bottles) for each blood culture ordered	**Grade A**	This helps to identify contaminants and increases yield of positives[12,14,15,19]
Inoculate 8–12 ml blood into each bottle	**Grade B**	This maximizes yield of positives[12,14,15,19]
Hold the culture bottles for 14–21 days before issuing the final negative report in order to minimize "culture-negative" episodes (not recommended)	**Grade C**	The yield is very low after 5 days[12,27]
Draw an arterial blood sample for culture if venous blood samples are negative but the diagnosis of IE still seems likely (not recommended)	**Grade C**	The benefit of culturing arterial blood is none or very small[23,28]

in 1973. Several years later a report describing two dimensional transthoracic echocardiographic findings of vegetations was published. Since then there have been many reports on the use of this technology to assist in the diagnosis of endocarditis.[29–45] The sensitivity of the procedure for detection of vegetations is 60–75%.[29–32]

Transesophageal echocardiography (TEE) was initially described in the late 1980s, and has proved especially valuable in evaluating patients with suspected endocarditis. TEE is more sensitive than TTE for detection of vegetations, abscesses, valve perforations, and other complications of IE.[30,35] Because a TEE examination is more costly than a TTE examination, many comparative studies have been undertaken to determine which technology should be used in the initial diagnostic evaluation of a patient with suspected IE.

Evidence

Multiple studies have demonstrated the superior sensitivity of TEE when compared to TTE. However, this fact does not resolve the question of which is the most appropriate and cost effective test for IE in patients with different pretest probabilities of having that disease.

Transthoracic echocardiography (TTE) has an overall sensitivity for detection of intracardiac vegetations of 60–75%.[32] Transesophageal echocardiography (TEE) has greater sensitivity – 95% or better overall, although the sensitivity in an individual case varies depending upon factors such as the location and size of the vegetations.[30,35–40]

TEE is far superior to TTE in detecting abscesses in patients with both native and prosthetic valve endocarditis (PVE), with a sensitivity of detection of 87%, as compared to 28% with TTE in one study.[41] Because patients with PVE are more likely than those with native valve endocarditis (NVE) to have perivalvular abscesses, it is now accepted that TEE is the technique of choice in evaluating a patient with suspected PVE. TEE should also be applied in cases of NVE where there is a prolonged clinical course of infection, as well as those patients who do not respond to adequate medical therapy.

The need for TEE in the initial evaluation of patients with NVE, however, is not so clear. In a retrospective analysis of 180 patients referred for echocardiography for suspected infective endocarditis, in whom both TTE and TEE were done, the TTE was reported as technically inadequate in 46 patients (25%). In the remaining 134 patients, there was an almost equal distribution of patients who had a positive TTE (41 patients), a negative TTE (46 patients), and an abnormal but non-diagnostic TTE (47 patients). All patients who had a positive TTE were subsequently found to have a positive TEE, while only two patients with a negative TTE were found to have a positive TEE, yielding a sensitivity of 100% and a specificity of 96%. The principal value of the TEE was in the non-diagnostic group, as well as those with a technically inadequate TTE. In the non-diagnostic group, 9 patients (41%) were found to have positive TEE results for vegetations or abscesses. The study concluded that for initial evaluation of suspected native valve endocarditis, a TTE should be the first echocardiographic study. If the TTE is technically inadequate, then a TEE should be performed. If the TTE is clearly positive, or clearly negative, no additional echocardiographic study should be performed, as there was no incremental diagnostic value with TEE. A TEE, however, should be routinely performed if the TTE is abnormal but non-diagnostic.

Another study analyzed the diagnostic value of echocardiography in suspected infective endocarditis, based on the pretest probability of disease.[42] In this study, both TTE and TEE were performed on 105 consecutive patients with suspected endocarditis. On the basis of clinical criteria and (separately) echocardiography, patients were classified as having either low, intermediate, or high probability of endocarditis. Echocardiography had low diagnostic value in patients with a low clinical probability of endocarditis, using either TTE or TEE. The authors concluded that echocardiography

Conclusions	Grading	Comments/references
Echocardiography should not be used routinely as a screening test to "rule out endocarditis" in patients with fever and murmur	**Grade B**	Not cost effective unless there is other evidence of IE, raising the pretest probability[30,32,42]
For suspected native valve infective endocarditis, TTE should be the initial echocardiographic study	**Grade A**	This is the most cost effective approach[32,42]
If the TTE is technically inadequate in a patient with intermediate or high clinical probability of IE, then TEE should be performed	**Grade A**	Otherwise the diagnosis may be missed[32,42]
If the TTE is abnormal but non-diagnostic in a patient with intermediate or high pretest clinical probability of IE, then TEE should be performed	**Grade B**	TEE is more sensitive[32,42]
If the TTE is negative or abnormal but non-diagnostic in a patient with high pretest clinical probability of IE, then TEE should be performed	**Grade B**	TEE is more sensitive[32,42]
If the TTE is technically adequate and positive, no additional echocardiographic studies are warranted initially – that is, it is not necessary to "confirm" a positive TTE with a TEE study	**Grade B**	Note however that TEE may be performed for other reasons, such as to detect abscesses[32,42]
In patients with suspected prosthetic valve endocarditis, TEE should be performed	**Grade A**	TEE is best for detection of abscesses[30,32,41,42]

should not be used to make a diagnosis of IE in patients with a low clinical probability of disease. In addition, for those patients with an intermediate or high clinical probability of IE, TTE should be the initial echocardiographic procedure, reserving TEE for those patients with prosthetic valves and those with either a technically inadequate TTE, or a TTE which indicates an intermediate probability of endocarditis.[42]

How can the diagnosis of suspected IE be confirmed?

Background

The vegetations of IE are located in an inaccessible site, and can be visualized directly only at surgery or autopsy. Therefore, for purposes of initial diagnosis of IE they must be visualized indirectly, usually by means of echocardiography. Positive findings on echocardiography are a major criterion for diagnosis of IE, but they are not definitive because of possible false positive or false negative results.[43–45] Likewise, blood cultures, which constitute the second major criterion for diagnosis of IE, also can yield false positive or false negative results.

Evidence

In 1981, von Reyn and colleagues[46] published a paper on infective endocarditis in which they proposed a set of diagnostic criteria which designated cases as definite, probable, possible, or rejected. These criteria, however, contained some confusingly worded definitions and did not utilize findings from echocardiography, which had only recently come into general use. In 1994, Durack and colleagues from the Duke Endocarditis Service published improved criteria which introduced the concept of major and minor diagnostic criteria and included echocardiographic findings.[13] (Tables 57.2 and 57.3). Subsequently, multiple studies have analyzed cases diagnosed by the gold standard of pathologic confirmation at surgery or autopsy, comparing both sets of criteria. In each of these studies the Duke criteria were found to be notably more sensitive than the von Reyn criteria.[47–51] In most of these studies, it was felt that the inclusion of echocardiographic data was the primary factor resulting in the increased sensitivity, although even when compared with a modified von Reyn classification with addition of echocardiographic data, there still was an increase in sensitivity. Often increased sensitivity is associated with a concomitant decrease in specificity, but two studies indicate that the Duke criteria have good specificity.[52,53] These criteria

Table 57.2   Criteria for diagnosis of infective endocarditis

Definite infective endocarditis

Pathologic criteria

Micro-organisms: demonstrated by culture or histology in a vegetation, or in a vegetation that has embolized, or in an intracardiac abscess, *or*

Pathologic lesions: vegetation or intracardiac abscess present, confirmed by histology showing active endocarditis

Clinical criteria (use specific definitions listed in Table 57.3)

2 major criteria, *or*

1 major and 3 minor criteria, *or*

5 minor criteria

Possible infective endocarditis

Findings consistent with infective endocarditis that fall short of "Definite," but not "Rejected"

Rejected

Firm alternative diagnosis for manifestations of endocarditis, *or*

Resolution of manifestations of endocarditis, with antibiotic therapy for 4 days or less, *or*

No pathologic evidence of infective endocarditis at surgery or autopsy, after antibiotic therapy for 4 days or less

Adapted from Durack *et al*[13] with permission

Conclusions	Grading	Comments/references
The diagnosis of IE is certain only if confirmed by suitable pathologic specimens and/or cultures obtained at surgery or autopsy	**Grade A**	Echocardiography can yield false positives[13]
A "definite" diagnosis of IE (more than 95% confidence) can be made without surgical or autopsy specimens if defined major and minor criteria (the Duke criteria) are properly applied	**Grade A**	13,47–50
The diagnosis of IE can be rejected with high specificity if defined clinical criteria are properly applied, but this usually requires some delay to allow a period of observation	**Grade A**	52,53
The decision as to whether or not to begin antibiotics should be made on the overall clinical assessment as to the likelihood of IE, not based solely upon the Duke criteria	**Grade B**	Treatment decisions often need to be made before all diagnostic information is available[13,53]

should be useful to specify patient entry criteria for epidemiologic studies and clinical trials involving IE.

Can IE be cured with bacteriostatic antimicrobials?

Background

Antimicrobial agents are traditionally classified as bactericidal or bacteriostatic, according to whether they kill or inhibit growth, respectively. In fact, this classification is an oversimplification because an antimicrobial drug may be partially bactericidal, or may be bacteriostatic for one species of bacteria and bactericidal for another. There is a widely quoted "general rule" that IE should be treated only with bactericidal drugs. The rationale often given to support this "rule" is that colonies of bacteria within a vegetation are protected from host defenses, especially neutrophils, which in other sites would usually eliminate organisms that had been inhibited by bacteriostatic antibiotics.

Table 57.3 Definitions of terminology used in the diagnostic criteria for endocarditis

Major criteria

Positive blood culture for infective endocarditis

Typical micro-organism for infective endocarditis from two separate blood cultures:
   Viridans streptococci,[a] *Streptococcus bovis*, HACEK group, or community
   acquired *Staphylococcus aureus* or enterococci, in the absence of a primary focus, *or*

Persistently positive blood culture, defined as recovery of a micro-organism consistent with
   infective endocarditis from:
   (i) Blood cultures drawn more than 12 hours apart, *or*
   (ii) All of three or a majority of four or more separate blood cultures, with first
        and last drawn at least 1 hour apart

Evidence of endocardial involvement

Positive echocardiogram for infective endocarditis
   (i) Oscillating intracardiac mass, on valve or supporting structures, or in the path
        of regurgitant jet, *or* on implanted material, in the absence of an alternative
        anatomic explanation, *or*
   (ii) Abscess, *or*
   (iii) New partial dehiscence of prosthetic valve, *or*

New valvular regurgitation (increase or change in pre-existing murmur not sufficient)

Minor criteria

● Predisposition: predisposing heart condition *or* injection drug use
● Fever: ≥ 38·0 °C (100·4 °F)
● Vascular phenomena: major arterial emboli, septic pulmonary infarcts, mycotic aneurysm,
  intracranial hemorrhage, conjunctival hemorrhages, Janeway lesions
● Immunologic phenomena: glomerulonephritis, Osler's nodes, Roth spots, rheumatoid
  factor
● Microbiologic evidence: positive blood culture, but not meeting major criterion as
  previously defined[b] *or* serologic evidence of active infection with organism consistent with
  infective endocarditis[c]
● Echocardiogram: consistent with infective endocarditis but not meeting major criterion as
  previously defined

[a] Including nutritional variant strains.
[b] Excluding single positive cultures for coagulase-negative staphylococci or organisms that do not cause endocarditis.
[c] Positive serology for *Coxiella burnetii* or *Bartonella* spp may be used as a major criteria.
HACEK, *Haemophilus* spp, *Actinobacillus actinomycetemcomitans*, *Cardiobacterium hominis*, *Eikenella* spp, and *Kingella kingae*
Source: adapted from Durack *et al*[13]

Evidence

In the early days of antimicrobial therapy before penicillin was available, patients with IE were often treated with prolonged courses of sulfonamides. This nearly always failed. For example, in one study none of 42 patients with streptococcal IE treated with sulfonamides survived.[54] On the other hand, sulfonamide therapy occasionally cured a fortunate patient.[55] Sulfonamides were most likely to succeed in the small subgroup of cases of IE caused by *Haemophilus* spp, which are especially susceptible to sulfonamides. In the special case of IE caused by *Coxiella burnetii* (the organism causing Q fever) bacteriostatic antibiotics such as tetracyclines are generally used for lack of better alternatives. In most cases they suppress but do not cure the endocardial infection; valve replacement surgery is required to increase the likelihood of cure. Similarly, few antibiotics are available to treat IE caused by resistant Gram-negative bacilli such as *Pseudomonas cepacia* or *Stenotrophomonas maltophilia*, in these the combination of a (bacteriostatic) sulfonamide plus trimethoprim has been used with some success.[56]

Should combinations of antimicrobials be used to treat IE?

Background

IE is generally regarded as being difficult and/or slow to cure. Therefore, many attempts have been made to improve cure rates by using optimal antimicrobial regimens, even more so than in most other infections. In the course of this effort, many combinations of antibiotics have been tried,

Conclusions	Grading	Comments/references
Bacteriostatic antibiotics often fail when used to treat IE	**Grade A**	There are animal data and case reports to show this[54,55]
Bacteriostatic antibiotics may be used to treat IE in a few special cases, for example, Q fever, resistant organisms like *Pseudomonas cepacia* or *Stenotrophomonas maltophilia*, or suppressive therapy for organisms not likely to be curable, such as *Pseudomonas* on a prosthetic valve	**Grade B**	Uncontrolled case reports show that cure or useful suppression can be achieved in some patients[56,57]

and a general impression exists that combination therapy is optimal for treatment of IE. This is only partly true.

Evidence

There is excellent documentation that enterococcal endocarditis usually is best treated with a combination of two antibiotics. The primary reason for this is that most strains of *Enterococcus faecalis* are relatively resistant to antibiotics, but are killed synergistically by a combination of a penicillin and an aminoglycoside.[58] This does not hold true, however, if the strain shows high level resistance to aminoglycosides (defined as resistance to 2000 micrograms/ml of streptomycin or 500 micrograms/ml of gentamicin). In the latter case, vancomycin should be substituted,[59] except for strains that are vancomycin resistant.[60] Ample documentation for the value of combination therapy has been published, based upon *in vitro* studies, and *in vivo* treatment of both animals and humans. Unfortunately, the frequency of high level resistance among enterococci has greatly increased over the past 15 years, making the choice of optimal therapy more difficult.[65]

Even when streptococci are fully sensitive to penicillin, combinations of a penicillin and an aminoglycoside or vancomycin act synergistically against them, so long as the strain is not vancomycin resistant (VRE) or has high level resistance to aminoglycosides.[61] This has been convincingly demonstrated both *in vitro* and in experimental animals.[62,63] The human correlate is found in the fact that combination therapy cures more than 97% of cases caused by penicillin-sensitive viridans streptococci within 2 weeks, whereas penicillin alone cures only 80–85% in the same interval, and requires 4 weeks to reach 97% cure or better. This fact has been well proven.[54,64]

What is the optimal duration of treatment for IE?

Background

Early experience established that endocarditis could not be cured by short courses of antibiotics (7–10 days) that would

have been adequate to cure other common infections such as pneumonia or gonorrhea. Trials of longer duration were more successful, eventually leading to the widely followed practice of treating IE for 6 weeks. This remains common practice today, despite the fact that more than half of all cases of IE could be reliably cured by 2–4 weeks of treatment.

Evidence

Before 1950 it was reported that IE could not be cured with 10 days of treatment, even when the organisms were highly susceptible to penicillin and/or high doses were given.[56,74,75] Subsequently, high cure rates were achieved by extending treatment to 4–6 weeks. For many years, 6 weeks of therapy was regarded as the standard duration for treatment of IE. In fact, this "rule" often led to overtreatment because 4 weeks would have been adequate for the majority of these cases.[55] Because of number preferencing for even numbers, 3 and 5 week regimens have not been studied, even though intuitively it seems likely that these durations would work as well as 4 and 6 week regimens, respectively.

Some cases of endocarditis can be cured with treatment for only 2 weeks. This is well supported by clinical experience for two important groups of patients: uncomplicated penicillin sensitive streptococcal native valve endocarditis,[55,76] and intravenous drug addicts with right-sided *S. aureus* endocarditis.[70]

It should be noted that outpatient parenteral antibiotic therapy (OPAT) is appropriate for selected patients with IE.[76–79] In most cases, these will be patients without serious complications who have responded promptly to standard therapy begun in hospital. When OPAT is employed for treatment of IE, the total duration of therapy should normally be the same as if the patient had been hospitalized throughout the course of treatment.

The **B** ratings listed in the conclusions below could be improved by publication of larger numbers of cases or by randomized controlled studies.

Conclusions	Grading	Comments/references
Combination therapy should be used for IE caused by enterococci	**Grade A**	60, 66
A combination of at least two antibiotics (a β lactam plus an aminoglycoside) should be used for IE caused by coagulase-negative staphylococci	**Grade A**	67, 68
A combination of three antibiotics (a β lactam plus an aminoglycoside plus rifampin) should be used for IE caused by coagulase-negative staphylococci	**Grade C**	Limited number of patients reported; no comparative trials[67,68]
An aminoglycoside should be added to a β lactam for the first few days of therapy for IE caused by *S. aureus*	**Grade C**	A definitive outcome study has not been done[68,69]
Combination therapy should be used for right-sided IE caused by *S. aureus* if a short course (2 week) regimen is used	**Grade B**	Only one major study available[70,71,72]
Addition of an aminoglycoside for IE caused by penicillin sensitive streptococci is beneficial and cost effective if a short course (2 week) regimen is used	**Grade A**	73
Addition of an aminoglycoside for IE caused by penicillin sensitive streptococci is beneficial and cost effective if a standard (4 week) regimen is used	**Grade C**	No modern cost effectiveness study has been done[73]

Conclusions	Grading	Comments/references
Penicillin sensitive IE can be cured in 2 weeks by combined penicillin plus aminoglycoside, or in 4 weeks by penicillin alone	**Grade A**	73, 80
Enterococcal endocarditis should be treated for at least 4 weeks	**Grade B**	59, 73, 81, 82
Most cases of HACEK endocarditis can be cured in 3–4 weeks (*Haemophilus, Actinobacilllus, Cardiobacterium, Eikenella, Kingella* spp)	**Grade B**	Total number of reported cases is small[73,83,84]
Most cases of tricuspid valve *S. aureus* IE in intravenous drug users can be cured in 2 weeks	**Grade B**	Only one major study done[70]
Results of treatment for IE in HIV infected patients with >200 CD4 lymphocytes/mm^3 are similar to results in non-HIV patients	**Grade B**	72
HIV infected patients with <200 CD4 lymphocytes and IE have a worse prognosis, and therefore should not receive short-course (2 week) antibiotic therapy for IE	**Grade C**	This has not been formally studied[72]
Most cases of left-sided native valve *S. aureus* IE can be cured in 4 weeks	**Grade B**	Controlled study not done[73]

What are the main indications for surgical intervention during management of IE?

Background

The introduction of valve replacement, valve repair, and other surgical procedures has revolutionized the management of IE, being second in importance only to the advent of antibiotic therapy for IE. Many studies have indicated that surgical intervention improves the prognosis of IE over medical therapy alone.[85–87] The benefits of early rather than late surgical intervention have been appropriately emphasized.[86–88] However, surgical placement of artificial cardiac valves is associated with high costs, significant morbidity, especially in the form of late complications, and some mortality. Furthermore, about two thirds of all patients with IE can be cured without any surgical intervention. Therefore, correct selection of the subgroup of about one third of patients who will benefit from surgery becomes of critical importance.

Evidence

Many hundreds of publications have reported on experience with surgery for IE, beginning in 1965[89] and continuing unabated today. The cumulative experience is based upon thousands of patients. However, this extensive experience does not include randomized studies of medical versus surgical therapy, primarily because selection bias (that is, choosing more seriously ill patients for surgery) is virtually impossible to overcome. Therefore, the conclusions which have emerged, although often well supported by case studies, can only be rated **B** in terms of evidence-based analyses.

What is the correct timing for valve replacement during management of IE?

Background

In the past, it was often stated on empirical grounds that valve replacement surgery should be postponed until the patient had been cured by antibiotics. If the patient could not survive until cure, it was believed that surgery should be delayed as long as possible to allow suppression of the number of remaining bacteria to the lowest possible level to reduce the risk of relapse or infection of the new prosthetic valve. The available evidence does not support these widely held views.

Evidence

Actual experience showed that the frequency of relapse and/or infection of the prosthesis after surgery for IE is low,

Conclusions I: Strong indications for surgical intervention during IE	Grading	Comments/references
Heart failure unresponsive to medical therapy	Grade B	7, 8, 87, 90
Presence of a valve ring abscess	Grade B	7, 8, 90, 91, 92
Early prosthetic valve infection (onset within 60 days of surgery)	Grade B	7, 8, 90, 93
Prosthetic valve infection caused by *S. aureus*	Grade B	7, 8, 68, 71, 92, 93
Prosthetic valve infection caused by Gram-negative bacilli (not HACEK group)	Grade B	7, 8, 93
Endocarditis caused by filamentous fungi (not yeasts)	Grade B	94, 95
Prosthetic valve infection caused by yeasts	Grade B	93, 96
Development of a sinus of Valsalva aneurysm	Grade B	97
Occlusion of valves by very large vegetations	Grade B	7, 8, 98

Conclusions II: Relative (less strong) indications for surgical intervention during IE	Grading	Comments/references
Recurrent arterial emboli	Grade C	7, 8, 99, 100
Native left-sided valve infection caused by *S. aureus*	Grade C	7, 8, 68, 71
Apparent failure of medical therapy (persistent bacteremia, persistent fever, increase in size of vegetation during treatment)	Grade C	7, 8, 90
Native valve infection caused by Gram-negative bacilli (not HACEK)	Grade C	7, 8
Large-sized left-sided vegetations by echo (greater than 15–20 mm)	Grade C	7, 8
Native valve infection caused by yeasts	Grade C	95, 96, 101–103
Late onset prosthetic valve infection	Grade C	7, 8, 93
Development of cardiac conduction abnormality during IE, but no abscess identified by TEE	Grade C	7, 8, 91

whether or not antibiotics had been given for long periods before operation. For patients with a good indication for valve replacement early in the course of active endocarditis, many authors have strongly advocated early surgery, before antibiotics have cured the patient, to avoid deaths and complications that might occur during antibiotic treatment.[85–88]

Can IE be prevented?

Background

IE sometimes develops as a complication of bacteremias associated with medical and dental procedures, such as urinary catheterizations or tooth extractions. Although these cases represent only a small proportion – about 5% – of all cases of IE, much effort has been made to prevent them because IE carries high associated morbidity and mortality. Soon after antibiotics became available, various attempts were made to prevent bacteremias and/or IE by giving antibiotics before dental extractions or other procedures.[104–108] Subsequently, the American Heart Association[109] and many other groups[110–112] have issued recommendations for prevention of IE by this means.

Evidence

The evidence that bacteremias induced by medical and dental procedures can cause IE in patients with predisposing heart lesions consists of many uncontrolled case reports. There are sufficient numbers of these to support the conclusion that there is a real risk after tooth extractions and procedures involving an infected genitourinary tract.[113–115] The evidence that lower-risk procedures such as gastrointestinal endoscopy, procedures on the uninfected urinary tract, and biopsies and other minor surgical procedures cause a significant number of cases of IE is sketchy.[108,116–114]

Prophylaxis of IE has been proven unequivocally to be effective in experimental animal models of endocarditis by giving antibiotics before injecting bacteria intravenously.[125–132] However, there has been no definitive study to demonstrate efficacy of antibiotic prophylaxis for infective endocarditis in humans.[116] One review of patients with prosthetic heart valves indicated that antibiotic prophylaxis before dental and urogenital procedures was effective,[133] but this study was retrospective, unrandomized, and unblinded. Analysis of prospectively collected cases in the Netherlands indicated that prophylaxis was either ineffective or, at best, only

Conclusions	Grading	Comments/references
If there is no indication for early surgery, complete a standard course of antibiotic treatment before valve replacement.	Grade B	No randomized studies available[90]
If there is an adequate indication for early surgery, proceed to valve replacement without regard to the duration of antibiotic treatment already given. Delay can result in avoidable complications or death.	Grade A	Many uncontrolled reports support early surgery[85–88,90]

Conclusions	Grading	Comments/references
Bacteremias following tooth extraction or surgical procedures involving an infected genitourinary tract can cause endocarditis	Grade B	137
Bacteremias following gastrointestinal endoscopy or surgical procedures involving an uninfected genitourinary tract can cause endocarditis	Grade C	124, 137, 138
Prevention of IE by giving antibiotics before medical and dental procedures that cause bacteremia is an empiric practice which has been proven effective in animal models but not in humans	Grade A	116, 129
Attempted prevention of IE in selected high-risk groups undergoing high-risk procedures such as tooth extraction is probably effective	Grade C	133
Attempted prevention of IE in selected high-risk groups undergoing high-risk procedures such as tooth extraction is recommended	Grade B	110–112
Extensive practice of attempted prophylaxis for IE is probably not cost effective	Grade B	139, 140

marginally effective.[134] Other analyses have indicated that even if prophylaxis is effective, it would probably not be cost effective as a general strategy.[135,136] Despite all this uncertainty, most authorities continue to recommend selective use of prophylaxis for patients with higher risk cardiac lesions undergoing higher risk procedures.[109,116]

References

1. Durack DT, Beeson PB. Experimental bacterial endocarditis. I. Colonization of a sterile vegetation. *Br J Exp Pathol* 1972;**53**:44–9.

2. Angrist A, Oka M, Nakao K. Vegetative endocarditis. *Pathol Ann* 1967;**2**:155–212.

3. Blanchard DG, Ross RS, Dittrich HC. Nonbacterial thrombotic endocarditis. *Chest* 1993;**102**:954–6.

4. Rodbard S, Yamamoto C. Effect of stream velocity on bacterial deposition and growth. *Cardiovasc Res* 1969;**3**:68–74.

5. Grant RT, Wood JE, Jr, Jones TD. Heart valve irregularities in relation to subacute bacterial endocarditis. *Am Heart J* 1928;**14**:247–61.

6. Moreillon P, Que YA, Bayer AS. Pathogenesis of streptococcal and staphylococcal endocarditis. *Infect Dis Clin North Am* 2002;**16**:297–318.

7. Durack DT. Infective and noninfective endocarditis. In: Hurst JW, ed. *The heart, arteries and veins*, 7th edn. New York: McGraw-Hill, 1990.

8. Scheld WM, Sande MA. Endocarditis and intravascular infections. In: Mandell GL, Douglas RG, Jr, Dolin R, eds. *Principles and practice of infectious diseases*, 4th edn. New York: Churchill Livingstone, 1995.

9. Cabell CH, Abruytn E. Progress toward a global understanding of infective endocarditis: early lessons from the International Collaboration on Endocarditis investigation. *Infect Dis Clin North Am* 2002;**16**:255–72.

10. Houpikian P, Raoult D. Diagnostic methods: current best practices and guidelines for identification of difficult-to-culture pathogens in endocarditis. *Infect Dis Clin North Am* 2002;**16**:377–92.

11. Schwartzman WA, Marchevsky A, Meyer RD. Epithelioid angiomatosis or cat scratch disease with splenic and hepatic abnormalities in AIDS: case report and review of the literature. *Scand J Infect Dis* 1990;**22**:121–33.

12. Towns ML, Reller LB. Diagnostic methods: current best practices and guidelines for isolation of bacteria and fungi. *Infect Dis Clin North Am* 2002;**16**:363–76.

13. Durack DT, Bright DK, Lukes AS, Duke Endocarditis Service. New criteria for diagnosis of infective endocarditis: utilization of specific echocardiographic findings. *Am J Med* 1994;**96**:200–9.

14. Washington JA, II. The role of the microbiology laboratory in the diagnosis and antimicrobial treatment of infective endocarditis. *Mayo Clin Proc* 1982;**57**:22–32.

15. Washington JA. The microbiological diagnosis of infective endocarditis. *J Antimicrob Chemother* 1987;**20**:29–39.

16. Maki DG, Agger WA. Enterococcal bacteremia: clinical features, the risk of endocarditis, and management. *Medicine* 1988;**67**:248–69.

17. Gullberg RM, Homann SR, Phair JP. Enterococcal bacteremia: analysis of 75 episodes. *Rev Infect Dis* 1989;**11**:74–85.

18. Beeson PB, Brannon ES, Warren JV. Observations of the sites of removal of bacteria from the blood in patients with bacterial endocarditis. *J Exp Med* 1945;**81**:9–23.

19. Weinstein M, Reller L, Murphy J, Lichtenstein K. Clinical significance of positive blood cultures: a comprehensive analysis of 500 episodes of bacteremia and fungemia in adults. I. Laboratory and epidemiologic observations. *Rev Infect Dis* 1983;**5**:35–53.

20. Towns M, Quartey S, Weinstein M *et al.* Clinical significance of positive blood cultures: a prospective, multicenter investigation. ASM 1993; Abstract No. C232: Abstract.

21. Weinstein M, Murphy J, Reller L, Lichtenstein K. Clinical significance of positive blood cultures: A comprehensive analysis of 500 episodes of bacteremia and fungemia in adults. II. Clinical observations, with special reference to factors influencing prognosis. *Rev Infect Dis* 1983;**5**:54–70.

22. Belli J, Waisbren BA. The number of blood cultures necessary to diagnose most cases of bacterial endocarditis. *Am J Med Sci* 1956;**232**:284–8.

23. Mallen MS, Hube EL, Brenes M. Comparative study of blood cultures made from artery, vein, and bone marrow in patients with subacute bacterial endocarditis. *Am Heart J* 1946;**XX**:692–5.

24. Geraci JE, Wilson WR. Endocarditis due to gram-negative bacteria: report of 56 cases. *Mayo Clin Proc* 1982;**57**:145–8.

25. Chen YC, Chang SC, Luh KT, Hsieh WC. *Actinobacillus actinomycetemcomitans* endocarditis: a report of four cases and review of the literature. *QJM* 1992;**81**:871–8.

26. Drancourt M, Birtles R, Chaumentin G, Vandenesch F, Etienne J, Raoult D. New serotype of *Bartonella henselae* in endocarditis and cat-scratch disease. *Lancet* 1996;**347**:441–3.

27. Doern GV, Davaro R, George M, Campognone P. Lack of requirement for prolonged incubation of Septi-Chek blood culture bottles in patients with bacteremia due to fastidious bacteria. *Diagn Microbiol Infect Dis* 1996;**24**:141–3.

28. Murray M, Moosnick F. Arterial vs venous blood cultures. *J Lab Clin Med* 1940;**26**:382–7.

29. Gilbert BW, Haney RS, Crawford F *et al.* Two-dimensional echocardiographic assessment of vegetative endocarditis. *Circulation* 1977;**55**:346–53.

30. Sachdev M, Peterson G, Jollis JG. Diagnostic methods: imaging techniques for diagnosis of endocarditis. *Infect Dis Clin North Am* 2002;**16**:319–38.

31. Stewart JA, Silimperi D, Harris P, Wise NK, Fraker TD, Jr, Kisslo JA. Echocardiographic documentation of vegetative lesions in infective endocarditis: clinical implications. *Circulation* 1980;**61**:374–80.

32. Irani WN, Grayburn PA, Afridi I. A negative transthoracic echocardiogram obviates the need for transesophageal echocardiography in patients with suspected native valve active infective endocarditis. *Am J Cardiol* 1996;**78**:101–3.

33. Jaffe WM, Morgan DE, Pearlman AS, Otto CM. Infective endocarditis, 1983–1988: echocardiographic findings and factors influencing morbidity and mortality. *J Am Coll Cardiol* 1990;**15**:1227–33.

34. Martin RP. The diagnostic and prognostic role of cardiovascular ultrasound in endocarditis: bigger is not better. *J Am Coll Cardiol* 1990;**15**:1234–7.

35. Taams MA, Gussenhoven EJ, Bos E *et al.* Enhanced morphological diagnosis in infective endocarditis by transesophageal echocardiography. *Br Heart J* 1990;**63**:109–13.

36. Rohmann S, Erbel R, Gorge G *et al.* Clinical relevance of vegetation localization by transoesophageal echocardiography in infective endocarditis. *Eur Heart J* 1992;**12**:446–52.

37. Shapiro SM, Bayer AS. Transesophageal and Doppler echocardiography in the diagnosis and management of infective endocarditis. *Chest* 1991;**100**:1125–30.

38. Pedersen WR, Walker M, Olson JD *et al.* Value of transesophageal echocardiography as an adjunct to transthoracic echocardiography in evaluation of native and prosthetic valve endocarditis. *Chest* 1991;**100**:351–6.

39. Morguet AJ, Werner GS, Andreas S, Kreuzer H. Diagnostic value of transesophageal compared with transthoracic echocardiography in suspected prosthetic valve endocarditis. *Herz* 1995;**20**:390–8.

40. Anders K, Foley K, Stern WE, Brown WJ. Intracranial sparganosis: an uncommon infection. Case report. *J Neurosurg* 1984;**60**:1282–6.

41. Daniel WG, Mugge A, Martin RP *et al.* Improvement in the diagnosis of abscesses associated with endocarditis by transesophageal echocardiography. *N Engl J Med* 1991;**324**: 795–800.

42. Lindner JR, Case RA, Dent JM *et al.* Diagnostic value of echocardiography in suspected endocarditis. An evaluation based on the pretest probability of disease. *Circulation* 1996;**93**:730–6.

43. Hickey AJ, Wolfers J. False positive diagnosis of vegetations on a myxomatous mitral valve using two-dimensional echocardiography. *Aust NZ J Med* 1982;**12**:540–2.

44. Mintz GS, Kotler MN. Clinical value and limitations of echocardiography. Its use in the study of patients with infectious endocarditis. *Arch Intern Med* 1980;**140**:1022–7.

45. Sokil AB. Cardiac imaging in infective endocarditis. In: Kaye D, ed. *Infective endocarditis. 2nd edn.* New York: Raven Press, 1992.

46. von Reyn CF, Levy BS, Arbeit RD, Friedland G, Crumpacker CS. Infective endocarditis: an analysis based on strict case definitions. *Ann Intern Med* 1981;**94**:505–17.

47. Bayer AS, Ward JI, Ginzton LE, Shapiro SM. Evaluation of new clinical criteria for the diagnosis of infective endocarditis. *Am J Med* 1994;**96**:211–19.

48. Del Pont JM, De Cicco LT, Vartalitis C *et al.* Infective endocarditis in children: clinical analyses and evaluation of two diagnostic criteria. *Pediatr Infect Dis* 1995;**14**:1079–86.

49. Fournier PE, Casalta JP, Habib G, Messana T, Raoult D. Modification of the diagnostic criteria proposed by the Duke Endocarditis Service to permit improved diagnosis of Q fever endocarditis. *Am J Med* 1996;**100**:629–33.

50. Cecchi E, Parrini I, Chinaglia A *et al.* New diagnostic criteria for infective endocarditis. A study of sensitivity and specificity. *Eur Heart J* 1997;**18**:1149–56.

51. Olaison L, Hogevik H. Comparison of the von Reyn and Duke criteria for the diagnosis of infective endocarditis: a critical analysis of 161 episodes. *Scand J Infect Dis* 1996;**28**: 399–406.

52. Hoen B, Beguinot I, Rabaud C *et al.* The Duke criteria for diagnosing infective endocarditis are specific: analysis of 100 patients with acute fever or fever of unknown origin. *Clin Infect Dis* 1996;**23**:298–302.

53. Dodds GA, Sexton DJ, Durack DT, Bashore TM, Corey GR, Kisslo J. Negative predictive value of the Duke criteria for infective endocarditis. *Am J Cardiol* 1996;**77**:403–7.

54. Galbreath WR, Hull E. Sulfonamide therapy of bacterial endocarditis: results in 42 cases. *Ann Intern Med* 1943;**18**:201–3.

55. Durack DT. Review of early experience in treatment of bacterial endocarditis, 1940–1955. In: Bisno AL, ed. Treatment of infective endocarditis. New York: Grune & Stratton, 1981.

56. Speller DCE. *Pseudomonas cepacia* endocarditis treated with co-trimazole and kanamycin. *Br Heart J* 1972;**35**:47–8.

57. Street AC, Durack DT. Experience with trimethoprim-sulfamethoxazole in treatment of infective endocarditis. *Rev Infect Dis* 1988;**10**:915–21.

58. Wilson WR, Wilkowske CJ, Wright AJ, Sande MA, Geraci JE. Treatment of streptomycin-susceptible and streptomycin-resistant enterococcal endocarditis. *Ann Intern Med* 1984; **100**:816–23.

59. Watanakunakorn C, Bakie C. Synergism of vancomycin–gentamicin and vancomycin–streptomycin against enterococci. *Antimicrob Agents Chemother* 1973;**4**:120–4.

60. Caron F, Lemeland JF, Humbert G, Klare I, Gutmann L. Triple combination penicillin–vancomycin–gentamicin for experimental endocarditis caused by a highly penicillin- and glycopeptide-resistant isolate of *Enterococcus faecium. J Infect Dis* 1993;**168**:681–6.

61. Watanakunakorn C, Glotzbecker C. Synergism with aminoglycosides of penicillin, ampicillin and vancomycin against non-enterococcal group-D streptococci and viridans streptococci. *J Med Microbiol* 1976;**10**:133–8.

62. Sande MA, Irvin RG. Penicillin-aminoglycoside synergy in experimental *Streptococcus viridans* endocarditis. *J Infect Dis* 1974;**129**:572–6.

63. Fantin B, Carbon C. *In vivo* antibiotic synergism: contribution of animal models. *Antimicrob Agents Chemother* 1992;**36**: 907–12.

64. Geraci JE. The antibiotic therapy of infective endocarditis: therapeutic data on 172 patient seen from 1951 through 1957: additional observations on short-term therapy (two weeks) for penicillin-sensitive streptococcal endocarditis. *Med Clin North Am* 1958;**42**:1101–48.

65. Hoen B. Special issues in the management of infective endocarditis caused by gram-positive cocci. *Infect Dis Clin N Am* 2002;**16**:437–52.

66. Rice LB, Calderwood SB, Eliopoulos GM, Farber BF, Karchmer AW. Enterococcal endocarditis: a comparison of prosthetic and native valve disease. *Rev Infect Dis* 1991; **13**:1–7.

67. Karchmer AW, Archer GL, Dismukes WE. *Staphylococcus epidermidis* causing prosthetic valve endocarditis: microbiologic and clinical observations as guides to therapy. *Ann Intern Med* 1983;**98**:447–55.

68. Karchmer AW. Staphylococcal endocarditis. In: Kaye D, ed. *Infective endocarditis, 2nd edn.* New York: Raven Press, 1992.

69. Sande MA, Courtney KB. Nafcillin-gentamicin synergism in experimental staphylococcal endocarditis. *J Lab Clin Med* 1976;**88**:118–24.

70. Chambers HF, Miller RT, Newman MD. Right-sided *Staphylococcus aureus* endocarditis in intravenous drug abusers: two-week combination therapy. *Ann Intern Med* 1988;**109**:619–24.

71. Petti CA, Fowler VG. *Staphylococcus aureus* bacteremia and endocarditis. *Infect Dis Clin North Am* 2002;**16**: 419–36.

72. Miro JM, del Rio A, Mestres CA. Infective endocarditis in intravenous drug abusers and HIV-1 infected patients. *Infect Dis Clin North Am* 2002;**16**:273–96.

73. Wilson WR, Karchmer A, Dajani A *et al.* Antibiotic treatment of adults with infective endocarditis due to viridans streptococci, enterococci, staphylococci and HACEK microorganisms. *JAMA* 1995;**274**:1706–13.

74. King FH, Schneierson SS, Sussman ML, Janowitz HD, Stollerman GH. Prolonged moderate dose therapy versus intensive short term therapy with penicillin and caronamide in subacute bacterial endocarditis. *J Mt Sinai Hosp* 1949; **16**:35–46.

75. Bloomfield AL, Armstrong CD, Kirby WMM. The treatment of subacute bacterial endocarditis with penicillin. *J Clin Invest* 1945;**24**:251–67.

76. Kwon-Chung KJ, Hill WB. Studies on the pink, adenine-deficient strains of *Candida albicans*. I. Cultural and morphological characteristics. *Sabouraudia* 1970;**8**:48–59.

77. Francioli P, Etienne J, Hoigne R, Thys J, Gerber A. Treatment of streptococcal endocarditis with a single daily dose of ceftriaxone sodium for 4 weeks. Efficacy and outpatient treatment feasibility. *JAMA* 1992;**267**:264–7.

78. Francioli P, Ruch W, Stamboulian D, International Infective Endocarditis Study Group. Treatment of streptococcal endocarditis with a single daily dose of ceftriaxone and netilmicin for 14 days: a prospective multicenter study. *Clin Infect Dis* 1995;**21**:1406–10.

79. Stamboulian D, Bonvehi P, Arevalo C *et al.* Antibiotic management of outpatients with endocarditis due to penicillin-susceptible streptococci. *Rev Infect Dis* 1991;**13**:S160–S3.

80. Wilson WR, Geraci JE, Wilkowske CJ, Washington JA. Short-term intramuscular therapy with procaine penicillin plus streptomycin for infective endocarditis due to viridans streptococci. *Circulation* 1978;**57**:1158–61.

81. Geraci JE, Martin WJ. Antibiotic therapy of bacterial endocarditis. VI. Subacute enterococcal endocarditis: clinical, pathologic and therapeutic consideration of 33 cases. *Circulation* 1954;**10**:173–94.

82. Moellering RC, Jr, Wennersten C, Weinstein AJ. Penicillin–tobramycin synergism against enterococci: a comparison with penicillin and gentamicin. *Antimicrob Agents Chemother* 1973;**3**:526–9.

83. Shorrock PJ, Lambert PA, Aitchison EJ, Smith EG, Farrell ID, Gutschik E. Serological response in *Enterococcus faecalis* endocarditis determined by enzyme-linked immunosorbent assay. *J Clin Microbiol* 1990;**28**:195–200.

84. Bieger RC, Brewer NS, Washington JA, II. *Haemophilus aphrophilus*: a microbiologic and clinical review and report of 42 cases. *Medicine* 1978;**57**:345–55.

85. Bogers AJJC, van Vreeswijk H, Verbaan CJ *et al.* Early surgery for active infective endocarditis improves early and late results. *Thorac Cardiovasc Surg* 1991;**39**:284–7.

86. Aranki SF, Adams DH, Rizzo RJ *et al.* Determinants of early mortality and late survival in mitral valve endocarditis. *Circulation* 1995;**92**:143–9.

87. Middlemost S, Wisenbaugh T, Meyerowitz C *et al.* A case for early surgery in native left-sided endocarditis complicated by heart failure: results in 203 patients. *J Am Coll Cardiol* 1991;**18**:663–7.

88. Jubair KA, Al Fagih MR, Ashmeg A, Belhaj M, Sawyer W. Cardiac operations during active endocarditis. *J Thorac Cardiovasc Surg* 1992;**104**:487–90.

89. Wallace AG, Young G, Jr, Osterhout S. Treatment of acute bacterial endocarditis by valve excision and replacement. *Circulation* 1965;**31**:450–3.

90. Olaison L, Pettersson G. Current best practices and guidelines: indications for surgical intervention in infective endocarditis. *Infect Dis Clin North Am* 2002;**16**:453–76.

91. DiNubile MJ, Calderwood SB, Steinhaus DM, Karchmer AW. Cardiac conduction abnormalities complicating native valve active endocarditis. *Am J Cardiol* 1986;**58**:1213–17.

92. Tucker KJ, Johnson JA, Ong T, Mullen WL, Mailhot J. Medical management of prosthetic aortic valve endocarditis and aortic root abscess. *Am Heart J* 1993;**125**:1195–7.

93. Karchmer AW, Longworth DL. Infections of intracardiac devices. *Infect Dis Clin North Am* 2002;**16**:477–506.

94. Woods GL, Wood P, Shaw BW, Jr. *Aspergillus* endocarditis in patients without prior cardiovascular surgery: report of a case in a liver transplant recipient and review. *Rev Infect Dis* 1989;**II**:263–72.

95. Fowler VG, Durack DT. Infective endocarditis. *Curr Opin Cardiol* 1994;**9**:389–400.

96. Guzman F, Cartmill I, Holden MP, Freeman R. Candida endocarditis: report of four cases. *Int J Cardiol* 1987;**16**: 131–6.

97. Scully RE, Mark EJ, McNeely WF, McNeely BU. Case records of the Massachussetts General Hospital. *N Engl J Med* 1996;**334**:105–11.

98. Khan SS, Gray RJ. Valvular emergencies. *Cardiol Clin* 1991; **9**:689–709.

99. Steckelberg JM, Murphy JG, Ballard D *et al.* Emboli in infective endocarditis: the prognostic value of echocardiography. *Ann Intern Med* 1991;**114**:635–40.

100. Sexton DJ, Spelman D. Current best practices and guidelines: assessment and management of complications of infective endocarditis. *Infect Dis Clin North Am* 2002;**16**:507–22.

101. Kawamoto T, Nakano S, Matsuda H, Hirose H, Kawashima Y. Candida endocarditis with saddle embolism: a successful surgical intervention (abstract). *Ann Thorac Surg* 1989; **48**:723–4.

102. Tanka M, Toshio A, Hosokawa S, Suenaga Y, Hikosaka H. Tricuspid valve *Candida* endocarditis cured by valve-sparing debridement. *Ann Thorac Surg* 1989;**48**:857–8.

103. Isalska BJ, Stanbridge TN. Fluconazole in the treatment of candidal prosthetic valve endocarditis. *BMJ* 1988;**297**:178–9.

104. Rhoads PS, Schram WR, Adair D. Bacteremia following tooth extraction: prevention with penicillin and N U 445. *J Am Dent Assoc* 1950;**41**:55–61.

105. Pressman RS, Bender IB. Antibiotic treatment of the gingival sulcus in the prevention of bacteremia. *Antibiotics Annual* 1954;92–104.

106. Northrop PM, Crowley MC. Further studies on the effect of the prophylactic use of sulfathiazole and sulfamerazine on bacteremia following extraction of teeth. *J Oral Surg* 1944;**2**:134.

107. Budnitz E, Nizel A, Berg L. Prophylactic use of sulfapyridine in patients susceptible to subacute bacterial endocarditis following dental surgical procedures. *J Am Dent Assoc* 1942;**29**:346.

108. Camara DS, Gruber M, Barde CJ, Montes M, Caruana JA, Jr, Chung RS. Transient bacteremia following endoscopic injection sclerotherapy of esophageal varices. *Arch Intern Med* 1983;**143**:1350–2.

109. Dajani AS, Taubert KA, Wilson WR *et al.* Prevention of bacterial endocarditis. Recommendations by the American Heart Association. *Circulation* 1997;**96**:358–66.

110. Delaye J, Etienne J, Feruglio A *et al.* Prophylaxis of infective endocarditis for dental procedures. Report of a working party of the European Society of Cardiology. *Eur Heart J* 1985;**6**:826–8.

111. Michel MF, Thompson J, Boering G, Hess J, Van Putten PL. Revision of the guidelines of the Netherlands Heart Foundation for the prevention of endocarditis. *Geneesmiddelen-bull* 1986;**20**:53–6.

112. Shanson DC. Antibiotic prophylaxis of infective endocarditis in the United Kingdom and Europe. *J Antimicrob Chemother* 1987;**20**:119–31.

113. Meneely JK. Bacterial endocarditis following urethral manipulation. *N Engl J Med* 1948;**239**:708–9.

114. Slade N. Bacteriaemia and septicaemia after urological operations. *Proc R Soc Med* 1958;**51**:331–4.

115. Sullivan NM, Sutter VL, Mims MM, Marsh VH, Finegold SM. Clinical aspects of bacteremia after manipulation of the genitourinary tract. *J Infect Dis* 1973;**127**:49–55.

116. Durack D. Prevention of infective endocarditis. *N Engl J Med* 1995;**332**:38–44.

117. Shorvon PJ, Eykyn SJ, Cotton PB. Gastrointestinal instrumentation, bacteraemia, and endocarditis. *Gut* 1983;**24**:1078–93.

118. Edson RS, Van Scoy RE, Leary FJ. Gram-negative bacteremia after transrectal needle biopsy of the prostate. *Mayo Clin Proc* 1980;**55**:489–91.

119. Livengood CH, III, Land MR, Addison WA. Endometrial biopsy, bacteremia, and endocarditis risk. *Obstet Gynecol* 1985;**65**:678–81.

120. Mellow MH, Lewis RJ. Endoscopy-related bacteremia. Incidence of positive blood cultures after endoscopy of upper gastrointestinal tract. *Arch Intern Med* 1976;**136**:667–9.

121. Yin TP, Dellipiani AW. Bacterial endocarditis after Hurst bougienage in a patient with a benign oesophageal stricture. *Endoscopy* 1983;**15**:27–8.

122. Giglio JA, Rowland RW, Dalton HP, Laskin DM. Suture removal-induced bacteremia: a possible endocarditis risk. *J Am Dent Assoc* 1992;**123**:65–70.

123. Ho H, Zuckerman MJ, Wassem C. A prospective controlled study of the risk of bacteremia in emergency sclerotherapy of esophageal varices. *Gastroenterology* 1991;**101**:1642–8.

124. Low DE, Shoenut JP, Kennedy JK *et al.* Prospective assessment of risk of bacteremia with colonoscopy and polypectomy. *Dig Dis Sci* 1987;**32**:1239–43.

125. Glauser MP, Bernard JP, Morceillon P, Francioli P. Successful single-dose amoxicillin prophylaxis against experimental streptococcal endocarditis: evidence for two mechanisms of protection. *J Infect Dis* 1983;**147**:568–75.

126. Bernard J, Francioli P, Glauser MP. Vancomycin prophylaxis of experimental *Streptococcus sanguis*; inhibition of bacterial adherence rather than bacterial killing. *J Clin Invest* 1981;**68**:1113–16.

127. Moreillon P, Francioli P, Overholser P, Meylan P, Glauser MP. Mechanisms of successful amoxicillin prophylaxis of experimental endocarditis due to *Streptococcus intermedius*. *J Infect Dis* 1986;**154**:801–7.

128. Malinverni R, Overholser CD, Bille J, Glauser MP. Antibiotic prophylaxis of experimental endocarditis after dental extractions. *Lab Invest* 1988;**77**:182–7.

129. Glauser MP, Francioli P. Relevance of animal models to the prophylaxis of infective endocarditis. *J Antimicrob Chemother* 1987;**20**(Suppl. A):87–93.

130. Durack DT, Petersdorf RG, Beeson PB. Penicillin prophylaxis of experimental *S. viridans* endocarditis. *Trans Assoc Am Phys* 1972;**85**:222–30.

131. Durack DT, Petersdorf RG. Chemotherapy of experimental streptococcal endocarditis. I. Comparison of commonly prophylactic regimens. *J Clin Invest* 1973;**52**:592–8.

132. Pelletier LL, Durack DT, Petersdorf RG. Chemotherapy of experimental streptococcal endocarditis. IV. Further observations on antimicrobial prophylaxis. *J Clin Invest* 1975;**56**:319–30.

133. Horstkotte D, Friedrichs W, Pippert H, Bircks W, Loogen F. Benefits of endocarditis prevention in patients with prosthetic heart valves. [German]. *Z Kardiol* 1986;**75**:8–11.

134. Van Der Meer JTM, Van Wijk W, Thompson J, Vandenbroucke JP, Valkenburg HA, Michel MF. Efficacy of antibiotic prophylaxis for prevention of native-valve endocarditis. *Lancet* 1992;**339**:135–40.

135. Patton JP. Infective endocarditis: economic considerations. In: Kaye D, ed. *Infective endocarditis, 2nd edn.* New York: Raven Press, 1992.

136. Imperiale TF, Horwitz RI. Does prophylaxis prevent post-dental infective endocarditis? A controlled evaluation of protective efficacy. *Am J Med* 1990;**88**:131–6.

137. Everett ED, Hirschmann JV. Transient bacteremia and endocarditis prophylaxis. A review. *Medicine* 1977;**56**:61–77.

138. Biorn CL, Browning WH, Thompson L. Transient bacteremia immediately following transurethral prostatic resection. *J Urol* 1950;**63**:155–61.

139. Clemens JD, Ransohoff DF. A quantitative assessment of pre-dental antibiotic prophylaxis for patients with mitral-valve prolapse. *J Chron Dis* 1984;**37**:531–44.

140. Bor DH, Himmelstein DU. Endocarditis prophylaxis for patients with mitral valve prolapse: a quantitative analysis. *Am J Med* 1984;**76**:711–17.

58 Antithrombotic therapy after heart valve replacement

Alexander GG Turpie, Walter Ageno

Introduction

Despite improvements in prosthetic materials and valve design, thromboembolism remains a serious complication in patients following heart valve replacement. It is generally agreed that lifelong oral anticoagulants are indicated in patients with mechanical prosthetic valves and in patients with tissue valves, if they have atrial fibrillation or a history of thromboembolism.[1–3] In the absence of antithrombotic therapy, systemic embolism and stroke have been reported in between 5% and 50% of patients, depending upon the valve site, the type of valve replacement and the presence of comorbid conditions.[2,3] With the use of anticoagulants, the rate of systemic embolism has been reduced to 1–3% per year.[4] Antithrombotic therapy, however, carries an important risk of bleeding, which is related to the level of anticoagulation used.[5] Studies of long-term oral anticoagulant therapy for deep vein thrombosis have shown that a less intense regimen (INR 2·0–3·0) is as effective but safer than the more intense regimen (INR 3·0–4·5) that was standard until recently.[6–8] Subsequently, studies in patients following either bioprosthetic or mechanical heart valve replacement have shown reduced bleeding with a lower intensity of anticoagulants without loss of efficacy,[9–11] and based on these studies there has been marked improvement in the safety of the long-term anticoagulant regimens used following heart valve replacement.

Bioprosthetic heart valves

The risk of thromboembolism is less with uncomplicated bioprosthetic valves than with mechanical valves.[12–15] Oral anticoagulants, including warfarin, have been shown to be effective and safe when used at a targeted INR of 2·0–3·0 in such patients based on the results of one prospective clinical trial.[9] This study compared two intensities of anticoagulation to determine the safety and efficacy of a less intense anticoagulant regimen in patients following tissue valve replacement. One hundred and eight patients were randomized to standard anticoagulant control (INR 3·0–4·5), and 102 patients to a less intensive regimen (INR 2·0–2·5). Treatment was continued for 3 months. In this study there

was no difference in the frequency of major systemic emboli (1·8% *v* 1·8%) between the two treatment groups, but there were significantly fewer major hemorrhagic complications (0·0% *v* 4·5%; *P* = 0·034) and total hemorrhagic complications (5·4% *v* 14·6%; *P* = 0·042) in the low intensity group (INR 2·0–3·0) compared to the high intensity group, respectively. This level of anticoagulation (INR 2·0–3·0) is now recommended by the American College of Chest Physicians (ACCP) for patients with tissue valve replacement.[4] **Grade A1a**

The risk of thromboembolism is limited mainly to the first 3 months postoperatively in uncomplicated patients with tissue valves, but is present indefinitely in patients with atrial fibrillation.[16] A low ejection fraction, an enlarged left atrium, previous history of venous thromboembolism, and the presence of a pacemaker also increase the risk of thromboembolic complications.[17,18] Consequently, in uncomplicated patients with mitral bioprosthetic valves, anticoagulant therapy is recommended for 3 months while long-term therapy is indicated in patients with atrial fibrillation, those with an atrial thrombus detected at echocardiography, and those who develop a systemic embolus.[4] **Grade B3** Patients with uncomplicated bioprosthetic valves in the aortic position are at very low risk of systemic embolism and some authorities therefore suggest they do not require anticoagulant therapy, although this recommendation remains controversial.[4,19] Long-term treatment with aspirin 80 mg/day following 3 months of oral anticoagulant therapy is likely to be beneficial to prevent subsequent thromboembolic events in patients with uncomplicated bioprosthetic valves.[4] **Grade B4** The current recommendations by the ACCP for patients with tissue valves are shown below.

Mechanical prosthetic heart valves

Patients with mechanical heart valve prostheses require lifelong anticoagulation therapy. The optimal level of anticoagulation in patients with mechanical heart valve replacements has been placed on a scientific footing based on the results of recent studies. Randomized trials have shown that oral anticoagulants are effective in reducing the risk of systemic embolism in patients with mechanical prosthetic valves

Antithrombotic therapy in bioprosthetic heart valve replacement: recommendations			
	INR	Duration	Grade of recommendation
Mitral	2·0–3·0	3 mth	**Grade B3**
Aortic	2·0–3·0	3 mth	**Grade B3**
Atrial fibrillation	2·0–3·0	Long-term	**Grade B3**
Left atrial thrombosis	2·0–3·0	Long-term (duration uncertain)	**Grade B3**
Permanent pacemaker	2·0–3·0	Optional	**Grade B4**
Systemic embolism	2·0–3·0	3–12 mth	**Grade B4**
Normal sinus rhythm	Long-term aspirin (80 mg/day)		**Grade B4**

From Stein *et al.*[4]

when given at lower intensity than has been used in the past. The 2001 guidelines of the ACCP[4] recommend two intensity regimens of long-term oral anticoagulant treatment according to the site of the mechanical prosthesis and the presence of concomitant risk factors. A lower INR range between 2·0 and 3·0 is now recommended for patients with a bileaflet valve (St Jude Medical or Carbomedics) or a tilting disc valve (Medtronic–Hall) in the aortic position who are in normal sinus rhythm and have a left atrium of normal size. These newer recommendations, which are levels of evidence **Grade A2** for the St Jude Medical valves and **Grade B2** for Carbomedics and Medtronic–Hall, are based on the results of long-term follow up studies.[20–23] In particular, a study from France[20] has confirmed the efficacy of a less intense level of anticoagulation following mechanical heart valve replacement. In this study 433 patients with mechanical prostheses were randomized to anticoagulant therapy monitored to achieve an INR of 2·0–3·0 or 3·0–4·5 and followed for 2·2 years. Thromboembolic outcome events, either clinical events or asymptomatic CNS abnormalities proven on CT scan, occurred in 10 of 185 (5·3%) patients in the low intensity group and 9 of 192 (4·7%) patients in the high intensity group ($P = 0.78$). Importantly, there was a statistically significant difference in the rate of bleeding complications between the two groups. Bleeding events occurred in 34 patients (18·1%) in the low intensity group compared with 56 patients (29·2%) in the high intensity group ($P < 0.01$). The majority of patients in this trial, however, had aortic valve replacements and were in sinus rhythm, which limits the generalizability of the results.

An INR range between 2·5 and 3·5 is still recommended for mechanical valves in the mitral position.[4] This recommendation was based on two prospective studies that demonstrated that anticoagulant therapy maintained within this target INR range was as effective as a more intense level of anticoagulation, but with less bleeding. In the first study[10] there was no difference in the frequency of major embolic events in the patients treated with a high intensity regimen (INR 9·0) compared with patients treated with a less intense (INR 2·65) anticoagulant regimen (4·0 v 3·7 embolic episodes per 100 patient years, respectively). However, there was significantly less bleeding in the less intense group (6·2 v 12·1 hemorrhagic episodes per 100 patient years; $P < 0.02$). The second study[11] compared low intensity (INR 2·0–2·99) with high intensity (INR 3·0–4·5) oral anticoagulants in patients with mechanical valves, all of whom were treated with aspirin (330 mg twice per day) in combination with dipyridamole (75 mg per day). In this study one transient ischemic attack occurred in the low intensity group and two in the high intensity group. There were significantly fewer bleeding events in the low intensity group, in which three episodes occurred compared with 12 in the high intensity group ($P < 0.02$).

Although these studies form the basis for the recommendations for a less intense level of anticoagulation, they have a number of limitations. In the first study a very high intensity anticoagulant regimen was compared with a moderately high intensity anticoagulant regimen. The mean daily dose of warfarin in the high intensity group was 8·5 mg and in the low intensity group the mean daily dose of 5·9 mg was similar to the average daily dose of 5·4 mg used in the high intensity group in three venous thrombosis studies,[6–8] and in the randomized study in patients with tissue valves.[9] This suggests that the low intensity group in the first mechanical valve study[10] may have been equivalent to the standard intensity group in the venous thromboembolism studies.[8] The second study[11] was small, and therefore the claim that the two regimens were identical in efficacy is questionable. This latter study does, however, confirm the marked difference in bleeding between high intensity and low intensity anticoagulant regimens. The ACCP recommendations for mechanical valves are shown below.

The ACCP recommendation of an INR target of 2·5–3·5 is lower than that reported in a study conducted in Europe which has recommended a target range of 3·0–4·0.[24] However, the European recommendation is based on retrospective data and largely on events that occurred in patients with older caged ball valve prostheses. Thus recommendations based on these data are unlikely to be applicable for use in patients with the modern bileaflet and tilting disc valves that are currently in use.

Of interest, two recent studies have reported a high sensitivity to warfarin in the immediate postoperative phase during oral anticoagulation induction and suggested the

Antithrombotic therapy in mechanical heart valve replacement: recommendations

	INR	Grade of recommendation
Uncomplicated bileaflet aortic	2·0–3·0	Grade A1a
Uncomplicated tilting disc aortic	2·0–3·0	Grade B3
Bileaflet aortic and atrial fibrillation	2·5–3·5 or 2·0–3·0 + aspirin 80 mg to 100 mg/day	Grade B3/4
Uncomplicated bileaflet mitral	2·5–3·5	Grade B3
Uncomplicated tilting disc mitral	2·5–3·5	Grade B2
Additional risk factors	2·5–3·5 + aspirin 80 mg to 100 mg/day	Grade B2
Systemic embolism	2·5–3·5 + aspirin 80 mg to 100 mg/day	Grade B2
Caged ball or caged disc valve	2·5–3·5 + aspirin 80 mg to 100 mg/day	Grade A/C

From Stein *et al.*[4]

need for lower starting doses of warfarin to regularly achieve the therapeutic range (that is, 2·5–3·0 mg instead of 5·0 mg) in most patients.[25,26]

Combination antithrombotic therapy

A major limitation to the current approach used to treat high-risk patients with prosthetic heart valves is that systemic embolism, which may result in disabling stroke, still occurs at a rate of approximately 2–3% per year, despite the use of anticoagulants.[4] The addition of antiplatelet agents to oral anticoagulants has been advocated as an improved approach to the treatment of patients with mechanical valves, or high-risk patients with tissue valves, to reduce further the risk of major systemic embolism. In an early study[27] the combination of dipyridamole and oral anticoagulants significantly reduced mortality in patients with early models of the Starr–Edwards prosthesis compared with anticoagulants alone. A subsequent study from the Mayo Clinic[28] reported that the addition of dipyridamole to oral anticoagulants significantly reduced the risk of thromboembolic events in patients with mechanical heart valve prostheses. A recent meta-analysis of the dipyridamole studies (Table 58.1) has confirmed improved outcomes with combined therapy compared with anticoagulants alone.[29] The routine use of dipyridamole in combination with oral anticoagulants is, however, not widely accepted for the treatment of patients with mechanical valves or high-risk patients with tissue valves, because of the frequency of adverse effects, including intractable headache, dizziness, nausea, flushing, and syncope.

The combination of aspirin and oral anticoagulants has also been used in the treatment of patients with heart valve replacement with a significant reduction in embolic complications, but with an increased risk of bleeding complications.[30] In the early studies reported to date, aspirin was used in high doses (approximately 1 g/day), and in most cases the bleeding with the combination of high-dose aspirin and high-dose oral anticoagulants was gastrointestinal.[31] There is good evidence that gastrointestinal irritation and hemorrhage is dose-dependent over a range of 100–1000 mg of aspirin per day and that the antithrombotic effects of aspirin are independent of the dose over this range.

One completed study[32] compared low-dose aspirin combined with warfarin in the treatment of patients with mechanical heart valve replacements to determine whether low-dose aspirin would result in an improved antithrombotic effect, without the same high risk of bleeding that has

Table 58.1 Dipyridamole plus anticoagulants following heart valve replacement

	Oral A/C alone	Oral A/C + dipyridamole	% RR	2*P*
Thromboembolism	69/582 (11·9%)	31/559 (5·5%)	56	0·007
Non-fatal T/E	48/582 (8·2%)	24/559 (4·3%)	50	0·005
Fatal T/E	21/582 (3·6%)	7/559 (1·3%)	64	0·008
Death	67/582 (11·5%)	40/559 (7·2%)	40	0·013
Hemorrhage	87/539 (16·1%)	80/501 (16·0%)	−1	0·94

Abbreviations: A/C, anticoagulants; T/E, thromboembolism
From Pouleur and Buyse[29]

Table 58.2 Effect of aspirin combined with antithrombotic therapy following heart valve replacement

	Aspirin + warfarin ($n = 186$)	Placebo + warfarin ($n = 184$)	RR% (95% CI)	2P
Systemic embolism	1·6	4·6	65·0 (1·8–37·5)	0·037
Vascular death	0·6	4·4	85·5 (36·0–96·7)	0·003
Death	2·8	7·4	61·7 (16·8–82·3)	0·009

Figures represent % annualized rates.
From Turpie *et al.*[32]

been reported for the combination of oral anticoagulants with high-dose aspirin. This was a double-blind, randomized trial to compare the relative efficacy and safety of aspirin (100 mg per day) with placebo in the prevention of systemic embolism or vascular death in patients with mechanical heart valve replacement or high-risk patients with tissue valves who had atrial fibrillation or a history of thromboembolism. Three hundred and seventy patients were treated with oral anticoagulant therapy (warfarin: INR 3·0–4·5) and randomized to receive aspirin (186 patients) or placebo (184 patients) and followed for up to 4 years (average 2·5 years). The outcomes of the study were systemic embolism, valve thrombosis, vascular death, and hemorrhage. Systemic embolism or vascular death occurred in 6 (3·2%) of the aspirin-treated patients and 24 (13·0%) of the placebo-treated patients (RR 77·2%; 90% CI 51·7–89·2; $P = 0·0002$). The corresponding rates for systemic embolism or death from any cause were 13 (7·0%) and 33 (17·9%), respectively (RR 64·7%; 90% CI 39·6–79·5; $P = 0·0005$); for vascular death 2 (1·1%) and 13 (7·1%), respectively (RR 85·4%; 90% CI 49·8–95·9; $P = 0·0015$); and for death from any cause 9 (4·8%) and 22 (12·0%), respectively (RR 62·7%; 90% CI 44·5–80·5; $P = 0·0048$). Major bleeding events occurred in 24 (12%) of the aspirin-treated patients compared with 19 (10·3%) in the placebo-treated patients (absolute difference 2·6%; 90% CI − 8·3–3·4; $P = 0·2710$).

The results of this study, the annualized rates of which are summarized in Table 58.2, demonstrated that in patients with mechanical valve replacement or high-risk patients with tissue valve replacement, the addition of aspirin (100 mg per day) to oral anticoagulation therapy (warfarin: INR 3·0–4·5) reduced mortality, vascular mortality, and systemic embolism, but with some increase in minor bleeding. In a recent study in patients with mechanical prostheses,[33] it was shown that low-dose aspirin (100 mg/day) was as effective as high-dose aspirin (650 mg/day) in combination with oral anticoagulants at a target INR of 2·0–3·0, but with a reduced risk of bleeding. Therefore, the addition of low-dose aspirin (80–100 mg/day) is now recommended for patients with concomitant atrial fibrillation or other additional risk factors and patients

who had thromboembolic events despite adequate oral anticoagulant therapy.

Ticlopidine may also be useful as an adjunct to oral anticoagulants, but the data are less solid since the one study in which it has been evaluated was not randomized.[34] There are currently no available data on the association of aspirin and clopidogrel in this setting.

Summary

The demonstration that, for most indications for oral anticoagulant therapy, less intense anticoagulation (INR 2·0–3·0) is as efficacious as standard intensity anticoagulation (INR 3·0–4·5) but with significantly less bleeding is an important advance in antithrombotic therapy. It has greatly improved safety of long-term oral anticoagulant therapy and has resulted in its more widespread use in the prevention and treatment of thromboembolism. It is the level of choice in uncomplicated patients with tissue prostheses. Further evidence is required, however, before this less intense regimen is routinely adopted for patients with mechanical valves and for high-risk patients with tissue valves. The addition of low-dose aspirin to anticoagulants may be more efficacious in the prevention of systemic embolism and vascular death in heart valve replacement patients than anticoagulants alone and may permit a lower intensity of anticoagulation to be used.

References

1. Starr A. Late complications of aortic valve replacement with cloth-covered composite-seat prostheses. *Ann Thorac Surg* 1975;**19**:289.
2. Larsen GL, Alexander JA, Stanford W. Thromboembolic phenomena in patients with prosthetic aortic valves who did not receive anticoagulants. *Ann Thorac Surg* 1977;**12**:323.
3. Limet R, Lepage G, Grondin CM. Thromboembolic complications with the cloth-covered Starr–Edwards aortic prosthesis in patients not receiving anticogulants. *Ann Thorac Surg* 1977;**23**:529.

4. Stein PD, Alpert JS, Bussey HI *et al.* Antithrombotic therapy in patients with mechanical or biological prosthetic heart valves. *Chest* 2001;**119**:220S–7S.

5. Levine MN, Hirsh J, Landefeld S *et al.* Hemorrhagic complications of anticoagulant treatment. *Chest* 1992;**102** (Suppl. 4):352–63.

6. Hull R, Delmore T, Genton E *et al.* Warfarin sodium versus low-dose heparin in the long-term treatment of venous thrombosis. *N Engl J Med* 1979;**301**:855–8.

7. Hull R, Hirsh J, Jay R *et al.* Different intensities of oral anticoagulant therapy in the treatment of proximal vein thrombosis. *N Engl J Med* 1982;**307**:1676–81.

8. Hull R, Delmore T, Carter C *et al.* Adjusted subcutaneous heparin versus warfarin sodium in the long-term treatment of venous thrombosis. *N Engl J Med* 1982;**306**:189–94.

9. Turpie AGG, Gunstensen J, Hirsh J *et al.* A randomized trial comparing two intensities of oral anticoagulant therapy following tissue heart valve replacement. *Lancet* 1988;**i**:1242–5.

10. Saour JN, Sieck JO, Gallus AS. Trial of different intensities of anticoagulation in patients with prosthetic heart valves. *N Engl J Med* 1990;**332**:428–32.

11. Altman P, Rouvier J, Gurfinkel E *et al.* Comparison of two levels of anticoagulant therapy in patients with substitute heart valves. *J Thorac Cardiovasc Surg* 1991;**101**:427–31.

12. Cevese PG. Long-term results of 212 xenograft valve replacements. *J Cardiovasc Surg* 1975;**16**:639–42.

13. Pipkin RD, Buch WS, Fogarty TS. Evaluation of aortic valve replacement with a porcine xenograft without long-term anticoagulation. *J Thorac Cardiovasc Surg* 1976;**71**:179–86.

14. Stinson EB, Griepp RB, Oyer PE *et al.* Long-term experience with porcine aortic valve xenografts. *J Thorac Cardiovasc Surg* 1977;**73**:54–63.

15. Ionescu MI, Pakrashi BC, Mary DAS *et al.* Long-term evaluation of tissue valves. *J Thorac Cardiovasc Surg* 1974;**68**:361–79.

16. Cohn LH, Collins JJ Jr, Rizzo RJ *et al.* Twenty-year follow-up of the Hancock modified orifice porcine aortic valve. *Ann Thorac Surg* 1998;**66**(Suppl):S30–S41.

17. Horstkotte D, Scharf RE, Schulteiss HP. Intracardiac thrombosis: patient-related and device-related risk factors. *J Heart Valve Dis* 1995;**4**:114–20.

18. Lonuagie YA, Jamart J, Enucher P *et al.* Mitral valve Carpentier–Edwards bioprosthetic replacement, thromboembolism, and anticoagulants. *Ann Thorac Surg* 1993;**56**:931–37.

19. Moinuddeen K, Quin J, Shaw R *et al.* Anticoagulation is unnecessary after biological aortic valve replacement. *Circulation* 1998;**98**:II-95–II-99.

20. Acar J, Iung B, Boissel JP *et al.* AREVA: multicenter randomized comparison of low-dose versus standard-dose anticoagulation in patients with mechanical prosthetic heart valves. *Circulation* 1996;**94**:2107–12.

21. Horstkotte D, Schulte HD, Birks W *et al.* Lower intensity anticoagulation therapy results in lower complication rates with the St Jude Medical Prosthesis. *J Thorac Cardiovasc Surg* 1994;**107**:1136–45.

22. David TE, Gott VL, Harker LA *et al.* Mechanical valves. *Ann Thorac Surg* 1996;**62**:1567–9.

23. Akins CW. Long term results with the Medtronic–Hall valvular prosthesis. *Ann Thorac Surg* 1996;**61**:806–13.

24. Cannegieter SC, Rosendaal FR, Wintzen AR *et al.* Optimal oral anticoagulant therapy in patients with mechanical heart valves. *N Engl J Med* 1995;**333**:11–17.

25. Ageno W, Turpie AGG. Exaggerated initial response to warfarin following heart valve replacement. *Am J Cardiol* 1999;**84**:905–8.

26. Ageno W, Turpie AGG, Steidl L *et al.* Comparison of a daily fixed 2·5 mg warfarin dose with a 5 mg, INR adjusted, warfarin dose initially following heart valve replacement. *Am J Cardiol* 2001;**88**:40–4.

27. Sullivan JM, Harken DE, Gorlin R. Pharmacologic control of thromboembolic complications of cardiac valve replacement. *N Engl J Med* 1971;**284**:1391–4.

28. Chesebro JG, Fuster V, Elveback LR *et al.* Trial of combined warfarin plus dipyridamole or aspirin therapy in prosthetic heart valve replacement: danger of aspirin compared with dipyridamole. *Am J Cardiol* 1983;**51**:1537–41.

29. Pouleur H, Buyse M. Effects of dipyridamole in combination with anticoagulant therapy on survival and thromboembolic events in patients with prosthetic heart valves. A meta-analysis of the randomized trials. *J Thorac Cardiovasc Surg* 1995;**110**:463–6.

30. Dale J, Myhre E, Storstein O *et al.* Prevention of arterial thromboembolism with acetylsalicylic acid: a controlled clinical study in patients with aortic ball valves. *Am Heart J* 1977;**94**:101–11.

31. Patrono C, Coller B, Dalen JE *et al.* Platelet-active drugs. The relationship among dose, effectiveness and side effects. *Chest* 2001;**119**:39S–63S.

32. Turpie AGG, Gent M, Laupacis A *et al.* A double-blind randomized trial of acetylsalicylic acid (100 mg) versus placebo in patients treated with oral anticoagulants following heart valve replacement. *N Engl J Med* 1991;**329**:1365–9.

33. Altman R, Rouvier J, Gurfinkel E, Scazziota A, Turpie AGG. Comparison of high-dose with low-dose aspirin in patients with mechanical heart valve replacement treated with oral anticoagulant. *Circulation* 1996;**94**:2113–16.

34. Hayashi JI, Nakazawa S, Oguma F, Miyamura H, Eguchi S. Combined warfarin and antiplatelet therapy after St Jude mechanical valve replacement for mitral valve disease. *J Am Coll Cardiol* 1994;**23**:672–7.

Part IIIh

Specific cardiovascular disorders: Other conditions

Bernard J Gersh and Salim Yusuf, Editors

Grading of recommendations and levels of evidence used in *Evidence-based Cardiology*

GRADE A

Level 1a   Evidence from large randomized clinical trials (RCTs) or systematic reviews (including meta-analyses) of multiple randomized trials which collectively has at least as much data as one single well-defined trial.

Level 1b   Evidence from at least one "All or None" high quality cohort study; in which ALL patients died/failed with conventional therapy and some survived/succeeded with the new therapy (for example, chemotherapy for tuberculosis, meningitis, or defibrillation for ventricular fibrillation); or in which many died/failed with conventional therapy and NONE died/failed with the new therapy (for example, penicillin for pneumococcal infections).

Level 1c   Evidence from at least one moderate-sized RCT or a meta-analysis of small trials which collectively only has a moderate number of patients.

Level 1d   Evidence from at least one RCT.

GRADE B

Level 2   Evidence from at least one high quality study of non-randomized cohorts who did and did not receive the new therapy.

Level 3   Evidence from at least one high quality case–control study.

Level 4   Evidence from at least one high quality case series.

GRADE C

Level 5   Opinions from experts without reference or access to any of the foregoing (for example, argument from physiology, bench research or first principles).

A comprehensive approach would incorporate many different types of evidence (for example, RCTs, non-RCTs, epidemiologic studies, and experimental data), and examine the architecture of the information for consistency, coherence and clarity. Occasionally the evidence does not completely fit into neat compartments. For example, there may not be an RCT that demonstrates a reduction in mortality in individuals with stable angina with the use of β blockers, but there is overwhelming evidence that mortality is reduced following MI. In such cases, some may recommend use of β blockers in angina patients with the expectation that some extrapolation from post-MI trials is warranted. This could be expressed as Grade A/C. In other instances (for example, smoking cessation or a pacemaker for complete heart block), the non-randomized data are so overwhelmingly clear and biologically plausible that it would be reasonable to consider these interventions as Grade A.

Recommendation grades appear either within the text, for example, **Grade A** and **Grade A1a** or within a table in the chapter.

The grading system clearly is only applicable to preventive or therapeutic interventions. It is not applicable to many other types of data such as descriptive, genetic or pathophysiologic.

59 Treatment of patients with stroke

Craig S Anderson

The increasing burden of stroke

Stroke is a major global healthcare problem.[1] In most Western countries, stroke is the third leading cause of death after heart disease and cancer, and is a major cause of long-term disability and a significant cost to health and social services.[2] The majority (about 75%) of new cases of stroke occur in people over the age of 65 years,[2–4] and about one third of them are dead within one year.[5,6] In addition to concerns about dependency and being a burden to others, survivors hope to remain free of recurrent stroke (and other serious vascular events), estimated at about 30–40% over the first five years after the onset of stroke.[7,8]

After a long period of neglect and an attitude to stroke that has been one of therapeutic nihilism, the past few decades has seen growing interest in the area of stroke medicine and considerable advances in the epidemiology and therapeutics of stroke. This can be explained by a number of factors, such as the ready availability of non-invasive diagnostic technology and an increase in evidence from randomized controlled trials. Computerized tomography (CT) and magnetic resonance imaging (MRI) provide the clinician with the ability to confirm the bedside diagnosis of stroke and transient ischemic attack (TIA), differentiate accurately intracerebral hemorrhage (and subarachnoid hemorrhage) from infarction, and distinguish the cerebral lesions underlying several distinct stroke syndromes in life. In comparison to ischemic heart disease, stroke is a heterogeneous clinical syndrome that encompasses a number of pathological entities that are not necessarily related to atherosclerosis, have different patterns of occurrence and outcome, and may require different management. However, it is often difficult to assign a specific cause for the different types of cerebral infarction (that is, large artery atherothrombosis, cardioembolism, and "small vessel" lacunes) in a particular individual due to the non-specific and overlapping nature of risk factors and other features. Modern neuro-imaging has also allowed a greater awareness of the importance of "silent strokes" and of the broader effects of strokes on the mind and emotion. Depression is an important sequela of stroke,[9] while cerebrovascular disease and Alzheimer's disease often coincide in older people. Indeed, evidence is accumulating that cerebrovascular disease may play a role in the etiology of Alzheimer's disease as well as vascular dementia.[10]

Although the continuous decline in mortality and incidence from stroke in some populations over recent decades is an encouraging trend,[11–17] there is still no general consensus about the factors responsible, or their relative contributions, to these trends. It is unclear, for example, whether there has been a change in the natural history with fewer and less severe strokes, either of which could be related to the better control of blood pressure and other risk factors; or whether there has been an improvement in survival following stroke related to improvements in acute and long-term medical care. It is also uncertain why there has been recent trend of a slowdown in the decline,[15,18,19] or even an increase in mortality rates from stroke in some Eastern European countries.[20] One possible explanation is that this is related to the decline in mortality from coronary artery disease and consequent rising prevalence of chronic ischemic heart disease and heart failure, which increase the pool of persons at high risk of stroke. Other potential candidates include changes in the prevalence of risk factors, in particular diabetes, obesity and smoking, and the recognized failure of hypertension detection and control programs.

Untangling the puzzle of trends in stroke is a matter of pressing importance because the elderly, the most stroke-prone age group, constitute the fastest growing segment of the population. If the incidence of stroke were to stabilize rather than fall, there will soon be an absolute increase in the numbers of disabled survivors of stroke, with major consequences for the health system and informal caregivers. In developed countries, at least, it has been suggested that early death from stroke in patients who were already "handicapped" from other causes may contribute to these communities avoiding an overall increase in the burden of care related to long-term survivors of stroke.[21] Even so, country-specific data on trends in the cause-specific incidence of stroke provide important local feedback on the success (or failure) of preventative strategies, while patterns of case fatality and outcome should bear a closer relationship to the management of acute stroke. Both are required for the planning of services that will inevitably come under increasing pressure from the aforementioned demographic changes. The burden of stroke, in particular, is projected to increase dramatically in developing countries, due to rapid changing population demographics and a shift from traditional, rural

Table 59.1 Summary of effectiveness and costs of acute treatment for stroke each year in a large population. (Modified with permission from Hankey GJ, Warlow CP. Treatment and secondary prevention of stroke: evidence, costs, and effects on individuals and populations. *Lancet* 1999;354:1457–63.)

Intervention	Death or dependency		RRR (95% CI)	ARR	Deaths/dependents avoided per 1000 treated (n)	NNT	Target population (% of all 2400 strokes)	Deaths/dependents avoided in 1 million population with 2400 strokes (n, (%))	Approximate cost per death or dependency avoided (Aus $)
	Control	Intervention							
Stroke unit	62·0%	56·4%	9% (4–14)	5·6%	56	18	1920 (80%)	107 (8·3%)	? Nil additional
Aspirin	47·0%	45·8%	3% (1–5)	1·2%	12	83	1900 (80%)	23 (1·8%)	$83
Thrombolysis	62·7%	56·4%	10% (5–15)	6·3%	63	16	240 (10%)	15 (1·2%)	$36 000 (t-PA) $3200 (streptokinase)

Table 59.2 Summary of secondary stroke prevention strategies and their cost effectiveness for patients with stroke or TIA each year in a large population. (Reproduced with permission from Hankey GJ, Warlow CP. Treatment and secondary prevention of stroke: evidence, costs, and effects on individuals and populations. *Lancet* 1999;354:1457–63.)

Strategy/ intervention	Stroke risk per year		RRR (95% CI)	ARR	Strokes avoided per 1000 treated per year (n)	TIA/ stroke patients needed to treat to avoid one stroke per year	Target population (% of all prevalent TIA and stroke survivors)	Strokes avoided per year among target population (n)	% of all 2400 strokes avoided each year in population of 1 million	Approximate cost per stroke avoided (Aus $)
	Control	Intervention								
Blood pressure lowering drugs	7·0%	4·8%*	28% (15–38)[a]	2·2%	22	45	6000 (50%)	132	5·5%	1 350 (diuretic) 18 000 (ACE inhibitor)
Smoking cessation	7·0%	4·7%	33% (29–38)	2·3%	23	43	3600 (30%)	84	3·5%	0 (voluntary) <19 600 (patches for all)
Cholesterol lowering drugs	7·0%	5·3%	24% (8–38)	1·7%	17	59	4800 (40%)	81	3·4%	41 000
Antiplatelet drugs							8000 (75% of 10 650 TIA/ischemic strokes)			
Aspirin	7·0%	6·0%	13% (4–21)	1·0%	10	100		80[b]	3·3%[b]	2000
Clopidogrel	7·0%	5·4%	10% (2–17)[b]	1·6%	16	62 (166[b])		128 (48[b])	5·3% (2·0[b])	74 400
Aspirin + dipyridamole	7·0%	5·1%	15% (5–26)[a, b]	1·9%	19	53 (111[b])		152 (72[b])	6·3% (3·0%[b])	18 500
Anticoagulants	12·0%	4·0%	67% (43–80)	8·0%	80	12	2130 (20% of 10 650 TIA/ischemic strokes) realistically but only up to 1065 (50%)	85	3·5%	1200
Carotid endarterectomy Symptomatic	8·8%	5·0%	44% (21–60)	3·8%	38	26	850 (8% of 10 650 TIA/ischemic strokes)	32	1·3%	182 000

[a] Size of effect remains to be confirmed in ongoing trials.
[b] Compared with aspirin (ie, over and above effect of aspirin).

to urban lifestyles.[1,22] It is imperative, then, that researchers, healthcare providers and policy makers develop appropriate and cost effective interventions for the prevention, treatment and management of stroke. Hankey and Warlow[23] provide an excellent overview of the effectiveness and costs of such strategies, and this is summarized in Tables 59.1 and 59.2.

Stroke units and stroke services

Arguably the single most important therapeutic advance during the past decade in the treatment of patients with acute stroke has been the development of stroke services and stroke units. Strong evidence exists from pooled clinical trial data that well coordinated multidisciplinary, inpatient, stroke unit care can significantly improve the likelihood of returning home and retaining independence after stroke.[24]

Grade A1c

Compared with conventional care in a general medical ward, stroke units are associated with a relative risk reduction (RRR) of 9% and an absolute risk reduction (ARR) of 5·6%. Thus, the number of patients with stroke that need to be treated (NNT) on a stroke unit to prevent one from dying or becoming dependent is an impressive 18.[23] The benefit of stroke units applies across all subgroups of patients including those who are old, severely disabled, or are admitted late to hospital.[24] While it is uncertain which part of this expert care is important, there is broad consensus that stroke services, both in the acute and rehabilitation phases, need to be well coordinated and include a multidisciplinary team approach, active participation of family, and special education and training of staff (see Table 59.3). In common with coronary care units, stroke units also facilitate the conduct of randomized trials and allow the development of protocols and practices to facilitate rapid, early and thorough evaluation, treatment and rehabilitation.

There is much interest in extending the "black box" package of stroke unit care into the community. In the past decade, there have been an increasing number of trials of specialist domiciliary (home-based) stroke care and rehabilitation schemes, with the aim of either avoiding the need for admission to hospital, or enabling earlier and more effective discharge and follow up. Although there may be scope to prevent some admissions to hospital after stroke, it is not an easy task, not least because stroke is a frightening illness, with most patients disabled at onset. In most countries, hospitals offer a safe and secure environment for intensive nursing care and rehabilitation. Patients with stroke, therefore, conventionally receive a substantial part of their acute care and rehabilitation in hospitals or in other institutions that offer a 24 hour stay. This emphasis on hospital care, together with greater public and professional education on acute symptoms and the need to regard stroke as an emergency,[25,26] mean that it is probably unrealistic to anticipate major service development to the area of "hospital avoidance" for patients with stroke in the future.

Conversely, there is much interest in the development of services that allow patients with stroke to be sent home from hospital earlier than usual and receive domiciliary rehabilitation. Advocates of early discharge schemes suggest several advantages: satisfying patient choice, reducing risks associated with prolonged inpatient care, the home setting

Table 59.3   Organization of stroke services – evidence grades

Recommendation	Evidence grade
1. Every health care organization involved in the care of patients with acute stroke should ensure that the there are specialty service(s) responsible for the management of these patients which comprise the following factors: • A geographically defined unit as the inpatient service base • A well coordinated multidisciplinary team • Staff with special training and expertise in stroke care and rehabilitation • Educational programs for staff, patients and caregivers • Agreed-on protocols for common problems	**Grade A1c**
2. Specialist stroke services can be delivered to patients, following the acute phase, equally effectively in hospital or the community	**Grade A1c**
3. Rehabilitation can be provided to patients within a specialist outpatient or domiciliary setting with equal effect	**Grade A1c**
4. Patients with acute stroke who are not admitted to hospital can benefit from a domiciliary rehabilitation team that includes an occupational therapist.	**Grade A1c**

being more focused toward rehabilitation outcomes, and savings in costs.[27] Since 1997, several randomized trials of early hospital discharge and domiciliary stroke rehabilitation have been published.[28] These data are consistent with regard to no adverse impact on patient outcomes and a reduction in hospital length of stay, and the limited economic analyses available indicate potential cost-savings with such schemes.[29,30] There is high quality evidence that allows some broad recommendations to be made regarding the organization of stroke care[31] (see Table 59.1).

Treatment of ischemic stroke

Another major therapeutic landmark in the management of stroke is the use of thrombolytic therapy for acute ischemic stroke. Most acute strokes are due to cerebral infarction following occlusion of arterial blood vessels. The pathogenesis of resulting brain damage can be separated into two sequential processes:

1. the vascular and hematological events that produce occlusion and reduce blood flow in the affected area
2. ischemic necrosis of brain cells.

Surrounding blood vessels in the brain may partly maintain blood flow into the damaged area and therefore, the outer regions of the damaged area are less severely affected than within the core. This process produces an area of irreversible severe ischemia surrounded by an area of moderate ischemia, known as the "penumbra". The recognition that further death of neurons in the penumbra may be prevented has focused attention on treatments to minimize, or even reverse, the damaging effects of ischemia provided they can be initiated within a short period of time after the onset of stroke. This "therapeutic window" may be divided into two partly overlapping components: the "reperfusion window" related to the restoration of blood flow and the "neuroprotective window" related to damaging effects within brain cells. Studies in various animal models and clinical trials suggest that the reperfusion window is very short, perhaps only a few hours, while the neuroprotective window may be much longer, maybe up to 48 hours. While an effective neuroprotective agent for acute stroke has yet to be identified, considerable progress has been made in therapies aimed at restoring blood flow to prevent or lessen the spreading ischemia within the penumbra.

In 1996, the United States Food and Drug Administration (FDA) approved intravenous recombinant tissue plasminogen activator (rt-PA) in selected patients with acute ischemic stroke, provided treatment can begin within 3 hours of the onset of symptoms. The approval was based largely on the results of two combined, National Institute of Neurologic Disease and Stroke (NINDS) Acute Stroke Studies, where all patients were treated within 3 hours of the onset of symptoms

and half of the patients were treated within 90 minutes.[32] Subsequent individual trials of rt-PA (and streptokinase) with time windows extending up to 6 hours after the onset of stroke have failed to show a definite positive benefit on their own, but several meta-analyses of the trials indicate a large beneficial effect of treatment, albeit with significant risk, mainly intracerebral hemorrhage.[33,34] Risk of intracerebral hemorrhage is estimated to be 5–10%, and appears more likely to occur in patients with evidence of a large visible infarct on CT, and concurrent use of aspirin among other factors. Despite this risk, use of intravenous rt-PA appears to result in at least a 30% RRR in disability from stroke. The benefits (about 65 patients per 1000 treated avoid "death or long-term dependence") appear to be several times greater than for aspirin, the only other proven effective medical treatment used early after the onset of stroke.[35,36] **Grade A1a**

Although licenses have been granted for the use of rt-PA in several countries and subsequent consensus statements from lead professional organizations such as the American Heart Association[37] endorsing the use of intravenous rt-PA. The uptake of this therapy in clinical practice is extremely limited, even despite intensive community and professional awareness campaigns.[38] In addition, there has been criticism of editorial format of certain consensus statements[39] and concerns raised about the randomization process in the NINDS trial and failure to adjust for imbalance in baseline variables (J Wardlow, personal communication). Thus, there is a long way to go before we can use thrombolysis *widely* in patients with acute ischemic stroke. Despite the published data, consensus statements, and guidelines, only a very small minority of patients with acute ischemic stroke currently receive intravenous rt-PA, mainly due to various educational barriers and delays in getting people to hospital quickly after the onset of symptoms. Much more data is required to establish reliably the balance of benefits and risks of thrombolysis across different groups of patients, even those patients treated after the 3 hour time window.[33,34] A large multicenter trial (International Stroke Trial (IST) – 3) has commenced to address these issues and influence clinical practice.

Apart from rt-PA, two very large trials have established that aspirin 300 mg, administered within the first 48 hours after the onset of ischemic stroke, reduce the risk of death or dependency at 6 months by 1·3%, mainly by reducing early recurrent ischemic stroke.[35,36] **Grade A1a**

Despite a long history of use as standard therapy for established or threatened acute ischemic stroke, a large number of trials individually, and when combined in a meta-analysis,[35,40] have established beyond doubt that heparin in any form, dose or route of administration has no benefit. Even among patients with presumed cardio-embolic stroke, the modest potential benefit is counterbalanced by a significant excess risk of symptomatic hemorrhage, of which the most lethal is intracerebral hemorrhage.[35,40,41] **Grade A1a**

Prevention of stroke

The most realistic approach to lessen the burden of stroke is prevention, with both population-based strategies and the targeting of high-risk individuals being advocated. Epidemiologic studies suggest that significant reductions in the incidence of stroke, as with coronary heart disease, can be expected by reducing the prevalence or shifting the distribution of risk factors across the entire population.[42] Thus, identifying risk factors and intervening to control or modify them remains the most important means of reducing the burden of stroke. Favorable lifestyle behaviors, including weight reduction, diets that are high in fish, fruit and vegetables, and increased physical activity, are based on sound epidemiologic data. Although direct evidence is lacking, observational studies suggest that stopping smoking decreases the risk of stroke by at least 30%.[43] A substantial reduction in the incidence of stroke has been noted following cessation of smoking, even in older people and in those who have been heavy smokers for many years.[44] **Grade B2**

The "high risk" strategy involves the identification and management of people at high risk of developing stroke. Therapies of proven benefit in the prevention of stroke among certain individuals are blood pressure lowering therapy, antiplatelet therapy, cholesterol lowering therapy, anticoagulation, and carotid endarterectomy. Evidence is mounting that aggressive treatment of hyperglycemia among patients with diabetes mellitus is also effective in reducing the risk of stroke.[45] The absolute benefits of these interventions appear to be greater in subjects in whom the absolute risk is particularly high, notably older people. Effective prevention of stroke in individuals depends on the efficient identification and management of these subjects, particularly in primary care.

Blood pressure reduction strategies

Blood pressure is the single most important reversible risk factor for stroke. Pivotal data about the relationship between blood pressure and stroke comes from both prospective observational studies and clinical trials. Observational studies provide information from which the effects of prolonged blood pressure differences can be estimated,[46] while trials provide data about the effects of short-term blood pressure reduction.[47] Four major overviews of observational studies on blood pressure and stroke have been conducted to date. Such analysis overcomes many of the limitations of individual studies, which have frequently failed to adjust the size of the association for measurement error, in particular regression dilution bias.[46,48–50] A consistent finding of these overviews is a continuous, approximately log linear relationship

between usual levels of blood pressure and the primary incidence of stroke, with no evidence of an upper or lower threshold level of blood pressure and stroke risk. On the basis of this relationship, it is estimated that a 5 mmHg lower diastolic blood pressure (or 10 mmHg lower systolic blood pressure) is associated with a 30–40% lower risk of stroke, and there is no evidence that these associations differ between men and women.

Most of the trial data is on the primary prevention of stroke, confirming beyond doubt the benefits of blood pressure lowering in preventing first-ever stroke in middle-aged men and women. Several meta-analyses of trials[51–53] demonstrate that lowering blood pressure in this age group is effective in preventing stroke, with risk reductions commensurate with predictions based on non-experimental epidemiologic studies of 30–40%. **Grade A1a**

Moreover, the Heart Outcomes Prevention Evaluation (HOPE) trial[54] results suggest that activation of the renin–angiotensin system is an independent risk factor for stroke. In this study of 9297 patients with a history of symptomatic vascular disease (mainly coronary artery disease), who were randomized to either ramipril 10 mg daily or placebo on top of best medical therapy, there was a significant reduction in the rate of the combined end point cluster of stroke, myocardial infarction, or death from vascular causes in the patients allocated ramipril (14·0%) compared with those given placebo (17·8%). This RRR of 22% (95% CI 14–30) and an ARR of 3·8% over about 5 years of follow up was much greater than could be expected from the size of the reductions in blood pressure (3 mmHg systolic, 1 mmHg diastolic). The effects of treatment on the end point of any stroke, a RRR of 32% (95% CI 16–44), were consistent across baseline blood pressures, concurrent medication use, and important patient subgroups including those with and without a history of hypertension.[55] Moreover, these data support the hypothesis that angiotensin converting enzyme (ACE) inhibition has beneficial effects independent of blood pressure reduction.

Existing data from randomized controlled trials and a systematic review including patients with cerebrovascular disease suggested that blood pressure lowering therapy may reduce the risk of recurrent stroke by an equivalent amount to that of primary stroke prevention.[56] However, this evidence has not been compelling enough to influence clinical practice. In fact, the approach to blood pressure control among clinicians involved in the care of patients with stroke, and particularly those who are old and normotensive, has been conservative, due in part to concerns about the adverse effects of aggressive blood pressure lowering in this setting. The Perindopril Protection Against Recurrent Stroke Study (PROGRESS) undertaken in over 6000 patients was designed to address this issue by determining the effects of a flexible ACE-inhibitor based blood pressure lowering regimen (perindopril with or without the addition of the diuretic, indapamide) on the risks of stroke and other major vascular events in patients with a history of stroke or TIA.[57] Overall, blood pressure was reduced by an average of 9·0/4·0 mmHg (SE 0·3/0·2) among patients assigned active treatment compared with those assigned placebo during the trial. Compared with those assigned to placebo, the blood pressure reductions among those treated with combination therapy (12·3/5·0 mmHg, SE 0·5/0·3) were about twice as high as those treated with single-drug therapy (4·9/2·8 mmHg, SE 0·6/0·3). The study showed that treatment reduced the incidence of stroke, coronary events and major vascular events by 28%, 26% and 26%, respectively. Active treatment reduced the risks of ischemic stroke by around one quarter and hemorrhagic stroke by one half, and was equally effective in patients with and without a history of hypertension. Combination perindopril and indapamide provided even greater benefits.

Thus, blood pressure lowering therapy should now be regarded as the most important measure for both the primary and secondary prevention of stroke. **Grade A1a**

Although the choice of therapy will depend on the degree of acceptance of direct evidence, as well as on regulations and prescribing patterns, the evidence is strong for therapy that includes an ACE inhibitor and maximizes the degree of blood pressure reduction, such as a combination of perindopril and indapamide. Moreover, effective implementation of such therapy in high-risk groups in combination with population-wide blood pressure lowering strategies, provides one of the most meaningful, practical, and effective ways of controlling the looming epidemic of cardiovascular disease and stroke, worldwide.

Antiplatelet therapy

In the late 1950s and mid-1960s two research paths converged. The first involved the identification of platelet fibrin thrombogenesis as a cause of retinal and hemispheric TIAs. The other involved investigators in Toronto, New York, and Oxford who coincidently determined that several drugs – sulfinpyrazone, aspirin, and dipyridamole – altered platelet responsiveness both in the test tube and in experimentally injured arteries.[58–60] Clinical trials of platelet inhibitors were subsequently undertaken for the prevention of stroke, interestingly before being tested in other vascular diseases. The first was a small trial of dipyridamole involving only 169 patients, which showed no benefit.[61] Next, the Canadian Cooperative Study was undertaken using a factorial study design in which patients received aspirin 1300 mg daily, sulfinpyrazone 800 mg, both or neither in patients with a recognizable arterial origin for their TIA or non-disabling stroke.[62] After 585 patients, two thirds male and one third female, had been followed for an average of 28 months, the investigators reported that patients in the two arms of the trial containing aspirin compared with those

not on aspirin had a RRR of 31% for the combined end point of stroke and death. No benefit was detected in the sulfinpyrazone arm. A subgroup analysis reported no benefit for the 200 women in the trial and when the results for men alone were analyzed in a data generated subgroup, a 48% benefit in stroke and death was observed in the aspirin containing groups.

Since the publication of that important study there has been a flurry of activity. Most importantly, the mode of action and effectiveness of aspirin has been well elucidated, and several new antiplatelet agents identified and tested. Aspirin inhibits thromboxane A_2 formation by irreversibly acetylating the platelet enzyme cyclo-oxygenase. Thromboxane A_2 is an important stimulus for platelet aggregation and release. Platelet aggregation is thus inhibited for up to 10 days after exposure to aspirin. Absorption of aspirin occurs rapidly and peak plasma concentrations are reached within 1–3 hours. Even though the plasma half life of aspirin is short, antiplatelet activity is prolonged, but bleeding times return to normal within two days of cessation of aspirin. In a meta-analysis of 145 randomized trials of antiplatelet therapy, aspirin was shown to be associated with a RRR of all vascular events (including stroke) of about 22%.[63] **Grade A1a**

Aspirin is, therefore, appropriate for all patients with ischemic stroke unless there is specific contraindication, such as aspirin sensitivity. Aspirin given to patients with a history of stroke or TIA reduces the relative risk of stroke and other important vascular events by about 14% (95% CI 4–21),[64] from about 7% to 6% per year. This equates to an ARR of 1·0% and an NNT of 100. Aspirin is also beneficial in such patients who also have atrial fibrillation (AF). The annual risk of stroke has been shown to be reduced from 12% to 10%, a RRR of 14% (95% CI 15–36) and an ARR of 2·0%.[65]

In the mid-1990s, there was much controversy over the most effective dose of aspirin.[66–68] The optimal dose for efficacy and tolerability is low dose aspirin (100–300 mg daily). Gastrointestinal side effects such as gastritis and hemorrhage are more common in older people and are dependent on the dose and duration of treatment. The small risk of intracerebral hemorrhage with prolonged use of aspirin is outweighed by the benefits in high-risk patients.

Among the other antiplatelet agents, dipyridamole, ticlopidine and clopidogrel have all been shown to be beneficial in the secondary prevention of stroke. Compared with aspirin, clopidogrel reduces the relative risk of stroke and other major vascular events by about 10% (95% CI 3–17)[69,70] from about 6·0% (aspirin) to 5·4% (clopridogrel) per year, which is an ARR of 0·6% compared with aspirin, and equates to about a NNT of 166 compared with aspirin, and probably 62 compared with aspirin. **Grade A1a**

Although expensive, clopidogrel is as safe as aspirin and, unlike the closely related agent ticlopidine, is not known to cause an excess of neutropenia and thrombocytopenia.[70,71] In the European Stroke Prevention Study 2 (ESPS 2),[72] 6602 patients were given aspirin (25 mg twice daily), modified-release dipyridamole (200 mg twice daily), the combination or placebo. The RRR for the combined end points of stroke and death were 13·2% for aspirin, 15·4% for dipyridamole, and 24·4% for the combination of aspirin and dipyridamole. An update of the data indicates that compared with aspirin, the combination of aspirin and modified-release dipyridamole reduces the risk of stroke by about 23% (95% CI 7–37), and that this effect is greater for stroke than other serious vascular events.[73,74] **Grade A1c**

Anticoagulants

AF is a major risk factor for stroke. It predisposes to the formation of intracardiac thrombi, mainly within the atria, that may embolize to the brain and other organs. The prevalence of AF increases with age, from 0·5% in patients aged 50–59 years to about 9% in patients over the age of 70 years.[75] With an aging population, it is likely that AF will become an increasingly important public health problem. Overall, the annual risk of stroke is about 5%, but rates vary from less than 2% to more than 10% according to the presence of one or more clinical characteristics such as congestive cardiac failure, hypertension, older age (≥75 years), diabetes and previous history of stroke or TIA.[76] **Grade A1a**

There is good evidence that warfarin and aspirin are both highly efficacious in preventing stroke (and other vascular and embolic events) in patients with AF. Six randomized trials have evaluated warfarin with placebo,[77–82] two other trials have compared warfarin with aspirin,[83,84] and a meta-analysis[85] indicates a 64% RRR of stroke favoring warfarin over placebo and a 48% RRR favoring warfarin over aspirin. Aspirin is associated with a RRR of 22%.[86,87] Given the consistency of the treatment effects across subgroups of patients, the absolute benefits of antithrombotic therapy is high in those patients who are at highest risk of stroke. Thus, the decision to commence warfarin anticoagulation therapy is usually based on an evaluation of the risks and benefits in an individual patient. Bleeding is the main risk associated with warfarin. Results of the pooled analyses of the major studies show a slightly higher frequency of major bleeding events in warfarin treated groups compared with placebo (1·3% v 1·0% per year). On the basis of these data, a target international normalized ratio (INR) of between 2·0 and 3·0 is generally recommended as a safe and effective level of anticoagulation.[88] These recommendations are further supported by the results of the Stroke Prevention in Reversible Ischemic Trial (SPIRIT),[89] which involved 1316 patients with TIA or minor stroke in which aspirin (30 mg daily) was compared with warfarin and a target INR of 3·0 to 4·5. The trial was stopped after the first scheduled interim analysis due to an excess of major bleeding in the warfarin group, and no significant difference between groups in the incidence of the non-hemorrhagic end points (hazard ratio 1·03, 95% CI 0·6–1·75).

Based on small studies only, warfarin (or heparin) appears to reduce the incidence of stroke in patients with recent anterior myocardial infarction.[90] Patients who have had a recent stroke or TIA in conjunction with a recent myocardial infarction should be given heparin therapy followed by 3–6 months of warfarin therapy.[91] In the setting of acute ischemic stroke attributed to cardio-embolism, though, it is often advisable to wait at least a week before commencing anticoagulation, in order to prevent hemorrhagic transformation of the infarct. **Grade B2**

In the absence of a potential cardiac source for the stroke, such as AF, recent transmural, anterior, myocardial infarction, dilated cardiomyopathy, valvular heart disease, there are presently no other clear indications for warfarin therapy for the prevention of stroke. In the recently completed Warfarin-Aspirin Recurrent Stroke Study (WARSS), there was no significant difference in the prevention of recurrent ischemic stroke, death or intracranial hemorrhage between the groups, although there was a slight trend for aspirin superiority.[92] **Grade A1a**

There may be benefit of warfarin in certain other subgroups of patients with vascular disease. On the basis of retrospective observational data, the Warfarin-Aspirin Symptomatic Intracranial Disease study[93] a clinical trial has commenced comparing warfarin with aspirin in patients with severe intracranial arterial stenosis.

Cholesterol lowering therapy

The relation between diet, serum cholesterol levels and ischemic heart disease is relatively well understood but the evidence is less reliable and more complex for stroke. This reflects, in part, the diversity of stroke pathogenesis, with qualitatively different associations of serum cholesterol with the risks of ischemic and hemorrhagic stroke.[94–98] High serum cholesterol is considered an important risk factor for ischemic stroke, more so in Western societies than in Asian populations,[99] whereas a weak inversion association is apparent between serum cholesterol and the risk of intracerebral hemorrhage. Although there have been no completed randomized trials of cholesterol lowering therapy in patients with stroke or TIA alone, several large scale, randomized trials have established that long-term use of certain 3-hydroxy-3-methylglutaryl co-enzyme A reductase inhibitors (statins) results in significant reductions in the risk of major cardiovascular events in patients with a wide range of lipid levels, both[100] with[101–103] and without,[104,105] a history of coronary artery disease. The evidence suggests that lowering serum cholesterol with statins can reduce the risk of stroke by about 25% (95% CI 14–41) over just a few years of therapy.[106] **Grade A1a**

Carotid endarterectomy

Symptomatic disease

Atherosclerotic disease of the carotid artery is an important cause of stroke. The risk of recurrent stroke in recently symptomatic patients with severe carotid stenosis is as high as 28% over 2 years. The introduction of carotid artery surgery in 1954 by Eastcott, Pickering, and Rob heralded a new era in stroke prevention. In 1967 a randomized trial was launched to evaluate this exciting prospect of carotid endarterectomy, with results published in 1970.[107] The trial, despite its merits, was not supportive of the procedure due to a number of problems including the small sample size of only 316 randomized patients and relatively high perioperative complication rate of 11%. In addition, almost half of the patients had symptoms only in the vertebral basilar vascular territory and too many patients were lost to follow up (12% in the surgical and 1·3% in the medical group). A second small trial conducted at the same time but reported much later, was overwhelmingly negative due to a high perioperative complication rate.[108]

These negative trials did not reduce the enthusiasm for the procedure. By 1985 a total of 107 000 endarterectomies were being carried out annually in the United States and it was estimated that a cumulative total of one million endarterectomies had been conducted for both symptomatic and asymptomatic disease. The appropriateness of patient selection and the awareness that in many centers, a forbiddingly high level of operative morbidity and mortality existed, led to a requirement for high quality clinical trials.

The two major trials for symptomatic disease are the North American Symptomatic Carotid Endarterectomy Trial (NASCET) and the European Carotid Surgery Trial (ECST), which between them included nearly 6000 patients, and they have demonstrated convincingly the benefits of carotid endarterectomy.[109,110] A third smaller trial, when stopped,

had a trend towards the same result but involved only 189 patients.[111] NASCET and ECST required angiography for entry and demanded focal hemisphere or retinal minor stroke or TIAs within 180 days. Both stopped the randomization of patients with severe stenosis because of compelling evidence on interim analyses demonstrating a clear reduction in ipsilateral strokes with endarterectomy. Both trials also showed no net benefit of surgery for all patients with mild-moderate grades of stenosis.[112,113] NASCET and ECST used measurements of the narrowest diameter of the stenosed segment as the numerator based on angiographic criteria. The results from NASCET demonstrated a 2 year 65% relative and a 17% absolute risk reduction favoring endarterectomy (Table 59·2). When the ECST angiograms were remeasured by the NASCET method and the results calculated for the reduced number of patients who would be "severe" by NASCET criteria, the favorable results in the survival curves for surgery were very similar.[114] **Grade A1a**

The compelling results in favor of endarterectomy for severe stenosis in NASCET and ECST are dependent on two important caveats. First, the surgical complication rate undertaken by experienced surgeons was low. In NASCET the occurrence of any stroke, disabling or mild, lasting more than 24 hours or death in the 30 day period was 5·8%. For disabling stroke and perioperative death, the complication rate was 2·1%. The long-term benefits of endarterectomy are abolished as the complication rate exceeds 10%. Surgeons must therefore be highly skilled.

Second, the results relate to a measurement of the degree of stenosis from conventional carotid angiograms. Conventional angiography carries a 1% risk of stroke; one stroke in five is disabling.[115] In NASCET, from 2929 angiograms performed in 100 centers, the minor and non-disabling stroke rate was 0·6%, the disabling stroke rate 0·1%. While this rate was high, it was only one tenth the risk of stroke from

Table 59.4 Risk of ipsilateral stroke or any perioperative stroke or perioperative death – NASCET. (Reproduced with permission from *Neurology* 1996;46:605)

Study time	Risk (%) medical	Risk (%) surgical	Risk (%) difference	RRR (%)	NNT
30 days	3·3	5·8	−2·5	—	—
1 year	17·3	7·5	9·8	57	10
2 years	26·0	9·0	17·0	65	6

From the North American Symptomatic Carotid Endarterectomy Trial (NASCET), the risk of stroke for 331 medically treated and 328 surgically treated patients with symptoms appropriate to severe stenosis are given at 30 days, 1 and 2 years. To prevent one stroke in 2 years, six patients need to have endarterectomy.
Abbreviations: NNT, number needed to treat by endarterectomy to prevent one stroke within the specified study time; RRR, relative risk reduction

endarterectomy: 5·8% for any stroke or death and 2·1% for disabling stroke or death. Modern non-invasive carotid imaging such as MRI, spiral CT and duplex and Doppler ultrasound avoids the risk associated with conventional intra-arterial catheter carotid angiography. However, it is important that the reliability of images obtained are well established in order to avoid operating on patients with false-positive scans, or denying benefits of the intervention in those with false-negative scans.[116] Moreover, carotid ultrasound alone will not identify important lesions of the intracranial arteries. Aneurysms and stenosis of intracranial vessels exists in about 2% and 5% of patients symptomatic with extracranial stenosis, respectively. If such lesions are identified, the benefit:risk ratio of endarterectomy will be reduced.

Although endarterectomy remains the standard treatment for a well defined group of high-risk patients, there is growing interest in the use of percutaneous, transluminal angioplasty (PTA) and stenting for carotid stenosis to avoid the significant risk of stroke or death of between 6% and 8% associated with surgery. In the Carotid and Vertebral Artery Transluminal Angioplasty Study (CAVATAS) involving over 500 patients, almost all with symptomatic carotid stenosis, randomized to PTA and surgery, the 30 day outcomes were almost identical for the groups.[117] The rate of death or any major stroke was 9·9% after surgery and 10·0% after angioplasty. Analysis of the other risks of treatment confirmed that PTA was safer than surgery in terms of minor morbidity, reduced hospital length of stay, but was associated with a higher rate of (asymptomatic) restenosis during follow up. Stents suitable for carotid use have only been available in recent years and few were used in CAVATAS. Given advances in technology in this area, further clinical trials are underway to evaluate whether primary carotid stenting should be the surgical procedure of choice for carotid stenosis based on effectiveness, lower risks and reduced costs.

Asymptomatic disease

Design flaws in early trials prevented conclusive evidence being gained about the benefit of endarterectomy in patients with asymptomatic carotid stenosis. In the Carotid Artery Stenosis with Asymptomatic Narrowing: Operation Versus Aspirin (CASANOVA) trial, patients with greater than 90% stenosis were excluded and crossovers were common between the medical and surgical groups, while in the Mayo Asymptomatic Carotid Endarterectomy (MACE) trial, standard medical care including use of aspirin, was not extended to the surgical arm. The United States Veterans Administration (VA) trial was small, with only 444 patients, and reported a perioperative complication rate of 4·4%, but the stroke-free survival curves were similar in patients receiving endarterectomy to those given best medical care alone.[118] A fourth trial, the Asymptomatic Carotid Atherosclerosis Study (ACAS), used a more robust design and randomized 1662 patients. A significant benefit was demonstrated in favor of endarterectomy with a RRR of 53% after 2·7 years of average follow up.[119] However, there are reservations about the clinical significance of this result (see Table 59.5). The absolute benefits of the procedure in this setting are small, RRR of 1% per year, so that 67 patients are required to undergo endarterectomy to prevent one stroke in 2 years. This is in contrast to the six symptomatic patients required to derive benefit with similarly severe disease. When the perioperative complication rate exceeds 3%, the benefits are negated. A higher figure is known to be common. Thus, endarterectomy for all patients with asymptomatic carotid stenosis is not a cost effective procedure. **Grade A1c**

All of the symptomatic trials and major observational case-series studies have observed a worsening of prognosis with increasing degrees of carotid stenosis.[120,121] However, there is also a strong association between cardiovascular risk

Table 59.5   Risk of ipsilateral stroke or any perioperative stroke or perioperative death (based upon 825 patients randomized to CEA) — ACAS. (Reproduced with permission from *Neurology* 1996;46:605)

Study time	Risk (%) medical	Risk (%) surgical	Risk (%) difference	RRR (%)	NNT
30 days	0·4	2·3	−1·9	–	–
1 year	2·4	3·0	−0·6	–	–
2 years	5·0	3·5	1·5	30	67
5 years	11·0	5·1	5·9	53	17

From the Asymptomatic Carotid Atherosclerosis Study (ACAS), the risk of stroke is compared between the medically and surgically treated patients. To prevent one stroke in 2 years, 67 patients need to have endarterectomy. Adjusting the surgical arm to include only the patients who had endarterectomy, the 30 day surgical risk becomes 2·6% and the 1, 2 and 5 year risks rise to 3·3%, 3·8% and 5·4% respectively. The number needed to treat to prevent one stroke in 2 years becomes 83.
Abbreviations: NNT, number needed to treat by endarterectomy to prevent one stroke within the specified study time; RRR, relative risk reduction

factors and carotid stenosis in all age groups.[122] Thus, although the reduction in strokes after endarterectomy is found to be greatest in those with the most severe stenosis, there remains uncertainty about the benefits of endarterectomy in the elderly, including those with asymptomatic disease.[123] In view of this uncertainty, a fifth and largest trial is being conducted in Europe, the Asymptomatic Carotid Surgery Trial (ACST).[124] It is possible that a high-risk patient subgroup, for example those with high grade stenosis (85–99%) and a high vascular risk profile, will be identified in which endarterectomy is definitely cost effective for asymptomatic carotid disease. In the meantime, only carefully selected high risk patients should be recommended for endarterectomy, conducted by the most expert of surgeons.

Conclusions

Four decades of clinical observation and randomized controlled trials in stroke prevention have provided very positive and promising results. Several key points emerge:

- Modifiable risk factors for stroke have been identified. From a public health viewpoint, risk factors of greatest importance in the prevention of stroke are those that carry a high population-attributable risk, such as high blood pressure, obesity, high cholesterol levels, physical inactivity, and cigarette smoking. Stroke prevention in the community requires manipulation of these risk factors in individuals at high risk and in the whole population.

- Given the continuous relationship between levels of risk factors and stroke risk, effective prevention of stroke involves the management of the patient as a *whole* person defined by their absolute risk of future major vascular events rather than by a single variable such as the level of blood pressure or serum cholesterol.

- On the basis of a large body of direct and indirect evidence, clinicians should now consider blood pressure lowering therapy as pivotal to the prevention of recurrent stroke in all patients with cerebrovascular disease, irrespective of blood pressure levels, age and other characteristics. Although there is no evidence at present to guide the timing of blood pressure lowering therapy after the onset of stroke, pragmatically it is probably wise to wait until patients are clinically stable. The evidence is strong for therapy that maximizes the degree of blood pressure reduction using an ACE inhibitor-based regimen.

- Aspirin is cheap, safe, familiar and acceptable as the antiplatelet agent of first choice for patients with vascular disease. The optimal dose of aspirin is 100–300 mg. Aspirin is also the first choice for patients with acute ischemic stroke, commencing within 48 hours of onset. Clopidogrel is more expensive and combination aspirin

and modified-release dypridamole is less well tolerated but both agents offer modest benefits over aspirin.

- Warfarin is indicated only for patients with a proven or potential, cardiac (embolic) source of stroke. Warfarin is favored when the risk of stroke is high and aspirin is favored when the risk of stroke is low. Various clinical parameters have been well identified that allow clinical stratification of risk.

- Carotid endarterectomy is indicated for patients with severe carotid artery stenosis who have had symptoms of retinal or brain ischemia appropriate to the stenosis, and are willing to undergo a small but definite risk of death or disability related to the procedure undertaken by an experienced surgeon. PTA may be undertaken as an alternative to carotid endarterectomy in experienced hands. There remains uncertainty about the cost effectiveness of endarterectomy in patients with high grade asymptomatic stenosis and that of carotid stenting.

- Cholesterol lowering therapy with statins is safe, well tolerated and cost effective in preventing major vascular events including stroke in all high-risk individuals irrespective of baseline cholesterol levels.

- Well organized care and rehabilitation within stroke units or services has been shown to save lives and reduce long-term dependency. The key components of such care should include multidisciplinary team approach, active participation of family, special education and training of staff, and early commencement of rehabilitation.

- The primary focus of thrombolytic therapy is to restore, preserve and improve circulation to acute focal brain ischemia. Although rt-PA remains the only approved hyperacute stroke therapy, all other data suggest that other thrombolytic or neuroprotective approaches are likely to have very short time-windows for efficacy and safety. While the risk of bleeding is significant, it is comparable with the risks associated with other procedures such as carotid endarterectomy. Effective community and professional education, motivation and training are likely to be important for more widespread application as acute stroke treatment.

References

1. Murray CJL, Lopez AD. *Global Health Statistics*. Geneva: World Health Organization, 1996.
2. Warlow CP. Epidemiology of stroke. *Lancet* 1998;**352** (Suppl. 3):SIII 1–4.
3. Bonita R, Anderson C, Broad J, Jamrozik K, Stewart-Wynne E, Anderson N. Stroke incidence and case-fatality in Australasia: a comparison of the Auckland and Perth population-based stroke registers. *Stroke* 1994;**25**:552–7.
4. Bonita R, Broad J, Beaglehole R, Anderson N. Changes in incidence and case-fatality in Auckland, New Zealand, 1981–1991. *Lancet* 1993;**342**:1470–3.

5. Anderson CS, Jamrozik KD, Broadhurst RJ, Stewart-Wynne EG. Predicting survival for 1 year among different subtypes of stroke. Results from the Perth Community Stroke Study. *Stroke* 1994;**25**:1935–44.

6. Bonita R, Stewart AWS, Ford M. Predicting survival after stroke: a three-year follow up. *Stroke* 1988;**19**:669–73.

7. Hankey G, Jamrozik K, Broadhurst R *et al.* Long-term risk of recurrent stroke in the Perth Community Stroke Study. *Stroke* 1998;**29**:2491–500.

8. Burn J, Dennis M, Bamford J, Sandercock P, Wade D, Warlow C. Long-term risk of recurrent stroke after a first-ever stroke: The Oxfordshire Community Stroke Project. *Stroke* 1994;**25**:333–7.

9. House A. Mood disorders after stroke: a review of the evidence. *Int J Geriatric Psychiatry* 1987;**2**:211–21.

10. De la Torre JC. Alzheimer Disease as a vascular disorder: nosological evidence. *Stroke* 2002;**33**:1152–62.

11. Thom JT. Stroke mortality trends: an international perspective. *Ann Epidemiol* 1993;**3**:509–18.

12. Bonita R, Beaglehole R. Monitoring stroke: an international challenge. *Stroke* 1995;**26**:541–2.

13. Bonita R, Broad JB, Beaglehole R. Changes in stroke incidence and case-fatality Auckland, New Zealand in 1981–1991. *Lancet* 1993;**342**:1470–2.

14. Stegmayr B, Asplund K, Wester PO. Trends in incidence, case fatality rate, and severity of stroke in Northern Sweden, 1985–1991. *Stroke* 1994;**25**:1738–45.

15. Brown RD, Whisnant JP, Sicks JD, O'Fallon WM, Wiebers DO. Stroke incidence, prevalence, and survival: secular trends in Rochester, Minnesota, through 1989. *Stroke* 1996;**27**:373–80.

16. Jamrozik K, Broadhurst RJ, Lai N, Hankey GJ, Burvill PW, Anderson CS. Trends in the incidence, severity, and short-term outcome of stroke in Perth, Western Australia. *Stroke* 1999;**30**:2105–11.

17. Thorvaldsen P, Davidsen M, Brønnum-Hansen H, Schroll M, for the Danish MONICA Study Group. Stable stroke occurrence despite incidence reduction in an aging population: stroke trends in the Danish Monitoring trends and determinants in cardiovascular disease (MONICA) population. *Stroke* 1999;**30**:2529–34.

18. Gillum RF, Sempos CT. The end of the long-term decline in stroke mortality in the United States. *Stroke* 1997;**28**:1527–9.

19. Sarti C, Tuomilehto J, Sivenious J *et al.* Declining trends in incidence, case-fatality and mortality of stroke in three geographical areas of Finland during 1983–1989: results from the FINMONICA stroke register. *J Clin Epidemiol* 1994;**47**:1259–69.

20. Ryglewicz D, Polakowska M, Lechowicz W *et al.* Stroke mortality rates in Poland did not decline between 1984 and 1992. *Stroke* 1997;**28**:752–7.

21. Malmgren R, Bamford J, Warlow C, Sandercock P, Slattery J. Projecting the number of patients with first ever strokes and patients newly-handicapped by stroke in England and Wales. *BMJ* 1989;**298**:656–60.

22. Reddy KS, Yusuf S. Emerging epidemic of cardiovascular disease in developing countries. *Circulation* 1998;**97**:596–601.

23. Hankey GJ, Warlow CP. Treatment and secondary prevention of stroke: evidence, costs, and effects on individuals and populations. *Lancet* 1999;**354**:1457–63.

24. Stroke Unit Trialists' Collaboration. Collaborative systematic review of the randomised trials of organised in-patient (stroke unit) care after stroke. *BMJ* 1997;**314**:1151–9.

25. The European Ad Hoc Consensus Group. European strategies for early intervention in stroke. A report of an ad hoc consensus group meeting. *Cerebrovasc Dis* 1996;**6**:315–24.

26. Organising Committees. Asia Pacific Consensus Forum on Stroke Management. *Stroke* 1998;**29**:1730–6.

27. Young J. Is stroke better managed in the community? *BMJ* 1994;**309**:1356–8.

28. Langhorne P, Dennis MS and collaborators. Services for reducing duration of hospital care for acute stroke patients (Cochrane Review). In: The Cochrane Library, 1, 1999. Oxford: Update Software.

29. Beech R, Rudd AG, Tilling K, Wolfe CDA. Economic consequences of early inpatient discharge to community-based rehabilitation for stroke in an inner-London teaching hospital. *Stroke* 1999;**30**:729–35.

30. Anderson C, Ni Mhurchu C, Rubenach S, Clark M, Spencer C, Winsor A. Home or hospital for stroke rehabilitation? Results of a randomised controlled trial. II: Cost minimisation analysis at 6 months. *Stroke* 2000;**31**:1032–7.

31. Intercollegiate Working Party for Stroke. *National Clinical Guidelines for Stroke*. London, England: Royal College of Physicians; 2000.

32. National Institute of Neurological Disorders and Stroke r-tPA Stroke Study Group. Tissue plasminogen activator for acute ischemic stroke. *N Engl J Med* 1995;**333**:1581–7.

33. Wardlaw J, del Zoppo G, Yamaguchi T. Thrombolysis for acute ischemic stroke (Cochrane review). Cochrane Database Syst Rev. 2000;(2):CD000213.

34. Ringleb PA, Schellinger PD, Schranz C, Hacke W. Thrombolytic therapy within 3 to 6 hours after onset of ischemic stroke: useful or harmful? *Stroke* 2002;**33**:1437–41.

35. International Stroke Trial Collaborative Group. The International Stroke Trial (IST): a randomized trial of aspirin, subcutaneous heparin, both, or neither among 19 435 patients with acute ischemic stroke. *Lancet* 1997;**349**:1569–14.

36. CAST (Chinese Acute Stroke Trial) Collaborative Group. CAST: randomized placebo-controlled trial of early aspirin use in 20 000 patients with acute ischemic stroke. *Lancet* 1997;**349**:1641–9.

37. Adams HP, Brott TG, Furlan AJ *et al.* Guidelines for thrombolytic therapy for acute stroke: a supplement for the guidelines for the management of patients with acute ischemic stroke: a statement for healthcare professionals from a special writing group of the Stroke Council, American Heart Association. *Circulation* 1996;**94**:1167–74.

38. Morgenstern LB, Staub L, Chan E *et al.* Improving delivery of acute stroke therapy: the TLL Temple Foundation Stroke Project. *Stroke* 2002;**33**:160–6.

39. Caplan LR, Moht JP, Kistler JP, Koroshetz W. Should thrombolytic therapy be the first-line treatment of acute ischemic stroke? Thrombolysis: not a panacea for ischemic stroke. *N Engl J Med* 1997;**337**:1309–10.

40. Gubitz G, Counsell C, Sandercock P. Anticoagulants for acute ischemic stroke (Cochrane Review). In The Cochrane Library. Issue 4. Oxford, UK: Update Software, 2001.

41. Adams HP. Emergent use of anticoagulation for treatment of patients with ischemic stroke. *Stroke* 2002;**33**:856–61.

42. Rose G. Sick individuals and sick populations. *Int J Epidemiol* 1985;**14**:32–8.

43. Hankey GJ. Smoking and risk of stroke. *J Cardiovasc Risk* 1999;**5**:207–11.

44. Wolf PA. Epidemiology and risk factor management. In: Welch KMA, Caplan LR, Reis DJ, Siesjö BK, Weir B, eds. *Primer on cerebrovascular diseases*. San Diego: Academic Press, 1997.

45. The Diabetes Control and Complications Trial Research Group. The effect of intensive treatment of diabetes on the development and progression of long-term complications in insulin-dependent diabetes mellitus. *N Engl J Med* 1993; **329**:977–86.

46. MacMahon S, Peto R, Cutler J, Collins R, Sorlie Pea. Blood pressure, stroke, and coronary heart disease. Part 1, prolonged differences in blood pressure: prospective observational studies corrected for regression dilution bias. *Lancet* 1990;**335**:765–74.

47. Collins R, Peto R, MacMahon S *et al.* Blood pressure, stroke, coronary heart disease. Part 2, short-term reductions in blood pressure: overview of randomised drug trials in their epidemiological context. *Lancet* 1990;**336**:827–38.

48. Prospective Studies Collaboration. Cholesterol, diastolic blood pressure and stroke; 13 000 strokes in 45 000 people in 45 prospective cohorts. *Lancet* 1995;**346**:1647–53.

49. Eastern Stroke and Coronary Heart Disease Collaborative Research Group. Blood pressure, cholesterol and stroke in Eastern Asia. *Lancet* 1998;**352**:1801–7.

50. Asia Pacific Cohort Studies Collaboration. Determinants of Cardiovascular Disease in the Asia Pacific region: Protocol for a Collaborative Overview of Cohort Studies. *CVD Prevention* 1999;**2**:281–9.

51. MacMahon S, Rodgers A. The effects of antihypertensive treatment on vascular disease: reappraisal of the evidence in 1994. *J Vasc Med Biology* 1993;**4**:265–71.

52. Insua JT, Sacks HS, Lau TS *et al.* Drug treatment of hypertension in the elderly: a meta-analysis. *Ann Int Med* 1994;**121**: 355–62.

53. Staessen JA, Gasowski J, Wang JG *et al.* Risks of untreated and treated isolated systolic hypertension in the elderly: meta-analysis of outcome trials. *Lancet* 2000;**355**:865–72.

54. The Heart Outcomes Prevention Evaluation (HOPE) Study Investigators. Effects of an angiotensin-converting-enzyme inhibitor, ramipril, on cardiovascular events in high-risk patients. *N Engl J Med* 2000;**342**:145–53.

55. Bosch J, Yusuf S, Progue J *et al.* on behalf of the HOPE Investigators. Use of ramipril in preventing stroke: double blind randomized trial. *BMJ* 2002;**324**:1–5.

56. Rodgers A, Neal B, MacMahon S. The effects of blood pressure lowering in cerebrovascular disease: an overview of randomized controlled trials. *Neurol Rev Int* 1997; **12**:12–15.

57. PROGRESS Collaborative Group. Randomized trial of a perindopril-based blood-pressure-lowering regimen among 6105 individuals with previous stroke or transient ischemic attack. *Lancet* 2001;**358**:1033–41.

58. Mustard JF, Rowsell HC, Smythe HA, Senyi A, Murphy EA. The effect of sulfinpyrazone on platelet economy and thrombus formation in rabbits. *Blood* 1967;**29**:859–66.

59. Weiss HJ, Aledort LM. Impaired platelet/connective-tissue reaction in man after aspirin ingestion. *Lancet* 1967;**ii**:495–7.

60. Emmons PR, Harrison MJ, Honour AJ, Mitchell JR. Effect of a pyrimido pyrimidine derivative on thrombus formation in the rabbit. *Nature* 1965;**208**:255.

61. Acheson J, Danta G, Hutchinson EC. Controlled trial of dipyridamole in cerebral vascular disease. *BMJ* 1969;**1**:614–5.

62. The Canadian Cooperative Study Group. A randomized trial of aspirin and sulfinpyrazone in threatened stroke. *N Engl J Med* 1978;**299**:53–9.

63. Antiplatelet Trialists' Collaboration. Collaborative overview of randomised trials of antiplatelet therapy in various categories of patients. *BMJ* 1994;**308**:81–106. [Published erratum appears *BMJ* 1994;**308**:1540.]

64. Alga A, van Gijn J. Cumulative meta-analysis of aspirin efficacy after cerebral ischaemia of arterial origin. *J Neurol Neurosurg Psychiatry* 1999;**66**:255.

65. European Atrial Fibrillation Trial Study Group. Secondary prevention in nonrheumatic atrial fibrillation after transient ischemic attack or minor stroke. *Lancet* 1993; **342**: 1255–62.

66. Barnett HJM, Kaste M, Meldrum HE, Eliasziw M. Aspirin dose in stroke prevention: beautiful hypotheses slain by ugly facts. *Stroke* 1996;**27**:588–92.

67. Hart RG, Harrison MJG. Aspirin wars: the optimal dose of aspirin to prevent stroke. *Stroke* 1996;**27**:585–7.

68. Patrono C, Roth GJ. Aspirin in ischemic cerebrovascular disease: how strong is the case for a different dosing regimen? *Stroke* 1996;**27**:756–60.

69. CAPRIE Steering Committee. A randomized, blinded, trial of clopidogrel versus aspirin in patients at risk of ischemic events (CAPRIE). *Lancet* 1996;**348**:1329–39.

70. Hankey GJ, Sudlow CLM, Dunbabin DW. Thienopyridines or aspirin to prevent stroke and other serious vascular events in patients at high risk of vascular disease. *Stroke* 2000; **31**:1779–84.

71. Hankey GJ. Clopidogrel and thrombotic thrombocytopenic purpura. *Lancet* 2000;**356**:269–270.

72. Diener HC, Cunha L, Forbes C *et al.* European Stroke Prevention Study 2. Dipyridamole and acetylsalicylic acid in the secondary prevention of stroke. *J Neurol Sci* 1996;**143**:1–13.

73. Wilterdink JL, Easton JD. Dipyridamole plus aspirin in cerebrovascular disease. *Arch Neurol* 1999;**56**:1087–92.

74. De Schryver ELLM on behalf of the European. Australian Stroke Prevention in Reversible Ischaemia Trial (ESPRIT) Group. Design of ESPRIT: an international randomized trial for secondary prevention after non-disabling cerebral ischaemia of arterial origin. *Cerebrovasc Dis* 2000;**10**: 147–50.

75. Kannel WB, Abbott RD, Savage DD, McNamara PM. Coronary heart disease and atrial fibrillation: the Framingham Study. *Am Heart J* 1983;**106**:389–96.

76. Cage BF, Waterman AD, Shannon W, Boechler M, Rich MW, Radford MJ. Validation of clinical classification schemes for

predicting stroke: results from the National Registry of Atrial Fibrillation. *JAMA* 2001;**285**:2864–70.

77.Petersen P, Godtfredsen J, Boysen G. Placebo-controlled, randomized trial of warfarin and aspirin for prevention of thromboembolic complications in chronic atrial fibrillation. The Copenhagen AFASAK study. *Lancet* 1989;**i**:175.

78.The Boston Area Anticoagulation Trial for Atrial Fibrillation Investigators. The effect of low-dose warfarin on the risk of stroke in patients with nonrheumatic atrial fibrillation. *N Engl J Med* 1990;**323**:1505–11.

79.Connolly SJ, Laupacis A, Gent M *et al.* Canadian atrial fibrillation anticoagulation (CAFA) study. *J Am Coll Cardiol* 1991; **18**:349–55.

80.Stroke Prevention in Atrial Fibrillation Investigators. Stroke Prevention in Atrial Fibrillation Study: final results. *Circulation* 1991;**84**:527–39.

81.Ezekowitz MD, Bridgers SL, James KE *et al.* Warfarin in the prevention of stroke associated with nonrheumatic atrial fibrillation. *N Engl J Med* 1992;**327**:1406–12. (Erratum, *N Engl J Med* 1993;**328**:148.)

82.EAFT (European Atrial Fibrillation Trial) Study Group. Secondary prevention in non-rheumatic atrial fibrillation after transient ischemic attack or minor stroke. *Lancet* 1993; **342**:1255–62.

83.Stroke Prevention in Atrial Fibrillation Investigators. Warfarin versus aspirin for prevention of thromboembolism in atrial fibrillation: Stroke Prevention in Atrial Fibrillation II Study. *Lancet* 1994;**343**:687–91.

84.Stroke Prevention in Atrial Fibrillation Investigators. Adjusted-dose warfarin versus low-intensity, fixed-dose warfarin plus aspirin for high-risk patients with atrial fibrillation: Stroke Prevention in Atrial Fibrillation III randomized clinical trial. *Lancet* 1996;**348**:633–8.

85.The Atrial Fibrillation Investigators. Risk factors for stroke and efficacy of antithrombotic therapy in atrial fibrillation. Analysis of pooled data from five randomised controlled trials. *Arch Intern Med* 1994;**154**:1449–57. (Published erratum appears in *Arch Intern Med* 1994;**154**:2254.)

86.Hart RG, Benavente O, McBride R, Pearce LA. Antithrombotic therapy to prevent stroke in patients with atrial fibrillation: a meta-analysis. *Ann Intern Med* 1999;**131**: 492–501.

87.Laupacis A, Boysen G, Connolly S *et al.* The efficacy of aspirin; in patients with atrial fibrillation: analysis of pooled data from 3 randomised trials. *Arch Intern Med* 1997;**157**: 1237–40.

88.Ezekowitz MD, Levine JA. Preventing stroke in patients with atrial fibrillation. *JAMA* 1999;**281**:1830–5.

89.The Stroke Prevention in Reversible Ischemia Trial (SPIRIT) Study Group. A randomised trial of anticoagulants versus aspirin after cerebral ischemia of presumed arterial origin. *Ann Neurol* 1997;**42**:857–65.

90.Cerebral Embolism Task Force. Cardiogenic brain embolism: the second report of the Cerebral Embolism Task Force. *Arch Neurol* 1989;**86**:727.

91.Turpie AGG, Robinson JG, Doyle DJ *et al.* Comparison of high-dose with low-dose subcutaneous heparin to prevent left ventricular mural thrombosis in patients with acute transmural anterior myocardial infarction. *N Engl J Med* 1989;**320**:352–7.

92.Mohr JP, Thompson JL, Lazar RM *et al.* for the Warfarin-Aspirin Recurrent Stroke Study Group. A comparison of warfarin and aspirin for the prevention of recurrent ischemic stroke. *N Engl J Med* 2001;**345**:1444–51.

93.Chimowitz MI, Kokkinos J, Strong J *et al.* The Warfarin-Aspirin Symptomatic Intracranial Disease Study. *Neurology* 1995;**45**:1488–51.

94.Neaton JD, Blackburn H, Jacobs D. Serum cholesterol level and mortality findings for men screened in the Multiple Risk Factor Intervention Trial. *Arch Int Med* 1992;**152**: 1490–500.

95.Yano K, Reed DM, MacLean CJ. Serum cholesterol and hemorrhagic stroke in the Honolulu Heart Program. *Stroke* 1989;**20**:1460–5.

96.Iribarren C, Jacobs DR, Sadler M, Claxton AJ, Sidney S. Low total serum cholesterol and intracerebral hemorrhagic stroke: is the association confined to elderly men? The Kaiser Permanente Medical Care Program. *Stroke* 1996;**27**:1993–8.

97.How Lin C, Shimzu Y, Kato H *et al.* Cerebrovascular diseases in a fixed population of Hiroshima and Nagasaki, with special reference to relationship between type and risk factors. *Stroke* 1984;**15**:653–60.

98.Iso H, Jacobs DRJ, Wentworth D, Neaton JD, Cohen JD. Serum cholesterol levels and six-year mortality from stroke in 350 977 men screened for the Multiple Risk Factor Intervention Trial. *N Engl J Med* 1989;**320**:904–10.

99.Eastern Stroke and Coronary Heart Disease Collaborative Research Group. Blood pressure, cholesterol, and stroke in eastern Asia. *Lancet* 1998;**352**:1801–7.

100.The Heart Protection Study. Presented at the Scientific Sessions of the American Heart Association; 2001. Available at: http://www.ctsu.ox.ac.uk/~hps/.

101.Scandinavian Simvastatin Survival Study Group. Randomised trial of cholesterol lowering in 4444 patients with coronary heart disease: the Scandinavian Simvastatin Survival Study (4S). *Lancet* 1994;**344**:1383–9.

102.Sacks FM, Pfeffer MA, Moyé LA *et al.* The effect of pravastatin on coronary events after myocardial infarction in patients with average cholesterol levels. *N Engl J Med* 1996;**335**:1001–9.

103.The Long-term Intervention with Pravastatin in Ischemic Disease (LIPID) Study Group. Prevention of cardiovascular events and death with pravastatin in patients with coronary heart disease and a broad range of initial cholesterol levels. *N Engl J Med* 1998;**339**:1349–57.

104.Shepherd J, Cobbe SM, Ford I *et al.* Prevention of coronary heart disease with pravastatin in men with hypercholesterolaemia. *N Engl J Med* 1995;**333**:1301–7.

105.Downs JR, Clearfield M, Wies S *et al.* Priimary prevention of acute coronary events with lovastatin in men and women with average cholesterol levels: results of AFCAPS/Tex CAPS. *JAMA* 1998;**279**:1615–22.

106.Sandercock P. Statins for stroke prevention? *Lancet* 2001; **357**:1548–9.

107.Fields WS, Maslenikov V, Meyer JS *et al.* Joint study of extracranial arterial occlusion. V. Progress report of prognosis following surgery or nonsurgical treatment for transient cerebral ischemic attacks and cervical carotid artery lesions. *JAMA* 1970;**211**:1993–2003.

108.Shaw DA, Venables GS, Cartlidge NEF, Bates D, Dickinson PH. Carotid endarterectomy in patients with transient cerebral ischaemia. *J Neurol Sci* 1984;**64**:45–53.

109.North American Symptomatic Carotid Endarterectomy Trial Collaborators. Beneficial effect of carotid endarterectomy in symptomatic patients with high-grade carotid stenosis. *N Engl J Med* 1991;**325**:445–3.

110.European Carotid Surgery Trialists' Collaborative Group. MRC European Carotid Surgery Trial: interim results for symptomatic patients with severe (70–99%) or with mild (0–29%) carotid stenosis. *Lancet* 1991;**337**:1235–43.

111.Mayberg MR, Wilson SE, Yatsu F *et al.* Carotid endarterectomy and prevention of cerebral ischemia in symptomatic carotid stenosis. *JAMA* 1991;**266**:3289–94.

112.European Carotid Surgery Trialists' Collaborative Group. Randomised trial of endarterectomy for recently symptomatic carotid stenosis: final results of the MRC European Carotid Surgery Trial (ECST). *Lancet* 2000;**351**: 1379–87.

113.North American Symptomatic Carotid Endarterectomy Trial Collaborators. Benefit of carotid endarterectomy in patients with symptomatic, moderate or severe stenosis. *New Engl J Med* 1998;**339**:1415–25.

114.Barnett HJM, Warlow CP. Carotid endarterectomy and the measurement of stenosis. *Stroke* 1993;**24**:1281–4.

115.Hankey GJ, Warlow CP, Molyneuz AJ. Complications of cerebral angiography for patients with mild carotid territory ischaemia being considered for carotid endarterectomy. *J Neurol Neurosurg Psychiatr* 1990;**53**:542–8.

116.Eliasziw M, Rankin RN, Fox AJ, Haynes RB, Barnett HJM, for the North American Symptomatic Carotid Endarterectomy Trial (NASCET) Group. Accuracy and prognostic consequences of ultrasonography in identifying severe carotid artery stenosis. *Stroke* 1995;**26**:1747–52.

117.CAVATAS Investigators. Endovascular versus surgical treatment in patients with carotid stenosis in the Carotid and Vertebral Artery Transluminal Angioplasty Study: a randomised trial. *Lancet* 2001;**357**:1729–37.

118.Hobson RW II, Weiss DG, Fields WS *et al.* Efficacy of carotid endarterectomy for asymptomatic carotid stenosis. *N Engl J Med* 1993;**328**:221–7.

119.Executive Committee for the Asymptomatic Carotid Atherosclerosis Study. Endarterectomy for asymptomatic carotid artery stenosis. *JAMA* 1995;**273**:1421–8.

120.Hennerici M, Hulsbomer HB, Hefter H, Lemmerts D, Rautenberg W. Natural history of asymptomatic extracranial arterial disease: results of a long-term prospective study. *Brain* 1987;**110**:777–91.

121.Norris JW, Zhu CZ, Bornstein NM, Chambers BR. Vascular risks of asymptomatic carotid stenosis. *Stroke* 1991;**22**: 1485–90.

122.Lernfelt B, Forsberg M, Blomstrand C, Mellström D, Volkmann R. Cerebral atherosclerosis as predictor of stroke and mortality in representative elderly population. *Stroke* 2002;**33**:224–9.

123.Rothwell P. Carotid endarterectomy and prevention of stroke in the very elderly. *Lancet* 2001;**357**:1142–3.

124.Halliday AW, Thomas D, Mansfield A. The Asymptomatic Carotid Surgery Trial (ACST) rationale and design. *Eur J Vasc Surg* 1994;**8**:703–10.

60 Heart disease and pregnancy

Samuel C Siu, Jack M Colman

Introduction

Women with heart disease comprise approximately 1% of the population in obstetric referral centers,[1] though they are less frequently seen in general obstetric practice. Current data on pregnancy outcomes of women with heart disease are primarily from studies that were retrospective, focused on a particular cardiac lesion, or examined populations managed at a single institution or from an earlier era. Treatment recommendations are usually based on institutional experience or extrapolation from observational studies.

Pregnancy in most women with heart disease has a favorable outcome for both mother and fetus. With the exception of patients with Eisenmenger syndrome, pulmonary vascular obstructive disease and Marfan syndrome with aortopathy, maternal death during pregnancy in women with heart disease is rare.[1–5] However, pregnant women with heart disease do remain at risk for other complications, including heart failure, arrhythmia and stroke.

Women with congenital heart disease comprise the majority of pregnant women with heart disease seen at referral centers.[1,5] The next largest group includes women with rheumatic heart disease. Other important conditions less frequently encountered include peripartum dilated cardiomyopathy, hypertrophic cardiomyopathy and coronary artery disease. Gestational hypertension, arising de novo or superimposed on pre-existing hypertension, is responsible for around 15% of all maternal mortality and considerable morbidity.[6]

Cardiovascular physiology and pregnancy

Pregnancy is characterized by hormonally mediated changes in blood volume, red cell mass and heart rate, resulting in a 50% increase in cardiac output during the antepartum period.[7] Increases in LV end-diastolic dimension and volume are present by 14 weeks' gestation and reach maximum levels early in the third trimester.[8–12] Preload- and afterload-adjusted indices of contractility remain in the normal range during the antepartum period.[13] LV mass increases during pregnancy as a consequence of increased LV wall thickness. Gestational hormones, circulating prostaglandins and the low-resistance vascular bed in the placenta result in decreases in peripheral vascular resistance and blood pressure (BP). These physiological changes are exacerbated in multifetal gestations. During labor and delivery there are additional increases in cardiac output and oxygen consumption.[7,14] Immediately following delivery, relief of caval compression and autotransfusion from the emptied uterus result in a transient increase in cardiac output. Most of the hemodynamic changes of pregnancy have resolved by the second postpartum week, but complete return to normal does not occur until 6 months after delivery.[15,16] LV diastolic dimension, volume and mass also return to preconception levels by the sixth postpartum month.

Outcomes associated with specific cardiac lesions

Congenital heart lesions

Left to right shunts

The effect of increase in cardiac output on the volume-loaded right ventricle in *atrial septal defect* (ASD), or the left ventricle in *ventricular septal defect* (VSD) and *patent ductus arteriosus* (PDA), is counterbalanced by a decrease in peripheral vascular resistance. Consequently, the increase in volume overload is attenuated. In the absence of pulmonary hypertension, pregnancy, labor and delivery are well tolerated.[1,4,5,17] **Grade B2** However, arrhythmias, ventricular dysfunction and progression of pulmonary hypertension may occur, especially when the shunt is large or when there is pre-existing elevation of pulmonary artery pressure. Infrequently, particularly in ASD, paradoxical embolization may be encountered if systemic vasodilatation and/or elevation of pulmonary resistance promote transient right to left shunting.

Left ventricular outflow tract obstruction

When *aortic stenosis* (AS) complicates pregnancy it is usually due to congenital bicuspid aortic valve, which may also be associated with aortic coarctation and/or ascending aortopathy. Other causes of left ventricular (LV) outflow tract obstruction at, below and above the valve have similar hemodynamic consequences. Women with symptomatic aortic stenosis should delay pregnancy until after surgical correction.[18] **Grade B4** However, the absence of symptoms is not sufficient assurance that pregnancy will be well tolerated. In a pregnant woman with severe AS the limited ability to augment cardiac output may result in abnormal elevation of LV systolic and filling pressures, which in turn precipitate or exacerbate heart failure or ischemia. In addition the non-compliant, hypertrophied ventricle is sensitive to falls in preload. The consequent exaggerated drop in cardiac output may lead to hypotension. In a compilation of many small retrospective series, 65 patients were followed through 106 pregnancies with a maternal mortality of 11% and a perinatal mortality of 4%.[19] In 25 of the same 65 pregnancies managed more recently there was no maternal mortality, although maternal functional deterioration occurred in 20% of pregnancies.[19] Women with moderate or severe aortic stenosis continue to be at increased risk for pulmonary edema or arrhythmia during pregnancy.[1,5,19] **Grade B2** Intrapartum palliation by balloon valvuloplasty may be helpful in selected cases. **Grade C5**

In the absence of prosthetic dysfunction or residual aortic stenosis, patients with bioprosthetic aortic valves usually tolerate pregnancy well. Although it had been stated that pregnancy might accelerate the rate of degeneration of bioprosthetic or homograft valves, recent studies have shown that this is not the case.[20] **Grade B2** A study of 14 pregnancies in women who underwent pulmonary autograft aortic valve replacement (Ross procedure) reported favorable maternal and fetal outcomes except in one woman who developed postpartum LV dysfunction.[21] **Grade B4** Pregnancy in a woman with a mechanical valve prosthesis carries an increased risk of valve thrombosis as a result of the hypercoagulable state. The magnitude of this increased risk (3–14%) is greater if subcutaneous unfractionated heparin rather than warfarin is used as the anticoagulant agent; this may be the result of inadequate dosing, insufficient monitoring or reduced efficacy of heparin[18,22] **Grade B4** (see anticoagulation section under antepartum management).

Coarctation of the aorta

Maternal mortality with uncorrected coarctation was 3% in an early series; the risk was higher in the presence of associated cardiac defects, aortopathy or long-standing hypertension; aortic rupture accounted for 8 of the 14 reported deaths and occurred in the third trimester as well as in the postpartum period.[23] **Grade B4** The results of recent studies have been more encouraging. In 182 pregnancies reported in three recent studies, the only maternal death occurred in a woman with Turner syndrome who had previously undergone coarctation repair.[1,5,24] **Grade B2** The management of hypertension in uncorrected coarctation is particularly problematic in pregnancy, because satisfactory control of upper body hypertension may lead to excessive hypotension below the coarctation site, thereby compromising the fetus. Intrauterine growth restriction and premature

labor and delivery are more common. Following coarctation repair, the risk of dissection and rupture is reduced but not eliminated. Pregnant women with repaired coarctation are at increased risk for pregnancy-induced-hypertension, probably as a result of residual abnormalities in aortic compliance.[1,5,24] **Grade B2**

Pulmonary stenosis

Mild pulmonic stenosis, or pulmonic stenosis that has been alleviated by valvuloplasty or surgery, is well tolerated during pregnancy and fetal outcome is favorable.[1,5] **Grade B2** Although a woman with severe pulmonic stenosis may be asymptomatic, the increased hemodynamic load of pregnancy may precipitate right heart failure or atrial arrhythmias; such a patient should be considered for correction prior to pregnancy. **Grade C5** Even during pregnancy, balloon valvuloplasty may be feasible if symptoms of pulmonary stenosis progress.

Cyanotic heart disease: unrepaired and repaired

In uncorrected or palliated pregnant patients with cyanotic congenital heart disease, such as tetralogy of Fallot, single ventricle etc., the usual pregnancy-associated fall in systemic vascular resistance and rise in cardiac output exacerbate right to left shunting, leading to increased maternal hypoxemia and cyanosis. A study examining the outcomes of 96 pregnancies in 44 women with a variety of cyanotic congenital heart defects reported a high rate of maternal cardiac events (32%, including one death), prematurity (37%) and a low livebirth rate (43%).[25] **Grade B4** The lowest livebirth rate (12%) was observed in mothers with arterial oxygen saturation ≤85%.

Tetralogy of Fallot is the most common form of cyanotic congenital heart disease. Pregnancy risk is low in women who have had successful correction of tetralogy.[1,4,5] **Grade B2** However, residua and sequelae, such as residual shunt, right ventricular outflow tract obstruction, arrhythmias, pulmonary regurgitation, right ventricular systolic dysfunction, pulmonary hypertension (owing to the effects of a previous palliative shunt) or LV dysfunction (owing to previous volume overload), increase the likelihood of pregnancy complications and require independent consideration.

Atrial repair (that is Mustard or Senning procedure) was developed for the surgical correction of complete transposition of the great arteries. The anatomic right ventricle supports the systemic circulation. Late adult complications following atrial repair include sinus node dysfunction, atrial arrhythmias and dysfunction of the systemic ventricle. In 43 pregnancies in 31 women described in recent reports, there was one late maternal death.[26,27] **Grade B4** There was a 14% incidence of maternal heart failure, arrhythmias or cardiac deterioration. There have been no studies of pregnancy outcome in women who received the current repair of choice for complete transposition, the arterial switch procedure. However, in the absence of ventricular dysfunction, coronary obstruction or other important residua or sequelae, a good outcome is expected. **Grade C5**

The Fontan operation eliminates cyanosis and volume overload of the functioning systemic ventricle, but patients have a limited ability to increase cardiac output. In a review of 33 pregnancies in 21 women who were doing well after the Fontan operation there were 15 (45%) term pregnancies with no maternal mortality, although two women had cardiac complications and the incidence of first-trimester miscarriage was high (39%).[28] **Grade B4** As the 10 year survival following the Fontan operation is only 60–80% it is important that information regarding long-term maternal prognosis be discussed during preconception counseling.

Marfan syndrome

Life-threatening aortic complications of Marfan syndrome are due to medial aortopathy resulting in dilatation, dissection and valvular regurgitation. Risk is increased in pregnancy owing to hemodynamic stress and perhaps hormonal effects. Although older case reports suggested a very high mortality risk in the range of 30%, a subsequent study found an overall maternal mortality of 1% and fetal mortality of 22%.[29] A prospective study of 45 pregnancies in 21 patients reported no increase in obstetric complications or significant change in aortic root size in patients with normal aortic roots. Importantly, in the eight patients with a dilated aortic root (>40 mm) or prior aortic root surgery, three of nine pregnancies were complicated by either aortic dissection (2) or rapid aortic dilatation (1).[30] Thus, patients with aortic root involvement should receive preconception counseling emphasizing their risk, and in early pregnancy should be offered termination. In contrast, women with little cardiovascular involvement and with normal aortic root diameter may tolerate pregnancy well, though there remains a possibility of dissection even without prior evidence of aortopathy. **Grade B4** The likelihood of aortic dilatation increases with increasing maternal age, so that advice to complete families at a younger age is appropriate. Serial echocardiography should be used to identify progressive aortic root dilatation during pregnancy and for 6 months postpartum; prophylactic β blockers should be administered.[31] **Grade C5**

Congenitally corrected transposition of the great arteries

Many adult patients will have had surgical interventions, primarily VSD closure and relief of pulmonic stenosis, sometimes requiring a valved conduit from the LV to the pulmonary artery. Potential problems in pregnancy include dysfunction of the systemic right ventricle and/or increased

systemic AV valve regurgitation, with heart failure, atrial arrhythmias and AV block. In two recent reports on 41 patients there were 105 pregnancies, with 73% live births and no maternal mortality, although seven patients developed heart failure, endocarditis, stroke or myocardial infarction.[32,33] **Grade B4**

Eisenmenger syndrome and pulmonary vascular obstructive disease

Maternal mortality in Eisenmenger syndrome is approximately 30% in each pregnancy.[34] **Grade B4** The majority of complications occur at term and during the first postpartum week. Preconception counseling should stress the extreme pregnancy-associated risks. Termination should always be offered to such patients, as should sterilization. The vasodilatation associated with pregnancy will increase the magnitude of right to left shunting in patients with Eisenmenger syndrome, resulting in worsening of maternal cyanosis and adverse effects on fetal outcome. Spontaneous abortion is common, intrauterine growth restriction is seen in 30% of pregnancies, and preterm labor is frequent. The high perinatal mortality rate (28%) is due mainly to prematurity.

Pregnancy may accelerate the progression of pulmonary vascular disease by increasing the risk of *in-situ* thrombosis and/or thromboembolism; other mechanisms may be operative as well. **Grade C5**

A recent review of outcome of 125 pregnancies in patients with Eisenmenger syndrome, primary pulmonary hypertension and secondary pulmonary hypertension reported poor outcomes in all three groups.[35] **Grade B4** The maternal mortality observed in the various groups was 36%, 30% and 56%, respectively. The overall neonatal mortality was 13%.

Mitral valve prolapse

Isolated mitral valve prolapse has an excellent outcome in pregnancy[36–38] **Grade B4** and affects management only as a possible indication for endocarditis prophylaxis, or if severe mitral regurgitation has led to symptomatic deterioration or left ventricular dysfunction.

Rheumatic heart disease

Mitral stenosis is the most common rheumatic valvular lesion encountered during pregnancy. The hypervolemia and tachycardia associated with pregnancy exacerbate the impact of mitral valve obstruction. The resultant elevation in left atrial pressure increases the likelihood of atrial fibrillation. Thus, even patients with mild to moderate mitral stenosis who are asymptomatic prior to pregnancy, may develop atrial fibrillation and heart failure during the ante- and peripartum periods. Atrial fibrillation is a frequent precipitant of heart failure in pregnant patients with mitral stenosis, owing primarily to uncontrolled ventricular rates; equivalent tachycardia of any cause may produce the same detrimental effect. Earlier studies examining a pregnant population comprised predominantly of women with rheumatic mitral disease showed that mortality rate increased with worsening antenatal maternal functional class.[3] More recent studies found no mortality, but described substantial morbidity from heart failure and arrhythmia.[1,5] The risk for complications was especially high in those women with moderate or severe mitral stenosis.[1,5,39] **Grade B2** Percutaneous mitral valvuloplasty should be considered in patients with functional class III or IV symptoms despite optimal medical therapy and hospitalization.[40–42] **Grade B4**

Pregnant women whose dominant lesion is rheumatic aortic stenosis have a similar outcome to those with congenital aortic stenosis. Aortic or mitral regurgitation is generally well tolerated during pregnancy even if severe, although deterioration in maternal functional class has been observed.

Peripartum cardiomyopathy

Peripartum cardiomyopathy is a form of idiopathic dilated cardiomyopathy diagnosed by otherwise unexplained LV systolic dysfunction, confirmed echocardiographically, presenting during the last antepartum month or in the first 5 postpartum months.[43] It usually manifests as heart failure, although arrhythmias and embolic events also occur. Many affected women will show improvement in functional status and ventricular function postpartum, but others may have persistent or progressive dysfunction. The relapse rate during subsequent pregnancies is substantial in women with evidence of persisting cardiac enlargement or LV dysfunction. However, pregnancy may not be risk free even in those with recovery of systolic function, as subclinical abnormalities may persist.[44] In a recently published multicenter survey examining the outcomes of 60 pregnancies in women with peripartum cardiomyopathy diagnosed during a prior pregnancy, 44% of women with LV ejection fraction <0·50 developed symptoms of congestive heart failure during subsequent pregnancies, with an associated mortality rate of 19%. In contrast, symptoms of congestive heart failure developed in 21% of women with LV ejection fraction ≥0·50, and none of this group died (Figure 60.1).[45] **Grade B4**

Hypertensive disorders in pregnancy

Hypertensive disorders of pregnancy are the second most common cause of maternal mortality, accounting for 15% of all obstetric deaths.[6] They also predispose to other complications, such as placental abruption, stroke, disseminated intravascular coagulation, renal and/or hepatic failure and congestive heart failure.[46] The fetus is at increased risk for intrauterine growth restriction, prematurity and intrauterine death.

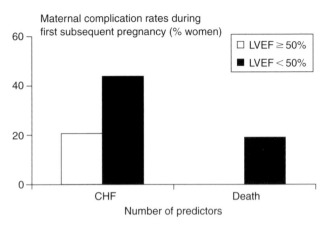

Figure 60.1 The frequency of maternal heart failure (CHF) and death during the first subsequent pregnancy in women with peripartum cardiomyopathy as stratified by preserved (LVEF ≥50%) versus reduced left ventricular ejection fraction (LVEF <50%). In the group with preserved left ventricular ejection fraction there were no deaths during the first subsequent pregnancy. (From Elkayam *et al.*[45])

Several guidelines and consensus documents have been developed which attempt to standardize definitions and criteria for diagnosis.[46–49] Unfortunately, terminology and definitions vary slightly, but importantly in these documents this compromises clarity. The recommendations of the Canadian Hypertension Society and the Society of Obstetricians and Gynaecologists of Canada define hypertension in pregnancy as *pre-existing hypertension* (elsewhere called chronic hypertension, renal hypertension, underlying hypertension, essential hypertension or secondary hypertension), *gestational hypertension without proteinuria and other adverse conditions* (elsewhere called pregnancy-induced hypertension, transient hypertension) or *gestational hypertension with proteinuria or other adverse conditions* (elsewhere called pre-eclampsia, eclampsia, HELLP [*h*emolysis, *e*levated *l*iver enzymes, *l*ow *p*latelets] syndrome, gestational proteinuric hypertension).[46,48,49] The recent American guidelines set criteria for the diagnosis of hypertension in pregnancy as seated systolic blood pressure ≥140 and/or diastolic blood pressure ≥90 mmHg (using Korotkoff phase V (disappearance of sound) to determine diastolic pressure).[6] The BP elevation should be noted on repeated measurements. Proteinuria in pregnancy is significant when there is >0·3 g protein in a 24 hour urine collection. Severe hypertension is defined as a systolic blood pressure ≥160 and/or a diastolic blood pressure ≥110 mmHg and severe proteinuria as a 24 hour urine protein excretion >2 g. Gestational hypertension may be *superimposed* on pre-existing hypertension. In the absence of proteinuria and other adverse conditions, gestational hypertension that resolves postpartum is called *transient hypertension* or *benign gestational hypertension*, whereas if it persists postpartum it is understood as pregnancy-induced unmasking of pre-existing (or chronic) hypertension.

The pathophysiology of gestational hypertension with proteinuria or other adverse conditions (pre-eclampsia) differs from other forms of hypertension. As a result of placental dysfunction, the normal cardiovascular adaptations to pregnancy (increased plasma volume and decreased peripheral resistance) do not occur. There is reduced perfusion to the placenta, liver, kidneys and brain. It is thought that endothelial dysfunction, perhaps a consequence of the decreased perfusion, results in excessive vasoactive toxins, which produce most if not all the manifestations of gestational hypertension. Thus, hypertension is but one effect, not a cause, of the clinical syndrome.

Certain adverse conditions are associated with worse outcomes. Frontal headache, severe nausea and vomiting, visual disturbances, chest pain and shortness of breath, and right upper quadrant pain are significant symptoms. The components of the HELLP syndrome may be found, either individually or combined. Other adverse maternal manifestations are severe hypertension, severe proteinuria, hypoalbuminemia (<18 g/l) oliguria, pulmonary edema and convulsions. Fetal compromise may be revealed by oligohydramnios, absent or reversed umbilical artery end-diastolic flow, and abnormalities in fetal biophysical profile. Intrauterine growth restriction, prematurity and placental abruption are the serious adverse fetoplacental consequences.

Hypertrophic cardiomyopathy

Hypertrophic cardiomyopathy is a disorder with distinct genetic abnormalities and a diverse clinical profile. Morphologically there is unexplained ventricular hypertrophy, which is usually asymmetric and predominantly involves the interventricular septum. Obstruction to left ventricular outflow is a common but not invariable feature. Diastolic function abnormalities are important determinants of the clinical manifestations.

In patients with dynamic left ventricular outflow tract obstruction, increases in preload tend to reduce the severity of obstruction, whereas increases in contractility and decreases in afterload tend to worsen it. Diastolic dysfunction magnifies the preload dependence on cardiac output. As a consequence, pregnancy may be associated with worsening symptoms. Maternal outcome is often good, although at least two deaths have been reported, and serious complications (congestive heart failure, supraventricular tachyarrhythmias, ventricular tachycardia, syncope) may occur, especially in women who already have symptoms prior to pregnancy, and in those with substantial LV diastolic and/or systolic dysfunction.[50,51] **Grade B4** Fetal outcomes are good. β Blockers may be used, as in the non-pregnant state. Dual chamber pacing may be of value in patients with symptoms refractory to medical therapy. **Grade C5** The role of septal alcohol ablation or surgical myectomy during pregnancy has not been defined.

Coronary artery disease

Symptomatic coronary artery disease (CAD) is an uncommon accompaniment of pregnancy. Major predisposing factors for atherosclerotic CAD include long-standing diabetes mellitus,[52] familial hypercholesterolemia and tobacco abuse. In addition, some non-atherosclerotic causes of CAD, though also rare, are more frequent in or aggravated by pregnancy, such as coronary artery dissection, coronary artery embolism, vascular complications of vasoactive obstetric therapies (for example ergot derivatives, prostaglandins), and collagen vascular diseases. The long-term residua of childhood Kawasaki disease include coronary artery stenoses and aneurysms, which may become symptomatic during pregnancy. Cocaine abuse must be considered in any young person with an acute coronary event.[53]

Diagnosis of infarction may be confounded peripartum because of the release of CK-MB isoenzyme from the uterus.[54] Because of the possibility of unusual causes of ischemia and infarction, coronary angiography should be considered early. Fetal exposure to radiation from routine coronary angiography is <5 mGy (<500 mrad).[55] Adverse fetal consequences of this amount of radiation are extremely small or negligible[55] **Grade B4**, and pregnancy should not be seen as a contraindication to a clinically necessary study.[56] Thrombolysis is not contraindicated,[53] but the diagnosis of coronary thrombosis as opposed to other causes of coronary occlusion cannot be routinely assumed; if immediately available, coronary angiography with the option of primary angioplasty can immediately confirm the diagnosis and thus increase the likelihood of providing appropriate therapy.

Management

Risk stratification and counseling

Risk stratification and counseling of women with heart disease is best accomplished prior to conception. The data required for risk stratification can be readily acquired from a thorough cardiovascular history and examination, 12-lead electrocardiogram (ECG) and transthoracic ECG. In patients with cyanosis, arterial oxygen saturation should be assessed by percutaneous oximetry. In counseling, the following areas should be considered: the underlying cardiac lesion; maternal functional status; the possibility of further palliative or corrective surgery; additional associated risk factors; maternal life expectancy and ability to care for a child; and the risk of congenital heart disease in the offspring.

Defining the *underlying cardiac lesion* is an important part of stratifying risk and determining management. Review of prior catheterization and operative reports may be necessary to clarify the diagnosis. The nature of residua and sequelae should be clarified, especially ventricular function, pulmonary pressure, severity of obstructive lesions, persistence of shunts and the presence of hypoxemia.

Almost all patients can be stratified into low-, intermediate- or high-risk groups (Box 60.1). *Maternal functional status* is widely used as a predictor of outcome, and most often defined by NYHA functional class. In a study of 482 pregnancies in women with congenital heart disease, cardiovascular morbidity was less (8% *v* 30%) and livebirth rate higher (80% *v* 68%) in mothers with NYHA functional class I than in the others.[2] **Grade B2** In two studies examining the outcomes of 851 pregnancies, poor functional status (NYHA > II) or cyanosis, left ventricular systolic dysfunction, left heart obstruction, and history of cardiac events prior to pregnancy (arrhythmia, stroke or pulmonary edema) were independent predictors of maternal cardiac complications.[1,5] **Grade B2** Poor maternal functional class or cyanosis was also predictive of adverse neonatal events.

Box 60.1   Maternal cardiac lesion and cardiac risk during pregnancy

Low risk

Left to right shunts

Repaired lesions without residual cardiac dysfunction

Isolated mitral valve prolapse without significant regurgitation

Bicuspid aortic valve without stenosis

Mild–moderate pulmonic stenosis

Valvular regurgitation with normal ventricular systolic function

Intermediate risk

Unrepaired or palliated cyanotic congenital heart disease

Uncorrected coarctation of the aorta

Mitral stenosis

Mild or moderate aortic stenosis

Mechanical prosthetic valves

Severe pulmonic stenosis

Moderate to severe systemic ventricular dysfunction

Systemic right ventricle or single ventricle

Hypertrophic cardiomyopathy

History of peripartum cardiomyopathy with no residual
  ventricular dysfunction

Symptomatic arrhythmia

Pre-existing hypertension

Gestational hypertension without pre-eclampsia

Stable coronary artery disease

High risk

New York Heart Association (NYHA) class III or IV symptoms

Significant pulmonary hypertension with or without right to
  left shunt

Marfan syndrome with aortic root or major valvular involvement

Severe aortic stenosis

History of peripartum cardiomyopathy with residual ventricular
  dysfunction

Recent myocardial infarction or unstable angina

Gestational hypertension with proteinuria or other adverse
  conditions (pre-eclampsia)

In a recently published prospective study the four independent risk factors described above (poor functional status or cyanosis, left ventricular systolic dysfunction, left heart obstruction, and history of cardiac events prior to

pregnancy) were incorporated into a revised risk index. The risk of a cardiac event (cardiac death, stroke, pulmonary edema or arrhythmia) during pregnancy increased with the number of predictors present during the antepartum evaluation. This risk index was derived using two thirds of the study sample and then validated in the remaining pregnancies. For each risk category there was excellent agreement between the expected and the observed rate of events in both the derivation and the validation set (Figure 60.2).[1] **Grade B2** The above-mentioned predictors were also predictive of the combined likelihood of cardiac event (as defined above), deterioration of maternal functional class during pregnancy, or need for an urgent cardiac intervention during the ante- or postpartum periods (Figure 60.3). This index, together with lesion-specific risk estimates, aids the risk stratification of women with heart disease at preconception counseling, and also during pregnancy.

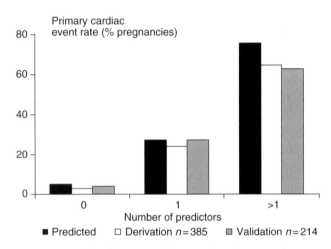

Figure 60.2 The frequency of maternal cardiac complications (pulmonary edema, cardiac arrhythmia, stroke or cardiac death) as predicted by the risk index and observed in the derivation and validation groups, as a function of the number of cardiac predictors (*n* denotes number of pregnancies). (From Siu *et al.*[1])

Further palliative or corrective surgery. Both maternal and fetal outcomes are improved by surgery to correct cyanosis, which should be undertaken prior to conception when possible.[4] **Grade B2** Similarly, patients with symptomatic obstructive lesions should undergo intervention prior to pregnancy.[18] **Grade B4** A systematic overview of the outcome of cardiovascular surgery performed during pregnancy reported a maternal and fetal mortality of 6% and 30%, respectively.[57] **Grade B4** Planning for valve replacement prior to pregnancy requires the need for ongoing anticoagulation with a mechanical valve to be weighed against the likelihood of early reoperation if a tissue valve is used. For aortic stenosis, an attractive alternative is

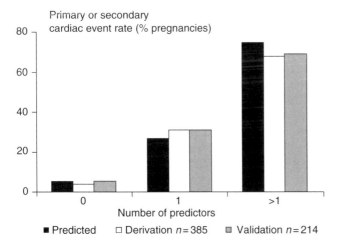

Primary or secondary
cardiac event rate (% pregnancies)

Number of predictors

■ Predicted □ Derivation *n* = 385 ▨ Validation *n* = 214

Figure 60.3 The frequency of any primary or secondary cardiac events (deterioration in maternal functional class, need for urgent cardiac interventions during the ante- or postpartum periods, pulmonary edema, cardiac arrhythmia, stroke, death) as predicted by the risk index and observed in the derivation and validation groups, as a function of the number of cardiac predictors (*n* denotes number of pregnancies). (From Siu *et al.*[1])

the pulmonary autograft. The lack of ideal choices once severe valve disease is present argues for completing families earlier, before the age-dependent progression of valve disease necessitates valve replacement surgery.

Additional associated risk factors that may complicate pregnancy include a history of arrhythmia or heart failure, prosthetic valves and conduits, anticoagulant therapy, and the use of teratogenic drugs such as warfarin or angiotensin-converting enzyme inhibitors.

Maternal life expectancy and ability to care for a child. A patient with limited physical capacity or with a condition that may result in premature death should be advised of her potential inability to look after her child. Women whose condition imparts a high likelihood of fetal complications, such as those with cyanosis or on anticoagulants, must be apprised of these added risks.

The *risk of recurrence of congenital heart disease in offspring* should be addressed in the context of a 0·4–0·6% risk in the general population. The risk with an affected first degree relative increases about 10-fold. A multicenter study examining the offspring of patients with major congenital heart defects who survived cardiac surgery described an overall recurrence rate of 4% in the offspring.[58] **Grade B2** Obstructive left heart lesions have a higher recurrence rate. Certain conditions, such as Marfan syndrome and the 22q11 deletion syndromes, are autosomal dominant, conferring a 50% risk of recurrence in an offspring. Patients

with congenital heart disease who reach reproductive age should be offered genetic counseling so that they are fully informed of the mode of inheritance and recurrence risk, as well as the prenatal diagnosis options available to them. **Grade C5** Preventative strategies to decrease the incidence of congenital defects, such as preconception use of multivitamins containing folic acid, can be discussed at the time of such counseling.[59] **Grade A1d**

Antepartum management

Pregnant women with heart disease may be at particular risk for one or more of congestive heart failure; arrhythmias; or thrombosis, emboli and adverse effects of anticoagulants. Pre-existing and/or gestational hypertension/pre-eclampsia may also require management.

When ventricular dysfunction is a concern, limitation of activity is helpful, and in severely affected women with class III or IV symptoms hospital admission by mid second trimester may be advisable. Gestational hypertension, hyperthyroidism, infection and anemia should be identified early and treated vigorously. For patients with functionally significant mitral stenosis, β adrenergic blockers should be used to control heart rate. Digitalis, although a time-honored treatment for the same purpose, is often ineffective in blunting pregnancy-induced tachycardia. We also offer empiric therapy with β adrenergic blockers to patients with coarctation and to Marfan patients. **Grade C5**

Arrhythmias

Arrhythmias in the form of premature atrial or ventricular beats are common in normal pregnancy; sustained tachyarrhythmias have also been reported. In those with pre-existing arrhythmias, pregnancy may exacerbate their frequency or hemodynamic severity. Pharmacologic treatment is usually reserved for patients with severe symptoms, or when sustained episodes are poorly tolerated in the presence of ventricular hypertrophy, ventricular dysfunction or valvular obstruction. Sustained tachyarrhythmias, such as atrial flutter or atrial fibrillation, should be treated promptly, avoiding teratogenic antiarrhythmic drugs. Digoxin and β adrenergic blockers are the antiarrhythmic drugs of choice, in view of their known safety profiles.[60] **Grade B4** Quinidine, adenosine, sotalol and lidocaine are also "safe", but published data on their use during pregnancy are more limited. Amiodarone is more problematic and standard texts classify it as contraindicated in pregnancy, although there are case reports describing its successful use with careful follow up; it is not teratogenic, but may impair neonatal thyroid function.[61,62] **Grade B4** Electrical cardioversion is safe in pregnancy. A recent report of 44 pregnancies in women with implantable cardioverter defibrillators reported favorable maternal and fetal outcomes.[63] **Grade B4**

Anticoagulation

When a pregnant woman with a mechanical heart valve requires anticoagulation heparin and warfarin are used, but controversy continues as to which is better at different stages of pregnancy. Oral anticoagulation with warfarin is better accepted by patients and is effective. However, warfarin embryopathy may be produced during organogenesis, and fetal intracranial bleeding can occur throughout pregnancy. A recent study of 58 pregnancies reported that a daily warfarin dose of ≤5 mg was associated with no cases of embryopathy.[22] **Grade B4** Fetal intracranial hemorrhage during vaginal delivery is a risk with warfarin unless it has been stopped at least 2 weeks prior to labor. Adjusted-dose subcutaneous heparin has no teratogenic effects as the drug does not cross the placenta, but heparin may cause maternal thrombocytopenia and osteoporosis. Claims of inadequate effectiveness of heparin in patients with mechanical heart valves have been countered by arguments that inadequate doses were used. In a systematic overview of prior studies examining the relationship between anticoagulation regimen and pregnancy outcome in women with prosthetic heart valves, the overall pooled maternal mortality was 2·9%.[64] **Grade B4** The use of oral anticoagulants throughout pregnancy was associated with the lowest rate of valve thrombosis/systemic embolism (4%). The use of unfractionated heparin between 6 and 12 weeks' gestation only was associated with an increased risk of valve thrombosis (9%). Recent practice guidelines have favored the use of either warfarin plus low-dose aspirin during the entire pregnancy, or warfarin substituted by heparin only during the peak teratogenic period (6–12 weeks' gestation).[18] **Grade B4** Low molecular weight heparin is easier to administer and has been suggested as an alternative to adjusted-dose unfractionated heparin. The adjunctive use of low-dose acetyl salicylic acid with heparin should also be considered.[65,66] **Grade C5** ASA in low dose is safe for the fetus, even at term[67] **Grade A1a**, although high maternal doses may promote premature duct closure.

Clinical trials are needed to better define the optimal anticoagulation strategy.

Eisenmenger syndrome

If a woman with Eisenmenger syndrome does not accept counseling to terminate, or presents late in pregnancy, meticulous antepartum management is necessary, including early hospitalization, supplemental oxygen, and possibly empiric anticoagulation. **Grade C5** The efficacy of nitric oxide therapy in these patients has yet to be demonstrated.

Hypertension in pregnancy

Mild pre-existing hypertension may not require pharmacotherapy in pregnancy, as fetal outcomes are unaffected, maternal blood pressure falls lower than baseline during the first 20 weeks of gestation, and excessive lowering of maternal blood pressure may compromise placental perfusion, with no proven maternal benefit.[6] Therapy should be initiated or reinstituted if moderate–severe hypertension develops (systolic BP ≥150–160; diastolic BP ≥100–110; or both), or there is target organ damage. It is not clear whether treatment of mild–moderate pre-existing (chronic) hypertension reduces the risk of developing superimposed gestational hypertension with proteinuria (pre-eclampsia). If treatment is indicated, drug therapy established as safe includes methyldopa, hydralazine, labetalol and other β-blockers[68] **Grade B4**, and nifedipine.[69] **Grade B4** Diuretics are indicated for the management of volume overload in renal failure or heart failure, may be used as adjuncts in the management of pre-existing (chronic) hypertension, but should be avoided in gestational hypertension (pre-eclampsia), which is a volume contracted state.[6,70] **Grade A1c** Angiotensin-converting enzyme inhibitors and angiotensin receptor blocking agents are contraindicated after the first trimester of pregnancy, and so should be stopped either before conception or in the first trimester as soon as pregnancy is diagnosed.[71,72] **Grade B4**

Gestational hypertension with proteinuria (pre-eclampsia) is treated effectively only by delivery of the fetus and placenta. Delay in delivery to allow maturation of the fetus can often be accomplished if the syndrome is mild, the patient is under very close surveillance in a hospital or obstetric day unit, and pregnancy is terminated as soon as further benefit to the fetus is unlikely or maternal safety is compromised.[6]

Multidisciplinary approach and high-risk pregnancy units

Women with heart disease who are at intermediate or high risk for complications should be managed in a high-risk pregnancy unit by a multidisciplinary team from obstetrics, cardiology, anesthesia and pediatrics (Box 60.2). **Grade C5** When dealing with a complex problem the team should meet early in the pregnancy. At this time the nature of the cardiac lesion, the anticipated effects of pregnancy and potential problems should be explored. As it is often not possible for every member of the team to be at the patient's bedside at a moment of crisis, it is helpful to develop and distribute widely a written management plan for foreseeable contingencies. Women with heart disease in the "low-risk" group can be managed in a community hospital setting. However, if there is doubt about the mother's status or the risk, consultation at a regional referral center should be arranged.

Box 60.2   Management of pregnancy in women with heart disease

All patients

- Define the lesion, the residua and the sequelae
- Assess functional status
- Determine predictors of risk: general and lesion specific
- Eliminate teratogens
- Arrange genetic counseling when relevant
- Consider consultation with a regional center
- Assess need for endocarditis prophylaxis during labor and delivery

Intermediate and high-risk patients

- Arrange management at a regional center for high-risk pregnancy
- Consider antepartum interventions to reduce pregnancy risk
- Engage a multidisciplinary team, as appropriate
- Consider a multidisciplinary case conference
- Develop and disseminate a management plan
- Anticipate vaginal delivery in almost all cases, unless there are obstetric contraindications
- Consider early epidural anesthesia
- Modify labor and delivery to reduce cardiac work
- Plan postpartum monitoring

Labor and delivery

Vaginal delivery is recommended, with very few exceptions. The only cardiac indications for cesarean section are aortic dissection, Marfan syndrome with dilated aortic root, and failure to switch from warfarin to heparin at least 2 weeks prior to labor. **Grade C5** Preterm induction is rarely indicated, but once fetal lung maturity is assured a planned induction and delivery in high-risk situations will ensure the availability of appropriate staff and equipment. Although there is no consensus on the use of invasive hemodynamic monitoring during labor and delivery, we commonly utilize intra-arterial monitoring and often central venous pressure monitoring as well in cases where there are concerns about the interpretation and deleterious effects of a sudden drop in systemic blood pressure (for example in patients with severe aortic stenosis, pulmonary hypertension, or more than moderate systemic ventricular systolic dysfunction). **Grade C5** The need for an indwelling pulmonary artery catheter is contentious and has not been studied during pregnancy. Its value has not been shown in several studies of unselected patients with heart disease monitored through non-cardiac surgical procedures. It may be considered when the information sought is not available otherwise and warrants the risk of the procedure; risk may be increased because of complex anatomy, such as atrial baffles, or in the setting of pulmonary hypertension, because of possible pulmonary infarction or rupture.

Heparin anticoagulation is discontinued at least 12 hours prior to induction, or reversed with protamine if spontaneous labor develops, and can usually be resumed 6–12 hours postpartum.

Endocarditis prophylaxis is initiated at the onset of active labor when indicated. The American Heart Association recommendations state that delivery by cesarean section and vaginal delivery in the absence of infection do not require endocarditis prophylaxis except, perhaps, in patients at high risk.[73] **Grade B2** Although many centers with extensive experience in caring for pregnant women with heart disease utilize endocarditis prophylaxis routinely, there is no evidence to support this common practice.

Epidural anesthesia with adequate volume preloading is the technique of choice. Epidural fentanyl is particularly advantageous in cyanotic patients with shunt lesions as it does not lower peripheral vascular resistance. In the presence of a shunt, air and particulate filters should be placed in all intravenous lines. **Grade C5**

Labor is conducted in the left lateral decubitus position to attenuate hemodynamic fluctuations associated with contractions in the supine position. Forceps or vacuum extraction will shorten the latter part of the second stage of labor and reduce the need for maternal expulsive effort. As hemodynamics do not approach baseline for many days after delivery, those patients at intermediate or high risk may require monitoring for a minimum of 72 hours postpartum. **Grade C5** Patients with Eisenmenger syndrome require longer close postpartum observation, as mortality risk persists for 7 days or more.

References

1. Siu SC, Sermer M, Colman JM *et al*. Prospective multicenter study of pregnancy outcomes in women with heart disease. *Circulation* 2001;**104**:515–21.
2. Whittemore R, Hobbins J, Engle M. Pregnancy and its outcome in women with and without surgical treatment of congenital heart disease. *Am J Cardiol* 1982;**50**:641–51.
3. McFaul P, Dornan J, Lamki H, Boyle D. Pregnancy complicated by maternal heart disease. A review of 519 women. *Br J Obstet Gynaecol* 1988;**95**:861–7.
4. Shime J, Mocarski E, Hastings D, Webb G, McLaughlin P. Congenital heart disease in pregnancy: short- and long-term implications. *Am J Obstet Gynecol* 1987;**156**:313–22.
5. Siu SC, Sermer M, Harrison DA *et al*. Risk and predictors for pregnancy-related complications in women with heart disease. *Circulation* 1997;**96**:2789–94.
6. Report of the National High Blood Pressure Education Program Working Group on High Blood Pressure in Pregnancy. *Am J Obstet Gynecol* 2000;**183**:S1–S22.
7. Elkayam U, Gleicher N. Hemodynamics and cardiac function during normal pregnancy and the puerperium. In: Elkayam U, Gleicher N, eds. *Cardiac Problems in Pregnancy: Diagnosis and Management of Maternal and Fetal Disease*, 3rd edn. New York: Wiley-Liss, 1998.
8. Rubler S, Damani P, Pinto E. Cardiac size and performance during pregnancy estimated with echocardiography. *Am J Cardiol* 1977;**40**:534–40.

9. Katz R, Karliner J, Resnik R. Effects of a natural volume overload state (pregnancy) on left ventricular performance in normal human subjects. *Circulation* 1978;**58**:434–41.

10. Robson S, Dunlop W, Moore M, Hunter S. Combined Doppler and echocardiographic measurement of cardiac output: theory and application in pregnancy. *Br J Obstet Gynaecol* 1987;**94**:1014–27.

11. Vered Z, Poler S, Gibson P, Wlody D, Perez J. Noninvasive detection of the morphologic and hemodynamic changes during normal pregnancy. *Clin Cardiol* 1991;**14**:327–34.

12. Sadaniantz A, Kocheril A, Emaus S, Garber C, Parisi A. Cardiovascular changes in pregnancy evaluated by two-dimensional and Doppler echocardiography. *J Am Soc Echocardiogr* 1992;**5**:253–8.

13. Geva T, Mauer M, Striker L, Kirshon B, Pivarnik J. Effects of physiologic load of pregnancy on left ventricular contractility and remodeling. *Am Heart J* 1997;**133**:53–9.

14. Robson S, Dunlop W, Boys R, Hunter S. Cardiac output during labour. *BMJ* 1987;**296**:1169–72.

15. Robson S, Hunter S, Moore M, Dunlop W. Haemodynamic changes during the puerperium: a Doppler and M-mode echocardiographic study. *Br J Obstet Gynaecol* 1987;**94**:1028–39.

16. Hunter S, Robson SC. Adaptation of the maternal heart in pregnancy. *Br Heart J* 1992;**68**:540–3.

17. Zuber M, Gautschi N, Oechslin E, Widmer V, Kiowski W, Jenni R. Outcome of pregnancy in women with congenital shunt lesions. *Heart* 1999;**81**:271–5.

18. Bonow RO, Carabello B, de Leon AC Jr *et al.* ACC/AHA Guidelines for the management of patients with valvular heart disease: A report of the American College of Cardiology/ American Heart Association Task Force on Practice Guidelines (Committee on Management of Patients with Valvular Heart Disease). *J Am Coll Cardiol* 1998;**32**:1486–588.

19. Lao T, Sermer M, MaGee L, Farine D, Colman J. Congenital aortic stenosis and pregnancy – a reappraisal. *Am J Obstet Gynecol* 1993;**169**:540–5.

20. North RA, Sadler L, Stewart AW, McCowan LM, Kerr AR, White HD. Long-term survival and valve-related complications in young women with cardiac valve replacements. *Circulation* 1999;**99**:2669–76.

21. Dore A, Somerville J. Pregnancy in patients with pulmonary autograft valve replacement. *Eur Heart J* 1997;**18**:1659–62.

22. Vitale N, De Feo M, De Santo LS, Pollice A, Tedesco N, Cotrufo M. Dose-dependent fetal complications of warfarin in pregnant women with mechanical heart valves. *J Am Coll Cardiol* 1999;**33**:1637–41.

23. Deal K, Wooley CF. Coarctation of the aorta and pregnancy. *Ann Intern Med* 1973;**78**:706–10.

24. Beauchesne LM, Connolly HM, Ammash NM, Warnes CA. Coarctation of the aorta: outcome of pregnancy. *J Am Coll Cardiol* 2001;**38**:1728–33.

25. Presbitero P, Somerville J, Stone S, Aruta E, Spiegelhalter D, Rabajoli F. Pregnancy in cyanotic congenital heart disease. Outcome of mother and fetus. *Circulation* 1994;**89**:2673–6.

26. Clarkson P, Wilson N, Neutze J, North R, Calder A, Barratt-Boyes B. Outcome of pregnancy after the Mustard operation for transposition of the great arteries with intact ventricular septum. *J Am Coll Cardiol* 1994;**24**:190–3.

27. Genoni M, Jenni R, Hoerstrup SP, Vogt P, Turina M. Pregnancy after atrial repair for transposition of the great arteries. *Heart* 1999;**81**:276–7.

28. Canobbio M, Mair D, van der Velde M, Koos B. Pregnancy outcomes after the Fontan repair. *J Am Coll Cardiol* 1996;**28**:763–7.

29. Pyeritz R. Maternal and fetal complications of pregnancy in the Marfan syndrome. *Am J Med* 1981;**71**:784–90.

30. Rossiter J, Repke J, Morales A, Murphy E, Pyeritz R. A prospective longitudinal evaluation of pregnancy in the Marfan syndrome. *Am J Obstet Gynecol* 1995;**173**:1599–606.

31. Shores J, Berger K, Murphy E, Pyeritz R. Progression of aortic dilatation and the benefit of long-term β-adrenergic blockade in Marfan's syndrome. *N Engl J Med* 1994;**330**:1335–41.

32. Connolly HM, Grogan M, Warnes CA. Pregnancy among women with congenitally corrected transposition of great arteries. *J Am Coll Cardiol* 1999;**33**:1692–5.

33. Therrien J, Barnes I, Somerville J. Outcome of pregnancy in patients with congenitally corrected transposition of the great arteries. *Am J Cardiol* 1999;**84**:820–4.

34. Gleicher N, Midwall J, Hochberger D, Jaffin H. Eisenmenger's syndrome and pregnancy. *Obstet Gynecol Surv* 1979;**34**:721–41.

35. Weiss B, Zemp L, Seifert B, Hess O. Outcome of pulmonary vascular disease in pregnancy: a systematic overview from 1978 through 1996. *J Am Coll Cardiol* 1998;**31**:1650–7.

36. Rayburn WF, Fontana ME. Mitral valve prolapse and pregnancy. *Am J Obstet Gynecol* 1981;**141**:9–11.

37. Tang LC, Chan SY, Wong VC, Ma HK. Pregnancy in patients with mitral valve prolapse. *Int J Gynecol Obstet* 1985;**23**:217–21.

38. Chia YT, Yeoh SC, Lim MC, Viegas OA, Ratnam SS. Pregnancy outcome and mitral valve prolapse. *Asia Oceania J Obstet Gynaecol* 1994;**20**:383–8.

39. Hameed A, Karaalp IS, Tummala PP *et al.* The effect of valvular heart disease on maternal and fetal outcome of pregnancy. *J Am Coll Cardiol* 2001;**37**:893–9.

40. Mangione JA, Lourenco RM, dos Santos ES *et al.* Long-term follow-up of pregnant women after percutaneous mitral valvuloplasty. *Catheter Cardiovasc Interv* 2000;**50**:413–17.

41. Desai DK, Adanlawo M, Naidoo DP, Moodley J, Kleinschmidt I. Mitral stenosis in pregnancy: a four-year experience at King Edward VIII Hospital, Durban, South Africa. *Br J Obstet Gynaecol* 2000;**107**:953–8.

42. de Souza JAM, Martinez EE, Ambrose JA *et al.* Percutaneous balloon mitral valvuloplasty in comparison with open mitral valve commissurotomy for mitral stenosis during pregnancy. *J Am Coll Cardiol* 2001;**37**:900–3.

43. Pearson GD, Veille JC, Rahimtoola S *et al.* Peripartum cardiomyopathy: National Heart, Lung, and Blood Institute and Office of Rare Diseases (National Institutes of Health) workshop recommendations and review. *JAMA* 2000;**283**:1183–8.

44. Lampert MB, Weinert L, Hibbard J, Korcarz C, Lindheimer M, Lang RM. Contractile reserve in patients with peripartum cardiomyopathy and recovered left ventricular function. *Am J Obstet Gynecol* 1997;**176**:189–95.

45. Elkayam U, Tummala PP, Rao K *et al.* Maternal and fetal outcomes of subsequent pregnancies in women with peripartum cardiomyopathy. *N Engl J Med* 2001;**344**:1567–71.

46. Helewa M, Burrows R, Smith J, Williams K, Brain P, Rabkin S. Report of the Canadian Hypertension Society Consensus Conference: 1. Definitions, evaluation and classification of hypertensive disorders in pregnancy. *Can Med Assoc J* 1997;**157**:715–25.

47. Brown MA, Hague WM, Higgins J *et al.* The detection, investigation and management of hypertension in pregnancy: full consensus statement. *Aust NZ J Obstet Gynaecol* 2000;**40**:139–55.

48. Moutquin J, Garner P, Burrows R *et al.* Report of the Canadian Hypertension Society Consensus Conference: 2. Non-pharmacologic management and prevention of hypertensive disorders in pregnancy. *Can Med Assoc J* 1997;**157**:907–19.

49. Rey E, LeLorier J, Burgess E, Lange I, Leduc L. Report of the Canadian Hypertension Society Consensus Conference: 3. Pharmacologic treatment of hypertensive disorders in pregnancy. *Can Med Assoc J* 1997;**157**:1245–54.

50. Elkayam U, Dave R. Hypertrophic cardiomyopathy and pregnancy. In: Elkayam U, Gleicher N, eds. *Cardiac Problems in Pregnancy*, 3rd edn. New York: Wiley-Liss, 1998.

51. Benitez RM. Hypertrophic cardiomyopathy and pregnancy: maternal and fetal outcomes. *J Maternal–Fetal Invest* 1996; **6**:51–5.

52. Gordon MC, Landon MB, Boyle J, Stewart KS, Gabbe SG. Coronary artery disease in insulin-dependent diabetes mellitus of pregnancy (class H): a review of the literature. *Obstet Gynecol Surv* 1996;**51**:437–44.

53. Roth A, Elkayam U. Acute myocardial infarction associated with pregnancy. *Ann Intern Med* 1996;**125**:751–62.

54. Leiserowitz GS, Evans AT, Samuels SJ, Omand K, Kost GJ. Creatine kinase and its MB isoenzyme in the third trimester and the peripartum period. *J Reprod Med* 1992;**37**:910–6.

55. Wagner LK, Lester RG, Saldana LR. *Exposure of the pregnant patient to diagnostic radiations: A guide to medical management*, 2nd edn. Madison, WI: Medical Physics Publishing, 1997.

56. Colletti PM, Lee K. Cardiovascular imaging in the pregnant patient. In: Elkayam U, Gleicher N, eds. *Cardiac problems in pregnancy*, 3rd edn. New York: Wiley-Liss, 1998.

57. Weiss BM, von Segesser LK, Alon E, Seifert B, Turina MI. Outcome of cardiovascular surgery and pregnancy: a systematic review of the period 1984–1996. *Am J Obstet Gynecol* 1998;**179**:1643–53.

58. Burn J, Brennan P, Little J *et al.* Recurrence risks in offspring of adults with major heart defects: results from first cohort of British Collaborative study. *Lancet* 1998;**351**:311–16.

59. Czeizel A. Reduction of urinary tract and cardiovascular defects by periconceptional multivitamin supplementation. *Am J Med Genet* 1996;**62**:179–83.

60. Chow T, Galvin J, McGovern B. Antiarrhythmic drug therapy in pregnancy and lactation. *Am J Cardiol* 1998;**82**:58I–62I.

61. Magee LA, Downar E, Sermer M, Boulton BC, Allen LC, Koren G. Pregnancy outcome after gestational exposure to amiodarone in Canada. *Am J Obstet Gynecol* 1995;**172**: 1307–11.

62. Bartalena L, Bogazzi F, Braverman LE, Martino E. Effects of amiodarone administration during pregnancy on neonatal thyroid function and subsequent neurodevelopment. *J Endocrinol Invest* 2001;**24**:116–30.

63. Natale A, Davidson T, Geiger M, Newby K. Implantable cardioverter-defibrillators and pregnancy: a safe combination? *Circulation* 1997;**96**:2808–12.

64. Chan WS, Anand S, Ginsberg JS. Anticoagulation of pregnant women with mechanical heart valves: a systematic review of the literature. *Arch Intern Med* 2000;**160**:191–6.

65. Turpie AG, Gent M, Laupacis A *et al.* A comparison of aspirin with placebo in patients treated with warfarin after heart-valve replacement. *N Engl J Med* 1993;**329**:524–9.

66. Ginsberg JS, Greer I, Hirsh J. Use of antithrombotic agents during pregnancy. *Chest* 2001;**119**:122S–131S.

67. CLASP: a randomised trial of low-dose aspirin for the prevention and treatment of pre-eclampsia among 9364 pregnant women. CLASP (Collaborative Low-dose Aspirin Study in Pregnancy) Collaborative Group. *Lancet* 1994;**343**:619–29.

68. Magee LA, Ornstein MP, von Dadelszen P. Fortnightly review: management of hypertension in pregnancy. *BMJ* 1999; **318**:1332–6.

69. Magee LA, Schick B, Donnenfeld AE *et al.* The safety of calcium channel blockers in human pregnancy: a prospective, multicenter cohort study. *Am J Obstet Gynecol* 1996;**174**:823–8.

70. Collins R, Yusuf S, Peto R. Overview of randomised trials of diuretics in pregnancy. *BMJ (Clin Res)* 1985;**290**:17–23.

71. Hanssens M, Keirse MJ, Vankelecom F, Van Assche FA. Fetal and neonatal effects of treatment with angiotensin-converting enzyme inhibitors in pregnancy. *Obstet Gynecol* 1991; **78**:128–35.

72. Piper JM, Ray WA, Rosa FW. Pregnancy outcome following exposure to angiotensin-converting enzyme inhibitors. *Obstet Gynecol* 1992;**80**:429–32.

73. Dajani A, Taubert K, Wilson W *et al.* Prevention of bacterial endocarditis: recommendations by the American Heart Association. *JAMA* 1997;**277**:1794–801.

61 Venous thromboembolic disease

Clive Kearon, Jeffrey S Ginsberg, Jack Hirsh

There are three main aspects to the management of venous thromboembolism (VTE): diagnosis, prevention, and treatment. Prior to focusing on these, relevant aspects of the pathogenesis and natural history of VTE will be reviewed.

Pathogenesis of VTE

Virchow is credited with identifying stasis, vessel wall injury, and hypercoagulability as the pathogenic triad responsible for thrombosis. This classification of risk factors for VTE remains valuable.

- *Venous stasis.* The importance of venous stasis as a risk factor for VTE is demonstrated by the fact that most deep vein thrombosis (DVT), associated with stroke, affect the paralyzed leg,[1] and most DVT which are associated with pregnancy affect the left leg,[2] the iliac veins of which are prone to extrinsic compression by the pregnant uterus and the right common iliac artery.
- *Vessel damage.* Venous endothelial damage, usually as a consequence of accidental injury, manipulation during surgery (for example, hip replacement), or iatrogenic injury, is an important risk factor for VTE. Hence, 75% of proximal DVT complicating hip surgery occur in the operated leg,[3] and thrombosis is common with indwelling venous catheters.[4,5]
- *Hypercoagulability.* A complex balance of naturally occurring coagulation and fibrinolytic factors, and their inhibitors, serve to maintain blood fluidity and hemostasis. Inherited, or acquired, changes in this balance predispose to thrombosis. The most important inherited biochemical disorders associated with VTE are due to defects in the naturally occurring inhibitors of coagulation: deficiencies of antithrombin, protein C or protein S, and resistance to activated protein C caused by factor V Leiden. The first three of these disorders are rare in the normal population (combined prevalence of <1%), have a combined prevalence of about 5% in patients with a first episode of VTE,[6] and are associated with a 10- to 40-fold increase in the risk of VTE.[7] The factor V Leiden mutation is common, occurring in about 5% of Caucasians and about 20% of patients with a first episode of VTE (that is, fourfold increase in VTE risk).[7,8]

Hyperhomocysteinemia, owing to hereditary and acquired factors, is also a risk factor for VTE.[9]

Elevated levels of a number of coagulation factors (I, II, VIII, IX, XI) are associated with thrombosis in a "dose-dependent" manner.[10–12] It is probable that such elevations are often inherited, with strong evidence for this with factor VIII.[10] A mutation in the 3' untranslated region of the prothrombin gene (G20210A), which is associated with about 25% increase in prothrombin levels, occurs in about 2% of Caucasians and about 5% of those with a first episode of VTE (that is, about a 2·5-fold increase in risk).[7,8,13] Prothrombotic abnormalities of the fibrinolytic system have questionable importance.

Acquired hypercoagulable states include estrogen therapy, antiphospholipid antibodies (anticardiolipin antibodies and/or lupus anticoagulants), systemic lupus erythematosus, malignancy, combination chemotherapy, and surgery.[14] Patients who develop immunologically-related heparin-induced thrombocytopenia also have a very high risk of developing arterial and venous thromboembolism.[15] Unlike the congenital abnormalities, acquired risk factors are often transient, which has important implications for the duration of anticoagulant prophylaxis and treatment.

- *Combinations of risk factors and risk stratification.* The risk of developing VTE depends on the prevalence and severity of risk factors (Box 61.1).[14] Accordingly, by assessment of these factors, surgical patients can be categorized as having a low, moderate, or high risk of VTE (Table 61.1).

Prevalence and natural history of VTE

VTE is rare before the age of 16 years, probably because the immature coagulation system is resistant to thrombosis. However, the risk of VTE increases exponentially with advancing age (1·9-fold per decade), rising from an annual incidence of approximately 30/100 000 at 40 years, to 90/100 000 at 60 years, and 260/100 000 at 80 years.[14,16] Clinically important components of the natural history of VTE are summarized in Box 61.2.[17]

Box 61.1   Risk factors for venous thromboembolism[a]

- *Patient factors*
  - Previous VTE[b]
  - Age over 40
  - Pregnancy, purpureum
  - Marked obesity
  - Inherited hypercoagulable state
- *Underlying condition and acquired factors*
  - Malignancy[b]
  - Estrogen therapy
  - Cancer chemotherapy
  - Paralysis[b]
  - Prolonged immobility
  - Major trauma[b]
  - Lower limb injuries[b]
  - Heparin-induced thrombocytopenia
  - Antiphospholipid antibodies
- *Type of surgery*
  - Lower limb orthopedic surgery[b]
  - General anesthesia >30 min

[a] Combinations of factors have at least an additive effect on the risk of VTE.
[b] Common major risk factors for VTE.
Abbreviation: VTE, venous thromboembolism

Diagnosis of VTE

Objective testing for DVT and pulmonary embolism (PE) is important because clinical assessment alone is unreliable, failure to diagnose VTE is associated with a high mortality, and inappropriate anticoagulation needs to be avoided.

Diagnosis of DVT

Venography is the criterion standard for the diagnosis of DVT.[18,19] However, because of its invasive nature, technical demands, costs, and the risks associated with contrast media, non-invasive tests have been developed, of which venous ultrasound imaging (VUI) and, more recently, D-dimer testing, are the most important (Box 61.3).

Clinical assessment

Although clinical assessment cannot unequivocally confirm or exclude DVT, clinical evaluation with empiric assessment or a structured clinical model (Table 61.2), can stratify patients as having a low (≤10% prevalence), moderate (~25% prevalence) or high (≥60% prevalence) probability

---

Table 61.1   Risk stratification for postoperative VTE, frequency of VTE without prophylaxis, and recommended methods of prophylaxis.

	Venographic DVT[a]		Pulmonary embolism		Recommended prophylaxis
	Calf (%)	Proximal (%)	Symptomatic (%)	Fatal (%)	
Low risk less than 40 years and uncomplicated surgery and no additional risk factors	2	0·4	0·2	<0·01	Early mobilization
Moderate risk more than 40 years or prolonged/complicated surgery or additional "minor" risk factors	20	5	2	0·5	Low-dose UFH[b] LMWH (~3000 U daily)[c] GC stockings[d]
High risk major surgery for malignancy or previous VTE or knee/hip surgery or heparin-induced thrombocytopenia	50	15	5	2	LMWH (>3000 U per day)[c] Warfarin (INR 2–3)[f] Adjusted-dose UFH[g] IPC devices[e]

[a] Asymptomatic DVT detected by surveillance bilateral venography.
[b] Low-dose UFH: 5000 U of subcutaneous unfractionated heparin preoperatively, and twice or three times daily postoperatively.
[c] LMWH: subcutaneous low molecular weight heparin; higher doses (for example, ~4000 U once daily with a preoperative start [Europe], or ~3000 U twice daily with a postoperative start [North America]) are used in high-risk patients; in moderate-risk patients ~3000 U daily with a preoperative start is used.
[d] GC stockings: graduated compression stockings, alone or in combination with pharmacologic methods.
[e] IPC devices: intermittent pneumatic compression devices, alone or in combination with graduated compression stockings and/or pharmacologic methods.
[f] Warfarin: usually started postoperatively and adjusted to achieve an International Normalization Ratio (INR) of 2·0–3·0.
[g] Adjusted-dose UFH: preoperative start with an adjusted, three times daily, dose to raise the activated partial thromboplastin time to the upper limit of the normal range.
Abbreviations: DVT, deep vein thrombosis; VTE, venous thromboembolism

Box 61.2 Natural history of venous thromboembolism (VTE)

- Clinical factors can identify high-risk patients[14]
- VTE usually starts in the calf veins[112]
- Over 80% of symptomatic DVTs are proximal[19,112]
- Two thirds of asymptomatic DVT detected postoperatively by screening venography are confined to the distal (calf) veins[19]
- About 20% of symptomatic isolated calf DVTs subsequently extend to the proximal veins, usually within a week of presentation[113]
- PE usually arises from proximal DVT[114]
- The majority (~70%) of patients with symptomatic proximal DVT have asymptomatic PE (high probability lung scans in ~40%),[115] and vice versa[43,116]
- Only one quarter of patients with symptomatic PE have symptoms or signs of DVT[117]
- About 50% of untreated symptomatic proximal DVTs are expected to cause symptomatic PE[83]
- About 10% of symptomatic PE are rapidly fatal[118]
- About 30% of untreated symptomatic non-fatal PE will have a fatal recurrence[74,119]
- The risk of recurrent VTE is lower if risk factors are reversible than if there is no apparent, or a persistent, risk factor[90–93,96]

Abbreviations: DVT, deep vein thrombosis; PE, pulmonary embolism

of DVT.[20] **Grade A** Such categorization is useful in guiding the performance and interpretation of objective testing.[20–22]

Venous ultrasound imaging

VUI has a sensitivity for proximal DVT of about 97% and a specificity of 94% in symptomatic patients, which, on average, translates into a positive predictive value of 97% and a negative predictive value of 98% for proximal DVT.[19] The essential component of VUI is assessment of venous compressibility of the common femoral and popliteal veins (down to the calf vein trifurcation), with application of ultrasound probe pressure.[19] **Grade A** VUI is much more difficult to perform and less accurate in the calf (sensitivity of ~70%).[19] For these reasons, and because isolated calf DVT is uncommon and of limited importance, VUI of the calf veins is often not performed. Instead, if DVT cannot be excluded by a normal proximal VUI in combination with other results (for example, low clinical probability or normal D-dimer [see Box 61.3]), a follow up VUI is performed after 1 week to detect extending calf vein thrombosis (~2% of patients).[19] If the second VUI examination is normal, the risk of symptomatic VTE during the next 6 months is less than 2%.[19]

Box 61.3 Test results which effectively confirm or exclude DVT (deep vein thrombosis)

- *Diagnostic for first DVT*
  - Venography: intraluminal filling defect
  - Venous ultrasound: non-compressible proximal veins at two or more of the common femoral, popliteal, and calf trifurcation sites[19]
- *Excludes first DVT*
  - Venography: all deep veins seen, and no intraluminal filling defects[18]
  - D-dimer: normal test, which has a very high sensitivity (≥98%) and at least a moderate specificity (≥40%)[27]
  - Venous ultrasound or impedance plethysmography: normal and
    (a) low clinical suspicion for DVT at presentation,[29,120] or
    (b) normal D-dimer test, which has a moderately high sensitivity (≥85%) and specificity (≥70%) at presentation,[29,120] or
    (c) normal serial testing (venous ultrasound at 7 days; impedance plethysmography at 2 and 7 days)
- Low clinical suspicion for DVT at presentation and a normal D-dimer test, which has a moderately high sensitivity (≥85%) and specificity (≥70%) at presentation[29]
- *Diagnostic for recurrent DVT*
  - Venography: intraluminal filling defect
  - Venous ultrasound:
    (a) a new non-compressible common femoral or popliteal vein segment,[19] or
    (b) a ≥4.0 mm increase in diameter of the common femoral or popliteal vein compared to a previous test[19,37a]
  - Impedance plethysmography:
    (a) conversion of a normal test to abnormal[121,122a]
    (b) an abnormal test 1 year after diagnosis[19a]
- *Excludes recurrent DVT*
  - Venogram: all deep veins seen and no intraluminal filling defects
  - Venous ultrasound or impedance plethysmography: normal, or ≤1 mm increase in diameter of the common femoral or popliteal veins on venous ultrasound compared to a previous test, and remains normal (no progression of venous ultrasound) at 2 and 7 days[19,37,121,122]
  - D-dimer: normal test, which has a very high sensitivity (≥98%) and at least a moderate specificity (≥40%)[27]

[a] If other evidence is not consistent with recurrent DVT (for example, venous ultrasound, impedance plethysmography, clinical assessment, D-dimer), venography should be considered. (Adapted from Kearon *et al.*[19])

Table 61.2 Clinical model for determining clinical suspicion of deep vein thrombosis (Wells *et al.*[20])

Variables	Points
Active cancer (treatment ongoing or within previous 6 months or palliative)	1
Paralysis, paresis, or recent plaster immobilization of the lower extremities	1
Recently bedridden >3 days or major surgery within 4 weeks	1
Localized tenderness along the distribution of the deep venous system	1
Entire leg swollen	1
Calf swelling 3 cm > asymptomatic side (measured 10 cm below tibial tuberosity)	1
Pitting edema confined to the symptomatic leg	1
Dilated superficial veins (non-varicose)	1
Alternative diagnosis as likely or greater than that of DVT	−2

Total points
Pretest probability calculated as follows:

High	>2
Moderate	1 or 2
Low	<1

Note: In patients with symptoms in both legs, the more symptomatic leg is used.

The accuracy of VUI is substantially lower if its findings are discordant with the clinical assessment[22,23] and/or if abnormalities are confined to short segments of the deep veins;[24] in about 25% of such cases, the results of venography differ with VUI or reveal calf vein thrombosis.

The accuracy of VUI in asymptomatic postoperative patients who have a high risk for DVT is poor with a sensitivity for proximal DVT of only about 62%,[19] and such screening is not recommended in patients who have received prophylaxis.[25] **Grade A**

D-dimer blood testing

D-dimer is formed when cross-linked fibrin is broken down by plasmin and levels are usually elevated with DVT and/or PE. Normal levels can help to exclude VTE but elevated D-dimer levels are non-specific and have low positive predictive value.[26] D-dimer tests differ markedly as diagnostic tests for VTE. **Grade A** A normal result with a very sensitive (≥98%) D-dimer assay excludes VTE on its own.[26,27] However, very sensitive D-dimer tests have low specificities (~40%), which limits their usefullness because of high false-positive rates.[27] In order to exclude DVT and/or PE, a normal result with a less sensitive D-dimer assay (≥85%) needs to be combined with either a low clinical probability or another objective test that has negative predictive but is also

non-diagnostic on its own (see Box 61.4).[28–32] As less sensitive D-dimer assays are more specific (~70%), they yield fewer false-positive results. Specificity of D-dimer decreases with aging[33] and with comorbid illness such as cancer.[34] Consequently, D-dimer testing has limited value as a diagnostic test for VTE in hospitalized patients and is unhelpful in the early postoperative period.

Diagnosis of DVT in pregnancy

Pregnant patients with suspected DVT can generally be managed in the same way as non-pregnant patients, although except for serial impedance plethysmography[19,35,36] diagnostic approaches have not been evaluated in this population. **Grade B** In pregnant patients with normal non-invasive tests who have a high clinical suspicion of isolated iliac or calf DVT, venography (a complete study or a limited study using abdominal shielding, respectively) should be considered. Alternatively, normal magnetic resonance imaging, a normal D-dimer, or normal Doppler ultrasound imaging of the iliac veins, are likely to helpful for excluding DVT.

Diagnosis of recurrent DVT

Persistent abnormalities of the deep veins are common following DVT.[19,37] **Grade B** Therefore, diagnosis of recurrent DVT requires evidence of new clot formation. Tests that can diagnose or exclude recurrent DVT are noted in Box 61.3.[19,37]

Magnetic resonance imaging (MRI)

A recent small but rigorous study suggests that direct MRI of thrombus is very accurate for the diagnosis of DVT, including thrombosis in the calf and pelvis, and in asymptomatic or pregnant patients.[38] The technique does not require radiographic contrast and has the potential to differentiate acute from old thrombus.

Diagnosis of PE

Pulmonary angiography is the criterion standard for the diagnosis of PE, but has similar limitations as venography.[39] As with suspected DVT, clinical assessment is useful for categorizing probability of PE (Table 61.3 and Box 61.4).[40] **Grade A**

Ventilation–perfusion lung scanning

The usual initial investigation in patients with suspected PE is a ventilation–perfusion lung scan. A normal perfusion scan excludes PE,[41] but is found in a minority (10–40%) of patients.[33,42–44] Perfusion defects are non-specific; only about one third of patients with defects have PE.[42,45] The probability that a perfusion defect is due to PE increases

Table 61.3 Model for determining a clinical suspicion of pulmonary embolism (Wells et al[123])

Variables	Points
Clinical signs and symptoms of deep vein thrombosis (minimum leg swelling and pain with palpation of the deep veins)	3·0
An alternative diagnosis is less likely than pulmonary embolism	3·0
Heart rate >100 beats/min	1·5
Immobilization or surgery in the previous 4 weeks	1·5
Previous deep vein thrombosis/pulmonary embolism	1·5
Hemoptysis	1·0
Malignancy (treatment ongoing or within previous 6 months or palliative)	1·0

Total points

Pretest probability calculated as follows:

High	>6
Moderate	2–6
Low	<2

with size and number, and the presence of a normal ventilation scan ("mismatched" defect).[42,45] A lung scan with mismatched segmental or larger perfusion defects is termed "high probability".[45] A single mismatched defect is associated with a prevalence of PE of about 80%.[46] Three or more mismatched defects are associated with a prevalence of PE of ≥90%.[46] Lung scan findings are highly age dependent with a relatively high proportion of normal scans and a low proportion of non-diagnostic scans in younger patients.[33]

Lung scanning and clinical assessment

Clinical assessment of PE is complementary to ventilation–perfusion lung scanning; a moderate or high clinical suspicion in a patient with a high probability lung scan is diagnostic (prevalence of PE of ≥90%); however, a low clinical suspicion with a high probability defect requires further investigation because the prevalence of PE with these findings is only about 50%.[42,45] **Grade A** The prevalence of PE with subsegmental, matched, perfusion defects ("low probability" scan) and a low clinical suspicion is expected to be less than 10% (see below).[27,30,42]

Helical (spiral) computerized tomography (CT)

Helical CT following intravenous injection of radiographic contrast can be used to visualize the pulmonary arteries. Although widely used to diagnose PE, the technique has yet to be definitively evaluated for this purpose.[47,48] **Grade B**

Current evidence suggests that helical CT can be interpreted as follows:

- Intraluminal filling defects in lobar or main pulmonary arteries are likely to be associated with a probability of PE of at least 85%, similar to a high-probability ventilation–perfusion scan.[48]
- Intraluminal defects confined to segmental or subsegmental pulmonary arteries are non-diagnostic, and patients with such findings require further testing.[48]
- A normal helical CT substantially reduces the probability of PE but does not exclude the diagnosis (that is, similar to a "low probability" ventilation–perfusion scan).[47,48]

Although this statement is largely based on extrapolation from experience with patients who have non-diagnostic lung scans, patients with helical CT scans that are not diagnostic for PE can be managed as outlined in Box 61.4. **Grade C**

Box 61.4 Test results which effectively confirm or exclude pulmonary embolism (PE)

- *Diagnostic for PE*
  - Pulmonary angiography: intraluminal filling defect
  - Helical CT: intraluminal filling defect in a lobar or main pulmonary artery[47,48]
  - Ventilation–perfusion scan: high probability scan and moderate/high clinical suspicion[42,43]
  - Diagnostic for DVT: with non-diagnostic ventilation–perfusion scan or helical CT[124]
- *Excludes PE*
  - Pulmonary angiogram: normal[39]
  - Perfusion scan: normal[41]
  - D-dimer: normal test, which has a very high sensitivity (≥98%) and at least a moderate specificity (≥40%)[27]
  - Non-diagnostic ventilation–perfusion scan, or normal helical CT, and normal proximal VUI and
    (a) low clinical suspicion for PE[30,50 a]
    (b) normal D-dimer test, which has at least a moderately high sensitivity (≥85%) and specificity (≥70%)[30,32 a]
  - Low clinical suspicion for PE and normal D-dimer, which has at least a moderately high sensitivity (≥85%) and specificity (≥70%)[30,32]

a If serial VUI (venous ultrasound imaging) is performed it is expected to become abnormal in 1–2% of these patients and reduce the frequency of symptomatic VTE (venous thromboembolism) during 3 months of follow up from ~1.5% to ~0.5%.

(Adapted from Kearon[40])

D-dimer testing

As previously discussed when considering diagnosis of DVT, a normal D-dimer result, alone[27] or in combination with another negative test,[30,32] can be used to exclude PE (Box 61.4). **Grade A**

> **Box 61.5 Management of patients with non-diagnostic non-invasive tests for PE**
>
> - *Serial VUI of the proximal veins after 1 and 2 weeks*
>   Suitable for most such patients,[30,44] although pulmonary angiography is preferred for the subgroups outlined below. This approach can be supplemented with bilateral venography (for patients that might otherwise be considered for pulmonary angiography).[116]
> - *Pulmonary angiography preferred option if:*
>   - segmental intraluminal filling defect on helical CT[a,b]
>   - subsegmental intraluminal filling defect and high clinical suspicion
>   - high probability ventilation–perfusion scan and low clinical suspicion[b]
>   - symptoms are severe, post-test probability is high but non-diagnostic, and PE needs to be excluded from the differential diagnosis
>   - serial testing is not feasible (for example, scheduled for surgery, geographic inaccessibility)
>
> [a] A segmental intraluminal filling defect with a high clinical suspicion is likely to have a positive predictive value of ≥85% and could be considered diagnostic for PE.
> [b] Ventilation–perfusion scanning can be performed after these findings have been obtained with helical CT; or helical CT may be performed after these findings have been obtained with ventilation–perfusion scanning;[47,48] If the second test is also non-diagnostic for PE, serial ultrasounds may be reconsidered.
> Abbreviations: DVT, deep vein thrombosis; LMWH, low molecular weight heparin; PE, pulmonary embolism; VTE, venous thromboembolism; VUI, venous ultrasound imaging, (Adapted from Kearon[40])

Tests for DVT in patients with suspected PE

Testing for DVT is an indirect way to diagnose PE (see Box 61.4).[49] VUI of the proximal veins is the usual method, although bilateral ascending venography, or CT or MRI of the legs at the same time as examination of the pulmonary veins, can also be used. Negative tests for DVT do not rule out PE but they reduce the probability, and suggest that the short-term risk of recurrent PE is low.[49] Because the prevalence of PE is expected to be less than 5% in patients with a non-diagnostic lung scan, a low clinical suspicion of PE, and a normal VUI of the proximal veins, it is reasonable to exclude PE with these findings.[27,30,44,50] **Grade B**

Management of patients with non-diagnostic combinations of non-invasive tests for PE (Box 61.5)

Patients with non-diagnostic test results for PE at presentation have, on average, a prevalence of PE of 20%.[42,49] Two management approaches are reasonable in such patients. The first is the performance of pulmonary angiography, which is usually definitive. The second is the withholding of anticoagulants and performance of serial VUI to detect evolving proximal DVT, the forerunner of recurrent PE. If serial VUI for DVT (two additional tests a week apart) is negative, the subsequent risk of recurrent VTE during the next 3 months is less than 1%,[30,44,51] which is similar to that after a normal pulmonary angiogram.[39] As an additional precaution, patients who have had PE and/or DVT excluded should routinely be asked to return for re-evaluation if symptoms of PE and/or DVT persist or recur.

Diagnosis of PE in pregnancy

Pregnant patients with suspected PE can be managed similarly to non-pregnant patients, with the following modifications: **Grade B**

- VUI can be performed first and lung scanning performed if there is no DVT; patients with unequivocal evidence of DVT can be presumed to have PE.
- The amount of radioisotope used for the perfusion scan can be reduced and the duration of scanning extended.
- If pulmonary angiography is performed, the brachial approach with abdominal screening is preferable.
- In the absence of safety data relating to helical CT in pregnancy, this is discouraged (if it is necessary, abdominal screening should be used). Consistent with other young patients who are suspected of having PE, a high proportion of pregnant patients have normal scans and a small proportion have high probability scans.[33,52] These recommendations are based on a belief that the risk of inaccurate diagnosis of suspected PE during pregnancy is greater than the risk of radioactivity to the fetus.[52,53]

Algorithms for the diagnosis of PE

Local availability of methods of testing and differences among patient presentations influence the diagnostic approach to PE. A number of prospectively validated algorithms have been published, which emphasize the use of different initial non-invasive tests in conjunction with ventilation–perfusion lung scanning including:

- structured clinical assessment and serial VUI;[44]
- sensitive D-dimer assay, empiric clinical assessment, and single bilateral VUI;[27]
- clinical assessment, moderately sensitive D-dimer assay and serial VUI.[30]

Prevention of VTE (Box 61.6)

In a non-randomized trial, oral anticoagulation was shown to prevent PE in patients with fractured hips, without causing an unacceptable increase in bleeding.[54] **Grade A** Subsequently, low-dose unfractionated heparin was shown to reduce postoperative DVT and fatal PE by two thirds.[55,56] Further studies have demonstrated that the efficacy of

Box 61.6 Prevention and treatment of venous thromboembolism

- Primary prophylaxis with anticoagulants and/or mechanical methods should be used in hospitalized patients who have a moderate or high risk of VTE. **Grade A**
- Acute VTE (DVT and/or PE) should be anticoagulated with:
  - Heparin (unfractionated or LMWH) for a minimum of 4–5 days. **Grade A** If unfractionated heparin is used, a dose of at least (a) 30 000 U/day or 18 U/kg/h by intravenous infusion; or (b) 33 000 U/day, by twice daily, subcutaneous, injection, should be administered. **Grade A** Dose of unfractionated heparin should be adjusted to achieve "therapeutic" APTT results. **Grade C**
  - Oral anticoagulation for 3–6 months, **Grade A** with a dose adjusted to achieve an INR of 2.0–3.0. **Grade A** Prolonged unfractionated heparin or LMWH at therapeutic, or near therapeutic, doses is a satisfactory alternative. **Grade A** Anticoagulation should be continued for longer than 3 months in patients with a first episode of idiopathic VTE, **Grade B** and when VTE is associated with a risk factor, for as long as such factors are active. **Grade C**

See Box 61.5 for abbreviations

low-dose unfractionated heparin can be improved either by increasing the dose so as to minimally prolong the activated partial thromboplastin time (APTT),[57] or by combining its use with graduated compression stockings[58] or intermittent pneumatic compression devices.[59]

Meta-analyses support that, at doses that are associated with equivalent efficacy (odds ratio 1·03) following general surgery, low molecular weight heparins (LMWH) are associated with less bleeding (odds ratio 0·68) than low-dose unfractionated heparin.[60] **Grade A** Used at higher dose than for general surgery, LMWH is more effective (odds ratio 0·83) that unfractionated heparin following orthopedic surgery and is associated with a similar frequency of bleeding.[60] An additional 3 or 4 weeks of LMWH after hospital discharge further reduces the frequency of symptomatic VTE after orthopedic surgery (from 3·3% to 1·3%[61]). Warfarin (target INR 2–3 for about 7 to 10 days) is less effective that LMWH at preventing DVT detected by venography soon after orthopedic surgery,[62] but appears to be similarly effective at preventing symptomatic VTE over a 3 month period.[62,63] **Grade A** There is evidence that aspirin reduces the risk of postoperative VTE by one third.[64] **Grade A** A study of over 17 000 patients, mostly following hip fracture repair, confirmed these findings, including a reduction in fatal PE (0·27% *v* 0·65%) during the month following surgery.[65] However, as warfarin and LMWH are expected to be more effective (at least a two thirds

reduction in VTE), aspirin alone is not recommended during the initial postoperative period.[62] It may be a reasonable alternative to LMWH or warfarin for the weeks following hospital discharge, particularly if patients do not have additional risk factors for VTE. **Grade B** Recently, hirudin[66] (a direct thrombin inhibitor) and fondaparinux[67,67a,67b] (the pentasaccharide of heparin that binds antithrombin) have been shown to be more effective than LMWH following major orthopaedic surgery; fondaparinux may cause marginally more bleeding. **Grade A**

The evidence that short-term prophylaxis (for example, low-dose unfractionated heparin) prevents clinically important VTE in immobilized medical patients is less convincing, partly because it has been less extensively studied in this population, and because there is concern that medical patients remain at high risk of VTE after prophylaxis is stopped.[62,68]

In addition to augmenting the efficacy of pharmacologic methods of prophylaxis, mechanical methods are effective on their own. Graduated compression stockings prevent postoperative VTE in moderate-risk patients (risk reduction of 68%),[62,69] and intermittent pneumatic compression devices prevent postoperative VTE in high-risk orthopedic patients.[62,70,71] The relative efficacy of graduated compression stockings and intermittent pneumatic compression devices is uncertain. No difference in efficacy was evident in neurosurgical patients;[72] however, pneumatic compression devices are expected to be superior to graduated compression stockings in high-risk patients.[62] Mechanical methods of prophylaxis should be used in patients who have a moderate or high risk of VTE if anticoagulants are contraindicated (for example, neurosurgical patients).[62] **Grade A**

Because postoperative fatal PE is rarely preceded by symptomatic DVT,[55] prophylaxis is the best way to prevent it. Use of primary prophylaxis is strongly supported by cost effectiveness analyses, which indicate that it reduces overall costs in addition to reducing morbidity.[73]

Treatment of VTE

Heparin therapy

In 1960, Barritt and Jordan established that heparin (1·5 days) and oral anticoagulants (2 weeks) reduced the risk of recurrent PE and associated death.[74] Based on expert opinion, 10–14 days of heparin therapy, and 3 months of oral anticoagulation became widely adopted in clinical practice. It was subsequently shown that 4 or 5 days of intravenous heparin is as effective as 10 days of therapy for the initial treatment of VTE.[75,76] Comparatively recently, the need for an initial course of heparin therapy was verified.[77] Many trials have established that weight-adjusted LMWH (without laboratory monitoring) is as safe and effective as adjusted-dose unfractionated heparin for the treatment of acute VTE;[78] it can be used to treat patients without hospital admission[79] and need only be injected subcutaneously once daily.[80] Danaparoid, hirudin, and argatroban can be used to treat heparin induced thrombocytopenia, with or without associated thrombosis.[81,82]

Oral anticoagulant therapy

A randomized trial of patients with DVT, comparing 3 months of warfarin (International Normalization Ratio (INR) ~3·0–4·0) with low-dose heparin after initial treatment with full-dose intravenous heparin, established the necessity for prolonged oral anticoagulation after initial heparin therapy.[83] **Grade A** Prolonged high-dose subcutaneous heparin[84] and, subsequently, LMWH (50–75% of acute treatment dose) was subsequently shown to be equally effective.[85] **Grade A** In the 1970s it was recognized that, because of differences in the responsiveness of thromboplastins to oral anticoagulants, a prothrombin time ratio of 2·0 reflected a much more intense level of anticoagulation in North America than in Europe. This prompted a comparison of two intensities of warfarin therapy (corresponding to mean INRs of ~2·1 and ~3·2) for the treatment of DVT.[86] This study found that the lower intensity of oral anticoagulation was as effective as the higher intensity but caused less bleeding. The trials showing that heparin therapy could be reduced to 5 days also showed that warfarin could be started at the same time as heparin.[75,76] A recent series of small studies support starting warfarin with the expected daily dose rather than a loading dose (for example, 5 mg *v* 10 mg),[87,88] and managing over-anticoagulation without bleeding (for example, INRs ≥ 6) with small oral rather than subcutaneous doses of vitamin K (for example, 1 mg).[89]

During the last decade, a series of well-designed studies have helped to define the optimal duration of anticoagulation. Their findings can be summarized as follows:

- Shortening the duration of anticoagulation from 3[90,91] or 6[92] months to 4[90,91] or 6[92] weeks results in a doubling of the frequency of recurrent VTE during 1[90,91] to 2[92] years of follow up. **Grade A**
- Patients with VTE provoked by a transient risk factor have a lower (about one third) risk of recurrence than those with an unprovoked VTE or a persistent risk factor.[90–94]
- Three months of anticoagulation is adequate treatment for VTE provoked by a transient risk factor; subsequent risk of recurrence is ≤3% per patient-year.[90,91,94–96] **Grade A**
- Three months of anticoagulation may not be adequate treatment for an unprovoked ("idiopathic") episode of VTE; subsequent early risk of recurrence has varied from 5% to 25% per patient-year.[92,95,97,98]
- After 6 months of anticoagulation, recurrent DVT is at least as likely to affect the contralateral leg; this suggests that "systemic" rather than "local" (including inadequate treatment) factors are responsible for recurrences after 6 months of treatment.[99]

- There is a persistently elevated risk of recurrent VTE after a first episode; this appears to be 5–12% per year after 6 or more months of treatment for an unprovoked episode.[92,95,98]
- Oral anticoagulants targeted at an INR of ~2·5 are very effective (risk reduction ≥90%) at preventing recurrent unprovoked VTE after the first 3 months of treatment.[97,100] **Grade A**
- Indefinite anticoagulation is an option for patients with a first unprovoked VTE who have a low risk of bleeding. **Grade B**
- A second episode of VTE does not necessarily indicate a high risk of recurrence or the need for indefinite anticoagulation.[97]
- Risk of bleeding on anticoagulants differs markedly among patients depending on the prevalence of risk factors (for example, advanced age; previous bleeding or stroke; renal failure; anemia; antiplatelet therapy; malignancy; poor anticoagulant control).[101]
- Risk of recurrence is lower (about half) following an isolated calf (distal) DVT; this favors a shorter duration of treatment.[92,95] **Grade B**
- Risk of recurrence is higher with antiphospholipid antibodies (anticardiolipin antibodies and/or lupus anticoagulants),[97,102] homozygous factor V Leiden[103] cancer[93] and, probably, antithrombin deficiency; these favor a longer duration of treatment. **Grade B**
- Heterozygous factor V Leiden and the G20210A prothrombin gene mutations do not appear to be clinically important risk factors for recurrence.[103] **Grade B**
- Other abnormalities, such as elevated levels of clotting factors VIII, IX, XI, and homocysteine, and deficiencies of protein C and protein S, may be risk factors for recurrence; they have uncertain implications for duration of treatment.

Thrombolytic therapy

Systemic thrombolytic therapy accelerates the rate of resolution of DVT and PE at the cost of around a fourfold increase in frequency of major bleeding, and about a 10-fold increase in intracranial bleeding.[104–107] This can be life-saving for PE with hemodynamic compromise.[106,108] **Grade A** Thrombolytic therapy may reduce the risk of the prothrombotic syndrome following DVT but this does not appear to justify its associated risks[104,105] Catheter-based treatments (that is, thrombolytic therapy or removal of thrombus) require further evaluation before they can be recommended.

Inferior vena caval filters

A recent randomized trial demonstrated that a filter, as an adjunct to anticoagulation, reduced the rate of PE (asymptomatic and symptomatic) from 4·5% to 1·0% during the

12 days following insertion, with a suggestion of fewer fatal episodes (0% *v* 2%).[109] However, after 2 years, patients with a filter had a significantly higher rate of recurrent DVT (21% *v* 12%) and a non-statistically significant reduction in the frequency of PE (3% *v* 6%). This study supports the use of vena caval filters to prevent PE in patients with acute DVT and/or PE who cannot be anticoagulated (that is, they are bleeding), but does not support more liberal use of filters. **Grade A** Patients should receive a course of anticoagulation if this subsequently becomes safe.

Treatment of VTE during pregnancy

Unfractionated heparin and LMWH do not cross the placenta and are safe for the fetus, whereas oral anticoagulants cross the placenta and can cause fetal bleeding and malformations.[110,111] Therefore, pregnant women with VTE should be treated with therapeutic doses of subcutaneous heparin (unfractionated heparin or, increasingly, LMWH) throughout pregnancy. **Grade B** Care should be taken to avoid delivery while the mother is therapeutically anticoagulated; one management approach involves stopping subcutaneous heparin 24 hours prior to induction of labor and switching to intravenous heparin if there is a high risk of embolism. After delivery, warfarin, which is safe for infants of nursing mothers, should be given (with initial heparin overlap) for 6 weeks and until a minimum of 3 months of treatment has been completed. **Grade B**

The future

There are many questions relating to currently available antithrombotic agents and diagnostic techniques that need answering, and many new antithrombotic agents under development that will require clinical evaluation. In addition, future studies are expected to focus on clinical and genetic subgroups that may benefit from tailored management, such as different intensities or durations of prophylaxis or treatment. Thrombolytic therapy deserves further evaluation, particularly systemic therapy for severe PE without overt hemodynamic compromise (for example, with echocardiographic right ventricular dysfunction), and catheter-directed therapy for iliofemoral DVT. Safer thrombolytic regimens might also broaden indications. In order to provide clear directions for clinical management, future studies need to focus on clinically important outcomes (that is, symptomatic VTE, major bleeding).

References

1. Turpie AGG, Levine MN, Hirsh J *et al.* Double blind randomised trial of Org 10172 low-molecular-weight heparinoid in the prevention of deep vein thrombosis in thrombotic stoke. *Lancet* 1987;**1**:523–6.

2. Ginsberg J, Brill-Edwards P, Burrows RF *et al.* Venous thrombosis during pregnancy: leg and trimester of presentation. *Thromb Haemost* 1992;**67**:519–20.

3. Cruickshank MK, Levine MN, Hirsh J *et al.* An evaluation of impedance plethysmography and ^{125}I-fibrinogen leg scanning in patients following hip surgery. *Thromb Haemost* 1989;**62**:830–4.

4. Bern MM, Lokich JJ, Wallach SR *et al.* Very low doses of warfarin can prevent thrombosis in central venous catheters. *Ann Intern Med* 1990;**112**:423–8.

5. Merrer J, De Jonghe B, Golliot F *et al.* Complications of femoral and subclavian venous catheterization in critically ill patients: a randomized controlled trial. *JAMA* 2001;**286**:700–7.

6. Heijboer H, Brandjes PM, Buller HR, Sturk A, ten Cate JW. Deficiencies of coagulation-inhibiting and fibrinolytic proteins in outpatients with deep-vein thrombosis. *N Engl J Med* 1990;**323**:1512–16.

7. Kearon C, Crowther M, Hirsh J. Management of patients with hereditary hypercoagulable disorders. *Ann Rev Med* 2000;**51**:169–85.

8. Emmerich J, Rosendaal FR, Cattaneo M *et al.* Combined effect of factor V Leiden and prothrombin 20210A on the risk of venous thromboembolism – pooled analysis of 8 case–control studies including 2310 cases and 3204 controls. Study Group for Pooled-Analysis in Venous Thromboembolism. *Thromb Haemost* 2001;**86**:809–16.

9. Cattaneo M. Hyperhomocysteinemia, atherosclerosis and thrombosis. *Thromb Haemost* 1999;**81**:165–76.

10. Rosendaal FR. High levels of factor VIII and venous thrombosis. *Thromb Haemost* 2000;**83**:1–2.

11. Meijers JC, Tekelenburg WL, Bouma BN, Bertina RM, Rosendaal FR. High levels of coagulation factor XI as a risk factor for venous thrombosis. *N Engl J Med* 2000;**342**:696–701.

12. van Hylckama Vlieg A, van der Linden IK, Bertina RM, Rosendaal FR. High levels of factor IX increase the risk of venous thrombosis. *Blood* 2000;**95**:3678–82.

13. Poort SR, Rosendaal FR, Reitsma PH, Bertina RM. A common genetic variation in the 3′-untranslated region of the prothrombin gene is associated with elevated plasma prothrombin levels and an increase in venous thrombosis. *Blood* 1996;**88**:3698–703.

14. Kearon C. Epidemiology of venous thromboembolism. *Sem Vasc Med* 2001;**1**:7–25.

15. Warkentin TE, Levine MN, Hirsh J *et al.* Heparin-induced thrombocytopenia in patients treated with low-molecular-weight heparin or unfractionated heparin. *N Engl J Med* 1995;**332**:1330–5.

16. Anderson FA, Wheeler HB, Goldberg RJ *et al.* A population-based perspective of the hospital incidence and case-fatality rates of deep vein thrombosis and pulmonary embolism. *Arch Intern Med* 1991;**151**:933–8.

17. Kearon C. Natural history of venous thromboembolism. *Sem Vasc Med* 2001;**1**:27–37.

18. Hull R, Hirsh J, Sackett DL *et al.* Clinical validity of a negative venogram in patients with clinically suspected venous thrombosis. *Circulation* 1981;**64**:622–5.

19. Kearon C, Julian JA, Newman TE, Ginsberg JS, for the McMaster Diagnostic Imaging Practice Guidelines Initiative. Non-invasive diagnosis of deep vein thrombosis. *Ann Intern Med* 1998;**128**:663–77.

20. Wells PS, Hirsh J, Anderson DR *et al.* A simple clinical model for the diagnosis of deep-vein thrombosis combined with impedance plethysmography: potential for an improvement in the diagnosis process. *J Intern Med* 1998;**243**:15–23.

21. Anand SS, Wells PS, Hunt D, Brill-Edwards P, Cook D, Ginsberg JS. Does this patient have deep vein thrombosis? *JAMA* 1998;**279**:1094–9.

22. Wells PS, Anderson DR, Bormanis J *et al.* Value of assessment of pretest probability of deep-vein thrombosis in clinical management. *Lancet* 1997;**350**:1795–8.

23. Wells PS, Hirsh J, Anderson DR *et al.* Accuracy of clinical assessment of deep-vein thrombosis. *Lancet* 1995;**345**: 1326–30.

24. Wells PS, Hirsh J, Anderson DR *et al.* Comparison of the accuracy of impedance plethysmography and compression ultrasonography in outpatients with clinically suspected deep vein thrombosis. A two center paired-design prospective trial. *Thromb Haemost* 1995;**74**:1423–7.

25. Robinson KS, Anderson DR, Gross M *et al.* Ultrasonographic screening before hospital discharge for deep venous thrombosis after arthroplasty: the Post-Arthoplasty Screening Study. A randomized, controlled trial. *Ann Intern Med* 1997;**127**: 439–45.

26. Lee AYY, Ginsberg JS. Laboratory diagnosis of venous thromboembolism. *Bailliere's Clin Haematol* 1998;**11**:587–604.

27. Perrier A, Desmarais S, Miron MJ *et al.* Non-invasive diagnosis of venous thromboembolism in outpatients. *Lancet* 1999; **353**:190–5.

28. Bernardi E, Prandoni P, Lensing AWA *et al.* D-dimer testing as an adjunct to ultrasonography in patients with clinically suspected deep vein thrombosis: prospective cohort study. *BMJ* 1998;**317**:1037–40.

29. Kearon C, Ginsberg JS, Douketis J *et al.* Management of suspected deep venous thrombosis in outpatients by using clinical assessment and D-dimer testing. *Ann Intern Med* 2001; **135**:108–11.

30. Wells PS, Anderson DR, Rodger M *et al.* Excluding pulmonary embolism at the bedside without diagnostic imaging: management of patients with suspected pulmonary embolism presenting to the emergency department by using a simple clinical model and d-dimer. *Ann Intern Med* 2001;**135**: 98–107.

31. Anderson DR, Wells PS, Stiell I *et al.* Thrombosis in the emergency department: use of a clinical diagnosis model to safely avoid the need for urgent radiological investigation. *Arch Intern Med* 1999;**159**:477–82.

32. Ginsberg JS, Wells PS, Kearon C *et al.* Sensitivity and specificity of a rapid whole-blood assay for D-dimer in the diagnosis of pulmonary embolism. *Ann Intern Med* 1998; **129**:1006–11.

33. Righini M, Goehring C, Bounameaux H, Perrier A. Effects of age on the performance of common diagnostic tests for pulmonary embolism. *Am J Med* 2000;**109**:357–61.

34. Lee A, Julian J, Levine M *et al.* Clinical utility of a rapid whole-blood D-dimer assay in patients with cancer who present with suspected acute deep venous thrombosis. *Ann Intern Med* 2000;**131**:417–23.

35. Hull RD, Raskob GE, Carter CJ. Serial impedance plethysmography in pregnant patients with clinically suspected deep-vein thrombosis. Clinical validity of negative findings. *Ann Intern Med* 1990;**112**:663–7.

36. de Boer K, Buller HR, ten Cate JW, Levi M. Deep vein thrombosis in obstetric patients: diagnosis and risk factors. *Thromb Haemost* 1992;**67**:4–7.

37. Prandoni P, Cogo A, Bernardi E *et al.* A simple ultrasound approach for detection of recurrent proximal vein thrombosis. *Circulation* 1993;**88**:1730–5.

38. Fraser DG, Moody AR, Morgan PS, Martel AL, Davidson I. Diagnosis of lower-limb deep venous thrombosis: a prospective blinded study of magnetic resonance direct thrombus imaging. *Ann Intern Med* 2002;**136**:89–98.

39. Stein PD, Athanasoulis C, Alavi A *et al.* Complications and validity of pulmonary angiography in acute pulmonary embolism. *Circulation* 1992;**85**:462–8.

40. Kearon C. Diagnosis of pulmonary embolism. *Can Med Ass J* 2002 (in press).

41. Hull RD, Raskob GE, Coates G, Panju AA. Clinical validity of a normal perfusion lung scan in patients with suspected pulmonary embolism. *Chest* 1990;**97**:23–6.

42. The PIOPED investigators. Value of the ventilation perfusion scan in acute pulmonary embolism. *JAMA* 1990;**263**:2753–9.

43. Hull RD, Hirsh J, Carter CJ *et al.* Pulmonary angiography, ventilation lung scanning, and venography for clinically suspected pulmonary embolism with abnormal perfusion lung scan. *Ann Intern Med* 1983;**98**:891–9.

44. Wells PS, Ginsberg JS, Anderson DR *et al.* Use of a clinical model for safe management of patients with suspected pulmonary embolism. *Ann Intern Med* 1998;**129**:997–1005.

45. Hull RD, Hirsh J, Carter CJ *et al.* Diagnostic value of ventilation–perfusion lung scanning in patients with suspected pulmonary embolism. *Chest* 1985;**88**:819–28.

46. Stein PD, Henry JW, Gottschalk A. Mismatched vascular defects. An easy alternative to mismatched segmental equivalent defects for the interpretation of ventilation/perfusion lung scans in pulmonary embolism. *Chest* 1993;**104**:468–72.

47. Rathbun SW, Raskob GE, Whitsett TL. Sensitivity and specificity of helical computed tomography in the diagnosis of pulmonary embolism: a systematic review. *Ann Intern Med* 2000;**132**:227–32.

48. Perrier A, Howarth N, Didier D *et al.* Performance of helical computed tomography in unselected outpatients with suspected pulmonary embolism. *Ann Intern Med* 2001;**135**:88–97.

49. Kearon C, Ginsberg JS, Hirsh J. The role of venous ultrasonography in the diagnosis of suspected deep venous thrombosis and pulmonary embolism. *Ann Intern Med* 1998; **129**:1044–9.

50. Perrier A, Miron MJ, Desmarais S *et al.* Using clinical evaluation and lung scan to rule out suspected pulmonary embolism: Is it a valid option in patients with normal results of lower-limb venous compression ultrasonography? *Arch Intern Med* 2000;**160**:512–16.

51. Hull RD, Raskob GE, Ginsberg JS *et al.* A noninvasive strategy for the treatment of patients with suspected pulmonary embolism. *Arch Intern Med* 1994;**154**:289–97.

52. Chan WS, Ray JG, Murray S, Coady GE, Coates AL, Ginsberg JS. Suspected pulmonary embolism in pregnancy: Clinical presentation, results of lung scan, subsequent maternal and pediatric outcomes. *Arch Intern Med* 2002 (in press).

53. Ginsberg JS, Hirsh J, Rainbow AJ, Coates G. Risks to the fetus of radiologic procedures used in the diagnosis of maternal venous thromboembolic disease. *Thromb Haemost* 1989;**61**:189–96.

54. Sevitt S, Gallagher NG. Prevention of venous thrombosis and pulmonary embolism in injured patients. *Lancet* 1959;**ii**:981–9.

55. Kakkar VV, Corrigan TP, Fossard DP. Prevention of fatal postoperative pulmonary embolism by low doses of heparin. An international multicenter trial. *Lancet* 1975;**ii**:45–51.

56. Collins R, Scrimgeour A, Yusuf S, Peto R. Reduction in fatal pulmonary embolism and venous thrombosis by perioperative administration of subcutaneous heparin. *N Engl J Med* 1988;**318**:1162–73.

57. Leyvraz PF, Richard J, Bachmann F. Adjusted versus fixed dose subcutaneous heparin in the prevention of deep vein thrombosis after total hip replacement. *N Engl J Med* 1983;**309**:954–8.

58. Wille-Jorgensen P, Thorup J, Fischer A, Holst-Christensen J, Flamsholt R. Heparin with and without graded compression stockings in the prevention of thromboembolic complications of major abdominal surgery: a randomized trial. *Br J Surg* 1985;**72**:579–81.

59. Ramos R, Salem BI, De Pawlikowski MP, Coordes C, Eisenberg S, Leidenfrost R. The efficacy of pneumatic compression stockings in the prevention of pulmonary embolism after cardiac surgery. *Chest* 1996;**109**:82–5.

60. Koch A, Bouges S, Ziegler S, Dinkel H, Daures JP, Victor N. Low molecular weight heparin and unfractionated heparin in thrombosis prophylaxis after major surgical intervention: update of previous meta-analyses. *Br J Surg* 1997;**84**:750–9.

61. Eikelboom JW, Quinlan DJ, Douketis JD. Extended-duration prophylaxis against venous thromboembolism after total hip or knee replacement: a meta-analysis of the randomised trials. *Lancet* 2001;**358**:9–15.

62. Geerts WH, Heit JA, Clagett GP *et al.* Prevention of venous thromboembolism. *Chest* 2001;**119**:132S–75S.

63. Colwell CW Jr, Collis DK, Paulson R *et al.* Comparison of enoxaparin and warfarin for the prevention of venous thromboembolic disease after total hip arthroplasty. *J Bone J Surg* 1999;**81-A**:932–40.

64. "Antiplatelet trialists' collaboration". Collaborative overview of randomised trials of antiplatelet therapy-III: reduction in venous thrombosis and pulmonary embolism by antiplatelet prophylaxis among surgical and medical patients. *BMJ* 1994;**308**:235–46.

65. Prevention of pulmonary embolism and deep vein thrombosis with low dose aspirin: Pulmonary Embolism Prevention (PEP) trial. *Lancet* 2000;**355**:1295–302.

66. Eriksson BI, Wille-Jorgensen P, Kalebo P *et al.* A comparison of recombinant hirudin with a low-molecular weight heparin to prevent thromboembolic complications after total hip replacement. *N Engl J Med* 1997;**337**:1329–35.

67. Turpie AG, Gallus AS, Hoek JA. A synthetic pentasaccharide for the prevention of deep-vein thrombosis after total hip replacement. *N Engl J Med* 2001;**344**:619–25.

67a. Eriksen BI, Bauer KA, Lassen MR, Turpie AG. Fondaparinux compared with enoxaparin for the prevention of venous thromboembolism after hip-fracture surgery. *N Engl J Med* 2001;**345**:1298–304.

67b. Bauer KA, Eriksson BI, Lassen MR, Turpie AG. Fondaparinux compared with enoxaparin for the prevention of venous thromboembolism after elective major knee surgery. *N Engl J Med* 2001;**345**:1305–10.

68. Gårdlund for the Heparin Prophylaxis Group. Randomised, controlled trial of low-dose heparin for prevention of fatal pulmonary embolism in patients with infectious diseases. *Lancet* 1996;**347**:1357–61.

69. Wells PS, Lensing AWA, Hirsh J. Graduated compression stockings in the prevention of postoperative venous thromboembolism: a meta-analysis. *Arch Intern Med* 1994;**154**:67–72.

70. Hull R, Delmore T, Hirsh J *et al.* Effectiveness of an intermittent pulsatile elastic stocking for the prevention of calf and thigh vein thrombosis in patients undergoing elective knee surgery. *Thromb Res* 1979;**16**:37–45.

71. Hull RD, Raskob GE, Gent M *et al.* Effectiveness of intermittent pneumatic leg compression for preventing deep vein thrombosis after total hip replacement. *JAMA* 1990;**263**:2313–17.

72. Turpie AGG, Hirsh J, Gent M, Julian DH, Johnson J. Prevention of deep vein thrombosis in potential neurosurgical patients: a randomized trial comparing graduated compression stockings alone or graduated compression stockings plus intermittent pneumatic compression with control. *Arch Intern Med* 1989;**149**:679–81.

73. Salzman EW, Davies GC. Prophylaxis of venous thromboembollism: analysis of cost effectiveness. *Ann Surg* 1980;**191**:207–18.

74. Barritt DW, Jordan SC. Anticoagulant drugs in the treatment of pulmonary embolism: a controlled trial. *Lancet* 1960;**1**:1309–12.

75. Gallus AS, Jackaman J, Tillett J, Mills W, Sycherley A. Safety and efficacy of warfarin started early after submassive venous thrombosis or pulmonary embolism. *Lancet* 1986;**2**:1293–6.

76. Hull RD, Raskob GE, Rosenbloom D *et al.* Heparin for 5 days as compared with 10 days in the initial treatment of proximal venous thrombosis. *N Engl J Med* 1990;**322**:1260–4.

77. Brandjes DPM, Heijboer H, Buller HR, de Rijk M, Jagt H, ten Cate JW. Acenocoumarol and heparin compared with acenocoumarol alone in the initial treatment of proximal-vein thrombosis. *N Engl J Med* 1992;**327**:1485–9.

78. Dolovich LR, Ginsberg JS, Douketis JD, Holbrook AM, Cheah G. A meta-analysis comparing low-molecular-weight heparins with unfractionated heparin in the treatment of venous thromboembolism: examining some unanswered questions regarding location of treatment, product type, and dosing frequency. *Arch Intern Med* 2000;**160**:181–8.

79. Koopman MMW, Prandoni P, Piovella F *et al.* Treatment of venous thrombosis with intravenous unfractionated heparin administered in the hospital as compared with subcutaneous low-molecular-weight heparin administered at home. *N Engl J Med* 1996;**334**:682–7.

80. Couturaud F, Julian JA, Kearon C. Low molecular weight heparin administered once versus twice daily in patients with venous thromboembolism: a meta-analysis. *Thromb Haemost* 2001;**86**:980–4.

81. Hirsh J, Warkentin TE, Shaughnessy SG *et al.* Heparin and low-molecular-weight heparin: mechanisms of action,

pharmacokinetics, dosing, monitoring, efficacy, and safety. *Chest* 2001;**119**:64S–94S.

82. Chong BH, Gallus AS, Cade JF *et al*. Prospective randomized open-label comparison of danaparoid with dextran 70 in the treatment of heparin-induced thrombocytopenia with thrombosis. *Thromb Haemost* 2001;**86**:1170–5.

83. Hull R, Delmore T, Genton E *et al*. Warfarin sodium versus low-dose heparin in the long-term treatment of venous thrombosis. *N Engl J Med* 1979;**301**:855–8.

84. Hull R, Delmore T, Carter C *et al*. Adjusted subcutaneous heparin versus warfarin sodium in the long-term treatment of venous thrombosis. *N Engl J Med* 1982;**306**:189–94.

85. Hyers TM, Agnelli G, Hull RD *et al*. Antithrombotic therapy for venous thromboembolic disease. *Chest* 2001; **119**:176S–93S.

86. Hull R, Hirsh J, Jay R *et al*. Different intensities of oral anticoagulant therapy in the treatment of proximal-vein thrombosis. *N Engl J Med* 1982;**307**:1676–81.

87. Harrison L, Johnston M, Massicotte MP, Crowther M, Moffat K, Hirsh J. Comparison of 5-mg and 10-mg loading doses in initiation of warfarin therapy. *Ann Intern Med* 1997; **126**:133–6.

88. Crowther MA, Ginsberg JS, Kearon C *et al*. A randomized trial comparing 5 mg and 10 mg warfarin loading doses. *Arch Intern Med* 1999;**159**:46–8.

89. Crowther MA, Julian J, McCarty D *et al*. Treatment of warfarin-associated coagulopathy with oral vitamin K: a randomised controlled trial. *Lancet* 2000;**356**:1551–3.

90. Research Committee of the British Thoracic Society. Optimum duration of anticoagulation for deep-vein thrombosis and pulmonary embolism. *Lancet* 1992;**340**:873–6.

91. Levine MN, Hirsh J, Gent M *et al*. Optimal duration of oral anticoagulant therapy: a randomized trial comparing four weeks with three months of warfarin in patients with proximal deep vein thrombosis. *Thromb Haemost* 1995;**74**:606–11.

92. Schulman S, Rhedin A-S, Lindmarker P *et al*. A comparison of six weeks with six months of oral anticoagulant therapy after a first episode of venous thromboembolism. *N Engl J Med* 1995;**332**:1661–5.

93. Prandoni P, Lensing AWA, Cogo A *et al*. The long-term clinical course of acute deep venous thrombosis. *Ann Intern Med* 1996;**125**:1–7.

94. Pini M, Aiello S, Manotti C *et al*. Low molecular weight heparin versus warfarin the prevention of recurrence after deep vein thrombosis. *Thromb Haemost* 1994;**72**:191–7.

95. Pinede L, Ninet J, Duhaut P *et al*. Comparison of 3 and 6 months of oral anticoagulant therapy after a first episode of proximal deep vein thrombosis or pulmonary embolism and comparison of 6 and 12 weeks of therapy after isolated calf deep vein thrombosis. *Circulation* 2001;**103**:2453–60.

96. Pinede L, Duhaut P, Cucherat M, Ninet J, Pasquier J, Boissel JP. Comparison of long versus short duration of anticoagulant therapy after a first episode of venous thromboembolism: a meta-analysis of randomized, controlled trials. *J Intern Med* 2000;**247**:553–62.

97. Kearon C, Gent M, Hirsh J *et al*. A comparison of three months of anticoagulation with extended anticoagulation for a first episode of idiopathic venous thromboembolism. *N Engl J Med* 1999;**340**:901–7.

98. Agnelli G, Prandoni P, Santamaria MG *et al*. Three months versus one year of oral anticoagulant therapy for idiopathic deep vein thrombosis. *N Eng J Med* 2001;**345**:165–9.

99. Lindmarker P, Schulman S. The risk of ipsilateral versus contralateral recurrent deep vein thrombosis in the leg. The DURAC Trial Study Group. *J Intern Med* 2000;**247**:601–6.

100. Schulman S, Granqvist S, Holmstrom M *et al*. The duration of oral anticoagulant therapy after a second episode of venous thromboembolism. *N Engl J Med* 1997;**336**:393–8.

101. Beyth RJ, Quinn LM, Landefeld S. Prospective evaluation of an index for predicting the risk of major bleeding in outpatients treated with warfarin. *Am J Med* 1998;**105**:91–9.

102. Schulman S, Svenungsson E, Granqvist S. Anticardiolipin antibodies predict early recurrence of thromboembolism and death among patients with venous thromboembolism following anticoagulant therapy. *Am J Med* 1998;**104**:332–8.

103. Lindmarker P, Schulman S, Sten-Linder M, Wiman B, Egberg N, Johnsson H. The risk of recurrent venous thromboembolism in carriers and non-carriers of the G1691A Allele in the coagulation factor V gene and the G20210A Allele in the prothrombin gene. *Thromb Haemost* 1999;**81**:684–9.

104. Hirsh J, Lensing A. Thrombolytic therapy for deep vein thrombosis. *Int Angiol* 1996;**5**:S22–S25.

105. Schweizer J, Kirch W, Koch R *et al*. Short- and long-term results after thrombolytic treatment of deep vein thrombosis. *J Am Coll Cardiol* 2000;**36**:1336–43.

106. Blackmon JR, Sautter RD, Wagner HN. Uokinase pulmonary embolism trial: phase I results. *JAMA* 1970;**214**:2163–72.

107. Dalen JE, Alpert JS, Hirsh J. Thrombolytic therapy for pulmonary embolism. Is it effective? Is it safe? When is it indicated? *Arch Intern Med* 1997;**157**:2550–6.

108. Jerjes-Sanchez C, Ramirez-Rivera A, de Lourdes Garcia M *et al*. Streprokinase and heparin versus heparin alone in massive pulmonary embolism: a randomized controlled trial. *J Thromb Thrombolys* 1995;**2**:227–9.

109. Decousus H, Leizorovicz A, Parent F *et al*. A clinical trial of vena caval filters in the prevention of pulmonary embolism in patients with proximal deep-vein thrombosis. *N Engl J Med* 1998;**338**:409–15.

110. Ginsberg JS, Hirsh J, Levine MN, Burrows R. Risks to the fetus of anticoagulant therapy during pregnancy. *Thromb Haemost* 1989;**61**:197–203.

111. Ginsberg JS, Greer I, Hirsh J. Use of antithrombotic agents during pregnancy. *Chest* 2001;**119**:122S–31S.

112. Cogo A, Lensing AWA, Prandoni P, Hirsh J. Distribution of thrombosis in patients with symptomatic deep-vein thrombosis: Implications for simplifying the diagnostic process with compression ultrasound. *Arch Intern Med* 1993;**153**:2777–80.

113. Lagerstedt CI, Olsson CG, Fagher BO, Oqvist BW, Albrechtsson U. Need for long-term anticoagulant treatment in symptomatic calf-vein thrombosis. *Lancet* 1985;**ii**:515–18.

114. Moser KM, LeMoine JR. Is embolic risk conditioned by location of deep venous thrombosis? *Ann Intern Med* 1981;**94**: 439–44.

115. Moser KM, Fedullo PF, LittleJohn JK, Crawford R. Frequent asymptomatic pulmonary embolism in patients with deep venous thrombosis. *JAMA* 1994;**27**:223–5.

116. Kruit WHJ, de Boer AC, Sing AK, van Roon F. The significance of venography in the management of patients with clinically

suspected pulmonary embolism. *J Intern Med* 1991;**230**: 333–9.

117.Hull RD, Raskob GE, Coates G, Panju AA, Gill GJ. A new non-invasive management strategy for patients with suspected pulmonary embolism. *Arch Intern Med* 1989;**149**:2549–55.

118.Stein PD, Henry JW. Prevalence of acute pulmonary embolism among patients in a general hospital and at autopsy. *Chest* 1995;**108**:978–81.

119.Bell WR, Simon TL. Current status of pulmonary embolic disease: pathophysiology, diagnosis, prevention, and treatment. *Am Heart J* 1982;**103**:239–61.

120.Ginsberg J, Kearon C, Douketis J *et al.* The use of D-dimer testing and impedance plethysmographic examination in patients with clinical indications of deep vein thrombosis. *Arch Intern Med* 1997;**157**:1077–81.

121.Hull RD, Carter CJ, Jay RM *et al.* The diagnosis of acute recurrent deep vein thrombosis: a diagnostic challenge. *Circulation* 1983;**67**:901–6.

122.Huisman MV, Buller HR, ten Cate JW. Utility of impedance plethysmography in the diagnosis of recurrent deep-vein thrombosis. *Arch Intern Med* 1988;**148**:681–3.

123.Wells PS, Anderson DR, Rodger M *et al.* Derivation of a simple clinical model to categorize patients probability of pulmonary embolism: increasing the models utility with the SimpliRED D-dimer. *Thromb Haemost* 2000;**83**:416–20.

124.Turkstra F, Kiujer PMM, van Beek E Jr, Brandjes DPM, ten Cate JW, Buller HR. Diagnostic utility of ultrasonography of leg veins in patients suspected of having pulmonary embolism. *Ann Intern Med* 1997;**126**:775–81.

62 Peripheral vascular disease

Jesper Swedenborg, Jan Östergren

Epidemiology

The prevalence of lower extremity arterial occlusive disease as judged by history has been examined in several studies. Large cohorts of patients have been questioned about symptoms of intermittent claudication. This has mostly been done using a questionnaire initially designed by Rose.[1] The method has an acceptable specificity but lacks sensitivity and, for obvious reasons, it does not detect asymptomatic arterial occlusive disease.[2] The prevalence of peripheral arterial occlusive disease varies between studies, with high figures reported from Russia and Finland.[3,4] With large and reliable studies, it is likely that the prevalence at the age of 60 is 3–6%.[5] Most studies report a prevalence of less than 5% at 50 years.

In order to detect lower extremity arterial occlusive disease more specifically, studies have been performed measuring ankle pressure with non-invasive techniques. In general it can be said that the prevalence of disease increases by a factor of 3 compared with studies based on questionnaires. There is a significant correlation between the ankle brachial pressure index (ABI) and the symptom of intermittent claudication, although the correlation is modest with r values between 0·1 and 0·2.[6] Based on such objective methods, 11·7% of the population in the Framingham study had peripheral arterial disease. Thus assessment of peripheral arterial disease by the symptom of intermittent claudication underestimates the true prevalence,[7] but the cut off points determining what is considered to be a pathologic ABI is of great importance for the estimation of the prevalence using objective methods.[8]

The prevalence is greatly influenced by age as pointed out in one of the major studies, the Framingham study.[9] Other important factors are cigarette smoking and sex. Thus non-smoking women in the age group 55–64 years showed a prevalence by history of 3·9% compared with smoking men in the age group 75–84 years where the prevalence was 14·5%. Additional factors increasing the risk are diabetes and fibrinogen levels.[10]

Few studies have examined the incidence of peripheral arterial occlusive disease by following normal subjects and determining when claudication appears. In the Framingham study, the yearly incidence increases from 0·2% in 45–55 year old men to 0·5% in 55–65 year old men.[9] In the last follow up after 38 years, the yearly rates were found to increase until the age 75 and then declined. The statistical analyses revealed that those with intermittent claudication were significantly older, had higher cholesterol levels, higher blood pressure, higher frequency of diabetes, and smoked more cigarettes.[11] The Edinburgh artery study provides similar figures with an annual incidence of 1·8 per 1000 randomly selected patients from general practitioners.[12]

Long-term outcome

The natural history of patients with lower extremity arterial disease has been studied regarding both the fate of the limb and mortality. Among patients with peripheral arterial occlusive disease, at most one in five will require surgical correction for their vascular disease[13] and 2–5% will undergo amputation.[5,9] The risk for amputation decreases if the patients can stop smoking.[14] Patients with peripheral arterial occlusive disease have a decreased life expectancy compared with the normal population. This is almost solely explained by cardiovascular disease in general and coronary artery disease in particular. After 10 years, only 52% of claudicants are still alive.[15] The relative risk of dying from cardiovascular disease and coronary heart disease (CHD) is reported to be 5–6 times that of the normal population over 10 years.[16] The severity of the peripheral arterial occlusive disease is associated with the risk of dying, since the lower extremity arterial disease is a surrogate variable reflecting the severity of atherosclerosis affecting the coronary arteries.[17] Smoking is also an important predictor of the risk of dying in these patient groups.[18] The greatest threat to the patient with peripheral arterial disease is thus death from cardiac causes. Patients with peripheral arterial disease and concomitant three vessel coronary artery disease (CAD) have an improved survival after coronary artery bypass grafting (CABG).[19] The natural course of intermittent claudication on the other hand is relatively benign in terms of limb survival as reflected by the low risk of amputation. This may, however, partly be explained by the fact that the mortality among patients with severe disease and high risk of amputation is considerably higher than for patients with mild disease.

Investigation of the patient with peripheral vascular disease

An adequate history and physical examination provide the basis for proper management of patients with peripheral vascular disease. The history should include a survey of relevant risk factors and possible symptoms of concomitant cardiovascular disease (for example, angina pectoris). Palpation of pulses and auscultation in the groin and over the femoral arteries may reveal signs of occlusion or stenoses in the vessels from the iliac artery down to the lower leg. The popliteal artery is best evaluated with the knee slightly elevated from the support and the tissue in the distal popliteal fossa pressed against the tibia. Palpation at this location is particularly important when a popliteal aneurysm is suspected. In cases with more severe ischemia, inspection may reveal a diminished growth of hair and nails, and distal ischemic ulcers often located on toes and heels. Elevation of the legs will cause a whitening of the most affected foot, which in the dependent position typically is more red than the contralateral one, owing to an increase of blood in the superficial venous plexa.

Measurement of the ankle pressure is of value as a quantitative estimate of the degree of arterial insufficiency. This is easily done with a continous wave pen-doppler detecting the pulse either in the posterior tibial or the dorsal pedal artery when a blood pressure cuff around the ankle is slowly deflated from a suprasystolic pressure. By dividing the measured value with the brachial pressure the ABI is determined. An index below 0·9 is considered pathologic. In patients with diabetes mellitus, the ABI may be falsely elevated owing to sclerosis of the media of the arteries, which resists compression by the cuff.

Further anatomic evaluation of the arterial system is needed only when invasive procedures are indicated. Duplex sonography is the method of choice, but in most cases has to be followed by angiography, when surgery is planned.

All patients with peripheral vascular disease should have blood tests to detect other treatable risk factors such as blood lipids, blood or plasma glucose, and serum creatinine. Systemic blood pressure is also a treatable risk factor that should be measured.

Intermittent claudication

Pathophysiology

Intermittent claudication is caused almost exclusively by atherosclerotic lesions in the arteries to the legs. The lesion causing the symptoms may be located above the inguinal ligament (the aorta, iliac artery, or the common femoral artery) or below, in such cases often in the distal part of the superficial femoral artery. Combinations of series of stenosis or occlusions also involving the popliteal and lower leg vessels are not uncommon.

The evolution of the disease may be slow with gradual onset of symptoms but in many cases the occurrence of a thrombus in a severely stenosed area or overlying a ruptured atherosclerotic plaque may cause an acute onset of symptoms.

The most common location of pain is in the calf, since the majority of vascular occlusions occur in the superficial femoral artery. When the main lesion is in the iliac region, pain and muscular dysfunction may also be located in the gluteal muscles and the thigh. The symptoms are caused by an inappropriate blood supply in relation to the metabolic needs of the muscles during exercise. When occlusion of the artery occurs gradually, collaterals, often from the deep femoral artery, may compensate for the limited arterial supply through the natural artery.

Therapy

General measures

The aim of therapy for intermittent claudication is twofold:

- to reduce risk factors associated with the disease and thereby improving the long-term prognosis of the patient;
- to improve walking distance and thus the quality of life for the patient.

In the general management of the patient it is mandatory to screen for risk factors associated with atherosclerosis. Smoking should be stopped immediately as the risk for the patient with claudication for having an amputation in the future is reduced to virtually zero.[14] **Grade B** Hyperlipidemia and hypertension should be treated according to guidelines outlined in other sections of this book. A meta-analysis of lipid lowering therapy in 698 patients with peripheral arterial disease indicated that active therapy reduced disease progression and the severity of claudication.[20] Recently the Heart Protection Study including 20 000 patients with coronary or non-coronary artery disease or diabetes was reported, showing that simvastatin 40 mg/day reduced cardiovascular mortality and morbidity. The 24% decrease of vascular events was consistent in all subgroups including patients with peripheral vascular disease and regardless of cholesterol levels.[21] **Grade A** Thus, a statin should be given as first-line therapy, but niacin could also be valuable since it increases serum HDL (high density lipoproteins) concentrations and lowers serum triglyceride concentrations, which are the most common lipid disturbances in patients with intermittent claudication.

A fear of reducing distal perfusion pressures in patients with claudication by antihypertensive treatment has sometimes prevented doctors from instituting adequate treatment of hypertension. In particular, β blockers have been considered by some to be contraindicated in this situation. Controlled studies have, however, shown that treatment of claudicants with β blockers only reduces walking capacity marginally or not at all.[22] Therefore, if strong indications, such as heart failure, or a previous myocardial infarction exist, β blockers should also be used in claudicants. **Grade A**

The HOPE study investigated the effect of the ACE inhibitor ramipril 10 mg/day compared with placebo.[23] The study included 1715 patients with symptomatic peripheral vascular disease and 3099 patients with an ABI < 0·9. These subgroups benefitted at least equally well as the entire study population from the treatment. The beneficial effect was seen even among patients who already had adequate blood pressure control. Treatment with an ACE inhibitor should thus be strongly considered in patients with peripheral arterial disease. **Grade A**

If symptoms of increased ischemia of the legs occur during treatment for hypertension, this strengthens the indication for an invasive procedure in order to relieve the symptoms of leg ischemia. If this is not possible, the antihypertensive therapy should be reduced with caution.

Since patients with intermittent claudication have an increased risk for major cardiovascular events because of their generalized atherosclerotic disease, antiplatelet therapy should be given prophylactically, preferably with aspirin, based on conclusions from meta-analysis.[24] **Grade A** Although major studies on the effect of aspirin in patients with claudication are lacking, the effect in subgroups with claudication (*n* = 3295; risk reduction from 11·8% to 9·7% over 27 months) seems to be equivalent to the reduction seen in the atherosclerotic population as a whole.[24] The combination with dipyridamole may provide an additional

preventive effect,[25] but so far only one study has shown an effect on major end points by this combination in the case of the secondary prevention of stroke.[26] In 687 claudicants studied over a 7 year period, ticlopidine 250 mg ×2/day reduced the need for vascular reconstructive surgery by 51% compared to placebo.[27] In the same trial, the mortality rate was 29.1% lower (64 *v* 89 cases) in the ticlopidine group compared with the placebo group.[28] The same dose of ticlopidine may also produce some increase in walking capacity in comparison with placebo.[29] The disadvantage of this compound is the risk of adverse effects and the need for laboratory control of white blood cell counts. A better and safer alternative to ticlopidine for patients who cannot tolerate aspirin is clopidogrel, which was studied in the CAPRIE trial.[30] In the 6452 patients with peripheral arterial disease, clopidogrel 75 mg/day showed a relative risk reduction of 23·8% in ischemic stroke, myocardial infarction, or death from other vascular causes compared to aspirin 325 mg/day.[30]

Exercise

Patients with claudication should be instructed to walk as much as possible and, when pain occurs, they should try to walk despite the pain.[31] Training by intensive walking on treadmill or outdoors has been shown to be as effective or even better than other programs of physical training and, in most cases, will improve walking capacity by 100–200%.[31] In some cases the symptoms of claudication may even disappear completely. The optimal exercise program includes walking to near maximal pain for more than 30 minutes per session at least three times weekly during at least a 6 month period.[32]

Pharmacologic treatment to increase walking capacity

Different pharmacologic agents have been evaluated for improvement of walking distance in addition to physical training. Most of these treatments have been inconsistent in their effect and of marginal benefit. Generally, vasodilators have not been shown to be effective. The agent so far most extensively studied has been pentoxifylline, which is available in most countries for the treatment of intermittent claudication. The patients most likely to respond are those with a history of claudication over 1 year and an ABI of <0·8.[33] A meta-analysis of the pentoxifylline studies has shown an increase of 44 meters in maximal walking distance on the treadmill compared with placebo.[34] The phosphodiesterase inhibitor cilostazol was approved in 1999 by the FDA for treatment of claudication. Cilostazol is primarily a platelet inhibitor and a vasodilator that has been shown to increase the walking distance compared with placebo and also with pentoxifylline.[35] However, the use of the drug is hampered by the risk for worsening heart failure.[36] A randomized but open study[37] indicates that prostaglandin E1 given intravenously may be more effective than pentoxifylline (60·4% compared with 10·5% increase in walking capacity), but further studies are needed to establish the role of prostaglandins in this context.

> ## Key points
> - Quit smoking!
> - Regular exercise – walking until intolerable pain.
> - Intervention against other cardiovascular risk factors; treat hypertension and institute a statin to all patients with a normal or high cholesterol level.
> - Antiplatelet therapy and ACE inhibitor to be considered for all patients.
> - Other pharmacologic therapy of very limited benefit.

Critical ischemia

Pathophysiology

When the distal pressure in the leg is too low to provide sufficient perfusion in order to meet the metabolic demands of the tissue, pain will also occur in the resting situation, particularly in the supine position when there is no contribution to distal pressures by hydrostatic forces. Subsequently ulcers in the apical parts of the extremity may develop owing to an insufficient nutritional blood flow in the skin.

According to the European Consensus Document on chronic lower limb ischemia, critical ischemia is defined as "persistently recurring rest pain requiring regular analgesia for more than 2 weeks and/or ulceration or gangrene of the foot and toes in combination with an ankle systolic pressure less than 50 mmHg". In the case of diabetes, where the measurements of ankle pressures are unreliable because of incompressible arteries, the absence of palpable pulses are sufficient.[38] The definition has been criticized because many patients with critical limb ischemia according to the above definition still have an intact lower extremity after 1 year. This is exemplified by the findings in control groups of randomized trials regarding non-surgical treatment of critical limb ischemia.[39] Furthermore, some patients who do not fit into this definition may lose their legs because of ischemia.[40] A recent consensus document was made more practical. A patient with critical limb ischemia is defined as "a patient with chronic ischemic rest pain, ulcers and gangrene attributable to objectively proven arterial disease".[41]

The crucial factor regarding tissue nutrition is the flow through the capillary bed, which is dependent not only on the pressure in the arteries but also on other factors, such as blood viscosity and distribution of flow between nutritional and non-nutritional vessels – that is, arteriovenous shunts. Intravital capillaroscopy and transcutaneous oxygen tension are methods that can assess tissue nutrition, thereby offering additional prognostic information in these patients.[38] Patients with critical ischemia should be evaluated for possible vascular reconstructive surgery or endovascular treatment (see below).

General measures

When invasive procedures to restore blood flow (see below) are not possible or have failed, several therapeutic measures should be considered. Optimization of the hemodynamic situation is one aim. Heart failure and edema should be treated vigorously. Lowering the foot end of the bed at night may improve distal perfusion pressure and relieve symptoms. Shoes should be well fitting to avoid the risk of pressure against the skin. Ulcers should be treated with care, and more often dry dressings are preferable in order not to moisturize intact skin around the ulcer area.

Though not scientifically proven in this situation, anticoagulation may be of benefit. Thus, oral anticoagulants or low molecular weight heparin should be considered as an alternative or an addition to aspirin, since both arterial and venous thrombi are common in the severely ischemic leg.[42] Warfarin has been shown to lower the risk of occlusion in femoropopliteal vein grafts.[43] Pain should be treated by pharmacologic measures. Spinal cord stimulation could be used since this method has been shown to decrease pain possibly by increasing microvascular blood flow.[44]

The only pharmacologic agent so far convincingly shown to have a positive influence on the prognosis of patients with critical limb ischemia is a synthetic prostacyclin (Iloprost), which is given intravenously daily for a period of 2–4 weeks. In a meta-analysis, rest pain and ulcer size were found to improve in comparison with placebo and, more importantly, the probability of being alive with both legs still intact after 6 months was 65% in the Iloprost-treated group compared to 45% in the placebo-treated patients.[39] **Grade A** Pentoxifylline has been shown to be of benefit in a short-term perspective as a pain reliever but no long-term trials have been performed.[45] Spinal cord stimulation has been used to avoid amputations, but so far it has not benefitted patients with critical limb ischemia as a preventive treatment.[46]

> ## Key points
> - Evaluate possibilities for revascularization.
> - Optimize cardiac hemodynamics.
> - Avoid hypotension – lower foot end of bed at night.
> - Provide adequate pain relief.
> - Optimize local skin and wound care.
> - Consider anticoagulation or antiplatelet therapy.
> - Consider Iloprost treatment when revascularization is not possible or has failed.

Surgical treatment of intermittent claudication and critical ischemia

In this chapter both open surgery and endovascular treatment are considered. In the latter group percutaneous transluminal angioplasty (PTA) in combination with both thrombolysis and stenting are included. The major indications for reconstructive procedures for lower extremity ischemia are critical ischemia and claudication.

Preoperative cardiac evaluation

Since patients with peripheral vascular disease have a high frequency of cardiac comorbidity, the perioperative mortality and morbidity is dominated by cardiac problems. Many attempts have been made to identify patients with a high risk of perioperative cardiac complications. The rationale for such a strategy is to identify patients in need of coronary artery revascularization before the vascular procedure, and also to provide a basis for more intensive cardiac monitoring during peripheral vascular surgery. Although not specifically designed for peripheral vascular surgery, clinical risk scores according to Goldman[47] or Detsky[48] have been used. Further tests include ambulatory ECG, dipyridamole thallium scintigraphy, ejection fraction estimation by radionuclide ventriculography, and stress echocardiography. All these tests are effective in predicting perioperative cardiac mortality and morbidity, but dobutamine stress echocardiography seems to be most promising in a meta-analysis.[49] Patients who have reversible defects on preoperative thallium scintigraphy are at a high risk of perioperative cardiac mortality and morbidity,[50] and successful coronary revascularization decreases this risk following vascular surgery.[51] Nevertheless, routine evaluation of all patients scheduled for peripheral vascular surgery with thallium scintigraphy is not warranted.[52] The reason for this is that both coronary angiography and coronary revascularization add to the risk.[53] Today it can therefore be concluded that patients with a low risk, as reflected by either absence of angina pectoris or only mild disease, do not benefit from further evaluation aiming at coronary angiography.[54] Patients with high risk according to clinical scoring systems or careful history should be evaluated with dipyridamole thallium scintigraphy or dobutamin stress echocardiography. **Grade B** The use of bisoprolol, a β1 selective inhibitor, reduced the 30 day combined cardiac morbidity and mortality from 34% to 3·4% in high-risk patients undergoing peripheral vascular surgery.[55] Whether other β blockers have the same effect remains to be shown. **Grade B**

Open surgical vascular reconstructions

The vascular reconstructions for lower limb ischemia are mainly divided into supra- and infrainguinal reconstructions.

Suprainguinal vascular reconstructions

In the aortoiliac segment, vascular reconstructive procedures were initially dominated by thromboendarterectomy (TEA); this, however, requires large dissections. After the introduction of bypass grafting with synthetic materials TEA was largely abandoned except for short localized lesions. The results of aortobifemoral bypass with Dacron grafts for arterial occlusive disease are usually good with 1 year patency rates in the range of 95%. The patency rates are influenced by the outflow bed, so that patients with a patent superficial femoral artery (SFA) have better patency rates than those with an occluded SFA. There are no prospective randomized trials comparing TEA and aortofemoral bypass. TEA is said to have lower long-term patency rates, and another disadvantage is that the surgical procedure is more extensive. Aortofemoral bypass with a synthetic graft, however, has the disadvantage of risk of infection. Although this is an infrequent complication, it is associated with major morbidity and mortality, since an infected graft has to be removed.

During recent years the number of aortobifemoral reconstructions have declined owing to the more frequent use of endovascular methods, particularly PTA with or without stenting. Thus the extensive procedure of aortobifemoral bypass can be converted into a lesser procedure if at least one iliac artery can be opened with PTA. In such cases the contralateral leg can be revascularized with the aid of an extra-anatomic procedure – that is, femorofemoral bypass. The latter procedure has good patency rates, approximately 90% at 1 year and 65% at 5 years.[56–58] In patients who are unfit for major surgery and where the iliac arteries cannot be opened up with endovascular procedures another extra-anatomic bypass can be employed. In such patients axillo-bifemoral bypass can be used, but this type of extra-anatomic bypass is a compromise, since it has lower patency rates than aortobifemoral bypass.[59]

Infrainguinal vascular reconstructions

The standard procedure for infrainguinal occlusive disease is femoropopliteal bypass or bypass to the crural arteries. Bypass to the crural arteries is often performed in people with diabetes since their occlusive disease is in many cases more peripherally located than in non-diabetic patients with atherosclerosis. The most commonly used graft material is the saphenous vein but, if this is unavailable, arm veins or synthetic grafts may be used. In general it has been stated that use of autologous material is superior in infrainguinal reconstructions.[60] Some randomized studies have failed to detect a difference in long-term patency between synthetic grafts and saphenous vein grafts. One study did not show a significantly different patency at 2 years follow up, but after 4 years there was a significant difference in favor of saphenous vein grafts, 68% patency versus 47%.[61] **Grade A** For bypass grafts with the lower anastomosis below the knee, autologous material is clearly preferred. This is particularly true when bypass procedures are done to the crural arteries where the use of synthetic grafts produces dismal results.

When an autologous vein is used, the original procedure implies excision and reversal of the vein so that the blood can flow freely across the valves. The "*in situ*" technique, originally introduced by Hall, has, however, in recent years gained more popularity:[62] the saphenous vein is left in its bed and the valves are destroyed by special instruments; tributaries are identified and tied off. Some prospective randomized trials have been performed comparing the two methods but no definitive advantage with either method has been shown.[63] Therefore the personal preference of the surgeon often decides which method should be used. The advantage with the *in situ* method is that the larger end of the vein is anastomosed to the larger artery, and the smaller end of the vein to the small distal artery. With meticulous technique it is said that the vein is exposed to less trauma, but the valve destruction definitely induces some damage to the vein.

In order to improve long-term patency rates, two methods have been employed: graft surveillance and pharmacologic treatment. Postoperative surveillance of vein grafts is used by many surgeons in order to detect a failing graft, defined as a graft with a developing stenosis that threatens to reduce the blood flow below a critical level. Only few randomized studies have been done examining the effect on long-term patency rates in surveillance programs identifying and treating critical graft stenosis. Conflicting results regarding the effectiveness of such programs have been obtained. One study reported a patency rate of 78% in an intensive surveillance program including duplex scanning of the graft after 3 years versus 53% without such a program.[64] Other studies, however, have failed to demonstrate an advantage of duplex scanning over clinical surveillance with measurements of ankle pressure.[65] Whether a graft surveillance program has a beneficial effect upon amputation rate also remains to be shown.

The effect of antiplatelet therapy on total mortality has been studied in several trials and it seems to reduce cardiovascular mortality.[66] There is only one trial that has studied the similar effects of oral anticoagulants, and this trial suggested that they both prevent graft occlusion and diminish the risk of cardiovascular death.[43] Pharmacologic therapy seems to improve the patency rate for infrainguinal vascular reconstructions. Most centers use antiplatelet therapy with acetylsalicylic acid, and a meta-analysis of randomized trials has indicated that such treatment improves the patency rate.[67] **Grade A** Oral anticoagulants are not used as widely as antiplatelet therapy but many surgeons use it selectively in patients where the prognosis for graft patency for some reason is bad. Whether antiplatelet therapy or oral anticoagulants differ in their effectiveness against graft

occlusion is not known. Only one study has addressed this question and no significant difference in graft patency was found between patients treated with warfarin or acetyl salicylic acid. Subgroup analysis, however, revealed that oral anticoagulants seemed to be more effective in patients receiving autologous grafts and antiplatelet therapy in those receiving synthetic grafts.[68] **Grade B**

Key points

- For bilateral suprainguinal occlusions aortofemoral bypass is the standard procedure, but endovascular methods are used at an increasing rate.
- For unilateral suprainguinal occlusions femorofemoral bypass can be used.
- For infrainguinal occlusions saphenous vein bypass is the standard procedure, but synthetic grafts can be used if suitable veins are lacking.
- Bypass to infragenicular arteries using synthetic grafts produces inferior results compared to saphenous vein bypass.

Endovascular procedures

Since the introduction of transluminal dilation by Dotter, this field has grown enormously.[69] The introduction of PTA has resulted in more indications for endovascular procedures to some extent at the expense of open surgical reconstructions.

Percutaneous transluminal angioplasty

In common with other vascular reconstructive procedures the success rate of PTA is highly dependent upon various factors. In general it can be said that proximal lesions – that is, iliac lesions – have a better success rate than distal ones – that is, femoropopliteal lesions. The chance of a successful outcome is higher for stenoses rather than occlusions, irrespective of the site of the lesion. In common with surgical vascular reconstructions, the outflow determines the outcome also for PTA. Thus, in cases of a good outflow, the results are better than if the outflow is poor.[70] In summary, the chance of success is much higher when a short iliac stenosis is dilated in a patient with patent superficial femoral and profunda femoris arteries than after dilation of a popliteal occlusion in a patient with occlusions of two out of three crural arteries.

The indications for this procedure need to be considered. PTA of an iliac stenosis in a patient with claudication has a low risk and a high chance of success and may, therefore, be perfectly appropriate, even if the severity of the disease state is relatively mild, as compared with a patient with critical limb ischemia and a threat of amputation. On the other hand, a patient with an occluded popliteal artery and poor leg run-off with ischemic ulceration has a strong indication for the procedure and, in such a patient, it may also be perfectly appropriate to make an attempt at PTA, even though the success rate is relatively low. For patients with critical ischemia, PTA of infrapopliteal vessels has also been performed successfully and could even be used for short occlusions.[71,72]

Subintimal angioplasty has been advocated.[73] The method implies that a guidewire enters the subintimal space and then re-enters the vessel distal to the occlusion, and the subintimal space is then dilated with the balloon. In the femoropopliteal segment, occlusions longer than 20 cm can be treated, whereas intraluminal angioplasty is generally not advocated for occlusions longer than a few centimeters. Patency rates of approximately 60% at 3 years for femoropopliteal occlusions have been reported after subintimal angioplasty.[74] The reported figures are patency rates for technically successful procedures, but in 20% the procedure cannot be performed. The method has also been used for infrapopliteal arteries.[75] Subintimal angioplasty, if proven successful, could be a future alternative to femoropopliteal bypass.

Formal comparisons in prospective randomized trials between PTA and surgery are relatively scarce. Such trials are difficult because, in order for a patient to be included, the lesion has to be suitable for PTA – that is, it should be either a stenosis or a short occlusion. Knowing that the treatment of a stenosis with PTA is relatively successful with less risk and shorter hospital stay, it is sometimes considered ethically questionable to include patients in a trial between PTA and surgery. In a study including 263 patients with lesions in the iliac, femoral, or popliteal arteries comparing bypass surgery and PTA, primary success favored surgery, while limb salvage favored PTA, but the differences were not statistically significant. After 4 years there was no significant difference in outcome.[76]

Randomized trials comparing angioplasty with non-surgical treatment for intermittent claudication have, however, been performed, but they are relatively small and the results are to some extent contradictory. In one study the treadmill distances improved in both groups but were superior in those undergoing an exercise program, and after 6 years there was no benefit in treadmill walking distance after angioplasty.[77] In another study, an improvement in ABI was shown 6 months following angioplasty, which could not be found in patients undergoing exercise programs. Significantly more patients were asymptomatic after 6 months in the angioplasty group compared with those treated with exercise programs. This study, however, had a shorter follow up, and the conservative treatment was not as active as in the study where no difference could be seen between exercise program and PTA.[78] It can still be concluded that PTA is suitable for stenoses or short occlusions in claudicants, but few claudicants have discrete lesions suitable for PTA.

Stenting has been used at an increasing rate over the last few years. It is generally advised not to use stents in smaller arteries, and this implies that stents are used relatively seldom in the femoropopliteal region. Stents, however, are used in the iliac arteries after PTA, particularly when there is recoil or dissection. Several types of stents have been used, both self-expandable and balloon-expandable ones. Stenting below the inguinal ligament is not generally recommended.

Thrombolysis

Thrombolysis of peripheral arterial occlusive disease is recommended for acute arterial occlusions, but it also has a place in subacute occlusions. Thrombolysis should be intra-arterial and preferably the thrombolytic agent should be delivered into the clot, either with an end hole catheter or a catheter with multiple side holes. Today recombinant tissue plasminogen activator (rtPA) is used most commonly. Other thrombolytic agents are, however, being developed and have been tried for indications other than peripheral arterial occlusive disease. The dosage and rate of administration of thrombolytic agents varies in different reports and makes comparisons difficult. There are, however, some prospective randomized trials comparing surgery with intra-arterial thrombolytic therapy. In one representative study, the mean duration of ischemia was almost 2 months and patients were included if the duration was less than 6 months. Overall the study favored surgery. Patients randomized to catheter-directed thrombolysis had significantly greater ongoing or recurrent ischemia, life-threatening hemorrhage, and vascular complications compared with surgical patients. Stratification by duration of ischemia, however, showed that patients treated within 14 days of onset of symptoms had an amputation rate after thrombolysis of 6% compared to 18% for those undergoing surgery. Patients treated with thrombolysis in this group also had a shorter hospital stay. In patients with acute ischemia the amputation-free survival at 6 months follow up was also better in those treated with thrombolysis.[79] Further analysis of this material reveals that thrombolysis provides a reduction of the predetermined surgical procedure in 50–60% of the cases.[80] **Grade B**

Key points
- PTA is more successful for stenoses than for occlusions.
- PTA is more successful for short than for long occlusions.
- PTA may be combined with stent if recoil occurs or if PTA produces dissection with intimal flaps.
- Thrombolysis should be performed by local intrathrombal administration of the drug.
- PTA may be preceded by thrombolysis in cases with recent occlusions.

Inflammatory vascular diseases – thromboangitis obliterans (Buerger's disease)

Temporal arteritis, Takayashu's disease of the aortic arch, and several diseases affecting the arterioles and microcirculatory vessels have an inflammatory or immunogenic origin. In this chapter these diseases are not considered.

Thromboangitis obliterans, or Buerger's disease, also has an inflammatory component, although the pathophysiology is still not fully known. The major pathogenetic factor, tobacco smoke, has been clearly established, however, for a long time. The patient is usually a young or middle aged man with excessive smoking habits. The disease is segmental and affects both veins and arteries leading to recurrent thrombophlebitis and, in more severe cases, to multiple ulcerations of toes and fingers owing to occlusion of distal arteries. Larger arteries are often affected, which in part may be due to concomitant atherosclerotic disease.

The treatment is based on total avoidance of tobacco smoke. Treatment with prostaglandins, especially the synthetic prostacyclin analog Iloprost (see critical ischemia above), has been shown to have positive effects regarding pain alleviation and healing of ulcers.[81]

References

1. Rose G. The diagnosis of ischaemic heart pain and intermittent claudication in field surveys. *Bull WHO* 1962;**27**:645–58.
2. Fowkes F. The measurement of atherosclerotic peripheral arterial disease in epidemiological surveys. *Int J Epidemiol* 1988;**17**:248–54.
3. Bothig S, Metelisa V, Barth W *et al.* Prevalence of ischaemic heart disease, arterial hypertension and intermittent claudication, and distribution of risk factors among middle-aged men in Moscow and Berlin. *Cor Vasa* 1976;**18**:104–18.
4. Heliovaara M, Karvonen W, Vilhunden R, Punsar S. Smoking, carbon monoxide and atherosclerotic diseases. *BMJ* 1978;**I**:268–70.
5. Dormandy J, Heeck L, Vig S. The natural history of claudication: risk to life and limb. *Semin Vasc Surg* 1999;**12**:123–37.
6. Feinglass J, McCarthy W, Slavensky R, Manheim L, Martin G. Effect of lower extremity blood pressure on physical functioning in patients who have intermittent claudication. *J Vasc Surg* 1996;**24**:503–12.
7. Criqui M, Fronek A, Barrett-Connor E, Klauber M, Gabriel S, Goodman D. The prevalence of peripheral arterial disease in a defined population. *Circulation* 1985;**71**:510–15.
8. Hiatt W. Effect of diagnostic criteria on the prevalence of peripheral arterial disease. The San Luis Valley Diabetes Study. *Circulation* 1995;**91**:1472–9.
9. Kannel W, McGee D. Update on some epidemiological features of intermittent claudication. *J Am Geriat Soc* 1985;**33**:13–18.
10. Dormandy J, Heeck L, Vig S. Predictors of early disease in the lower limbs. *Semin Vasc Surg* 1999;**12**:109–17.
11. Murabito JM, D'Agostino RB, Silbershatz H, Wilson WF. Intermittent claudication. A risk profile from The Framingham Heart Study. *Circulation* 1997;**96**:44–9.
12. Leng GC, Lee AJ, Fowkes FG *et al.* Incidence, natural history and cardiovascular events in symptomatic and asymptomatic peripheral arterial disease in the general population. *Int J Epidemiol* 1996;**25**:1172–81.
13. McGrath M, Graham A, Hill D *et al.* The natural history of chronic leg ischaemia. *Wld J Surg* 1983;**7**:314–18.
14. Jonason T, Bergstrom R. Cessation of smoking in patients with intermittent claudication: effects on the risk of peripheral vascular complications, myocardial infarction and mortality. *Acta Med Scand* 1987;**221**:253–60.
15. Kallero K. Mortality and morbidity in patients with intermittent claudicationas defined by venous occlusion plethysmography: a ten year follow up. *J Chron Dis* 1981;**34**:445–62.
16. Criqui M, Langer R, Fronek A *et al.* Mortality over a period of 10 years in patients with peripheral arterial disease. *N Engl J Med* 1992;**326**:381–5.
17. Leng G, Fowkes F, Lee A, Dunbar J, Housley E, Ruckley C. Use of ankle brachial pressure index to predict cardiovascular events and death: a cohort study. *BMJ* 1996;**313**:1440–4.
18. Reunanen A, Takkunen H, Aromaa A. Prevalence of intermittent claudication and its effect on mortality. *Acta Med Scand* 1982;**211**:249–56.
19. Rihal S, Eagle K, Mickel C *et al.* Surgical therapy for coronary artery disease among patients with combined coronary artery and peripheral vascular disease. *Circulation* 1995;**91**:46–53.
20. Leng GC, Price JF, Jepson RG. Lipid-lowering for lower limb atherosclerosis. *Cochrane Database Syst Rev* 2000;**2**.
21. The Heart Protection Study Presentation at AHA, 2001. www.heart-protection.com
22. Hiatt W, Stoll S, Nies A. Effect of beta-adrenergic blockers on the peripheral circulation in patients with peripheral vascular disease. *Circulation* 1985;**72**:1226–31.
23. Yusuf S, Sleight P, Pogue J, Bosch J, Davies R, Dagenais G. Effects of an angiotensin-converting-enzyme inhibitor, ramipril, on cardiovascular events in high-risk patients. The Heart Outcomes Prevention Evaluation Study Investigators. *N Engl J Med* 2000;**342**:145–53.
24. Antiplatelet Trialists' Collaboration. Collaborative overview of randomised trials of antiplatelet therapy-I: Prevention of death, myocardial infarction, and stroke by prolonged antiplatelet therapy in various categories of patients. *BMJ* 1994;**308**:81–106.
25. Hess H, Mietaschik A, Deichsel G. Drug induced inhibition of platelet function delays progression of peripheral occlusive arterial disease: a prospective double blind arteriographic controlled trial. *Lancet* 1985;**1**:416–19.
26. Diener F, Coccheri S, Libretti A *et al.* European stroke prevention study 2. Dipyridamole and acetylsalicylic acid in the secondary prevention of stroke. *J Neurolog Sci* 1996;**143**:1–13.
27. Bergqvist D, Almgren B, Dickinson J. Reduction of requirement for leg vascular surgery during long-term treatment of claudicants patients with Ticlopidine: Results from the Swedish Ticlopidine Multicenter Study (STIMS). *Eur J Vasc Endovasc Surg* 1995;**10**:69–76.

28. Janzon L, Bergqvist D, Boberg J *et al.* Prevention of myocardial infarction and stroke in patients with intermittent claudication: effects of ticlopidine, results from STIMS, the Swedish Ticlopidine Multicenter Study. *J Intern Med* 1990;**227**: 301–8.

29. Balsano F, Coccheri S, Libretti A *et al.* Ticlodipine in the treatment of intermittent claudication. A 21-month double-blind trial. *J Lab Clin Med* 1989;**114**:84–91.

30. CAPRIE Steering Committee. A randomised, blinded, trial of clopidogrel versus aspirin in patients at risk of ischemic events (CAPRIE). *Lancet* 1996;**348**:1329–39.

31. Hiatt W, Wolfel E, Meire R, Regesteiner J. Superiority of treadmill walking exercise versus strength training for patients with peripheral arterial disease. Implications for the mechanism of the training response. *Circulation* 1994;**90**:1866–74.

32. Gardner A, Poehlman E. Exercise rehabilitation programs for the treatment of claudication pain. A meta-analysis. *JAMA* 1995;**274**:975–80.

33. Lindgärde F, Jelnes R, Björkman H *et al.* Conservative drug treatment in patients with moderately severe chronic occlusive peripheral arterial disease. *Circulation* 1989;**80**:1549–56.

34. Girolami B, Bernardi E, Prins MH *et al.* Treatment of intermittent claudication with physical training, smoking cessation, pentoxifylline, or nafronyl: a meta-analysis. *Arch Intern Med* 1999;**159**:337–45.

35. Dawson DL, Cutler BS, Hiatt WR *et al.* A comparison of cilostazol and pentoxifylline for treating intermittent claudication. *Am J Med* 2000;**109**:523–30.

36. Hiatt WR. Medical treatment of peripheral arterial disease and claudication. *N Engl J Med* 2001;**344**:1608–21.

37. Scheffler P, de la Hamette D, Gross J, Müller H, Schieffer H. Intensive vascular training in stage IIb of peripheral arterial occlusive disease. The additive effects of intravenous prostaglandin E1 or intravenous pentoxiphylline during training. *Circulation* 1994;**90**:818–22.

38. The European Working Group on Critical Leg Ischaemia. Second European consensus document on chronic critical leg ischaemia. *Circulation* 1991;**84**(Suppl. 4):1–22.

39. Loosemore T, Chalmers T, Dormandy J. A meta-analysis of randomized placebo control trials in Fontaine stages III and IV peripheral occlusive arterial disease. *Int Angiol* 1994;**13**: 133–42.

40. Thompson M, Sayers R, Varty K, Reid A, London M, Bell P. Chronic critical leg ischaemia must be redefined. *Eur J Vasc Surg* 1993;**7**:420–6.

41. Group TW. Management of peripheral Arterial Disease. *J Vasc Surg* 2000;**31**(1, part 2).

42. Conrad M. Abnormalities of the digital vasculature as related to ulceration and gangrene. *Circulation* 1968;**49**:1196–201.

43. Kretschmer G, Herbst F, Prager M *et al.* A decade of oral anticoagulant treatment to maintain autologous vein grafts for femoropopliteal atherosclerosis. *Arch Surg* 1992;**127**:1112–15.

44. Jivegård LE, Augustinson LE, Holm J *et al.* Effects of spinal cord stimulation (SCS) in patients with inoperable severe lower limb ischemia: a prospective randomised controlled study. *Eur J Vasc Endovasc Surg* 1995;**9**:421–5.

45. The European Study Group. Intravenous pentoxiphylline for the treatment of chronic critical limb ischemia. *Eur J Vasc Endovasc Surg* 1995;**9**:426–36.

46. Klomp HM, Spincemaille GH, Steyerberg EW, Habbema JD, van Urk H. Spinal-cord stimulation in critical limb ischaemia: a randomised trial. ESES Study Group. *Lancet* 1999;**353**:1040–4.

47. Goldman L, Caldera D, Nussbaum S. Multifactorial index of cardiac risk in noncardiac surgical procedures. *N Engl J Med* 1977;**297**:845–50.

48. Detsky A, Abrams H, Forbath N, Scott J, Hilliard J. Cardiac assessment for patients undergoing noncardiac surgery: a multifactorial clinical risk index. *Arch Intern Med* 1986;**146**: 2131–4.

49. Mantha S, Roizen M, Barnard J, Thisted R, Ellis J, Foss J. Relative effectiveness of four preoperative tests for predicting adverse cardiac outcome after vascular surgery: a meta-analysis. *Anaesth Analg* 1994;**79**:422–33.

50. Eagle K, Singer D, Brewster D, Darling R, Mulley A, Boucher C. Dipyridamole-thallium scanning in patients undergoing vascular surgery. *JAMA* 1987;**257**:2185–9.

51. Hertzer N, Beven E, Young J *et al.* Coronary artery disease in peripheral vascular patients. A classification of 1000 coronary angiograms and results or surgical management. *Ann Surg* 1984;**199**:222–3.

52. Mangano D, London M, Tubau J *et al.* Dipyridamole thallium-201 scintigraphy as a preoperative screening test. *Circulation* 1991;**84**:493–502.

53. Mason J, Owens D, Harris D, Ryan A, Cooke J, Hlatky M. The role of coronary angiography and coronary revascularization before noncardiac vascular surgery. *JAMA* 1995;**273**: 1919–25.

54. Wong T, Detsky A. Preoperative cardiac risk assesment for patients having peripheral surgery. *Ann Intern Med* 1992;**116**:743–53.

55. Poldermans D, Boersma E, Bax JJ *et al.* The effect of bisoprolol on perioperative mortality and myocardial infarction in high-risk patients undergoing vascular surgery. Dutch Echocardiographic Cardiac Risk Evaluation Applying Stress Echocardiography Study Group. *N Engl J Med* 1999;**341**:1789–94.

56. Mason R, Smirnov V, Newton G, Giron F. Alternative procedures to aortobifemoral bypass grafting. *J Cardiovasc Surg (Torino)* 1989;**30**:192–7.

57. Becker GJ, Katzen BT, Dake MD. Noncoronary angioplasty. *Radiology* 1989;**170**:921–40.

58. Johnston KW. Iliac arteries: reanalysis of results of balloon angioplasty. *Radiology* 1993;**186**:207–12.

59. Swedenborg J, Bergmark C. Is there a place for primary axillofemoral bypass? In: Greenhalgh R, Fowkes F, eds. *Trials and tribulations of vascular surgery*. London: WB Saunders Company Ltd, 1996.

60. Michaels J. Choice of material above-knee femoropopliteal bypass graft. *Br J Surg* 1989;**76**:7–14.

61. Veith F, Gupta S, Ascer E *et al.* Six-year prospective multicenter randomised comparison of autologous saphenous vein and expanded polytetrafluoroethylene grafts in infrainguinal arterial reconstruction. *J Vasc Surg* 1986;**3**:104–14.

62. Hall K, Rostad H. *In situ* vein bypass in the treatment of femoropopliteal atherosclerotic disease. A ten year study. *Am J Surg* 1978;**136**:158–61.

63. Moody A, Edwards P, Harris P. *In situ* versus reversed femoropopliteal vein grafts long-term follow-up of a prospective, randomized trial. *Br J Surg* 1992;**79**:750–2.

64. Lundell A, Lindblad B, Bergqvist D, Hansen F. Femoropopliteal-crural graft patency is improved by an intensive surveillance program: a prospective randomized study. *J Vasc Surg* 1996; **21**:26–33.

65. Ihlberg L, Luther M, Alback A, Kantonen I, Lepantalo M. Does a completely accomplished duplex-based surveillance prevent vein-graft failure? *Eur J Vasc Endovasc Surg* 1999;**18**: 395–400.

66. Tangelder MJ, Lawson JA, Algra A, Eikelboom BC. Systematic review of randomized controlled trials of aspirin and oral anti-coagulants in the prevention of graft occlusion and ischemic events after infrainguinal bypass surgery. *J Vasc Surg* 1999;**30**:701–9.

67. Antiplatelet Trialists' Collaboration. Collaborative overview of randomised trials of antiplatelet therapy-II: maintenance of vascular graft or arterial patency by antiplatelet therapy. *BMJ* 1994;**308**:159–68.

68. The Dutch Bypass Oral Anticoagulants or Aspirin Study. Efficacy of oral anticoagulants compared with aspirin after infrainguinal bypass surgery: a randomised trial. *Lancet* 2000;**355**:346–51.

69. Dotter C, Judkins M. Transluminal treatment of arteriosclerotic obstructions. *Circulation* 1964;**30**:654–70.

70. Johnston K, Rae M, Hogg-Johnston S *et al.* 5-year results of a prospective study of percutaneous transluminal angioplasty. *Ann Surg* 1987;**206**:403–12.

71. Dorros G, Lewin R, Jamnadas P *et al.* Below-the-knee angioplasty: Tibioperoneal vessels, the acute outcome. *Catheter Cardiovasc Diag* 1990;**19**:170–8.

72. Sivananthan U, Browne T, Thorley P *et al.* Percutaneous transluminal angioplasty of the tibial arteries. *Br J Surg* 1994;**81**:1282–5.

73. Bolia A, Miles K, Brennan J, Bell P. Percutaneous transluminal angioplasty of occlusions of the femoral and popliteal arteries by subintimal dissection. *Cardiovasc Interven Radiol* 1990; **13**:357–63.

74. London N, Srinivasan R, Naylor A *et al.* Subintimal angioplasty of femoropopliteal artery occlusions: the long-term results. *Eur J Vasc Surg* 1994;**8**:148–55.

75. Nydahl S, London N, Bolia A. Technical report: recanalisation of all three infrapopliteal arteries by subintimal angioplasty. *Clin Radiol* 1996;**51**:366–7.

76. Wolf G. Surgery or balloon angioplasty for peripheral vascular disease: a randomized clinical trial. Principal investigators and their Associates of Veterans Administration Cooperative Study Number 199. *J Vasc Intervent Radiol* 1993;**4**:639–48.

77. Perkins J, Collin J, Creasy T, Fletcher E, Morris P. Exercise training versus angioplasty for stable claudication. Long and medium results of a prospective, randomised trial. *Eur J Vasc Endovasc Surg* 1996;**12**:167–72.

78. Whyman M, Fowkes F, Kerracher E *et al.* Randomised controlled trial of percutaneous transluminal angioplasty for intermittent claudication. *Eur J Vasc Endovasc Surg* 1996;**12**: 167–72.

79. The STILE Investigators. Results of a prospective randomized trial evaluating surgery versus thrombolysis for ischemia of the lower extremity. The STILE Trial. *Ann Surg* 1994;**220**: 251–68.

80. Weaver F, Comerota A, Youngblood M *et al.* Surgical revascularization versus thrombolysis for nonembolic lower extremity native artery occlusions: Results of a prospective randomized trial. *J Vasc Surg* 1996;**24**:513–23.

81. Fiessinger J, Schäfer M. Trial of Iloprost versus aspirin treatment for critical limb ischemia of thromboangitis obliterans. *Lancet* 1990;**335**:556–7.

Index

Note: *v* denotes differential diagnosis or comparisons.